Clinical MR Imaging

Peter Reimer
Paul M. Parizel
James F. M. Meaney
Falko A. Stichnoth (Eds.)

Clinical MR Imaging

A Practical Approach

3rd Edition

Springer

Prof. Dr. Peter Reimer
Städtisches Klinikum
Dept. Radiology
Moltkestraβe 90
76133 Karlsruhe
Germany
peter.reimer@klinik.uni-karlsruhe.de

Prof. James F. M. Meaney
St. James' Hospital/Trinity College Dublin
James's Street
Dublin 8
Ireland
jmeaney@meaneys.com

Prof. Dr. Paul M. Parizel
University Hospital Antwerpen
Dept. of Radiology
Wilrijkstraat 10
2650 Edegem
Belgium
paul.parizel@ua.ac.be

Dr. Falko A. Stichnoth
Radiologie München Zentrum
Sonnenstr. 17
80331 München
Germany
stichnothfa@t-online.de

ISBN 978-3-662-49598-8 ISBN 978-3-540-74504-4 (eBook)

DOI 10.1007/978-3-540-74504-4

Springer Heidelberg Dordrecht London New York

Cover design: eStudio Calamar, Figures/Berlin

Printed on acid-free paper

Springer is part of Springer Science+Business Media (www.springer.com)

Foreword I

This is the third edition of this very popular general textbook on MRI, with the previous editions having been published in English and German in 1999 and 2003. Since the last edition, MRI advances and developments have continued to occur regularly and rapidly, with MRI continuing to be the most complex imaging technique available in medicine. At the same time, MRI has proven to be the single most useful imaging method for a whole host of diseases and organ systems. Hence the publication of the third edition of this very practical book now, in 2009, is very appropriate, timely, and welcome. It makes the reader up to date and has been revised extensively.

The three introductory chapters of the previous editions have been combined in a single chapter covering the principles of MR Imaging. This overview is followed by chapters on each of the major human organ systems with chapters on brain, spine, head and neck, MSK, abdomen, retroperitoneum, pelvis, chest, heart, angiography, breast, pediatric MRI, and whole-body MRI. All chapters have been extensively revised by including new figures. Most chapters have been re-written, many with new co-authors, broadening the scope of each individual chapter, and covering the new technical and clinical developments in these areas.

As with the first two editions, all the chapters are written by recognized authorities renowned for their subject expertise, and all are tied into a single, excellent, very readable volume by editors Peter Reimer, Paul Parizel, James Meaney, and Falko A. Stichnoth. The editors and authors are to be commended for achieving the proper balance of the technical and clinical aspects of MRI. The book is very practical, and is both comprehensive and concise. Every chapter is up-to-date with the latest techniques, and very well illustrated with key diagrams and case material. The entire book can be easily read in a few days, and at the same time held as a handy and authoritative reference text. Trainees, technologists, and especially practicing radiologists will find this an extremely useful book.

Walter Kucharczyk, MD, FRCPC

Professor, Departments of Medical Imaging
and Surgery
University of Toronto, Canada
Princess Margaret Hospital
610 University Avenue
Toronto, ON M5G 2M9, Canada

Foreword II

When I was asked by the authors to write a foreword to the third edition of their acclaimed book *Clinical MR Imaging: A Practical Approach*, I was very honored and I immediately accepted. Indeed, I know the second edition well and use it extensively for teaching purposes. So I went to my bookshelf to look into it once more, now in more detail, but I couldn't find it. Suddenly, I remembered lending it to one of my research fellows when he started working with magnetic resonance (MR) imaging. I told him that this was the best book for learning the basics in a comprehensive, practical fashion. But apparently this fellow liked the book so much that I never got it back! I decided to buy a new book, but was informed by the publisher that the second edition is completely sold out. Medical books that completely sell out in their second edition must have certain characteristics: high quality, practical approach, comprehensive overview, up-to-date information, and a strong feeling for clinically relevant developments. This describes this multiauthor book perfectly.

Over the past 30 years since its introduction to medicine, MR imaging has developed into one of the most versatile tools of daily diagnostic imaging. However, the end of its technological advancement has by far not yet been reached. MR imaging is one of the most highly used imaging modalities in fundamental and translational research, while new clinical applications pop up almost on a weekly basis. These clinical applications reach from screening for breast cancer in high-risk patients, to morphologic and functional diagnosis of brain or cardiac diseases, to therapy monitoring and follow-up of arthritis. Especially in an area undergoing such a tremendous and rapid advancement, one might assume that a textbook like this one is not needed, and that practical knowledge can be better obtained by reading the newly published literature. I think the contrary is true: A comprehensive, practical overview of the established knowledge helps a lot more than studying confusing new results derived from recently developed pulse sequence modifications, in areas where a lot of studies are needed to establish the necessary clinical evidence. Those who are less interested in fancy new developments but rather are looking for practical explanations of established applications in all relevant parts of medicine will find this book particularly helpful.

Peter Reimer, Paul M. Parizel, James F. M. Meaney and Falko A. Stichnoth, the editors of *Clinical MR Imaging: A Practical Approach*, are well-known experts in the field of *clinical MR* imaging. Their affiliations with a university medical center, a large community hospital, and a private practice respectively guarantee that the book highlights all the different perspectives of clinical MR imaging from primary to tertiary care. The authors of the different chapters are the finest and most renowned experts in Europe in their respective fields. Most of them have been involved in major new developments in MR imaging and have extensively contributed to the advancement of the technology as well as its clinical use. The European "flavor" of the book is especially recognizable in some of the described indications. High-quality figures illustrate extensively each of the applications, and a short overview of the relevant literature concludes each of the chapters.

I am firmly convinced that the third edition of this book will have the same success as the previous editions and will be soon sold out. So get ahold of it quickly or you will have to wait for the fourth edition.

Gabriel P. Krestin

Professor and Chairman
Department of Radiology
Erasmus MC, University Medical Center Rotterdam
The Netherlands

Preface

Magnetic resonance (MR) imaging has developed into the most versatile cross-sectional imaging method in clinical practice. Improvements in both hardware and sequences are broadening the scope of clinical applications with breathtaking speed. From the start MR gained an early foothold in neuroradiology and musculoskeletal radiology; however, recent developments have widened its application to include abdominal, cardiovascular, breast, chest and whole-body applications.

As a result of novel technical developments, MR imaging offers to medical practitioners a palette of high-quality anatomical imaging, and, more recently broader functional imaging applications. Diffusion-weighted imaging, a technique for the detection of early cerebral ischemia, is no longer regarded as a brain only study and offers advantage for anatomical and functional assessment of tumours outside the nervous system. The many paradigm shifts in MR imaging frequently present an obstacle not only to beginners who may find it difficult to get started while the goal-posts are changing so rapidly, but also to more experienced users who find it hard to keep abreast of recent advances and new applications. Comprehensive information about all aspects of MR imaging can be found in many excellent textbooks and reference works, several of which have become encyclopaedic in scope and sheer volume, and examining the subject matter in such detail is beyond the scope of this textbook. However, in recognition of the fact that routine diagnostic questions account for more than 90% of examinations in most departments, the editors and authors of this book, endeavoured to present a more clinically relevant approach. This lead to a practical protocol-based approach to the routine workflow in the MR unit, which can be streamlined considerably, which is increasingly critical in today's economic environment. We have aimed to equip the reader with such information, to allow best use of MR technology and capability, based on our collective experience gleaned from years of cutting-edge clinical practice.

The third edition of this book thus offers practical guidelines for efficient and cost-effective MR imaging examinations in daily practice. The authors and editors have rewritten all chapters, included new techniques where appropriate, added new figures and replaced older ones, reflecting best clinical practice. Major changes include new chapters on whole-body imaging and on the technical background of MR imaging, a new subchapter on the GI tract within the abdominal chapter, a combined chapter on musculoskeletal MR, in addition to complete revisions of all other chapters.

As editors, we hope that this book will lead to a better practical understanding of MR imaging and improved appreciation of new sequences and protocols, which will contribute to enhanced clinical problem solving. As such, we believe this book will continue to help beginners to advance their starting point in tailoring protocols and aiding more experienced users in updating their knowledge.

Karlsruhe, Germany Prof. Dr. Peter Reimer
Edegem, Belgium Paul M. Parizel
Dublin, Ireland James F.M. Meaney
München, Germany Falko A. Stichnoth

Contents

Contributors

Thomas Allkemper Department of Clinical Radiology, University of Muenster, Albert-Schweitzer-Straβe 33, 48129 Münster, Germany

Thomas Balzer Bayer Health Care Pharmaceuticals Inc., P.O. Box 1000, Montville, NJ 07045, USA

Matthias Boos Institut für Radiologie und Nuklearmedizin, Krankenhausstraβe 70, 85276 Pfaffenhofen, Germany

Christoph Bremer Department of Clinical Radiology, St. Franziskus-Hospital, Hohenzollernring 72, 48145 Münster, Germany

Jan W. Casselman Department of Radiology, A.Z. St. Jan, Ruddershove 10, 8000 Brugge, Belgium

Eva Coppenrath Department of Clinical Radiology, LMU-University of Munich, Innenstadt Campus, Ziemssenstraße 1, 80336 München, Germany

Arthur M. de Schepper Department of Radiology, Universitair Ziekenhuis Antwerpen, Wilrijkstraat 10, 2650 Edegem, Belgium

Frank De Belder Department of Radiology, Universitair Ziekenhuis Antwerpen, Wilrijkstraat 10, 2650 Edegem, Belgium

Bert De Foer Department of Radiology, AZ Sint–Augustinus Hospital, Oosterveldlaan 24, 2610 Wilrijk, Belgium

Dietmar Dinter Institute of Clinical Radiology and Nuclear Medicine, University Medical Center Mannheim, Theodor–Kutzer–Ufer 1-3, 68167 Mannheim, Germany

Uwe Fischer Diagnostisches Brustzentrum Göttingen, Bahnhofsallee 1d, 37081 Göttingen, Germany

Jan Gielen Department of Radiology, Universitair Ziekenhuis Antwerpen, Wilrijkstraat 10, 2650 Edegem, Belgium

Daniel S. Grosu Bayer Health Care Pharmaceuticals Inc., P.O. Box 1000, Montville, NJ 07045, USA

Gertraud Heinz-Peer Department of Radiology, Medical University of Vienna, Allgemeines Krankenhaus (AKH), Währinger Gürtel 18–20, 1090 Wien, Austria

Hermann Helmberger Zentrum für Radiologie und Nuklearmedizin Nymphenburg, Klinikum Dritter Orden, Menzinger Straße 44, 80638 München, Germany

Birgit Kammer Pediatric Radiology, Dr. von Haunersches Kinderspital, LMU-University of Munich, Innenstadt Campus, Lindwurmstrasse 4, 80337 Munich, Germany

Hans-Ulrich Kauczor Department of Diagnostic and Interventional Radiology, University of Heidelberg, Im Neuenheimer Feld 110, 69120 Heidelberg, Germany

Claudia M. Keser Department of Anesthesiology, Dr. von Haunersches Kinderspital, LMU-University of Munich, Innenstadt Campus, Nussbaumstraße 20, 80336 München, Germany

Dow-Mu Koh Department of Diagnostic Radiology, The Royal Marsden NHS Foundation Trust, Downs Road, Sutton, Surrey SM2 5PT, UK

Thomas Lauenstein Department of Radiology, University Hospital Essen, Hufelandstraße 55, 45122 Essen, Germany

David MacVicar Department of Diagnostic Radiology, The Royal Marsden Hospital, Downs Road, Sutton, Surrey, SM2 5PT, UK

James F. M. Meaney MRI Department, St. James's Hospital, St. James's Street, Dublin 8, Ireland

Wolfgang R. Nitz University Hospital of Regensburg, Franz-Josef Strauss Allee 1, 93053 Regensburg, Germany

Paul M. Parizel Department of Radiology, Antwerp University Hospital and University of Antwerp, Wilrijkstraat 10, 2650 Edegem, Belgium

Bernard Pilet Department of Radiology, AZ Turnhout, Steenweg op Merksplas 44, 2300 Turnhout, Belgium

Peter Reimer Department of Radiology, Klinikum Karlsruhe, Moltkestrasse 90, 76133 Karlsruhe, Germany

Maximilian Reiser Department of Clinical Radiology, LMU-University of Munich, Großhadern Campus, Marchioninistraße 15, 81377 München, Germany

Sanjay Saini Department of Radiology, Massachusetts General Hospital, 32 Fruit Street, Boston, MA 02114, USA

Rodrigo Salgado Department of Radiology, Universitair Ziekenhuis Antwerpen, Wilrijkstraat 10, 2650 Edegem, Belgium

Wolfgang Schima Abteilung für Radiologie, Krankenhaus Göttlicher Heiland, Dornbacherstraße 20-28, 1170 Wien, Austria

Gerwin Schmidt Department of Clinical Radiology, LMU-University of Munich, Grosshadern Campus, Marchioninistrasse 15, 81377 Munich, Germany

Karl Schneider Pediatric Radiology, Dr. von Haunersches Kinderspital, LMU-University of Munich, Innenstadt Campus, Lindwurmstraße 4, 80337 München, Germany

Stefan Schoenberg Institute of Clinical Radiology and Nuclear Medicine, University Medical Center Mannheim, Theodor–Kutzer–Ufer 1-3, 68167 Mannheim, Germany

John Sheehan Departments of Neuroradiology, Musculoskeletal, Body and Cardiovascular Imaging, Northwestern Memorial Hospital and Northshore Healthcare University System, 251 East Huron Street, Chicago, IL 60611, USA

Falko A. Stichnoth Radiologie München Zentrum, Sonnenstraße 17, 80331 München, Germany

Hervé Tanghe Department of Radiology, Academisch Ziekenhuis Rotterdam, Dr. Molewaterplein 40, 3015 GD Rotterdam, The Netherlands

Edwin J. R. Van Beek University of Edinburgh, Clinical Research Imaging Centre CO.19, Queen's Medical Research Institute, 47 Little France Crescent, Edinburgh EH16 4TJ, UK

Luc van den Hauwe Department of Radiology, AZ Klina, Augustijnslei 100, 2930 Brasschaat, Belgium

Wim Van Hecke Department of Radiology, Universitair Ziekenhuis Antwerpen, Wilrijkstraat 10, 2650 Edegem, Belgium

Pieter Van Dyck Department of Radiology, Universitair Ziekenhuis Antwerpen, Wilrijkstraat 10, 2650 Edegem, Belgium

Johan W. M. Van Goethem Department of Radiology, Universitair Ziekenhuis Antwerpen, Wilrijkstraat 10, 2650 Edegem, Belgium

Filip M. Vanhoenacker Department of Radiology, Universitair Ziekenhuis Antwerpen, General Hospital Sint-Maarten Duffel-Mechelen, Wilrijkstraat 10, 2650 Edegem, Belgium

Caroline Venstermans Department of Radiology, Universitair Ziekenhuis Antwerpen, Wilrijkstraat 10, 2650 Edegem, Belgium

Maurits Voormolen Department of Radiology, Universitair Ziekenhuis Antwerpen, Wilrijkstraat 10, 2650 Edegem, Belgium

Abbreviations

ADC	Analog to digital converter (in conjunction with data acquisition)
ADC	Apparent diffuson coefficient (in conjunction with DWI)
ASL	Arterial spin labeling
b	*b*-value in s/mm^2 indicative for the diffusion weighting
B_0	Field strength of the main magnetic field in Tesla (T)
B_1	Magnetic field component of an RF pulse
bEPI	Echo-planar imaging sequence with "blipping" phase encoding gradient pulses
bFFE	Balanced fast field echo sequence
BLADE	Data acquisition with a radial trajectory within k-space
BOLD	Blood oxygenation level dependent
bSSFP	Balanced steady state free precession sequence (trueFISP)
CASL	Continuous arterial spin labeling
ceMRA	Contrast-enhanced magnetic resonance angiography
CHESS	Chemical shift selective pulse
CISS	Constructive interference steady-state sequence
CNR	Contrast-to-noise ratio
CP	Circular polarization (in conjunction with transmitting and receiving coils)
CSF	Cerebrospinal fluid
CSI	Chemical shift imaging
CUBE	3D FSE imaging sequence with variable refocusing angle (SPACE)
DESS	Double-echo steady-state sequence
DRIVE	DRIVE sequence ("driving" the longitudinal magnetization)
DSC	Dynamic susceptibility contrast
DTI	Diffusion tensor imaging (illustration of directional diffusion)
DWI	Diffusion weighted imaging
DW-SE-EPI	Diffusion weighted spin-echo echo-planar-imaging sequence
EPI	Echo planar imaging
EPISTAR	Echo-planar imaging with signal targeting using alternating RF
ETL	Echo train length: number of phase encoded echoes used in a multi-echo sequence
FA	Fractional anisotropy
FAIR	Flow alternated inversion recovery
FFE	Fast-field echo sequence
FFT	Fast Fourier transformation

FID	Free induction decay
FIESTA	Fast imaging employing steady state acquisition sequence
FISP	Fast imaging with steady-state precession sequence
FLAIR	Fluid attenuated inversion recovery
FLASH	Fast low-angle shot sequence
fMRI	Functional magnetic resonance imaging
FoV	Field of view
FRFSE	Fast recovery fast spin echo sequence
FS	Fat saturation
FSE	Fast spin-echo sequence
FSPGR	Fast spoiled GRASS sequence
GBP	Global bolus plot
GMR	Gradient motion rephasing
GRAPPA	Generalized autocalibrating partially parallel acquisition
GRASE	Gradient and spin echo sequence
GRASS	Gradient recalled acquisition in the steady state sequence
GRE	Gradient echo sequence
GSP	Graphical slice positioning
HASTE	Half Fourier acquired single-shot turbo spin-echo sequence
HASTIRM	Half Fourier acquired single-shot turbo spin-echo sequence using inversion recovery and only the signal magnitude
HYPR	Highly contrained backprojection for time-resolved MRI
IR FSE	Inversion-recovery fast spin-echo sequence
IR	Phase sensitive inversion-recovery sequence
IRM	Inversion-recovery sequence that utilizes only the magnitude
k-t BLAST	k-t broad-use linear acquisition speed-up technique
LAVA-XV	Volume interpolated sequence
LOTA	Long time averaging
MEDIC	Multi-echo-data image-combination
MERGE	Synonym for MEDIC
MIP	Maximum intensity projection
MPR	Multi planar reconstruction
MP-RAGE	Magnetization-prepared rapid acquired gradient echo sequence
MR	Magnetic resonance
MRA	Magnetic resonance angiography
MRCP	MR cholangiopancreatography
MRS	Magnetic resonance spectroscopy
mSENSE	Modified SENSE
MT	Magnetization transfer
MTC	Magnetization transfer contrast
MTS	Magnetization transfer saturation
MTT	Mean transit time
MultiVane	Data acquisition with a radial trajectory within k-space
NATIVE	Gated sequences for nonenhanced MRA of the signal
PACE	Prospective acquisition correction
PASL	Pulsed arterial spin labeling
PAT	Parallel acquisition techniques
PBP	Percentage of baseline at peak
PC-MRA	Phase contrast MR angiography

PD	Proton density
PD-W	Proton density weighted
PILS	Partially parallel imaging with localized sensitivities
PPA	Partially parallel acquisition
PROPELLER	Data acquisition with a radial trajectory within k-space
PSIF	A backwards-running FISP sequence
PWI	Perfusion weighted imaging
QUIPSS	Quantitative imaging of perfusion using a single subtraction
RA	Relative anisotropy
RARE	Rapid acquisition with relaxation enhancement
rCBF	Regional cerebral blood flow
rCBV	Regional cerebral blood volume
RESTORE	RESTORE sequence ("restoring" longitudinal magnetization)
RF	Radio frequency
rMTT	Regional mean transit time
ROI	Region of interest
SAR	Specific absorption rate
SE	Conventional spin-echo sequence
SENSE	Sensitivity encoding
sEPI	Spiral echo-planar imaging sequence
SMASH	Simultaneous acquisition of spatial harmonics
SPACE RIP	-Sensitivity profiles from an array of coils for encoding and reconstruction in parallel
SPACE	Sampling perfection with application optimized contrast by using different flip angle evolutions sequence
SPAIR	Spectral inversion using an adiabatic RF pulse sequence
SPGR	Spoiled GRASS sequence
SPIR	Spectral inversion recovery sequence
SR	Saturation recovery sequence
SSD	Surface shaded display
SSFSE	Single-shot fast spin-echo sequence
STEAM	Stimulated echo acquisition mode
STIR	Short tau inversion recovery sequence
SVS	Single voxel spectroscopy
SWI	Susceptibility weighted imaging
T1	Tissue-specific spin-lattice relaxation time
T1-W	Contrast is weighted by the T1 relaxation time
T2	Tissue-specific spin-spin relaxation time
T2*	Relaxation time T2 plus additional dephasing mechanism (signal decay) due to local field inhomogeneities or chemical shift
T2-W	Contrast is weighted by the T2 relaxation time
TE	Echo time
TFE	Turbo field echo sequence
TFL	TurboFLASH
TGSE	Turbo gradient and spin-echo sequence
THRIVE	Volume interpolated sequence
TIR	Turbo inversion recovery sequence
TIRM	Turbo inversion recovery sequence that utilizes only the magnitude of the signal

ToF-MRA	Time of flight MR angiography
TONE	Tilted optimized non-saturating excitation
TR	Repetition time
TRACE	Trace of the diffusion tensor (sum of the diagonal elements)
TRAPS	Transition between pseudo steady-state sequence
TREAT	Time-resolved echo-shared angiography technique
TRICKS	Time-resolved imaging of contrast kinetics
trueFISP	True fast imaging with steady precession
TSE	Turbo spin-echo sequence
TTP	Time to peak
turboFLASH	Fast low angle shot sequence with preceeding inversion pulse
TWIST	3D time-resolved angiography with interleaved stochastic trajectories
VENC	Velocity encoding
VERSE	Variable-rate selective excitation
VIBE	Volume interpolated breathhold examination sequence
VIPR	Vastly undersampled isotropic projection imaging sequence
VISTA	3D TSE imaging sequence with variable refocusing angle (SPACE)
VR	Volume ratio
VRT	Volume rendering technique

Principles of Magnetic Resonance

1

Wolfgang R. Nitz, Thomas Balzer, Daniel S. Grosu, and Thomas Allkemper

Contents

W. R. Nitz (✉)
University Hospital of Regensburg, Franz-Josef Strauss Allee 1, 93053 Regensburg, Germany
e-mail: wolfgang.nitz@siemens.com

The Chapter "Principles of Magnetic Resonance" has been divided into three sections for the reader's convenience. The first section deals with the absolute basics, the second section covers topics that were rated essential to address the 20% of information necessary to cover 80% of common clinical questions, and the third section contains more details and addresses more sophisticated methods.

1.1 The Basics

1.1.1 Spin and Resonance

The atom as introduced by Demokrit (400 BC) was considered the smallest particle that could not be split further by chemical means. But it was later found that the atom could be shattered by physical means and it turned out to consist of a negatively charged shell, the electrons, and a positive charged core, the protons and the neutrons. Bohr postulated in 1913 that the electrons circulate around the positively charged nucleus where the coulomb attraction of particles of opposite charge would be compensated by the centripedal force. He solved the minor problem that a charged particle on a circular path should emit electromagnetic waves, loosing energy, and in a spiral movement collide with the nucleus, by simply making the statement that the atomic system can only exist in particular stationary or quantized states. This was one of the statements that led to the field of quantum mechanics. Sommerfeld later (1916) introduced a more general quantization rule allowing elliptical pathways for the electrons. This theoretical model was able to predict the spectral lines of burning hydrogen. Even the spectral splitting when

P. Reimer et al. (eds.), *Clinical MR Imaging*,
DOI: 10.1007/978-3-540-74504-4_1, © Springer-Verlag Berlin Heidelberg 2010

introducing a magnetic field was predictable (Zeeman effect – coupling with the magnetic moment generated by the circulating electron). Unfortunately, there were sublevels (anomalous Zeeman effect) that could not be explained with the existing theory at that point in time. Uhlenbeck and Goudsmit solved that dilemna in 1925 by introducing the concept of a rotating electron, a further quantized state named a *Spin*. A particle property that looked like a magnetic moment correlated with an angular momentum. The nuclear spin (e.g., the *Spin* of the proton) was introduced by Wolfgang Pauli in 1924 to explain the hyperfine structure of atomic spectra. According to the quantization rule, a particle with a spin of ½ (as is the case for the electron as well as the proton) can only have two energy states, a lower energy state where the angular momentum and its correlated magnetic moment is aligned parallel to an external magnetic field and a higher energy state where the angular momentum and its correlated magnetic moment is aligned antiparallel to the external magnetic field B_0 (Fig. 1.1). The energy difference between these two possible positions can be written as the quantized energy of a photon

$$\Delta E = \gamma \cdot \eta \cdot B_0,$$

with γ is the gyromagnetic ratio and $h = h/2\pi$ with h as Planck's constant.

The spin system will absorb energy, if the energy introduced by an electromagnetic radiation (RF pulse) is matching

$$E_{\mathrm{RF}} = h \cdot \nu = \gamma \cdot \eta \cdot B_0,$$

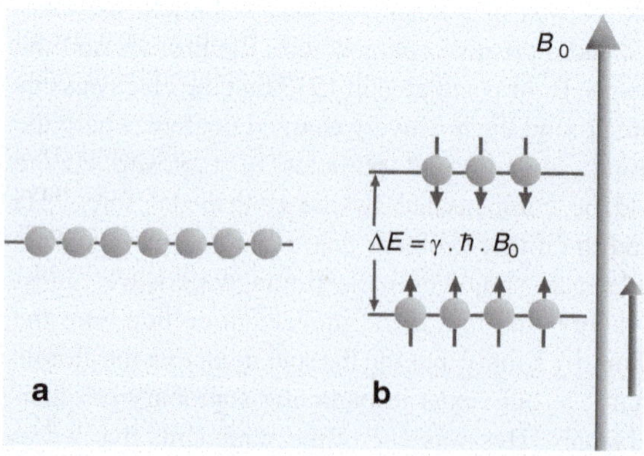

Fig. 1.1 (**a**) No nuclear magnetization in the absence of an external magnetic field. (**b**) Exposed to an external field, the spins and their correlated magnetic moments will align preferably parallel to the external field causing the buildup of a nuclear magnetization M_0

The energy is proportional to the frequency of the RF pulse and will cause some of the parallel aligned nuclear spins to temporarily assume an antiparallel position, only if the energy of the introduced RF pulse is matching the energy difference of the two positions. The frequency describing the energy difference between parallel and antiparallel spin alignment is called the Larmor frequency. Using an RF pulse with that frequency means being in resonance with the spin system. This phenomenon was named nuclear magnetic resonance (NMR). With the nuclear spins turning into the old position after excitation, the energy is emitted as magnetic resonance (MR) signal. In 1946, Edwards Mills Purcell was successful in demonstrating NMR via absorption, whereas Felix Bloch's experimental evidence was based on spontaneous RF emission (detecting an MR signal). For these experimental proofs, Bloch and Purcell shared the Nobel Prize in physics in 1952. In view of public opinions with respect to nuclear bombs and nuclear power plants, the term "nuclear" was dropped later and today the method is referred to as MR. To explain a 90° RF excitation pulse and the 180° RF refocusing pulse using equations with flipping spins is somewhat cumbersome. An elegant solution is offered by Ehrenfest: "The behavior of a large number of spins can be considered equivalent to a quantum average or expectation and, fortunately, can be treated as a macroscopic nuclear magnetization M_0 following the laws of classical electrodynamics." As more spins are aligned parallel to the externally applied magnetic field as compared to the antiparallel aligned state, a macroscopic nuclear magnetization is building up that can be dealt with like a spinning magnetic rod. As illustrated in Fig. 1.1, the hydrogen nuclei will provide a macroscopic nuclear magnetization when exposed to an external magnetic field, aligned in the direction of the main static field, usually referred to as the z-direction. This magnetization is also called longitudinal (nuclear) magnetization. Using the perspective of classical physics, the magnetic moment and the angular momentum of the nuclear magnetization will cause a precession around the direction of the magnetic field with a frequency of 42.58 MHz/T, the Larmor frequency as previously introduced. The precession will not only appear around the direction of the main magnetic field B_0, but also around the magnetic component B_1 of an RF pulse. But this will take place only if the B_1 component rotates with the same precessional frequency around the direction of the main magnetic field, in which case, we are in resonance. In such a case, the nuclear magnetization is turned for the duration of the RF pulse (Fig. 1.2). Converting the longitudinal nuclear magnetization into a transverse magnetization is called a 90° excitation.

With the B_1 field switched off, the nuclear magnetization continues to rotate with the specific frequency of 42.58 MHz/T (a function of the current locally experienced magnetic field strength), and will induce a signal in a nearby coil, the MR signal, as indicated in Fig. 1.3.

The signal will vanish over time as the transverse magnetization is dephasing and the magnetization will slowly return to its original position. Both processes are called relaxation.

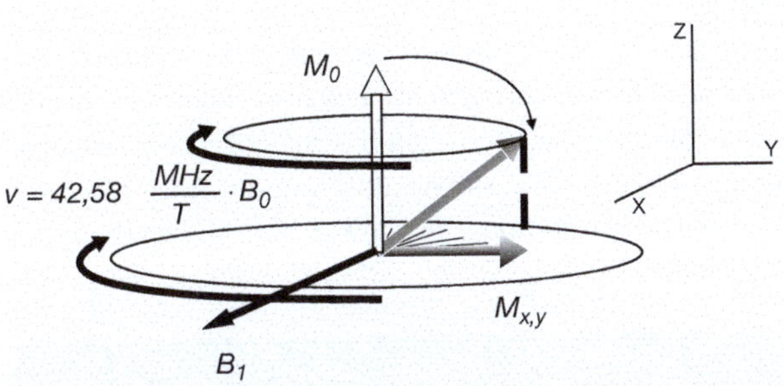

Fig. 1.2 The "resonance" phenomenon: A B_1 field perpendicular to the main field (z-direction) causes the macroscopic magnetization to flip toward the x-y plane. Any attempt to turn the macroscopic magnetization away from the direction of the main magnetic field will cause a rotation around the z-direction. If the B_1 component of the electromagnetic field is rotating at the same frequency, the situation is called "on resonance" and the B_1 field will continue to turn the macroscopic magnetization

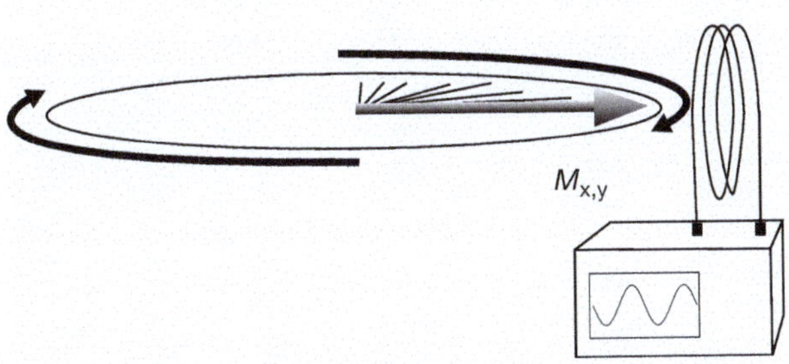

Fig. 1.3 The induction of the MR signal: If the macroscopic magnetization is not aligned with the direction of the main field, the magnetization continues to rotate around the z-axis and will induce a signal in a nearby coil

1.1.2 Tissue-Specific Parameters: PD, T1, T2, χ and T2*

The amplitude of the induced signal is a composition of all signals from each voxel within the excited slice. A voxel is the smallest selected spatial dimension that is planned to be identified. The voxel is given by the selected slice thickness, the field of view, and the selected matrix size. A spatial encoding will allow resolving the composition of the signals coming simultaneously from all voxels, and will enable to identify the signal amplitude coming from each individual voxel to be assigned to the according pixel brightness on the display.

1.1.2.1 Proton Density, PD

For a first excitation following rapid data sampling, the signal amplitude that is emitted from a single voxel is proportional to the number of hydrogen nuclei (protons) that are involved in the excitation process (PD). An imaging protocol, where the parameters of an imaging sequence are selected to show a difference in signal contributions for tissues with different PD, is called a PD-weighted (PD-W) protocol.

1.1.2.2 T1 Relaxation Time

The course in time for the imaging actions like slice selective excitation and the spatial encoding followed by the recording of the signal is called a sequence, or better, an imaging sequence. With the exception of a few exotic imaging sequences, several excitations are necessary to encode enough spatial information to reconstruct an image. Each time the actual longitudinal magnetization is flipped, it is converted to a signal inducing rotating transverse magnetization. Time is necessary to allow the recovery of the longitudinal magnetization prior to the next repetition of an excitation. The recovery is a function of the tissue-specific relaxation rate, describing the time needed for the realignment of the magnetization with the main magnetic field. That time is called the T1-relaxation time.

The amplitude of the induced signal depends on the actual amount of longitudinal magnetization "flipped" into the transverse plane. An imaging protocol, where the parameters of an imaging sequence are selected to show a difference in signal contributions for tissues with different T1-relaxation times, is called a T1-weighted (T1-W) protocol (e.g., short time between repetitions of the excitation). In order to "flip" or turn the magnetization, the generated B_1-field has to be "in resonance" with the rotating magnetization. A similar rule is influencing the relaxation process responsible for the realignment of the magnetization with the main magnetic field B_0, the "recovery" of the longitudinal magnetization. For tissue, where the "tumbling" water molecules causing field fluctuations close to the Larmor frequency, the T1-relaxation time will be short. If the molecules are very small and mobile (free water), the tumbling frequency will be higher than the Larmor frequency, causing a slow T1-relaxation process. If the water molecules are motion restricted, the tumbling frequency may be below the Larmor frequency, and the result will be the same: a slow T1-relaxation process. The time for the recovery process, the T1-relaxation time, is also called the longitudinal relaxation time or spin-lattice relaxation time, since it depends on how fast the stored energy (of the spin system) can be returned to the surrounding environment (the "lattice"). The mechanism is also called spin-lattice interaction. As a rule, the higher the mobility of the water molecules (the "squishier" the tissue), the longer the T1-relaxation time. Tissues with a long T1-relaxation time show up hypointense on T1-W images — T1-WIs (Sect. 1.1.3.7).

Since the Larmor frequency depends on the field strength whereas the "tumbling" frequency of common water molecules within the human tissue remains the same, T1-relaxation times are field strength-dependent, as listed in Table 1.1.

The majority of MR contrast agents utilize the paramagnetic properties of gadolinium (Gd). Gadolinium has a powerful magnetic moment and is chelated to a reasonably mobile ligand. The magnetic moment interacts with the resonating magnetizations of the hydrogen nuclei, allowing the magnetizations to relax more rapidly – leading to a significant shortening of T1-relaxation times. As a result, tissues with increased uptake of the contrast media will show up hyperintense on T1-W images.

1.1.2.3 T2 Relaxation Time

The rotating transverse magnetization is the result of a significant number of individual magnetic moments of hydrogen nuclei (protons). Primarily, the intramolecular dipole-dipole interaction between all these magnetic moments will cause a "dephasing" of the transverse magnetization. The slower the data are acquired after the initial excitation, the lower the induced signal

Table 1.1 Relaxation parameters for various tissues

Region		Longitudinal relaxation times			Transverse relaxation times
		T1 (ms)			T2 (ms)
		1.5 T	1.0 T	0.2 T	
Brain	Gray matter (GM)	921	813	495	101
	White matter (WM)	787	683	390	92
	Cerebrospinal fluid (CSF)	3,000	2,500	1,200	1,500
	Edema	1,090	975	627	113
	Meningioma	979	871	549	103
	Glioma	957	931	832	111
	Astrocytoma	1,109	1,055	864	141
	Misc. tumors	1,073	963	629	121
Liver	Normal tissue	493	423	229	43
	Hepatomas	1,077	951	580	84
	Misc. tumors	905	857	692	84
Spleen	Normal tissue	782	683	400	62
Pancreas	Normal tissue	513	455	283	
	Misc. tumors	1,448	1,235	658	
Kidney	Normal tissue	652	589	395	58
	Misc. tumors	907	864	713	83
Muscle	Normal tissue	868	732	372	47
	Misc. tumors	1,083	946	554	87

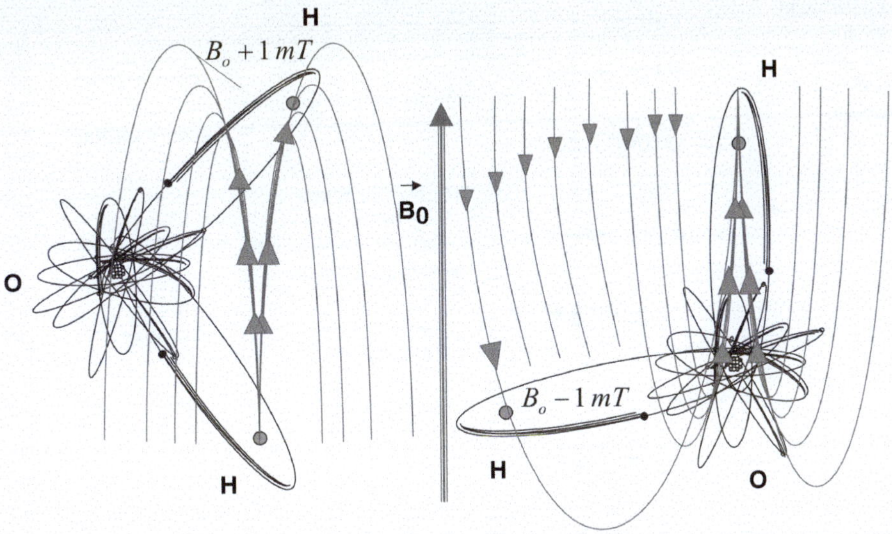

Fig. 1.4 The dipole–dipole interaction as a main source for relaxation: Intramolecular dipole–dipole interactions are the dominant factors for T1 and T2 relaxation times. The spin of a single hydrogen nucleus, aligned parallel to an external field B_0, has a correlated magnetic moment indicated by the field lines. That field is superimposed on the external field experienced by the neighboring hydrogen nuclei. Depending on the orientation of the water molecule within the external field, the effective field is diminished or increased. This will lead to significant differences in resonance frequencies on the molecular level

detected. The relaxation rate assigned to the phenomenon of this "dephasing" is tissue-specific and is called T2-relaxation. A simple dipole–dipole interaction is illustrated in Fig. 1.4. Depending on the orientation of the two protons relative to the main magnetic field B_0, the field of the first proton may either augment or oppose the main magnetic field at the location of the second proton. The difference in field strength can be approximately as high as 2 mT. Such a difference in field strength on a molecular level would lead to a difference in resonance frequencies of approximately 85 kHz, and the transverse magnetization would dephase within 12 μs. Fortunately, the majority of water molecules in human soft tissue are highly mobile, tumbling around, and the averaging over the fluctuating fields leads to a slower dephasing of the transverse magnetization. The time for the dephasing process, the T2-relaxation time, is also called the transverse relaxation or spin-spin relaxation time. As a rule, the higher the mobility of the water molecules (the "squishier" the tissue), the longer the T2-relaxation time. An imaging protocol, where the parameters of an imaging sequence are selected to show a difference in signal contributions for tissues with different T2-relaxation times, is called a T2-W protocol (e.g., a long time between excitation and data acquisition, Sect. 1.1.3.7). Ice cubes will have a very short T2 relaxation time and the signal will not be observed with conventional imaging. Tissue with a long T2-relaxation time will show up hyperintense on T2-W images.

1.1.2.4 The Three-Compartment Model

Although the simple dipole–dipole interactions are the most important processes for the T1- and T2-relaxation process, a variety of other mechanisms may be important in certain tissues. Sophisticated theories have been developed to explain the relaxation properties of even simple solutions. Figure 1.5 illustrates a three-compartment model, and even this more complicated perspective is only a crude approximation of "reality."

1.1.2.5 Magnetic Susceptibility χ

The magnetic susceptibility, often referred to simply as susceptibility in magnetic resonance imaging (MRI), is the degree of magnetization of a material in response to an externally applied magnetic field, in this case B_0. The magnetization of the material is superimposed to the external field and the resulting local effective magnetic field strength $B_{0\,(\mathrm{eff})}$ is responsible for the Larmor frequency

$$\nu = \frac{\gamma}{2\pi} \cdot B_{0(\mathrm{eff})} = \frac{\gamma}{2\pi} \cdot (1+\chi) B_0.$$

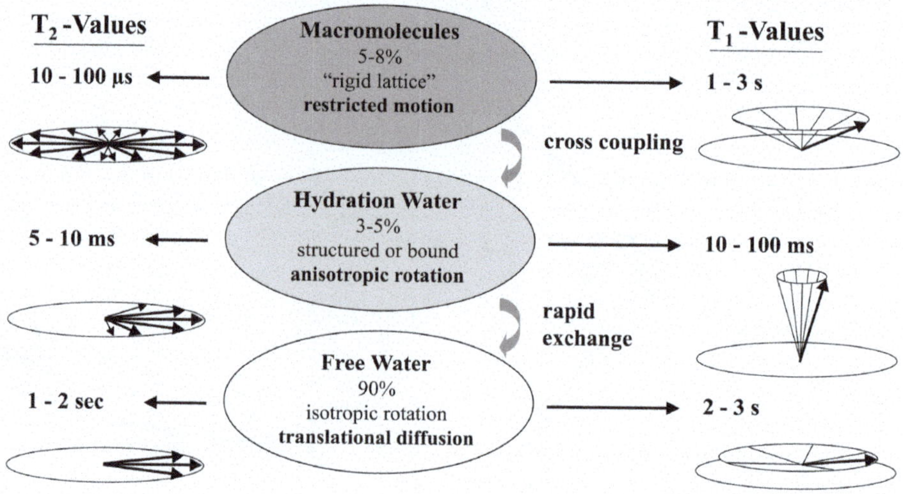

Fig. 1.5 A three-compartment model as an example for approximation of T1 and T2 relaxation times for different tissue hydrogen fractions

The material reducing an externally applied field is called diamagnetic. The material that is weakly enhancing the magnetic field up to 1% is called paramagnetic and the material that is increasing the field beyond 1% is called ferromagnetic. Biological tissue, in general, is diamagnetic. For example, measuring the magnetic field strength within the liver of a patient positioned in a 1.5 T magnet will likely return the value of 1.49999 T. At first glance this may sound negligible, but it is not. Changes in magnetic susceptibility, even in the diamagnetic region, can cause severe artifacts (Sect. 1.3.7).

1.1.2.6 T2* Relaxation Time

Tissues with different values of the magnetic susceptibility χ within a voxel or within the vicinity of a voxel will cause local magnetic field inhomogeneities. As an example, there might be a magnetic field strength of 1.4995 T in one corner of the voxel as compared to 1.4996 T in the opposite corner. As the Larmor frequency is a function of field strength, the generated transverse magnetization at the location of the first corner will rotate with 63.8487 MHz, whereas the transverse magnetization within the opposite corner will rotate with 63.8529 MHz. As a consequence, the transverse magnetization within the voxel will be completely dephased within 0.234 ms using the above example. Field inhomogeneities, e.g., based on magnetic susceptibility gradients, cause a rapid dephasing of the transverse magnetization. The relaxation time taking into account the dephasing due to T2-relaxation as well as the local field inhomogeneities is called T2*:

$$\frac{1}{T_2^*} = \frac{1}{T_2} + \gamma \cdot \Delta B.$$

γ is the magnetogyric ratio, ΔB represents the field inhomogeneity across half a pixel.

1.1.3 Excitation, Image Formation and Image Contrast

Excitation as well as spatial encoding utilizes the linear relation of Larmor frequency and magnetic field strength. In order to have the magnetic field strength as a function of location, a magnetic field gradient is superimposed during excitation and during data acquisition for the purpose of spatial encoding. This magnetic field gradient is generated by a so-called gradient coil located inside the bore of the magnet. The referred gradient coil is actually a construct of three gradient coils, which are perpendicular to each other in order to serve, for example, the direction *x*, *y*, and *z* or any combination of those (Fig. 1.6).

Contrary to CT, there is an unlimited freedom to select any imaging plane, as the plane will be defined by the direction of the magnetic field gradient during

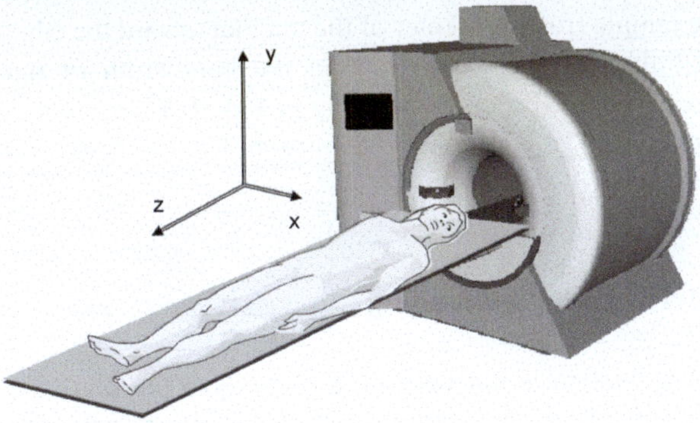

Fig. 1.6 The labeling of directions with x, y and z has historic reasons and is just used in this case as it keeps the indices conveniently short. For a patient in supine position with head first toward the magnet, the x-direction becomes left–right, the y-direction becomes anterior-posterior, and the z-direction becomes inferior-superior or caudocranial

excitation. If a sagittal plane is desired, the magnetic field gradient will be established in the x-direction. If a coronal plane is to be imaged, a magnetic field gradient will be established in the y-direction prior and during the excitation. For a transverse plane, a magnetic field gradient in the z-direction is applied. As magnetic field gradient coils (dedicated to the three directions x, y and z) can be combined, the user can select any double-angled imaging plane (usually via a graphical user interface with the aid of previously acquired multiplanar localizers).

There is a default for the directions of frequency-encoding and phase-encoding, partially for historical but more important, also for practical reasons. Frequency-encoding direction and phase-encoding direction can be swapped by the user prior to execution of the imaging sequence. For a transverse plane, the phase-encoding direction is usually anterior–posterior and the frequency-encoding direction is left–right correspondingly. For a sagittal plane, the phase-encoding direction is usually anterior–posterior and the frequency-encoding direction is caudocranial. For a coronal plane, the phase-encoding direction is usually anterior–posterior and the frequency-encoding direction is caudocranial. As will be explained later in more detail, flow- and motion-artifacts are always propagating along the direction of phase encoding. The measurement time is proportional to the number of necessary phase-encoding steps, and reducing the field-of-view (FoV) in the direction of phase-encoding will require fewer phase-encoding steps while keeping the same spatial resolution. All these are practical reasons for the selection of the direction of phase-encoding.

1.1.3.1 Excitation

With the magnetic field strength being a function of location, the Larmor frequency also becomes a function of location, allowing a spatially selective excitation. For example, in order for the excitation of a 5 mm thick sagittal slice positioned in the center of the magnet, a magnetic field gradient of e.g., 4.8 mT/m is turned on from left to right prior to the RF excitation and is left on for the duration of the excitation pulse. The Larmor frequency at the center of the magnet (location 0.0) with a field strength of 1.5 T will be 63.87 MHz. At location −2.5 mm, the magnetic field strength will be 12 μT lower (4.8 mT/m*2.5 mm) and the Larmor frequency will be at 63.86995 MHz. At location +2.5 mm, the local magnetic field strength will be 12 μT higher and the Larmor frequency will be at 63.87005 MHz. Applying an RF excitation pulse with a frequency range from 63.86995 to 63.87005 MHz in the presence of the applied magnetic field gradient will cause the excitation of a 5 mm thick region at the center of the magnet. The Larmor frequency is also called the resonance frequency, as the frequency of the excitation pulse has to exactly match the Larmor frequency of the location that is to be excited. The Larmor frequency is indicative of the energy difference between the parallel and antiparallel alignment of the nuclear spins of the hydrogen atoms, and it also describes the precessional frequency of the nuclear magnetization as it is turned away from the parallel alignment in the presence of another magnetic field B_1 produced by the RF excitation pulse. If B_1 rotates with the same frequency than the rotational frequency of the nuclear magnetization, we have a "resonance." The RF pulse causes a so-called 90° excitation if the product of B_1 amplitude and RF pulse duration is flipping the longitudinal magnetization completely into the transverse plane, converting M_0 to M_{xy}.

1.1.3.2 Frequency Encoding

Spatial encoding utilizes the linear relation of Larmor frequency and magnetic field strength. Paul Lauterbur, who received the Nobel Prize for medicine in 2003, suggested a procedure in 1973 which is fundamental to MRI. In order to have the magnetic field strength as a function of location, a magnetic field gradient is superimposed during data acquisition for the purpose of spatial encoding. This magnetic field gradient is generated by a so-called gradient coil located inside the bore of the magnet. With the magnetic field strength being a function of location, the Larmor frequency also becomes a function of location, allowing to retrieve a spatial information from the signal. For example, in order to identify inferior and superior in a sagittal slice with a field-of-view (FoV) of 230 mm, a magnetic field gradient of 5.973 mT/m is turned on in the direction of frequency encoding at the beginning of the data acquisition. The measured MR signal from tissue at position −165 mm will have a frequency of 63.86999996 MHz in this case, whereas the signal at position +165 mm will have a frequency of 63.87000004 MHz. Analyzing the incoming data for frequency components is called a Fourier transformation and frequency corresponds to location in this case (Fig. 1.7). The difference in frequency of 29.25 kHz in this example from the center of the magnet toward the edge of the field-of-view is called the bandwidth of the sequence (GE), corresponding to 195 Hz/pixel (in this example) as bandwidth definition for Siemens and Philips.

1.1.3.3 Phase Encoding

The system is not only able to analyze the digitized data for frequency components, it can also identify the phase of the signal. The phase corresponds to the position of the nuclear magnetization within the transverse plane. The preparation of this phase along the column of the tissue is done with a so-called phase encoding gradient. The column of the tissue has been identified with the previously explained frequency encoding, and the signal pattern within the column to be identified with phase encoding has already been indicated in Fig. 1.7. For example, in order to identify the anterior and posterior in a sagittal slice, a magnetic field gradient is established in that direction for a short duration

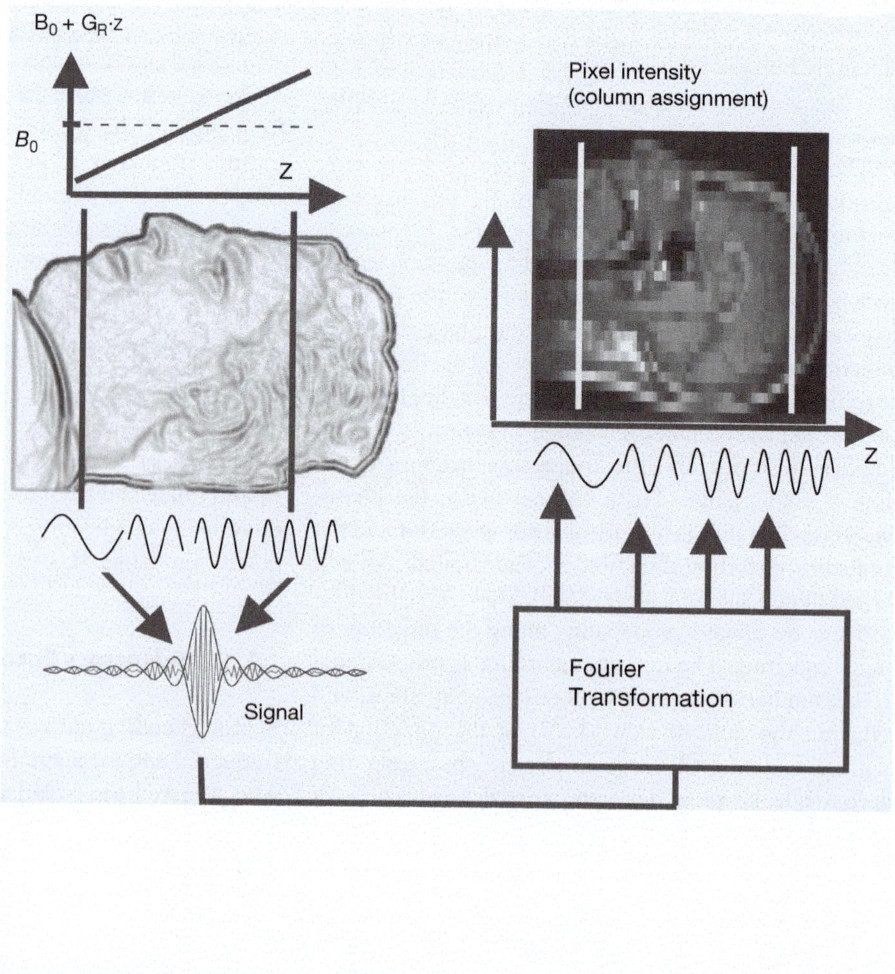

Fig. 1.7 The "frequency" encoding: all resonance frequencies resulting from a magnetic field gradient being switched on during data sampling are detected simultaneously. Sampling the signal while a field gradient is switched on will provide information on the location of the signal sources in one direction. The information is utilized to assign the signal intensity of a pixel on a monitor, corresponding to the signal magnitude received from a single voxel within the excited slice

so that the sum of all transverse magnetizations within the anterior half of the slice point to the opposite direction when compared to the sum of all transverse magnetizations of the posterior half of the slice. Such a step would be called a sampling of the low spatial frequency. This sampling is then repeated for higher spatial frequencies up to the point where the final high resolution information is collected, with a phase encoding gradient amplitude that causes the transverse magnetizations of adjacent voxels being of opposite polarity at the end of the phase encoding preparation.

1.1.3.4 The GRE Sequence

The sequence diagram is a graphical illustration of the temporal course of action for the magnetic field gradients, the RF, and the data acquisition (Fig. 1.8). The first action is to switch on a magnetic field gradient in the direction of slice selection (GS).

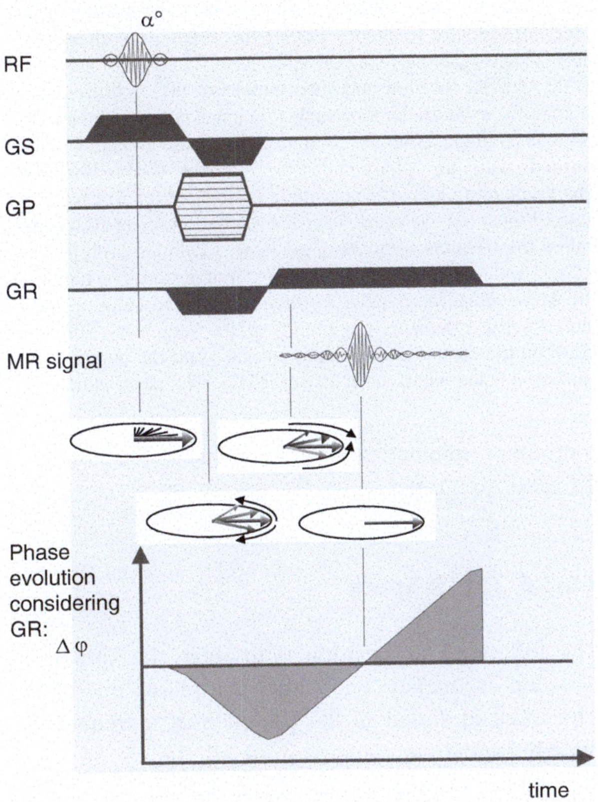

Fig. 1.8 The gradient-echo sequence - GRE. The two bipolar lobes of the frequency-encoding gradient GR recall a so-called gradient echo. *GP* phase-encoding gradient; *GR* read-out gradient; *GS* slice-selection gradient; *RF* radiofrequency

Once the magnetic field gradient is established, the RF pulse is applied with a frequency composition appropriate to excite the desired slice thickness at the desired location. As the frequency difference during the excitation process is causing a dephasing of the generated transverse magnetization toward the end of the RF excitation pulse, a "negative" magnetic field gradient is applied after the excitation to compensate that dephasing. Once the RF is switched off, the phase of the generated transverse magnetization will be prepared in the direction of phase encoding (GP). During data acquisition, an unwanted dephasing of the transverse magnetization is to be expected due to the desired difference in frequencies. That dephasing is compensated in advance by applying a frequency-encoding gradient of opposite polarity for half of the data sampling duration to follow later (GR). The sequence ends with ramping up the frequency-encoding gradient and collecting the MR signal (5). As bipolar magnetic field gradients are used to generate "an echo", such a sequence is called a gradient echo sequence (GRE). The dephasing of the observed transverse magnetization is characterized by T2*, which includes the dephasing due to T2 as well as the additional dephasing mechanisms based on susceptibility gradients and other reasons for local magnet field inhomogeneities. A disadvantage is the sensitivity to susceptibility gradients as they are found at bone/tissue or air/tissue interfaces, often leading to a total signal loss in the vicinity of these areas. This increased sensitivity turns into an advantage when looking for hemorrhagic lesions or perfusion studies in conjunction with paramagnetic contrast agents.

1.1.3.5 The SE Sequence

Erwin Hahn discovered that a 180° RF refocusing pulse applied between excitation and data acquisition will eliminate the dephasing caused by local field inhomogeneities (Fig. 1.9). Sequences utilizing such RF refocusing pulses are called spin echo sequences (SE).

Similar to the GRE sequence, the first action in a SE Sequence (Fig. 1.10) is to switch on a magnetic field gradient in the direction of slice selection. Once the magnetic field gradient is established, the RF pulse is applied with a frequency composition appropriate to excite the desired slice thickness at the desired location. The frequency difference during the excitation

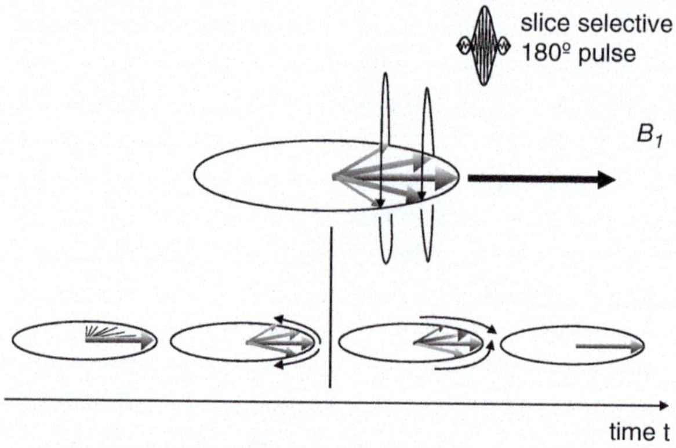

Fig. 1.9 The 180° refocusing pulse: the macroscopic magnetization within a voxel will not only undergo a dephasing due to spin–spin interaction (T2 decay) but will also experience a difference in resonance frequencies due to local variation of susceptibility, due to magnet inhomogeneities, or due to chemical shift. Most of these effects are fixed in location and stable over time. There will be components of the magnetization that experience a lower resonance frequency – falling behind in a rotating group of magnetizations – and there will be components that experience a higher field, a higher resonance frequency – speeding ahead. A 180° radiofrequency refocusing pulse will put the faster component behind the slower and vice versa. Since the effect remains that the faster component will still correspond to a higher magnetic field, the magnetization will be refocused, forming a so-called spin echo

process that is causing a dephasing of the generated transverse magnetization toward the end of the RF excitation pulse is usually compensated by a small extension of the slice-selection gradient that is used during the slice-selective RF refocusing.

Once the RF is switched off, the phase of the generated transverse magnetization can already be prepared in the direction of phase encoding (GP). During data acquisition, an unwanted dephasing of the transverse magnetization is to be expected due to the wanted difference in frequencies. That dephasing is compensated in advance by switching of a frequency-encoding gradient of the same polarity but for half the duration of the data acquisition window (GR) prior to the application of the 180° RF refocusing pulse. The application of the 180° RF refocusing pulse in the presence of the same slice-selection gradient will place any faster transverse magnetization behind the slower component, and at the time of data acquisition, the fast transverse magnetization will again coincide with the slower one. The sequence ends with ramping up the frequency-encoding gradient and collecting the MR signal (GR). The remaining observed dephasing of the

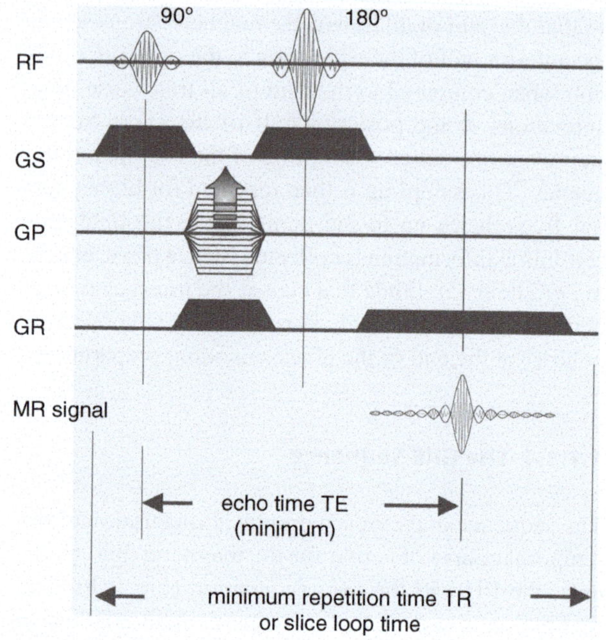

Fig. 1.10 The spin-echo sequence - SE: the sequence starts with ramping up the slice-selection gradient (GS) to establish a difference in resonance frequencies along the direction of slice selection. A slice-selective (center frequency and bandwidth according to the desired location and slice thickness) 90° radiofrequency (RF) pulse will turn the longitudinal magnetization into the transverse (*x-y*) plane. After the excitation, the phase encoding is performed with the phase-encoding gradient (GP). For each phase-encoding loop, the amplitude is changed (except for averaging loops). At the same time, the readout gradient (GR), also called the frequency-encoding gradient is compensating for the later expected dephasing during the readout period. The length of the data acquisition is given by the desired bandwidth per pixel and usually dominates the timing of the sequence. The time between the center of the excitation pulse and the center of the spin echo is known as the echo time (TE). *TR* repetition time

transverse magnetization is characterized by the T2-relaxation time.

1.1.3.6 The "k-Space"

The following explanation is to show the similarity between frequency encoding and phase encoding. The induced signal in the presence of a frequency-encoding gradient is the sum of all signals for each "frequency column." The signal within each "frequency column" is proportional to the proton density within each voxel along the "frequency column" and proportional to the other tissue-specific parameters as previously discussed. The transverse magnetization within each "frequency column" either speeds ahead or falls behind compared to the adjacent "frequency columns," depending on the difference in resonance frequency as given by the local field strength. This speeding ahead or falling behind is described as a phase shift φ_R (with R for readout). If, as an example, the frequency-encoding gradient is in the *z*-direction, the phase of the transverse nuclear magnetization for each position in the direction of frequency encoding would be:

$\varphi_R = \gamma \cdot GR_Z \cdot t_R \cdot z = k_R \cdot z$ with *z* being the distance to isocenter. The isocenter is the center of the magnet. The frequency difference between "columns" is $\Delta v \sim GR_z \cdot \Delta z$, with Δ_Z as the requested spatial resolution in the direction of frequency encoding, in this case, the *z*-direction. The phase difference between "frequency columns" is a function of the sampling time t_R. The product of gyromagnetic ratio γ, magnetic field gradient in the read-out direction GR_z, and sampling time t_R is denoted as *k*-value $k_R = \gamma \cdot GR_Z \cdot t_R$. The data sampled in the presence of a frequency-encoding gradient are stored along a data vector that has a *k*-index.

If, as an example, the phase-encoding gradient is in the *y*-direction, the phase of the transverse nuclear magnetization for each position in the direction of phase encoding would be:

$$\varphi_P = \gamma \cdot GP_y \cdot t_P \cdot y = k_P \cdot y.$$

While t_R is incremented during frequency encoding (sampling interval times sampling point), defining the k_R value, the GP_Y amplitude is commonly altered (phase encoding steps) to define the k_p value for phase encoding.

The string of sampled data (analog to digital converted induced voltages due to the MR signal at the time t_n, with index *n* from 0 to m, with m being the matrix size in the direction of frequency encoding) is called a Fourier-line. Each value has a k_R index, a reason to call a Fourier-line also a *k*-space line. Each Fourier-line has been acquired with a preceding phase-encoding step, giving the line also a k_P index. All data (acquired analog and converted to a digital value) are stored in a so-called raw data buffer.

As each of the data points is characterized by a k_R and k_P value, the raw data buffer is also called *k*-space (Fig. 1.11). In order to acquire the information from two adjacent voxels, it is necessary to switch on a large phase-encoding gradient. This measured line is stored at the beginning of *k*-space and contains the high spatial frequency information of the object. As the phase-encoding gradient is lowered with the next measurement, the next line contains a lower spatial frequency. The line where no phase-encoding gradient is switched on contains the projection; the very coarse structure of the object. This line is stored in the center of *k*-space. For conventional imaging, the lower part of *k*-space is again filled with information from higher spatial frequencies.

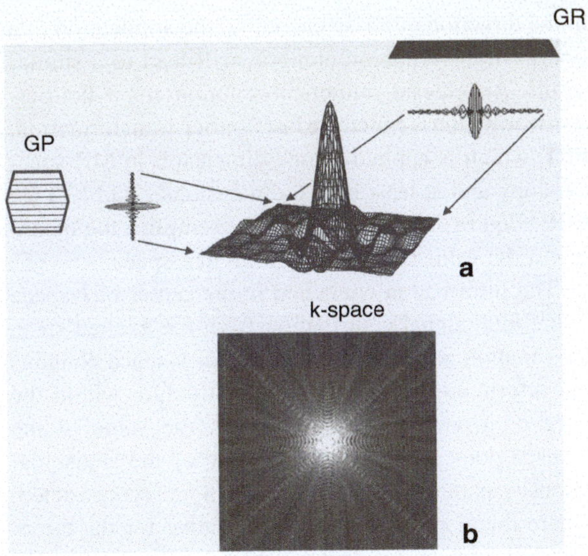

Fig. 1.11 The *k*-space. Prior to image reconstruction, each measured Fourier line (frequency-encoded data for each phase-encoding step) is stored in a raw data memory. GP indicates the address of the measured Fourier line as given by the amplitude of the phase-encoding gradient. GR is indicating the positions of the data points as a function of the duration of the frequency-encoding gradient. (**a**) Illustrates an amplitude representation of *k*-space. (**b**) It is a representation of *k*-space, where the amplitude has been converted to pixel intensity. *GP* phase-encoding gradient; *GR* readout gradient

The consideration of *k*-space is very helpful to discuss image appearance or artifacts as a consequence of irregularities during the measurement. The objective of the previous derivation of phase changes within *k*-space due to frequency-encoding and phase-encoding magnetic field gradients was to convince, that the structure of the information is equal, whether a *k*-space line is considered or a *k*-space column. Applying a Fourier-transformation along a *k*-space line will provide a frequency spectrum. As frequency has been a function of location during data sampling, the derived amplitudes can immediately be assigned to signal contributions as a function of geometry in the direction of frequency encoding. As the data structure is identical in the direction of phase encoding, the application of a Fourier-transformation along k_P will lead to a similar result. An elegant numerical solution for a Fourier-transformation is called the fast Fourier-transformation, FFT, which is applied in one dimension in MR spectroscopy and at least in two dimensions (2D FFT) for MRI. Figure 1.12 is provided to exemplify the meaning of the value of each data point in *k*-space.

The information contained in the center of *k*-space is the total signal contribution from the excited slice. Information adjacent to the center of *k*-space contains the information about the coarse structure within the slice or, from another perspective, the value of the *k*-space point defines the amplitude of the sinusoidal intensity pattern within the image to be reconstructed, where the *k*-space position is indicative for the direction and frequency of that pattern.

1.1.3.7 Image Contrast

In conventional spin-echo imaging, a 90° RF pulse is used to convert the longitudinal magnetization M_z to the transverse magnetization M_{xy}. This initial pulse is also called the excitation pulse. Immediately following the turning away from an alignment parallel to the direction of the magnetic field, the magnetization will rotate around that direction with the field strength specific Larmor frequency. The finally generated transverse magnetization will continue to rotate after the excitation pulse and will induce the MR signal in an adjacent coil. The amplitude of the induced signal is proportional to the amount of transverse magnetization. The transverse magnetization is proportional to the longitudinal magnetization prior to excitation. The longitudinal magnetization in turn is a function of the number of protons participating in the excitation process (PD), the time needed for the tissue to recover (T1) and the time between excitations (of the same slice), the repetition time (TR). The T2-relaxation, immediately following the RF excitation, will cause a dephasing of the transverse magnetization M_{xy}, leading to a decreased signal the later the data are acquired. Leaving ample room between excitations (long TR), the magnetizations of all tissues will be realigned with the main magnetic field, and no differences in T1-relaxation will be observed. The time between the center of the excitation pulse and the magnetization refocusing point within the data-acquisition window is called the echo time (TE). The shorter the TE, the less the

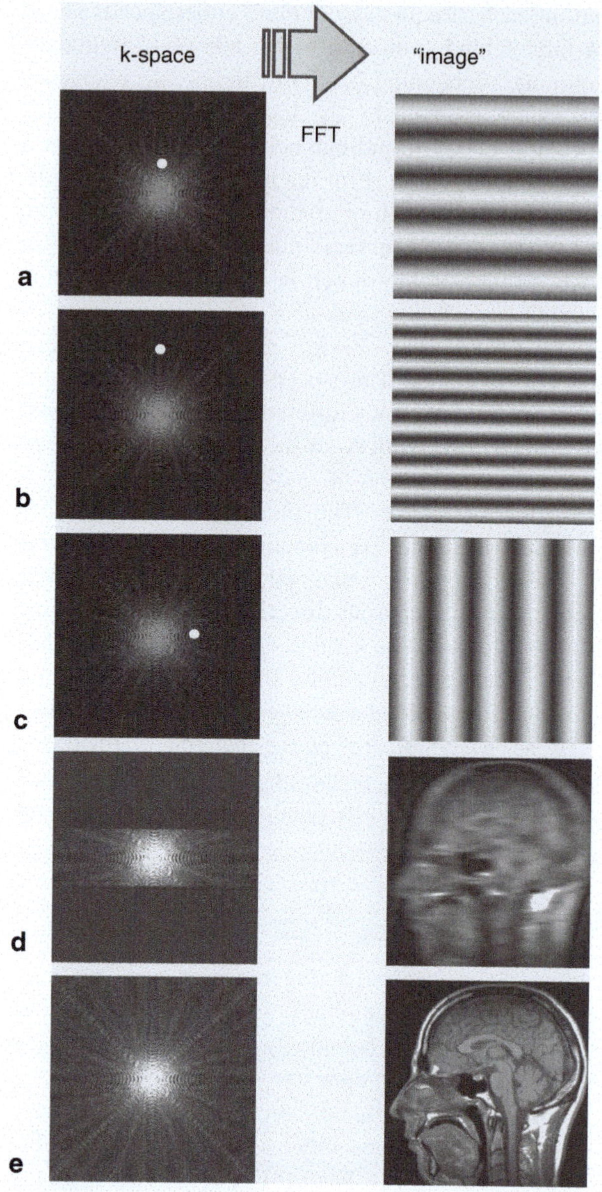

Fig. 1.12 *k*-space: Each data point in *k*-space represents direction and intensity of a "spatial frequency." (**a**) The value of a data point close to the center of *k*-space indicates the intensity of the frequency pattern as illustrated to the right (in the direction of phase encoding). (**b**) The value of a data point further distant from the center of *k*-space indicates the intensity of a pattern with a higher frequency. (**c**) The value of a data point close to the center of *k*-space along a Fourier line through the center of *k*-space indicates the intensity of the adjacent pattern to be used to compose an image. (**d**) A few Fourier lines around the center of *k*-space contain enough information to reconstruct a coarse image already demonstrating anatomy and weighting. (**e**) Considering all *k*-space lines while performing a 2D-FFT will lead to the image with the desired spatial resolution and with (usually) negligible artifacts

influence of the T2-related dephasing mechanism. A long TR, short TE generated image is called proton-density weighted (PD-W), since that is the main tissue parameter influencing the contrast (Fig. 1.13).

In order to differentiate tissues based on their T1-relaxation times, the TR has to be reduced, with the TE kept short, to acquire T1-WIs. In that case, the contrast is dominated by the difference in T1-relaxation times of the various tissue types. Cerebrospinal fluid (CSF) and "squishy" tissues with long T1-relaxation times will appear hypointense on T1-WIs (Fig. 1.14).

A T2-W contrast is achieved by using a long TR, similar to the PD-W approach, but instead of using a short TE, a long TE will provide a stronger signal amplitude dependence on the T2-relaxation time of the various tissues. CSF and "squishy" tissues with long T2-relaxation times will appear hyperintense on T2- WIs (Fig. 1.15).

1.1.4 Basic Elements of a Magnetic Resonance Scanner

The previous chapter already indicated the hardware needed for an MR scanner (Fig. 1.16).

1.1.4.1 The Magnet

A nuclear spin is only observable in the presence of a reasonably strong magnetic field. There are three possibilities to create the magnetic field for a whole body MR imager.

- Permanent magnet
- Resistive magnet
- Superconductive magnet

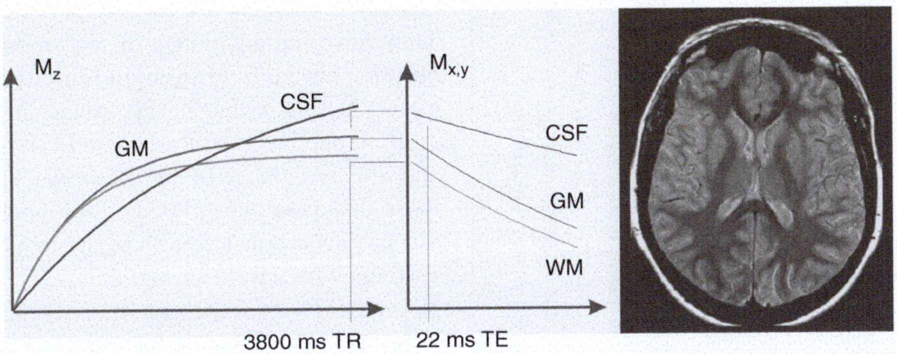

Fig. 1.13 Proton density weighting - PD-W: the *left graph* illustrates the recovery of the longitudinal magnetization (M_z) following excitation. The *right graph* demonstrates the dephasing of the generated transverse magnetization ($M_{x,y}$) due to the T2-decay. Cerebrospinal fluid (CSF) has a higher proton density than gray (GM) or white matter (WM) and should appear hyperintense on truly proton density-weighted (PD-W) images

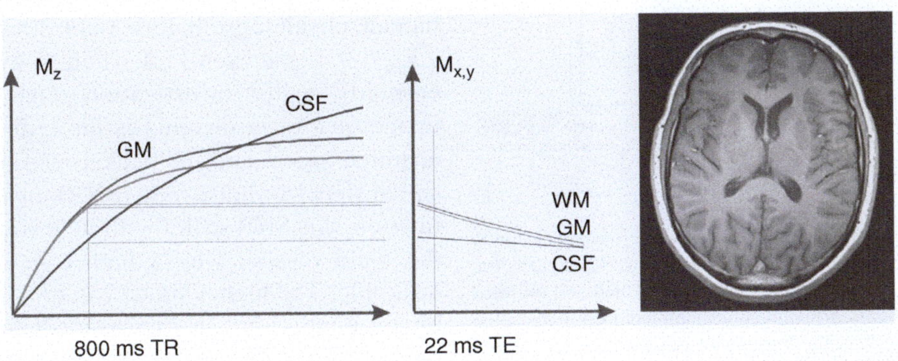

Fig. 1.14 T1 weighting - T1-W: the *left graph* illustrates the recovery of the longitudinal magnetization (M_z) following excitation. The *right graph* demonstrates the dephasing of the generated transverse magnetization ($M_{x,y}$) due to the T2-decay. For a 1.5-T system, the optimum TR for gray matter–white matter differentiation is 800 ms. The selected TE has to be sufficiently short in order to minimize the influence of the T2 relaxation on image contrast

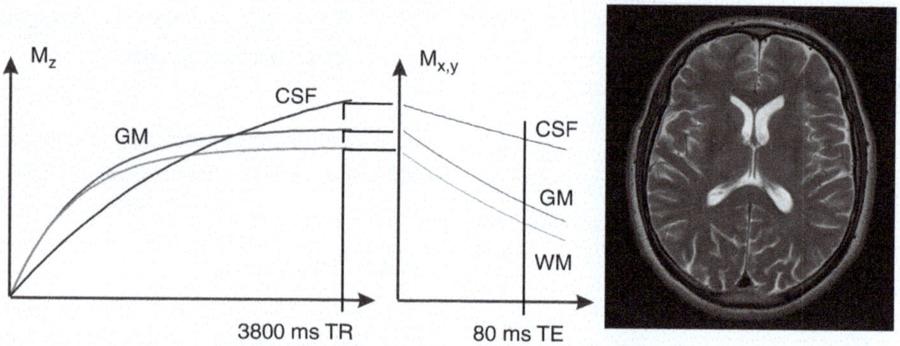

Fig. 1.15 T2 weighting - T2-W: the *left graph* illustrates the recovery of the longitudinal magnetization (M_z) following excitation. The *right graph* demonstrates the dephasing of the generated transverse magnetization ($M_{x,y}$) due to the T2-decay. A long TR and long TE protocol will result in a T2-W image. Image contrast is dominated by the contribution of proton density and T2 relaxation of the various tissues

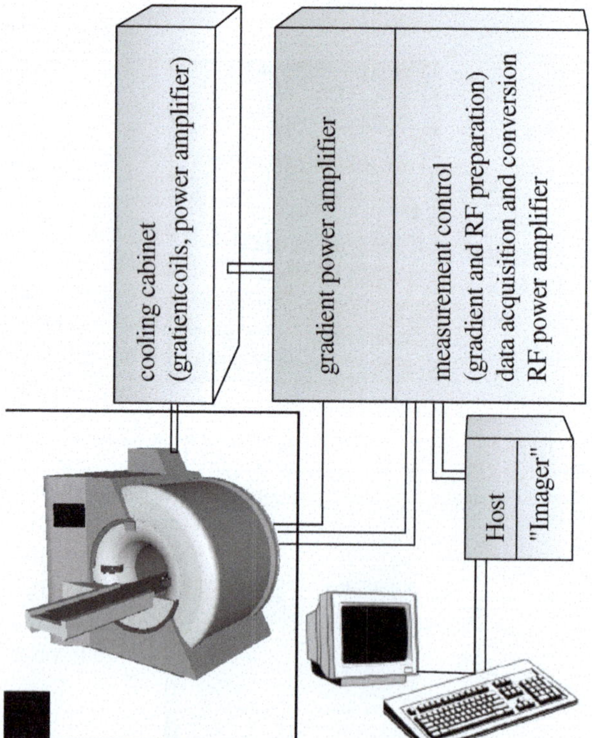

Fig. 1.16 Basic elements of a magnetic resonance scanner. Besides the magnet with the attached patient table, there is the operating console where the protocols are selected and initiated and where the images are viewed and archived on a so-called host computer. Besides the host, there is usually a specialized computer called an imager, which does nothing else but image reconstruction and inline postprocessing. The whole measurement is controlled by a so-called measurement control unit

C-shaped magnets are usually permanent magnets. They have the advantage of low operational costs, but they have a field strength limitation of approximately 0.35 T. Other disadvantages are the temperature dependence of the magnetic field (stability), and the weight (≥14 *t*). Resistive systems share these disadvantages plus the high operational costs due to power consumption of the magnet coils. MR systems with a field strength above 0.5 T utilize the phenomenon of superconductivity. Certain alloys loose any resistance, if they are kept cold enough. Superconductors use liquid Helium (−269°C = −452°F = 4K). The currently used, most common field strength is 1.5 T, with a significant increase in number of 3 T installations. Since the magnetic field strength seems to have no permanent effect on human physiology, higher field strength systems e.g., 7, 9.4, and even 11 T whole body imagers are currently under investigation. One measure of image quality in imaging is the ratio between the acquired signal and the background noise, the so-called signal-to-noise ratio (SNR). In a first approximation, this SNR scales with field strength. This is the main reason, why a higher field strength is desirable. The higher signal can be utilized to gain image quality for an increased diagnostic confidence, or to utilize methods for reducing measurement time (which is usually correlated with a loss in SNR).

1.1.4.2 The Gradient Coil

The Larmor frequency is a linear function of the magnetic field strength. To be able to excite a specific region, the magnetic field needs to be a function of location. This is achieved by sending electric currents through a so-called gradient coil, which in turn produces a magnetic field gradient. There are basically three physical orthogonal gradient coil arrangements each of which would allow a magnetic field gradient caudo-cranial, anterior posterior or left to right direction. In addition, as these coils can be combined, any arbitrary imaging plane can be selected. A typical value for the strength of a gradient system would be 45 mT/m and the combination of strength and speed is characterized by the so-called slew rate, e.g., 200 T/m/s. A further increase in amplitude and speed is technologically possible, but is unreasonable, as fast and large changes in the magnetic field induce currents within the patient's body, potentially causing peripheral nerve stimulations (PNS). This seems to be the current limitation for further increasing the performance of a conventional magnetic field gradient coil. The gradient coil is located behind the cover inside the bore of the magnet.

1.1.4.3 The Body Coil

The RF antenna that is in general producing the electromagnetic field for excitation or refocusing is situated between cover and gradient coil inside the bore of the magnet. This coil is called the body coil or transmit coil. The body coil can also be used as a receive coil, but is in this function not competitive to a small antenna placed close to the region to be imaged. Such an antenna is called a surface coil.

1.1.4.4 The Surface Coils

The dominant source of noise in the MR image is caused by the thermally driven Brownian motion of electrons within the patient's body conducting tissue. Even though a single slice is excited, a coil will pick up any noise that is within the coil range. The advantage of small surface coils is that they have a limited range and will, therefore, pick up less noise. The disadvantage of small surface coils is that they have a limited range and may not cover the whole area of interest. The solution is that several small coils can be connected with each other in a so-called phased-array concept. The closer an RF receiving coil can get to the origin of the MR signal, the better (the stronger the received signal). This is the reason for the significant number of coils designed for the various anatomical regions. Potentially, the head coil as well as the extremity coil may not only be able to receive the MR signal, but also serve as transmit coils. The advantage is that only the tissue inside the coil is exposed to the RF field. Distributed coil arrangements can also be utilized to retrieve spatial information that otherwise would have to be measured, thus potentially can be used to save measurement time. As all of these coils receive the MR signal "in parallel," such methods are called "parallel acquisition" techniques (Sect. 1.2.5). Various combinations of coil elements allow either a homogeneous appearance of signal intensities within the image or an optimal performance in parallel acquisition techniques.

1.1.4.5 The "Computers"

There are basically three main computational tasks to be performed

- Patient data and imaging protocol handling
- Measurement control and data reception
- Fourier transformation and (inline) image postprocessing.

Different vendors have different strategies and there are fast changes when it comes to computers. Patient data, imaging protocol handling, and measurement setup are usually done with a so-called "host," likely located close to the measurement console. The strategies have been changing from a single computer to distributed intelligence back to three computers, and they may eventually end up in one computer again, pending progress in technology. The computer in the background, which is mainly storing the raw data, performing Fourier transformations, and executing the inline postprocessing is called the "imager." The computer addressing the different hardware components based on the given imaging protocol is called the "measurement control."

1.2 The Essentials

While the previous chapter dealt with the absolute basics, the following section addresses the absolute essentials for clinical imaging, which is basically

- MR safety
- Basic preparation of the longitudinal magnetization like fat suppression and fluid-attenuated inversion recovery
- In-phase, opposed phase imaging with GREs
- Fast spin echo imaging
- Parallel imaging
- Imaging protocol parameter
- Contrast agents for MRI
- Appearance of hemorrhagic lesions
- Magnetic resonance angiography - MRA
- Diffusion-weighted imaging - DWI
- Perfusion-weighted imaging - PWI

1.2.1 MR Safety

For the year 1995–2005, the FDA database shows 389 reports on accidents related to MRI. Ten percentage of these accidents were related to ferromagnetic objects being sucked into the magnet. Seventy percentage were dealing with RF burns.

1.2.1.1 Attractive Forces

Ferromagnetic objects will become magnetized in a strong external magnetic field and they will be pulled toward the location with the highest magnetic field strength. The pulling force is proportional to the magnetic moment M of the ferromagnetic object and the experienced magnetic field gradient. The latter is given by the fringe field distribution of the magnet. The magnetic moment M of the ferromagnetic object is proportional to the experienced external field $M \sim x \,.\, B_0$. Thus the translational force depends on the fringe field and the field strength distribution in the vicinity of the magnet.

Illustrated in Fig. 1.17 is the fringe field distribution multiplied with the magnetic field strength distribution for the longitudinal axes and one lateral direction (distribution is symmetric with respect to the geometry of the magnet). For the magnet illustrated (3 T field strength), the maximum force is given at the location of 20 T²/m at the inside of the bore ~80 cm from the isocenter of the magnet. Once the ferromagnetic object is inside the magnet, no further pulling force is experienced. The boomerang effect reported in some accidents is based on the fact that the object is accelerating, gaining speed while approaching the isocenter, and will pass the same if there is no counterforce stopping the motion. The object then continues to fly through the magnet until its kinetic energy is compensated by

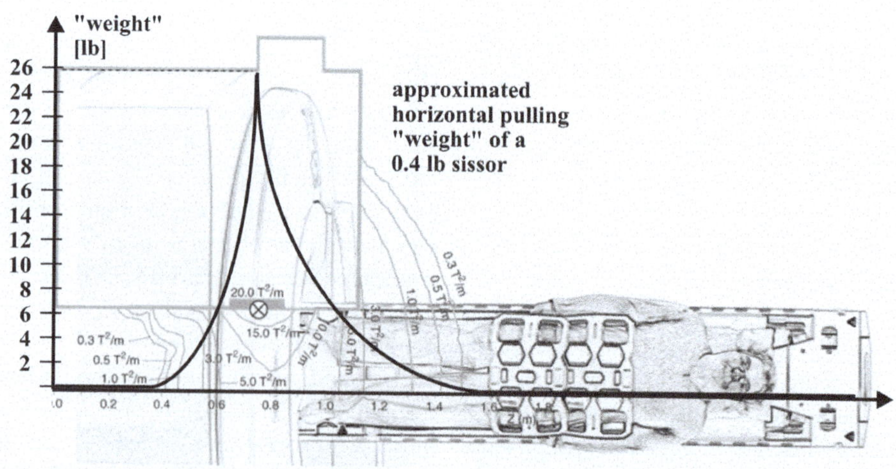

Fig. 1.17 The final horizontal pulling force is a function of the field strength distribution B_0, as this is defining the magnetic moment of the ferromagnetic object, and the fringe field, as this indicates the magnetic field gradient. The product of both distributions gives T²/m as factor for the pulling force. An approximation for a 0.4 lb sissor is shown for a 3 T magnet. The horizontal pulling force for the worst case (20 T²/m location) is equivalent to the gravitational force of a 26 lb weight (The graphic is just an illustration. The scaling is relatively arbitrary and does not represent the true course of the pulling force)

the potential energy of the force pulling the object back into the center of the magnet. At that point, the object will change directions and will fly back again toward the isocenter of the magnet. The illustrated maximum horizontal pulling force for a 0.4 lb sissor is comparable to a gravitational force of a 26 lb weight using a 3 T system. This pulling force will be reduced to approximately 8.5 lb in case of a 1.5 T system.

1.2.1.2 Torque

A ferromagnetic object exposed to a magnetic field will become magnetized. There will be no force and no attraction if the ferromagnetic object is symmetrical and if the experienced magnetic field is homogeneous within the geometric extension of the object. If the ferromagnetic object is asymmetric, the object will experience a significant torque, which is proportional to the magnetic field strength and the magnetic moment of the object. The latter is proportional to the ferromagnetic mass and the local experienced magnetic field strength. This torque will be greatest near the magnet center. Needle-shaped objects will tend to turn their long axis parallel to the field direction, and plate-like objects will tend to turn their flat surfaces parallel to the field lines. In many situations, the torque represents a greater hazard than the translational force.

1.2.1.3 Specific Absorption Rate: SAR

When tissue is exposed to a strong external magnetic field, the spins of the hydrogen atom nuclei (a single proton) are allowed to take two positions. They may align themselves parallel with the field, which is the low energy position, or they may align themselves antiparallel with the field, which is the less desired higher energy position. The difference in population, as more spins will be aligned parallel as compared to antiparallel, represents the longitudinal magnetization. To get a signal, a RF excitation pulse is required that provides exactly the energy difference between the parallel alignment and the antiparallel alignment of the nuclear spins. After excitation, the spins fall back into their original position, emitting a fraction of the energy with the MR signal. The RF pulse will also interact with water molecules. Since the weak molecular dipole moments of water try to align to the flux lines of the applied RF field, their rotational motion is accelerated. An increase in motion is equivalent to an increase in kinetic energy, and represents an increase in temperature. The energy per unit time (power) that is absorbed by the patient during MRI is characterized by the SAR. The order of magnitude of the power deposition during MRI is close to the human metabolic rate. An averaged sized person requires about 8,000 kJ/day to exist in a resting state. This translates into continuous power all day long of about 90 W. This power is known as the basal metabolic rate. The international guideline (IEC 60601–2–33) on safety requirements in MR assumes 2 W/kg whole-body SAR exposure as being no burden to the patient (normal mode), that is 160 W for a patient weight of 176 lbs for the duration of a scan.

The classical perspective of the SAR mechanism considers the interaction of the electrical component and the magnetic component of the RF field with the biological tissue of the patient's body. The RF frequency $\omega_0 = 2\pi\nu_0$ contributes with the power of two, as does the amplitude B_1 of the RF pulse. Various conductive pathways along soft tissue allow resistive losses, and multiple water molecules are craving for some guidance by rapidly changing RF flux lines. The likelihood of interaction, represented by the SAR value, scales with the fifth power of the patient's circumference b. The likelihood of interaction, represented by the SAR value, also scales with the conductivity ($1/\rho$) inside the patient.

$$\mathrm{SAR} \sim \frac{\omega_0^2 \cdot B_1^2 \cdot b^5}{\rho}.$$

The international standard (IEC 60601–2–33 (9 September 2001)) on "particular requirements for the safety of magnetic resonance equipment for medical diagnosis" considers the SAR threshold values for three different modes: the normal mode, the first level, and the "forbidden" second level. Exposure below the first mode SAR level (0 W/kg to 2 W/kg) is assumed to cause no physiological stress to the patient (~160 vs. 90 W). For SAR values within the range of the first level (0 W/kg to 2 W/kg), medical supervision of the patient is required. The energy per unit time at that level corresponds to the metabolic rate of a marathon runner. Specifically, the system has to indicate that it has to switch into first level in order to execute the requested protocol and the operator must acknowledge the instruction in order for the system to continue.

Normal mode:

- Up to 2 W/kg whole body exposure
- Up to 2–10 W/kg partial body exposure, depending on the ratio between exposed and unexposed patient mass
- Up to 3.2 W/kg for head exposure
- Up to 10 W/kg for local SAR within the head/trunk region
- Up to 20 W/kg for local SAR values within the extremities
- The increase in body core temperature is not to exceed 0.5°C.

First level mode:

- Up to 4 W/kg whole body exposure
- Up to 4–10 W/kg partial body exposure, depending on the ratio between exposed and unexposed patient mass
- Up to 3.2 W/kg for head exposure
- Up to 10 W/kg for local SAR within the head/trunk region
- Up to 20 W/kg for local SAR values within the extremities
- The increase in body core temperature is not to exceed 1°C.

Values are averaged over a 6-min time frame. For a period of 10 s, the averaged SAR is permitted to exceed up to three times the level of the current mode. These levels are valid for a bore temperature of up to 77°F. Beyond this temperature, the limit for the normal mode decreases linearly from 2 to 0 W/kg if the temperature inside the bore approaches 91.4°F.

The software on the MR system will calculate and compare all possible above-mentioned limits for the selected mode and will indicate the most critical value. If the critical value exceeds the level of the selected mode, suggestions are made to the operator regarding which scan parameters to change (and to what value) in order to stay within the guidelines. No MR system will allow the execution of a protocol that exceeds the guidelines of the country where the scanner is located.

SAR Management

SAR is primarily a function of field strength, amplitude of the RF pulse, patient conductivity, patient circumference, and finally, the patient's effective region within the RF field (transmitter coil design). The latter considers the patient position relative to the transmitter coil. As a safety precaution, vendors perform mathematical simulations using various human models to verify compliance with the safety guidelines. The various limits are checked prior to execution of the sequence. The user will have guided choices to start the measurement. All vendors must have at least a dual path to verify that the SAR limits are not exceeded. The first path consists of a direct measurement. The energy lost within the system is estimated during the adjustment. Based on these values, the energy absorbed by the patient is approximated. The second path will take the transmitter adjustment values and the results of the simulations, the patient's weight, age, height, and position in order to come up with an estimation of the energy likely to be absorbed by the patient. Whatever value is delivered by any of these paths, the most conservative is taken and displayed as the SAR value.

Any RF pulse within the protocol to be executed will contribute to the SAR. This can be spatial saturation pulses, fat saturation pulses, inversion pulses, magnetization transfer saturation (MTS) pulses, excitation, or refocusing pulses.

In cases where the SAR limit exceeds the guidelines, the following measures will help:

- Prolong the TR (prolonging the measurement time) will help to spread the energy over a longer time window.
- Reduce the number of slices, which will reduce the number of RF pulses for the same measurement time.
- Reduce the refocusing flip angle. That will decrease the B_1 field amplitude. That factor is contributing with a power of two to the SAR value.
- Reduce the echo train length (ETL). That will lead to fewer RF pulses for the same TR, spreading the delivered energy over a longer time window (to the expense of increased measurement time).
- Use low SAR pulses. The B_1 amplitude will dictate the speed of flipping. A short RF pulse with large B_1 field amplitude will have the same flipping or refocusing effect as a long RF pulse with smaller B_1 field amplitude. Since B_1 is contributing by the power of two to the SAR, a reduction in amplitude causes a significant reduction in the SAR value. On the other hand, longer RF pulses will lead to prolonged TEs, which prolong the length of echo trains, resulting in reduced signal. The latter is due to T2 decay. Longer echo trains or longer TEs will also

lead to a higher sensitivity to flow, motion, and susceptibility artifacts. In other words, the utilization of low SAR RF pulses may have a negative effect on image quality.

- Place a pause before or after the measurement. Some vendors provide the option to select in advance a pause at the end of the measurement. That pause will be considered in the SAR calculation, averaged over time, and may result in the scan being within SAR guidelines. The same is applicable for an alternative delay prior to executing multiple measurements in conjunction with contrast enhancement. Some vendors offer a SAR look ahead to avoid any enforced pausing between measurements.

1.2.1.4 Radio Frequency Interaction with the Patient

Besides the previously mentioned SAR, it has to be kept in mind that biological tissue is a conductor, although a poor conductor. Poor conducting loops build by the patient himself have to be avoided. Leaving a small gap inside a soft tissue loop may cause sparking and minor burns. A dry towel should be placed between legs, feet, hands, hand and hip in order to prevent sparking. The E-field distributions close to the RF transmitter coil may be significant and some vendors advice to avoid contact of bare skin with the cover of the magnet inside the bore.

1.2.1.5 Radio Frequency Interaction with Orthopedic (Passive) Implants

Considering the safety of passive implants, the following primary interactions with the MR system have to be discussed:

- Static magnetic field
- Magnetic gradient field
- Dynamic field changes
- RF field

Implants classified as "non ferromagnetic" are deemed safe. In most cases, these types of implants present no hazard to the patient. Implants are characterized as being MR safe using ex vivo testing as described by the ASTM (American Society for Testing and Materials). In the case of ferromagnetism, two interactions with the static magnetic field have to be considered:

- Torque, which is a function of the field strength
- Translational attraction, which is in addition a function of the fringe field distribution

Brain aneurysm clips represent a classic contraindication for MRI due to at least one reported fatality where a ferromagnetic aneurysm clip tore a middle cerebral artery. Recent publications have documented that at least those aneurysm clips made from titanium alloys can be considered MR safe. The translational attractive force on a ferromagnetic object is a function of the product of the local magnetic field strength and the magnetic gradient field. Orthodontic appliances pose a potential risk during MRI due to forces on metallic objects within the static magnetic field. Steel ligature wires and arch wires made of cobalt chromium, titanium molybdenum, nickel-titanium, and brass alloys have shown no or negligible forces within the magnetic field. Steel retainer wire bonds should be checked to ensure secure attachment prior to an MRI exam as translational forces are estimated to be 27–75 times as high as gravitational forces on these objects.

The switching of magnetic field gradients potentially causing PNS is of less concern for conductive implants. Heating of implants and similar devices may occur if they are made from conductive materials and have an elongated shape or are arranged in loops.

The coupling of conductive implants with the RF used for saturation, excitation, and refocusing is of greater concern. The voltage buildup along the implant may cause tissue heating in the vicinity as a consequence of resistive losses due to dissipating currents. The heating is approximately a function of the local SAR value and the geometric arrangement with respect to the RF transmitting coil.

Recent reports indicate that aneurysm coils for example may cause a noticeable heating of their environment. Conductive implant shapes with a dimension of about half the wave length of the basic frequency are considered a potential hazard, as they may permit the induced currents to get in resonance with the RF field. The RF wavelength in water is approximately 52 cm for a 1.5 T system. For a 3 T system, that wavelength is only 26 cm. A conductive structure as short as 13 cm may resonate with the RF field, causing currents within conductive implants that have the potential to heat the implant itself.

1.2.1.6 Radio Frequency Interaction with Body Piercings and Tattoos

Piercings can be treated similarly to passive implants. Their ferromagnetism is usually negligible and their size is usually too small to interact with the switching of the magnetic field gradients or with the RF field. They will cause significant artifacts but they do not present a potential hazard to the patient. There are no reports of body piercings being torn and pulled into the magnet and there are no reports of these piercings becoming hot. The discussion on tattoos and permanent cosmetics is somewhat controversial. Problems related to MR procedures and tattoos are reported to be associated with the use of iron oxide or other metal-based pigments. A few cases are published where patients with tattoos who underwent MR procedures experienced transient skin irritation, cutaneous swelling, or heating sensations. There are studies reporting that approximately 1.5% of patients with permanent cosmetics will experience problems associated with MRI.

It has also been reported that decorative tattoos tend to cause more severe problems, including first- and second-degree burns. Due to the relatively remote possibility of an incident occurring in a patient with permanent cosmetics or a tattoo and to the relatively minor short-term complications reported so far, the patient should be informed about a possible reaction, but then permitted to undergo MRI. The application of ice packs or a wet towel to the site of the tattoo has been suggested to reduce the possibility of thermal injury, although there are no empiric data to date to support this recommendation.

1.2.1.7 Radio Frequency Interaction with Active Implants

Cardiac pacemakers are the most common electronically activated implants found in patients. Similar to passive implants, in regard to possible interactions with the MR system, the static magnetic field, the fringe field, and the RF field must be considered.

Any ferromagnetic components within the pulse generator may result in a movement of the object. Reed switch function is usually unpredictable and may result in ventricular fibrillation, rapid pacing, asynchronous pacing, inhibition of pacing output, alteration of programming, or possible damage to the pacemaker circuitry. Several studies on non-pacemaker-dependent patients indicate that certain pacemakers may be MR safe. However, the majority of these studies are based on empirical and not analytical experiments.

The lateral course of the pacemaker lead may interact with the axial E-field component of the RF field. The craniocaudal extension of the lead will present no potential hazard as long as it is close to the isocenter of the magnet. If the latter is not the case, the lead may couple with horizontal E-field components found in the vicinity of the RF transmit coil. For non-pacemaker-dependent patients, this will, as empirically evaluated and published, not lead to any consequences, although a number of reports indicate a necessary readjustment of the pacing threshold values. Although the reported results are encouraging, clinicians must be aware that manufacturers do not claim that their devices are currently MR safe or MR compatible. There are no cardiac devices that have yet achieved FDA clearance for MR compatibility.

Addressing the same issue, there are a number of publications dealing with the safety of patients with neurostimulators during an MR examination, with the claim that MRI can be performed safely even at 3 T. According to the warning letter issued by the FDA in May 2005, the FDA received several reports of serious injury, including coma and permanent neurological impairment in patients with implanted neurological stimulators who underwent an MRI procedure. The statement continues that the mechanism for these adverse events is likely to involve heating of the surrounding tissue at the end of the lead wires, resulting in injury. Although these reports involved deep brain stimulators and vagus nerve stimulators, similar injuries could be caused by any type of implanted neurological stimulator, such as spinal cord stimulators, peripheral nerve stimulators, and neuromuscular stimulators.

The majority of publications, generating the impression that MRI of patients with active implants may be safe, point out that their findings are highly specific to the MR system, the software version running the scanner, types of pacemakers and lead system and the geometrical arrangement of the device, the leads and the patient within the RF resonator of the scanner.

1.2.1.8 Switching of Magnetic Field Gradients

In order to excite a specific location or to identify the geometric location of a signal based on its frequency and phase, the Larmor frequency has to be a function of location. As the Larmor frequency is proportional to magnetic field strength, the magnetic field strength has to become a function of location. Desired is a linear dependence throughout the imaging volume. This is established by sending electric currents through the windings of the previously mentioned gradient coils. The amplitudes of the desired magnetic field gradients increase in conjunction with an increase in spatial resolution or a higher imaging bandwidth. The time needed to achieve the nominal value of the desired amplitude is called gradient rise time. Short gradient rise times allow shorter TEs and shorter ETLs, often documented as an improvement in image quality. The slew rate represents the magnetic field gradient amplitude that can be achieved by the gradient system, divided by the gradient rise time necessary to achieve this maximum amplitude. Unfortunately, a strong slow gradient system will have the same slew rate as a weak but fast gradient system. The patient seems to be the limiting factor for further increasing the performance of conventional gradient coils.

- Stimulation

A change in magnetic field over time is termed d*B*/d*t*. According to Maxwell's law, this d*B*/d*t* will induce a current in a conductive loop. Since the patient represents multiple potential although weak conductive loops, at a certain d*B*/d*t* value (either large change in amplitude (d*B*) and/or in a very short time (d*t*), the induced current might be large enough to stimulate peripheral nerves (PNS). Since d*B*/d*t* values can be calculated prior to sequence execution, a software monitor compares the calculated value with the PNS threshold and prohibits the execution of a pulse sequence, will recalculate the sequence timing and will issue a warning if the threshold is within 20% of the PNS limit. As PNS is only a function of d*B*/d*t*, there is no dependence on the overall magnetic field strength.

- Acoustic noise

Hendrik Anton Lorentz, a Dutch physician, discovered and documented that a conductive wire bearing an electric current will experience a mechanical force in the presence of a magnetic field. The force is proportional to the magnetic field strength, the current, and the wire length. Considering a magnetic field strength of 1.5 T and approximately 600 A flowing through a single winding of a gradient coil with a radius of 0.5 m, the force on the single wire will be 2,827 N or approximately equivalent to a weight of 635 lbs. The force will remain for the time the current is flowing and will vanish as soon as the (magnetic field) gradient is switched off. The duration of a slice-selective gradient is e.g., 2.5 ms. The frequency of the pulling followed by no pulling would be 200 Hz. That would generate a tone between an "a (220 Hz)" and a "g (196 Hz)." For a 195 Hz/pixel bandwidth, the readout gradient has a duration of 5.128 ms. The frequency of pulling as the current is switched on followed by no pulling as the gradient is switched off is 97.5 Hz, which is close to a "G (98 Hz)." Unfortunately, the gradient switching is not sinusoidal in general and different tasks approximate different frequencies and therefore, the sound produced during MRI is not quite harmonic. The necessity of modifying the magnetic field locally in order to be able to selectively excite or for the purpose of spatial encoding is correlated with a sound production due to the vibration of the (magnetic field) gradient coil. The mechanical force on a wire carrying a current through a magnetic field is called the Lorentz force. For example, for a magnetic field gradient along the direction of the main field (*z*-direction), the Lorentz force will cause one end of the gradient coil to be compressed and the other end to be expanded. Although made out of solid material, the gradient coil will vibrate due to the fast switching of currents (creating magnetic field gradients), causing the noise heard during an MR examination. As the Lorentz force is proportional to the current through the wire and the strength of the main magnetic field, one would expect the generated acoustic noise at a higher field strength to be stronger, if no counteracting measures are performed (for example, additional damping or any action to keep the vibrating gradient coil from generating air pressure waves). Considering the above-mentioned forces, it becomes obvious that it is not a trivial task to avoid any noise production by limiting the twisting, the bending, and the vibration of a gradient coil in action during imaging. The amplitude of the noise is measured in dB(A) and no vendor is allowed to introduce a scanner capable of generating more than 140 dB(A). During MRI, it is required to stay below 99 dB(A) at the ear of the patient (with or without ear protection).

1.2.2 Adipose Tissue

Molecules containing aliphatic lipid protons are intermediate in size, and their motions are close to the Larmor frequency, causing short T1-relaxation times. As a consequence, fat appears bright on T1-W images. On the other hand, there are only a few "static" contributions in adipose tissue to allow a rapid dephasing due to T2-relaxation. As a result, fat also appears bright on T2-W images. Fat is the only tissue for which a long T2-relaxation time is not correlated with a prolonged T1-relaxation time.

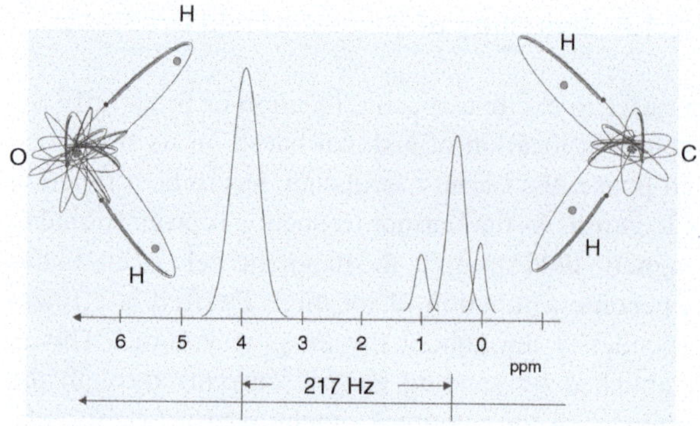

Fig. 1.18 Chemical shift: the electrons of oxygen-bounded hydrogen atoms are more drawn towards the oxygen atom than the electrons of carbon-bounded hydrogen. Hydrogen nuclei in adipose tissue are more "shielded," leading to a lower resonance frequency than free water. The term describing the effect of an electronic environment on the Larmor frequency is called "chemical shift"

1.2.2.1 Chemical Shift

The behavior of mobile fatty acids is slightly different compared to the oxygen-bounded hydrogens in water molecules as previously discussed. For the water molecule, the oxygen demands the single electron of the attached hydrogen, thus "deshielding" the proton. The carbon-bounded hydrogen nuclei are more "shielded" by the circulating single electron, thus experiencing an effective lower field than the water-bounded hydrogen nuclei. As a result, the Larmor frequencies of mobile fatty acids are below the water frequency. This phenomenon is called chemical shift (Fig. 1.18). The difference in resonance frequency scales with the strength of the main magnetic field and is approximately 3.5 ppm.

As the frequency information is utilized for spatial encoding, the chemical shift causes a pixel shift of the "water-image" vs. the "fat-image" (see also Sect. 1.3.7.2). The chemical shift enables a spectral suppression of the signal from fat as well as a utilization of in-phase vs. opposed-phase imaging for tumor characterization.

1.2.2.2 In-Phase, Opposed-Phase Imaging

The nuclei (protons) of fat and water-bounded hydrogen atoms have a slightly different resonance frequency. Starting with the excitation, the generated transverse macroscopic magnetization of the water will speed ahead in the transverse plane, while the fat-originated magnetization falls behind. In SE imaging, the 180° refocusing pulse will place the slower fat component in front of the faster water component. At the time the echo is acquired, they will both be in phase again. In that case, only the shift between the fat and water image remains, depending on the selected bandwidth per pixel. Avoiding the 180° refocusing, as done in GRE imaging, there will be a continuous dephasing of the water-originated magnetization and the fat-originated magnetization following the excitation. Depending on the TE, a situation will develop in which the magnetization of fat and water will point in the same direction. This situation is called in-phase. There will also be the other extreme, where the magnetization from fat is pointing in the opposite direction to that from water. This situation is called opposed phase. Depending on the content of fat and water in a single voxel, the residual magnetization from fat and water will be diminished, leading to a hypointense appearance, allowing the characterization of lesions with fatty infiltrations. The TE-dependent in-phase/opposed-phase situation in GRE imaging is a function of the difference in resonance frequencies between the magnetization of the fat-bounded hydrogen atoms (nuclei) and the water-bounded hydrogen atoms (nuclei). Depending on the type of fat molecule, this difference ranges from 3.2 to 3.5 ppm. Table 1.2 lists the standard suitable TEs to achieve an in-phase or opposed-phase situation, depending on the field strength of the MR system used.

Table 1.2 Echo times for in-phase and opposed-phase situation for different field strength. These are theoretical values based on a water-methylen two-component system. For some fat molecules and fat-infiltrated tissue, there may be a slight difference compared to these theoretical values, leading to a nonperfect in-phase or opposed-phase situation with increasing echo time and may require some tests for selecting the optimal echo time

Field strength (T)	Frequency shift (Hz)	First opposed-phase situation at a TE of (ms)	Second in-phase situation at a TE of (ms)	Second opposed-phase situation at a TE of (ms)
0.2	29	17.3	34.5	51.8
0.35	51	9.85	19.7	29.6
0.5	72	6.9	13.8	20.7
1.0	144	3.45	6.9	10.4
1.5	217	2.3	4.6	6.9

1.2.2.3 Spectral Suppression of Fat Signal

Fat usually appears hyperintense on PD-W and T1-W images. The high signal intensity often reduces the dynamic range for windowing the images, or it may obscure lesions. Artifacts due to respiratory motion usually originate within the subcutaneous fat. These are reasons why it is often desirable to eliminate or reduce the signal from fat. As mentioned above, the resonance frequency of fat-bounded hydrogen is approximately 3.5 ppm lower than the resonance frequency for water-bounded hydrogen, i.e., 217 Hz for a 1.5 T system or 147 Hz for a 1.0 T magnet. Applying a spectral saturation pulse prior to the imaging sequence, as indicated in Fig. 1.19, it is possible to suppress the signal from fat.

A frequency selective excitation pulse is used to excite all fat within the imaging volume. With this pulse, the longitudinal nuclear magnetization within adipose tissue is converted to a transverse magnetization. Immediately following is the application of "spoiler" gradients, which dephase the transverse magnetization. A dephased transverse magnetization will not induce any signal and will not interfere with the imaging sequence to follow. The fat saturation scheme can be combined with any imaging sequence. The time needed to excite the fat and to spoil the transverse magnetization will prolong the time needed to measure a single Fourier-line or an echo train. As the time needed per slice is increased, there will be fewer slices for a given TR when utilizing this fat saturation scheme. One approach to regain the possible number of slices for a given TR is to use a "fast fat saturation" scheme. In this case, the fat saturation scheme is only applied and repeated e.g., for the first slice, but not for the Fourier-lines for the slices to follow. Advantage of this method is that more slices can be measured within a given TR. The disadvantage is the increasing temporal distance from the fat excitation pulse to the excitation pulse of a given slice, resulting in a slice position dependent vanishing effectiveness of the fat saturation. The fast fat saturation scheme is usually only combined with gradient echo imaging. Challenging for these techniques is the fact that a good magnetic field homogeneity is required throughout the imaging volume in order for the resonance frequency of water and fat not to change with location. If this condition is not fulfilled, fat may appear unsaturated at one corner of the image and even water may become saturated. The process to establish a homogeneous field for the imaging volume is called "shimming." In this case, currents are sent through shim coils, or, as an offset, through the gradient coils, in order to have the same magnetic field everywhere within the volume of interest during the fat saturation process. It is also possible to define a "shimming volume" as a subregion within the imaging volume for a better and faster shimming procedure for a specific area of interest.

1.2.3 Inversion Recovery

The longitudinal nuclear magnetization can be "prepared" prior to imaging. These preparation schemes can be usually combined with any imaging sequence. The previously discussed fat saturation scheme can be considered one form of preparation. Another form of preparation is the inversion of the longitudinal nuclear magnetization prior to imaging - IR. This will allow the suppression of

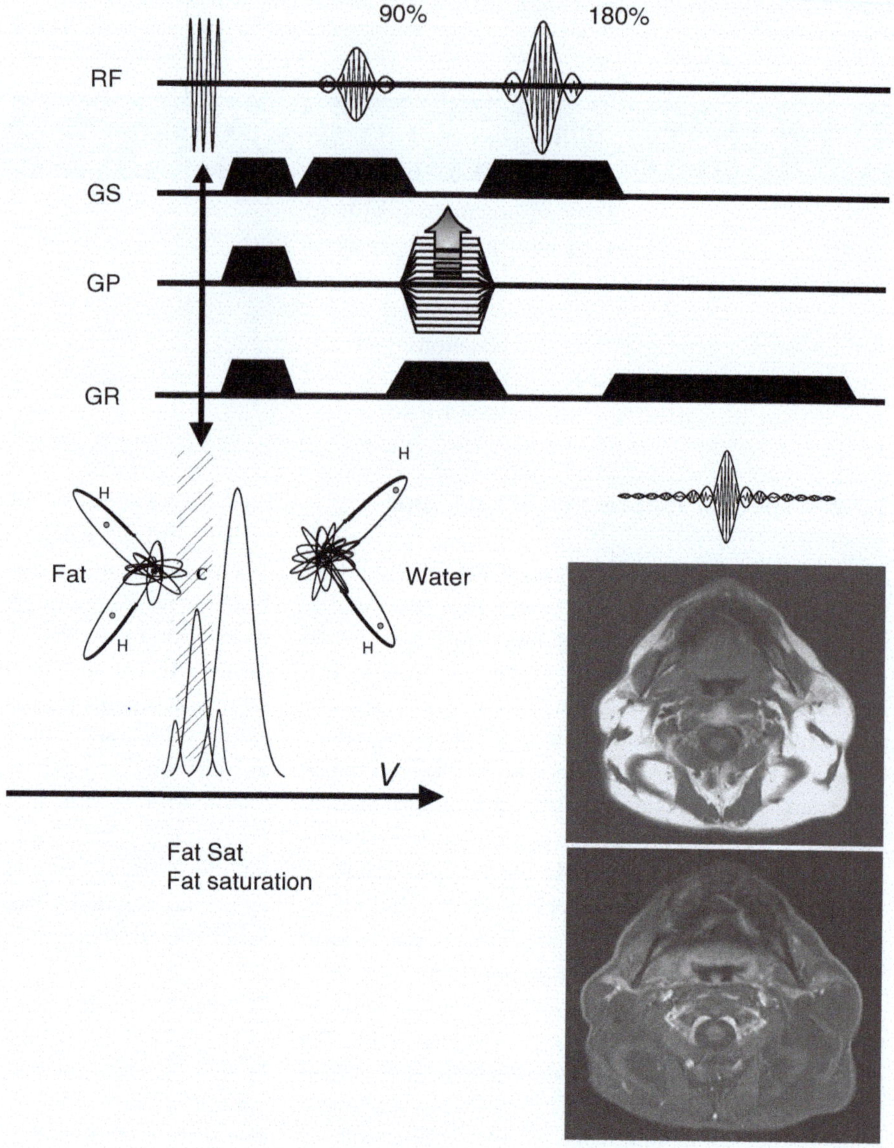

Fig. 1.19 Spectral fat suppression - FS: since the resonance frequencies of fat and water differ by about 3.5 ppm, a frequency-selective saturation pulse can be used to reduce the signal from fat. A frequency-selective excitation pulse converts the longitudinal nuclear magnetization of adipose tissue to a transverse magnetization, which is immediately dephased using "spoiler" gradients. The longitudinal magnetization within adipose tissue will have no time to recover prior to the imaging sequence to follow (e.g., a spin echo sequence as in this example), leading to a fat suppressed image

signal from tissue with a specific relaxation time like fat (short T1 relaxation time) or fluid (long T1 relaxation time), or can be used to improve T1-weighting.

The course of the longitudinal magnetization following inversion is

$$M_z = M_0 \cdot (1 - 2 \cdot e^{-T_I/T_1}),$$

with T_I as inversion time, the time between inversion of the longitudinal magnetization and the excitation pulse of the imaging sequence. The following recovery is a function of the tissue-specific T1 relaxation time. The above equation is only valid for a recovery that does not consider an influence of the imaging sequence. For a real imaging sequence, it has to be considered that the inversion is applied to a longitudinal magnetization that has only partially recovered, depending on the selected TR. It has also to be considered that each RF refocusing pulse of a spin echo sequence or a multi spin echo sequence is operating as an inversion pulse for the recovered longitudinal magnetization at that point and the course of the longitudinal nuclear magnetization becomes

$$M_z = M_0 \cdot \left(1 - 2 \cdot e^{-T_I/T_1} + 2 \cdot e^{-(T_R - T_E/2)/T_1} - e^{-T_R/T_1}\right).$$

Starting the imaging sequence at a point in time, where the longitudinal magnetization of a specific tissue is zero as it is in the transition from antiparallel orientation to parallel orientation, there will be no longitudinal magnetization to be converted to a transverse magnetization, thus there will be no signal generated within that tissue. As described previously, this is the method to suppress the signal from fat if the inversion time selected is short enough and the same method applies to suppressing the signal from fluid when selecting a long inversion time. As the recovery is dependent on T1 relaxation time, the method is also suitable to enhance T1-weighting. For example, selecting an inversion time at the point where the difference in longitudinal magnetization between gray and white matter is at its maximum will generate images with a superior contrast between gray and white matter as is mainly used to document the maturing brain.

1.2.3.1 Relaxation-Dependent Elimination of Fat Signal

Fat has a very short T1 relaxation time. Using an inversion pulse prior to the measurement, it is possible to apply the excitation pulse of the imaging sequence at the time the recovering longitudinal magnetization of fat is zero, which is at the point where the antiparallel aligned magnetization is changing to a parallel aligned magnetization (Fig. 1.20). In this case, fat will not be excited. Such a technique is called short tau inversion recovery - STIR, and is often used in conjunction with faster imaging techniques to be mentioned later. The inversion time for fat suppression on a 1.5-T system is approximately 150 ms when used in conjunction with a conventional imaging sequence. Used in conjunction with faster imaging techniques, the inversion time may have to be prolonged to 170 ms. A disadvantage of the STIR technique is that the inversion pulse affects all tissues, often reducing the SNR dramatically. That disadvantage can be compensated utilizing a spectral inversion (SPIR) or a spectral adiabatic inversion (SPAIR). As STIR will diminish the signal from tissue with a short T1 relaxation time (like fat), it is advised not to use STIR techniques after contrast administration, since the majority of contrast agents used in MR are T1-shortening agents. In which case, the signal from tissue of enhancing lesions (T1-reduced) may be reduced.

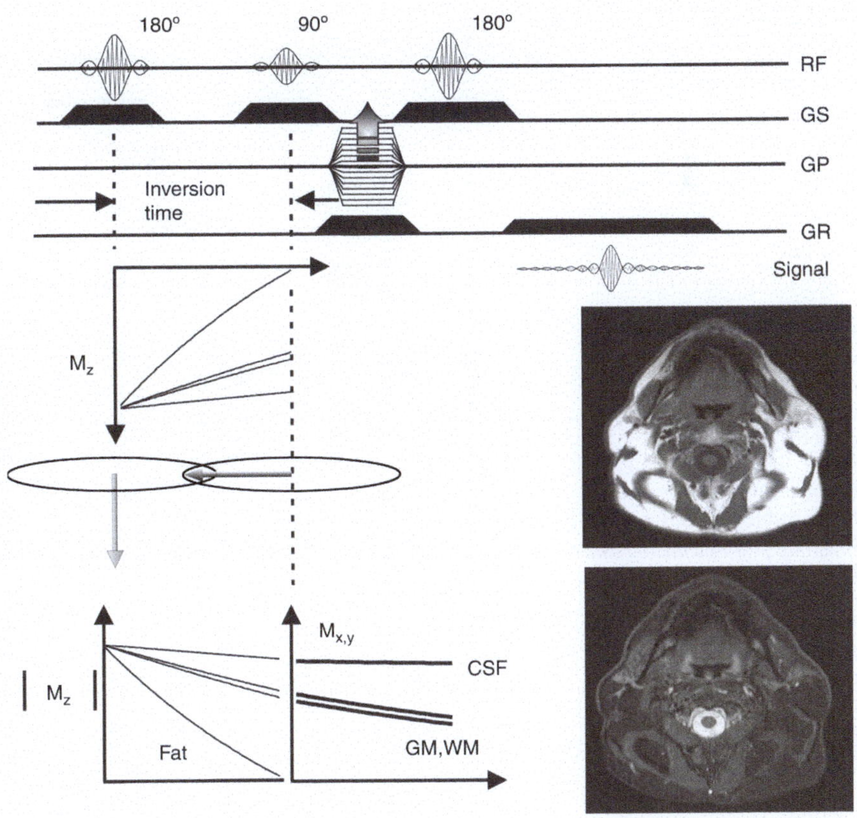

Fig. 1.20 The short tau inversion recovery (STIR) approach used for relaxation-dependent fat suppression. The equilibrium magnetization is inverted at the beginning of the sequence, and the longitudinal magnetization recovers depending on the tissue-specific relaxation time T1. The recovered longitudinal magnetization M_z is turned into the transverse plane, becoming M_{xy} after an inversion time T1. In STIR imaging, T_I is the selected time at which the fat is assumed to have no longitudinal component, and therefore no transverse component can be generated with the excitation. Only the magnitude of the longitudinal component is considered, not the direction. Such an approach is also called IRM (inversion recovery with magnitude reconstruction). *GP* phase-encoding gradient; *GR* readout gradient; *GS* slice-selection gradient; *RF* radiofrequency; *WM* white matter; *GM* gray matter

1.2.3.2 Relaxation-Dependent Elimination of Signal from Fluid

With the faster imaging techniques to be described later, the discussion of a suitable inversion time in conjunction with a reasonable measurement time becomes obsolete. In conjunction with fast imaging techniques, it becomes feasible to select an inversion period of, for example, 2 s, nullifying the signal of the CSF (Fig. 1.21). This technique is very useful when studying periventricular lesions, often obscured by the bright signal of adjacent CSF spaces. In conjunction with a conventional SE acquisition scheme, this technique has been introduced as fluid-attenuated inversion recovery - FLAIR.

1.2.3.3 Inversion Recovery to Improve T1-Weighting

The longitudinal nuclear magnetization will recover after inversion with the tissue-specific T1 relaxation as previously discussed. The nuclear magnetization within tissue with a relatively short T1 relaxation will recover fast, indicated with a steep recovery course of the longitudinal magnetization. The nuclear magnetization within tissue with a relatively long T1 relaxation time will recover slower indicated by a flat recovery course of the longitudinal magnetization. Consider a 90° RF excitation pulse causing a clockwise rotation of the longitudinal nuclear magnetization. Magnetization that is aligned parallel to the direction of the magnetic field will be flipped to the right whereas antiparallel aligned magnetization will be flipped to the left. Both longitudinal magnetizations will be converted to a signal inducing transverse magnetization. They will only have the opposite phase in the transverse plane. The above-mentioned inversion recovery methods like STIR and FLAIR only consider the magnitude and not the phase of the signal (inversion recovery with magnitude reconstruction - IRM). Inversion recovery imaging methods that also utilize the phase information are called phase sensitive. The phase of the induced signal indicates the parallel or antiparallel alignment of the longitudinal magnetization prior to the excitation pulse. For phase sensitive inversion recovery techniques, no

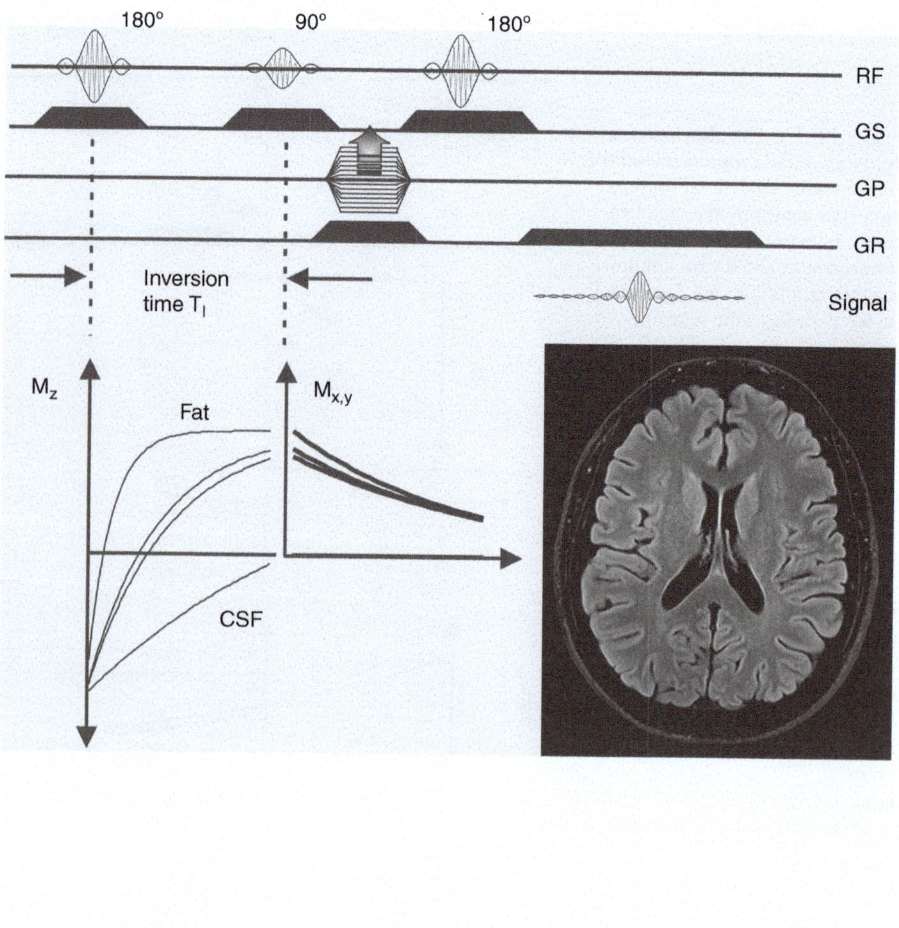

Fig. 1.21 The fluid-attenuated inversion recovery (FLAIR) approach used for relaxation-dependent suppression of the cerebrospinal fluid (CSF) signal. In FLAIR imaging, the inversion time T_I is the time at which the CSF has no longitudinal component, and therefore no transverse component can be generated with the excitation. *GP* phase-encoding gradient; *GR* readout gradient; *GS* slice-selection gradient; *RF* radiofrequency

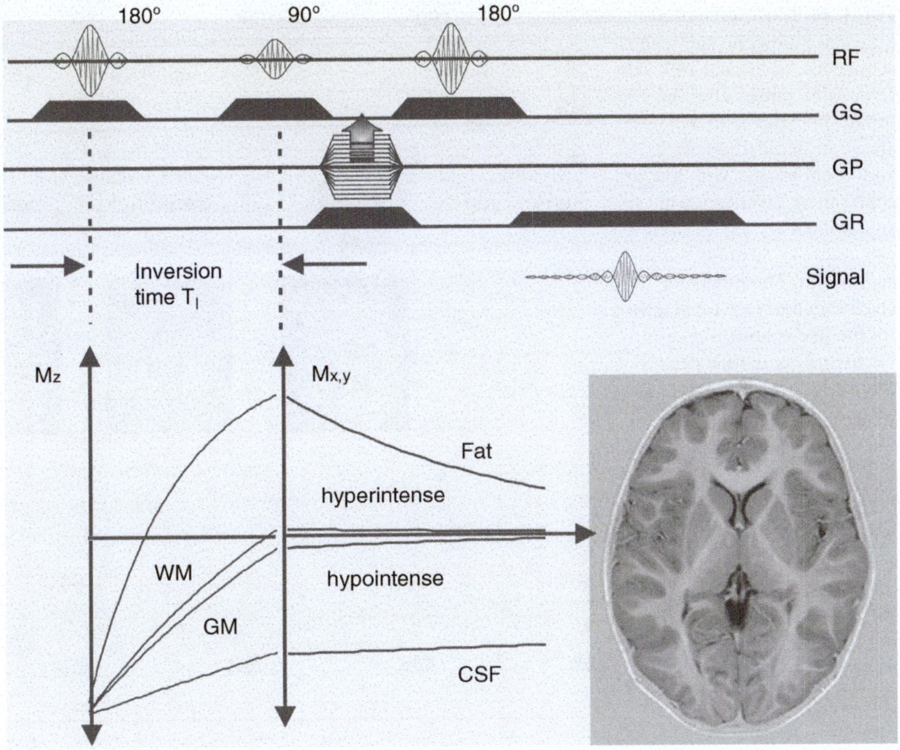

Fig. 1.22 The true inversion recovery technique (IR) provides an impressive differentiation between tissues with a small difference in T1 relaxation times. At an inversion time of approximately 350 ms, the longitudinal magnetization of white matter is already parallel aligned whereas the magnetization of gray matter is still antiparallel aligned to the direction of the main magnetic field. The excitation pulse generates a transverse magnetization within both tissues and the phase difference is utilized to display white matter hyperintense and gray matter hypointense. No signal is presented as intermediate gray. *GP* phase-encoding gradient; *GR* readout gradient; *GS* slice-selection gradient; *RF* radiofrequency

signal will be presented as an intermediate grey, signal of previously antiparallel aligned longitudinal magnetization will be presented hypointense, and signal of previously parallel aligned longitudinal magnetization will be presented hyperintense. This technique will allow a superior contrast between tissues with small differences in T1 relaxation time, like grey and white matter (Fig. 1.22).

1.2.4 Faster SE Imaging Using Multiple Phase Encoded Echoes

Using multiple 180° RF refocusing pulses following a single excitation will allow the acquisition of multiple images with different TEs, as indicated in Fig. 1.23. This technique is still used today for scientific reasons, as the signal course within each pixel permits the calculation of the T2 relaxation time at each location within the slice. A prerequisite is, of course, the use of a long TR in order to suppress the T1 influence on image contrast. Viewing these images, it is apparent that the shortest possible TE presents a PD-W image whereas the following images show just an increase in T2-weighting with an increase of the weighting with TE. The basic contrast, in this example, is identical: CSF is always hyperintense, followed by gray matter and white matter is hypointense. This appearance triggered the idea to phase encode the different echoes in order to acquire the *k*-space for a single image in a shorter time (Fig. 1.24). The potential reduction in measurement time is proportional to the utilized echoes, also called the echo train length - ETL. The sequence is named fast spin echo sequence - FSE or turbo spin echo sequence - TSE. This technique has replaced conventional SE imaging for PD-W and T2-W imaging. It is even sometimes utilized in T1-W imaging.

The theoretical penalty for each Fourier line having a different T2-weighting is well compensated as protocols involving TSE imaging techniques usually use a longer TR for an improved contrast compared to the conventional SE techniques, and they often utilize a larger matrix size, leading to improved spatial resolution. It has been documented that these measures

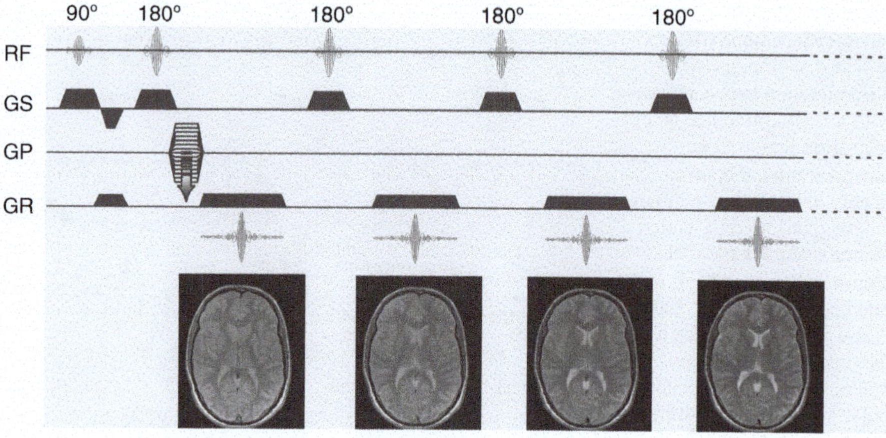

Fig. 1.23 Illustration of a classical multiecho spin-echo sequence. Additional 180° RF refocusing pulses after the initial first spin echo will allow the acquisition of additional images with longer echo times. The change in signal intensity can be used to calculate the T2 value within each voxel. The moderate change in contrast, especially for the late echoes, suggests the use of phase-encoded echoes in fast spin echo imaging

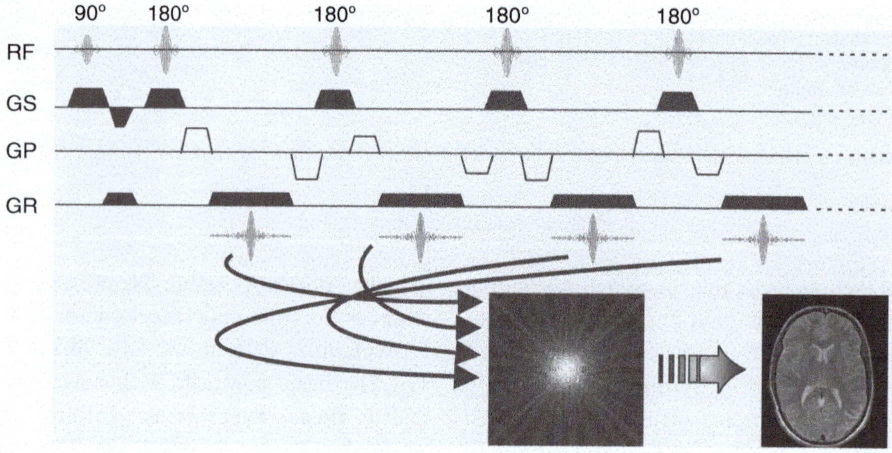

Fig. 1.24 Fast spin echo imaging (FSE, TSE) utilizes multiple echoes to fill the raw data matrix. Each echo has a different phase encoding. The possible reduction in measurement time is directly proportional to the number of echoes used. The effective echo time is given at the time the low spatial frequencies are acquired. Since the data acquisition is along a T2-relaxation curve, there is the potential of image blurring due to different weighting within *k*-space. For T2-W imaging, this effect is almost negligible. The illustration above only shows the first four echoes of a sequence design that usually utilizes 15–23 echoes for imaging. *GP* phase-encoding gradient; *GR* read-out gradient; *GS* slice-selection gradient; *RF* radiofrequency

overcompensate the risk of missing small lesions as a consequence of differently weighted Fourier lines. Other interesting observations of fast spin echo imaging, like the bright appearance of fat or the reduced sensitivity to hemorrhagic lesions, will be discussed in the "advanced" section of this chapter. T1-W protocols with fast spin echo imaging are less successful as the TR has to be kept short to achieve a T1-weighting and the use of multiple echoes per slice will prolong the time needed for a single slice, and thus, only a few slices can be acquired within the given TR. At the same point in time, only a few phase-encoded echoes can be utilized as not to contaminate the T1-weighting with the T2 relaxation process.

The previously mentioned IR techniques combined with the fast spin echo acquisition modes are called IR-FSE, TIR, or TIRM, similar to the acronym used in SE applications. Due to the potential savings in measurement time using TIRM imaging, the inversion time can be prolonged to more than 2 s to get even the zero crossing of the recovering magnetization within CSF. The latter technique has the potential for a better delineation of periventricular lesions, as already previously mentioned. In fact, all the inversion recovery techniques mentioned previously are usually combined with such a fast spin echo approach.

1.2.5 Faster Imaging Using Spatially Distributed Surface Coils (Parallel Acquisition Techniques)

The number of phase-encoding steps is one of the factors dictating the length of the measurement time. The number of phase-encoding steps is necessary to spatially encode the signal from an object for a desired field of view (FoV) and a requested spatial resolution. The maximum amplitude and duration of the phase-encoding gradient provide information about the highest spatial resolution causing a phase change of 180° for the transverse magnetization within adjacent voxels. Measuring with as many phase-encoding steps as there are matrix lines in the direction of phase encoding allows unequivocal assignment to the suitable spatial frequencies. Omitting every other phase-encoding step, as illustrated in Fig. 1.25c, corresponds to a reduction of the FoV in the direction of phase encoding by a factor of two. If the object extends beyond that FoV, an aliased image will be the result. Aliasing or wrap around corresponds to an overlapping representation of signal from tissue that is located outside the FoV at the opposite end.

An array of closely packed receiver coils surrounding the object has been suggested to reestablish the unequivocal assignment. As each coil has a defined location and "sensitivity profile," that information can be used to "unwrap" the image. Since each coil is separately receiving the signal from the object within the sensitivity region, but parallel to other adjacent coils, these methods are called parallel acquisition techniques. There are multiple strategies for image unwrapping, e.g., the method sensitivity encoding (SENSE) uses the image information for each coil channel, whereas the simultaneous acquisition of spatial harmonics (SMASH) performs the "unwrapping" within *k*-space. Other acronyms for different strategies in parallel acquisition reconstructions are "scissors methods," Roemer method, partially parallel imaging with localized sensitivities (PILS), sensitivity profiles from an array of coils for encoding and

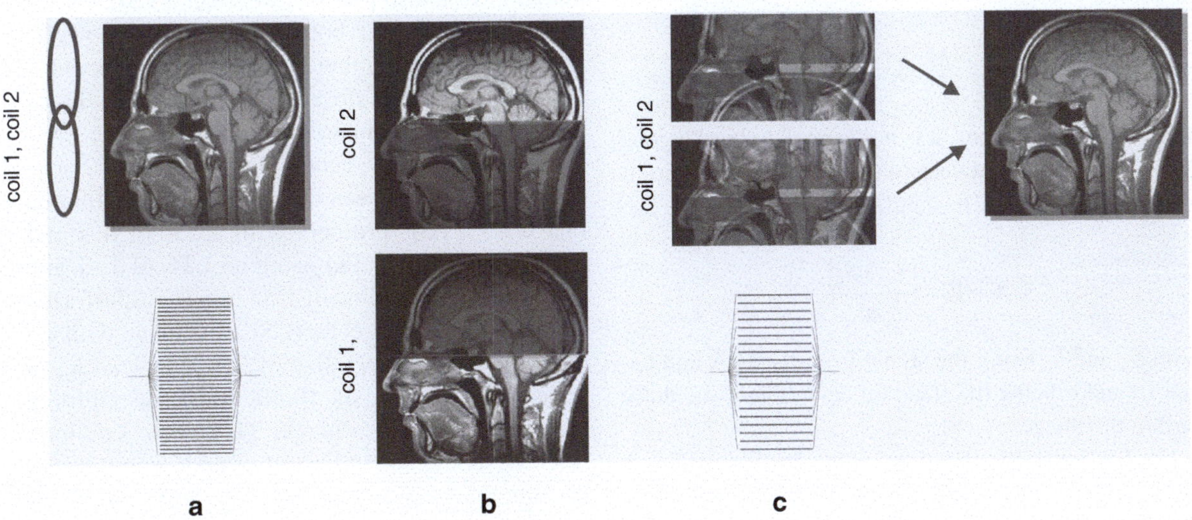

Fig. 1.25 Parallel acquisition techniques - PAT: These are graphical illustrations, not actual measurements. (**a**) A two-coil set-up illustration the acquisition of a sagittal image with a full *k*-space matrix. (**b**) Parallel acquisition and image reconstruction for each of the two coil channels. (**c**) Undersampling the data corresponds to a rectangular field of view, resulting in aliased images. Notice the aliasing artifact for the neck measured with coil 1 is stronger than the same region detected with coil 2. The aliasing artifact from the upper part of the brain has a stronger signal within the image of coil 2 than the appearance in the image of coil 1. Using this information (the sensitivity profiles of the coils), the image can be "unwrapped"

reconstruction in parallel (SPACE RIP), and generalized autocalibrating partially parallel acquisitions (GRAPPA).

1.2.6 Imaging Protocols and Image Quality

The task is obvious: It is desired to have the best spatial resolution with the optimum of contrast between lesion and normal parenchyma in the shortest possible measurement time.

1.2.6.1 Sequence Dependent Imaging Protocol Parameters

Sequence Type SE: T1-Weighting: Focus Central Nervous System

The signal generating transverse magnetization is proportional to the longitudinal magnetization at the time of the (90°) excitation pulse, and for SE, the course of the longitudinal magnetization is $M_z = M_0 \cdot (1 - e^{-T_R/T_1})$, and after excitation, the course of the transverse magnetization is $M_{x,y} = M_z \cdot e^{-T_E/T_2}$, and therefore, the induced signal follows

$$S \sim \frac{dM_{x,y}}{dt} \sim M_0 \cdot \left(1 - e^{-T_R/T_1}\right) \cdot e^{-T_E/T_2}.$$

To differentiate lesions, it is not enough to have a good SNR; the contrast between two different tissue types is also of importance. The contrast is given by

$$\mathrm{CNR} = \frac{|S_A - S_B|}{\sigma},$$

with S_A and S_B being the signal from tissue A and tissue B, and σ being the standard deviation of the noise within the image.

In SE imaging, the time between repetitions is used to excite and acquire data from adjacent slices. This is called multislice imaging. The time needed to acquire one Fourier-line in conventional imaging or multiple Fourier-lines in multi-echo imaging is called a slice-loop time. The number of selected slices times this slice-loop time has to be accommodated within the given TR. Optimizing the TR for T1-W imaging may lead to a TR, which is too short to do a multislice measurement with the necessary number of slices to cover the desired volume. The commonly used protocols tend to be a compromise between using as many slices as necessary to cover the region of interest and the selection of the shortest possible TR to still achieve an optimal T1-weighting.

Sequence Type FSE: PD and T2-Weighting

In order to suppress the influence of T1 recovery, the selection of a long TR is desired. Unfortunately, measurement time scales directly with TR. The established solution to this problem is to minimize the number of necessary repetitions by filling *k*-space with multiple phase-encoded echoes. The number of echoes used following an excitation is called ETL. The reduction in measurement time is proportional to the number of phase-encoded echoes. As the number of echoes increase the time needed to acquire the data for a single slice, this method is mainly suitable for applications that utilize a long TR (PD- or T2-weighting). For T2-weighting, an ETL between 7 and 15 is suitable. Due to the rapid signal changes for short TEs, a shorter ETL (≤7) is advised for PD-W imaging. It is also possible to select a FSE sequence protocol to provide both images, PD- as well as T2-weighting. Even though each Fourier line for this method will have a different T2-weighting, the contrast will be dominated by the weighting of the Fourlines around the center of *k*-space (coarse spatial resolution). It has been documented in the literature that e.g., a FSE protocol with a TR of 4 s and a matrix size of 512*384 using an ETL of 13 leading to a measurement time of 1:58 min is outperforming a conventional spin echo (CSE) sequence with a TR of 2.5 s and a matrix size of 256*256 leading to a measurement time of 10:40 min. The additional recovery following a longer TR and the commonly selected better spatial resolution is compensating for potential consequences of the different weighting within *k*-space (missing of small objects, edge enhancement, edge smoothing, or image blurring). The TE for the central *k*-space line is dominating the weighting of the image and is named the "effective TE."

Sequence Type GRE: T1-Weighting: Abdominal Imaging

Despite numerous techniques that allow abdominal imaging with free breathing, breath-hold imaging techniques still have their advantage and often provide superior image quality as compared to free breathing methods. In order to allow imaging for the duration of a suspended respiration, imaging time has to be shorter than 25 s. This is not quite achievable with T1-W SE imaging. GRE sequences turned out to be suitable. With the application of protocols using short TR in order to have a reasonable measurement time while keeping a 90° RF excitation pulse, the signal will be poor as the longitudinal magnetization does not have enough time to recover. A higher signal contribution can be achieved by utilizing a low flip angle excitation (as already known from MR spectroscopy). The excitation angle with a maximum signal response is also called the Ernst angle and is illustrated in Fig. 1.26. A GRE technique in conjunction with spoiling and a low angle excitation has been named "fast low angle shot" - FLASH. Various applications of this FLASH technique can be found throughout the book, primarily for musculoskeletal imaging, abdominal breath-hold techniques, dynamic imaging of the heart, studying the temporal course of enhancement after contrast media application, and MRA. The signal course of a spoiled gradient-echo sequence is as follows

$$S \sim M_{x,y} = M_0 \cdot \frac{(1-e^{-T_R/T_1})}{1-\cos\alpha \cdot e^{-T_R/T_1}} \cdot e^{-T_E/T_2^*} \cdot \sin\alpha$$

and the Ernst angle derived from this equation is

$$\alpha_{\text{Ernst}} = \arccos e^{-T_R/T_1}.$$

Sequence Type IR: Inversion Recovery

The recovery of the longitudinal magnetization following an inversion is leading to $M_z = M_0 \cdot \left(1-2\cdot e^{-T_I/T_1} + 2\cdot e^{-(T_R-T_E/2)/T_1} - e^{-T_R/T_1}\right)$. with the sequence-specific imaging parameter being the inversion time T_I. A short T_I (e.g., 150 ms for a STIR sequence) characterizes the utilization of a fat suppression technique based on the typical short T1 relaxation time within the adipose tissue, a long T_I (e.g., 2 s for a FLAIR approach) characterizes the utilization of a fluid attenuated method, and an inversion time of approximately 350 ms aims for a maximum contrast between gray and white matter using a phase sensitive inversion recovery method. The inversion can be combined with a fast spin echo imaging method leading to IR-FSE, TIRM, or TIR as already discussed in Sect. 1.2.3).

1.2.6.2 Sequence Independent Imaging Protocol Parameters

Number of Slices

There are a few imaging sequences that acquire slices sequentially. Those are easily identified as the measurement time will increase with the number of selected slices. The majority of imaging sequences acquire slices

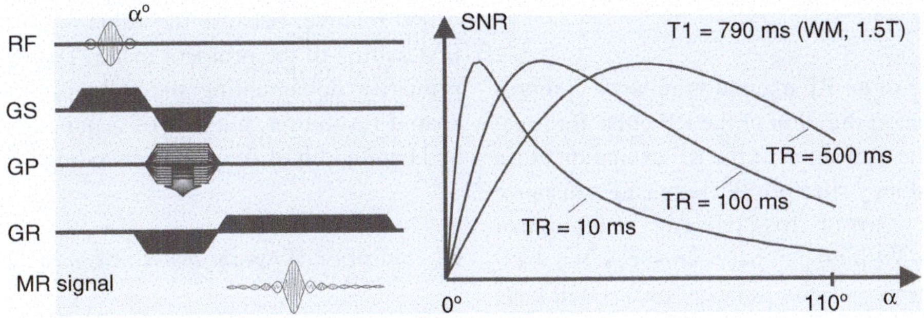

Fig. 1.26 The Ernst angle. For a given tissue (T1 relaxation time) and a given repetition time (TR), there is always one excitation angle where the signal response is maximal. This angle is called the Ernst angle. The above curves are normalized to the same measurement time (e.g., 10 ms TR, 50 acquisitions compared with 500 ms TR, 1 acquisition). For a TR of 10 ms, the optimal angle would be 10°, whereas for the 500 ms TR sequence, the maximal signal response would be achieved with an excitation angle of 58°. This Ernst angle approach is utilized in musculoskeletal imaging as well as for time-of-flight magnetic resonance angiography. *SNR* signal-to-noise ratio

in an interleaved fashion, that is one or more Fourier lines are acquired per slice and then other slices are addressed prior to getting back to the first slice as the selected TR expired. There is usually a warning issued and solutions are offered if the number of slices multiplied with the time needed to excite and acquire data from a single slice exceeds the selected TR. The three solutions offered are an extension of the TR, a reduction of the number of slices, or the selection of a concatenation. The latter means that the TR and the number of slices are kept as they are and the number of slices are distributed equally over more than one measurement.

It has also to be kept in mind that a number of tasks will extend the time needed to excite and acquire data from an individual slice:

- Prolonging the TE will proportionally increase the time needed for a single slice.
- Spectral saturation is usually done per slice and therefore will increase the time needed per slice.
- Any regional saturation pulse is usually applied prior to each excitation pulse and will increase the time needed per slice.
- Any additional phase-encoded echo (increase of ETL) will reduce the measurement time as the number of necessary excitations will decrease, but the time needed to address a single slice will increase, thus reducing the number of possible slices per selected TR.

There are exceptions, e.g., a so called fast fat saturation scheme, where the saturation of fat is not repeated for each slice (Sect. 1.2.2.3).

Distance Factor

The slice profile of an RF excitation pulse is compromised due to a short duration of the RF pulse for practical reasons. The truncation of the RF excitation pulse will result in a sloppy slice profile, requiring a distance factor in order to avoid cross talk (the saturation of adjacent slices). With no gap between slices, the excitation or refocusing pulse of adjacent pulses will have a decreasing effect on the longitudinal magnetization of adjacent slices, leading to a reduced signal. Thus, a reasonable gap (e.g., 10% of the selected slice thickness) between slices will improve image quality. With increasing gap size, the probability will increase that small lesions will be missed.

Interpolation

The Fourier transformation requires for the highest spatial resolution to be resolved, that the transverse magnetization of adjacent voxel in the direction of frequency encoding is of opposite sign at the beginning and at the end of a measured Fourier line. The same requirement applies for the transverse magnetization of adjacent voxel in the direction of phase encoding for the first and last Fourier line acquired. As transverse magnetizations identical in amplitude and opposite in sign will lead to a cancelled signal, the data values of outer *k*-space are of very low amplitude. An interesting approach is the so-called zero filling. The system is told that more *k*-space data points have been acquired (with no signal, zero value) than have actually been measured. For example, a 256*256 acquired *k*-space matrix is placed into the center of a 512*512 *k*-space matrix filled with zero values for the outer *k*-space data points. It can be derived mathematically that this zero filling corresponds to a voxel shifted interpolation, that is, the image appearance is improved (reduced partial volume effects) although the actually measured spatial resolution is still as poor as before. This method is also called Fourier-interpolation.

1.2.6.3 Sequence Independent Imaging Protocol Parameters that Are Documented with a Relative SNR Indicator

All major vendors have a relative SNR indicator for all imaging parameters where the influence on SNR can be unambiguously calculated. The SNR indicator is called relative, because the value is set to 1.0 for the first calling of the protocol menu. The relative SNR is primarily documenting the influence of changes in spatial resolution, number of acquisitions (averages), and bandwidth of frequency encoding.

n_{acq}: Number of Averages–Number of Excitations

The number of acquisitions, as they show up in the protocol dialog, contributes proportionally to the square root to the overall SNR. Intuitively, it can be assumed that each acquisition is collecting true signal as well as noise. With an additional acquisition, the signal is collected again, and the received noise may contain other frequencies as compared to the previous measurement. With each acquisition, the probability increases that the noise pattern has similarities with previous measurements. This is the intuitive explanation for the square root dependency.

$$\mathrm{SNR} \sim \sqrt{n_{\mathrm{acq}}}.$$

d: Slice Thickness

The amplitude of the received signal depends on how many nuclear spins are participating in the excitation and relaxation process, and how many have to be assigned to a single voxel. As the number of hydrogen nuclei increase with voxel size and as the voxel size is a linear function of the slice thickness, SNR increases proportional to the selected slice thickness. A thick slice is advantageous with respect to SNR and coverage but bears the potential of so-called partial volume effects. Lesions smaller than the slice thickness may be obscured by the signal from adjacent tissues. Tissue boundaries changing their course within the selected slice thickness will turn out blurred and smoothed. This is called the partial volume effect.

$$\mathrm{SNR} \sim d.$$

FoV: The Field of View

The spatial resolution of the measurement is given by the field of view divided by the selected matrix size. The spatial resolution is defining the voxel size and with this the number of protons involved in the imaging process. As the field of view defines the extent of the voxel in the two perpendicular directions, its influence is quadratic with respect to SNR. Halving the field of view will quarter the number of protons to generate the signal whose amplitude will be converted to a pixel intensity (representing the signal from the small voxel). As a consequence, 16 acquisitions ($\sqrt{16} = 4$) will be necessary to compensate the SNR loss when halving the FoV. As practical consequence: A small reduction in FoV of e.g., 10% will lead to a SNR decrease of 19%. This also indicates that a small sacrifice in spatial resolution will gain SNR, which in turn can be used to shorten the measurement time.

$$\mathrm{SNR} \sim \mathrm{FoV}^2.$$

$\mathrm{FoV_P}$: The Field of View in the Direction of Phase Encoding

The spatial encoding in the direction of phase encoding requires multiple excitations followed by the acquisition of one or more phase-encoded echoes, with the TR as waiting period in between excitations. Without any changes in spatial resolution, a smaller field of view will require fewer phase-encoding steps, thus saving measurement time. On the other hand, each measured Fourier line also presents an additional acquisition, as it contains information about all objects within the slice. For example, reducing the FoV in the direction of phase encoding by 50% will result in a decrease in SNR of 29% (while halving the measurement time).

$$\mathrm{SNR} \sim \sqrt{\frac{\mathrm{FoV_P}}{\mathrm{FoV}}}.$$

$\mathrm{Mat_b}$: Matrix (Base) Size

The voxel size and with this the number of protons contributing to the signal is given by the slice thickness and the field of view divided by the matrix size. With a few exceptions, the measurement time is proportional to the matrix size in the direction of phase encoding. Each measured Fourier line (phase encoded echo) can be seen as an additional acquisition. Halving the matrix size (e.g., 256–128) will increase the voxel size by a factor of four, will decrease the number of acquisitions by a factor of two, and the four fold gain in SNR due to changes in geometry will be diminished by a factor of 0.71 due to changes in the number of acquisitions (SNR(128) = 2.83*SNR(256)).

$$\mathrm{SNR} \sim \frac{\sqrt{Mat_b}}{Mat_b^2}.$$

$\mathrm{Mat_{asym}}$: Phase Resolution

The measurement time is primarily dictated by the number of phase-encoding steps necessary to achieve the spatial resolution in the direction of phase encoding. It is possible to have a different spatial resolution in the direction of frequency encoding as compared to the spatial resolution in phase encoding. In return, there will be a reduction in measurement time correlated with an unexpected gain in SNR. For example, selecting a 256*128 matrix (50% phase resolution, $Mat_{asym} = 0.5$) will increase the voxel size by a factor of two as compared to a 256*256 matrix (100% phase resolution). The number of phase-encoding steps (acquisitions) will decrease by a factor of two and as a consequence, a factor of 0.71 will have to multiplied with the twofold gain in SNR. (SNR(256*128) = 1.414* SNR(256*256)).

$$\text{SNR} \sim \frac{\sqrt{Mat_{asym}}}{Mat_{asym}}.$$

GP_{ov}: Oversampling

The number of sampling points during the duration of data acquisition defines the sampling interval and the range of frequencies that can be unambiguously identified. The amplitude of the identified frequencies is then, in conjunction with the phase encoding information, assigned to a pixel intensity representing the position of the signal source within the image. If there is signal generated outside the FoV, the sampling will identify a frequency pattern that fits inside the FoV. The result is a wraparound artifact (see also 1.3.7.3). Doubling the sampling rate in the direction of frequency encoding has no penalty and is usually done by default. That is why there are no wraparound artifacts in the direction of frequency encoding. Increasing the sampling rate in the direction of phase encoding will proportionally increase the measurement time and should only be done if needed. As each additional Fourier line corresponds to another acquisition, selecting oversampling will also improve SNR. (SNR(50%oversampling) = 1.23* SNR(no oversampling)).

$$\text{SNR} \sim \sqrt{1+\text{GP}_{ov}}.$$

GP_{PF}: Partial Fourier

In theory, the *k*-space is symmetric. One quadrant of *k*-space contains enough spatial information to reconstruct an image. In practice, the symmetry is slightly imperfect, potentially causing a blurred image appearance if only half of the *k*-space is used for image reconstruction. An easy and fast solution has been the acquisition of the whole *k*-space, mainly for historic reasons. It also has to be considered that every measured Fourier line contributes to the overall SNR. The selection of a partial acquisition of *k*-space will allow a reduction of measurement time to the expense of a drop in SNR, and a potential degradation in image quality. (SNR(50% partial Fourier) = 0.71*SNR(full *k*-space acquisition)).

$$\text{SNR} \sim \sqrt{\text{GP}_{PF}}.$$

PAT Factor, Utilization of Parallel Acquisition Techniques

As previously mentioned, the spatial distribution of surface coils can be used to retrieve spatial information that otherwise would have to be measured. A PAT factor of two indicates that the measurement of every other Fourier line is skipped (corresponding to a FoV reduction in the direction of phase encoding) and the resulting wrap around artifacts are eliminated prior to showing the images using the images or the *k*-space data from individual coils. As the measurement of half of the Fourier lines is skipped, there is an expected drop in SNR. (SNR(PAT = 2) = 0.71*SNR(noPAT)).

$$\text{SNR} \sim \frac{1}{\sqrt{\text{PAT}}}.$$

ν: Imaging Bandwidth

The frequency range per pixel, also called imaging bandwidth, is a parameter that dictates the length of the data acquisition window. The consequence of a low bandwidth is a prolonged minimum TE. Noise is to be found at every frequency. A high bandwidth corresponds to a large frequency range, and consequently more noise is picked up. As the MR signal drops exponentially following excitation, the strongest signal is picked up with the shortest possible TE. As short TE also means a possible short TR, the high signal for short TE, fast imaging techniques outperforms the additional noise to be picked up when using a larger bandwidth. For studying hemorrhagic lesions, a reasonably long TE is utilized to allow the dephasing mechanisms of susceptibility gradients to produce the desired signal voids. In this case, a lower bandwidth is advised. The following equation does not consider the SNR gain as a consequence of a shorter TE.

$$\text{SNR} \sim \frac{1}{\sqrt{\nu}}.$$

1.2.7 Contrast Agents for Magnetic Resonance Imaging

In the early days of MRI, many experts in the field were skeptical that there would be any utility for contrast media with this new imaging modality. T1, T2, and Pd weighting were believed to provide sufficient tissue contrast for the contemplated clinical applications. Over the following two decades, however, MRI contrast agents have become an indispensable adjunct for a significant proportion of MRI examinations, and have emerged as key enablers in modern diagnostic radiology. A January 2006 review found that the single most cited article in the 100-year history of the American Journal of Roentgenology was a milestone report from 1984 on "the characteristics of gadolinium-DTPA complex as a potential NMR contrast agent." Approximately one-third of all MRI examinations today are performed using injectable contrast agents, and over 150 million doses of these contrast agents have been administered to patients worldwide since the first MRI contrast agent, gadolinium-DTPA, became available for clinical use in 1988 under the brand name Magnevist®.

In current clinical practice, the most commonly used MRI contrast agents (in terms of both volume and breadth of clinical applications) are those that exhibit paramagnetic properties, in particular those that are based on gadolinium (Gd). Gadolinium-based contrast agents (GBCAs) have always accounted for the vast majority of contrast-enhanced MRI examinations and are currently used to image most body regions for a wide variety of pathological conditions. Manganese (Mn) is another paramagnetic element that has been employed in a contrast agent specifically designed for liver imaging. Superparamagnetic contrast agents are based on iron (Fe) oxides and are used in niche applications such as liver imaging. This chapter will only address contrast agents that have received regulatory approval or are in late phases of clinical development in the United States or the European Union.

1.2.7.1 Basic Principles and Properties

Mechanism of Action

The alteration of signal intensity in diseased tissue forms the basis for MRI. The tissue signal intensity observed in MR images is the result of a complex interaction of numerous factors, which can be classified as those that reflect intrinsic properties of biological tissues, e.g., T1 and T2 relaxation times and Pd, and those that are equipment related, e.g., field strength and pulse sequences. However, due to a wide biologic variation, the relaxation times of normal and abnormal tissues often overlap. This limits the ability of plain MRI to detect and characterize abnormal tissue. By using very specialized pulse sequences, some of these limitations can be overcome, but not all. A solution is provided by MR contrast agents, which alter the relaxation times of tissues into which they diffuse and therefore change the intrinsic tissue signal intensity, enhancing contrast.

Certain elements or molecules possess unique magnetic properties (e.g., paramagnetism and superparamagnetism) that arise from the particular composition of their nuclei (number of protons and neutrons) and from their electron configurations. These magnetic properties cause predictable magnetic field perturbations that impact the relaxation times of hydrogen protons in surrounding water molecules – the same protons that ultimately serve as the source of the detected signal in MRI. Thus, the fundamental mechanism of action for all injectable MRI contrast media is the shortening of relaxation times (T1 and T2) of hydrogen protons in water molecules, in tissues into which the contrast agent has diffused. This highly localized effect also means that the specific tissue distribution of a contrast agent directly impacts its observed effects in vivo.

Paramagnetic Contrast Media

Physical Properties

Paramagnetism arises in certain atoms or molecules owing to the presence of unpaired electrons in the atomic or molecular electron orbitals. As a result, these atoms or molecules have permanent magnetic moments (dipoles), which are randomly oriented in space in the absence of an external magnetic field. When placed in an external magnetic field, these atoms or molecules show a significant net magnetization because of the preferential orientation of the paramagnetic dipole moments parallel to the applied magnetic field; the magnitude of this net magnetic moment is proportional to the magnitude of the external magnetic field.

Paramagnetic contrast agents in current clinical use are based on the metal ions Mn^{2+} (manganese) and Gd^{3+} (gadolinium). Gadolinium, a rare earth metal in the lanthanide series, is one of the strongest paramagnetic compounds because of its seven unpaired electrons. Through interactions between the electron spins of the paramagnetic gadolinium and hydrogen protons in nearby water molecules, the relaxation rates T1 (and to a lesser extent T2) of the protons are increased, meaning that T1 and T2 times are decreased. Because tissue T1 relaxation is inherently slow compared with T2 relaxation, the predominant effect of paramagnetic contrast media is on T1 relaxation times. This results in an increase in signal that is visible on T1-WIs in tissues into which the contrast agent has diffused. At higher tissue concentrations, paramagnetic agents can also shorten the T2 relaxation time, resulting in signal loss on T2-WIs.

For T1 relaxation to occur, the absorbed energy introduced with the RF excitation pulse must be released. The release of energy involved in T1 relaxation is primarily stimulated. Stimulated transitions require interaction between excited nuclei and local electromagnetic fields, which are time-varying at the appropriate frequency, the Larmor frequency. These time-varying fields are produced by the translational and rotational movement of the molecular environment. For T1-shortening contrast agents, an effective dipole–dipole interaction requires the magnetic dipole of the contrast agent to be of sufficient magnitude and for the molecular tumbling to be sufficiently close to the Larmor frequency in order to stimulate a spin transition. The second dominant interaction between water protons and the unpaired electrons of a T1-shortening contrast agent that stimulate spin transition is called scalar interaction. This mechanism too scales with the magnitude of the relaxation agent's magnetic moment.

Paramagnetic contrast agents elevate the magnetic field locally due to the positive magnetic susceptibility. This will introduce local field inhomogeneities, resulting in a shorter T2* relaxation time for the surrounding environment.

The theory of weakly magnetized particles also causing a shortening of T2 relaxation time relates to chemical exchange and a variety of diffusion-related mechanism. It is obvious that the diffusion of excited water protons in random magnetic field gradients as produced by the paramagnetic contrast agent will cause temporary shifts in Larmor frequencies, causing alteration of phase position of the nuclear transverse magnetization. The latter results in random dephasing that cannot be refocused by an RF refocusing pulse, thus appearing as a signal loss characterized by a shorter T2 relaxation time.

Relaxation times and relaxivity

As described earlier, paramagnetic and superparamagnetic contrast agents shorten (to various degrees) both T1 and T2 relaxation times, which is equivalent to saying that these agents increase the T1 and T2 relaxation rates of tissues into which they diffuse. Relaxation rates are defined as 1/T1 and 1/T2, i.e., the reciprocals of the T1 and T2 relaxation times. The ability of a contrast agent to shorten the relaxation time of a tissue depends both on the agent's concentration in the respective tissue and on the intrinsic relaxation time of the tissue. For instance, a concentration of 0.1 mM of a Gd chelate is a powerful relaxation enhancer, sufficient to decrease the relaxation times of many biological fluids by 50%. However, to influence tissues of shorter intrinsic relaxation times to the same extent, a higher concentration of the same contrast agent would be required.

The efficacy of MRI contrast agents is determined not only by their pharmacokinetic properties (such as distribution and time dependence of their concentration in areas of interest) but also by their magnetic properties, described by their T1 and T2 relaxivities, r_1 and r_2. The ability of a contrast agent to enhance the relaxation rate (or shorten the relaxation time) is called "relaxivity." For example, the efficiency of Gd-DTPA at enhancing the longitudinal relaxation (shortening of T1) is expressed as its r_1 relaxivity and is approximately 4.1 L/mmol s (at 1.5 T in human plasma at 37°C). The effect of Gd-DTPA on transverse relaxation (shortening of T2) is similarly described by its r_2 relaxivity, and is approximately 4.6 L/mmol s (at 1.5 T in human plasma at 37°C).

The relaxivity of a contrast agent is determined by the molecular structure of its chelate, which dictates the interaction between the chelate's metal center and hydrogen protons in the surrounding water ("inner-sphere effects"), as well as by other factors such as molecular motion and "outer-sphere effects." In vivo, the observed relaxivity of certain contrast agents is further affected by transient binding to plasma proteins, which increases the rotational correlation time of the bound contrast agent molecule and may yield a considerable enhancement in relaxivity. Finally, GBCAs show considerable variation in their relaxivities depending on the field strength of the magnet used for MRI. Thus, at lower field strengths (e.g., below 0.5 T), considerable differences in both r_1 and r_2 relaxivity are noted between GBCAs that exhibit protein binding and those that do not bind to plasma proteins. However, at field strengths commonly used in clinical practice (1.5 T and especially 3 T), differences in relaxivity among GBCAs are significantly reduced, and the impact of the remaining differences on the clinical usefulness of the various GBCAs remains incompletely understood.

Chemical Properties

Paramagnetic contrast agents consist of the metal ion (Gd^{3+} or Mn^{2+}) chelated with an organic ligand that envelops the central metal ion through multiple ionic-like bonds. While the contrast generating effect is due solely to the central metal ion, the use of a metal-ligand complex (also known as a "chelate") is necessary for in vivo use. Chelation of Gd in particular is required to avoid acute toxicity, and in the case of both Gd and Mn, the use of a chelate renders the resulting contrast agent hydrophilic, affording clinically useful pharmacokinetic properties.

The ligand can be an open-ended molecule (as in linear GBCAs) or a closed ring structure (as in macrocyclic GBCAs). Both types of GBCAs exist in ionic and nonionic forms depending on the total number of negative charges present on the ligand: thus, the Gd^{3+} ion will form a "nonionic" (i.e., electrically neutral) chelate with a ligand that has three negative charges, or an "ionic" chelate (with a net charge of −2) with a ligand that has five negative charges. Ionic chelates are therefore formulated with a positively-charged excipient to balance the electrical charges. For instance, Gd-DTPA (gadopentetate) is an ionic Gd chelate with a −2 net charge and it is formulated with the excipient meglumine (which carries a +1 charge per molecule) to yield the final injectable product, gadopentetate dimeglumine.

Osmolality and viscosity

The osmolality of currently available GBCAs varies considerably, from 630 to 1970 mOsmol/kg H_2O. However, the volumes typically employed in MRI are small: 0.2–0.6 mL/kg body weight (BW) (0.1–0.3 mmol/kg BW), so that a 70 kg person receiving a standard dose of 0.1 mmol/kg BW of a GBCA will be injected with just 14 mL of the contrast medium. The amount of osmotically active contrast medium "particles," i.e., the "total osmotic load," of such small volumes of GBCAs are far lower than those seen with the much larger volumes of iodinated contrast agents routinely used in X-ray and computed tomography applications. Consequently, the osmolality of currently available GBCAs is not considered to have any appreciable effect on the safety or tolerability profiles of these agents. The viscosity of various GBCA formulations likewise shows considerable variation, but this does not have a significant impact on their method of administration or safety profile. Warming the contrast medium vial to body temperature (37°C) prior to injection is frequently done in clinical practice, as it lowers the viscosity of the injected fluid (compared to its value at room temperature) and allows the use of a range of injection rates (up to several mL/s) with or without a power injector; it also creates a better experience for the patient, who is less likely to experience a sensation of coldness in the injected arm during the infusion.

Complex stability

Mangafodipir trisodium, the sole Mn-based chelate in clinical use, is rapidly metabolized in vivo since the bond between the Mn^{2+} ion and its ligand (fodipir) is designed to break soon after injection through dephosphorylation followed by competitive exchange of Mn with plasma zinc (Zn). This allows the free Mn^{2+} ion to be taken up mainly by the liver, where it yields organ-specific enhancement.

By contrast, GBCAs are not metabolized at a detectable level in vivo as the bond between the Gd^{3+} ion and its ligand is designed to be very strong in all commercially available GBCAs. The "stability" of a Gd-ligand complex, often referred to as "complex stability," indicates the degree to which the Gd ion might dissociate from its ligand and can be described in a number of ways:

- Thermodynamic stability, measured at the dissociation equilibrium in idealized laboratory conditions at very high pH (e.g., pH 11).
- Conditional stability, measured at the dissociation equilibrium at a pH of 7.4 and thus "conditional" on the pH value commonly encountered in the human serum.
- Kinetic stability, measured as the rate at which the dissociation equilibrium is reached.

In general, ionic linear GBCAs tend to have higher thermodynamic and conditional stability constants than nonionic linear GBCAs. The latter are correspondingly formulated to include a larger amount of free ligand. Macrocyclic GBCAs have high kinetic stabilities compared to linear GBCAs, the result of reinforcing steric effects present in a completely closed molecular ring structure. In the complex physiological milieu of the human blood, a Gd chelate's stability may be further modulated by the presence of cations (i.e., zinc, copper) that compete for the ligand molecule, and of anions (i.e., phosphate, carbonate) that compete for the Gd^{3+} ion.

According to some investigators, differences in stability among currently available GBCAs may have an impact on clinically relevant issues such as nephrogenic systemic fibrosis (NSF) and contrast medium interference with colorimetric serum calcium measurements, both discussed later in this chapter.

Pharmacokinetics

While the Gd^{3+} ion is solely responsible for the paramagnetic effect of Gd chelates, it is the ligand that determines the pharmacokinetic behavior of each particular complex. Due to their high hydrophilicity and low molecular weight, most Gd chelates rapidly diffuse into the extracellular interstitial space after intravenous injection, with a very short intravascular phase; they do not cross the intact blood–brain barrier (BBB). Protein binding in plasma is negligible for most of these agents, with a few exceptions (e.g., gadofosveset, gadoxetic acid, gadobenate); in the case of gadofosveset, protein binding occurs to such an extent that this agent persists in the vasculature for a long period of time, which allows it to be used as a "blood pool" contrast agent. GBCAs are eliminated in most cases via passive glomerular filtration, with elimination half-lives typically shorter than 2 h. A few GBCAs have a secondary elimination pathway through the liver, such as to a lesser extent, gadofosveset and gadobenate; this property allow some of these Gd chelates (gadoxetic acid and gadobenate) to be used as liver-specific contrast agents. Most GBCAs are completely eliminated from the body within 24 h if glomerular filtration is not diminished; elimination half-life can be prolonged in patients with impaired renal function.

In the case of mangafodipir, the manganese ion and its ligand separate soon after injection and have different pharmacokinetic profiles. Manganese has an initial plasma half life of 20 min or less, with significant uptake into the liver, pancreas, kidneys, and spleen; about 15–20% of the manganese is eliminated in the urine within the first 24 h, and most of the remainder is excreted in the feces over the following 4 days. The ligand fodipir has an initial plasma half-life of about 50 min; following its metabolism, nearly all of the ligand is excreted in urine within 24 h, with negligible amounts being eliminated via the feces (Table 1.3).

Superparamagnetic Contrast Media

Superparamagnetism is induced by very small ferromagnetic particles that have only a single magnetic domain. In an external magnetic field, these particles show a magnetization curve similar to that of paramagnetic agents, but with a much stronger response, and saturation effects are readily attained. The increase in magnetization at escalating external field strengths is nonlinear. After removal of the applied magnetic field, no net magnetization is retained.

Superparamagnetic contrast agents in current clinical use consist of small particles containing magnetite (iron oxide) cores coated with polymers (e.g., dextran, carboxydextran) that ensure biocompatibility and prevent magnetic aggregation in vivo. The size of the particles is important as it dictates their biodistribution and relative impact on T1 and T2 relaxation times. Injectable SPIOs (superparamagnetic iron oxides) typically range in diameter from 60 to 150 nm and are avidly taken up by cells of the reticulo-endothelial system (RES) in the liver (Kupffer cells) and spleen within minutes of injection, resulting in a short half-life in the blood. SPIOs exert a strong T2 relaxation effect that predominates over their T1 effect (i.e., they have a high T2 relaxivity/T1 relaxivity ratio). Injectable USPIOs (ultrasmall superparamagnetic iron oxides) typically range in diameter from 10 to 40 nm and can cross capillary walls, whereupon they are sequestered by RES cells in lymph nodes and the bone marrow. They also have a much longer intravascular half-life compared to SPIOs. USPIOs have more balanced T2 relaxivity/T1 relaxivity ratios, which allows them to be used for both T2- and T1-W imaging. After phagocytosis by various cells of the RES, the iron in superparamagnetic contrast media becomes integrated into the physiological iron pool and is subject to normal physiological iron metabolism.

Table 1.3 Paramagnetic contrast agents in MRI

Trade name(s)	Generic name	Chemical abbreviation	Molecular structure and charge	Osmolality (mOsmol/kg H_2O) (at 37°C)	Viscosity (mPa·s) (at 37°C)	r_1 relaxivity[a] at 1.5 T (L/mmol s)	r_1 relaxivity[a] at 3T (L/mmol s)
Magnevist®, Magnograf®	Gadopentetate dimeglumine	Gd-DTPA	Linear Ionic	1,960	2.9	4.1	3.7
MultiHance®	Gadobenate dimeglumine	Gd-BOPTA	Linear Ionic	1,970	5.3	6.3	5.5
Primovist®, Eovist®	Gadoxetate disodium	Gd-EOB-DTPA	Linear Ionic	688	1.19	6.9	6.2
Vasovist®	Gadofosveset trisodium	Diphenylcyclohexyl phosphodiester-Gd-DTPA	Linear Ionic	825	3.0[b]	19.0	9.9
Omniscan®	Gadodiamide	Gd-DTPA-BMA	Linear Nonionic	789	1.4	4.3	4.0
OptiMARK®	Gadoverset-amide	Gd-DTPA-BMEA	Linear Nonionic	1,110	2.0	4.7	4.5
Dotarem®, Magnescope®	Gadoterate meglumine	Gd-DOTA	Macrocyclic Ionic	1,350	2.0	3.6	3.5
Gadovist 1.0®, Gadograf 1.0®	Gadobutrol	Gd-BT-DO3A	Macrocyclic Nonionic	1,603	4.96	5.2	5.0
ProHance®	Gadoteridol	Gd-HP-DO3A	Macrocyclic Nonionic	630	1.3	4.1	3.7
Teslascan®	Mangafodipir trisodium	Mn-DPDP	Linear Ionic	290	0.7	3.6	2.7

[a]Relaxivities measured at 37°C in plasma

[b]Viscosity for gadofosveset measured at 20°C

The biocompatibility of SPIOs and USPIOs makes them a popular choice among researchers for labeling cells (e.g., various stem cells), as these agents can be used for this purpose without significantly affecting cell viability or differentiation potential. However, this is not a clinically approved indication for any of the existing superparamagnetic contrast agents (Table 1.4).

Table 1.4 Superparamagnetic contrast agents in MRI

Trade name(s)	Generic name	Name during development	Class
Endorem®, Feridex®	Ferumoxide	AMI-25	SPIO
Resovist®, Cliavist®	Ferucarbotran	SHU 555 A	SPIO
Sinerem®, Combidex®	Ferumoxtran	AMI-227	USPIO
Supravist®	Ferucarbotran	SHU 555 C	USPIO

1.2.7.2 Clinical Applications

The range of clinical applications for MR contrast media has expanded tremendously since Gd-DTPA was first approved for visualization of central nervous system (CNS) lesions in 1988, and now comprises most body regions, most age groups (including pediatrics), and a broad range of pathological conditions. It should be noted that approved indications for the various MR contrast agents vary considerably around the world, and many agents are commercially available only in certain countries. Dosage, injection rate, and safety considerations may also vary from country to country. The reader is advised to consult and observe the appropriate prescribing information for locally approved contrast agents in making clinical decisions involving the use of these products. This section will focus on key indications that are approved in at least one major geographical region, and will briefly review the future potential of certain MR contrast agents in several new areas of application.

Neuroimaging

Well over 50% of contrast-enhanced MRI examinations today are performed in CNS indications, and historically this proportion has been even higher. One reason for this is that in the early days of MRI even the most basic sequences required many minutes of continuous imaging, so clinical applications of the new modality were limited to body areas for which motion or flow artifacts either did not exist or could be controlled to a considerable extent. Those areas are predominantly the CNS and the musculoskeletal system, with the latter being another important current indication for MRI. As a result, considerable experience has been gained over the years in imaging these body areas, with well-established protocols and extensive expertise in the user community. Another reason why CNS is the most common indication for MR contrast media is the existence of the BBB. In the healthy CNS, Gd chelates behave strictly as intravascular contrast agents, and only diffuse into the interstitial space (leading to enhancement) in the case of disruption in the BBB – such as caused by neoplasm, trauma, infarction, or inflammatory and demyelinating disease. Metastases do not have a BBB and enhance after injection of contrast media.

Body Imaging

The term "body imaging" has acquired a particular meaning in the idiom of modern radiology, and is now commonly understood to refer to imaging of the chest, abdomen, and pelvis. MR contrast agents are routinely used to evaluate tumors and other lesions with abnormal vascularity of the internal organs, using both anatomical and dynamic imaging sequences for fuller characterization of these lesions. Traditional extracellular (nontissue-specific) GBCAs are used in most contrast-enhanced body MRI examinations. However, contrast-enhanced MRI of the liver in particular has developed with a high degree of sophistication and has come to include specialized tissue-targeted contrast agents. Also, contrast-enhanced MRI of the breast has experienced rapid growth over the past few years. These specialized applications are therefore discussed in some detail below.

Liver Imaging

In the early years of contrast-enhanced MRI, non-tissue-specific extracellular Gd-based contrast agents were used with considerable success for structural and dynamic imaging of the liver, and many of these methods remain in clinical use today. In subsequent years, two different classes of specialized contrast media were developed to specifically target the liver in MRI: (1) paramagnetic contrast agents (based on Gd and Mn) that are taken up by healthy hepatocytes, are eliminated via the biliary route, and provide contrast by shortening T1, and (2) SPIO particles that are phagocytosed by cells of the RES in the liver and act as T2 contrast agents. The basic concept for both the hepatocyte-specific and the RES-specific contrast media is that they can only be taken up by liver tissue containing the respective type of cells. Lesions of nonhepatic origin, such as metastases, do not show any uptake and are visualized as a bright or dark area within the liver. In lesions of hepatic origin, the uptake of contrast medium depends on the number and functional integrity of the hepatocytes or RES cells. The variation among lesion types in the liver and the resulting differential uptake of contrast media provide clinically useful information. Lesion characterization is further enhanced by the ability of some contrast media to allow dynamic (time-resolved) imaging. This involves acquiring separate images at multiple time points following injection of the contrast medium; important information can be obtained from the observed time course of contrast enhancement.

Hepatocyte-specific contrast agents

Several paramagnetic contrast agents are now available for hepatobiliary imaging. Two (gadoxetic acid and gadobenate) are derived from Gd-DTPA, wherein a carboxyl group is replaced by a lipophilic moiety. This allows uptake of the contrast agent by healthy hepatocytes via an active transport mechanism mediated by the organic anion transporting polypeptide OATP1. This is followed by intracellular binding to transport proteins and finally secretion into the biliary system via the passive canalicular multi-organic anion transporter (cMOAT). These agents accumulate in healthy hepatocytes and subsequently in the biliary tree, causing signal enhancement in these tissues through T1 shortening effects. Lesions of the liver that lack functional hepatocytes (e.g., metastases or poorly differentiated hepatocellular carcinomas) do not take up these contrast agents and appear as hypointense areas on T1-WIs.

The degree of specific uptake of these agents by hepatocytes is species- and agent-dependent. Whereas both gadobenate and gadoxetic acid exhibit significant hepatic uptake in various animal species, in humans only 1–4% of the injected dose of gadobenate is specifically taken up by the liver and secreted into the biliary system. As a result, the accumulation of a sufficient amount of gadobenate in the liver is slow, requiring a waiting period of 60–120 min after injection for optimal MRI. With gadoxetic acid, approximately 50% of the injected dose is taken up by the human liver, so that the optimal imaging time point for the hepatobiliary phase is about 15–20 min after injection (Fig. 1.27), with an imaging window of up to 120 min. The rapid concentration of gadoxetic acid in hepatocytes also permits the use of a very low dose for effective enhancement (0.025 mmol/kg BW). Both gadoxetic acid and gadobenate have been shown to improve the detection of liver lesions. In both cases, the injected fraction not eliminated via the biliary route is excreted via the kidneys as with purely extracellular GBCAs.

Mangafodipir trisodium, the sole Mn-based chelate in clinical use, is another liver-specific contrast agent. The bond between the Mn^{2+} ion and its ligand (fodipir) is designed to break soon after injection, and Mn is preferentially taken up by normal liver parenchyma and the pancreas. As with Gd chelates, the effect is a

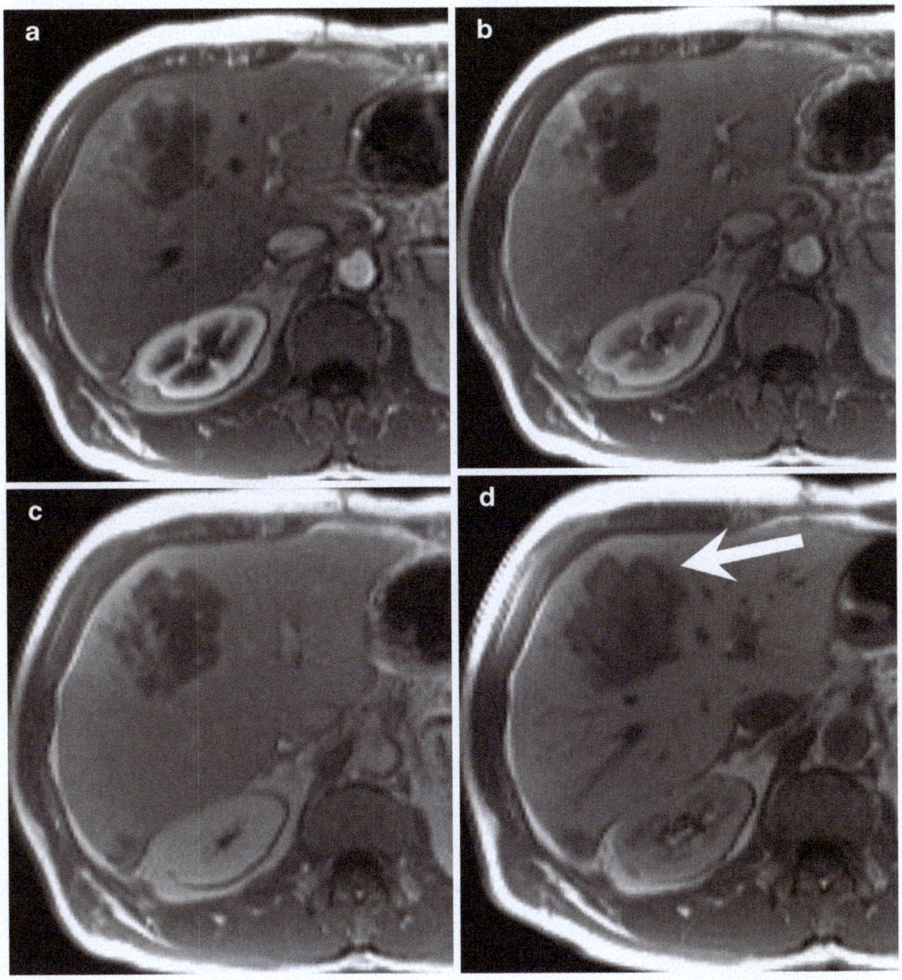

Fig. 1.27 Dynamic contrast-enhanced imaging of colorectal cancer metastatic to the liver, using gadoxetate disodium (0.025 mmol/kg). Similar degrees of enhancement are achieved in the first few minutes of imaging with 0.1 mmol/kg of gadopentetate dimeglumine (a nontissue-specific extracellular contrast agent) or 0.025 mmol/kg of gadoxetate disodium (a hepatocyte-specific high relaxivity contrast agent). However, lesion conspicuity is greater with gadoxetate disodium at 20 min because hepatocytes in healthy liver tissue accumulate this agent whereas cells of the metastatic lesion do not. (**a**) Arterial phase (20 s). (**b**) Portal-venous phase (50 s). (**c**) Equilibrium phase (1 min 30 s). (**d**) Hepatocyte phase (20 min). (Time intervals shown refer to time after injection of gadoxetate disodium). Reproduced with kind permission of Dr. Luigi Grazioli, Department of Radiology, University of Brescia, Italy

shortening of the T1 relaxation time of targeted tissues during MRI, leading to an increase in signal intensity of the liver parenchyma and the pancreas. Enhancement in both organs is near maximal for up to 4 h after administration of mangafodipir.

RES-specific contrast agents

Two SPIO agents, ferumoxide and ferucarbotran, are currently employed in MRI of the liver to exploit their affinity for cells of the reticuloendothelial system (RES). These agents differ in their hydrodynamic diameters (averaging 150 nm for ferumoxide and 60 nm for ferucarbotran). Both are coated, with dextran in the case of ferumoxide and with carboxydextran in the case of ferucarbotran, in order to prevent in vivo magnetic aggregation of the particles and to ensure biocompatibility (cardiovascular tolerability in particular). SPIOs are phagocytosed by RES cells in the liver (Kupffer cells), and to a lesser extent in the spleen, bone marrow, and lymph nodes. The half-life in plasma before phagocytosis is biphasic: there is a rapid uptake of the bigger particles with a half-life of about 5 min, and a slower uptake of the smaller particles with a longer half-life of about 2–3 h.

SPIO particles exert a strong magnetic susceptibility effect, reducing the T2 relaxation time and producing a drop in signal in areas where they accumulate. This is visualized as areas of decreased signal intensity in normal liver tissue with an intact reticuloendothelial system, which takes up the iron oxide particles. Lesions of the liver that are associated with an alteration in the RES (e.g., metastases, poorly differentiated hepatocellular carcinomas (Fig. 1.28)) do not exhibit this hypointensity on T2-WIs, and stand out as comparatively brighter areas against the background of normal liver tissue.

Ferumoxide has to be prepared for administration by dilution with a 5% dextrose solution, and must be infused slowly over a period of 20–30 min. Imaging can begin immediately after the dose is infused and may be performed up to 3.5 h after the end of the infusion. Ferucarbotran is a ready-to-use suspension that is injected intravenously as a bolus, thus allowing dynamic imaging.

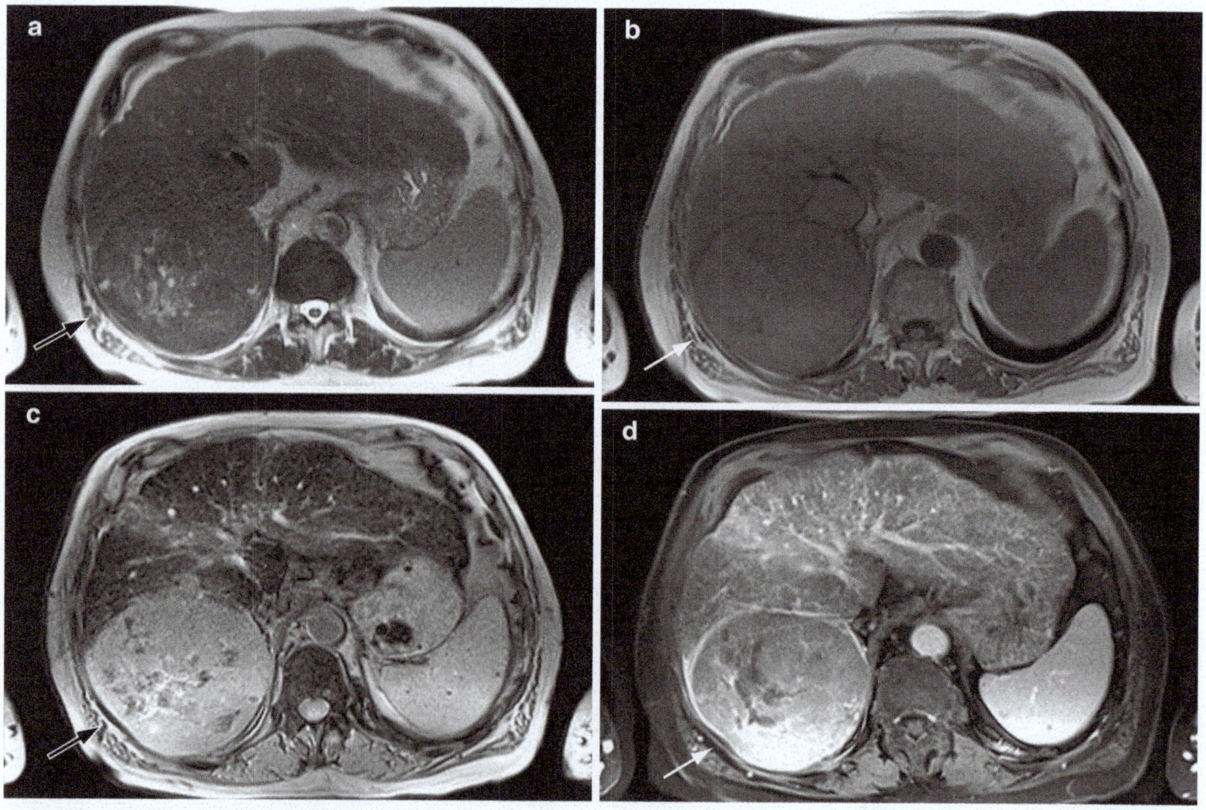

Fig. 1.28 Patient with a large HCC. (*arrows*) (**a**) T2-W image prior to contrast injection, (**b**) T1-W image prior to contrast injection, (**c**) T2-W image after Resovist (Ferucarbotran) administration, (**d**) GD portal venous phase after Resovist (Ferucarbotran) administration

Breast Imaging

MRI of the breast has experienced rapid growth in recent years, owing mainly to the evolving ability of this imaging method to detect neoplastic lesions at a relatively early stage. In most cases, breast MRI requires the use of an extracellular (nontissue-specific) Gd-based contrast agent for both structural and dynamic imaging of suspect lesions to facilitate fuller characterization of these lesions. In 2007, the American Cancer Society (ACS) issued formal guidelines for breast screening with MRI as an adjunct to mammography, noting that new evidence on breast MRI screening has become available since the ACS last issued guidelines for the early detection of breast cancer in 2003. The ACS expert panel noted that GBCA-enhanced MRI has been shown to have a high sensitivity for detecting breast cancer in high risk asymptomatic and symptomatic women, although reports of specificity have been more variable. The new guidelines recommended screening MRI for women with an approximately 20–25% or greater lifetime risk of breast cancer, including women with a strong family history of breast or ovarian cancer and women who were treated for Hodgkin disease. The ACS expert panel also noted that there are several risk subgroups for which the available data are insufficient to recommend for or against screening, including women with a personal history of breast cancer, carcinoma in situ, atypical hyperplasia, and extremely dense breasts on mammography.

ceMRA: Contrast Enhanced Magnetic Resonance Angiography

Three-dimensional contrast-enhanced magnetic resonance angiography (3D MRA) is a widely used technique that uses contrast agents together with very fast imaging sequences to produce detailed images of vascular structures throughout the body with relatively short imaging times. Pioneered in the early 1990s, contrast-enhanced MRA was originally developed using traditional extracellular Gd chelates. These agents distribute into the interstitial space within minutes of intravenous injection, allowing relatively little time for imaging vascular structures. For this reason, "first pass imaging" is typically employed with these agents, and accurate timing is critical in order to not miss the first pass of the injected bolus through the vessels of interest.

Blood-Pool Contrast Agents

In order to bypass some of the limitations of traditional GBCAs in MRA applications, specialized "blood-pool" contrast agents have been developed to offer longer intravascular half-lives. Gadofosveset is the representative member of this new class of agents. Its molecular structure allows it to bind extensively (though reversibly) to albumin, a protein that is present in higher concentration in the serum compared to the extravascular space. The resulting complex is much larger than the gadofosveset molecule itself and does not readily diffuse into the interstitial space. As a result, this contrast agent remains in the vascular space for an extended period of time, allowing for extended imaging time windows, higher spatial resolution, and larger anatomic coverage. The protein binding also greatly increases the rotational correlation time of gadofosveset, resulting in an effective r_1 relaxivity in plasma several times higher than that of GBCAs that do not exhibit protein binding. The long intravascular residence time and high relaxivity in plasma of gadofosveset allow it to be effective at a much lower dose (0.03 mmol/kg BW) than required of other GBCAs for vascular imaging. Both dynamic (first-pass) MRA and high-resolution steady-state vascular imaging (up to 60 min post injection) can be performed using gadofosveset (Fig. 1.29).

The prolongation of a contrast agent's half-life in the blood can be achieved by other approaches as well. The uptake of superparamagnetic iron-oxide particles by cells of the RES through phagocytosis is related to protein absorption on the particle surface and subsequent opsonization. Minimizing the particle surface will result in decreased protein absorption and hence will reduce phagocytosis, yielding a longer plasma half-life. USPIOs (e.g., SHU 555 C), with their long plasma half-life and T1 shortening effects, have the potential to become alternative blood pool agents in MRI. Gd-based polymeric macromolecules that are too large to readily diffuse into the interstitial space provide yet another possibility for the future of vascular imaging. Beyond macrovascular imaging, the evaluation of microvascular flow (mainly in tumors) might become a promising future application for blood-pool agents.

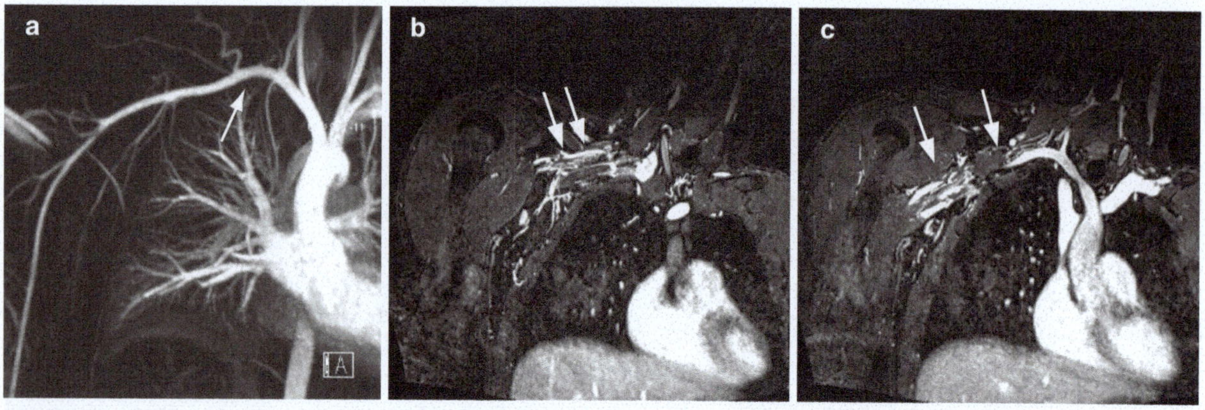

Fig. 1.29 Patient with thoracic inlet syndrome: (**a**) arterial phase (normal) (*long arrow*); (**b**) and (**c**) two high resolution sections of the venous phase with a thrombus in the subclavian vein (*arrowheads*) (Gadofosveset)

Other Applications

Other MRI applications that make use of contrast media include imaging of the head and neck; heart; musculoskeletal system, and lymph nodes. Tumors and other lesions of the head and neck are routinely evaluated using extracellular (nontissue-specific) GBCAs. Contrast-enhanced MRI of the heart includes delayed-enhancement with nontissue-specific GBCAs for assessment of myocardial viability, and coronary artery evaluation with blood-pool GBCAs. Certain musculoskeletal diseases (such as bone tumors or inflammatory conditions) are frequently evaluated with contrast-enhanced MRI, although much of musculoskeletal MRI today is done without contrast. Joint imaging is sometimes performed using intra-articular injections of small amounts of highly diluted GBCAs. Finally, USPIOs have shown promise for lymph node imaging; their small size allows them to evade the RES cells of the liver and spleen and to diffuse into the interstitium, where they are phagocytosed by RES cells in healthy lymph nodes and cause T2/T2* loss of signal. Metastatic lesions in lymph nodes commonly obliterate resident macrophage populations and therefore fail to accumulate USPIO particles.

1.2.7.3 Safety Considerations

General Safety

Gd-based contrast agents, by far the most commonly used MR contrast media, have established an excellent safety record in the general patient population over the past two decades and in more than 150 million cumulative administrations worldwide. The most commonly encountered adverse events following administration of GBCAs are headache, nausea, injection site coldness, and dizziness. These adverse events are usually mild to moderate in severity and are self-limiting, requiring no treatment. Less frequently encountered mild or moderate adverse events include hypersensitivity reactions (e.g., urticaria) and taste perversion. Serious adverse events, including deaths, have occurred after administration of GBCAs. These occurrences are extremely rare, and typically involve anaphylactoid or anaphylactic reactions during or immediately following injection; such reactions can also occur with mangafodipir and with iron oxide-based contrast agents. Prompt treatment in these situations can be life-saving. Patients with a history of drug reactions, allergy, or other hypersensitivity disorders are considered to be at increased risk for severe reactions.

A dose of 0.1 mmol/kg BW is often considered a "standard dose" for many GBCAs, but doses as low as 0.025 mmol/kg BW and as high as 0.3 mmol/kg BW are commonly employed depending on the particular GBCA, the clinical application, and locally approved labeling. For most adverse events and at clinically approved doses, there is no clear correlation between dose and incidence or severity of adverse events. One potential exception is the deterioration in renal function in patients with preexisting renal impairment following GBCA administration; although very rarely encountered, the risk for such deterioration appears to be higher with increasing doses of contrast medium.

Reported incidence rates for adverse events among GBCAs can vary considerably according to study phase, design, and location. As seen with many other pharmacological compounds, postmarketing surveillance studies for GBCAs typically report lower incidence rates compared to controlled clinical studies, and spontaneous reporting shows yet lower incidence rates. The few comparative studies among currently available GBCAs have failed to demonstrate any significant differences in the incidence or type of adverse events reported. Considered in the aggregate, the evidence available to date suggests that all GBCAs currently in use have very similar general safety profiles.

Adverse events most commonly reported after administration of mangafodipir include feeling of warmth/flushing, headache, nausea, vomiting, other gastrointestinal symptoms, and taste sensations; most of these were transient and of mild intensity. The frequency of mild and moderate adverse reactions, mainly transient warmth and flushing, is likely to increase if mangafodipir is administered faster than at the recommended rate of 2–6 mL/min.

The most commonly noted adverse events reported for SPIOs are back pain, leg pain, and vasodilation. The pain typically occurs during the infusion and resolves if the infusion is stopped, although some patients require treatment. Most other adverse reactions (e.g., nausea, urticaria) are mild to moderate in severity, of short duration, and resolve spontaneously without treatment.

Pediatric Safety

Perhaps as many as 10% of all contrast-enhanced MR examinations are currently performed in the pediatric population. A number of GBCAs have received approval for various indications in the pediatric age group on the basis of controlled clinical trials, and their safety in children from 0 to 18 years of age has also been documented through postmarketing surveillance studies, spontaneous reporting, and reviews of the scientific literature. The evidence to date indicates that the safety profiles of GBCAs in the pediatric population, in terms of type and incidence of reported adverse events, do not show appreciable differences compared to those observed in the adult population.

Interference with Colorimetric Calcium Assays

Literature reports dating back to the mid 1990s have raised awareness in the medical community about the potential of certain GBCAs to cause interference with colorimetric serum calcium (Ca) measurement methods, including the Arsenazo, methylthymol blue (MTB), and *o*-cresol-phthalein (OCP) assays. The OCP assay is the most commonly used method for routine measurements of serum calcium, wherein the OCP reagent binds the Ca^{2+} ion in the serum sample and yields a change in the color of the solution that is quantifiably related to the concentration of Ca^{2+} ions in the sample. The other colorimetric methods work along similar principles.

The Gd-based contrast agents gadodiamide and gadoversetamide, at clinical doses, have been shown to predictably alter the measured calcium values when colorimetric assays are used. In the case of OCP, the observed calcium values are artifactually decreased, so that a patient with a normal Ca level may be mistakenly thought to have a below-normal level of this important electrolyte. Such "spurious hypocalcemia" may trigger unnecessary clinical investigations and may even result in inappropriate treatment (e.g., intravenous calcium administration). In the case of patients with high serum calcium (e.g., patients with novel bone tumors), the interference of gadodiamide or gadoversetamide with the OCP assay may yield a spuriously normal calcium value, thus masking an important disease signal. It has been shown that the mechanism of action for this interference is the dissociation of the Gd^{3+} ion from its ligand in the Gd chelate and the formation of a new Gd-OCP complex. As a result, less OCP reagent is available to bind calcium in the sample, altering the change in color that forms the basis for this assay. The interference is more pronounced at higher GBCA doses and in renally impaired patients, who have longer elimination times.

The dissociation of the Gd-ligand complex in gadodiamide and gadoversetamide has been attributed to the lower complex stability of these agents, which have a nonionic linear molecular structure. These two GBCAs also interfere with the other two colorimetric methods (Arsenazo and MTB) but in the opposite direction, artifactually increasing the reported calcium value. Other calcium measurement methods, such as ion-selective electrode and atomic emission spectroscopic assays, are not subject to this interference but they have higher costs and are not widely available. Macrocyclic and ionic linear GBCAs do not interfere with any calcium measurement method, presumably as a result of their higher complex stability.

Use of GBCAs in Renally Impaired Patients

Renal Tolerance

Early experience with GBCAs in renally impaired patients showed that these agents had superior renal tolerance compared to iodinated contrast agents, leading some experts to conclude that GBCAs are essentially nonnephrotoxic. Extensive experience in this patient population has since accumulated to support the excellent renal tolerance profile of GBCAs, and contrast-induced nephropathy (CIN) remains much less frequently encountered after GBCA administration than after administration of iodinated contrast media. However, it should be noted that the volumes of GBCAs used in MRI (typically 10–30 mL per administration) are considerably lower than the volumes of iodinated contrast media required for X-ray and CT applications (commonly 100 mL and higher). In patients with renal insufficiency, acute renal failure requiring dialysis or worsening renal function have occurred, mostly within 48 h of GBCA injection. The risk of these events is higher with increasing dose of contrast. Documented instances of this type of adverse outcome are extremely rare. GBCAs are dialyzable, and three sessions of hemodialysis typically remove more than 95% of an injected dose; peritoneal dialysis is considerably slower at removing these agents from the body.

Nephrogenic Systemic Fibrosis (NSF)

The use of GBCAs in patients with severe renal impairment has recently come under scrutiny because of a previously unrecognized potential association between GBCA administration and the development of a serious condition called NSF in some of these patients.

NSF, previously known as nephrogenic fibrosing dermopathy (NFD), was first described in the medical literature in 2000, with the first reported case going back to 1997. To date, NSF has been reported only in patients with acute or chronic severe renal insufficiency (glomerular filtration rate <30 mL/min/1.73m^2) of various etiologies, or in patients with acute renal insufficiency of any severity due to the hepato-renal syndrome or in the perioperative liver transplantation period. The risk, if any, for developing NSF among patients with mild to moderate renal insufficiency, or with normal renal function, is unknown. NSF patients develop fibrosis of the skin and connective tissues. The skin thickening may inhibit flexion and extension of joints, resulting in contractures. In addition, patients may develop fibrosis of other organs. In its more severe forms, the disease can be highly debilitating, and in approximately 5% of patients, the course of the disease is rapidly progressive and may lead to a fatal outcome. It appears that males and females are affected in approximately equal numbers, with onset generally during middle age, although pediatric cases have also been reported. Currently, there is no known cure for NSF, although a number of treatment options have shown promise. In particular, improving renal function seems to slow or arrest the progression of NSF, and may even result in a gradual reversal.

The exact etiology of NSF remains unknown but is likely to be multifactorial. Specific triggers under scientific evaluation include recent surgery and the occurrence of thrombosis or other vascular injury; a proinflammatory state; the administration of high doses of erythropoietin; and more recently, the use of GBCAs. Several case series published in the scientific literature beginning with 2006 have identified at least one GBCA administration in all or most patients who subsequently developed NSF, suggesting an epidemiological association.

As a result, the prescribing information for GBCAs in major markets around the world has recently been updated to include warnings to healthcare professionals that exposure to GBCAs increases the risk for NSF in patients with acute or chronic severe renal insufficiency (glomerular filtration rate <30 mL/min/1.73 m^2).

Many of the current guidelines advise healthcare professionals to become familiar with the patient populations who are at known risk for NSF and avoid use of GBCAs in these patients unless the diagnostic information is essential and can not be obtained with non-contrast enhanced MRI or other diagnostic procedures; to screen all patients for renal dysfunction by obtaining a history and/or laboratory tests; to not exceed the dose recommended in product labeling, when administering a GBCA; and to allow sufficient time for elimination of the GBCA from the body prior to any readministration. For patients already on hemodialysis, prompt hemodialysis after administration of a

GBCA may be considered, as hemodialysis greatly enhances GBCA elimination.

Recent research into the pathophysiology of the disease suggests that in vivo dissociation of the gadolinium ion from its ligand may be one potential trigger, a phenomenon that may be linked in part to the complex stability of each GBCA formulation. Macrocyclic GBCAs have been associated with the lowest number of reports of NSF, considering their volume of use in the general patient population; furthermore, linear ionic agents have been associated with comparatively fewer reports than nonionic linear agents. The first research reports using animal models have shown that nonionic linear agents have the potential to induce NSF-like lesions in rodents whereas the other GBCA classes seem not to have this effect; furthermore, the presence of NSF-like lesions was associated with high levels of Gd in the skin of affected animals. However, these differentiating observations are confounded by lack of detailed statistical data on the at-risk patient population exposed to the various GBCAs, incomplete understanding of the pathophysiology of the disease, lack of an optimal animal model for NSF, and the difficulty of transferring findings from preclinical experimental models to the clinical setting. The fact that the majority of patients with severe renal impairment who were exposed to GBCAs never developed NSF underscores the likely multifactorial nature of this complex disease.

The association between NSF and GBCAs is currently an area of intense investigation in the scientific community, and significant advancements in knowledge are anticipated over the next few years. Healthcare professionals who make decisions about the use of GBCAs in renally impaired patients are encouraged to stay abreast of the scientific literature on this topic, and to observe the current prescribing information for locally approved GBCAs.

1.2.8 Hemorrhage

The identification of hemorrhage with MR is superior to other imaging modalities and may have important implications for the clinical management and outcome of a patient.

Hemorrhage is able to exhibit all possible MR signal patterns, depending on biological variables and imaging techniques. Hemorrhage therefore is an excellent tool for understanding the basic principles influencing MR contrast, furthermore giving the possibility to comprehend the signal characteristics of many other entities. Therefore, it is extremely helpful to gain a basic knowledge of the biological and physical processes underlying the signal changes of an evolving hematoma.

The appearance of hemorrhage mainly depends on the age of a hematoma and the type of MR contrast (T1-W or T2-W). The combination of a dark or bright appearance on T1-W or T2-W images offers the possibility to define five stages of the evolution of hemorrhage, which can be distinguished with MRI. These signal patterns evolve in an almost predictable temporal pattern within the brain, while the appearance of hemorrhage in other organs may vary. Therefore, MRI is able to show the extent of an intracerebral hematoma and may also provide information about the age of such a lesion.

1.2.8.1 Oxidation and Denaturation of Hemoglobin

An important factor influencing the MR appearance of hemorrhage on T1-W or T2-W images is the specific form of hemoglobin within a region of hemorrhage. As the hematoma ages, the hemoglobin passes through several forms (oxy-, deoxy- and methemoglobin) before red blood cell lysis occurs. To bind oxygen reversibly, the heme iron in the circulating form of hemoglobin (oxy- and deoxyhemoglobin) must be in the ferrous (Fe^{2+}) state. Being removed from the high oxygen level of the circulating blood, hemoglobin is denatured to methemoglobin and the heme iron becomes oxidized to the ferric (Fe^{3+}) form. As denaturation and oxidation continue, methemoglobin is converted to so-called hemichromes. The iron remains in the ferric state but the tertiary structure of the globin molecule is changed. Later on, the red blood cells become lysed and the hemichromes are broken down into the heme iron and the globin molecule. After phagocytosis by macrophages and intracranially by glial cells, the iron is stored as a derivative called ferritin, which consists of water-soluble ferric hydroxide-phosphate micelles attached to an iron storage protein (apoferritin), which keeps the iron in its hydrophobic centre. If there is a lack of apoferritin, hemosiderin is formed, which consists of water-insoluble clumps of ferritin (Table 1.5).

Table 1.5 Different derivatives during the denaturation of hemoglobin

Oxyhemoglobin
⬍
Deoxyhemoglobin
⬍
Methemoglobin
⬍
Hemichromes

These different oxidation and denaturation states of hemoglobin have certain magnetic properties, which have an influence on T1 and T2 relaxation times.

1.2.8.2 Magnetic Properties in Hemorrhage

Diamagnetism and Paramagnetism are two major types of magnetic properties of matter that are most relevant to the MR appearance of biological substances. Most substances consist of elements in which the electrons are paired in atomic and molecular orbitals. Such materials generate a magnetic field opposed to the applied magnetic field. The magnitude of the magnetic field within the material is reduced below that of the applied magnetic field. These materials are called diamagnetic.

Substances containing unpaired electrons have different magnetic properties due to resultant magnetic dipoles. If these dipoles are randomly orientated and separated, the resultant magnetization is zero, but after application of a magnetic field, these dipoles will align in a parallel or antiparallel manner, depending on the temperature of the material. At physiological temperatures, most electrons align parallel to the applied field, causing a magnification of the magnetic field. Materials without an intrinsic magnetic field that show an enhancement of an applied magnetic field are therefore called paramagnetic.

Oxyhemoglobin and hemichromes are diamagnetic; the heme iron contains paired electrons, whereas deoxy- and methemoglobin are paramagnetic because of unpaired electrons within the heme iron.

1.2.8.3 Relaxation Mechanisms

Diamagnetic Effects

Changes of the T1 or T2 relaxation times of an anatomical structure result in an alternated MR appearance. There are several mechanisms that may cause a T1 and T2 shortening in hemorrhage.

Protein Binding

Free water has very high motional frequencies, resulting in a very long and inefficient T1 relaxation of substances with high water content like CSF. Addition of protein causes an attraction of polar water molecules to charged protein groups, building a hydration layer. "Protein-bound-water" is almost prevented from free motion and has shorter T1 relaxation times than pure CSF, therefore the T1 relaxation time of proteinaceous, diamagnetic oxyhemoglobin is much less than that of CSF and is mostly similar to brain parenchyma.

Paramagnetic Effects

Paramagnetic substances offer considerably greater T1 shortening than that provided by protein binding effects. This is caused by dipole–dipole interaction between paramagnetic substances with unpaired electrons and the surrounding aqueous solution.

The magnitude of these effects mainly depends on the interaction of water molecules and hemoglobin – the hydrogen nuclei must be able to approach the heme iron, because the interaction falls off as the sixth power of the distance between them. Since the water molecules are not able to approach the heme iron closely enough, methemoglobin shows paramagnetic T1 shortening while deoxyhemoglobin does not.

The amount of T1 shortening also depends on the number of unpaired electrons of a substance; the greater the number of unpaired electrons, the greater the paramagnetic effect.

If sufficient amounts of water are bound by the proteinaceous solution, forming an almost mucinous gel, visible T2 shortening occurs. A similar mechanism for T2 shortening is encountered due to an increasing hematocrit as water is resorbed from hemorrhage.

Susceptibility Effects

Much greater T2* and T2 shortening occurs from the magnetic susceptibility effects resulting from compartmentalization of paramagnetic deoxy- or methemoglobin inside intact red blood cells.

The term "magnetic susceptibility" describes how magnetized a substance becomes when placed in a magnetic field, giving the ratio between the applied and the induced magnetic field.

Compartmentalization of paramagnetic substances with high magnetic susceptibility inside intact red blood cells causes a nonuniformity of the magnetic field in the imaging volume if the induced magnetic field inside the red blood cell is greater than that outside in the nonparamagnetic plasma. This leads to significant T2* shortening due to rapid spin dephasing and signal loss on T2*-W GRE images. Water protons diffuse through these nonuniform regions and loose phase coherence, resulting in decreased signal intensity on T2-W images.

The magnitude of the phase coherency loss depends on the time interval between two successive echoes (interecho time) and is proportionally increased when increasing the interecho time. Sequences using shorter interecho times than CSE like TSE sequences provide a decreased sensitivity to susceptibility effects. The decrease is proportional to the ETL of such sequences.

Susceptibility effects are increased when increasing the applied field strength because the induced field and therefore the induced nonuniformity is proportional to the applied magnetic field.

To summarize, the sensitivity to magnetic susceptibility increases with a decreasing number of 180° refocusing pulses from TSE to CSE to GRE, from T1 to T2 or T2* weighting and from lower to higher field strengths.

1.2.8.4 Evolving Parenchymal Hemorrhage

Considering the above-mentioned signal changes, the combination of T1-W and T2-W images allows the definition of five stages of evolution of a hematoma. Hyperacute (intracellular oxyhemoglobin, first few hours), acute (intracellular deoxyhemoglobin, 1–3 days), early subacute (intracellular methemoglobin, 3–7 days), late subacute (extracellular methemoglobin, older than 14 days), and chronic (intracellular hemosiderin and ferritin, older than 4 weeks) (Table 1.6). The exact times may vary.

Hyperacute

At the initial state, the hematoma consists of a liquid suspension of intact red blood cells containing a mixture of oxy- and deoxyhemoglobin. Later on, water is resorbed forming a more solid conglomerate of intact red blood cells. These few hours old hematomas mainly consist to 95% of oxyhemoglobin because most of nontraumatic intracranial hemorrhages result from an arterial bleeding (e.g., aneurysms). This stage of hemorrhage is very rarely seen in MRI.

These "hyperacute" hemorrhages often have a higher water content than normal brain tissue, which contributes to an iso- to hypointense signal behavior due to the longer T1 times of water on T1-W images and a hyperintense signal behavior on T2-W images.

Oxyhemoglobin is diamagnetic and unable to cause significant T2 shortening. Due to this reason, hyperacute hemorrhage without higher water content may exhibit signal characteristics on T2-W images, which cannot be distinguished from normal brain tissue.

It is important to remember that CT may be more sensitive during the first few hours, because high-oxygenated hemorrhages with little water content may be undetectable on MR-images.

Table 1.6 Evolution of intracerebral hemorrhage – signal intensities in correlation with different stages

Stage	Age	Red blood cells	Magnetic susceptibility	Compared to normal brain tissue	
				T1-W	T2-W
Hyperacute	Hours	Intact	–	⇔ / ⇓	⇑
Acute	Days	Intact	+	⇔ / ⇓	⇓⇓
Subacute	Weeks	Intact	+	⇑⇑	⇓⇓
	Months	Defect	–	⇑⇑	⇑⇑
Chronic	Years	Defect	++	⇔ / ⇓	⇓⇓

⇔ = isointense, ⇓ = hypointense, ⇑ = hyperintense when compared to normal brain tissue

Acute

After 24 h, almost all oxyhemoglobin has been deoxygenated to deoxyhemoglobin, while the red blood cells are still intact. As thromboses progresses, clot retraction occurs and an increasing hematocrit is observed, resulting in a progressive concentration of intact red blood cells, which causes further T2 shortening.

As noted earlier, deoxyhemoglobin is not able to cause significant T1 shortening. This results in signal intensities of the hemorrhage that could not be distinguished from surrounding brain tissue, as water is resorbed from the hematoma.

The compartmentalization of deoxyhemoglobin, which is magnetically susceptible, within intact red blood cells creates local nonuniformities in the magnetic field, resulting in T2 shortening due to dephasing of water molecules, which diffuse in and out of intact red blood cells. Both effects, increasing hematocrit due to clot retraction, and increasing susceptibility due to compartmentalization of deoxyhemoglobin lead to T2 shortening and apparent signal loss on T2-W images during the acute stage, while T1-W images may be slightly hypointense or show almost no signal change (Fig. 1.30).

Early Subacute

In the early subacute stage, the red blood cells are still intact, but deoxyhemoglobin undergoes permanent oxidization to methemoglobin. The dipole–dipole interaction between these paramagnetic molecules causes severe T1 shortening resulting in increased signal intensity on T1-W images. The oxidization of methemoglobin starts peripherally, because the oxygen level in the normal surrounding brain is higher than in the centre of the hemorrhage. Later on, the central deoxyhemoglobin becomes oxidized as well.

Since a great portion of red blood cells is still intact, the centre of these cells becomes more magnetized due to the magnetically susceptible methemoglobin than the surrounding plasma. These magnetic nonuniformities also cause severe T2 shortening and therefore strong signal loss on T2-W images.

Since methemoglobin has five unpaired electrons compared to deoxyhemoglobin (four unpaired electrons), these effects should be less apparent in the acute than in the early subacute stage of a hematoma.

However, the best way to distinguish between these two stages remains the hyperintense signal of methemoglobin in the early subacute stage on T1-W images (Fig. 1.31).

Late Subacute

The red blood cells undergo further degeneration by membrane lysis. Methemoglobin is now no longer compartmentalized and the T2 shortening resulting from compartmentalization is diminished.

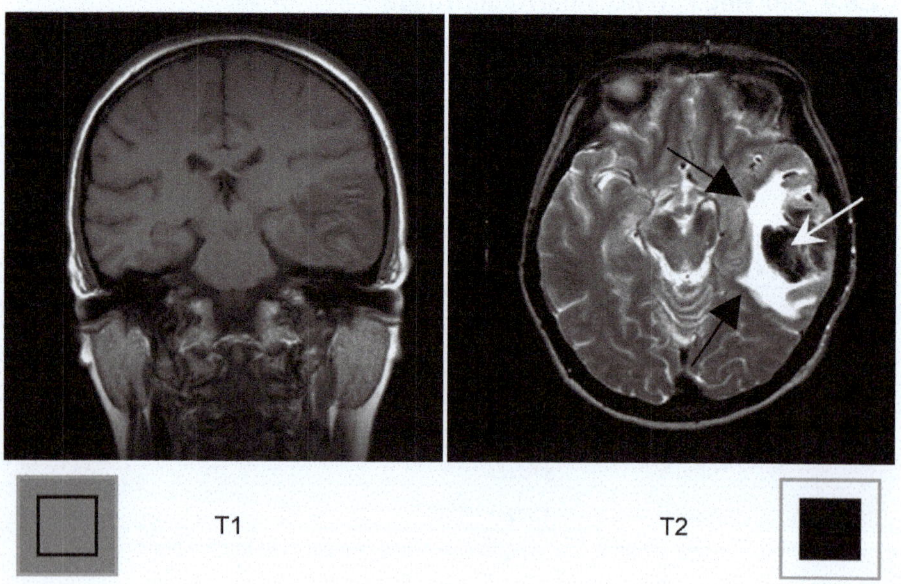

Fig. 1.30 Acute hematoma in a 50-year-old woman with a 3-day history of thrombosis of the left sinus sigmoideus. The T1-W coronal CSE image (TR 500, TE 15) demonstrates a slightly hypointense area compared to brain. The T2-W axial CSE image (TR 2000, TE 90) demonstrates the hypointense centre (*white arrow*) with a hyperintense surrounding edema (*black arrows*). The combination of T1-W and T2-W findings indicate that this hematoma mainly consists of intracellular deoxyhemoglobin

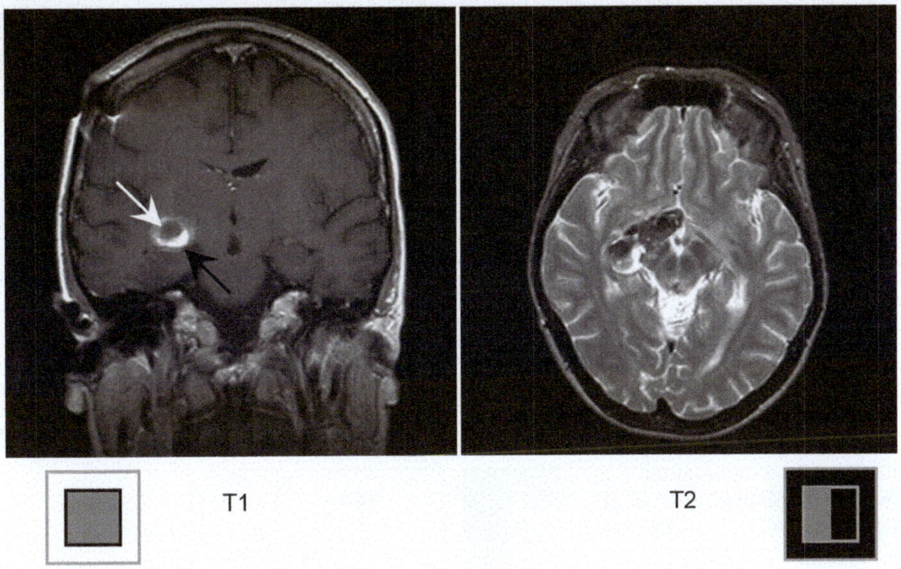

Fig. 1.31 Early subacute hematoma in a 35-year-old woman with a glioblastoma after radiotherapy. The T1-W coronal CSE image (TR 500, TE 15) demonstrates an isointense central (*white arrow*) area with a hyperintense rim (*black arrow*). T2-W CSE imaging (TR 2000 TE 90) shows the hypointense to isointense centre. These findings are typical for the early subacute stage and show the beginning oxidization of deoxyhemoglobin to methemoglobin at the rim

Late subacute stage hematomas are bright on T1-W and T2-W images as well. T2-W imaging is necessary to distinguish between early and late subacute hemorrhage (Fig. 1.32).

Chronic

After red blood cell lysis, paramagnetic hemosiderin and ferritin with high magnetic susceptibility is formed and stored inside macrophages surrounding the hematoma. The compartmentalization of these susceptible substances produces a great T2 shortening at the rim of a hematoma while the centre is filled with nonphagocytized and therefore not susceptible methemoglobin, which appears bright on T2-W images.

These hemichromes have little to no effect on T1-W images, which makes them appear almost brain isointense or slightly hypointense, caused by great

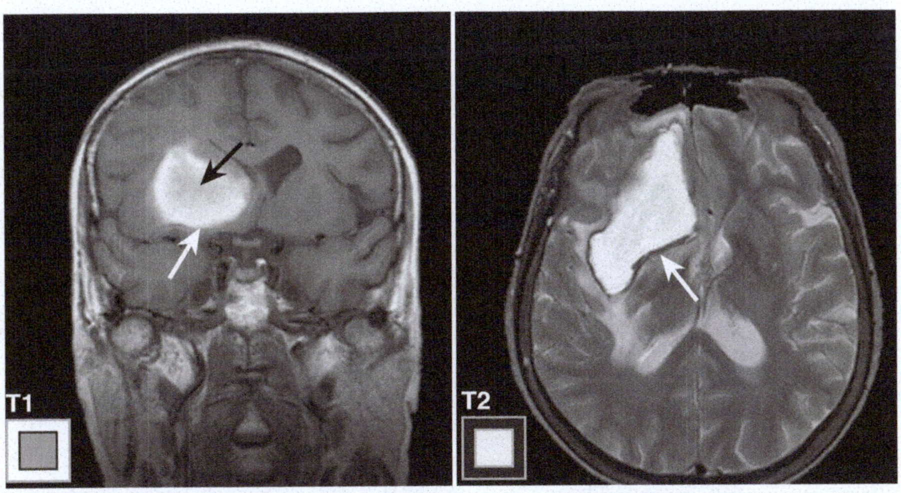

Fig. 1.32 Late subacute hematoma in a 74-year-old woman, 3 weeks after spontaneous hemorrhage. The T1-W coronal CSE image (TR 500, TE 15) demonstrates an isointense central area (*black arrow*) with a hyperintense rim (*white arrow*). T2-W CSE imaging (TR 2000 TE 90) shows the hyperintense centre with a slightly hypointense rim (*white arrow*) caused by beginning phagocytosis of methemoglobin and production of hemichromes. These findings are typical for the late subacute stage and show the prolonged T2 due to methemoglobin that is no longer compartmentalized within red blood cells

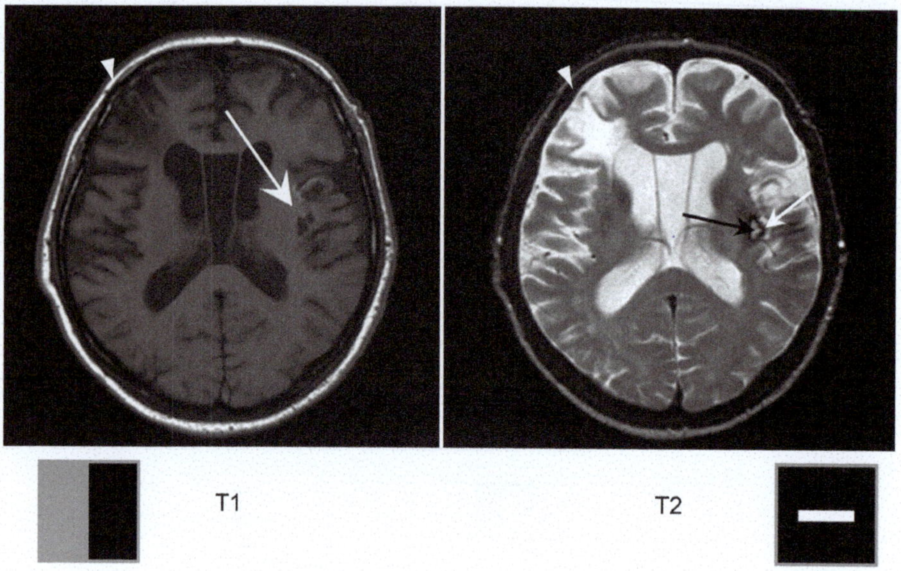

Fig. 1.33 Chronic hematoma in a 71-year-old man, 5 months after stroke in the left a cerebri media territory. The T1-W axial CSE image (TR 500, TE 15) demonstrates a hypointense to isointense central area (*white arrow*). T2-W CSE imaging (TR 2000 TE 90) shows the hyperintense centre (*black arrow*) with a hypointense rim (*white arrow*) caused by susceptibility effects of phagocytised hemosiderin. These findings may stay for a long time with an eventually further collapse of the lesion over years . Additional an old infarct in frontal lobe on the right side (*arrowheads*)

magnetic nonuniformities due to the strongly susceptible hemichromes, which may not only cause T2 shortening but also prolong T1 relaxation times (Fig. 1.33).

During a long time (in general years), hematomas may be completely resorbed or transformed to a collapsed scar and may then remain for a lifetime as a completely hypointense small lesion (Fig. 1.34).

1.2.8.5 Sub- and Epidural Hemorrhage

Epidural and subdural hematomas evolve almost like parenchymal hemorrhage in five stages. In contrast to parenchymal hemorrhage, they offer a slower progression to the next stage, caused by the very well vascularized dura mater.

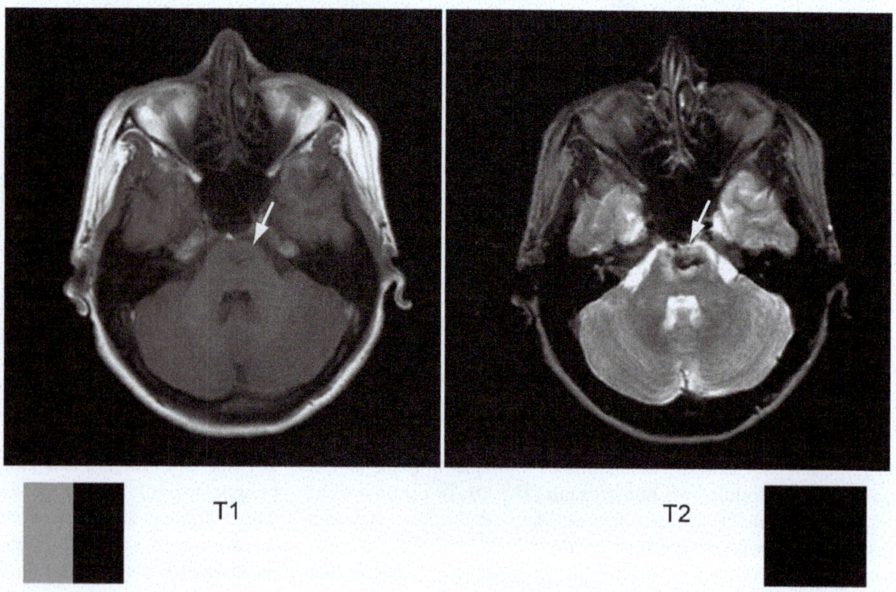

Fig. 1.34 Late chronic hematoma in a 31-year-old woman with a history of hemorrhage in the pons during childhood due to an AV malformation. T1-W axial CSE imaging (TR 500, TE 15) demonstrates a hypointense to isointense central area. T2-W CSE images (TR 2000 TE 90) show the collapsed, hypointense hematoma with susceptibility effects. These findings may remain for a lifetime (*arrows*)

The first four stages evolve in a similar pattern, but the chronic stage normally shows no dark rim, because there are no tissue macrophages. Since no phagocytosis takes place, no susceptibility effects caused by compartmentalization of hemichromes are visible. The chronic stage of sub- and epidural hematomas is characterized by continued oxidative denaturation of methemoglobin, which causes an increase of T1 times. Therefore, the signal intensity of chronic subdural hematoma may be somewhat lower than during the subacute stage.

Recurrent bleeding can sometimes cause "hemosiderin staining," which resembles the hemosiderin surrounding a parenchymal hematoma in the chronic phase.

These events may be distinguishable by the different signal intensities.

Epidural hematomas are distinguished from subdural hematomas by classic morphology that means concave vs. convex shape and by the low intensity of the dura mater between the hematoma and normal brain tissue.

1.2.8.6 Subarachnoid and Intraventricular Hemorrhage

Subarachnoid and intraventricular hemorrhages have high ambient oxygen levels and therefore, age more slowly compared to sub- and epidural hematomas. Acute subarachnoid and intraventricular hematomas may show higher signal intensities due to mixture with CSF.

Sometimes, the red blood cells may be resorbed; therefore the anticipated T1 shortening cannot be seen. In chronic, repeated subarachnoid hemorrhages, hemosiderin may stain the meninges, leading to a short T2 appearance (superficial siderosis).

1.2.8.7 Intratumoral Hemorrhage

Intratumoral hemorrhage may evolve more slowly due to the lower oxygen tension. Delayed evolution of hematoma is therefore visible at high oxygen levels (methemoglobin is deoxidized to deoxyhemoglobin by the methemoglobin reductase system) and comparatively low oxygen levels (deoxyhemoglobin is not oxidized to methemoglobin) at different stages in the evolution.

Intratumoral hemorrhage builds a hemosiderin membrane like parenchymal hemorrhage, but this membrane may become disrupted with renewed tumor growth. This sign is not necessarily tumor specific since any other rebleeding can cause a membrane rupture, too.

1.2.8.8 Technical Considerations

Operating Field Strength

Since the degree of para-/diamagnetic and susceptibility effects depends directly on the applied field strength, the operating field strength of an imaging unit has an important influence on the signal behavior of hemorrhage. Changing the operating field strength mostly affects the sensitivity of T2-W images to susceptibility effects, which causes a signal loss on T2-W images.

The contrast in acute hemorrhage on T2-W images, which is caused by T2 shortening arising from compartmentalized deoxyhemoglobin may not be detected at low field-strength systems using spin echo sequences. In vitro studies of deoxygenated erythrocytes showed a quadric dependence of T2 times on magnetic field strength, demonstrating that the minimal concentration of deoxyhemoglobin that produces visible T2 shortening therefore mainly depends on the applied field strength (Fig. 1.35).

On low field-strength systems, every stage seems to be prolonged since more time is required until appropriate amounts of deoxy-, methemoglobin, or hemosiderin have been formed.

Generally spoken, imaging at low field-strength systems will provide less lesion contrast and causes a virtual prolongation of the ageing process of a hematoma.

In recent years, whole-body MRI units with field strengths of 3.0 T have become available for clinical routine imaging. At 3.0 T, the central and peripheral part of acute and early subacute hemorrhage is markedly hypointense on T2-W MR images compared to imaging at 1.5 T (Figs. 1.36 and 1.37).

The central hypointensity of early subacute hemorrhage decreases but remains at 3.0 T, differing significantly from the central part of hemorrhage imaged at 1.5 T, which appears hyperintense during this stage on T2-W MR images. Since susceptibility effects depend on field strength, at 3.0 T, apparently minimal amounts of intracellular deoxyhemoglobin or methemoglobin suffice to evoke these effects and cause hypointensity or even reduce the signal intensity, and obviously greater amounts of extracellular

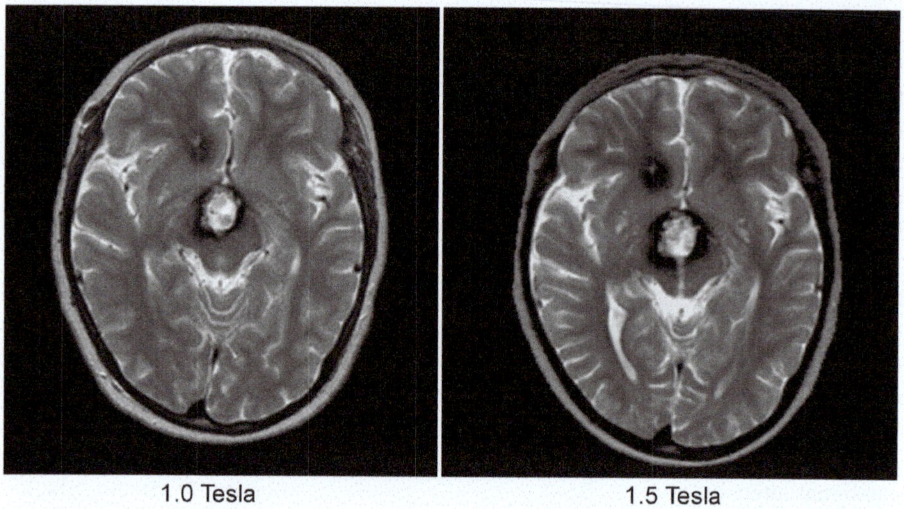

Fig. 1.35 T2-W CSE images (TR 2000, TE 90) of a 17-year-old patient with two cavernomas, acquired at the same level, but with different operating field strengths (*left*: 1.0 T, *right*: 1.5 T). Susceptibility effects (black area around the cavernoma) due to phagocytised hemichromes within macrophages are much more pronounced at higher field strengths and make the areas of hemorrhage appear bigger

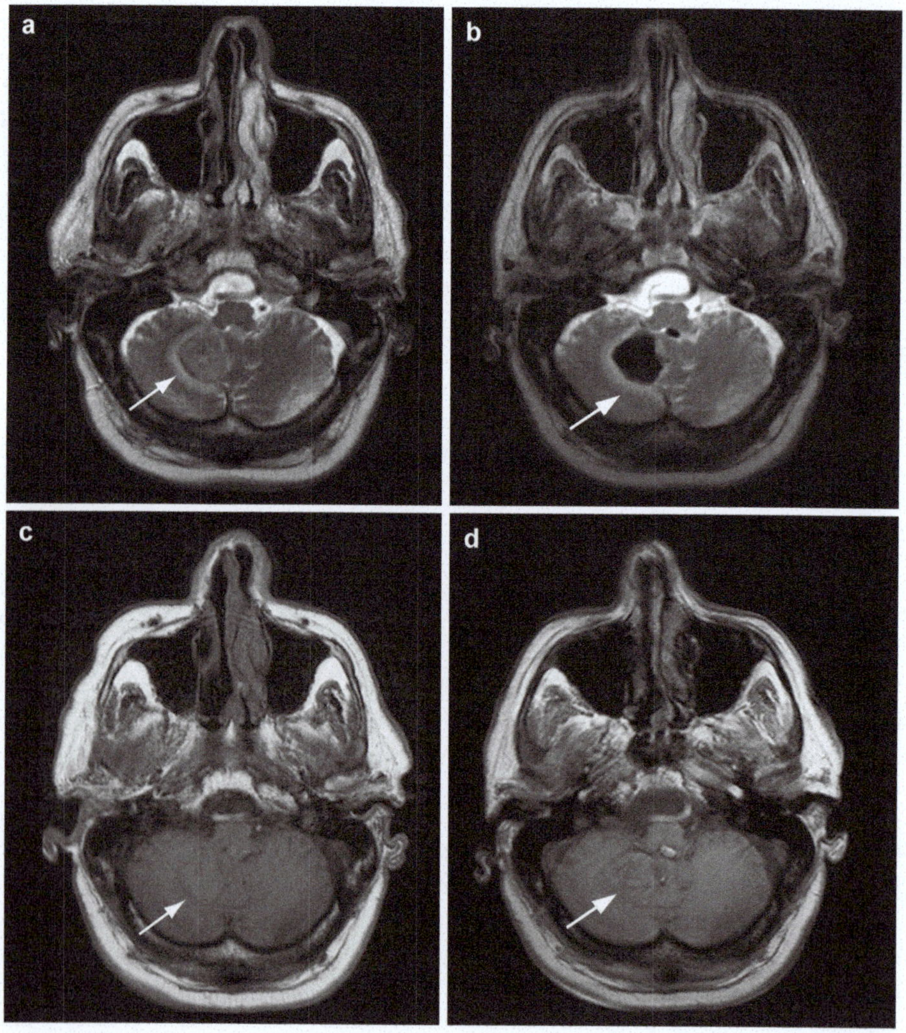

Fig. 1.36 Acute intracerebral hemorrhage: 77-year-old patient, receiving anticoagulative medication, imaged on the second day after onset of clinical symptoms (dizziness, nausea). Axial, T2-W (**a**, **b**) and T1-W (**c**, **d**) imaging at 1.5 T (*arrows*) (**a**, **c**) and 3.0 T (*arrowheads*) (**b**, **d**). On T2-W images, hemorrhage is depicted iso- to hyperintense at 1.5 T but markedly hypointense at 3.0 T

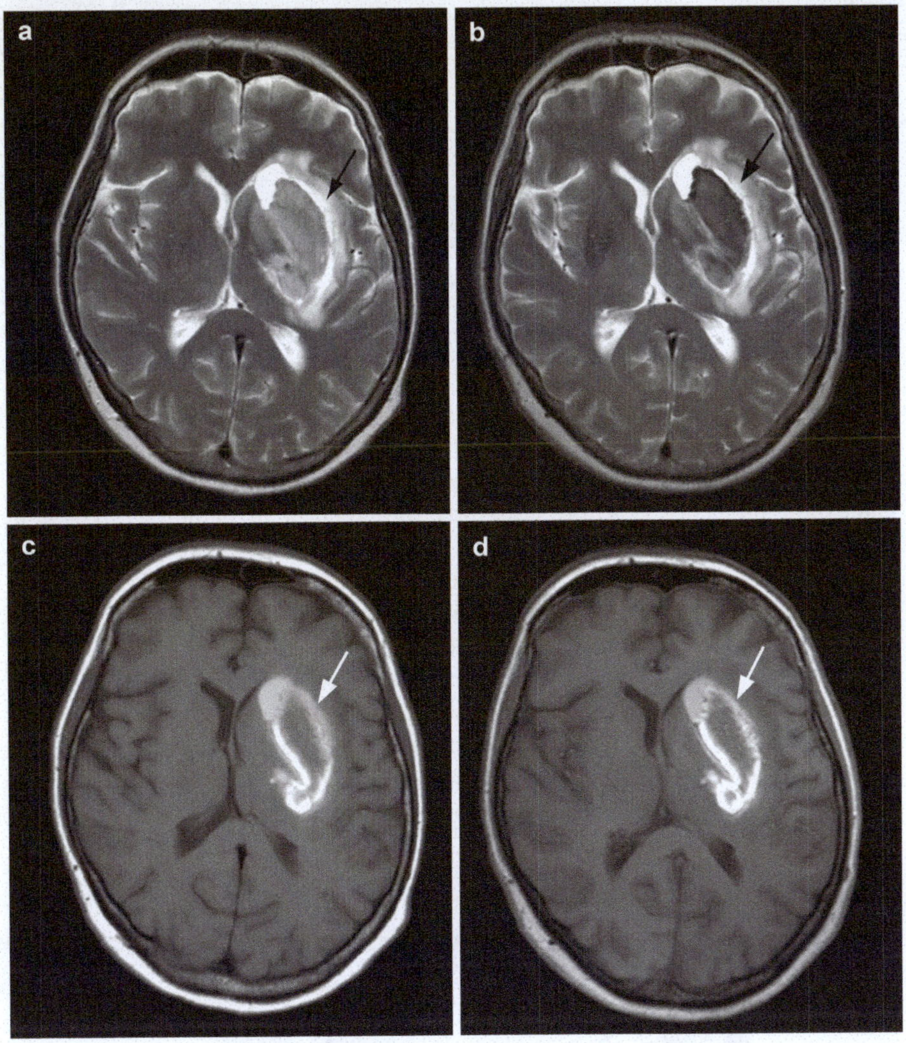

Fig. 1.37 Early subacute hemorrhage: 56-year-old patient, suffering from arterial hypertension, imaged on the sixth day after onset of clinical symptoms (hemiplegia on right hand side).T2-W (4,000/90) (**a**, **b**) and T1-W (**c**, **d**) imaging at 1.5 T (*arrow*) (**a**, **c**) and 3.0 T (*arrowheads*) (**b**, **d**). Hemorrhage is depicted hyperintense on T2-W images at 1.5 T but hypointense at 3.0 T

methemoglobin and higher water contents are required at 3.0 T to prevent susceptibility-induced effects and to alter the signal intensity of the periphery of early subacute hemorrhages so as to result in hyperintensity on T2-W MR images. Consequently, TSE sequences, which are known to provide reduced sensitivity to susceptibility effects, are able to depict small hemorrhagic lesions with increased hypointensity at 3.0 T, resembling T2-W CSE or even GRE imaging at 1.5 T (Fig. 1.38).

T1-W MRI does not provide significant differences between 1.5- and 3.0 T. Although formation of methemoglobin is expected to be better demonstrated at 1.5 T, since the paramagnetic T1 shortening caused by methemoglobin is supposed to inversely vary with field strength, the increased SNR at 3.0 T is responsible for the lack of differences in the depiction of methemoglobin between 1.5- and 3.0-T T1-W MRI (Figs. 1.36 and 1.37).

In summary, despite the fact that all parts of the acute and early subacute hemorrhage show significantly increased hypointensity on 3.0-T T2-W MR images, images obtained at 1.5 and 3.0 T are equivalent in age determination of acute to late subacute hemorrhage. However, knowledge of the image characteristics of hemorrhage at 1.5 and 3.0 T is required to compare and correctly appreciate the progression of these lesions.

Sequence Types

MR contrast of intracerebral hemorrhage highly depends on the used type of pulse sequence. Image

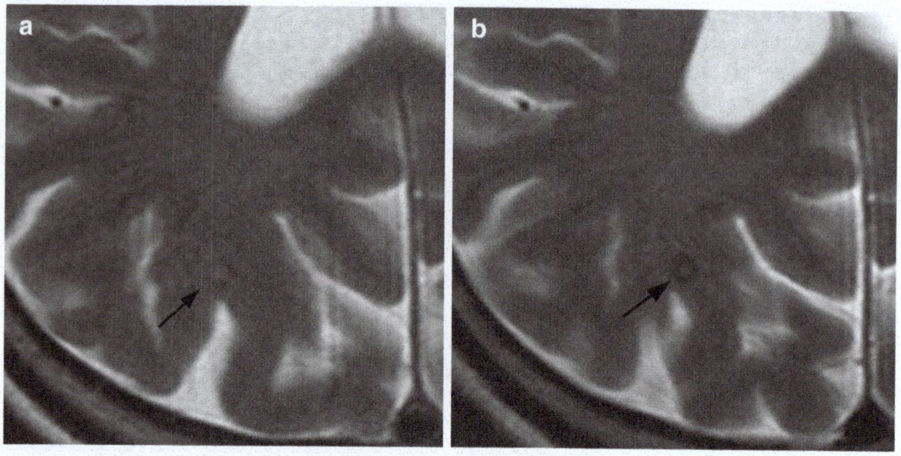

Fig. 1.38 Petechial hemorrhage: Detailed view of T2-W TSE imaging at 1.5 (*arrow*) (**a**) and 3.0 T (*arrowhead*) (**b**)

acquisition protocols generally use three different pulse sequences: GRE, CSE, and TSE.

GREs use a gradient reversal to rephase the spins to generate the echo, providing a very high sensitivity for susceptibility effects. Although sensitivity to paramagnetic constituents of the hematoma and magnetic susceptibility effects is increased, other border zones of different susceptibility (for example interfaces between air and tissue) also produce strong signal loss and geometric distortions, decreasing visualization of large regions of the brain. It is sometimes difficult not to interpret these artifacts on real pathology. These dephasing effects are voxel size dependent and can be reduced to a certain degree by reducing the voxel size, which reduces the magnitude of the magnetic gradient between two voxels.

GRE sequences are very sensitive for the detection of mild intracerebral hemorrhage, but they often show anatomical misregistrations, thus GREs should preferably be used at lower field strengths. They may also serve as a sequence type for very sensitive detection of mild or small intracranial hematomas, if other sequence types fail to detect them (Fig. 1.39).

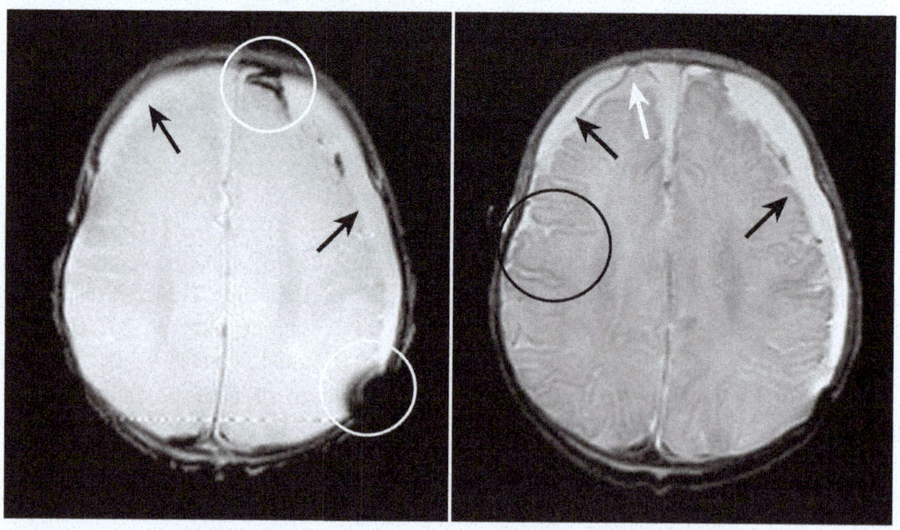

Fig. 1.39 T2-W images of the same level of a 8-month-old boy, suspicious for a battered child syndrome, with subdural fluid (*black arrows*), acquired with different sequence types (*left*: GRE, TR 150, TE 4.1; *right*: CSE, TR 2000, TE 90). CSE images provide much more anatomical information (e.g., edema in right frontal lobe (*white arrow*), differentiation between white and grey matter (*black circle*)), whereas susceptibility effects ("hemosiderin staining"), which proof the existence of hemorrhage, are much more pronounced on gradient echo images and almost invisible on spin echo images (*white circles*)

CSE sequences generate echoes in a different manner. They use a 180° radio frequency pulse to refocus the dephasing transversal magnetization to generate an echo. Due to this sequence design, they are able to correct the distorting effects of magnetic field inhomogeneities that normally cause rapid signal loss. However, if the lesion itself is identified by these distortions, as in hematomas, the contrast that is required for the detection of the lesion is also diminished.

Despite this, effects resulting from the diffusion of water through local field gradients are not considerably diminished unless the TE is made very short in relation to the correlation time of water diffusion, which means, no significant dephasing can occur.

TSE sequences differ from CSE sequences because they generate multiple spin echoes per TR, called echo train. The number of spin echoes per excitation cycle is also called ETL. In combination with a shortened interecho time, this sequence design significantly shortens the total acquisition time.

The use of multiple spin echoes in combination with a shortened interecho time results in a lower sensitivity of TSE sequences for magnetic susceptibility and diffusion effects compared to CSE. Several studies have shown that the sensitivity to these effects is proportionately reduced with increasing ETL (Fig. 1.40).

Gradient- and spin echo (GRASE) sequences, which are also called turbo gradient spin echo (TGSE) sequences are a hybrid technique mixing gradient- and spin echoes (Sect. 1.3.1.3).

GRASE was expected to provide higher sensitivity to susceptibility effects because of its gradient echo content in combination with a good anatomical

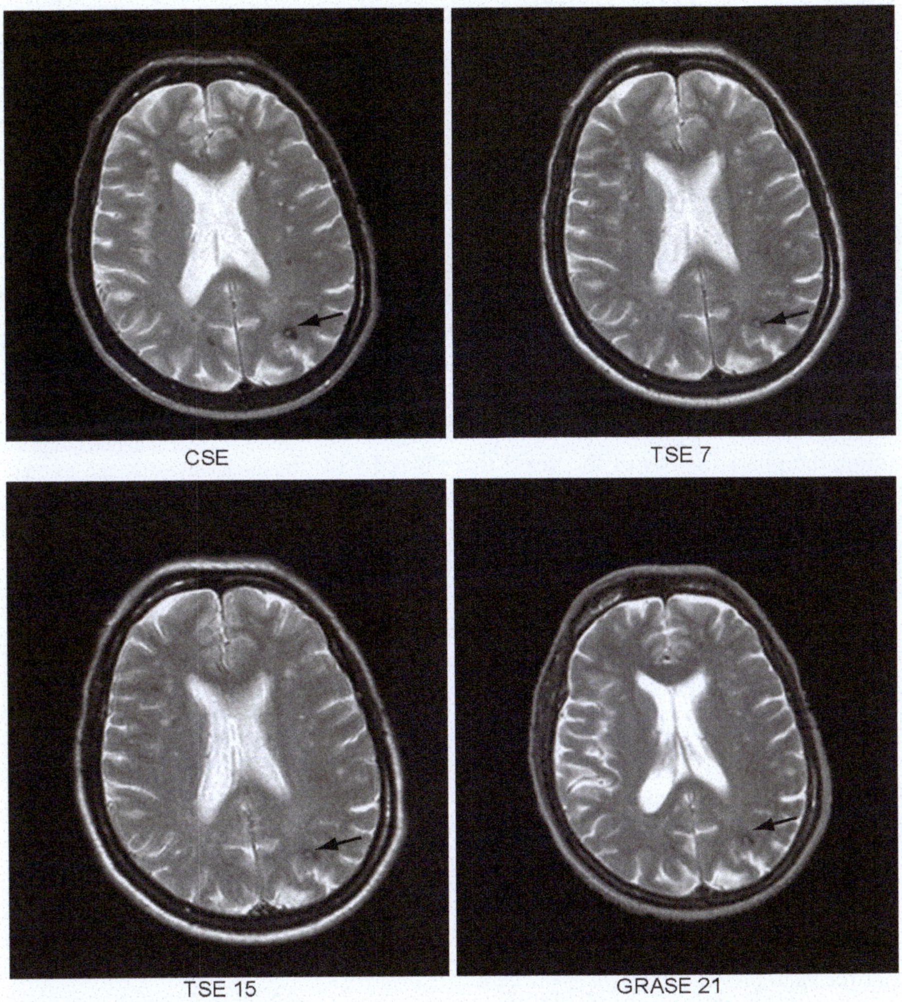

Fig. 1.40 Four T2-W images of a 54-year-old woman with multiple small hemorrhagic lesions, acquired at almost the same level, but with different sequence types (*upper left*: CSE, *upper right*: TSE with an ETL of 7, *lower left*: TSE with an ETL of 15, *lower right*: GRASE with an ETL of 21). These images demonstrate the decreased susceptibility-based contrast of small hemorrhagic lesions with increasing number of echoes per echo train because of decreasing sensitivity to susceptibility effects (*arrows*). This also accounts for the GRASE 21 sequence, although this sequence type should theoretically provide an increased susceptibility contrast compared to the TSE 7 counterpart. Conventional spin echo demonstrates the highest susceptibility contrast, whereas some smaller lesions are not detectable on TSE and GRASE images

resolution due to the spin echo content, but recent studies showed that TSE sequences are still more sensitive to susceptibility effects. The exact reason for the reduced sensitivity is unclear and remains to be investigated. GRASE sequences require very short acquisition times, but they are unable to provide proper detection of small parenchymal lesions (Fig. 1.40).

In conclusion, SE and TSE sequences with short ETLs are the sequence type of choice for the detection and classification of hemorrhage, although they are more time consuming than GRE or GRASE sequences. However, GRE sequences may serve for very sensitive detection of mild or small intracranial hematomas, if other sequence types fail to detect them.

1.2.9 Flow and Motion (MR Angiography, Diffusion and Perfusion)

Imaging sequences discussed up to this point are all flow sensitive. The phase of a generated transverse magnetization following excitation characterizes the position within the transverse plane, as illustrated in Fig. 1.41. Switching a field gradient for the purpose of spatial encoding will result in a different phase of magnetization within adjacent voxels. Switching the field gradient in the opposite direction with the same amplitude and duration will move the phase back to the same position for stationary tissue. For moving tissue, the phase history of the voxel that moved will be different than the phase history of a stationary voxel at the same location. If the phase information is just to be used for spatial encoding, this is an unwanted phenomenon. It can be shown that with an arrangement of three gradient lobes, a rephasing can be performed at the same location and the same time for the stationary tissue as well as the flowing blood (Fig. 1.42). This method is called gradient motion rephasing — GMR. GRE techniques utilizing this GMR have the advantage that the images have fewer artifacts for slices containing vascular structures. The disadvantage of the three-lobe arrangement is a prolonged TE. Including phase-encoding steps in the direction of slice selection will allow the slice (usually at this point called a slab) to be further "partitioned." This is called a 3D technique.

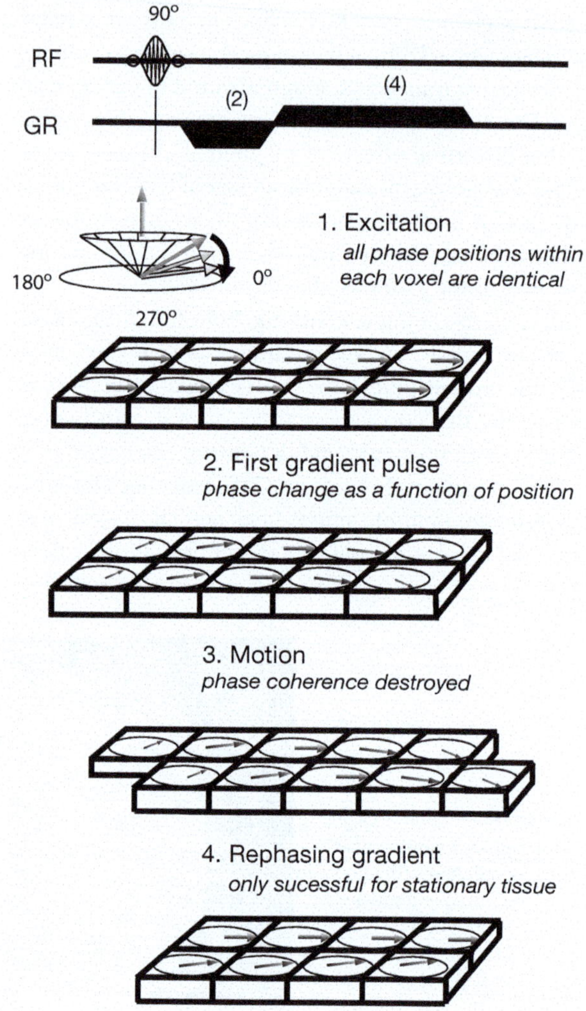

Fig. 1.41 The "phase" is defined as the position of the transverse nuclear magnetization within the *x*-*y* or transverse plane. Immediately after the excitation, all macroscopic magnetizations have the same phase position. The gradient GR preparing the gradient or spin echo will produce a phase difference in the direction of encoding. At the time the rephasing gradient is applied, parts of the voxel have moved, showing a different phase history as compared with the magnetization of stationary tissue. The rephasing gradient will rephase the magnetization within the stationary tissue, but the magnetization within moving structures will show a different phase. The phase difference may lead to a signal void and thus artifacts, since the phase information is also used for spatial encoding. The phase position can be evaluated to quantify the flow velocity

1.2.9.1 3D Time of Flight MR Angiography (3D-ToF-MRA)

Time of flight MR Angiography (3D-ToF-MRA) is based on the effect of unsaturated blood flowing into an imaging volume with primarily saturated stationary

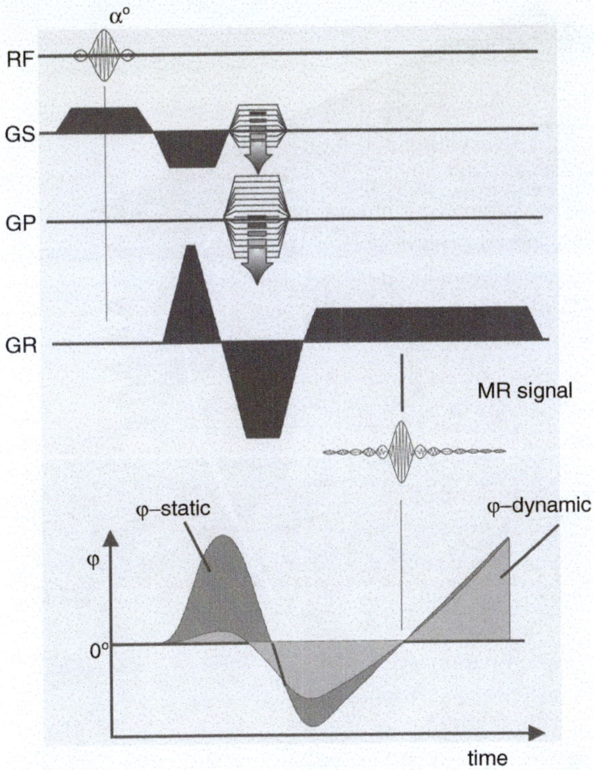

Fig. 1.42 3D Gradient echo sequence with gradient motion rephasing (GMR). The constant velocity of a moving structure causes the phase evolution to be quadratic in time. It can be shown that with a three-lobe gradient structure, as illustrated here, a rephasing can be achieved at the time of the echo for static tissue as well as for tissue that moves with a constant velocity. This phenomenon is called GMR. *GP* phase-encoding gradient; *GR* readout gradient; *GS* slice-selection gradient; *RF* radiofrequency

tissue. An additional phase encoding in the direction of slice selection allows a thick slice to be "partitioned". Minor obstacle is that for each in-depth phase-encoding step all in-plane phase-encoding steps have to be repeated. This explains why 3D techniques are only practical to be combined with short TR GRE sequences or SE multi-echo approaches. The combination of a 3D GRE method with the above GMR is the basis for a 3D-ToF-MRA as illustrated in Fig. 1.42. The unsaturated blood within the vessel appears hyperintense compared with the stationary surroundings. To visualize the vascular tree, projections are reconstructed, which assign the highest signal intensity found along a ray of the perspective to the signal intensity of the pixel, as illustrated in Fig. 1.43. Such a projection is called a maximum intensity projection — MIP. The disadvantage of this technique is that small vessels visible on the native slice will be obscured by the higher signal contribution of the noise contained in adjacent slices. Nevertheless, this technique has succeeded so far as a robust method for the visualization of the vascular system especially of the cerebral circulation. For the evaluation of questionable areas and for the smaller vessels, there is always the possibility of assessing the native images.

1.2.9.2 Contrast-Enhanced MR Angiography (ceMRA)

With the ability to acquire a 3D MRA within a breath-hold – or the passing of a contrast bolus – the so-called contrast-enhanced MRA techniques have outperformed the time-of-flight methods for the vasculature below the carotid bifurcation. A GRE technique is applied with the shortest suitable TE selected (no GMR), the shortest possible TR, and a moderate excitation angle. The aim is to provide an image of a passing contrast bolus. Figure 1.44 demonstrates an example of a so-called time-resolved ceMRA, where the measurement of the transit time is omitted and replaced by multiple sequential acquisitions of the same region. The T1 shortening of the blood as a consequence of administering a paramagnetic contrast agent will allow the imaging of the vascular tree with no saturation effects. There is no entry plane and no concern about saturation. Without a time-resolved method, the challenging part for the user is the timing between the injection of the bolus and the start of the breath-hold acquisition. The goal is to acquire the data at the time, where the contrast bolus is within the volume of interest. The timing of the measurement depends on the transit time of the bolus to the region of interest, the phase-encoding loop structure of the imaging sequence, and the duration of the injection time. The transit time, the time between intravenous injection of the contrast bolus and the appearance within the region on interest, can be evaluated prior to the ceMRA protocol by using a small test bolus and a fast imaging technique through the region of interest with an update of one image/s. An alternative is usually offered in the form of a combined protocol. The user can start a bolus tracking fast 2D technique, inject the contrast bolus, and semiautomatically can switch to the (3D) ceMRA technique as soon as the arrival of the bolus is noted within the region of interest (e.g., CARE bolus technique). To cover large regions as required in the ceMRA evaluation of the peripheral vasculature, protocols are offered that include automatic table feed to cover several vascular stations utilizing one single bolus injection.

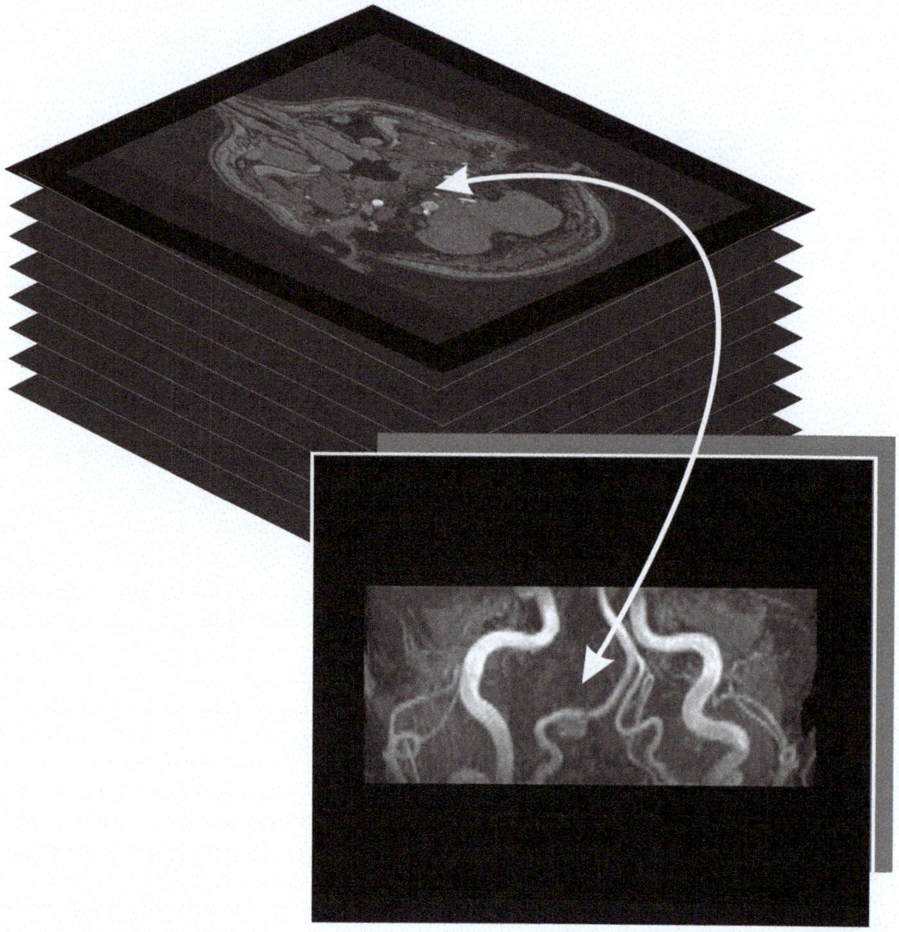

Fig. 1.43 The maximum intensity projection (MIP) projects the maximum intensity found in a stack of images to the pixel intensity on the screen, depending on the view, the perspective that the user defines. In this example, a transverse 3D ToF-MRA was performed to study the aneurysm in the right vertebral artery. A coronal MIP was applied to these transverse stack of images

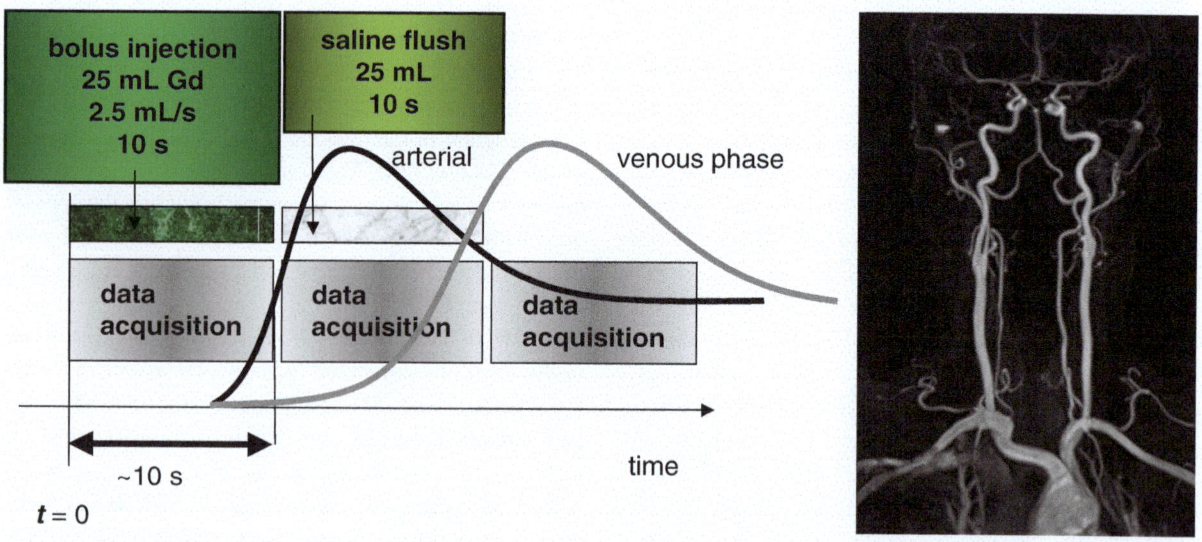

Fig. 1.44 ceMRA Principle. Contrast strongly depends on matching the arrival of the bolus within the region of interest and placing the *k*-space acquisition accordingly. Time-resolved imaging of the extracranial cerebral circulation will provide the native scan, the arterial phase, and images of the venous phase of the passing contrast media

1.2.9.3 Diffusion and Diffusion Weighting

Diffusion characterizes the arbitrary motion of water molecules within a given tissue and has recently attracted attention as a tool for the early detection of infarction, brain trauma, and tumor characterization. The ability of water molecules to perform random translational motion within a given tissue is described by the diffusion coefficient. The application of a magnetic field gradient for a short duration will cause a temporary change in resonance frequencies and a correlated dephasing of the transverse magnetization. Applying the same gradient for the same duration but of opposite polarity will result in a "rephasing" of the transverse magnetization - for stationary tissue. For molecules which have changed position in the meantime, the rephasing of the transverse magnetization will be incomplete (Fig. 1.41), causing a signal loss. In order to enhance this effect, relatively large magnetic field gradients are necessary. Diffusion weighted imaging - DWI, involves the application of large magnetic field gradients in addition to the field gradients used for spatial encoding. Tissue or tissue areas with an increased diffusion will appear as hypointense areas in DWI. The classical Stejskal-Tanner approach of diffusion weighting is illustrated in Fig. 1.45. The Stejskal-Tanner approach uses two large gradients around a 180° refocusing pulse. This gradient has no effect on stationary material but produces a significant sensitivity to flow, motion, and diffusion. Since physiological or global motion causes changes of magnitude higher than that of diffusion, DWI today is, with a very few exceptions (like diffusion-weighted SSFP), solely applied in conjunction with fast imaging techniques like echo planar (EPI). EPI enables an image acquisition within 80–120 ms. There are a few clinical applications in which EPI is the preferred imaging technique. These applications include the utilization of EPI read-out modules for a prepared magnetization that would otherwise be destroyed by a prolonged read-out period, like diffusion weighting in stroke imaging or tumor characterization. The classical form uses one excitation pulse and multiple phase-encoded echoes to generate an image, as illustrated in Fig. 1.45. The effect on transverse magnetizations that change position during the duration of the diffusion-weighting gradients is a function of the

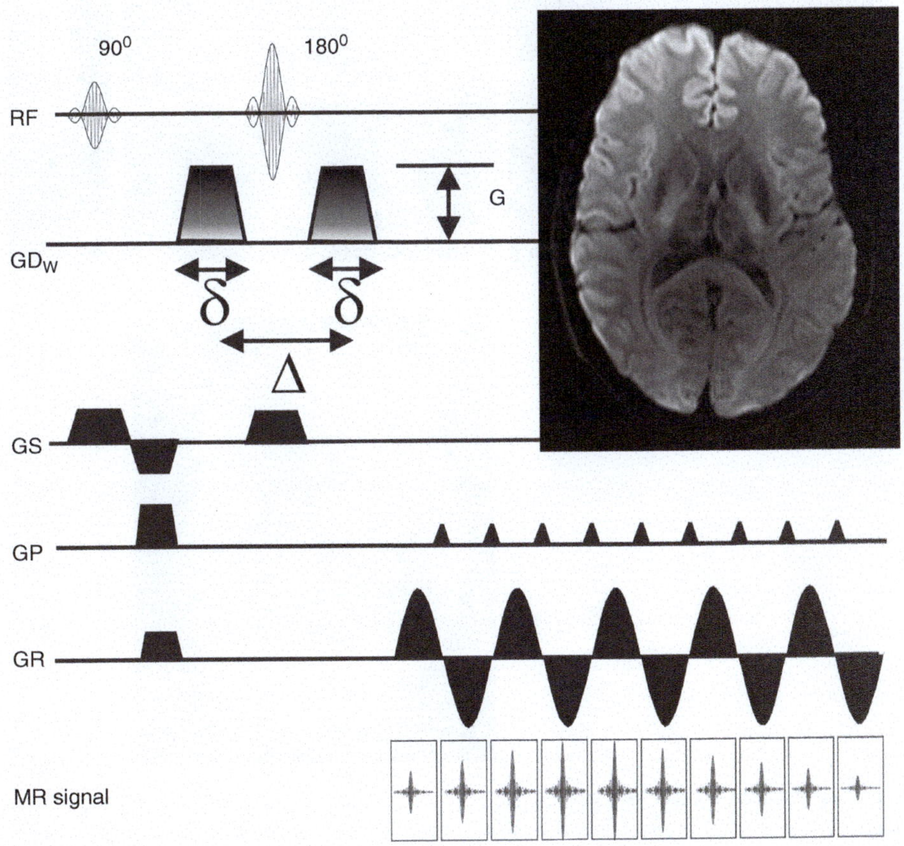

Fig. 1.45 The blipped spin-echo echo-planar imaging (SE-bEPI) sequence design with diffusion sensitization. In this example, the gradients providing the diffusion weighting are placed in the direction of slice selection. A spin-echo envelope is generated, containing multiple gradient echoes. In this example, the phase-encoding gradient is "blipped" between the readout gradient lobes. *GP* phase-encoding gradient; *GR* readout gradient; *GS* slice-selection gradient; *RF* radiofrequency

strength of the diffusion-weighting magnetic field gradient amplitude G_{DW}, the duration of these gradient pulses δ, and the time interval Δ between these diffusion gradients. Fortunately, all these functions can be summarized with a so-called b-value (in s/mm²), with the expected signal being $S \sim e^{-bD}$, where D is the apparent diffusion coefficient (ADC) and

$$b = \gamma^2 \cdot G_{DW}^2 \cdot \delta^2 \cdot \left[\Delta - \frac{\delta}{3}\right].$$

In clinical practice, b-values around 1,000 s/mm² are most commonly used. Tissues in which water mobility is restricted appear bright on DWI and dark on the calculated ADC maps. As the DWI are often contaminated with the effect of T2* relaxation (T2 shine through), it is advised to calculate the ADC images to increase the diagnostic confidence.

In practice, the diffusion-weighting gradient scheme has become more complex as compared to the illustrated two lobe approach. As diffusion weighting depends on the direction of the diffusion-weighted gradients, there are usually three measurements with orthogonal directions combined to create a "trace" image. That "trace" image represents the geometric mean of the diffusion measured with the individual DWI (Fig. 1.46), with the signal being proportional to

$$S \sim e^{-bD_{av}} \text{ with } D_{av} \sim \frac{1}{3} \cdot (D_{xx} + D_{yy} + D_{zz}).$$

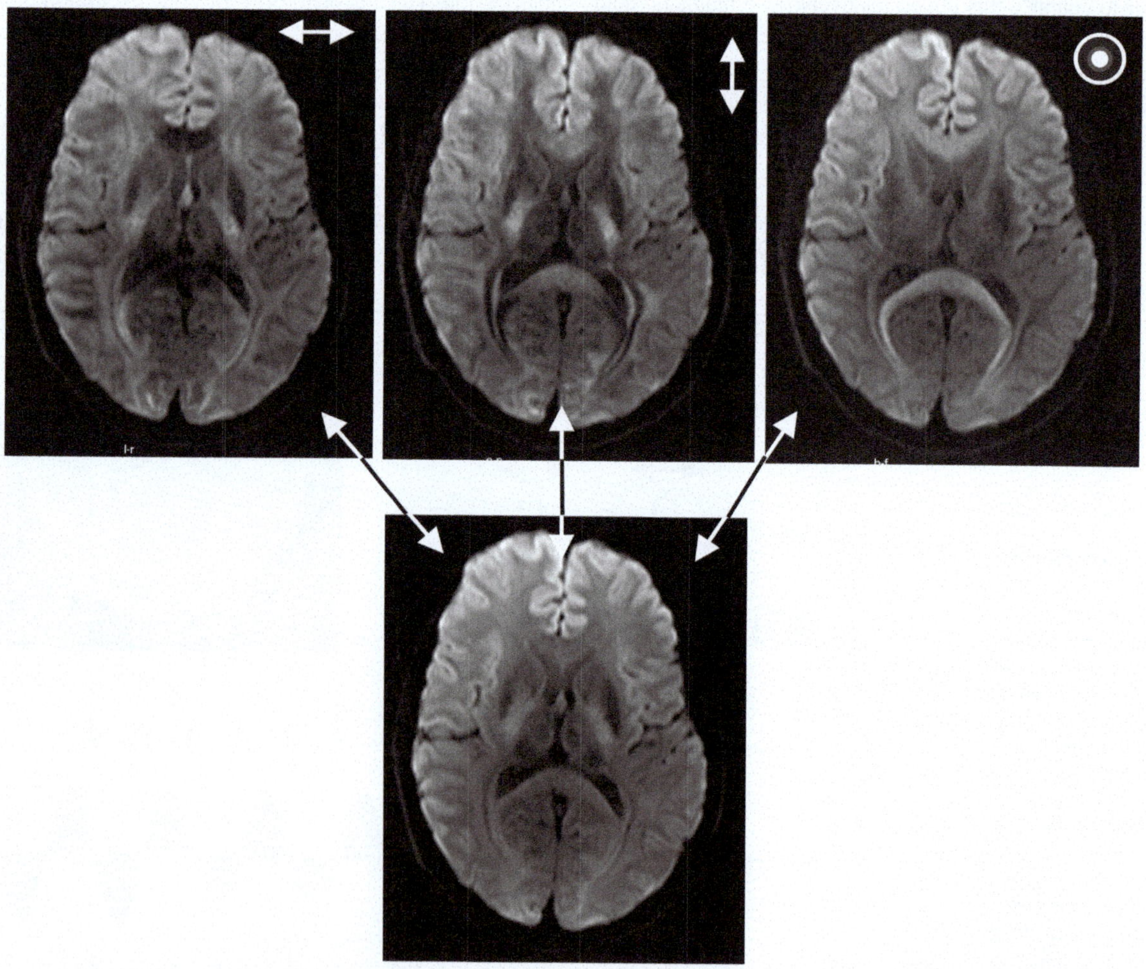

Fig. 1.46 Trace weighting: this case demonstrates the directional dependence of diffusion and diffusion-weighting magnetic field gradients (*arrows*). As the trace of the diffusion tensor is an invariant to directional dependence, a combined image that considers the averaged diffusion coefficients is called trace weighted

1.2.9.4 Perfusion-Weighted Imaging (PWI) Using Contrast Agents

Numerous techniques have been proposed to measure various perfusion-related parameters, mainly for the brain but also for other organs, e.g., the kidney. There are two main principal methods. One group of methods is relying on the administration of a contrast agent, where a second group of methods is focusing on arterial spin labeling. The latter seems to show some potential, especially in conjunction with high field systems, but as this observation is more recent and more sophisticated, it will be discussed in Sect. 1.3.4.3.

DSC: Dynamic Susceptibility Contrast

The magnetic field in a sample depends on the strength of the external magnetic field and the magnetic susceptibility constant of the sample

$$B_{0(\mathrm{eff})} = (1+\chi)B_0.$$

MRI contrast agents are either paramagnetic or superparamagnetic. The increase in blood susceptibility induced by the contrast agent is proportional to the concentration of the latter in the blood pool. Following the injection of an MR contrast agent, susceptibility differences will build up between vascular and extravascular compartments. This susceptibility difference causes magnetic field distortions in the vicinity of blood vessels, resulting in a decrease of the transverse relaxation times of protons in the extravascular compartment (spin dephasing – signal loss). The signal intensity over time (DSC, Fig. 1.47) can be converted to a relative measure of the contrast agent concentration, respectively a change in the local transverse relaxation rate.

$$\Delta R_2^* = -\ln\left[\frac{S(t)}{S_{\mathrm{baseline}}}\right] \Big/ \mathrm{TE}.$$

PBP: Percentage of Baseline at Peak

A PBP map gives a qualitative impression of perfusion irregularities. It is a pixel-by-pixel comparison of signal alterations caused by the first pass of a contrast bolus (Fig. 1.48). Areas where the signal is less affected by the passing contrast bolus appear as bright pixels in the PBP map.

TTP: Time to Peak

A TTP map gives a qualitative impression of perfusion irregularities. In this case, each pixel intensity scales with the time of duration between arterial injection and

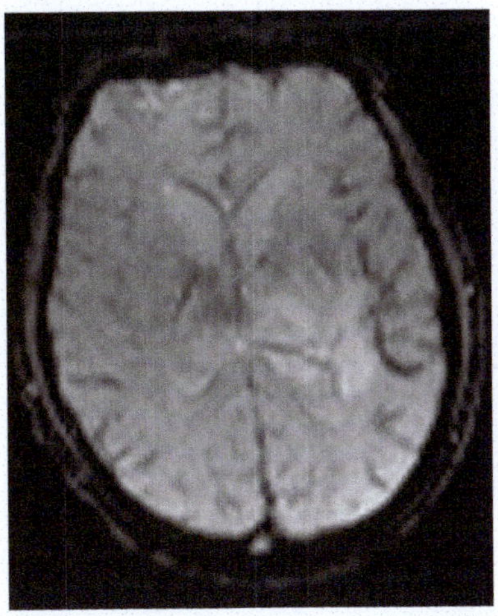

Fig. 1.47 DSC - dynamic susceptibility contrast: the arrival of the paramagnetic contrast bolus is demonstrated by the change in magnetic susceptibility within the (venous) vasculature – compared to the diamagnetic parenchyma causing a signal loss as characterized by the increase in local transverse relaxation rate

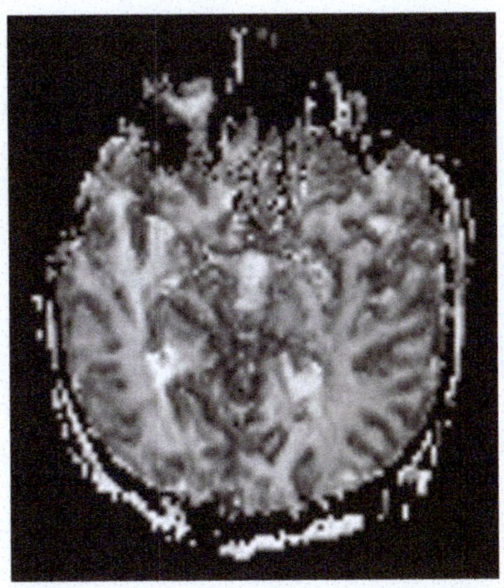

Fig. 1.48 PBP – percentage of baseline at peak: the ischemic region of this stroke patient is barely identified as compared to the following illustration of other indicative perfusion-related values

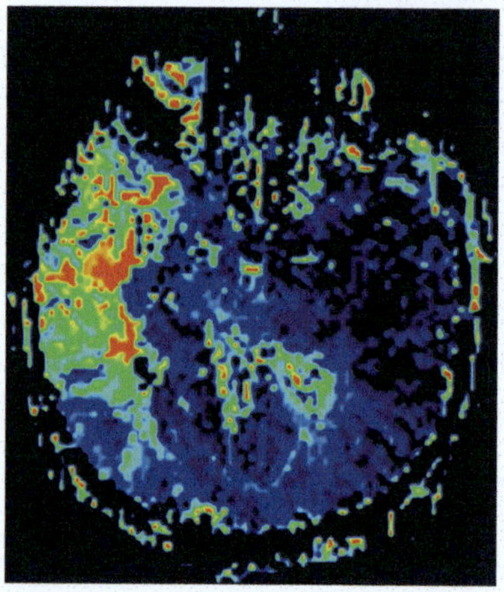

Fig. 1.49 TTP – time to peak: the delay in arrival time is assigned to specific color and a specific intensity and impressively illustrates the perfusion deficit in this stroke patient

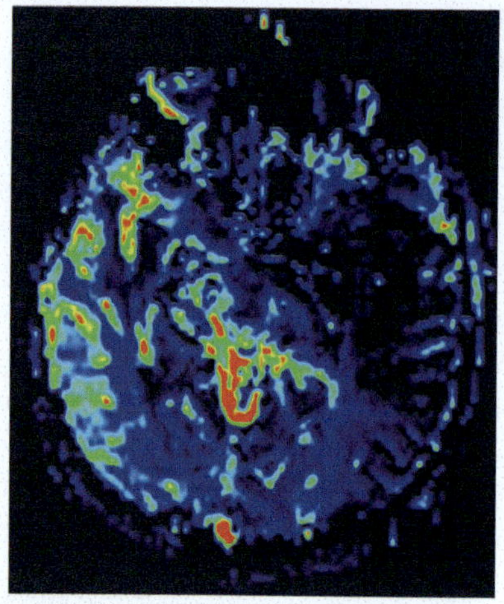

Fig. 1.50 rCBV – regional cerebral blood volume: the ischemic region is visualized by using color and intensity for the value of the ratio between the time-dependent concentration curve within the local region and the concentration curve within a feeding artery

bolus peak (Fig. 1.49). Areas with delayed arrival of the contrast bolus appear with brighter pixels in the TTP map.

rCBV: Regional Cerebral Blood Volume

rCBV is defined as the volume of blood in a brain voxel divided by the mass of the voxel

$$\mathrm{rCBV} = \frac{\text{Volume of blood in a voxel}}{\text{Mass of the voxel}}.$$

Calculation of rCBV from concentration-versus-time curves is based on the indicator dilution methods for nondiffusible tracers. rCBV maps are obtained from measuring the time dependence of the tracer concentration in the tissue $c_t(t)$ considering the time-dependent arterial concentration of the contrast agent $c_a(t)$, also called arterial input function (AIF). The latter function can be estimated by measuring signal changes inside a major blood vessel (Fig. 1.50).

$$\mathrm{rCBV} = \frac{\int_{-\infty}^{+\infty} C_t(t)\,\mathrm{d}t}{\int_{-\infty}^{+\infty} c_a(t)\,\mathrm{d}t}.$$

rCBF: Regional Cerebral Blood Flow

rCBF is defined as the net blood flow through the voxel divided by the mass of the voxel

$$\mathrm{rCBF} = \frac{\text{Net blood flow through the voxel}}{\text{Mass of the voxel}}.$$

Using a bolus tracking technique based on DSC, rCBF can be derived by tracking the tracer concentration in the tissue $C_t(t)$. The measured tissue concentration of contrast agent is the convolution of rCBF with the AIF $c_a(t)$ and a theoretical function representing the fraction of tracer still present in the tissue after time t after an ideal bolus injection $R(t)$ (Fig. 1.51).

$$C_t(t) = \int_0^t CBF \cdot c_a(\tau) \cdot \Re(t-\tau)\,\mathrm{d}\tau.$$

rMTT: Regional Mean Transit time

The rMTT describes the average amount of time it takes for the contrast agent to pass through the voxel vasculature (Fig. 1.52).

$$\mathrm{rMTT} = \frac{\mathrm{rCBV}}{\mathrm{rCBF}}.$$

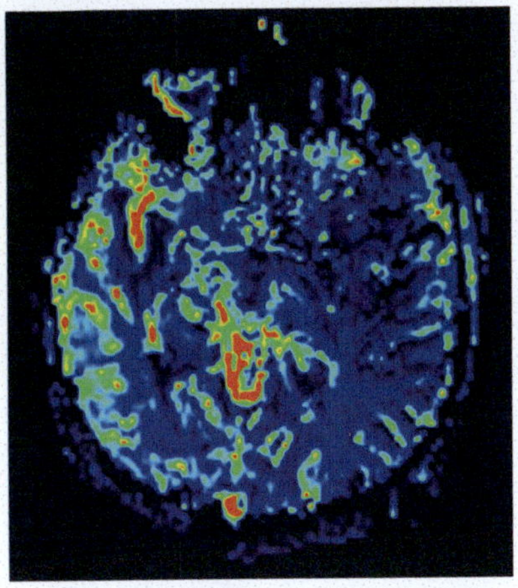

Fig. 1.51 rCBF – regional cerebral blood flow: the derived ratio between net blood flow through single voxel as compared to the mass of the voxel is assigned to a color with a specific intensity for visualization of ischemic regions

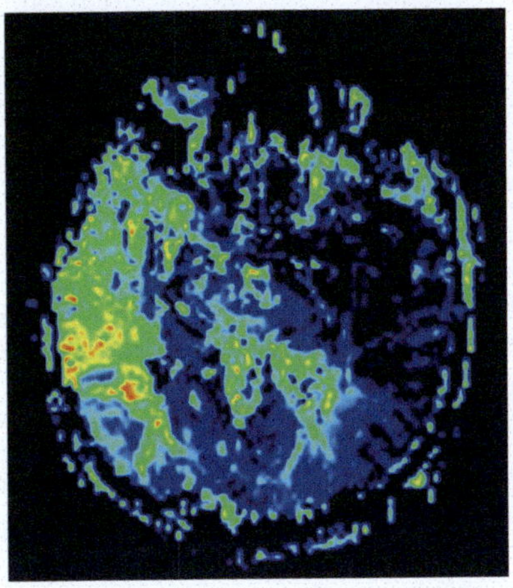

Fig. 1.52 rMTT – regional mean transit time: the average amount of time it takes for the contrast agent to pass through a single voxel is indicative for a specific color with a specific intensity illustrating the ischemic region for this stroke patient

Table 1.7 Pulse sequence classification scheme

	Spin-echo sequences	Hybrids	Gradient-echo sequences
Single echo techniques	CSE		GRE
			PSIF, trueFISP, CISS, DESS, FISP, FLASH, VIBE
Single echo techniques with magnetization preparation	IR IRM STIR SPIR, SPAIR		TFL MP-RAGE
Mulitecho techniques	TSE		MEDIC segmented FID-EPI
		TGSE segmented SE-EPI	
Multiecho techniques with magnetization preparation	STIR[a], TIR, TIRM SPIR, SPAIR[a] SPACE RESTORE		
Single-shot techniques	HASTE	SE-EPI	FID-EPI
Single-shot techniques with magnetization preparation	HASTIRM	DW-SE-EPI	

[a]Redundant listing indicates, that the preparation can be used for single echo techniques as well as for multi echo methods

1.3 The Advanced

The intention of the following section is to provide additional information for the advanced user.

1.3.1 *Sequence Acronyms, Characterization, Mechanism and Applications*

Imaging sequences can be assigned to a SE group and a GRE group (and the hybrids). Each of the group can be further divided into single-echo techniques (one Fourier line per excitation), multi-echo techniques (multiple Fourier lines per excitation) and single-shot techniques (one excitation and complete or partial filling of *k*-space with multiple phase-encoded echoes). Techniques within each of the six groups can be combined with a preparation of the nuclear magnetization prior to imaging.

Table 1.7 documents this classification scheme applied to the sequence acronyms used by the vendor "Siemens" and Table 1.8 shows the comparison chart with the sequence acronyms used by other vendors for the same or comparable methods.

1.3.1.1 The Spin Echo Family

CSE: The Conventional Spin Echo

The basic concept of SE imaging has been introduced in Sect. 1.1.3.5. A slice-select gradient is switched on prior to a slice-selective RF pulse. This is followed by

Table 1.8 Acronym comparison chart

Generic description	Siemens	GE	Philips
Spoiled gradient echo (spoiled GRE)	FLASH	SPGR	FFE-T1
Partial refocused GRE	FISP	GRASS	FFE
SE-acquisition of the SSFP signal	PSIF	SSFP	FFE-T2
Fully refocused GRE (bSSFP)	CISS, DESS trueFISP	3D-PC-FIESTA FIESTA	bFFE
Multiecho GRE	MEDIC	MERGE	mFFE
3D GRE with volume interpolation	VIBE	LAVA-XV	THRIVE
GRE with magnetization preparation	TFL MP-RAGE	FSPGR 3D-FSPGR	TFE 3D TFE
Fast spin echo	TSE	FSE	TSE
3D fast spin echo with variable refocusing angle	SPACE	CUBE	VISTA
Fast spin echo with flip back pulse	RESTORE	FRFSE	DRIVE
Gradient and spin echo	TGSE	GRASE	GRASE
SE-single-shot techniques	HASTE	SSFSE	SSTSE
SE-single-shot techniques with magnetization preparation	HASTIRM	SS-IR-FSE	SSTIR

the phase-encoding gradient, during which the dephasing in the direction of read-out is also prepared. The 180° slice-selective refocusing pulse inverts the accumulated dephasing, causing the appearance of a SE, usually in the middle of the acquisition window with the frequency-encoding gradient being activated. This step is repeated with different phase-encoding steps and as often as averages are requested by the user (Fig. 1.10).

IR, IRM: The Conventional Spin Echo Sequence Combined with a Preceding Inversion of the Magnetization

The IR techniques have already been discussed in Sect. 1.2.3. IR techniques use a 180°-inversion pulse prior to the SE imaging sequence to manipulate the contrast. The preparation is repeated prior to each Fourier line measurement. IR techniques that consider the position of the macroscopic magnetization (parallel or antiparallel to the direction of the main field) during image reconstruction are called true or phase sensitive IR techniques and are usually utilized to improve the T1-W contrast between gray and white matter. IR techniques that only take the absolute value of the prepared magnetization into account are called IR techniques with utilization of the magnitude of the signal (IRM). Sequences with a short inversion time for fat-suppressed imaging are called STIR techniques and the selection of a long T_I to suppress the signal from fluid does not present a new sequence but rather a "dark fluid protocol" (although it is sometimes referred to FLAIR (fluid attenuated inversion recovery).

TSE, FSE: Multi Echo Imaging with Spin Echoes

The multiecho spin echo concept has been introduced earlier ("Essentials," Sect. 1.2.4) as it is the common sequence utilized for PD and T2-W imaging. Multiple phase-encoded echoes are utilized to fill multiple *k*-space lines per excitation, causing a potential reduction in measurement time. The time savings is usually utilized to improve the contrast by selecting longer TR or to improve the spatial resolution by selecting a higher matrix size, or to utilize long inversion times T_I in order to suppress the signal from fluid within a reasonable measurement time.

There are several observations that have not been mentioned so far:

- The signal to noise ration in TSE imaging is better than predicted.
- The contrast between gray and white matter is better than expected.
- Fat appears bright compared to CSE imaging.
- The sequence is less sensitive to hemorrhagic lesions as compared to CSE imaging.

In a simplified perspective, a RF refocusing pulse will also excite (especially if a poor slice profile with an according flip angle distribution is considered). The next RF pulse will again refocus what has been generated with the first RF excitation pulse, but will also refocus what has been excited with the preceding RF refocusing pulse, and will excite too. This is the simplified perspective of stimulated echoes. Stimulated echoes contribute up to 30% to the SNR in fast spin echo imaging.

Another positive aspect of TSE imaging is the phenomenon of magnetization transfer (still to be discussed (Sect. 1.3.4.2)). Water molecules in the vicinity of macromolecules are called "bounded" and have a very short T2. A short T2 refers to a large difference in resonance frequencies, causing a rapid dephasing. They are not directly observable and have a very broad resonance frequency. Applying an RF excitation off resonance, those invisible molecules can be saturated. Since they communicate with their "free" partners via magnetization transfer, this off-resonance pulse has an effect on the image contrast. Multiple 180° refocusing pulses are used in fast spin echo imaging with a frequency range for one specific slice. Those frequencies act as off-resonance pulses for all adjacent slices and are, therefore, magnetization transfer saturation - MTS pulses. This is the explanation for the better contrast between gray and white matter in images acquired with a TSE method as compared to those acquired with conventional SE techniques.

The spins in hydrogen atoms bound to fat are coupled. Multiple hydrogen atoms belong to the same molecule, and the corresponding nuclear spins interact with each other via their electromagnetic fields. Such a coupling is referred to as J-coupling. This coupling leads to a slow dephasing mechanism in CSE imaging despite 180° refocusing pulses. This J-coupling is broken with a rapid application of a series of 180° refocusing pulses, as used in TSE imaging. The consequence is a hyperintense appearance of fat as compared with the images acquired with convention spin echo imaging, as the dephasing is finally refocused. If the bright fat is annoying, there is always the possibility of fat saturation.

Diamagnetic and paramagnetic properties in hemorrhagic lesions cause local field inhomogeneities with a rapid dephasing of the signal as a consequence. A RF refocusing pulse is supposed to refocus all dephasing mechanisms that are constant in time and fixed in location. Unfortunately, water molecules may move between the excitation and the refocusing RF pulse, a phenomenon called diffusion. This movement is causing an insufficient rephasing with a hypointense signal appearance of hemorrhagic lesions in CSE imaging. As diffusion time, the time between excitation and refocusing and between refocusing pulses in fast spin echo imaging is significantly reduced, the dephasing effects due to local susceptibility gradients are reduced. Thus, hemorrhagic lesions are less visible on fast spin echo images as compared to those acquired with CSE imaging. The solution is to apply a sequence and a protocol that is sensitive to T2* changes (conventional GRE with long TEs or a susceptibility weighted approach).

TIR, TIRM, RESTORE, SPACE: Magnetization Prepared Multiecho Imaging with Spin Echoes

TIR, TIRM, IR-FSE

The preparation of the longitudinal nuclear magnetization with a RF inversion pulse as discussed in Sect. 1.2.3 can be combined with the multiecho spin echo approach. If the phase of the generated transverse nuclear magnetization is considered, the IR technique is considered phase sensitive, and is sometimes also called true or real. The combination with the fast spin echo imaging sequence to follow is indicated by the T from TSE or by adding FSE to the IR acronym. The M in TIRM stands for "magnitude reconstruction". In this case the phase of the signal is ignored. No indication is given with respect to a potential parallel or antiparallel alignment of the longitudinal magnetization at the time the excitation pulse has been applied. The inversion is repeated prior to each echo train acquisition. Multiple phase-encoded echoes are utilized to fill multiple *k*-space lines per excitation, causing a potential reduction in measurement time and providing time for other sophisticated contrast manipulations. An impressive example is the fluid attenuated inversion recovery approach - FLAIR, where the reduction in measurement time based on the multiecho approach enables the acquisition within a reasonable measurement time despite inversion times of around 2 s.

RESTORE

At the end of the ETL, there is still residual transverse magnetization left for tissue with long T2 relaxation times (CSF and fluid-filled cavities). Applying a −90° RF pulse for the last echo will "restore" longitudinal magnetization for tissues with long T2 relaxation time, thus improving contrast-to-noise ratio (CNR) as compared to the "conventional" multiecho spin echo technique (Fig. 1.53).

SPACE

It has been discussed in Sect. 1.2.1.3 that the amplitude of the refocusing pulse significantly contributes to the SAR and that one measure to avoid the limitation would be the utilization of a small flip angle refocusing pulse (e.g., 120 vs. 180°). In conjunction with fast spin echo imaging, the application of multiple refocusing pulses with low refocusing angles will lead to a quite complex superimposition of multiple pathways. The effect is even amplified when combining the fast spin echo concept with a 3D acquisition. As the Fourier lines in and around the center of *k*-space are dominant for the SNR and CNR, it has been documented that focusing on the signal gain of those *k*-space lines using variable flip angle refocusing pulses throughout the acquisition may achieve a higher SNR as compared to a fully refocused fast spin echo method. Since the superimposition of multiple echo paths can be regarded as an echo of echoes, the term "hyperecho" has been introduced. Acronyms like TRAPS (transitions between pseudo steady state) and SPACE (sampling perfection with application optimized contrast by using different flip angle evolutions, Fig. 1.54) represent further extensions and refinements of these variable refocusing angle fast spin echo imaging methods. SPACE can be combined with a preceding inversion of the longitudinal magnetization and a long inversion time to achieve a dark appearance of fluid.

SS-FSE, SS-TSE, HASTE: Single Shot Imaging with Spin Echoes

Using only a single excitation followed by multiple phase-encoded spin echoes in order to fill *k*-space is called a single shot spin echo technique (SS-FSE, SS-TSE). To acquire the *k*-space for a matrix with 128 columns in the direction of phase encoding would

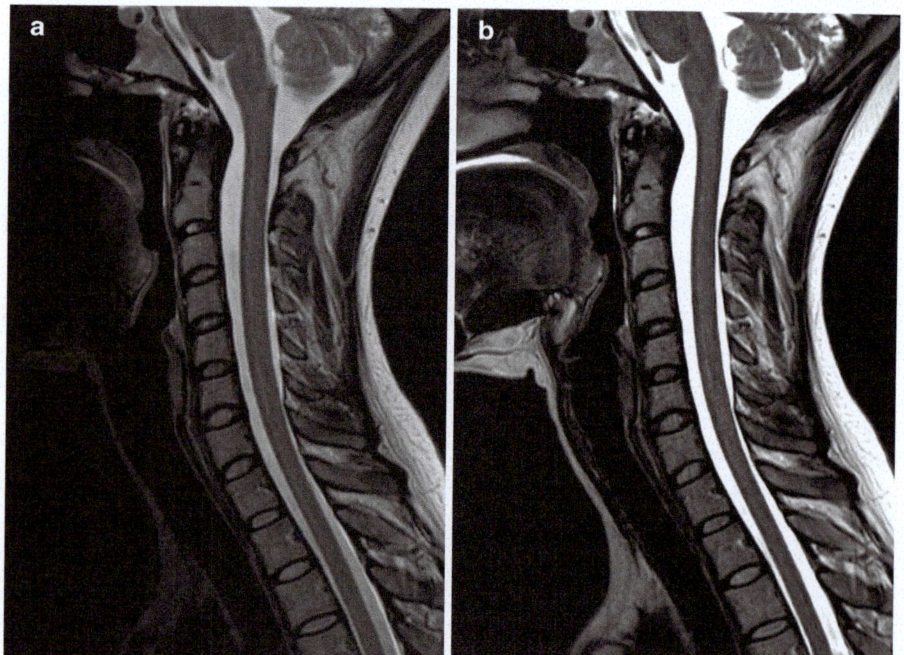

Fig. 1.53 The application of a flip back (−90°) pulse at the end of an echo train will force the remaining transerse magnetization back into the longitudinal direction, causing an improved signal for tissues with a long T2 relaxation time. (**a**) T2-W TSE image of a sagittal spine. (**b**) RESTORE image of a sagittal spine acquired with similar parameters, plus a flip back pulse

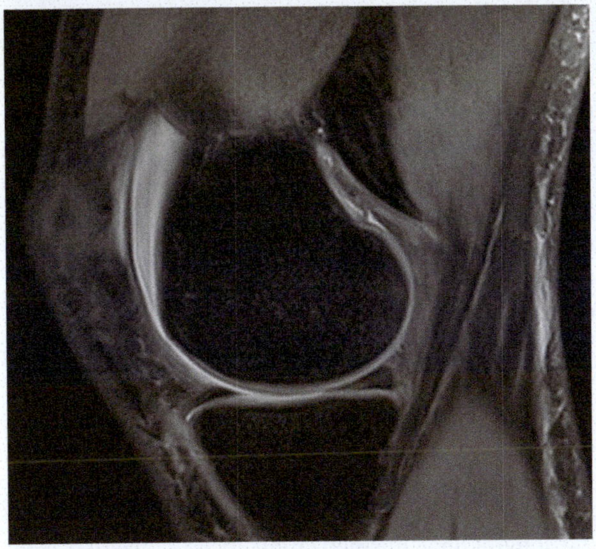

Fig. 1.54 SPACE is a 3D fast spin-echo acquisition scheme, where the refocusing angle of the RF refocusing pulse is less than 180° and is altered throughout the 3D acquisition (variable flip angle) to achieve an optimal contrast and a high spatial resolution while still exhibiting a low SAR value. The illustrated knee is using SPACE in conjunction with fat saturation using PD weighting and demonstrating a meniscal tear

require 128 phase-encoded spin echoes. The correlated long echo train implies that the contrast is solely T2-W. As indicated in Sect. 1.2.6.3, the *k*-space is symmetric. Utilizing partial Fourier and acquiring only half the *k*-space (plus a few Fourier lines beyond the center of *k*-space) is called Half Fourier. Combining single shot fast spin echo imaging with the Half-Fourier concept leads to Half Fourier Acquired Single Shot Turbo Spin Echo —HASTE. Prenatal imaging is a typical application for single shot fast spin echo imaging like HASTE. The different weighting of Fourier lines will cause a slight image blurring. The consequences of violation of *k*-space symmetry in half-Fourier imaging will have a similar appearance. Single shot techniques are sequential techniques. Previously mentioned sequences were multislice capable, that is within the selected TR, Fourier lines of multiple slices are acquired prior to returning to the first slice for starting the acquisition of the next Fourier line. As single shot techniques have no repetition, the acquisition is done slice by slice. In this case, the measurement time is a function of the number of selected slices. The correlated long echo trains indicate solely T2-weighting and a perfect method to visualize fluid-filled cavities as done in MR cholangiopancreatography (MRCP) (Fig. 1.55).

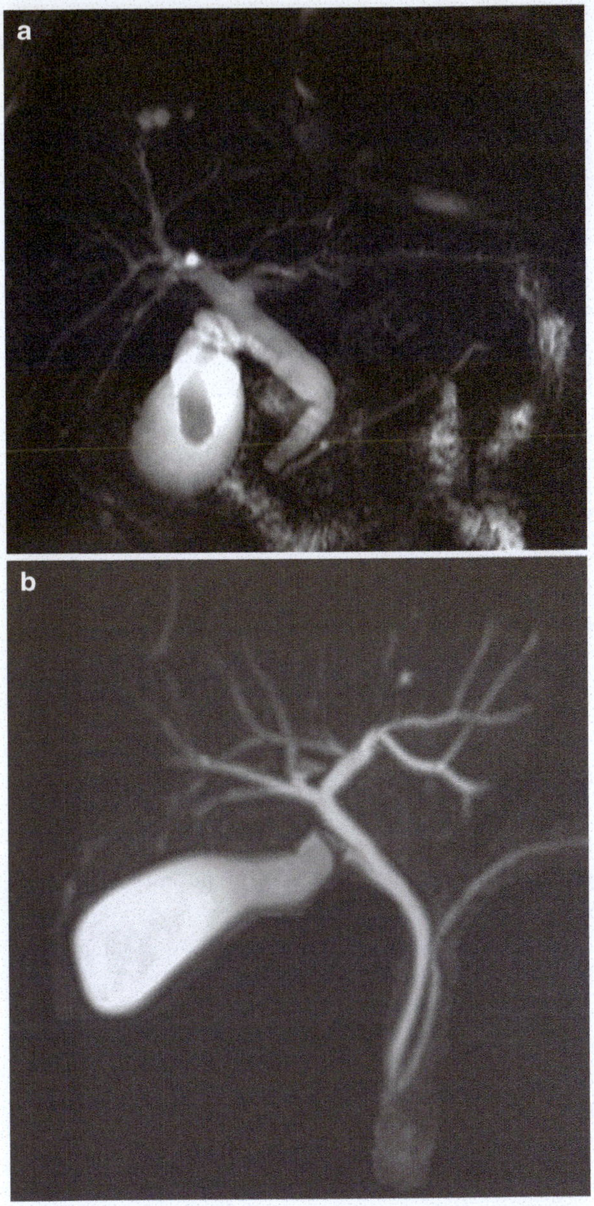

Fig. 1.55 (**a**) HASTE – half-Fourier acquired single-shot turbo spin echo allows the acquisition of an image within less than 600 ms. The contrast is always T2-W and a typical application is to be found in prenatal diagnostics – or MRCP; (**b**) The illustrated MRCP acquisition has been performed using SPACE with a RESTORE pulse and a GRAPPA algorithm for reducing measurement time

HASTIRM: Magnetization Prepared Single Shot Imaging with Spin Echoes

Any preceding manipulation of the longitudinal nuclear magnetization, e.g., like the IR preparation schemes as described in Sect. 1.2.3, can be combined with the

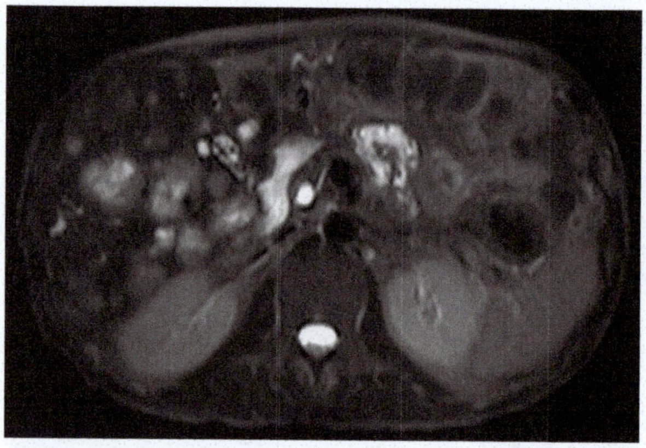

Fig. 1.56 HASTIRM: HASTE combined with a preceding inversion pulse and the utilization of a short inversion time permits a relaxation-time-dependent fat suppression

single shot spin echo acquisition like HASTE, sometimes leading to new imaging acronyms like HASTIRM (Fig. 1.56).

1.3.1.2 The Gradient Echo Family

GRE: The Conventional Gradient Echo

In conventional imaging, the measurement time is given by the TR multiplied by the number of desired Fourier lines times the number of acquisitions. Eliminating the RF refocusing pulse, as indicated in Fig. 1.8, will cause the imaging sequence to be T2* sensitive. This is desired for certain applications, but, as T2* is also a function of patient-related field inhomogeneities, represents a major obstacle in areas of large susceptibility gradients (e.g., base of the scull). Solely bipolar magnetic field gradients are used to generate the echo, suggesting the name GREs for these kind of methods. Due to the saved time slot, skipping the RF refocusing pulse will allow for shorter TE, which in turn provides a higher signal. The shorter TE is also potentially allowing a shorter TR, which is desired for dynamic or 3D imaging. With respect to the latter, the image reconstruction software does not care about the direction in which the phase-encoding step has been applied. The only prerequisite is, in order to distinguish two orthogonal phase-encoding directions, that for each phase-encoding step in one direction, all the encoding steps in the other direction have to be repeated, as already illustrated in Fig. 1.42. The advantage of 3D data acquisition is the gapless coverage of a volume of interest. As there is no gap between adjacent pixels within an image, there is also no gap from one slice to the next for a 3D sequence, in this case referred to as partition instead of slice. The other advantage is that each measured line contains information of the whole object and, therefore, contributes to a better SNR. The only prerequisite for 3D data acquisition is the possibility of a reasonably short TR (and/or the combination with a multiecho acquisition scheme) in order to acquire all the necessary phase-encoding steps in a reasonable measurement time.

FLASH: Fast Low Angle Shot or Spoiled GRE

A low angle excitation will cause only part of the existing longitudinal magnetization to be converted to a transverse magnetization. The latter is responsible for the strength, for the amplitude of the induced MR signal. The first excitation pulse will utilize the full magnetization. Since it is a low flip angle, the projection of the tilted magnetization onto the z-axis will remain as longitudinal magnetization and will grow pending the recovery or relaxation rate until the next excitation reduces the longitudinal magnetization even further, as illustrated in Fig. 1.57. The more the longitudinal magnetization is reduced, the higher the relaxation rate. After a few excitations, the relaxation rate will be high enough to compensate for the reduction of the longitudinal magnetization caused by the excitation pulse. The amount of longitudinal magnetization prior to excitation and the amount of generated transverse magnetization can, at that point, be considered constant for the duration of the remaining measurement time. They have reached a steady-state. If the remaining transverse magnetization after the measurement of the gradient echo is not purposefully made zero, the following RF low angle excitation will also operate as refocusing RF pulse (generating a spin echo), and part of the data acquisition to follow can be considered as containing spin-echo components. In which case, those techniques are considered, although not consequently throughout the literature, as hybrids, and will be discussed later (Sect. 1.3.1.3). The FLASH concept evolved while studying these steady-state techniques. The steady state for the FLASH concept refers to the longitudinal magnetization only. The remaining transverse magnetization at the end of the Fourier line acquisition is purposefully made zero by using

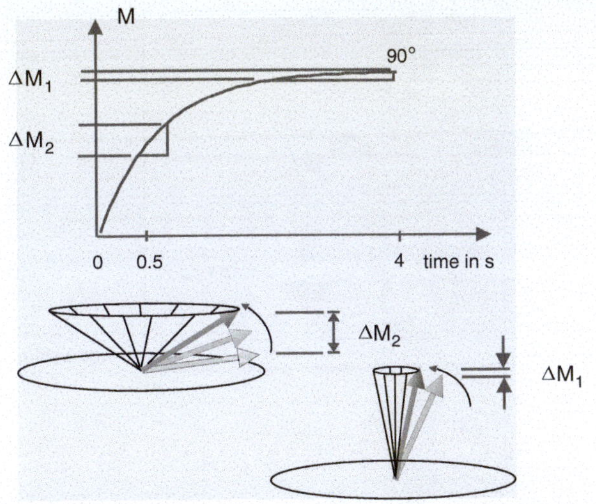

Fig. 1.57 The steady-state concept. The relaxation rate, the amount of recovery per unit time, depends on whether the longitudinal magnetization is far away from the fully relaxed state (ΔM_2) or close to equilibrium (ΔM_1). Between rapid excitations with low flip angle, the magnetization will recover with the relaxation rate at that position of the relaxation curve. If the amount of longitudinal magnetization that is reduced due to a low flip angle excitation is larger than the recovered magnetization between two excitations, the remaining longitudinal magnetization will be reduced, getting further away from equilibrium. The latter will increase the relaxation rate. This process will continue until the relaxation rate is high enough that the amount of recovered magnetization is identical to the amount of longitudinal magnetization reduced by the low-angle excitation. For each Fourier line, the same magnitude of transverse magnetization is now projected onto the *x-y* plane. That situation is called steady state

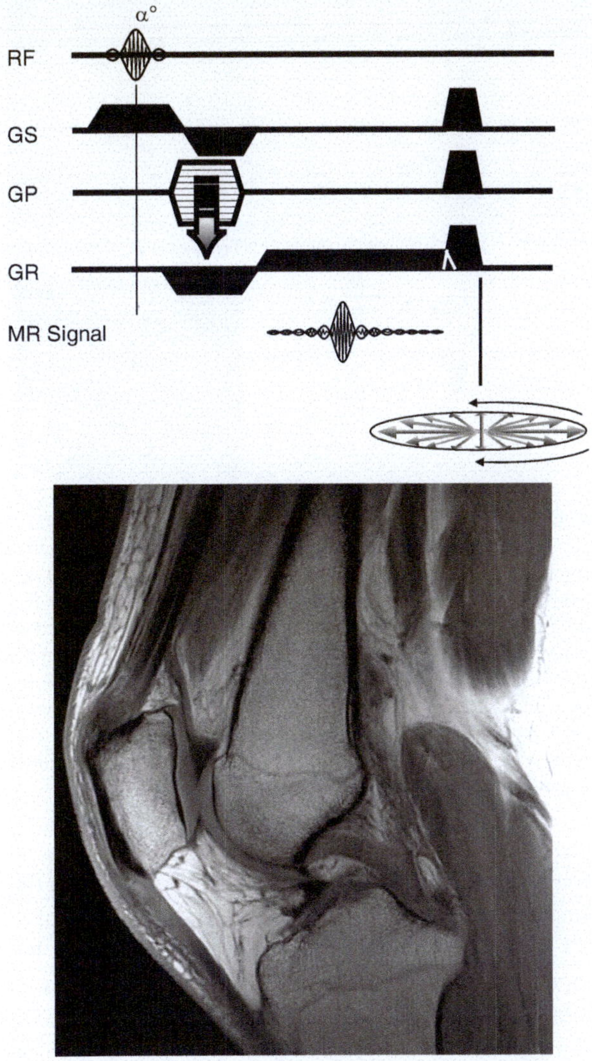

Fig. 1.58 Fast low angle shot — FLASH. After the measurement of a single Fourier line, the remaining transverse nuclear magnetization is purposefully made zero by applying spoiler gradients. In which case, only the steady state of the longitudinal nuclear magnetization has to be considered being responsible for the signal composition. *GP* phase-encoding gradient; *GR* read-out gradient; *GS* slice-selection gradient; *RF* radiofrequency

"spoilergradients" at the end of the Fourier line measurement as illustrated in Fig.1.58.

The steady state of the transverse nuclear magnetization can also purposefully made to zero by randomly changing the phase (the direction of flipping) of the low angle RF exaction pulse, also referred to as "RF spoiling."

Utilizing an even lower flip angle, the differences in T1-based recovery can be minimized, achieving a T2*-W impression even with a short TR (Fig. 1.59). Using a relatively small excitation angle, the macroscopic magnetization remains close to equilibrium, and the T1 relaxation rate is very small, almost independent of the T1 value. The T1 influence is then suppressed, and the T2* difference will dominate within the image contrast, as desired in T2(*)-WI.

TFL, MP-RAGE: Magnetization Prepared Gradient Echo Imaging

The fastest way to acquire an image with a conventional GRE sequence would be to select a high bandwidth, requesting only a small data acquisition window, selecting a minimum TE, and selecting the shortest possible TR. In order to achieve any signal at all, the Ernst angle needs to be selected. The inversion of the

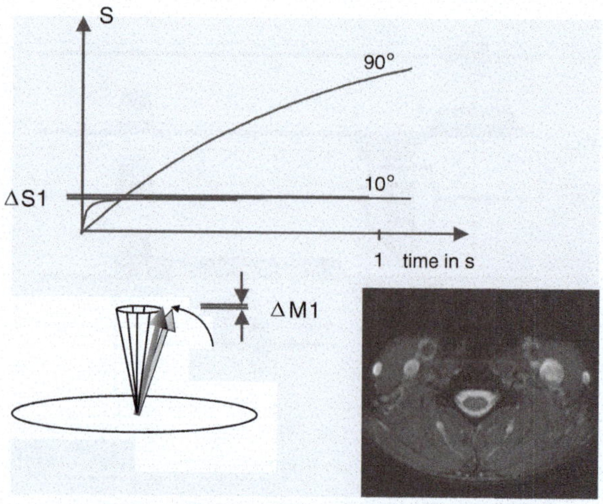

Fig. 1.59 T2*-W imaging with FLASH. Working with very low flip angle excitation, e.g., 10°, the longitudinal magnetization remains close to equilibrium even with TRs as short as 120 ms. Staying close to equilibrium means a small relaxation rate. The T1 influence is suppressed. The same situation is achieved in T2-W SE imaging. A long repetition time (TR) is selected in SE imaging to avoid the T1 influence in T2-W scans. As a consequence, low-angle GRE imaging allows T2*-W measurements with very short TRs. ΔM the recovered longitudinal magnetization; ΔS the signal induced by the projection of the longitudinal magnetization onto the x-y plane

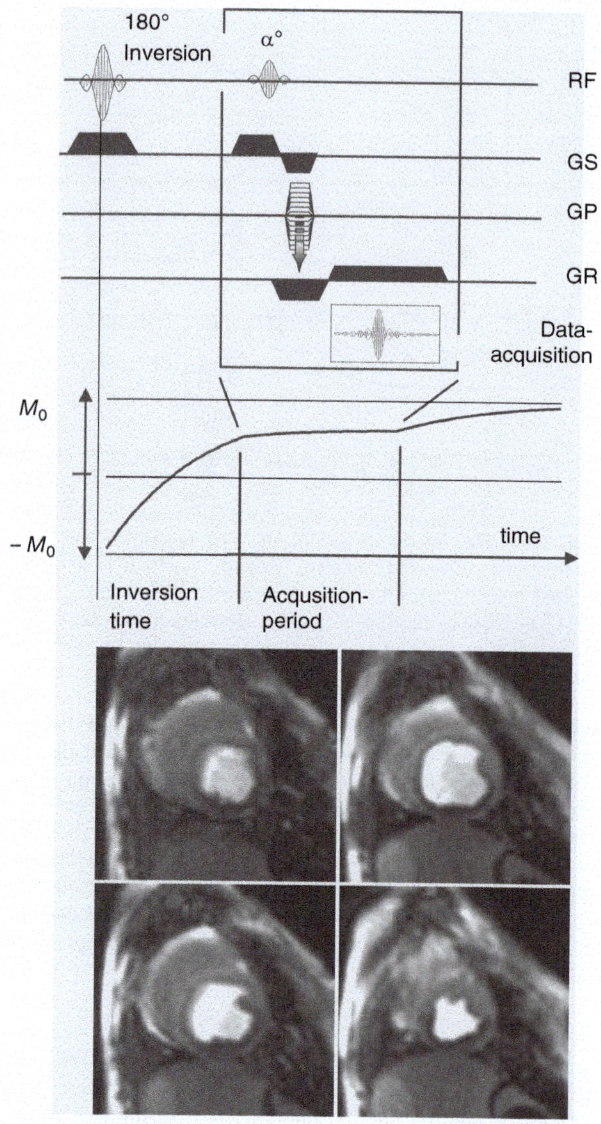

Fig. 1.60 The turbo fast low-angle shot sequence, turboFLASH — TFL: the classical TFL sequence has an inversion pulse at the beginning of the whole measurement to establish a T1-W contrast. After the inversion period, a rapid gradient-echo sequence acquires the data along a relaxation curve. The contrast is dominated by the position on the relaxation curve at the time the low spatial frequencies are measured. The clinical example illustrates one to the rare applications (although combining the inversion with a trueFISP approach, TFI). The inversion time is selected to null the signal from the native myocardium, to demonstrate perfusion deficits during the first pass of a T1-shortening contrast bolus. *GP* phase-encoding gradient; *GR* read-out gradient; *GS* slice-selection gradient; *RF* radiofrequency

longitudinal nuclear magnetization prior to starting the imaging sequence will allow the introduction of a T1-W contrast or will enable the elimination of the signal of a tissue with a specific T1 relaxation time, similar to the discussed STIR approach. The inversion does not take place prior to each Fourier line as in IR imaging, but as a preparation preceding the rapid acquisition of all Fourier lines, as illustrated in Fig. 1.60. Such an acquisition method has been named turboFLASH — TFL. Each Fourier line, each spatial frequency is measured at a different point in time along the relaxation curve following the inversion. The dominant contrast will be given by the time the low spatial frequencies are acquired (center of *k*-space). The TFL sequence is the only imaging technique, where the contrast might vary with a change in matrix size.

Since the higher spatial frequencies usually contribute significantly different signal amplitudes, turboFLASH images may appear slightly blurred. The technique is used today almost solely for the first pass perfusion measurement in cardiac imaging.

The time to acquire a 3D data set is too long in order for any preparation of the longitudinal nuclear magnetization to remain effective for the duration of a 3D measurement. The preparation scheme for a 3D approach is, therefore, slightly altered compared with the 2D method and is illustrated in Fig. 1.61. The preparation pulse is placed prior to each depth-encoding loop and repeated after a recovery time for the next depth-encoding loop with a different in-plane phase-encoding step. This technique has been named magnetization prepared rapid gradient-echo—MP-RAGE. This technique provides the possibility of achieving a better T1-W than with SE, covering the whole head in less than 5 min with no gap between partitions.

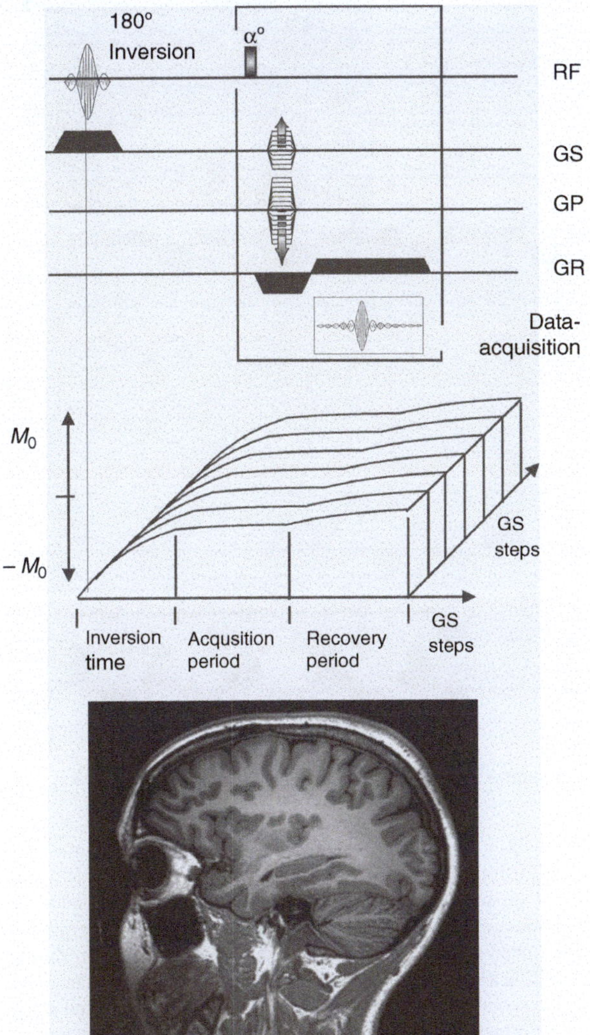

Fig. 1.61 MP-RAGE – The magnetization-prepared rapid-acquired gradient-echo sequence design. An inversion pulse is placed prior to each GP loop. The GS loops are then executed, collecting data along a relaxation curve. After a recovery time, the next GP value is selected, the inversion pulse applied, and the GS loops repeated. The classical MP-RAGE sequence uses a nonselective low flip angle excitation, allowing a further reduction in echo time and repetition time. *GP* phase-encoding gradient; *GR* read-out gradient; *GS* slice-selection gradient; *RF* radiofrequency

The advantage of MP-RAGE is that the signal contribution for each phase-encoding step in the plane is constant, presenting an artifact-free image similar to a conventional GRE technique. The signal variation due to the data collection along a relaxation curve is effective along the direction of depth encoding and only visible if a multiplanar reconstruction is performed in that direction. The other advantage of this technique is the control over the T1-weighting via the inversion time, providing a better contrast than possible in SE imaging. Despite the impressive performance of MP-RAGE, it has to be kept in mind that the underlying principle is a gradient-echo acquisition scheme with the correlated T2* sensitivity (Signal void at the base of the skull due to susceptibility gradients and a possible complex image contrast in conjunction with the uptake of paramagnetic contrast agents).

MEDIC, MERGE, Segmented EPI: Multi Echo Imaging with Gradient Echoes

There are basically two concepts in multiecho imaging. One concept as previously discussed utilizes additional phase-encoded echoes in order to reduce measurement time, the other concepts is utilizing additional echoes without applying a different phase encoding, but just to use the additional acquisition to improve SNR plus enhancement of T2-weighting (Fig. 1.62). Multiple echoes are used for improving image quality by averaging without increasing the measurement time, although to the expense of a larger slice-loop time (less slices for the same TR).

The later-to-be-mentioned single-shot gradient-echo approach has the disadvantage of loosing all preparations during a long echo train or having image quality problems due the dramatic T2* sensitivity of a long ETL. With the approach of "segmentation" the measurement time is again prolonged, but the shorter ETLs leading to a reduced T2* sensitivity, thus causing less artifacts and an improved image quality.

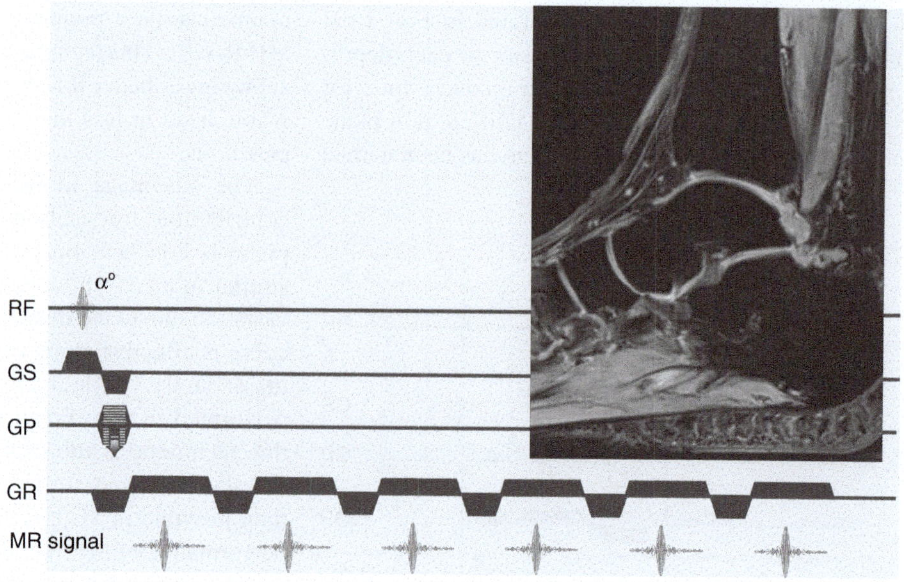

Fig. 1.62 MEDIC – multi-echo data image-combination. Multiple echoes are averaged in order to improve SNR and T2-weighting. *GP* phase-encoding gradient; *GR* read-out gradient; *GS* slice-selection gradient; *RF* radiofrequency

FID-EPI: Single Shot Gradient Echo Imaging

Echo Planar Imaging - EPI has been introduced 1977 and is considered the oldest proposed fast imaging technique, sometimes also referred to as ultra-fast imaging method. The classical form uses one excitation pulse and multiple phase-encoded echoes to generate an image, as illustrated in Fig. 1.63.

The signal loss immediately following an RF excitation due to the dephasing of the transverse nuclear magnetization is also called a free induction decay. A gradient echo formation is therefore referred to as measurement of the free induction decay. The data sampling with multiple phase-encoding echoes following a single excitation with no other preparation is usually called FID-EPI in order to differentiate from other EPI acquisition schemes. With EPI, it is possible to generate an image within 80–120 ms. The classical technique has intrinsic artifacts due to the length of the so-called echo train (ETL) of GREs as there are severe geometrical distortions for the regions of large susceptibility gradients such as the facial region or the base of the skull. The other disadvantage is the limited spatial resolution that competes with today's high-resolution TSE imaging. The applied low phase-encoding gradients correspond to a very low bandwidth. Good fat signal suppression is a prerequisite for EPI applications, otherwise the fat image will appear as an annoying ghost. Nevertheless, there are a few clinical applications in which EPI will be the only imaging technique of choice. These applications include the utilization of EPI read-out modules for a prepared magnetization that would otherwise be destroyed by a prolonged read-out period. Such preparations include the diffusion weighting in stroke imaging as indicated in Fig. 1.45. Other

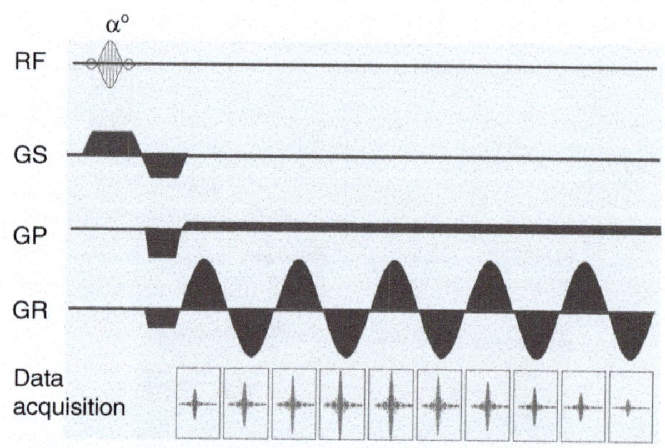

Fig. 1.63 FID-EPI – free induction decay echo-planar-imaging. This illustration is only one possible gradient arrangement that would be named echo planar imaging. Following a selective excitation, multiple gradient echoes are generated. In the version reproduced here, a small phase-encoding gradient is on during the whole measurement, providing a progressive phase encoding for the sequence of gradient echoes. The data are collected along a T2* relaxation curve. The effective echo time is the time at which the low spatial frequencies are acquired. *GP* phase-encoding gradient; *GR* read-out gradient; *GS* slice-selection gradient; *RF* radiofrequency

applications are rapid acquisition of large volumes as needed in functional MRI (fMRI) or imaging of the coronary vasculature.

1.3.1.3 The Hybrids

Gradient echo imaging techniques, where the signal may be a composition of multiple echo paths, are considered hybrids, as residual transverse nuclear magnetization, after completion of a Fourier line measurement, is refocused with the next RF excitation pulse and can be considered a spin echo.

FISP, trueFISP, CISS, DESS and PSIF

The FLASH technique is solely working with the steady state of the longitudinal nuclear magnetization by destroying the transverse nuclear magnetization at the end of the measurement of a single Fourier line by applying "spoiler" gradients or by avoiding a steady state of the transverse nuclear magnetization by using "RF spoiling". Changing this technique by rephasing the transverse nuclear magnetization at the end of the measurement of a single Fourier line will change the image contrast. Rephasing the part of the transverse nuclear magnetization that has been dephased for the purpose of spatial encoding will lead to a new sequence, which is called fast imaging with steady-state precession — FISP as illustrated in Fig. 1.64.

The original idea was to rephase all three dimensions, the phase-encoding direction, the slice-selection direction, and the frequency-encoding direction. However, this implementation is causing severe artifacts if the multiple echo paths are not in phase with each other; especially field inhomogeneities shifting the phase of these echo paths, causing black bands as a consequence of destructive interference. With improvements in hardware and software to follow, the implementation of the original idea was feasible, creating a new imaging sequence with the acronym trueFISP (Fig. 1.65).

In order to get a trueFISP contrast, a large flip angle and a short TR have to be selected, otherwise there will be no significant remaining transverse nuclear magnetization to make a difference in image contrast as compared to the FLASH contrast. The constructive interference steady-state (CISS) sequence has been and still is an

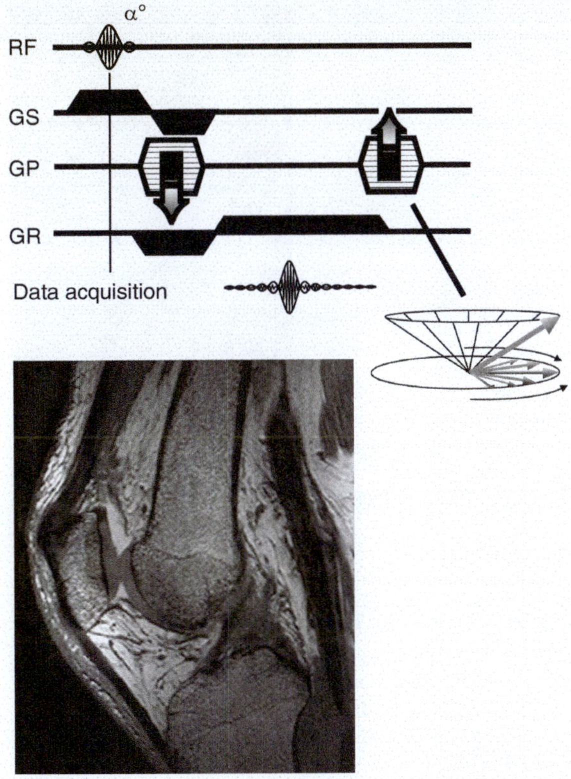

Fig. 1.64 FISP – Fast imaging with steady-state precession. The dephasing with the phase-encoding gradient, done for the purpose of spatial encoding, is rephased after data acquisition. A steady state will build up for the transverse component. Compared with FLASH, an improved signal contribution is achieved for tissue with a long T2, using a protocol with a short repetition time and a large flip angle. *GP* phase-encoding gradient; *GR* read-out gradient; *GS* slice-selection gradient; *RF* radiofrequency

attempt to eliminate the destructive interference artifacts in a nonperfect 3D trueFISP approach. Two 3D measurements are sampled and averaged, one measurement with alternation of the phase of the RF excitation pulse and one measurement without alternation. This will produce two sets of images (not shown to the user) with shifted patterns of the previously mentioned destructive interference bands. In merging these images, these patterns of destructive interference vanish. Thus, the acronym CISS.

Utilization of the SE part in steady-state approaches is possible using a PSIF technique (Fig. 1.66). This sequence is currently clinically not relevant. It is an interesting sequence as an alternative to be used with diffusion weighting. But in this context, it solely serves the purpose to explain the following sequence, double-echo

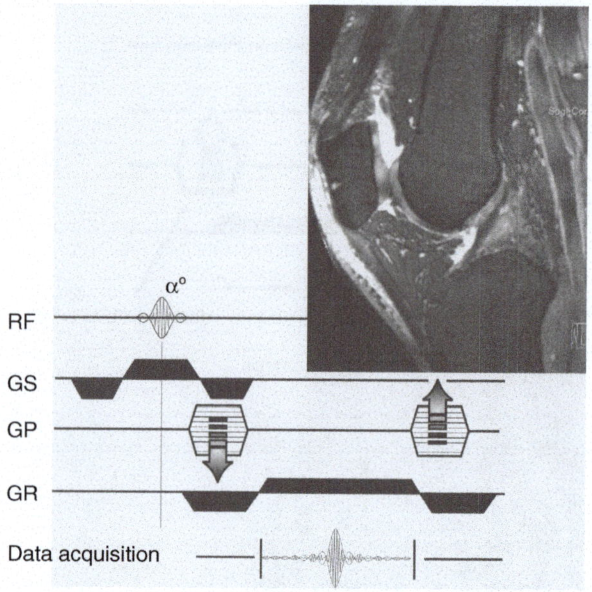

Fig. 1.65 trueFISP – the true fast imaging with steady-state precession is the originally published FISP. Rephasing all components within the direction of slice selection, the direction of phase encoding, and the direction of read out, the contribution of the steady state of the transverse magnetization is maximized. This sagittal image has been acquired within 4 s, using trueFISP. *GP* phase-encoding gradient; *GR* read-out gradient; *GS* slice-selection gradient; *RF* radiofrequency

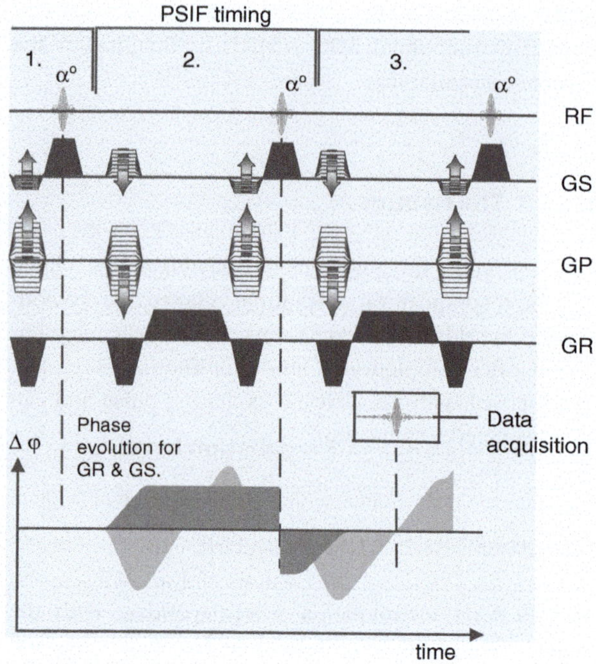

Fig. 1.66 PSIF – the backwards running fast imaging with steady-state precession sequence. The timing for the PSIF (2) sequence looks like a backwards running FISP. This fact is also the explanation for the acronym. First comes the phase encoding, then the data acquisition followed by the excitation – a violation of causality. In order to understand the signal generation, three consecutive loops (1–3) have to be discussed. The transverse magnetization is generated at the end of the first loop (1). For the readout period of the second loop, the transverse magnetization is dephased by the variable pulse GS at the beginning of the sequence. The RF pulse at the end of the second loop operates not only as an excitation pulse, but also as the refocusing pulse for the dephased transverse magnetization. The following variable pulse GS refocuses the dephasing in the direction of slice selection, and the GR gradient timing of the third loop (3) refocuses the echo in the center of the data acquisition window. Since a radiofrequency pulse has been used for refocusing, the acquired signal is a spin echo. The sequence provides a heavy T2 weighting. *GP* phase-encoding gradient; *GR* read-out gradient; *GS* slice-selection gradient; *RF* radiofrequency

steady state (DESS). It is also misleading to place the PSIF technique within the hybrid family of this section, as it is solely a spin-echo sequence. As the actual TE is the labeled TE plus the TR, PSIF images are always heavily T2-W (and not T2*-W). A separate acquisition of the GRE part and the SE part, combining both signal contributions during image reconstruction, is called DESS (Fig. 1.67) and is applied in musculoskeletal imaging.

An impressive documentation of the above-mentioned contributions is given in Fig. 1.68. Starting with the FLASH, the transverse component in FISP is adding to the signal of tissue with a long T2*, and DESS increases that signal intensity even further in adding a heavily T2-W SE component.

TGSE: Turbo Gradient and Spin Echo, SE-EPI

Hybrids are called imaging methods that utilize a mixture of gradient echoes and spin echoes. A classical example is GRASE – gradient and spin echo also called TGSE – turbo Gradient and Spin Echo. This technique combines gradient echoes with spin echoes by collecting gradient echoes within a spin-echo envelope, as illustrated in Fig. 1.69. Since this technique prolongs the distance between RF refocusing pulses, the J-coupling pattern, responsible for the bright appearance of fat in TSE imaging, is not broken, and fat appears similar as in images acquired with CSE. Since gradient echoes are sensitive to susceptibility differences and since the RF refocusing pulses are now further apart, allowing more time for diffusion, the sensitivity to hemorrhagic lesions is slightly improved as compared to TSE image acquisitions.

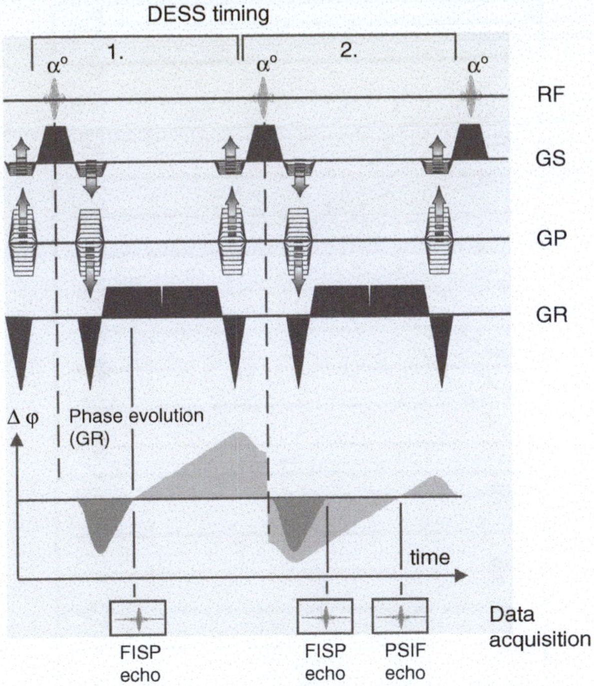

Fig. 1.67 DESS – the double-echo steady-state sequence. DESS combines the fast imaging with steady-state precession (FISP) echo with the backward running fast imaging with steady-state precession (PSIF) echo, collecting the data out of two directly adjacent acquisition windows. The first loop generates a FISP echo and the transverse magnetization for the PSIF echo, which is refocused with the excitation pulse of the next loop and read out within the second acquisition window. The two images are combined, to add the T2 weighting of the PSIF echo to the FISP image. *GP* phase-encoding gradient; *GR* readout gradient; *GS* slice-selection gradient; *RF* radiofrequency

A spin-echo EPI (SE-EPI) in comparison to the FID-EPI is also considered a hybrid as the gradient echoes are acquired under a SE envelope. The difference to TGSE is that only a 90–180° RF pair is used in EPI whereas 180° repetitions are used in TGSE. An example has already been presented with the introduction of DW-SE-EPI (Fig. 1.45). "Segmenting" the EPI approach by repeating the excitation and refocusing following shorter ETLs is finally leading to a sequence timing identical with TGSE.

1.3.2 k-Space Trajectories and Motion Compensation Strategies

Conventional *k*-space acquisition schemes apply a frequency encoding magnetic field gradient for the duration of data acquisition with a preceding preparation of the phase of the transverse magnetization in the direction of phase encoding. The phase preparation dictates the position of the measured Fourierline within *k*-space as indicated in Fig. 1.70a. This *k*-space acquisition scheme is representative for GRE (Fig. 1.8) as well as SE (Fig. 1.10), and even fast spin echo imaging (Fig. 1.24). In the latter case, the phase information is reset to zero prior to the next RF refocusing pulse. A low phase-encoding gradient measures the coarse object structures in the direction of phase encoding and the Fourierline is to be assigned around

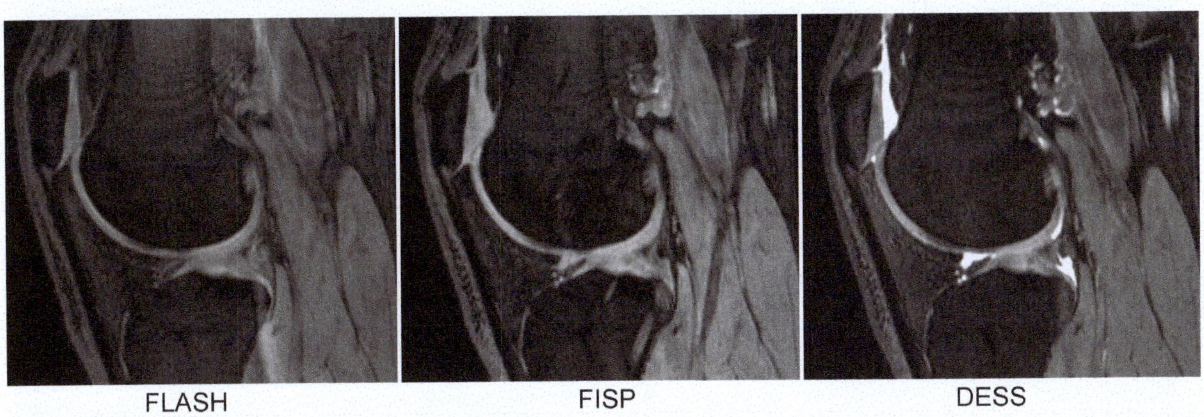

Fig. 1.68 FLASH, FISP, DESS comparison. Sagittal cuts of the knee demonstrate the clinically relevant difference between the fast low-angle shot sequence (FLASH), fast imaging with steady-state precession (FISP), and double-echo steady-state sequence (DESS). Starting with the FLASH, the transverse steady-state component of FISP provides a higher signal intensity for tissue with a longer T2*. The heavily T2-W spin-echo component of the DESS technique that is added to the FISP component acquired simultaneously clearly demonstrates the advantage of this technique. DESS apparently allows a better delineation between fat, cartilage, and joint effusion. *GP* phase-encoding gradient; *GR* read-out gradient; *GS* slice-selection gradient; *RF* radiofrequency

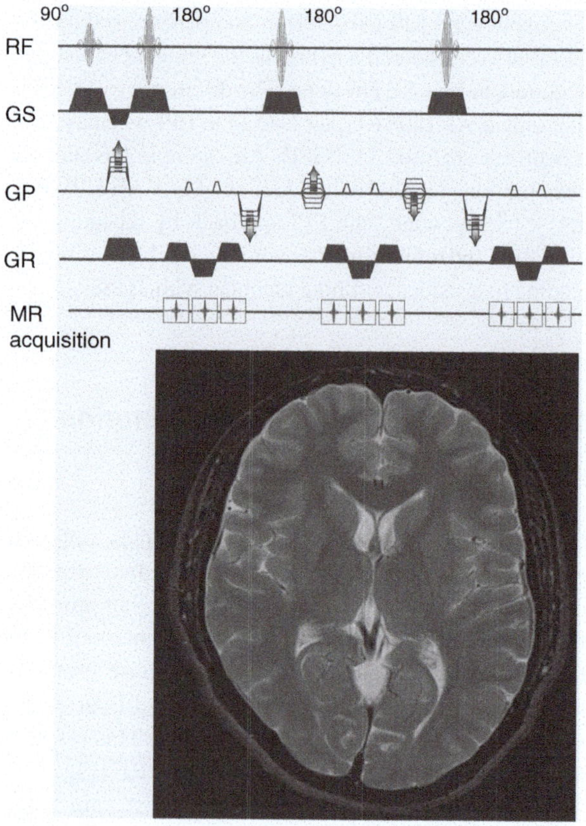

Fig. 1.69 TGSE – the turbo-gradient and spin-echo sequence. Multiple echoes with different phase-encoding steps are used to acquire all the data necessary to fill the raw data matrix. For each spin-echo envelope, multiple gradient echoes (in this case, three) are utilized, leading to a further possibility in reducing measurement time compared with the TSE sequence design. Other advantages are the unbroken J-coupling (fat appears similar to SE imaging) and the theoretical increase in sensitivity to susceptibility gradients (hemorrhagic lesions should appear similar to SE imaging). *GP* phase-encoding gradient; *GR* read-out gradient; *GS* slice-selection gradient; *RF* radiofrequency

the center of *k*-space. A high phase-encoding gradient provides information of the high spatial resolution details in the direction of phase encoding and the corresponding Fourierline is assigned to the outer *k*-space. For single shot techniques like bEPI as indicated in Fig. 1.45, the *k*-space is sampled according to the scheme illustrated in Fig. 1.70b. Finally, if a small phase-encoding gradient is left on for the duration of the data sampling, as indicated in Fig. 1.63 for the FID-EPI, the *k*-space trajectory follows the zig-zag pattern as indicated in Fig. 1.70c. At this point, it

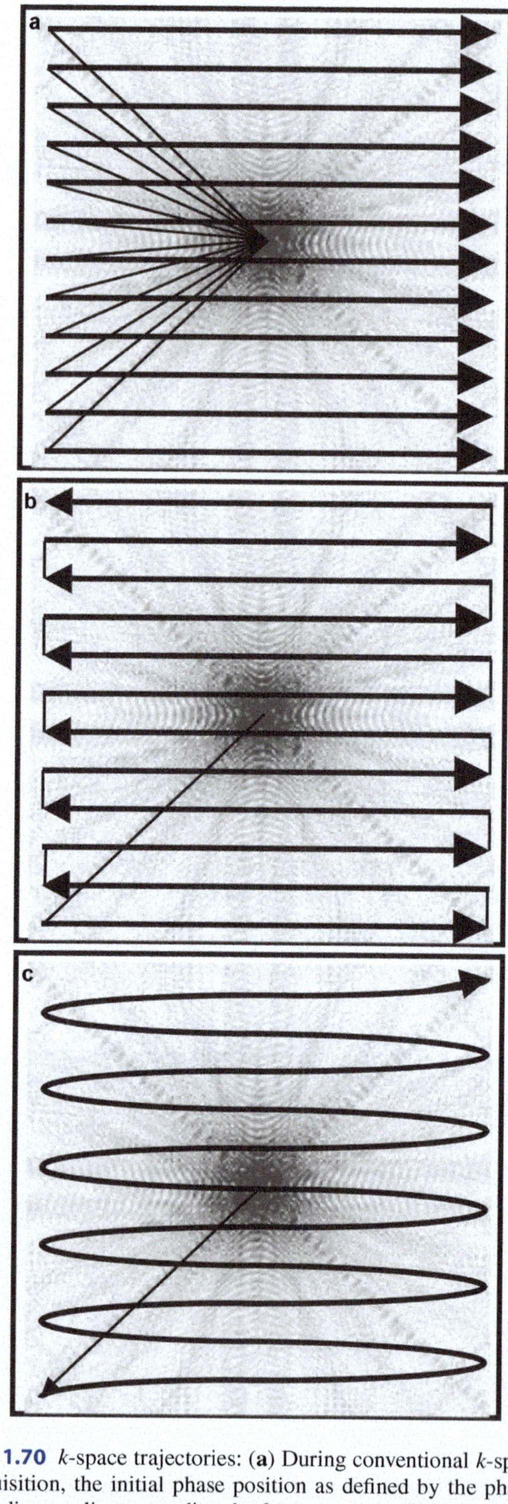

Fig. 1.70 *k*-space trajectories: (**a**) During conventional *k*-space acquisition, the initial phase position as defined by the phase-encoding gradient preceding the frequency encoding defines the Fourier line to be measured. (**b**) With bEPI, the phase encoding is advanced at the time the oscillating frequency encoding gradient changes polarity. (**c**) A continuous advancement of the phase is observed for the classical FID-EPI acquisition scheme

is obvious that the *k*-space trajectory is not in line with the cartesian grid as used for the fast fourier transformation. The process to calculate the potential signal value on the cartesian grid based on the values of the truly measured *k*-space trajectory is called "regridding."

In analyzing how the Fourier transformation identifies different frequencies, it becomes obvious that phase encoding is identical to frequency encoding. Both directions within *k*-space contain a time domain. While the frequency encoding direction contains at least as many values as dictated by the matrix size, the time between assignments of data points is given by the sampling rate of the analog-to-digital conversion. The frequency differences are identified in analyzing the phase evolution of the transverse magnetizations for the duration of the data acquisition of a single Fourierline. The data points in *k*-space characterizing the phase-encoding direction are separated by the repetition time in single echo imaging, respectively by the echo spacing in multiecho imaging. Similar to the frequency encoding, spatial information is contained in the phase evolution of the signal inducing transverse magnetizations for each Fourier line.

A displacement of the object or part of the object during phase- or frequency encoding or in between a pair of dephasing and rephasing gradient pulses will cause an incorrect phase assignment with respect to location and appearing as motion artifacts solely in the direction of phase encoding.

Spiral Data Acquisition Schemes

As indicated above, a spatial assignment is based on analyzing the phase evolution of the induced signal. Using an oscillating frequency-encoding gradient will lead to multiple gradient echoes. If a small phase-encoding gradient is provided at the same time, the course of the acquired data line will correspond to a zigzag trajectory in *k*-space. This is the classical acquisition scheme for an echo-planar-imaging sequence. If the phase evolution is provided by using a small blipped phase-encoding gradient at the time where the frequency-encoding gradient is changing polarity, the sequence is called a blipped EPI-bEPI. If oscillating magnetic field gradients with increasing amplitudes are used for the direction of phase encoding as well as the direction of frequency encoding, the path within *k*-space will follow a spiral trajectory causing the sequence to be named spiral EPI – sEPI (Fig. 1.71).

Radial Data Acquisition Schemes

In conventional Fourier-encoded imaging, the user usually selects, prior to executing the imaging protocol, not only the orientation of the imaging plane but also the direction of frequency and phase encoding. A novel acquisition scheme utilizes a rotation of the frequency-encoding gradient direction during imaging rather than stepping through phase-encoding lines (Fig. 1.72). This sampling strategy is close to the scheme used in

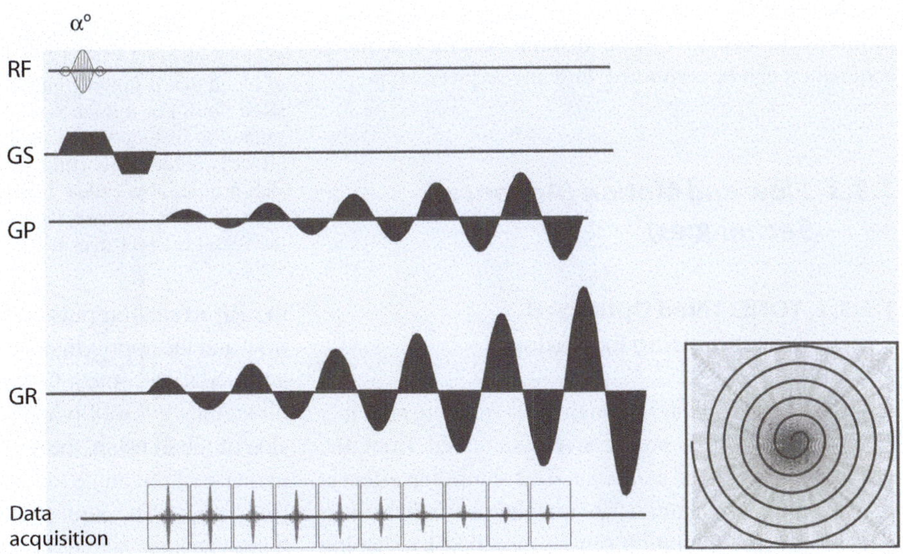

Fig. 1.71 sEPI – the spiral echo-planar imaging sequence. The readout gradient as well as the phase-encoding gradient oscillate with increasing amplitude. This causes a data trajectory that "spirals" through *k*-space, starting in the center of *k*-space with the acquisition of low spatial frequencies. *GP* phase-encoding gradient; *GR* read-out gradient; *GS* slice-selection gradient; *RF* radiofrequency

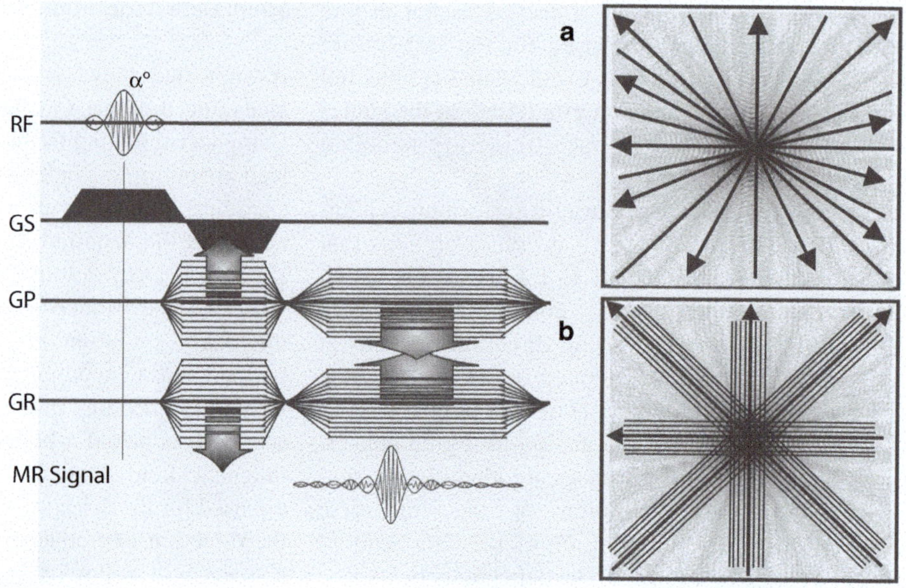

Fig. 1.72 Radial sampling is performed by rotating the frequency-encoding gradient direction around the object, similar to the rotating dector in CT. (**a**) There are some disadvantages, e.g., regridding challenges, if every measured Fourier line goes through the center of *k*-space. These disadvantages are reduced by implementing the acquisition scheme (**b**)

computer tomography and is called a radial acquisition (Fig. 1.72a). Image reconstruction usually follows the conventional Fourier transformation scheme and the correction of the data points to fit on the conventional *k*-space grid is called "regridding." Modification to this sampling scheme is the utilization of a few phase-encoding steps perpendicular to the direction of frequency encoding (Fig. 1.72b). This acquisition scheme is called BLADE, PROPELLER, or MultiVane. The method has some intrinsic advantages. Measurements in the vicinity of the center of *k*-space enable a relatively easy detection and correction of motion. Thus, this method has potential to generate images without motion artifacts despite significant movements. While spiral acquisition is primarily limited to EPI acquisition schemes, a radial acquisition can be combined with any sequence type.

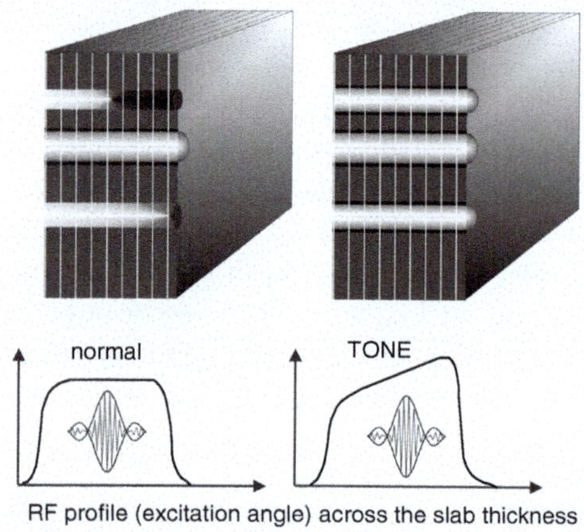

Fig. 1.73 The time-of-flight effect in 3D magnetic resonance angiography (3D ToF-MRA): the contrast is given by the amount of blood that is flowing into the excited slab, replacing the saturated fluid. For a thick slab and slow flow, there is a potential saturation of blood towards the distal portion of the slab. This effect is reduced by using an asymmetric radiofrequency (RF) slab profile, also called TONE (tilted optimized nonsaturating excitation). In that case, the excitation angle at the entry point of the vessel is lower than at the exit port

1.3.3 Flow and Motion (Advanced Techniques)

1.3.3.1 TONE: Tilted Optimized Nonsaturating Excitation

As blood flows into and through a 3D imaging slab in a 3D ToF-MRA, it is progressively saturated from the entry point toward the exit point. This saturation effect is causing artifacts in multislab imaging as indicated in Fig. 1.74a. This saturation can be modified by shaping the RF excitation pulse. Depending on the direction of flow and the approximated flow velocity, the flip-angle is adjusted to become a function of location along the flow direction. A low flip-angle excitation is applied at one side of the 3D slab, the entry point of the vessel, with an increase of flip angle toward the opposite side of the slab (Fig. 1.73). The aim of this procedure is to achieve a homogeneous signal contribution throughout the 3D volume and reduction of boundary artifacts in multislab ToF MRA imaging (Fig. 1.74b). The technique is also called tilted optimized nonsaturating excitation - TONE.

1.3.3.2 TWIST and TRICKS: Time Resolved ceMRA

Contrast-enhanced MRA has been introduced in Sect. 1.2.9.2, and the challenge to match the bolus arrival with the start of the imaging sequence has already been discussed. A different approach is the time-resolved acquisition of the 3D slab after contrast injection. The repeated sampling of the low-spatial-resolution *k*-space lines combined with temporal interpolation allows the generation of a series of time-resolved imaging of contrast kinetics — TRICKS. A different approach is the utilization of a 3D time-resolved angiography with interleaved stochastic trajectories – TWIST (Fig. 1.75). In both cases, 3D ceMRA can be performed with high temporal and spatial resolution without prior estimation of the bolus transit time. Other acronyms to refer to interpolation in space and time in order to become time resolved are TREAT – time-resolved echo-shared angiography technique, *k*-t BLAST – broad-use linear acquisition speed-up technique, HYPR – highly constrained backprojection

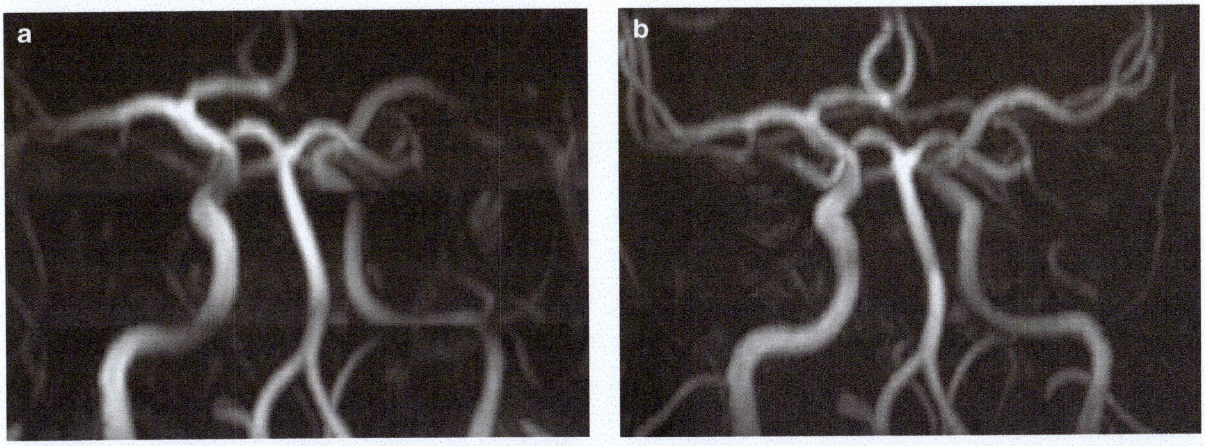

Fig. 1.74 Multi-slab 3D ToF-MRA (**a**) without modified RF excitation pulse (same flip angle distribution throughout the imaging slab). (**b**) With TONE (linear flip angle change in the direction of flow)

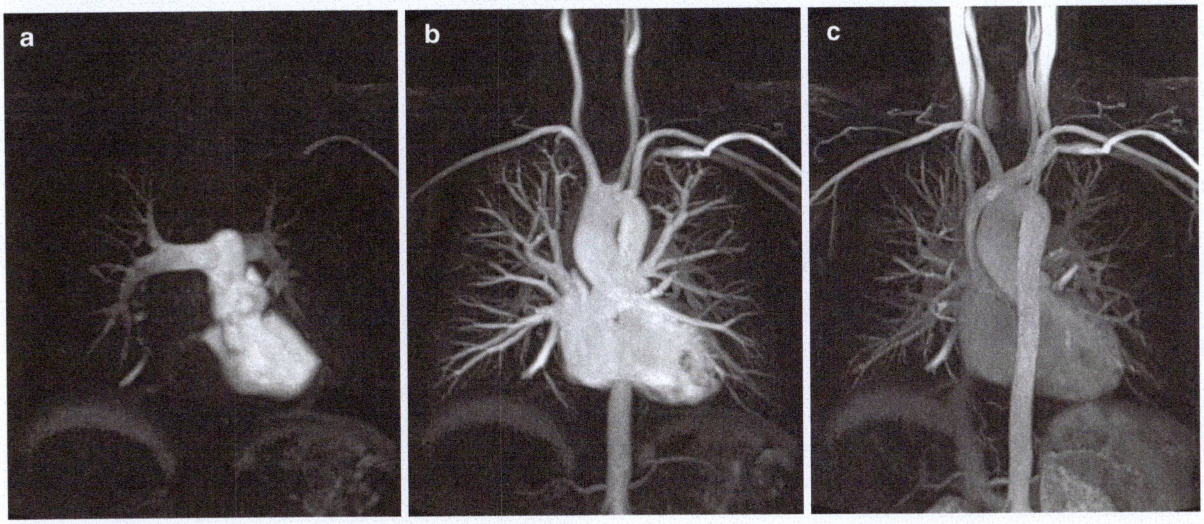

Fig. 1.75 TWIST – time-resolved contrast-enhanced MR angiography with interleaved stochastic trajectories (**a**) early bolus arrival in the pulmonary vasculature, (**b**) arterial phase, (**c**) venous phase

for time-resolved MRI and VIPR – vastly undersampled isotropic projection imaging. The latter utilize radial acquisition techniques as indicated in the acronym.

1.3.3.3 Flow Quantification

As previously discussed (Sect. 1.2.9), magnetic field gradients are used for the purpose of spatial encoding and if the tissue with the generated transverse magnetization is changing position during or between active magnetic field gradients, the phase position of the transverse magnetization is altered in comparison to stationary tissue at that location. This phase change is proportional to the velocity of the flowing blood. Comparing this phase with the phase of a flow desensitized sequence (Fig. 1.42), where the phase within the flow corresponds to the phase of a potential stationary tissue at that location, will allow the flow to be quantified. An example for a 2D GRE through plane flow desensitized/sensitized interleaved sequence is given in Fig. 1.76. Flow sensitization can also be generated in the direction of phase or frequency encoding, but is usually omitted due to a potential contamination via partial volume effects. Processing the phase information enables the direct visualization of flow direction and flow velocity (Fig. 1.77).

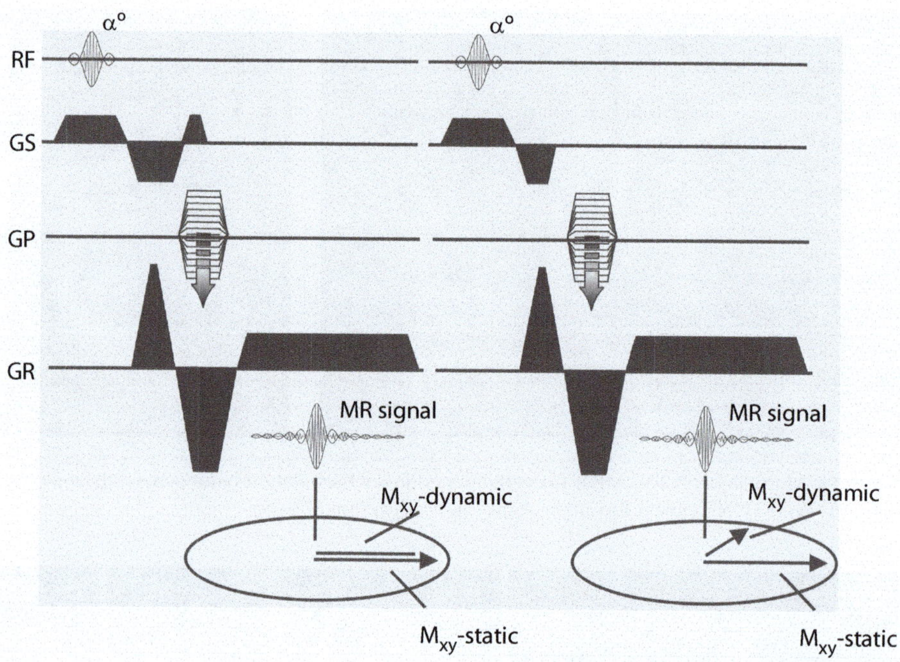

Fig. 1.76 Example of a sequence arrangement for flow quantification, in this case, sensitized for flow in the direction of slice selection. There are typically two interleaved measurements, separated by the selected repetitiontime. A first measurement serves as a reference and is flow insensitive, while the following measurement is flow sensitized, demonstrating a phase shift proportional to the flow velocity

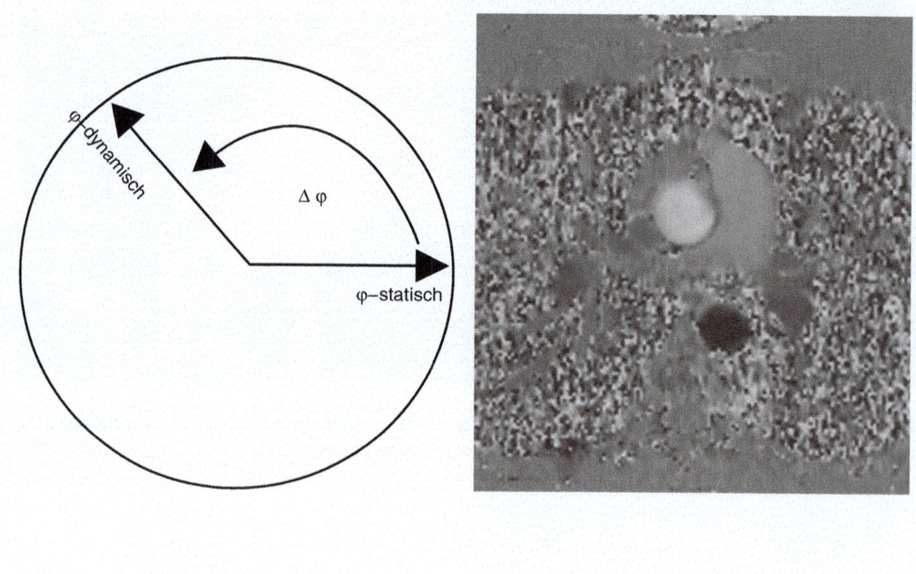

Fig. 1.77 Flow quantification - FQ: the phase difference between flow-sensitized and flow-desensitized transverse nuclear magnetization is converted to a signal intensity within the image. In this case, the gray scale corresponds directly to a measured velocity. Shown is the transverse cut through the aortic arch at the level of the pulmonary artery. The ascending aorta appears hyperintense whereas the descending aorta shows hypointensity according to flow direction and amplitude

Flow quantification with MRI has some potential in quantifying the flow through a dialysis shunt, investigating valvular insufficiencies, grading of shunts in congenital malformations of the heart, providing information on the extent to which flow in a false lumen supplies vital organs in aortic dissection, and investigating patent CSF channels in patients with hydrocephalus.

1.3.3.4 PC-MRA: Phase-Contrast MR Angiography

MRA techniques based on a velocity-dependent phase shift of the transverse magnetization, the phase-contrast - PC-MRA, use the "difference vector" between the transverse magnetization of the flow-compensated (desensitized) measurement and the transverse magnetization of the following flow-sensitized measurements for the visualization of the vascular tree (Fig. 1.78). In this case, the second sequence is usually sensitized in the direction of frequency encoding and is typically used as a fast localizer for the peripheral vasculature with the frequency-encoding direction being caudo cranial. The technique can also be structured as 3D measurement with an interleaved flow desensitized part for the creation of a reference and three sequences to follow with flow sensitization in the three orthogonal directions. The latter will lead to relatively long measurement times. The image quality of a 3D PC-MRA also depends on the selection of a suitable flow sensitivity. If the selected sensitivity is too high, corresponding to an underestimated velocity range, the contrast will be poor (due to multiple phase wraps). If the selected sensitivity is too low, corresponding to an overestimated velocity range, the contrast will be poor (due to just a small phase difference). In addition, this technique is sensitive to higher-order motion and apparently not as robust as the ToF techniques.

The advantages of this technique are the perfect background suppression and the adjustable sensitivity to slow velocities. The PC-MRA method is currently mainly utilized as 2D version providing a reasonable localizer for a contrast-enhanced MRA technique to follow.

1.3.3.5 Nonenhanced MR Angiography

Nonenhanced MR angiographic methods have been available prior to 1987, at which point in time ToF-MRA and PC-MRA where competing with respect to image quality, robustness, and speed. The introduction of gadolinium-enhanced MRA has been too promising with respect to speed and robustness and has replaced the above-mentioned nonenhanced MRA methods for all regions below the carotid bifurcation. 2D PC-MRA remains as a common technique for vessel localization. 3D ToF-MRA is still the method of choice for the intracranial cerebral vasculature mainly due to the currently still higher spatial resolution. Recent technical advances and new concerns about the safety of GBCAs have spurred a resurgence of interest in methods that

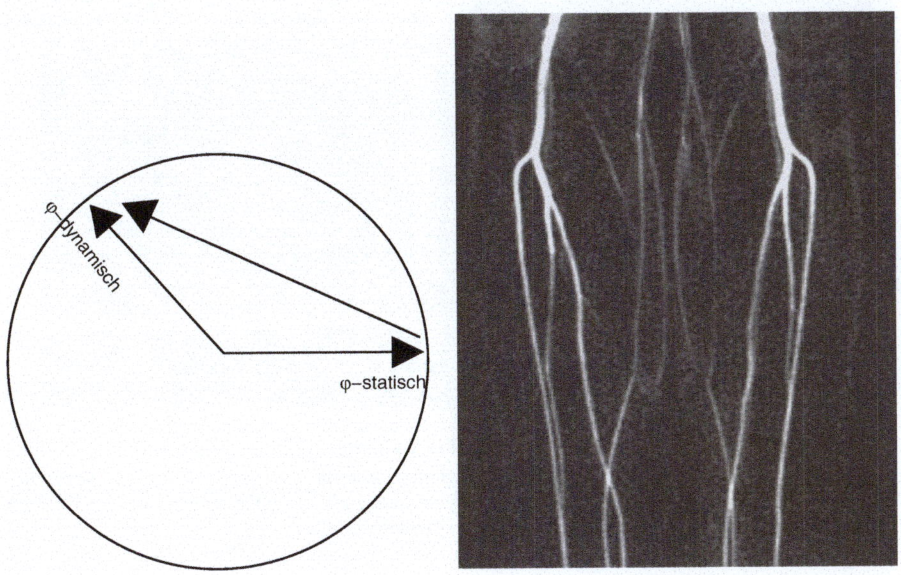

Fig. 1.78 Phase contrast MRA - PC-MRA: the length of the vector between the stationary reference and the signal from the moving blood is translated to a pixel intensity within the image

do not require exogenous contrast material. These additional "newer" techniques will be discussed as follows.

Electrocardiographically (ECG)-Gated 3D (Partial-Fourier) Fast Spin-Echo Methods

ECG triggered nonenhanced MRA techniques have been published as early as 1985. Recent improvements have made these methods clinically feasible on modern MR systems. One concept utilizes an ECG-gated fast spin-echo acquisition scheme in conjunction with a partial Fourier acquisition, e.g., HASTE or SS-FSE within a systolic and a diastolic time window. In combination with parallel imaging, the acquisition time is in the order of 350 ms per image. The method relies on loss of signal, or flow void, as a result of fast arterial flow during systole in contrast to the high signal intensity during diastole due to slow flow in the arteries. Due to the relative slow flow, venous blood is bright during both systole and diastole. MRA is achieved by subtracting systolic from diastolic images. As *k*-space symmetry is suffering due to T2-decay during sampling, vessels should be oriented parallel to the phase-encoding direction in order to minimize vessel blurring artifacts. Recent progress has been made to utilize SPACE (Sect. 1.3.1.1) together with the concept of triggered acquisitions. This method is also referred to as NATIVE SPACE (Fig. 1.79).

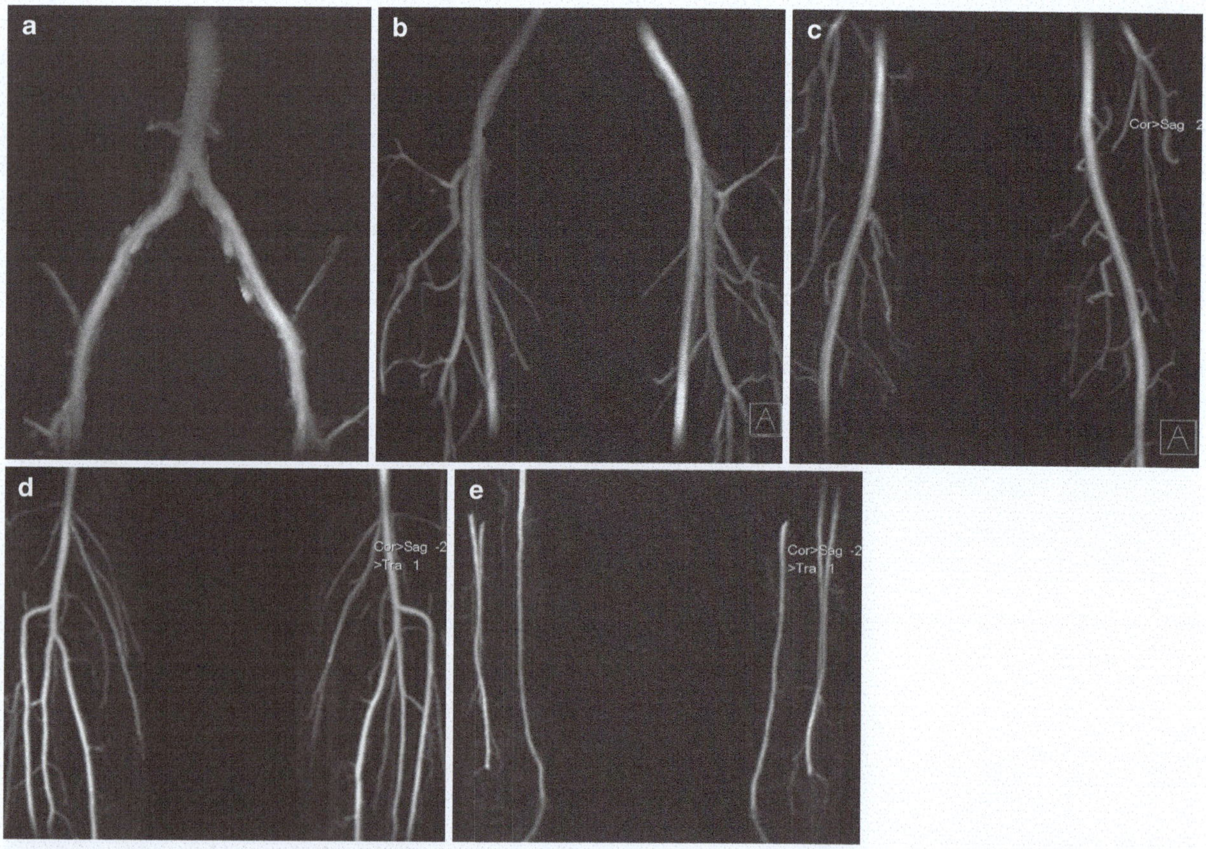

Fig. 1.79 MIP of the vasculature below the aortic bifurcation using NATIVE SPACE: Two 3D fast spin echo sequences with optimized arrangements of low angle refocusing pulses, image acquisition in systole and diastole with inline subtraction to follow (**a**) at the level of the iliac bifurcation, (**b**) at the upper level of the femoral artery, (**c**) at the lower level of the femoral artery, (**d**) at the level of the popliteal trifurcation, (**e**) at the level of the tibial arteries

Electrocardiographically (ECG)-Gated Balanced Steady-State Free Precession Techniques

With balanced SSFP like trueFISP, FIESTA, or bFFE, both the arteries and the veins have high signal intensity. In theory, image contrast is determined by T2/T1 ratios, which produce bright-blood imaging without reliance on inflow. TRs of less than 4 ms combined with high flip angles can produce high signal-to-noise-ratio MR angiographic images (Fig. 1.80). The sequence is susceptible to field inhomogeneities and a localized shimming may be advised.

ASL Related Methods

The combination of ASL with tagged and untagged balanced SSFP can provide bright arteries in venous-free angiographic images (Fig. 1.81). As an alternative to balanced SSFP, partial-Fourier fast spin-echo methods can also be used in conjunction with ASL. These methods have the advantage of less sensitivity to susceptibility artifacts in comparison with balanced SSFP.

1.3.3.6 Motion Compensation and Correction Techniques

Patient motion produces artifacts in MRI due to tissue displacement during and between excitation and data sampling and due to motion-induced phase shifts in the presence of magnetic field gradients.

GMR: Gradient Motion Rephasing

Flow- and motion-induced phase shifts of the transverse magnetization can be reduced by using GMR, also called gradient motion refocusing or gradient moment nulling. It is usually an option within the sequence menu and will initiate a three-lobe gradient structure in the direction of slice selection and readout, leading to a longer TE if selected (see also Fig. 1.42). The three-lobe magnetic field gradient structure will allow the compensation of first-order motion, that is a "constant velocity." Flow changes within a second due to the periodicity of the cardiac cycle can be approximated as being "constant," as the "constant" is referring to the time between excitation and data acquisition, which is typically only a few milliseconds.

For sequences and applications using very short TE, the motion-induced phase shifts may be negligible and a GMR selection may be an inappropriate choice. This is for example a valid conclusion for ceMRA applications.

Navigator

The term "navigator" is often used for different methods to monitor and compensate motion. A one-dimensional navigator is often referred to a pencil-shaped volume excitation that crosses the diaphragm (Fig. 1.82). A fast frequency encoded readout along the pencil excitation potentially allows the tracking of the liver-lung interface in between measurements, to trigger or gate the acquisition with the respiratory cycle.

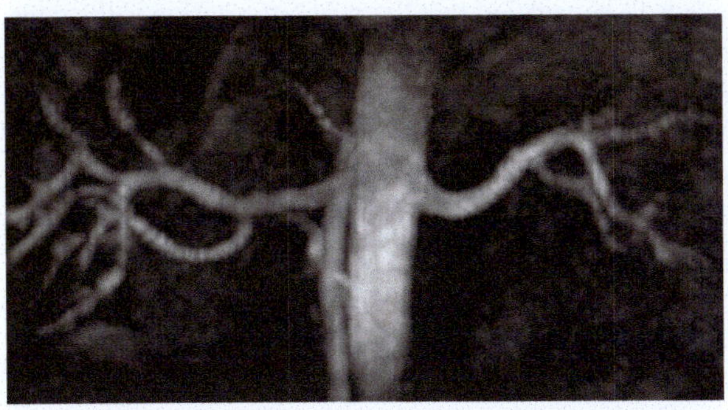

Fig. 1.80 MIP of the renal vasculature using NATIVE trueFISP: Two 2D or 3D trueFISP sequences acquire one set of images in systole and one set of images in diastole with inline subtraction to follow

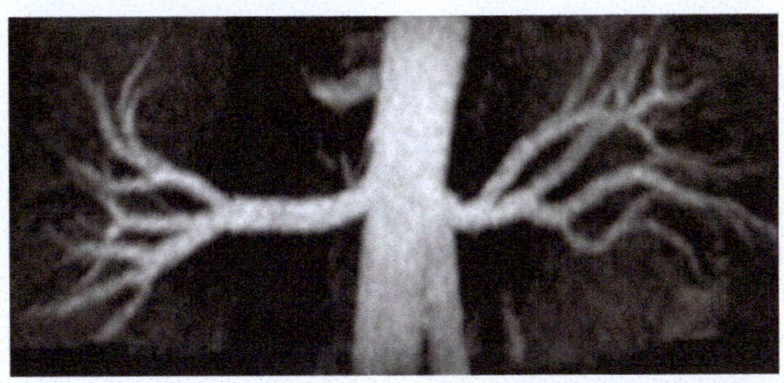

Fig. 1.81 MIP of the renal vasculature using NATIVE trueFISP and venous suppression: two 2D or 3D trueFISP sequences acquire one set of images in systole and one set of images in diastole with inline subtraction to follow and a preceding inversion of the magnetization within the imaging volume

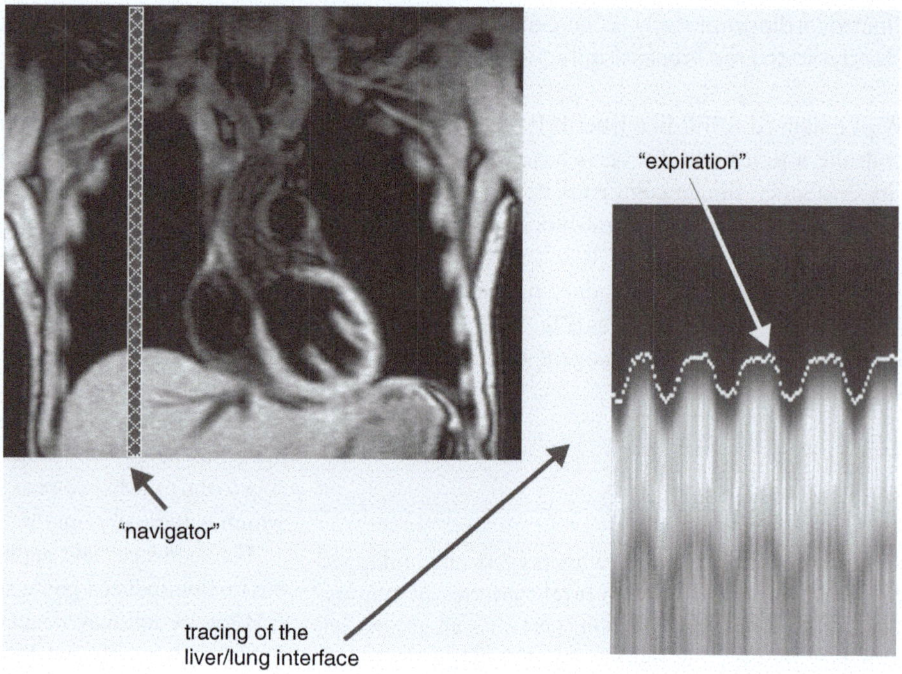

Fig. 1.82 The "navigator" technique. A 2D-slice or rod is placed across the liver/lung interface to monitor the respiratory cycle

A two-dimensional navigator is sometimes referred to a low-resolution image across the liver-lung interface. As this provides more information, this method is more robust than the one-dimensional navigator. A navigator scan may also refer to a repeated measurement of the central *k*-space line in order to detect and correct any system-related phase shifts of the signal or phase shifts due to object motion.

3D Motion Correction

fMRI is an application where motion detection and instantaneous adjustment of the acquisition according to this information is crucial. One method is a real-time statistical analysis of each 3D dataset acquired in rapid succession and the comparison of each data set with the previous to calculate and correct translation as well as rotation.

Radial Acquisition and Motion Correction

Imaging methods that repeatedly take measurement points close to the center of *k*-space, like projection-reconstruction, radial acquisition, and spiral MRI, have shown to reduce motion artifacts. This is partially related to the oversampling of the central *k*-space, similar to multiple averaging in conventional imaging. Motion artifacts related to motion-related phase shifts can be reduced by utilizing so-called navigator echoes, as previously mentioned. Rotated overlapping parallel *k*-space lines as measured with PROPELLER, BLADE, or MultiVane contain "navigator" information (Fig. 1.72), which in turn can be used to further reduce motion artifacts. The acquired Fourier line with a radial trajectory through *k*-space is also referred to as strip. Prior to combining strips, it needs to be verified that the point of rotation is the center of *k*-space. Removing the displacement of the *k*-space center will remove all low-frequency spatially varying phase in image space as well as related phase shifts due to bulk rigid body motions. The rotation of an object in image space produces identical rotations of its Fourier transform in *k*-space. A correlation analysis will allow to estimate and correct any bulk rotational motion. Linear spatial shifts in image space produce linear phase shifts in *k*-space. Comparing the data with the averaged data set (due to the oversampling of the center of *k*-space readily available) will allow the estimation and correction of bulk translational motion.

1.3.4 Advanced Contrast Mechanisms

The previously discussed tissue-specific contrast mechanisms have been PD – proton density, T1–relaxation, T2–relaxation, T2*–relaxation. In addition, perfusion, diffusion, and flow have been introduced. The following chapter addresses a few more sophisticated mechanisms to generate a specific image contrast.

1.3.4.1 BOLD: Blood Oxygenation Level Dependent Imaging

Imaging of susceptibility differences is utilized in the evaluation of hemorrhagic lesions and in fMRI, based on the blood oxygenation level-dependent (BOLD) contrast. Deoxyhemoglobin is paramagnetic, while oxyhemoglobin demonstrates diamagnetic properties. A relative decrease of the deoxyhemoglobin level, as an "overcompensation" reaction to oxygen consumption, will lead to a diminished microscopic susceptibility effect and is measured as a small increase in signal intensity - for imaging sequences sensitive to susceptibility gradients. The changes in signal intensities can be evaluated and displayed as color-encoded fMRI (Fig. 1.83).

1.3.4.2 Magnetization Transfer Contrast

Macromolecules have a layer of motion restricted water molecules also called "bound" water. Since static or slow changing magnetic fields are dominant in the vicinity of macromolecules, the associated hydrogen pool has a very short T2. The correlated fast dephasing of the transverse magnetization causes this pool of water to be "invisible." However, the magnetization of that "invisible" water pool is transferred to the visible pool of "free" water via various mechanisms like chemical exchange or cross-relaxation (Fig. 1.84). The term for these processes is called "magnetization transfer"— MT. Cross-relaxation is a special form of dipole–dipole interaction in which a proton on one molecule transfers its spin orientation to that of another molecule. A short T2 or fast dephasing is synonymous for a broad range of resonance frequencies, whereas a long T2 is indicative of a narrow range. If there are applicable magnetization transfer mechanisms within the tissue, a saturation of the "invisible" water pool will affect the "visible" water pool. Applying an RF saturation pulse off resonance, as illustrated, those invisible molecules can be saturated. Since they communicate with their "free" partners via magnetization transfer, this off-resonance

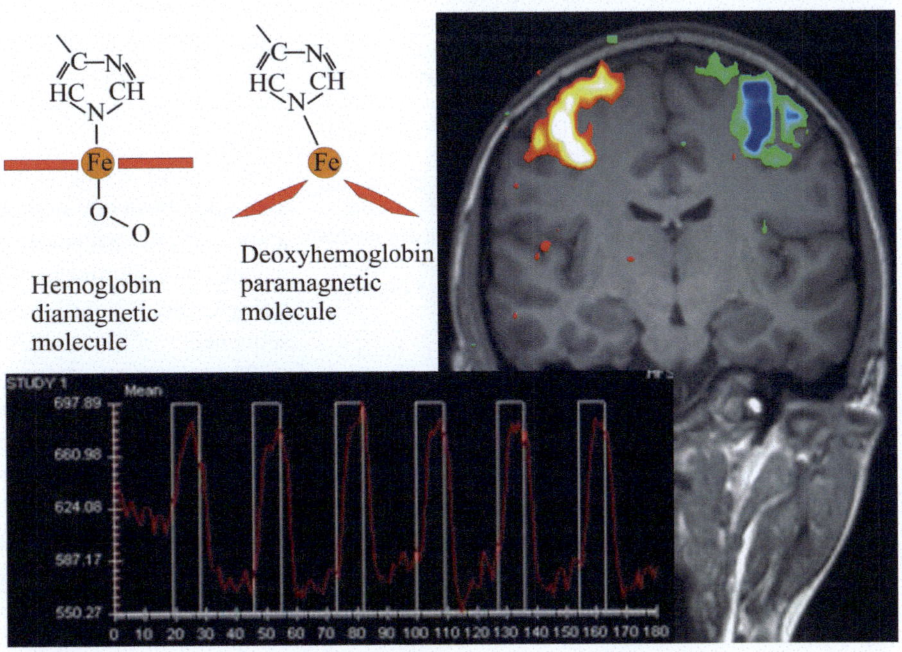

Fig. 1.83 The *upper left* graphic indicates the magnetic properties of oxyhemoglobin and dexoyhemoglobin. The stimulation paradigm is indicated in the *lower left* graph. The change in magnetic susceptibility within the blood containing lumen is causing a signal loss in the vicinity if the magnetic susceptibility is different as compared to the diamagnetic surrounding. The signal difference can be represented as colors with according intensities and mapped to an image representing the corresponding anatomy. The illustrated case represents a finger tapping experiment

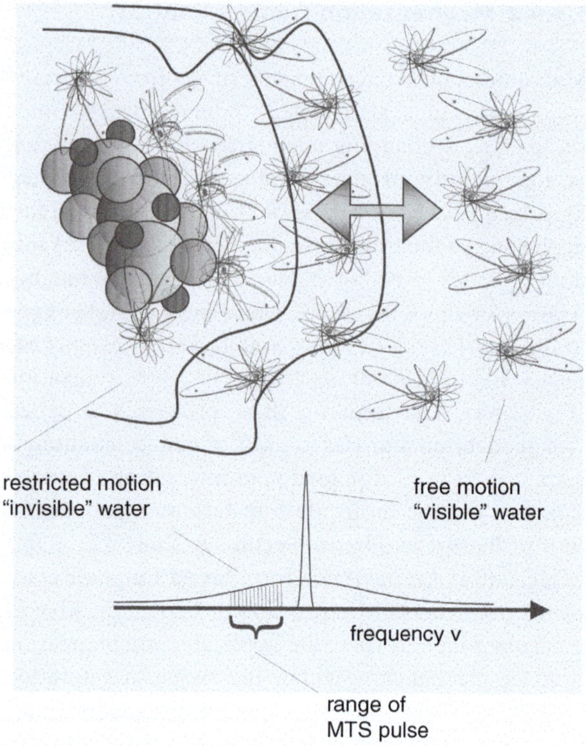

Fig. 1.84 Magnetization transfer - MT: water molecules that are closely associated with proteins and other macromolecules are restricted in motion. The resulting static dephasing mechanism leads to a very short T2, making these water molecules "invisible." A short T2 is also synonymous for a very broad range of resonance frequencies. In contrast, the "visible" water pool has a very narrow frequency range. Mechanisms like cross-relaxation between protons within the "invisible" water pool and protons within the "visible" water pool are called "magnetization transfer" (MT) mechanisms. Saturating the "invisible" water pool will result in a diminished signal within the "visible" water pool as a consequence of this magnetization transfer. The magnetization transfer saturation pulse (MTS) is an off-resonance pulse (e.g., 1 kHz below the resonance frequency of water), which does not directly affect the appearance of "free" water but does saturate the invisible "bounded" water molecules. Magnetization transfer mechanisms provide a transfer of this saturation to the visible pool of "free" water, leading to a lower signal in areas where "bounded" water exists in close vicinity to "free" water

pulse has an effect on the image contrast. The technique is called magnetization transfer saturation — MTS. The contrast achieved with this technique is often referred to as magnetization transfer contrast - MTC. MTS pulses are usually utilized to further suppress the background signal of stationary tissue in 3D ToF-MRA.

1.3.4.3 Perfusion-Weighted Imaging (PWI) Using Arterial Spin Labeling

There are two principal methods for measuring perfusion using MRI. One method is utilizing the bolus tracking of a contrast injection, primarily based on dynamically measuring the changes in magnetic susceptibility within the vascular supply. The second method is called arterial spin labeling - ASL, where the water molecules are "labeled" prior to arrival within the tissue of interest.

ASL can be accomplished using a variety of approaches. The two most common ASL approaches use either pulsed arterial spin labeling - PASL, with spatially selective saturation or inversion, or continuous arterial spin labeling - CASL, likely utilizing a flow-driven adiabatic passage. One example for a pulsed ASL technique is called echo-planar imaging with signal targeting using alternating RF - EPISTAR. In this case, tagging is accomplished using 90° slice-selective saturation pulse applied to the slice to be studied. A spatially selective inversion pulse inverts spins within a thick slab proximal to the imaging slice. A delay time prior to imaging allows inverted arterial spins to travel from the tagged slab to the imaging plane and to perfuse into the tissue. The control image without arterial tagging is acquired by placing the spatially selective inversion pulse distal to the imaging plane by equal distance. This procedure compensates for the expected off-resonance irradiation via the MT effect. The subtle difference between images acquired with and without ASL can be modeled to derive a calculated blood flow image showing perfusion at each voxel.

A second PASL technique is called FAIR (flow alternated inversion recovery), utilizing a selective and a nonselective inversion pulse to produce a tagged and a control image. Images are commonly acquired using a single-shot EPI pulse sequence following the tagging sequence.

The currently favored technique seems to be quantitative imaging of perfusion using a single subtraction - QUIPSS, respectively QUIPSS II. For this technique, a slice-selective saturation pulse is applied to the imaging slice, immediately followed by an inversion tag. In QUIPSS II, a second saturation pulse is applied to the tagging region after a delay. After an additional delay, an image is acquired using single-shot EPI. The utilization of multiple saturation pulses improves the degree of saturation considerably (Fig. 1.85).

1.3.4.4 DTI: Diffusion Tensor Imaging

Diffusion is a three-dimensional process. As diffusion is encoded in the MR signal by using magnetic field gradients, only molecular displacement along the direction of the gradient will have an impact on the diffusion-encoded component of the signal. The effect of diffusion anisotropy can easily be detected by changing the direction of the diffusion-encoding gradients. With the introduction of diffusion-weighted MRI, diffusion anisotropy has been documented at the end of the 1980s in spinal cord as well as brain white matter. Diffusion anisotropy in white matter originates more or less from the organization of myelinated axonal fibers running in parallel. Diffusion in the direction of the fibers is faster than in the perpendicular direction. With the introduction of the formalism of the diffusion tensor, diffusion anisotropy effects can be fully extracted, characterized, and exploited. The most advanced application is certainly that of fiber tracking in the brain. The diffusion tensor **D** fully describes molecular mobility along each direction and correlation between these directions.

$$\underline{D} = \begin{matrix} D_{xx} & D_{xy} & D_{xz} \\ D_{yx} & D_{yy} & D_{yz} \\ D_{zx} & D_{zy} & D_{zz} \end{matrix}$$

As the diffusion tensor is symmetric, containing only six independent values (e.g., $D_{yx} = D_{xy}$), measurements with diffusion weighting in at least six different directions are mandatory to retrieve the value of the elements of the tensor matrix. Determining the main direction of diffusivity with a respective rotation of the coordinate system leads to a "diagonalization" of the diffusion tensor.

$$\underline{D'} = \begin{matrix} D_{x'x'} & 0 & 0 \\ 0 & D_{y'y'} & 0 \\ 0 & 0 & D_{z'z'} \end{matrix} = \begin{matrix} \lambda_1 & 0 & 0 \\ 0 & \lambda_2 & 0 \\ 0 & 0 & \lambda_3 \end{matrix}$$

In this case, the remaining tensor elements are called eigenvectors and eigenvalues. From the diffusion tensor elements one may calculate indices that reflect either the average diffusion or the degree of anisotropy. Several scalar indices have been proposed. The most commonly used are the relative anisotropy (RA)

$$\mathrm{RA} = \sqrt{(\lambda_1 - \langle\lambda\rangle)^2 + (\lambda_2 - \langle\lambda\rangle)^2 + (\lambda_3 - \langle\lambda\rangle)^2} \Big/ \sqrt{3\langle\lambda\rangle},$$

with $\langle\lambda\rangle = \lambda_1 + \lambda_2 + \lambda_3/3$, the fractional anisotropy (FA)

$$\mathrm{FA} = \sqrt{3\left[(\lambda_1 - \langle\lambda\rangle)^2 + (\lambda_2 - \langle\lambda\rangle)^2 + (\lambda_3 - \langle\lambda\rangle)^2\right]} \Big/ \sqrt{2(\lambda_1^2 + \lambda_2^2 + \lambda_3^2)},$$

and the volume ratio (VR)

$$\mathrm{VR} = (\lambda_1 \cdot \lambda_2 \cdot \lambda_3) / \langle\lambda\rangle^3.$$

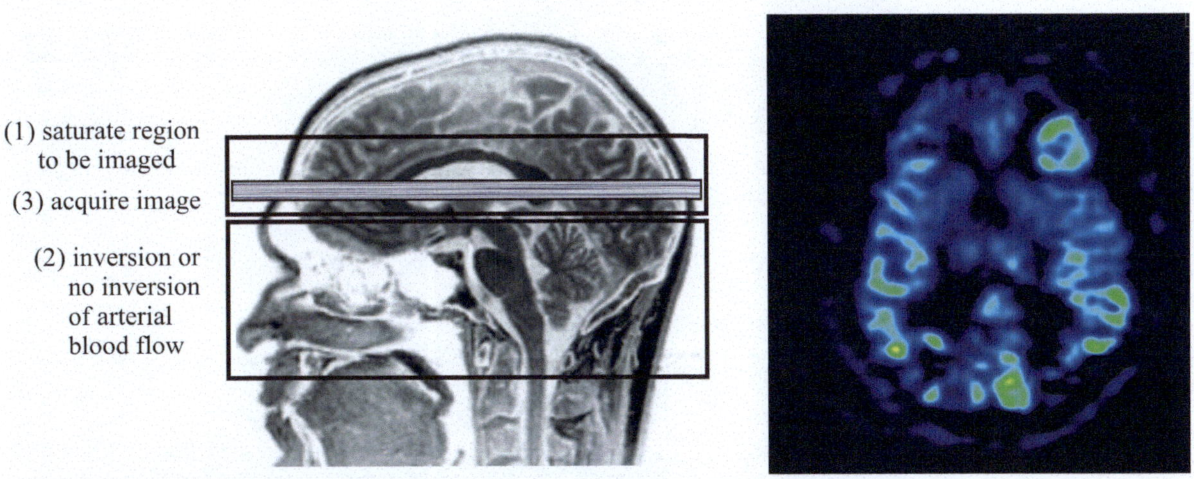

Fig. 1.85 Graphical illustration of QUIPSS II, including a clinical example

The eigenvalues utilized in the above equations are retrieved by diagonalizing the diffusion tensor. The diagonalization will cancel nondiagonal terms of the diffusion tensor, similar to the directional diffusion-weighting gradients coinciding with the diffusion frame of the tissue. The displaying options for diffusion tensor data on a voxel-by-voxel basis are color maps, diffusion ellipsoids (Fig. 1.86a), or vectors pointing in the fiber direction. The recent most impressive application of DTI is the demonstration of brain connectivity through fiber tracking (Fig. 1.86b).

1.3.4.5 Parametric Maps

There are a few recently introduced methods to enhance existing information or to use calculated parameters to define color and intensity of maps to be used as overlay on gray-scaled weighted anatomic images.

Susceptibility-Weighted Imaging (SWI)

Susceptibility differences between tissues (partially deoxgenated venous blood, blood clot, calcium or iron-laden tissue in comparison to parenchymal surrounding) will cause subtle differences in Larmor frequencies leading to a dephasing of the transverse magnetization and a difference in phase position of the transverse magnetization between voxels. The phase information can be used as a mask to enhance the contrast between tissues with different susceptibilities. This phenomenon is utilized in susceptibility-weighted imaging (SWI, Fig. 1.87b).

Fast T1-Mapping

In orthopedic imaging, several biochemical imaging techniques have been evaluated recently, to map biochemical changes within the cartilage. T1-mapping has been and is used in delayed Gadolinium Enhanced MRI of Cartilage - dGEMRIC, to measure the proteoglycan content of the cartilage. To calculate T1, two adjacent spoiled GREs can be utilized with the same TR but different excitation angles. In this case, the change in signal contribution is also a function of the differences in T1-relaxation time. The retrieved value can be used to control the color and the intensity of a T1-map (Fig. 1.88a), which can be fused with the anatomic image in order to enhance or outline the desired information (Fig. 1.88b).

T2-Mapping

The T2 relaxation time is commonly measured with a relatively time-consuming multiecho spin-echo

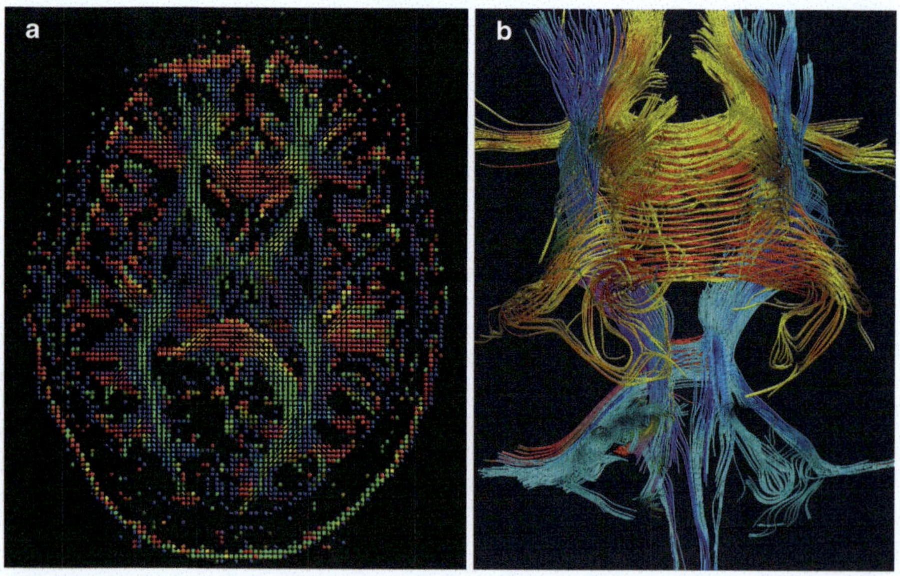

Fig. 1.86 (**a**) The tensor graphic demonstrates the direction of diffusion voxel-by-voxel. Degree and the direction of diffusion are shown as an ellipsoid. The color of the ellipsoid indicates the direction of diffusion; the elongated shape indicates the strength of the preferred direction. (**b**) Visualization of brain connectivity with color display of apparent fiber tracks through combination of preferred directions of diffusivity

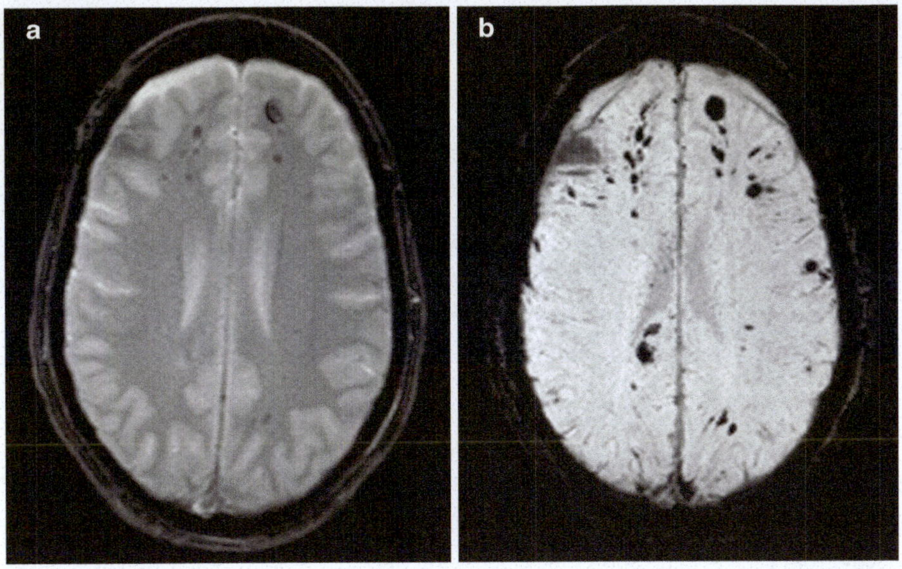

Fig. 1.87 Images of a patient involved in a car accident. (**a**) Low flip angle T2-W GRE protocol, designed to demonstrate signal void in case of susceptibility gradients due to hemorrhagic lesions. (**b**) Lesion enhancement using the phase information as a mask for the image (*SWI* susceptibility weighted imaging)

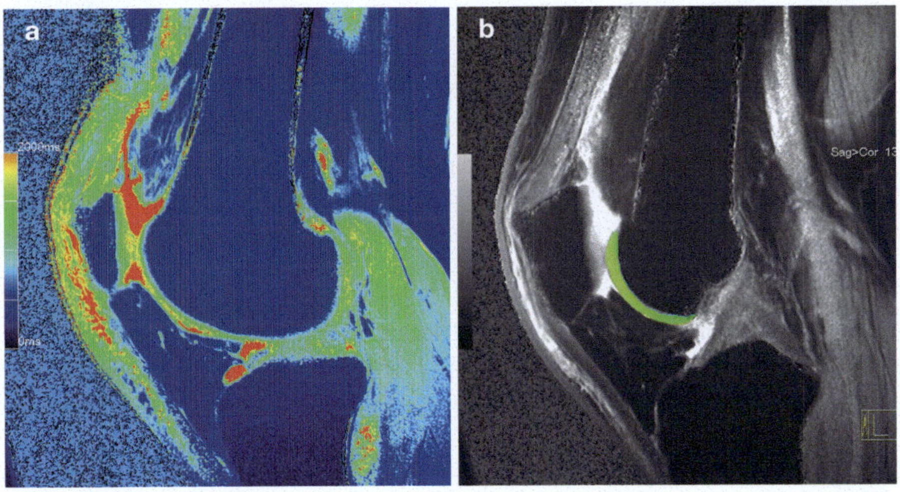

Fig. 1.88 (**a**) T1 map of a knee: color representing the calculated T1. (**b**) Color overlay on specified regions may add additional information to the acquired anatomic image

sequence. The signal decay analyzed pixel-by-pixel echo-by-echo will enable to calculate the average T2 value for each voxel (Fig. 1.89). The value can be used to control the color and intensity of a T2-map that can be fused with the anatomic image. The T2 value has been used to study cartilage repair therapies. T2 provides changes in the water content of the cartilage. Compressed areas show less water content (shorter T2) as compared to less compressed areas with higher water content (longer T2).

T2* Mapping

As introduced in Sect. 1.1.2.6, T2* is the apparent transverse relaxation rate when using spoiled gradient-echo techniques. Since T2* is also a function of T2, it can be used as a substitute for T2-mapping. A T2 estimation is usually correlated with a longer measurement time, as compared to the acquisition enabling a T2* estimation. Similar to the spin-echo approach, the technique utilizes a multiecho gradient-echo imaging sequence. The signal

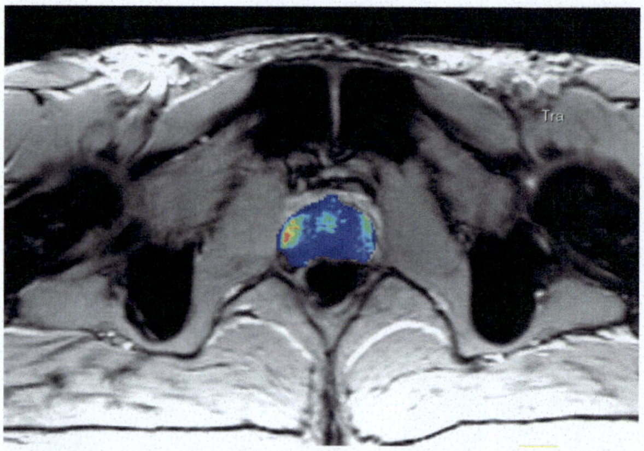

Fig. 1.89 T2 map through the prostate region, which can potentially be used as a colored overlay providing additional information or enhancing existing information

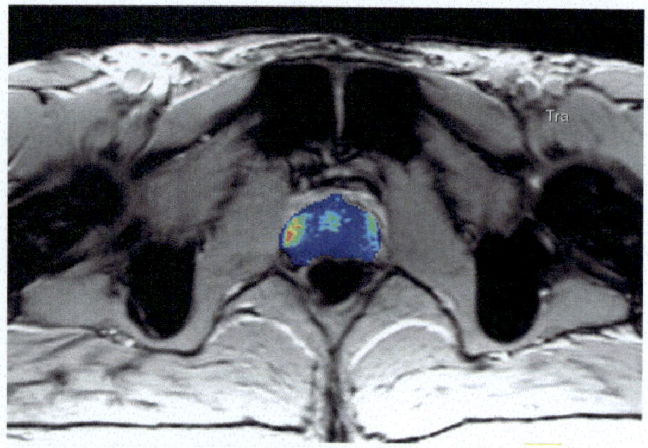

Fig. 1.90 T2* mapping of the prostate gland: a colored overlay representing the calculated T2* value provides additional information to the acquired image

decay from echo to echo allows the calculation of a T2* value on a voxel-by-voxel case. The retrieved value can be used to control the color and intensity of appropriate overlay (Fig. 1.90).

1.3.5 Techniques in Cardiac Imaging

The time-consuming acquisition of multiple Fourier lines usually takes too long to capture the motion of the beating heart. Exceptions are EPI techniques and recently developed "real-time" trueFISP sequences. For all other imaging techniques, image acquisition is triggered or gated with physiological signals from ECG electrodes or a pulse sensor. The advantage of the time-of-flight effect of inflowing blood, creating a hyperintense signal appreciated in MRA, turns into a disadvantage for certain cardiac applications and is compensated with a so-called "dark blood" magnetization preparation scheme.

1.3.5.1 ECG Gating: Prospective Triggering and Retrospective Cardiac Gating

In order to get a "frozen" image of the beating heart, the Fourier lines for the slices to be imaged have to be taken at the same point in time within the cardiac cycle. The starting point for a multislice measurement of T1-WIs acquired with conventional spin-echo sequences is estimated prospectively based on the advent of the ECG signal as illustrated in Fig. 1.91. As a practical hint, the acquisition of a stack of slices should be moved toward the end of the cardiac cycle in order to minimize motion artifacts.

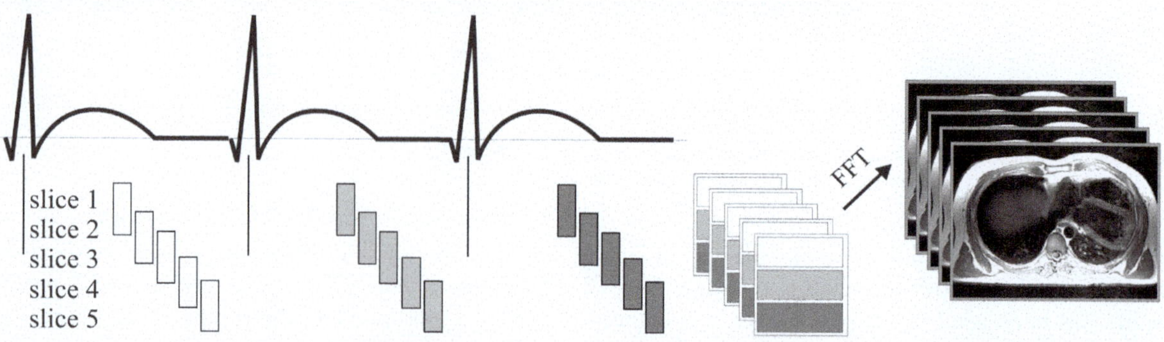

Fig. 1.91 Prospective ECG-triggered multislice acquisition. For simplicity, the *k*-space consists of only three Fourier lines (three different *gray-shaded boxes*) in this illustration. The usual matrix size requires 128 Fourier lines. One Fourier line is measured per heart beat. Multiple slices can be measured within one heart beat. Measurement should take place in end-diastole to minimize motion artifacts

With the introduction of fast low-angle shot imaging (FLASH) and other gradient-echo techniques, it became possible to reduce the TR to e.g., 40 ms and lower, allowing the acquisition of time-resolved images of the beating heart. Figure 1.92 illustrates the prospective triggering previously described as well as the retrospective cardiac gating approach. For the latter, Fourier lines are measured for the same phase-encoding step with the selected TR of the sequence and are stored together with a time stamp of the last ECG event. After completion of one or two cardiac cycles, the phase-encoding amplitude is advanced to measure the next Fourier line. Data are later normalized and resorted, and the user can select the temporal resolution, that is, the number of images that he would like to have calculated for one cardiac phase. The advantage of retrospective cardiac gating is that the cardiac cycle is covered completely, without any gap in time, whereas for prospective triggering there is a gap between the last measurement and the beginning of the next measurement with the next ECG event. The disadvantage of retrospective cardiac gating is the sensitivity to extrasystolic events and arrhythmic heart beats. The measurement may become invalid if such an event occurs when the center of *k*-space is being acquired.

1.3.5.2 Segmentation and Echo Sharing

In order to reduce the measurement time down to one breath-hold period, the concept of "segmentation" was introduced. Instead of measuring one Fourier line per heart beat per cardiac phase, multiple Fourier lines are measured (Fig. 1.93). For example, for a 126*256 matrix and a *k*-space that is split up into nine segments, nine Fourier lines are measured per heart beat per cardiac phase, one line for each *k*-space segment. The measurement time will last one heart beat for the preparation scan, and 14 heart beats are needed to fill up the *k*-space (14 × 9 = 126). Fifteen heart beats are well tolerated for a breath-hold period.

The benefit of suspended breathing will result in a crisper representation of the myocardial border, but there is a price to pay. For a gradient-echo sequence with a bandwidth of 195 Hz/pixel, the minimum measurement time for one Fourier line is approximately 9 ms. With nine segments to be measured, this represents a temporal resolution of 81 ms. In order to reestablish the temporal resolution, the measurement of one segment, the segment containing the low *k*-space frequencies, is placed between the measurements of

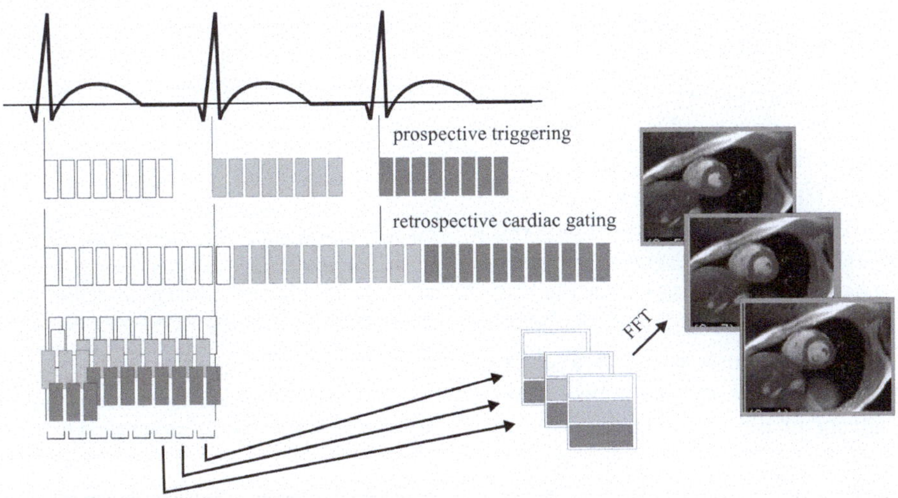

Fig. 1.92 Prospective ECG-triggered single-slice acquisition and retrospective cardiac gating. In this illustration, the *k*-space consists of only three Fourier lines (three different *gray-shaded boxes*). The usual matrix size requires 128 Fourier lines. In prospective triggering, one Fourier line is measured per heart beat per cardiac phase. In retrospective cardiac gating, the same Fourier line is measured continuously well beyond the time of a cardiac cycle. The Fourier lines are later normalized and resorted. The temporal resolution is given by the number of images per cardiac cycle as selected by the user. Images are reconstructed based on interpolated and weighted Fourier lines measured within the given time segment

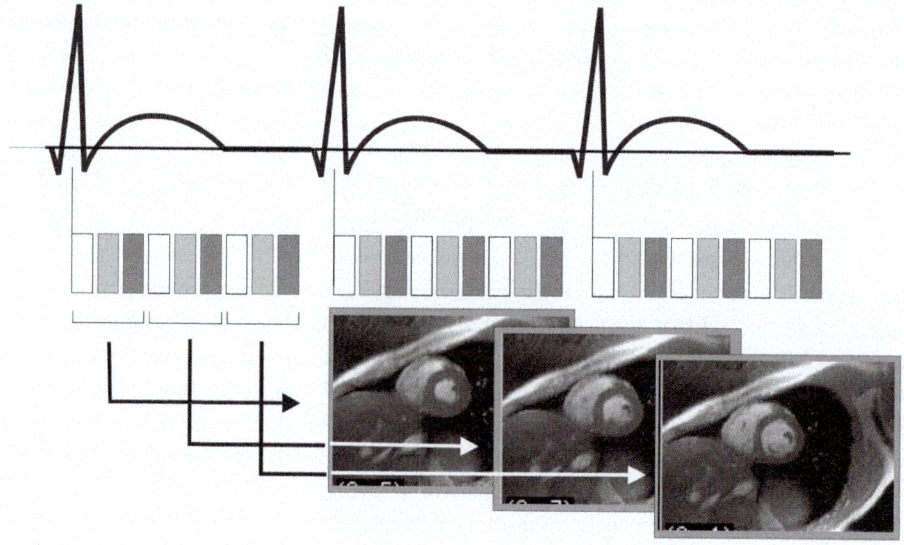

Fig. 1.93 Prospective ECG-triggered "segmented" acquisition within a breath-hold. For reasons of simplicity, the illustration shows a *k*-space divided into three segments. One Fourier line is measured per segment per heart beat per cardiac phase. The typical situation would be a *k*-space divided into nine segments. For a 126 matrix size, this would require 14 heart beats to fill the 14 Fourier lines within each of the nine segments (9*14 = 126)

adjacent cardiac phases as illustrated in Fig. 1.94, and while sharing the Fourier lines of adjacent measurements, a true image of another cardiac phase can be reconstructed. This leads to an overall temporal resolution of, e.g., 57 ms.

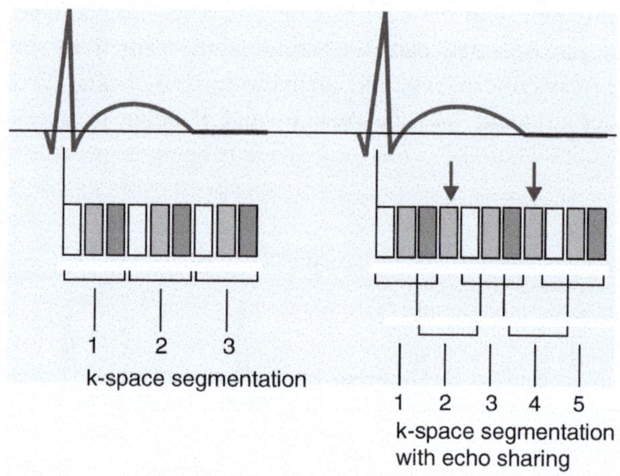

Fig. 1.94 Prospective ECG-triggered "segmented" acquisition within a breath-hold with "echo sharing." For reasons of simplicity, the illustration shows a *k*-space divided into three segments. One additional segment, containing the lower *k*-space frequencies, is measured in between the *k*-space segments of adjacent cardiac phases (indicated by the *arrows*). As illustrated, "sharing" the information contained in the adjacent cardiac phases will allow the reconstruction of an additional cardiac phase, leading to an improved temporal resolution

1.3.5.3 "Dark Blood" Preparation

The inflow of unsaturated blood into the imaging slice or slab has been utilized in MRA to display the vasculature. In cardiac imaging, the hyperintense blood in conjunction with phase changes due to motion and acceleration causes severe flow artifacts in conventional spin-echo imaging. With the introduction of T2-W imaging within a breath-hold with fast spin-echo, a sophisticated solution has been presented and dubbed "dark blood" preparation. As illustrated in Fig. 1.95, the sequence starts with a nonselective inversion of all the magnetization, followed immediately by a selective reinversion for the slice to be imaged. This all takes place with the advent of the ECG signal, where the heart is still in end-diastole. During the waiting period to follow, the reinverted blood is washed out of the slice and is replaced by inverted, saturated blood. As the heart is moving into diastole, the TSE acquisition starts, producing "dark blood" images. T2-W imaging of the beating heart within a breath-hold is a single-slice technique.

1.3.5.4 Coronary Artery Imaging

Coronary artery imaging started with a single-slice gradient-echo imaging approach, using the same effect as utilized in 2D-ToF-MRA. The sequence was triggered and segmented, and the data acquisition was placed in

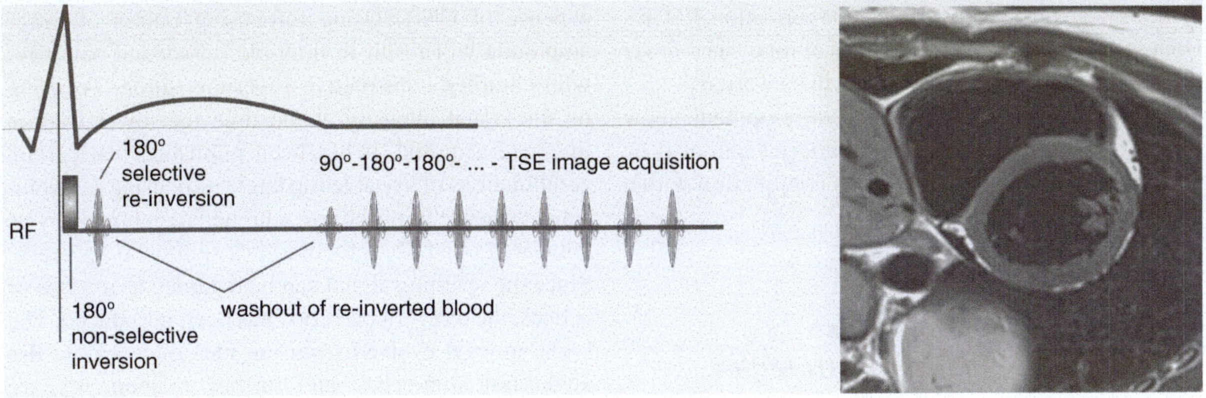

Fig. 1.95 "Dark blood" preparation scheme. With the detection of the QRS complex within the ECG signal, a nonselective RF inversion pulse is executed, immediately followed by a selective "reinversion" for the slice to be imaged. During a waiting period, the reinverted blood is washed out of the slice and is replaced by inverted blood. The TSE image acquisition to follow will produce a "dark blood" image. Shown is a short-axis perspective of the right and left ventricle surrounded by epicardial fat

end-diastole, where the heart moves less and where the flow within the coronaries is supposed to be maximal. The usual degree of segmentation allowed data acquisition within 11 heart beats. A further refinement was implemented using variable flip angles, that is, low flip angles for the first Fourier lines to be measured per heart beat followed by increased flip angles for the subsequent k-space segments. This approach compensated for saturation effects during data acquisition. Searching for coronary arteries with a single-slice approach is cumbersome, lengthy, and often not convincing. Questionable areas often remain questionable. A 3D approach is needed for retrospective reconstruction of the coronary vasculature. A 3D approach using similar parameters is too slow to be performed within one breath-hold period. A solution was presented using a so-called navigator technique as illustrated in Fig. 1.96. The "navigator," a sagittal 2D slice or rod is placed through the liver to monitor the position of the liver/lung interface, and a 3D gradient-echo sequence slab is placed where the proximal parts of the coronary arteries are expected. While the 3D data set is executing the measurement of the same Fourier line multiple times, the data for the "navigator" is collected immediately afterwards. If the position of the liver/lung interface indicates "close to expiration," the Fourier line of the 3D data set is accepted, otherwise it is waived. The position of the liver/lung interface can also be used prospectively to correct the position

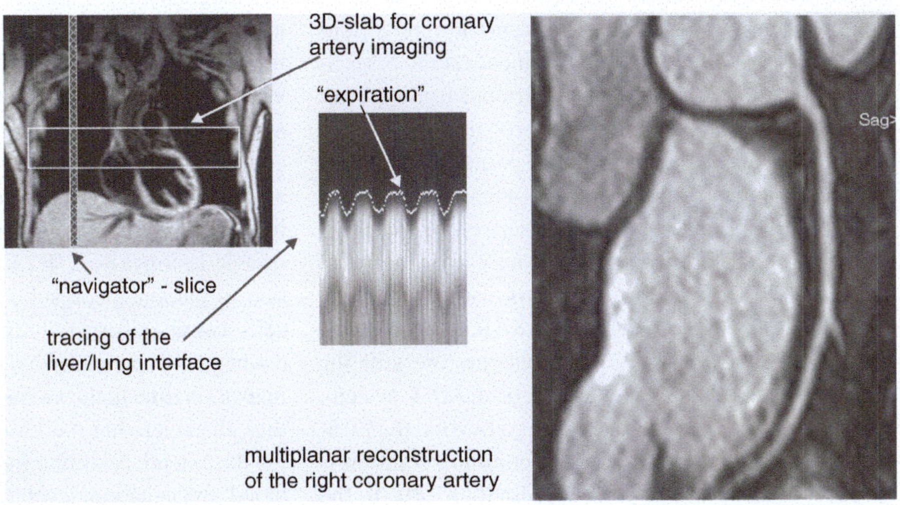

Fig. 1.96 The "navigator" technique. A 2D-slice or rod is placed across the liver/lung interface to monitor the respiratory cycle. A 3D-ToF-MRA slab is placed across the coronary arteries. The position of the liver/lung interface is evaluated, and the 3D slab is moved prospectively and/or is taken as information to reject/accept the Fourier line for the 3D data set

of the 3D slab (prospective acquisition correction, PACE). Doing so will reduce the measurement time since fewer Fourier lines of the 3D acquisition will be waived.

Recent advances in sequence development show that 3D imaging of the coronary arteries can also be performed within a breath-hold, in conjunction with a T1-shortening contrast agent.

1.3.6 High Magnetic Fields and SAR Reduction Strategies

As already indicated in Sect. 1.1.4.1, in a first approximation the SNR scales with the field strength. A more elaborate explanation, which finally leads to the same conclusion, is that the noise voltage spectral density coming from the patient is proportional to the field strength. The induced signal depends on the change of the magnetization d*M*/d*t* in front of the receiving coil. d*M*/d*t* is proportional to the resonance frequency and the amount of transverse nuclear magnetization *M*. The resonance frequency is proportional to field strength B_0 and the nuclear magnetization is proportional to field strength B_0, thus the signal increases with the square of the field strength. As the noise is proportional to field strength, the signal-to-noise scales linearly with field strength, which is the main reason why a higher field strength is desirable. There are some undesirable reasons to go to higher field strength, besides the correlated increase in cost for the system: As the SNR is improved, so is the signal intensity of motion-related artifacts of moving strong signal emitting structures like fat and blood flow. As the patient's geometry is getting close to the wavelength of the utilized RF, electromagnetic interactions are leading to B_1-field inhomogeneities. As the SAR as discussed in Sect. 1.2.1.3 is proportional to the power of two for the resonance frequency of the MR system utilized. The above mentioned three points are currently the focus of technological developments in order to make high field imaging more attractive. While imaging at 3 T can theoretically provide a twofold improvement in SNR compared to 1.5 T, it is also burdened by a fourfold increase in RF power (SAR). It has to be pointed out that the safety requirements are still the same whether it is a 1.5 T system or a 3.0 T system. Measures will have to be taken that go beyond the measures discussed in Sect. 1.2.1.3. A common solution is the use of refocusing pulses with less than 180° to the expense of CNR. Using refocusing pulses of lower amplitude will result in multiple refocusing pathways with complex constructive superimposition. Focusing on the signal intensity at the time the lower *k*-space lines are acquired, it has been published that certain combinations of variable flip angle refocusing fast spin-echo sequence may achieve a higher signal intensity as compared to a fully refocused fast spin-echo sequence. Since the resulting signal can be regarded as a echoe of echoes, the term "hyperecho" has been introduced. The basic concept evolved from the idea of "variable flip angle fast spin-echo" and further refinements are called TRAPS and SPACE (Sect. 1.3.1.1). Another approach to reduce the RF power has been named VERSE – variable-rate selective excitation. The "Low SAR" pulses mentioned in Sect. 1.2.1.3 have the disadvantage of significantly prolonging the RF duration leading to longer echo trains, fewer slices for a given TR, and image quality degradation. The basic idea of VERSE is to use "short" RF duration at the beginning and the end of the RF pulse and use "long" duration only at the time of the expected B_1 peak of RF pulse, which usually appears halfway through the duration of a normal RF pulse. This will reduce the RF amplitude at a point in time where the SAR contribution is significant otherwise.

1.3.7 Artifacts in MRI

Artifacts are misrepresentations of tissue structures seen in medical images produced by patient motion and tissue heterogeneity, by intrinsic limitations of utilized methods, by inappropriate user interactions, and sometimes by system insufficiencies. These artifacts are caused by a variety of mechanisms, such as underlying physics, data acquisition errors, undersampling, truncation or compromised reconstruction algorithms. A number of artifacts have already been mentioned as a helpful aid to increase diagnostic confidence. The appearance of hemorrhagic lesions (Sect. 1.2.8.3) due to compartmentalization of paramagnetic substances inside intact red blood cells cause a susceptibility gradient within otherwise diamagnetic parenchyma, leading to a shorter T2* relaxation time in the vicinity causing blooming artifacts, thus characterizing the lesion and potentially exaggerating the extend. A similar mechanism allows fMRI, as the blood oxygenation level (Sect. 1.3.4.1) changes from deoxyhemoglobin (paramagnetic) to oxyhemoglobin (diamagnetic), changing the susceptibility gradient with respect to the diamagnetic surrounding causing signal alteration based on changes in T2* relaxation time. The identification of microbleeding is only possible due to an exaggerated visualization based on susceptibility weighting (Sect. 1.3.4.5). Susceptibility changes are also utilized to mark stem cells or to trace the position of interventional tools. Perfusion measurements in conjunction with paramagnetic or superparamagnetic contrast agents (Sect. 1.2.9.4) are only possible due to the induced changes in susceptibility, thus causing dynamic signal changes that can be used to derive perfusion-related parameters. The difference in resonance frequencies between carbon-bounded hydrogen nuclei and oxygen-bounded hydrogen nuclei, referred to as chemical shift, is causing an artificial signal loss in opposed-phase images, useful to characterize fat-containing benign lesions. This is just to remind that "artifacts" are sometimes desired. The annoying artifacts to be discussed as follows are numerous and are assigned to their origins as being patient-related, method-related, user-related or system-related artifacts.

1.3.7.1 Patient-Related Artifacts

Artifacts introduced by the heterogenous tissue composition of the patients are unavoidable, but can sometimes be reduced with the utilization of appropriate techniques. The four main topics are changes in magnetic susceptibilities at tissue boundaries, drastic jumps in susceptibility with the introduction of ferromagnetic foreign bodies, motion (blood flow pulsation, respiratory displacement, and peristalsis), and fancy phenomenon like the "Magic Angle" effect.

Susceptibility Artifacts

The abbreviated title should have been "exaggerated signal voids due to artificial shortening of T2* relaxation time as a consequence of significant local magnetic field inhomogeneities due to local changes in tissue-related magnetic susceptibility." The local change in magnetic field strength is in this case also referred to as a susceptibility gradient. The Larmor frequency is used to identify the position of the signal. As the Larmor frequency is also changing with the locally experienced magnetic field strength, which in turn is a function of the local magnetic susceptibility of the tissue, the image will be distorted. The signal from tissue experiencing an elevated magnetic field will be misassigned the another location based on the frequency information, causing a hyperintense area in the direction of frequency encoding, as apparent in the orbital frontal areas as illustrated in Fig. 1.97. The significance of this part of the artifact is a function of the selected imaging bandwidth. The higher the bandwidth, the smaller the artifact. The second part of the artifact is presented by a signal void. This signal void is based on the previously mentioned misassignment using SE and GRE imaging techniques, plus an additional signal void in GRE imaging. The extent of the latter artifact is given by the T2* sensitivity of the imaging protocol and the selected spatial resolution. The signal void is a function of the dephasing of the signal based on the frequency range of the transverse magnetizations within the voxel due to the local magnetic field inhomogeneity. The signal within a smaller voxel will experience less dephasing as the frequency range covered will also be small. A high spatial resolution will cause a moderate appearance of the artificial signal void as compared to a

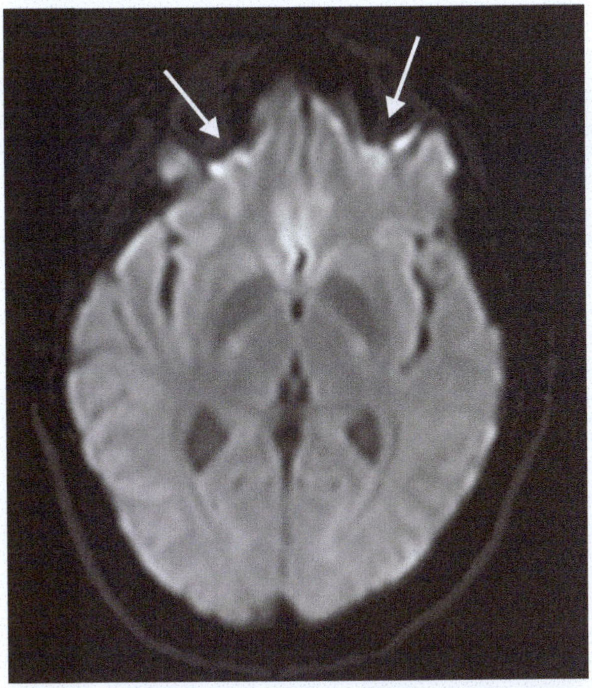

Fig. 1.97 Susceptibility gradients at the orbitofrontal cortex lead to signal void and distortions in heavily T2*-sensitive imaging methods. Arrows point to the artificial signal enhancement and incorrect assignment of location due to the susceptibility based shift in resonance frequency and the nonlinear representation of voxel size

protocol utilizing a low spatial resolution. A GRE with a short TE, usually correlated with a high bandwidth for the frequency encoding, will present only minor artifacts as compared to a GRE with a prolonged TE. The most T2*-sensitive imaging protocol is utilizing a single-shot multiecho gradient-echo sequence, also referred to as echo-planar imaging (EPI). As EPI is used as a readout module following the preparation of the transverse magnetization with diffusion-weighting magnetic field gradients, the significant signal voids at the base of the skull, as a consequence of significant magnetic susceptibility gradients, are well known (Fig. 1.98). A reduction in T2* sensitivity will also lead to an artifact reduction. Reducing the echo-train length of an EPI protocol by utilizing parallel imaging will help to reduce the artifacts.

Foreign Bodies

The introduction of foreign bodies always introduces susceptibility-related artifacts as the material is rarely diamagnetic. In general, the same discussion of susceptibility-related artifacts is applicable to foreign bodies. If the foreign bodies are of metallic nature, they will show different artifacts depending on whether they are only conductive or whether they are conductive and ferromagnetic. In the latter case, the effect of conductivity is usually negligible. It has been demonstrated that even "nonmagnetic," meaning only slightly paramagnetic, conductive material will demonstrate artifacts due to induced currents by switching of magnetic field gradients. The appearance of stent grafts as used in endovascular surgery has been changing over the last years to accommodate the increasing utilization of ceMRA not only for the diagnosis, but also for the follow-up examination to verify stent patency. Some older stents were clearly slightly ferromagnetic, causing a correlated signal void beyond the location of the stent graft. The next-generation stents were made of slightly paramagnetic material, barely visible mainly due to the RF shielding effect (Faraday shield), causing the lumen to appear slightly hypointense as compared to the bright vessel (Fig. 1.99). Newer stent generations are almost invisible on ceMRA studies, allowing an uncompromised diagnosis of vessel patency.

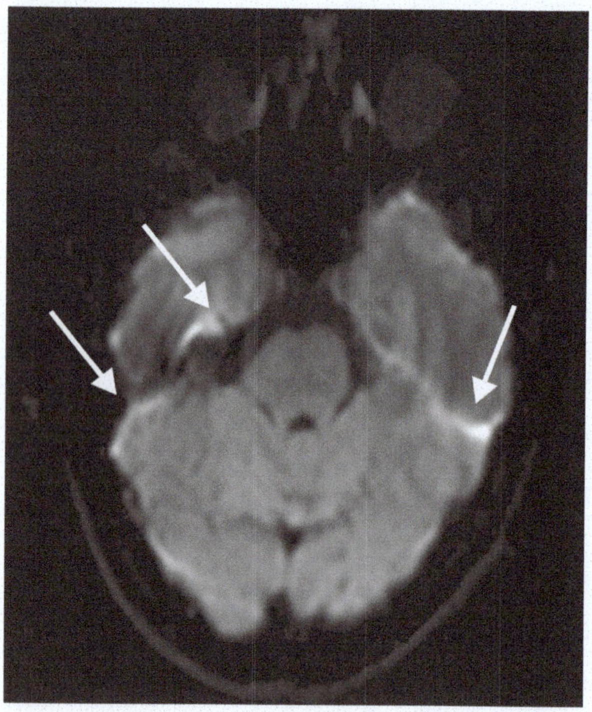

Fig. 1.98 Susceptibility gradients at the base of the skull lead to signal void and distortions in heavily T2*-sensitive imaging methods . Arrows point to the artificial signal enhancement and incorrect assignment of location due to the susceptibility based shift in resonance frequency and the nonlinear representation of voxel size

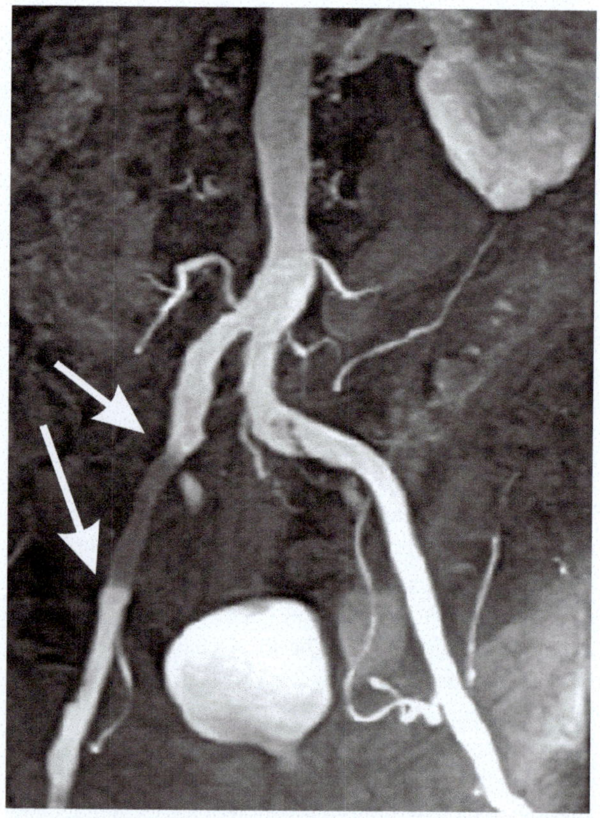

Fig. 1.99 Appearance of a nonferromagnetic but conductive stent in MRI (*arrows*)

Any foreign body comprising ferromagnetic material, whether as dental implant or bone screw, will locally increase the magnetic field strength and will distort the homogeneity of the magnetic field far beyond its origin. Correlated with the increase in field strength, the signal response will have an accordingly higher Larmor frequency being misassigned to a location of a frequency that the system expects in the presence of the applied magnetic field gradient. The consequence is the assignment of the signal to a wrong location as demonstrated in Fig. 1.100c (permanent ferromagnetic eye shadow). Less visible, but as dramatic, is the distortion of the selected slice. The excitation plane is defined by the frequency range of the excitation pulse and the linear course of the magnetic field established by the slice-select magnetic field gradient. This linearity is dramatically distorted by metallic foreign bodies. Ferromagnetic foreign bodies will slightly change the frequency distributions even for remote locations, causing steady-state free precession sequences like trueFISP, CISS, bFFE, or FIESTA to demonstrate complex destructive interference pattern within the image (Fig. 1.100a).

Flow and Motion

With no countermeasures, any motion in the presence of magnetic field gradients will induce phase shifts in the signal causing a local misassignment within the image. Any displacement of the signal origin during the measurement will conflict with the process of spatial encoding causing blurring or misassignment due to altered phase- or frequency information. Any repetition of signal pattern within *k*-space will produce a ghost of whatever is causing the repetition (Fig. 1.101). As the repetitive pattern usually takes place with respect to phase encoding, the ghosts will appear in the direction of phase encoding. Averaging will help, as long as the averaging procedure is not harmonic with the repetitive pattern (breathing or heart rate). Utilizing "long-term averaging" might be an alternative. In order to avoid motion artifacts due to breathing, use a respiratory belt for triggering or gating, or use the discussed navigator techniques (Sect. 1.3.3.6) for respiratory triggering or gating. The difference between triggering and gating is that triggering will start a partial measurement and will stop at the predefined measurement duration whereas gating usually continuously measures but executes data sampling only within a predefined window of the motion indicating scale.

The "Magic Angle"

The T2 relaxation time of tissue depends on the mobility of the signal contributing water molecules. Rapid tumbling tends to average out dipole–dipole (internuclear) interactions that otherwise can substantially shorten the T2 relaxation time, the reason why no signal is observed from an ice cube when using clinically feasible TEs. The level of interaction between the two

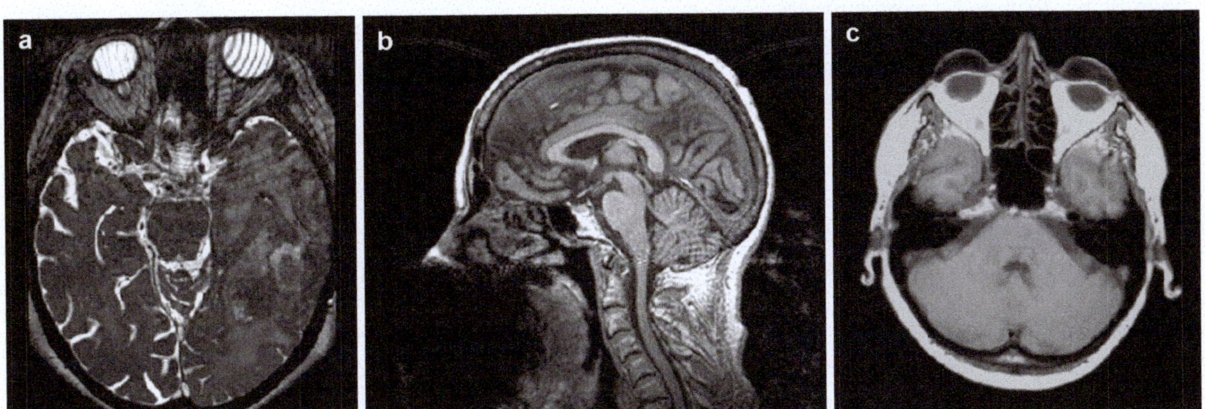

Fig. 1.100 "Metal" artifacts. (**a**) For trueFISP techniques, metal does not even have to be inside the imaging slice to cause severe artifacts. The *dark lines* are results of a destructive interference pattern caused by off-resonance effects due to ferromagnetic objects elsewhere. (**b**) The total signal void caused by ferromagnetic objects in conjunction with gradient-echo imaging is typical, as presented in this MP-RAGE case. (**c**) Even in spin-echo imaging, the displacement and distortion due to ferromagnetic components within the permanent eye shadow are obvious

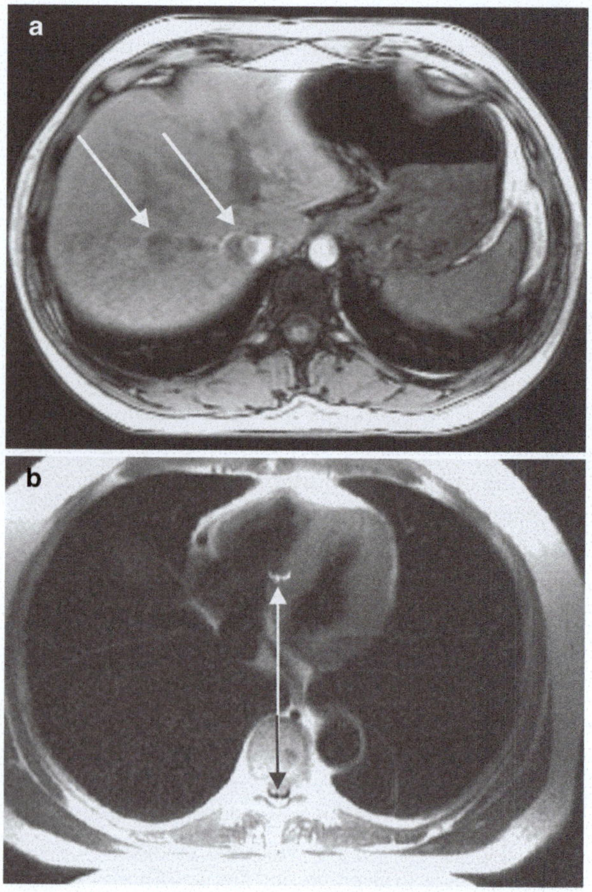

Fig. 1.101 The "pulsatility" artifact. Periodic pulsatile signal variations during data acquisition manifest themselves as multiple ghosts in the direction of phase encoding (**a**) demonstrates artifacts from pulsatile blood flow within the descending aorta. (**b**) shows a ghost originated within pulsatile liquor flow

dipols of the hydrogen nuclei attached to an oxygen atom (the internuclear interaction of the water molecule) can be calculated with respect to its orientation relative to the direction of the external magnetic field. It turns out that the term responsible for a signal reduction (short T2) disappears if the angle between the internuclear vector and the direction of the external magnetic field is equal to 54.74°. In the presence of highly ordered collagen microfibrils as to be found e.g., in tendons, the motion restriction will lead to an artificial signal increase (due to a prolonged T2 relaxation time) if the tendon or a tendon segment courses at or near 55° with respect to the direction of the main magnetic field. This angle is called the "magic angle." The magic angle effect is obvious on T1-WIs and is much less apparent on T2-W acquisitions. It is advised to prolong the TE to 35–45 ms in

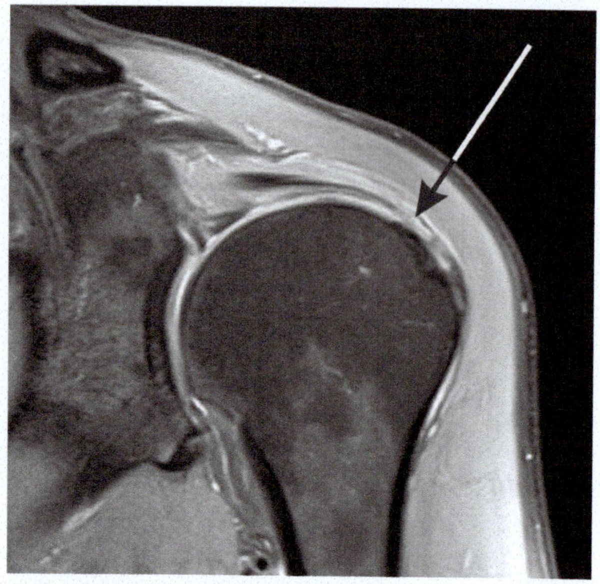

Fig. 1.102 The "Magic Angle" effect in musculoskeletal imaging might cause a hyperintense appearance of the distal portion of the supraspinatus tendon (*arrow*)

PD-W musculoskeletal imaging. This will allow a better visualization of fluid collections based on the slightly increased T2-W and it will reduce the appearance of the "magic angle" effect. Without this measure, e.g., the distal portion of a normal supraspinatus tendon may be presented with increased signal intensity (Fig. 1.102).

1.3.7.2 Method Related Artifacts

Chemical Shift

Chemical shift is the term for the frequency difference between the Larmor frequency of the spin of the hydrogen nuclei within a water molecule and the Larmor frequency of the spin of the carbon-bounded hydrogen nuclei within adipose tissue (Sect. 1.2.2). This difference in frequencies is utilized for spectral fat saturation (Sect. 1.2.3.3) or spectral inversion (Sect. 1.2.3.1) and in in-phase opposed-phase imaging, for the characterization of fat-containing lesions (Sect. 1.2.2.2). As the frequency information is used for spatial encoding, the "fat-image" is shifted relative to the "water-image." The shift is a function of the user-selected image bandwidth. The frequency difference for a 1.5 T system is about 217 Hz. The selection of an imaging bandwidth of 217 Hz/pixel, which is clinically reasonable, would

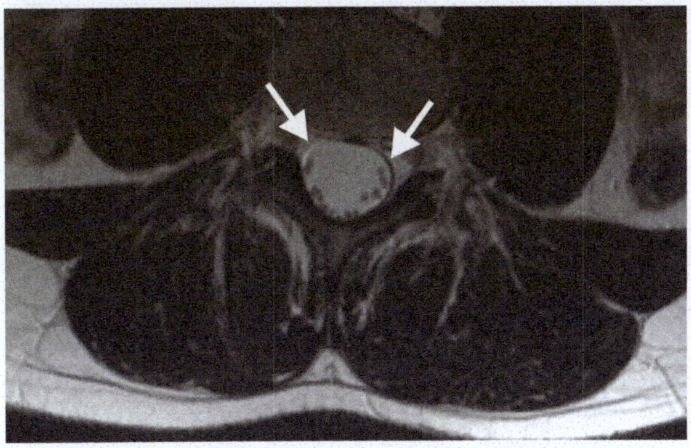

Fig. 1.103 Chemical shift artifact in transverse imaging of the lumbar spine

shift the fat image with respect to the water image exactly by one pixel. A bright rim will appear in the image, where the fat is assigned to a location that already contains signal contributions from the water image, and at the opposite end of the adipose tissue, a dark rim will indicate a location where no water signal is present and the fat at that location has been assigned to a different image position based on the received signal frequency (Fig. 1.103). These misassignments have been named “chemical shift artifacts.”

It might be confusing at first, but the phase-encoding direction has a bandwidth too. In fact, analyzing how frequency differences are identified by the system, it will become obvious that frequency encoding and phase encoding are basically the same. In EPI, the phase encoding is done with gradient blips of relatively low, constant gradient amplitude in the direction of phase encoding throughout the duration of the echo train. In both cases, the bandwidth in the direction of phase encoding is very low causing a significant chemical shift artifact in the direction of phase encoding. For this reason, a good fat suppression is mandatory in EPI protocols.

Truncation

The one-dimensional Fourier transformation of a rectangular object will give an infinite number of spatial frequencies that, combined again (another Fourier transformation) will reproduce the appearance of the (in this case, one-dimensional) rectangular object. As an infinite number is impractical, the truncation of the data or the incomplete sampling will have its consequences on the image appearance. If the selected spatial resolution is too poor to represent correctly high contrast transitions, there will be so called “edge ringing” as high spatial frequency components are missing. These artifacts are well understood and are called truncation artifacts. In general, today’s selected spatial resolution is high enough for truncation artifacts being negligible. Truncation artifacts have sometimes a renaissance in ceMRA. The selected spatial resolution may be high enough to accurately represent the vessels in question. But the truly measured spatial resolution depends on the time the contrast bolus has been present during data sampling, which might sometimes be the case only for part of the *k*-space, which is equivalent to a reduced or asymmetric matrix size. The often appearing “dissection” of, e.g., the pelvic arteries in ceMRA acquisitions is in fact a truncation artifact (Fig. 1.104).

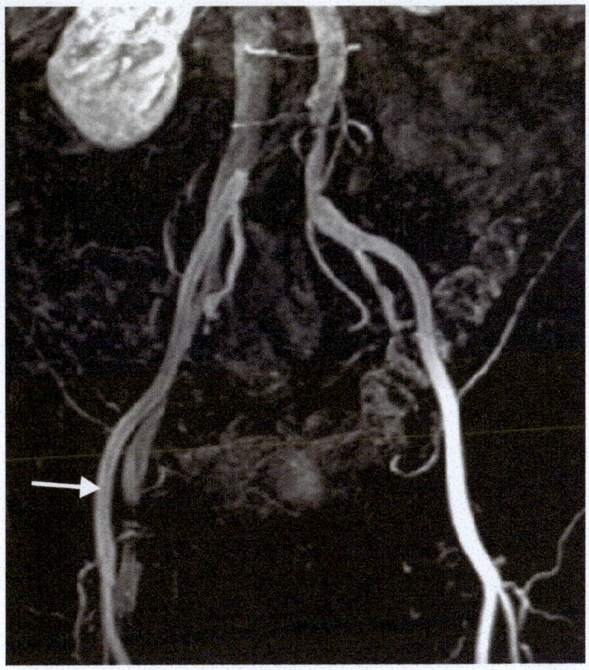

Fig. 1.104 The “truncation” artifact. A reduced matrix size and a suboptimal timing between bolus arrival and start of the ceMRA measurement may result in a “truncation” artifact mimicking a dissection

1.3.7.3 User Related Artifacts

Wrap-Around Artifacts

Data acquisition is done by sampling the induced voltage of the rotating transverse magnetization with

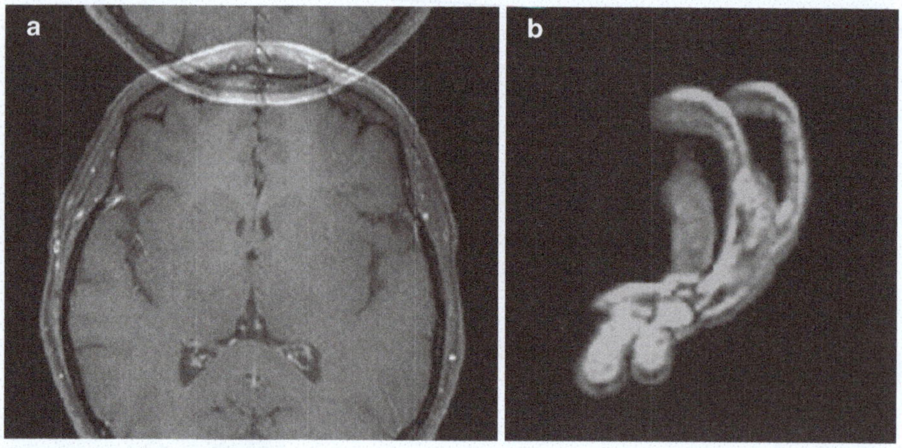

Fig. 1.105 "Aliasing" artifacts: for a selected FoV being smaller than the object (**a**), for an object that extends beyond the 3D slab of an MPRAGE measurement ((**b**), left and right ear show up as wrap-in-artifact into the outer partitions)

a sufficient temporal resolution in order to identify all frequencies to be assigned to a location within the field of view. It can easily be shown that the frequency of a signal source outside the field of view is crossing the identical sampling spots of a lower frequency (at the opposite end) within the field of view. As a result, the signal position outside the field of view will be assigned to the opposite position within the field of view, causing the so called wrap-around artifact or overfolding techniques (Fig. 1.105a). Doubling the sampling rate will allow the correct identification of the signal source of twice the field of view. As doubling the sampling rate in the direction of frequency encoding has no noticeable consequences (for the user), it is usually activated by default, the reason why an overfolding effect in the direction of frequency encoding is hardly observed. Any additional sampling in the direction of phase encoding will proportionally increase the measurement time, something less desired. Wrap-around artifacts are well understood and easily circumvented, but they have an interesting renaissance with the introduction of parallel imaging techniques. In this case we have more complex wrap-around artifacts within the image that are less easily identified as such.

External Interference

The signal induced by the rotation of transverse nuclear magnetizations within the patient's body is pretty weak and the RF coils have to be very sensitive. Unfortunately, the covered frequency range is close if not identical to the RF frequencies used for radio transmission or to frequencies sporadically emitted from any electrical device that is not shielded. For this reason, the room with the scanner has always a copper "wallpaper" and a door that is designed to block any RF. If the door is left open or if the door has a defect or somebody damaged the copper-shield, the incoming frequencies will show up as streak artifacts perpendicular to the direction of frequency encoding (Fig. 1.106). The same appearance might show up in case of a non-MR compatible electric device being moved into the RF cabin.

1.3.7.4 System Related Artifacts

Spikes

Every point within *k*-space represents a spatial frequency and the value of that point in *k*-space indicates the intensity of the spatial frequency within the image to be displayed. Any misrepresentation of any point within *k*-space will show up as a fish-bone appearance within the image. Misrepresentation of single *k*-space points are called "Spikes." They can be due to a discharge of loaded plastic material (patient clothing, support cushion, coil cover), a loose connection within the gradient or RF system, or an improper or defective room illumination. The image appearance depends on the time of spike occurrence in *k*-space. If the spike is located in the outer part of *k*-space, there will be a settle sometimes barely

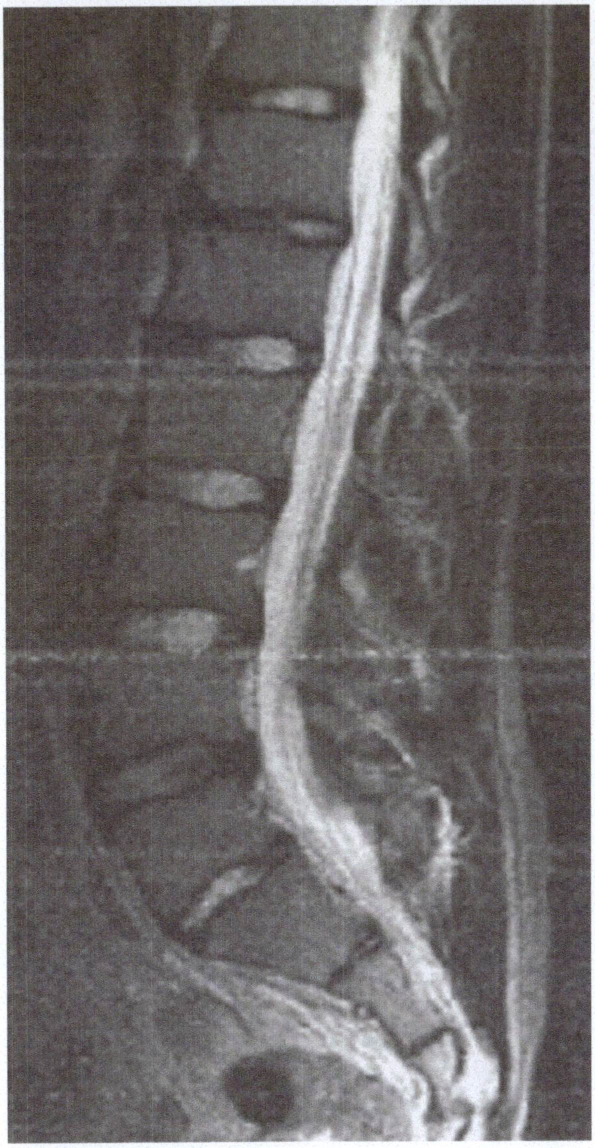

Fig. 1.106 Typical appearance of an external interference. The door has been left open and the detected frequencies have no phase correlation, thus appearing as streaks in the direction of phase-encoding

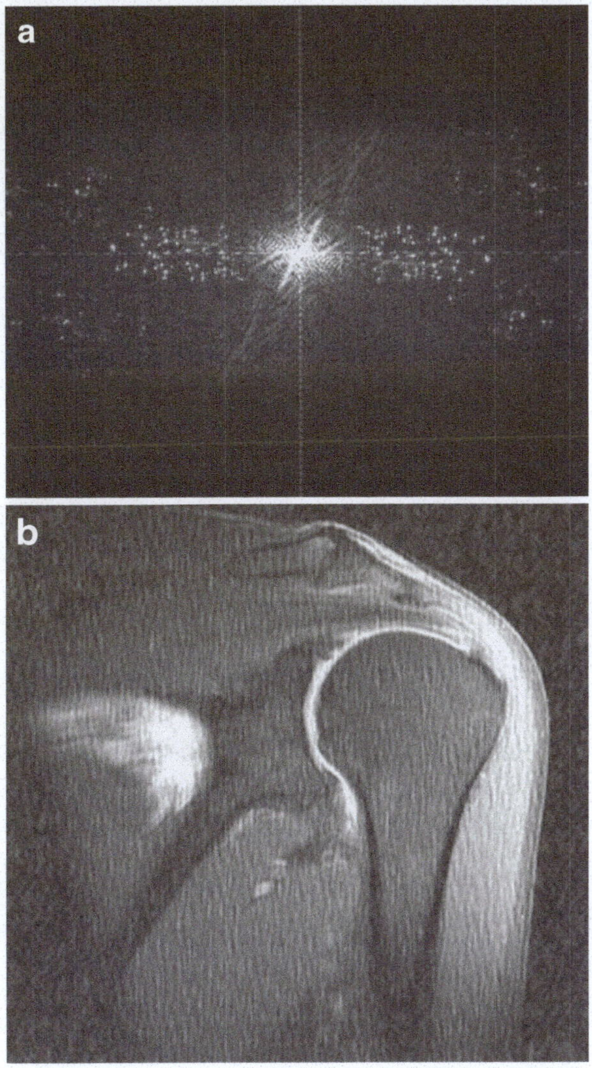

Fig. 1.107 "Spike" – or herring bone artifacts. (**a**) The *k*-space has been generated retrospectively by applying a Fourier-transformation to the image. As the *k*-space is symmetric any spike causing the artifact within the image will show up in all four quadrants, although might have appeared in only one of them (**b**) A coronal study of the shoulder with "spikes" within *k*-space (electrical discharge within RF cabin)

noticeable intensity oscillation across the image (Fig. 1.107). If the spike is appearing close to the center of *k*-space, the imaged anatomy will barely be identified.

Misadjustments

Considering the maturity of today's scanner, misadjustments are rare. With the significant increase in the utilization of steady-state free precession sequences like trueFISP, FIESTA, or bFFE, it should be noted that these imaging techniques are very sensitive to minor frequency misadjustments of the scanner. This might lead to the shown destructive interference pattern (Fig. 1.108). As for all artifacts, if the image appearance is suspected to be artificial, utilizing a different method to image the same region usually clarifies.

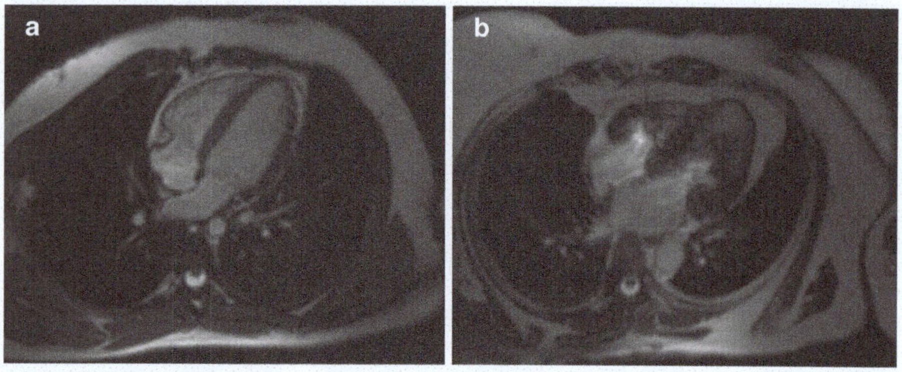

Fig. 1.108 (**a**) A trueFISP acquisition of the long axis of the heart, as it should appear. (**b**) A trueFISP image of a healthy volunteer, but with a slightly misadjusted frequency with the resulting image mimicking myocardial hypertrophy

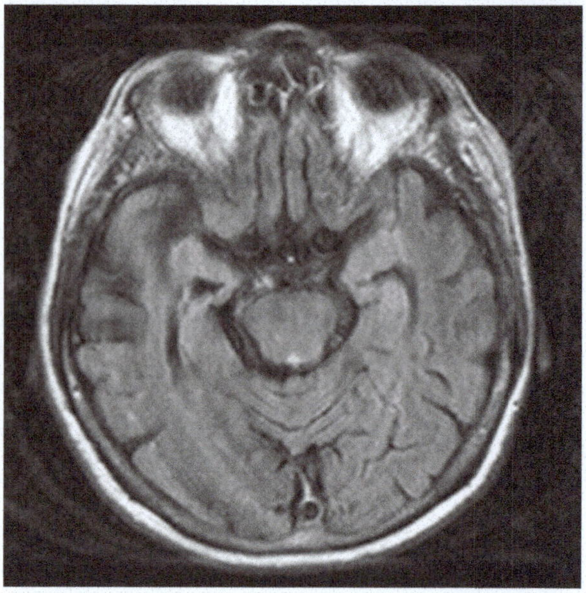

Fig. 1.109 System instabilities (e.g., sporadic changes in the RF excitation amplitude) mimicking an incooperative moving patient

System Instabilities

Theoretically, there are a significant number of potential system deficiencies. On the other hand, no vendor will survive in view of system insufficiencies that frequently interfere with image quality (or patient throughput). Unfortunately, the majority of malfunctions, e.g., inconsistent reproduction of magnet field gradient amplitudes or lack of RF amplitude reproducibility will cause image artifacts similar to incooperative moving patients (Fig. 1.109). Imaging the provided phantom will clarify the situation. If the stationary phantom shows breathing artifacts, a service call is justified.

Further Reading

American College of Radiology (2008) Manual on contrast media, version 6 www.acr.org/contrast-manual. Accessed 13 December 2009

Barbier EL, Laurant L, Décorps M (2001) Methodology of brain perfusion imaging. J Magn Reson Imaging 13:496–520

Boyden TF, Gurm HS (2008) Does gadolinium-based angiography protect against contrast-induced nephropathy? A systematic review of the literature. Catheter Cardiovasc Interv 71(5):687–693

Broome DR (2008) Nephrogenic systemic fibrosis associated with gadolinium-based contrast agents: a summary of the medical literature reporting. Eur J Radiol 66(2):230–234

Bui-Mansfield LT (2006) Top 100 cited AJR articles at the AJR's Centennial. AJR Am J Roentgenol 186(1):3–6

Edelman RR (2004) Contrast-enhanced MR imaging of the heart: overview of the literature. Radiology 232(3):653–668

Emerson J, Kost G (2004) Spurious hypocalcemia after Omniscan- or OptiMARK-enhanced magnetic resonance imaging: an algorithm for minimizing a false-positive laboratory value. Arch Pathol Lab Med 128(10): 1151–1156

European Society of Urogenital Radiology (2007) ESUR guidelines on contrast media, version 6.0. ESUR, Vienna

Goyen M, Debatin JF (2004) Gadopentetate dimeglumine-enhanced three-dimensional MR-angiography: dosing, safety, and efficacy. J Magn Reson Imaging 19(3): 261–273

Huppertz A, Balzer T, Blakeborough A, Breuer J, Giovagnoni A, Heinz-Peer G, Laniado M, Manfredi RM, Mathieu DG, Mueller D, Reimer P, Robinson PJ, Strotzer M, Taupitz M, Vogl TJ (2004) European EOB Study Group. Improved detection of focal liver lesions at MR imaging: multicenter comparison of gadoxetic acid-enhanced MR images with intraoperative findings. Radiology 230(1):266–275

Kanal E, Barkovich AJ, Bell C, Borgstede JP, Bradley WG Jr, Froelich JW, Gilk T, Gimbel JR, Gosbee J, Kuhni-Kaminski E, Lester JW Jr, Nyenhuis J, Parag Y, Schaefer DJ, Sebek-Scoumis EA, Weinreb J, Zaremba LA, Wilcox P, Lucey L, Sass N (2007) ACR Blue Ribbon Panel on MR Safety. ACR guidance document for safe MR practices. AJR Am J Roentgenol 188(6):1447–1474

Kanal E, Broome DR, Martin DR, Thomsen HS (2008) Response to the FDA's May 23, 2007, nephrogenic systemic fibrosis update. Radiology 246(1):11–14
Kirchin MA, Runge VM (2003) Contrast agents for magnetic resonance imaging: safety update. Top Magn Reson Imaging 14(5):426–435
Knopp MV, Balzer T, Esser M, Kashanian FK, Paul P, Niendorf HP (2006) Assessment of utilization and pharmacovigilance based on spontaneous adverse event reporting of gadopentetate dimeglumine as a magnetic resonance contrast agent after 45 million administrations and 15 years of clinical use. Invest Radiol 41(6):491–499
Kuhl C (2007) The current status of breast MR imaging. Part I. Choice of technique, image interpretation, diagnostic accuracy, and transfer to clinical practice. Radiology 244(2): 356–378
Kuhl CK (2007) Current status of breast MR imaging. Part 2. Clinical applications. Radiology 244(3):672–691
Le Bihan D, Mangin J-F, Poupon C et al (2001) Diffusion tensor imaging : concepts and applications. J Magn Reson Imaging 13:534–546
Lin SP, Brown JJ (2007) MR contrast agents: physical and pharmacologic basics. J Magn Reson Imaging 25(5):884–899
Miyazaki M, Lee VS (2008) Nonenhanced MR Angiography. Radiology 248:20–43
Prince MR, Arnoldus C, Frisoli JK (1996) Nephrotoxicity of high-dose gadolinium compared with iodinated contrast. J Magn Reson Imaging 6(1):162–166
Reiser MF, Semmler W, Hricak H (2007) Magnetic resonance tomography. Springer, Berlin
Rinck PA (2001) Magnetic resonance in medicine. Blackwell, Berlin
Rohrer M, Bauer H, Mintorovitch J, Requardt M, Weinmann HJ (2005) Comparison of magnetic properties of MRI contrast media solutions at different magnetic field strengths. Invest Radiol 40(11):715–724
Runge VM (2008) Notes on "characteristics of gadolinium-DTPA complex: a potential NMR contrast agent". AJR Am J Roentgenol 190(6):1433–1434
Saraste A, Nekolla S, Schwaiger M (2008) Contrast-enhanced magnetic resonance imaging in the assessment of myocardial infarction and viability. J Nucl Cardiol 15(1):105–117
Saslow D, Boetes C, Burke W, Harms S, Leach MO, Lehman CD, Morris E, Pisano E, Schnall M, Sener S, Smith RA, Warner E, Yaffe M, Andrews KS, Russell CA (2007) American Cancer Society Breast Cancer Advisory Group. American Cancer Society guidelines for breast screening with MRI as an adjunct to mammography. CA Cancer J Clin 57(2):75–89
Semelka RC, Helmberger TK (2001) Contrast agents for MR imaging of the liver. Radiology 218(1):27–38
Sieber MA, Pietsch H, Walter J, Haider W, Frenzel T, Weinmann HJ (2008) A preclinical study to investigate the development of nephrogenic systemic fibrosis: a possible role for gadolinium-based contrast media. Invest Radiol 43(1):65–75
Thomsen HS; European Society of Urogenital Radiology (ESUR) (2007) ESUR guideline: gadolinium-based contrast media and nephrogenic systemic fibrosis. Eur Radiol 17(10): 2692–2696
Weinmann HJ, Brasch RC, Press WR, Wesbey GE (1984) Characteristics of gadolinium-DTPA complex: a potential NMR contrast agent. AJR Am J Roentgenol 142(3):619–624
Zhang HL, Ersoy H, Prince MR (2006) Effects of gadopentetate dimeglumine and gadodiamide on serum calcium, magnesium, and creatinine measurements. J Magn Reson Imaging 23(3):383–387
Zhang Z, Nair SA, McMurry TJ (2005) Gadolinium meets medicinal chemistry: MRI contrast agent development. Curr Med Chem 12(7):751–778

Magnetic Resonance Imaging of the Brain

2

Paul M. Parizel, Luc van den Hauwe, Frank De Belder, J. Van Goethem, Caroline Venstermans, Rodrigo Salgado, Maurits Voormolen, and Wim Van Hecke

Contents

P. M. Parizel (✉)
Department of Radiology,
Antwerp University Hospital
and University of Antwerp,
Wilrijkstraat 10, 2650 Edegem, Belgium

P. Reimer et al. (eds.), *Clinical MR Imaging*,
DOI: 10.1007/978-3-540-74504-4_2,

2.1 Coils and Positioning

2.1.1 Coil Choice and Patient Installation

Magnetic resonance imaging (MRI) examinations of the brain can be performed with several coil types, depending on the design of the MRI unit and the information required.

- Traditionally, MRI examinations of the brain are performed with quadrature (i.e., circularly polarized) head coils. These volume coils are closely shaped around the head of the patient and usually present a so-called "bird-cage" configuration. Many coils are split in half, for easier patient access and positioning.
- Recently, phased-array head coils have become the standard of practice for state-of-the-art high-resolution MRI of the brain. Phased-array head coils contain multiple small coil elements, which are arranged in an integrated design which surrounds the head (e.g., 8-, 12- or even 32-channel head coils). Data from the individual coils are integrated by special software to compensate for the nonuniform distribution of the signal-to-noise ratio (SNR) between the peripheral and central parts of the brain. The major advantage of a multichannel, phased-array head coil is that it allows the application of parallel acquisition techniques (PAT), which can be used to speed up MRI. The concept is to reduce the number of phase-encoding steps by switching a field gradient for each phase-encoding step. Skipping, for example, every second phase-encoding line accelerates the acquisition speed by a factor of two. This is called the acceleration or PAT factor. The trade-off for this increased imaging speed is a decrease in SNR. Image reconstruction with PAT techniques is more complicated, and several algorithms have been described, depending on whether image reconstruction takes place before (SMASH, GRAPPA (generalized autocalibrating partially parallel acquisition)) or after (SENSE) Fourier transform of the image data.
- In MRI systems where the direction of the B_0 field is oriented perpendicular to the long axis of the body, e.g., open-design resistive or permanent magnet systems, solenoid head coils can be used. By diagonally crossing two solenoid wire loops, a CP head coil can be created to improve SNR.
- Surface coils are rarely used for brain imaging and are usually reserved for "special" applications: high-resolution imaging of the orbits or the temporomandibular joints (double-doughnut surface coil). One should keep in mind that phased-array coils are, in fact, a combination of multiple small surface coils.

For MRI examinations of the brain, the patient is placed in a supine position. Before the table is entered into the magnet, the patient must be correctly positioned in the head coil. Most MRI systems provide laser cross-hairs to assist in patient positioning. The narrow nature of the head coil may induce anxiety. Therefore, it is important that the patient feels comfortable. A pillow placed under the shoulders may be helpful. A wide field-of-view (FoV) mirror, placed on top of the coil allows the patient to see outside the magnet and reduces anxiety and claustrophobia. For some patients, sedation may be required and should be individually tailored.

2.1.2 Imaging Planes

An MRI examination of the brain begins with one (or more) fast localizer scans (also known as scout or survey images). For this purpose, we use fast sequences (obtained in seconds), and ideally obtain slices in three orthogonal imaging planes. On the basis of the initial localizer images, additional localizer scans are performed, if needed, until the operator is satisfied that imaging sequences can be started in true sagittal, coronal, or axial planes. On the coronal localizer image, a fast mid-sagittal acquisition is positioned. We then position our first series of axial scans on this image. Modern MRI scanners provide software that allows the user to position slices simultaneously on three localizer images. This permits multiple oblique slice orientations and obviates the need to obtain several sequential localizer scans.

The positioning of sagittal images is obvious, due to the left–right symmetry of the brain. Sagittal images are placed on a coronal localizer image if the head is not rotated. An axial plane can also be used, provided there is no left–right tilt of the head. In clinical practice, the positioning of sagittal images is self-explanatory. Ideally, on the midsagittal image, the following anatomical landmarks should be identified: corpus callosum (over its entire length), Sylvian aqueduct, fourth ventricle, and cervical spinal cord.

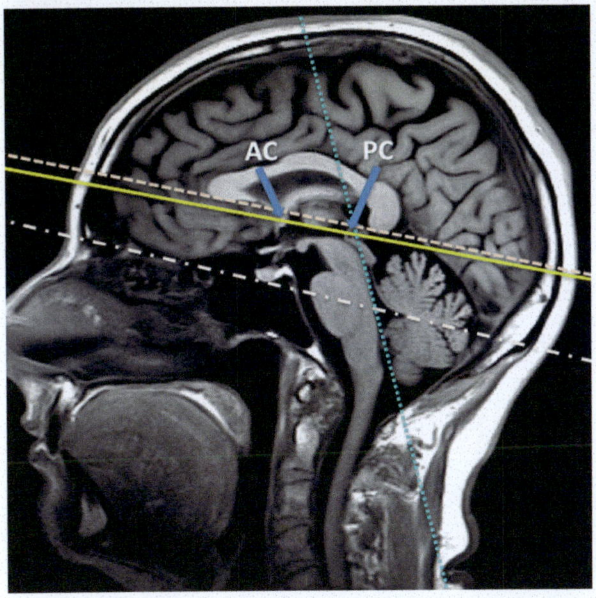

Fig. 2.1 Anatomic landmarks for positioning of axial slices. Axial slices should be positioned parallel to the bicommissural line, which links the anterior to the posterior commissure (*yellow line*). Alternatively, axial slices can be oriented parallel to a line linking the floor of the sella turcica to the fastigium of the fourth ventricle (*lower dotted line*). A third alternative solution is to position slices parallel to a line linking the inferior borders of the genu and splenium of the corpus callosum (*upper dotted line*). In most (adult) patients, these imaging planes differ by only a few degrees. For coronal scans, we prefer a plane parallel to the posterior surface of the brainstem (*blue dotted line*)

The plane of axial images should be parallel to the bicommissural line, which links the anterior to the posterior commissure (Fig. 2.1). Sometimes, this line may be difficult to identify on a low-resolution localizer image. There are two alternative solutions: (1) position the center of the slice group at the inferior borders of the genu and splenium of the corpus callosum or (2) use a plane parallel to a line linking the floor of the sella turcica to the fastigium (the highest point in the roof of the fourth ventricle). In most adults, these imaging planes differ only by a few degrees. It is important, however, to set a standard imaging plane, so that images obtained in follow-up examinations can be compared with the baseline study. Some vendors are nowadays implementing automatic alignment software, which provides reproducible slice positioning for the MRI of the head, without the need for manual adjustments. This maximizes standardization and comparability in follow-up MRI examinations of the same patient.

For coronal images, we typically choose a tilted plane, perpendicular to the long axis of the temporal lobes. This can be obtained by positioning the coronal slices on a midsagittal image, parallel to the posterior part of the brainstem (Fig. 2.1). For pituitary studies, the coronal images should be perpendicular to the sellar floor or tilted slightly backward (parallel to the pituitary stalk).

The choice of imaging planes should be determined by the clinical questions to be answered. For example, in a patient with optic neuritis, thin coronal fat-suppressed images through the orbits are useful for comparing the right and left optic nerves. To rule out hippocampal sclerosis in patients with intractable partial complex seizures, tilted coronal slices perpendicular to the long axis of the hippocampus are preferred; axial scans tilted parallel to the hippocampal axis may also be helpful. In a patient with multiple sclerosis (MS), subependymal white-matter lesions perpendicular to the ventricular surface ("Dawson's fingers") are particularly seen well on the sagittal images. Lesions within the corpus callosum are well depicted on the sagittal or coronal sections and may be difficult to see on axial scans.

2.1.3 Protocol for Routine MRI of the Brain

Imaging protocols for the brain should meet several criteria:

- They must address the clinical questions to be answered
- They must be complete and provide all the required information
- They must be as short as possible (to minimize the time the patient has to spend in the magnet and optimize patient throughput)
- They must be reproducible

Protocols should be standardized to ensure continuity over time. Frequent changes in imaging protocols should be avoided, since this may confuse the technologists operating the MRI equipment. Obviously, imaging protocols should be adapted to the equipment available.

As a general rule, MRI studies of the brain should include at least two imaging planes and two "weightings," and preferably more. Table 2.1 provides an overview of (some) standard sequences for MRI of the brain,

Table 2.1 Overview of some commonly used MRI sequences

FLAIR	• Standard sequence for lesion detection, especially in white matter • Less sensitive in the posterior fossa • Usually applied in axial and/or coronal imaging planes • Sagittal FLAIR is indicated in demyelinating disease • Often combined with fat saturation to avoid the "glare" of bright subcutaneous fat
FLAIR + Gd	• Indicated for the detection of leptomeningeal disease
PD/T2	• Proton density (first echo) can be used as an alternative to FLAIR, and is more sensitive for the detection of posterior fossa lesions • T2-WI (second echo) are a staple sequence for detection of long T2 lesions
DWI/ADC	• Is mandatory in all patients referred with a suspicion of stroke or cerebrovascular disease • Is indicated in the evaluation of cystic lesions (e.g., to differentiate abscess from necrotic tumor, or epidermoid from arachnoid cyst) • Is useful in trauma to detect diffuse axonal injury (DAI) and hemorrhagic lesions; findings on DWI are believed to correlate closely with outcome • Is indicated in brain tumors to assess cell density • The motto should be: "diffusion imaging for all patients"
SWI	• Sequence which combines magnitude and phase information • Useful for the detection of intracranial calcifications or hemosiderin deposits (cavernous malformations, hemosiderin deposits, DAI, …) • Is more sensitive for the detection of "microbleeds" than gradient echo T2*-WI
T2*	• Gradient echo sequence provides information about hemoglobin breakdown products and calcifications • Sensitivity to susceptibility effects is proportional to TE and field strength
T1±Gd	• Part of most routine brain imaging protocols • Usually applied in sagittal, axial or coronal imaging planes, depending on indication • Same imaging plane should be used before and after gadolinium-chelate injection
MP-RAGE, 3D SPGR (±Gd)	• Isotropic 3D T1-W sequence, allowing reformatting in other imaging planes • Provides excellent differentiation between gray and white matter • Indicated to detect migration disorders (e.g., gray matter heterotopia, etc.) • Less sensitive to enhancement as compared to SE or TSE T1-W sequences
Fat-sat T2, STIR	• Indicated to detect white matter-lesions in "difficult areas," e.g., in the optic nerve (optic neuritis)
TOF MRA	• Indicated to examine intracranial vessels and circle of Willis
Contrast-enhanced MRA	• Indicated in follow-up after endovascular aneurysm coiling • Allows for time-resolved angiography (separating afferent arteries and draining veins)

with their specific indications. The choice of the imaging sequence influences the look, signal intensity (SI), conspicuity, and even the size of a lesion. For example, vascular malformations or tumors can present a highly variable appearance, depending on the imaging parameters; this can be illustrated by applying different pulse sequences to a patient with a right parietal cavernous malformation (Fig. 2.2). Some clinically important lesions may remain undetected if the wrong imaging protocol is applied. Therefore, there is no such thing as an "ideal" imaging protocol, and there is not a single imaging protocol that befits all indications. The imaging strategy should be guided by the questions to be answered and the clinical information available. We use a set of standard imaging protocols for some of the most common indications (e.g., stroke, tumor, dementia, epilepsy, …). However, for difficult cases, or patients who do not fit into these broad categories, the imaging protocol should be individually tailored. Moreover, imaging protocols should be adapted to the available equipment (magnet, coils, sequences, software, etc.). Finally, there may be individual preferences.

A long repetition time (TR) sequence is still a standard part of most imaging protocols. This sequence can be obtained with either a spin-echo (SE) or turbo spin-echo (TSE) technique and provides proton-density weighted images (PD-WI) and T2-W images (T2-WI). They are used to detect intraparenchymal signal abnormalities. Most pathological processes in the brain result in increased water content (vasogenic edema, cytotoxic edema, necrosis, or cyst formation) and are therefore readily identified on T2-WI.

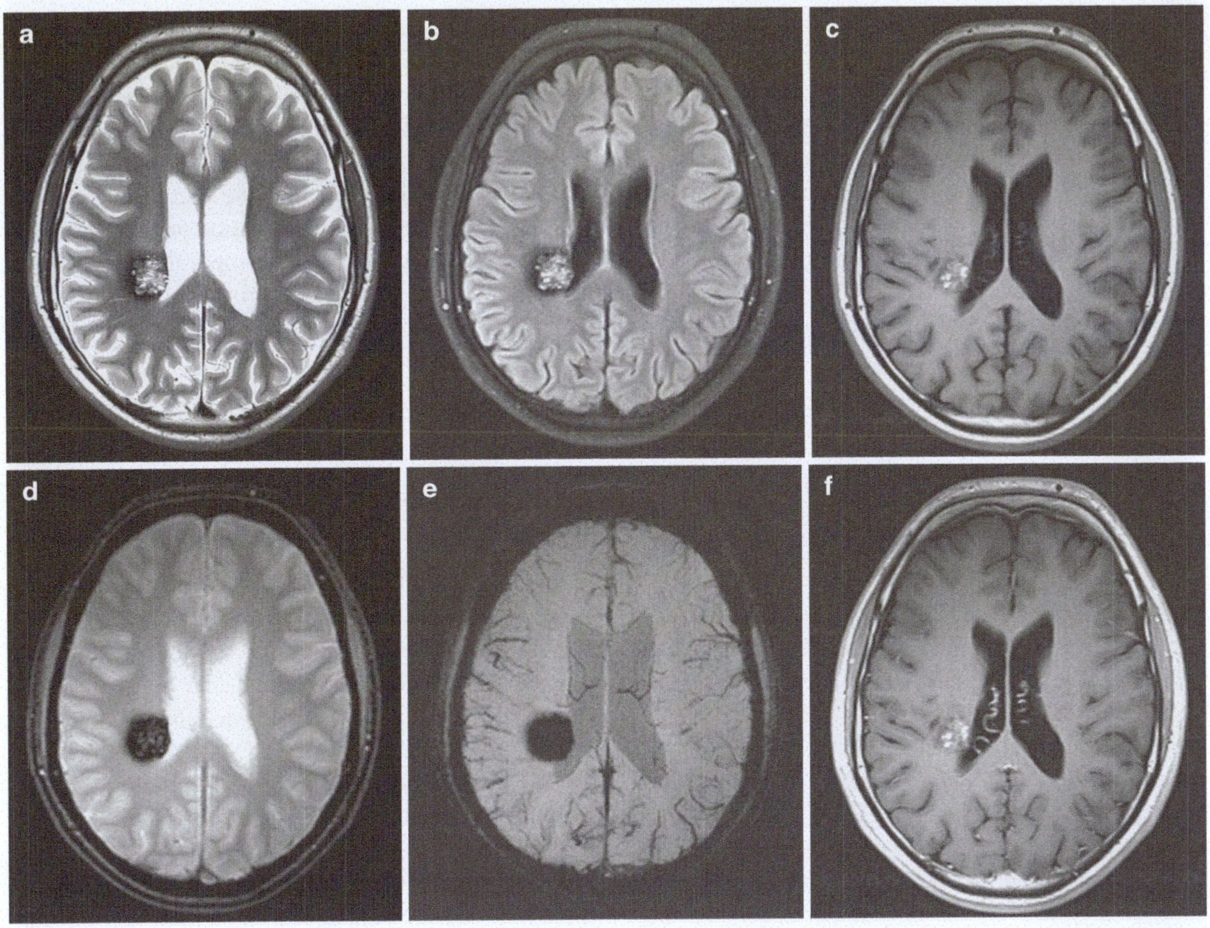

Fig. 2.2 Cavernous malformation: overview of imaging sequences. (**a**) Axial TSE T2-WI. (**b**) Axial fat-sat turbo FLAIR. (**c**) Axial TSE T1-WI. (**d**) Axial gradient echo FLASH T2*-WI. (**e**) Axial susceptibility-weighted image (SWI). (**f**) Gd-enhanced axial T1-WI. On T2 and FLAIR images, the cavernous malformation presents a characteristic "popcorn" appearance; the center of the lesion is inhomogeneous but predominantly hyperintense, and is surrounded by a hypointense halo, representing blood degradation products (hemosiderin). On TSE T1-WI, the cavernous malformation is predominantly hyperintense, and shows only minimal enhancement (compare (**c**) with (**f**)); the surrounding hypointense rim is not seen. On gradient echo T2*, and even more so on SWI, the lesion becomes almost completely hypointense; this is due to dephasing susceptibility effects caused by hemosiderin

Small high-SI lesions adjacent to the ventricles or subarachnoid spaces, e.g., periventricular white matter and cortical gray matter, may be missed on T2-WI, because they cannot be differentiated from the cerebrospinal fluid (CSF), which is also hyperintense. These lesions are better appreciated on PD-WI, where the lesions are hyperintense, but the SI from the CSF is diminished. An alternative is to use a T2-W sequence with dark CSF signal, such as fluid attenuated inversion recovery (FLAIR). In this T2-W sequence, the signal of CSF is attenuated by the use of a long inversion time, typically around 2,000 ms. FLAIR provides excellent contrast resolution at brain-CSF interfaces and improves the conspicuity of small white-matter lesions. Thus, in most modern imaging protocols, FLAIR and TSE T2-W sequences are used instead of the dual-echo PD-W and T2-W sequence.

The short TR/short echo time (TE) or T1-W sequence is used to evaluate the gross anatomy and structure of the brain. Moreover, T1-WI are often better for the anatomical definition of an underlying lesion (the increased signal of an intraparenchymal area of edema on T2-WI may obscure the underlying lesion). Following the intravenous injection of a paramagnetic contrast agent, T1-WI in two orthogonal planes should be obtained. Alternatively, a three-dimensional (3D) volume acquisition can be used, which permits reconstructions in multiple planes. Unenhanced and gadolinium (Gd)-enhanced images with the same thickness, positions, and parameters should be available for comparison in at least one imaging plane.

The effect of contrast agents can be potentiated using spectral fat-suppression techniques (e.g., in the orbit) or magnetization-transfer contrast techniques for background suppression (e.g., in MS). On most modern MRI equipment, magnetization transfer is a push-button option that is frequently used for most Gd-enhanced brain scans, except when thin slices are required, e.g., for the pituitary gland or internal auditory canal.

2.1.4 Spatial Resolution

Spatial resolution in an MR image is determined by slice thickness, FoV, and matrix size. These parameters define the size of a voxel (volume element). The slice thickness for routine MRI of the brain is usually between 3 and 5 mm, with an interslice distance of ≤1 mm. When imaging at 3 T, we routinely use 3 mm slices, whereas with a field strength of 1.5 T, a slice thickness of 5 mm is advocated to obtain sufficient SNR. Complete coverage of the brain, for example in the axial or sagittal plane, usually requires 25–35 slices. For a quantitative assessment of the number of lesions, as in MS trial protocols, a slice thickness of 3 mm or less is usually advocated. For a volumetric assessment of white-matter lesions or tumors, a 3D sequence should be employed.

In specific anatomic regions (pituitary gland, CP angle, and internal auditory canal), thin slices (0.5–3 mm) must be used. With 3D volume acquisitions, the dataset consists of a much larger number of thin slices (thickness ≤1.0 mm), e.g., magnetization-prepared rapid acquired gradient-echoes (MP-RAGE).

In-plane resolution is determined by FoV and matrix size. For routine adult MRI of the brain, we typically use an FoV of 230 mm (range 220–250 mm, depending on the size of the patient's head) and a matrix of 512 or 256, depending on sequence and equipment. Images with 512 matrix are preferable because they offer improved anatomic detail. More and more, for applications which require high spatial resolution, a matrix size of 1,024 is used. Images with higher in-plane spatial resolution can be obtained by increasing the matrix size (with constant FoV) or by decreasing the FoV (with constant matrix); however, increasing the spatial resolution results in decreased SNR, due to the smaller pixel size.

Rectangular FoV is routinely used in cerebral MRI in the axial and coronal imaging planes (*not* in the sagittal plane). In axial images, phase encoding is chosen left to right, to avoid superimposition of phase artifacts from eye movement on the temporal and occipital regions. The exception to this rule is axial diffusion-weighted images, where the phase encoding is placed in anterior to posterior direction.

2.1.5 Signal-to-Noise Ratio

Intrinsic SNR scales linearly with static magnetic field strength: high-field-strength magnets provide a proportionally higher SNR. However, due to hardware limitations, the actual SNR that can be achieved is somewhat lower than the intrinsic SNR gain. For a given magnetic field strength, the SNR can be improved by using state-of-the-art hardware. Phased-array head coils provide a higher SNR than quadrature CP head coils. SNR is also dependent on sequence parameters. For example, SNR is also proportional to the pixel size (FoV/matrix), slice thickness, and a number of acquisitions (N_{acq}), and is inversely proportional to the receiver bandwidth.

The SNR can be improved by increasing N_{acq}. SNR increases with $\sqrt{N_{acq}}$, whereas acquisition time increases linearly with N_{acq}. Thus, after increasing to four N_{acq}, it becomes relatively inefficient in terms of improving the SNR. Moreover, the probability of patient motion increases with longer imaging times.

The SNR for a particular examination can be optimized using sequences with a narrow bandwidth. This is commonly done at lower field strengths, where chemical-shift artifacts are less of a problem. At higher field strengths, mixed bandwidth sequences are useful with multi-echo sequences. The bandwidth for the second echo of a long TR sequence (T2-WI) is lower than that for the first echo (PD-WI). This improves the SNR on the longer TE images, where it is most needed.

Spatial resolution can be traded in for improvements in SNR. The larger the voxels, the better SNR is obtained. Therefore, in MR examinations of the brain, there is a trade-off between spatial resolution (slice thickness, FoV, matrix size) and SNR. The goal should be to find a voxel size that provides an adequate SNR for contrast resolution, yet is small enough to provide the necessary spatial resolution.

With phased-array head coils, the SNR is nonuniformly distributed throughout the volume examined, and a "normalization" process is required to compensate for SNR differences between the peripheral and central parts of the brain. When phased-array head coils are used in conjunction with PAT, the imaging speed increases, but SNR decreases by the square root of the acceleration factor. Furthermore, the image reconstruction process for a phased-array head coil with PAT may further reduce the SNR.

2.1.6 The Big Question: 1.5 or 3.0 T (or More)?

MRI of the brain at 3.0 T provides a higher signal-to-noise ratio and allows improved spatial resolution (thinner slices, higher matrix). A few years ago, when 3.0 T MRI of the brain was being assessed, there were some doubts whether the improvements in image quality had a clinically beneficial effect. These doubts have dissipated. MRI of the brain at 3 T is superior in detection and accurate characterization of structural brain lesions (Fig. 2.3). Compared with 1.5 T MR images, whole brain 3 T images are of better quality, can be performed with thinner slices, and offer superior SNR.

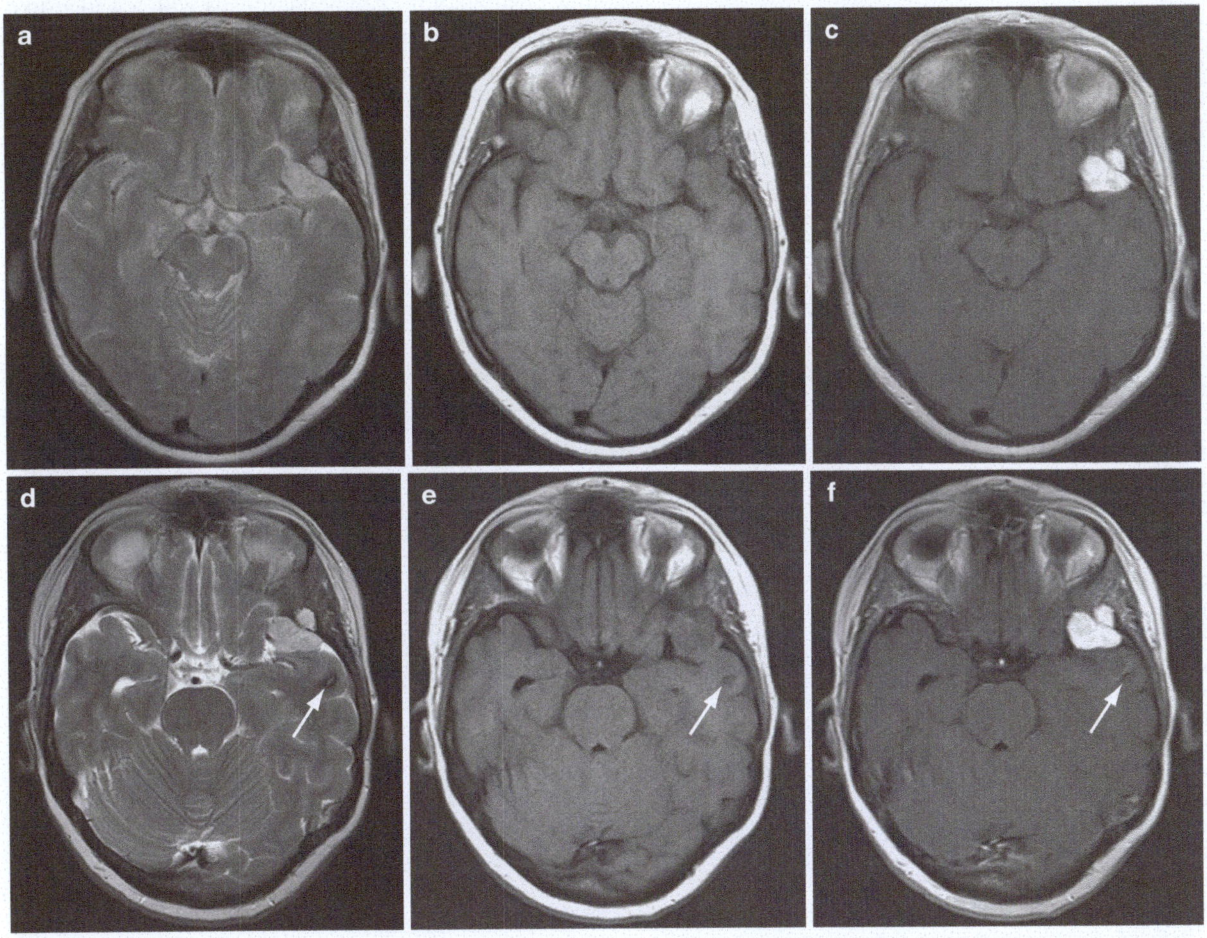

Fig. 2.3 Improved lesion detection on 3 T compared with 1.5 T MRI. (**a–c**) Imaging at 1.5 T, (**a**) Axial TSE T2-WI. (**b**) Axial TSE T1-WI. (**c**) Gd-enhanced axial T1-WI. (**d–f**) Imaging at 3.0 T, (**d**) Axial TSE T2-WI. (**e**) Axial TSE T1-WI. (**f**) Gd-enhanced axial T1-WI. The patient is a 50-year-old woman with a history of intractable focal epileptic seizures, originating in the left temporal lobe. MRI of the brain at 1.5 T, with a slice thickness of 5 mm, shows a sharply marginated and intensely enhancing meningioma of the greater wing of the sphenoid on the left, with intra-osseous extension. MRI of the brain at 3 T, with a slice thickness of 3 mm, reveals a small hypointense, nonenhancing cavernous malformation in the left temporal lobe, which is much more conspicuous at 3 T than at 1.5 T (*arrow*)

2.2 Congenital Disorders and Hereditary Diseases

Clinical suspicion of a developmental anomaly of the central nervous system (CNS) is a frequent indication for performing an MRI examination of the brain. For a more complete discussion of developmental abnormalities, the reader should consult Chap. 13.3.3. In the following paragraphs, we shall focus on practical guidelines for interpreting MRI studies in adult or adolescent patients with suspected congenital disorders.

2.2.1 Craniocervical Junction

The craniocervical junction (CCJ) is best appraised on sagittal images. Sagittal (T)SE T1-WI constitute an essential part of the imaging protocol, although sagittal T2-WI are also acceptable. Coronal sections are very useful as a second imaging plane for the CCJ.

On a midsagittal image, the level of the foramen magnum can be identified by drawing a line from the *basion* (lowermost portion of the clivus, anterior border of the foramen magnum) to the *opisthion* (free margin of the occipital bone which constitutes the posterior margin of the foramen magnum). Normally, the inferior pole of the cerebellar tonsils lies above or not more than 3 mm below this line. *Chiari type I* malformation is defined as a downward displacement of the cerebellar tonsils through the foramen magnum into the upper cervical spinal canal. When the tonsillar herniation is 5 mm or less, this condition is described as "tonsillar ectopia." In the true Chiari I malformation, tonsillar herniation exceeds 5 mm below the level of the foramen magnum. Sagittal MR images typically show a low position of the cerebellar tonsils with a wedge-like configuration of their most inferior aspect. The cisterna magna is obliterated. Cardiac-gated phase-contrast techniques are useful to assess the flow of CSF at the CCJ (Fig. 2.4). Chiari I malformation is commonly associated with syringohydromyelia (40–70%) and

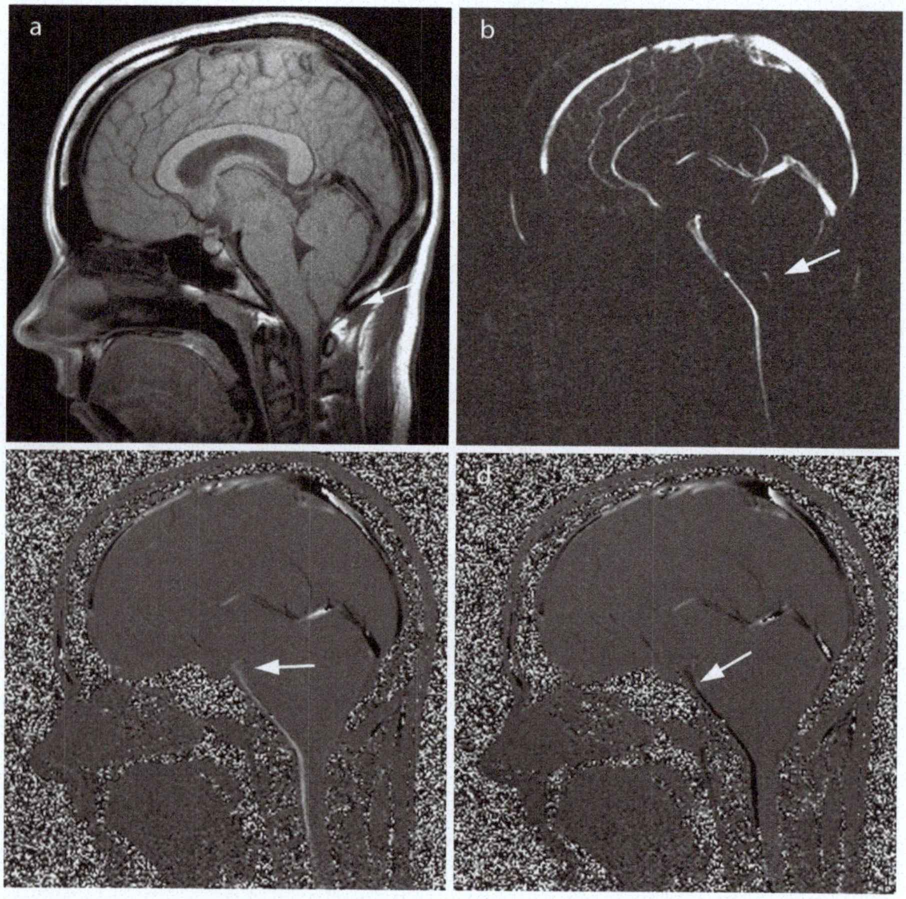

Fig. 2.4 Chiari I malformation with phase-contrast CSF flow study. (**a**) Midsagittal SE T1-WI. (**b**) Midsagittal ECG-triggered magnitude image. (**c**, **d**) Midsagittal ECG-triggered phase-contrast images during systole and diastole, providing directional flow information. There is a downward herniation of the cerebellar tonsils into the foramen magnum (*long arrow*) (**a**). The cisterna magna is obliterated and the magnitude image shows absence of CSF flow posteriorly (*short arrow*) (**b**). In the prepontine cistern and anterior cervical subarachnoid spaces, there is downward flow during systole and upward flow during diastole (*arrowhead*), as evidenced on the phase-contrast CSF flow quantification study

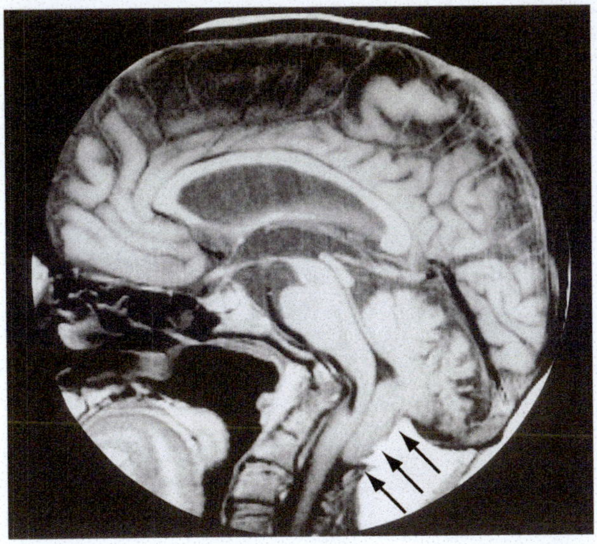

Fig. 2.5 Chiari I malformation with basilar invagination. This sagittal SE T1-WI shows downward displacement and peg-like configuration of the cerebellar tonsils (*arrows*). There is an associated osseous malformation of the skull base (platybasia). The tip of the odontoid is projected above the level of the foramen magnum

hydrocephalus (10–30%). The fourth ventricle is normal in size and position. In 20–30% of patients with Chiari I malformation, there is an associated osseous abnormality of the CCJ (platybasia or basilar invagination) (Fig. 2.5).

Chiari II malformation is a complex hindbrain-mesodermal malformation involving the entire neuraxis; it is most likely caused by a congenitally small posterior fossa (Fig. 2.6). The main imaging findings are: small posterior fossa with low tentorial attachment, compression of the hindbrain, indentation of the lower cerebellum by the foramen magnum or C1 and that of the upper cerebellum by the tentorium, and abnormality of the midbrain with tectal "beaking." Chiari II malformation is almost invariably associated with myelomeningocele. Hydrocephalus and a variety of other intracranial abnormalities are common.

Osseous abnormalities of the CCJ can be congenital (basilar invagination) or acquired (basilar impression). Primary developmental craniocervical dysgenesis includes conditions such as basiocciput hypoplasia, occipital condyle hypoplasia, abnormalities of C1–C2,

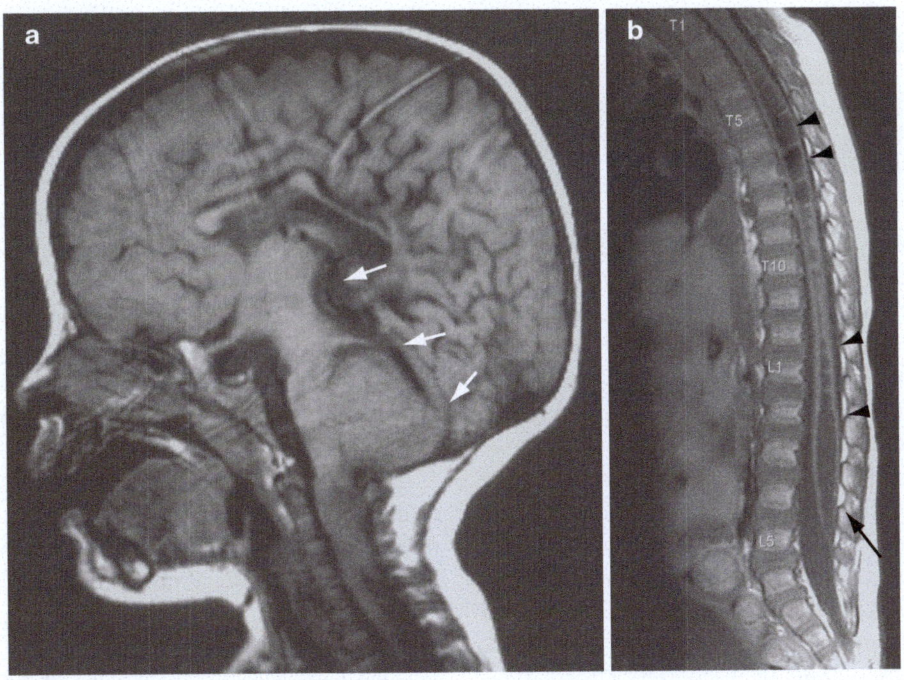

Fig. 2.6 Chiari II malformation. (**a**) Midsagittal SE T1-WI through the brain. (**b**) Midsagittal SE T1-WI through the thoraco-lumbar spine region. The patient is a 1-year-old boy after surgical repair of a myelomeningocele. At the level of the posterior fossa and craniocervical junction, the typical features of a Chiari II malformation are seen (*arrows*): beaking of the midbrain, small posterior fossa with low tentorial attachment, inferior displacement and narrowing of the fourth ventricle, downward displacement of the pons and medulla, and peg-like protrusion of the vermis with cervicomedullary kinking. The spinal cord is tethered by scar tissue (*long arrow*), and is widened by a segmented syringohydromyelia extending down to the low-lying conus medullaris (*arrowheads*)

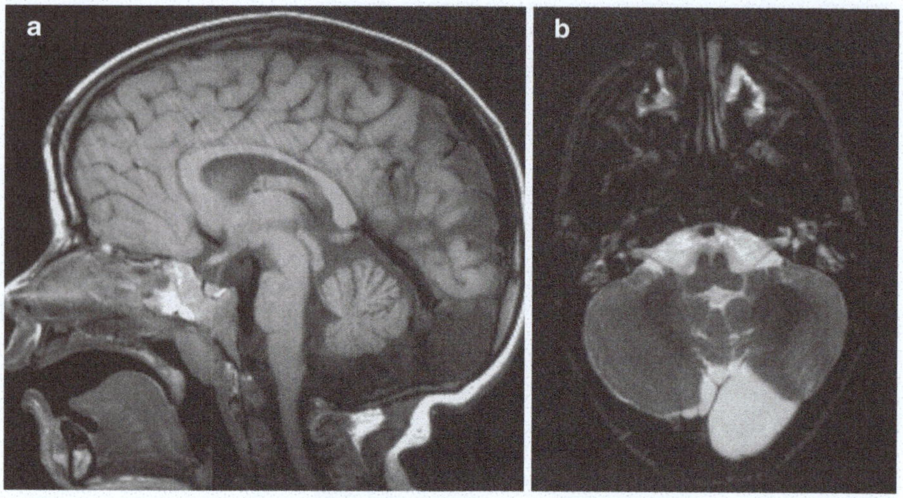

Fig. 2.7 Megacisterna magna or retrocerebellar arachnoid pouch. (**a**) Midsagittal SE T1-WI. (**b**) Axial SE T2-WI. The normally developed vermis and cerebellar hemispheres are associated with an enlarged cisterna magna, or retrocerebellar arachnoid pouch, which causes scalloping of the inner table of the occipital bone and mild enlargement of the posterior fossa. There is an incomplete and bifid falx cerebelli

Klippel-Feil syndrome, etc. Acquired basilar impression results from softening of the skull base, e.g., Paget's disease, osteomalacia, and rheumatoid arthritis. Achondroplasia is characterized by narrowing and deformation of the foramen magnum, short and vertical clivus, stenotic jugular foramina, hydrocephalus, and macrocephaly which occurs secondary to impaired venous outflow.

2.2.2 Posterior Fossa

The gross anatomic relationships of the posterior fossa contents are best evaluated on sagittal images. On a midsagittal image, the following anatomic landmarks should be recognized: mesencephalon, pons, medulla oblongata, fourth ventricle, cerebellar vermis, and foramen magnum, as defined by the line linking the basion to the opisthion.

Vermian-cerebellar hypoplasia is characterized by a small vermis and cerebellum with a prominent folial pattern, a large fourth ventricle, a large cisterna magna, and a wide vallecula. Vermian and/or cerebellar hypoplasia can be an isolated anomaly or occur in association with malformative syndromes.

Cystic malformations of the posterior fossa range from megacisterna magna, retrocerebellar arachnoid cyst, Dandy-Walker malformation, and Dandy-Walker variant. These entities may represent a continuum of posterior fossa developmental anomalies. They are sometimes referred to as the Dandy-Walker complex.

Megacisterna magna is a large CSF space posterior and inferior to the cerebellum, which is normally developed. There is no mass effect. It cannot be differentiated from a retrocerebellar arachnoid cyst (Blake's pouch), which is a collection of CSF not communicating with the fourth ventricle (Fig. 2.7). It is most commonly situated in the midline, behind the vermis. The thin membrane surrounding the cyst is usually not seen on imaging. The cerebellar hemispheres and vermis are normally developed, but may be compressed from behind. The inner table of the occipital bone may be scalloped. The size of the posterior fossa, the position of the tentorium and straight sinus are normal. However, the cyst, when large, may show a diverticulum-like extension through the splayed tentorium. In most instances, a retrocerebellar arachnoid cyst is an incidental imaging finding. The condition is usually asymptomatic.

Dandy-Walker malformation (Fig. 2.8) is characterized by three key features: (1) dysgenesis or agenesis of the cerebellar vermis, (2) cystic dilatation of the fourth ventricle, which balloons posteriorly, and (3) enlargement of the posterior fossa, with high position of the tentorial insertion ("torcular-lambdoid inversion"). Additional imaging features include scalloping of the inner table of the occipital bone and hypoplasia of the cerebellar hemispheres. Associated findings are: hydrocephalus, corpus callosum dysgenesis, and heterotopic gray matter.

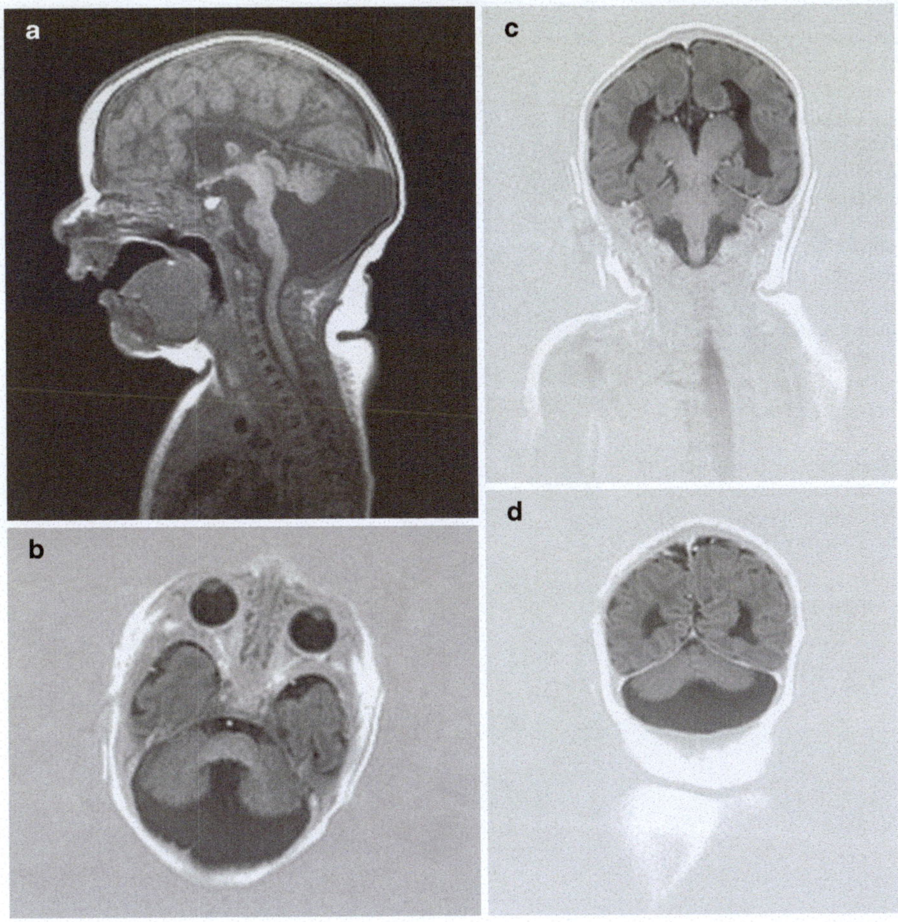

Fig. 2.8 Dandy-Walker malformation with agenesis of the corpus callosum. (**a**) Midsagittal TSE T1-WI. (**b**) Axial turbo IR T1-WI. (**c**, **d**) Coronal turbo IR T1-WI through the brainstem and posterior fossa. These images show the classic findings of a Dandy-Walker malformation: enlarged posterior fossa, high position of the tentorium, hypogenesis of the cerebellar vermis, and cystic dilatation of the fourth ventricle, extending below the cerebellum; which is pushed upward. Supratentorially, there is complete agenesis of the corpus callosum, with typical parallel orientation of the lateral ventricles, colpocephaly, and upward extension of the third ventricle into the interhemispheric fissure. The Dandy-Walker malformation is associated with 20–25% callosal agenesis

The term Dandy-Walker "variant" covers a heterogeneous group of atypical cystic posterior fossa malformations, for which common MRI findings include: cystic dilatation of the fourth ventricle, dysgenesis or hypoplasia of cerebellar hemisphere(s) and/or vermis. However, the posterior fossa is not enlarged, and the torcular is not elevated.

2.2.3 Supratentorial Midline Structures

On the midsagittal image, the corpus callosum constitutes an important anatomic landmark. It is the largest interhemispheric commissure and the most concentrated bundle of axons in the brain. It contains myelinated fibers linking left and right cerebral hemispheres. The corpus callosum is a firm structure and helps the ventricles maintain their normal size and shape. Anatomically, on the midsagittal image, four elements constituting the corpus callosum can be identified (from anterior to posterior): rostrum, genu, body (or truncus), and splenium. Embryologically, the corpus develops in anterior to posterior fashion (genu first, then body, then splenium), with the exception of the rostrum which forms last.

Agenesis of the corpus callosum can be partial or complete (Fig. 2.9–2.11). Axons that would normally cross the midline instead run along the medial wall of the lateral ventricles, and thereby form the bundles of Probst.

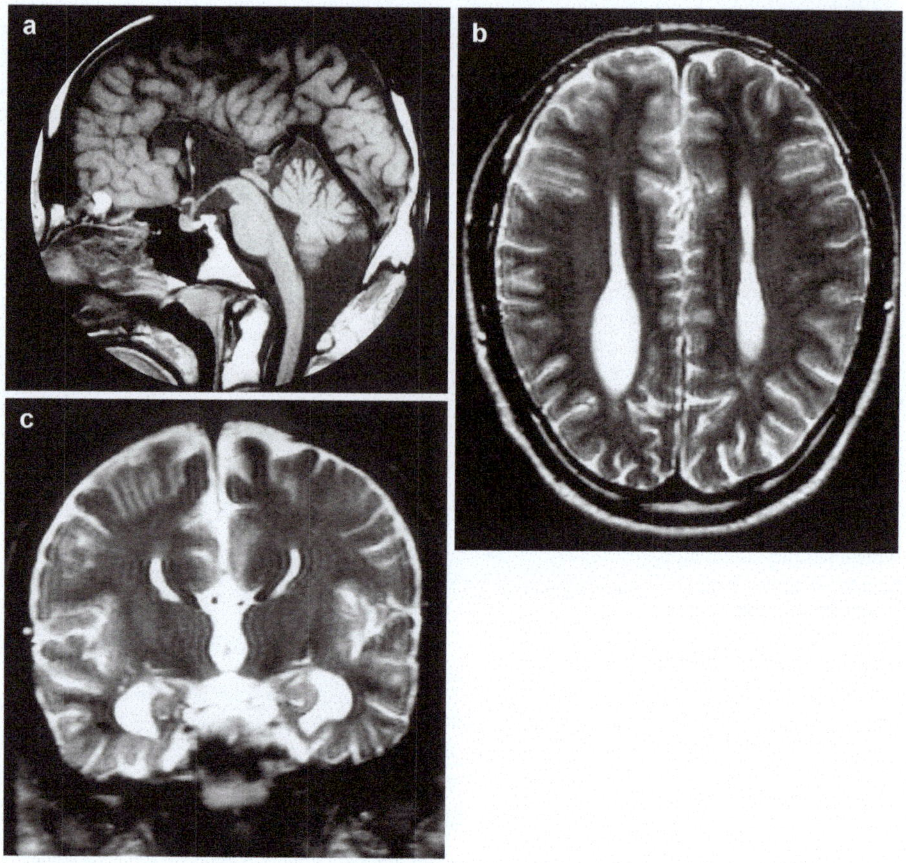

Fig. 2.9 Agenesis of the corpus callosum. (**a**) Midsagittal SE T1-WI. (**b**) Axial SE T2-WI. (**c**) Coronal SE T2-WI. There is a complete absence of the corpus callosum. In the axial imaging plane, there is a parallel orientation of the widely spaced lateral ventricles. Note the widening of the posterior section of the lateral ventricles; this is termed "colpocephaly". In the coronal plane, the high-riding third ventricle is in continuity with the interhemispheric fissure. The lateral ventricles are indented medially by Probst's bundles

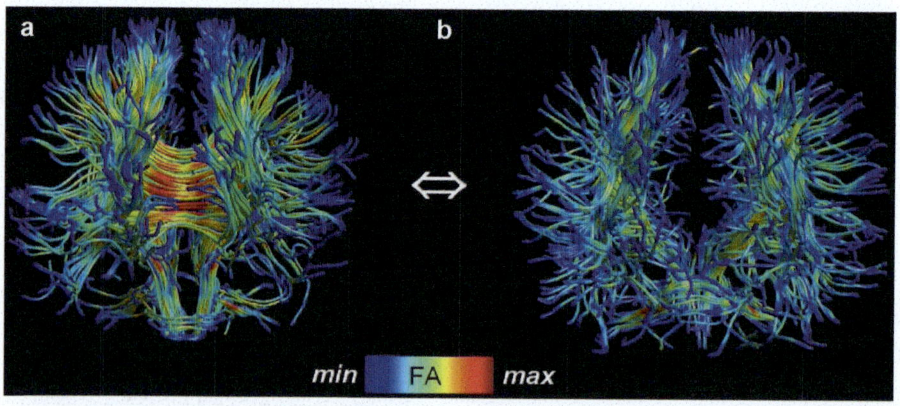

Fig 2.10 A,B. Fiber tractography of cerebral white-matter tracts, AP views. (**a**) Normal brain (*left*). (**b**) Agenesis of the corpus callosum (*right*). The color coding indicates the degree of anisotropy; *red* denotes a high fractional anisotropy (FA) and *blue* a low FA. In the normal brain of a 26-year-old man (**a**, *left*), the corpus callosum can be seen as a broad bundle of horizontal fibers, connecting both hemispheres. In the patient with complete agenesis of the corpus callosum (**b**, *right*), there is no connection between the right and left cerebral hemispheres

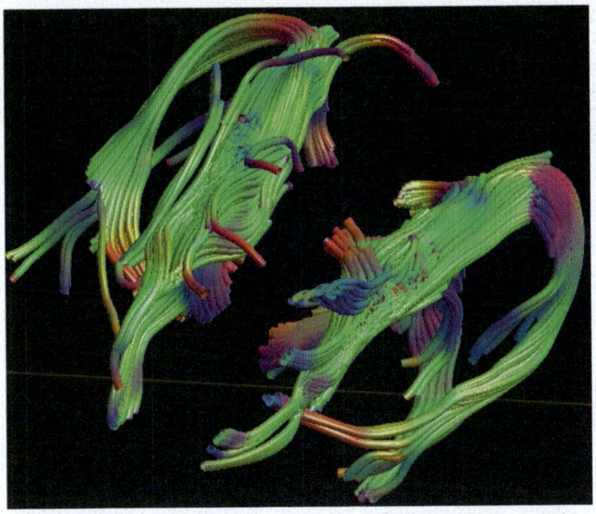

Fig. 2.11 Fiber tractography in complete agenesis of the corpus callosum (*right*), oblique superior view. In this graph, the color coding indicates the predominant diffusion direction. *Green* indicates anterior-posterior fibers, corresponding to the Probst and cingulate bundles, which course along the inner surface of the cerebral hemispheres. There is complete absence of the corpus callosum

MRI findings of corpus callosum agenesis include:

- Partial or complete absence of the corpus callosum (midsagittal image)
- Radial orientation of the gyri on the medial surface of the cerebral hemispheres (sagittal images) and eversion of the cingulate gyrus (coronal images)
- Parallel orientation of the lateral ventricles (axial images)
- Longitudinal white-matter tracts (Probst bundles) indent the superomedial walls of the lateral ventricles (axial and coronal images)
- Colpocephaly, i.e., dilatation of the trigones and occipital horns (from the Greek word "kolpos" meaning a fold, cleft, or hollow)
- Upward extension of the third ventricle between the lateral ventricles (coronal images)
- Crescent-shaped ("bull's horn") frontal horns
- Hypoplastic or dysgenetic anterior commissure and hippocampal formation

Agenesis of the corpus callosum can occur as an isolated finding, but is frequently associated with other congenital anomalies of the brain, including Chiari II, Dandy-Walker, interhemispheric cysts, migration disorders, and lipoma. Other midline structures that should be identified on the midsagittal image include the anterior commissure, the posterior commissure, the pineal gland, the pituitary and pituitary stalk, the aqueduct, the quadrigeminal plate, and the floor of the anterior fossa.

2.2.4 Cerebral Hemispheres

The symmetry of the cerebral hemispheres is best appreciated on axial and/or coronal scans. A sequence providing high contrast between white and gray matter is preferred. Our choice is a "true" turbo inversion recovery (IR), heavily T1-W sequence (Fig. 2.12), or a 3D

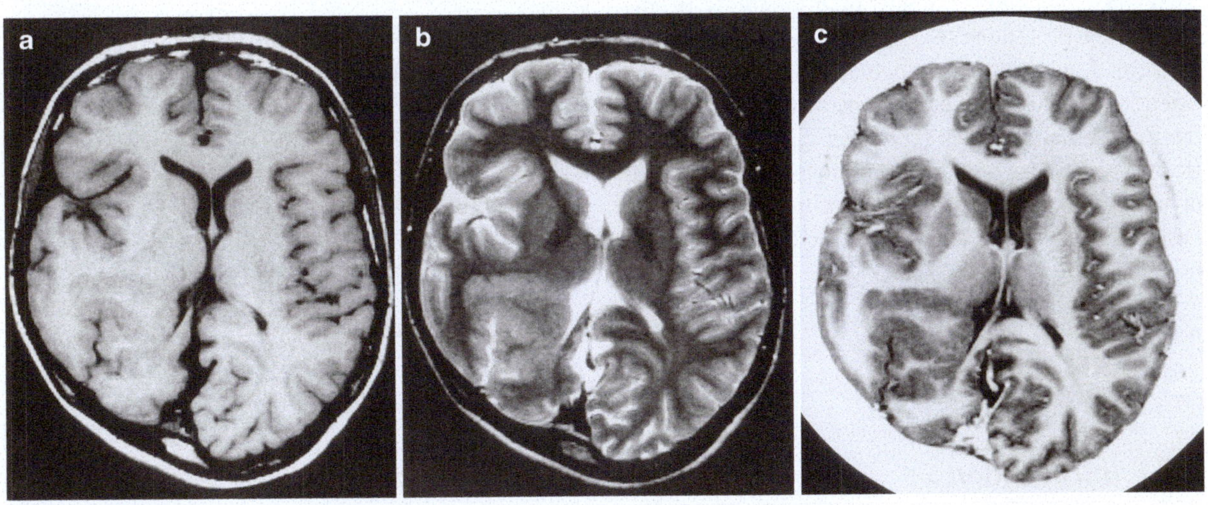

Fig. 2.12 Migrational disorder (gray matter heterotopia) in a patient with intractable seizures. (**a**) Axial SE T1-WI. (**b**) Axial TSE T2-WI. (**c**) Axial TIR T1-WI. The right occipital lobe contains dysplastic, disorganized gray matter. The heterotopic gray matter indents the right lateral ventricle. On all sequences, the heterotopic gray matter is isointense to cortex. TIR images provide the best contrast between gray and white matter and can be very helpful in the characterization of migrational disorders

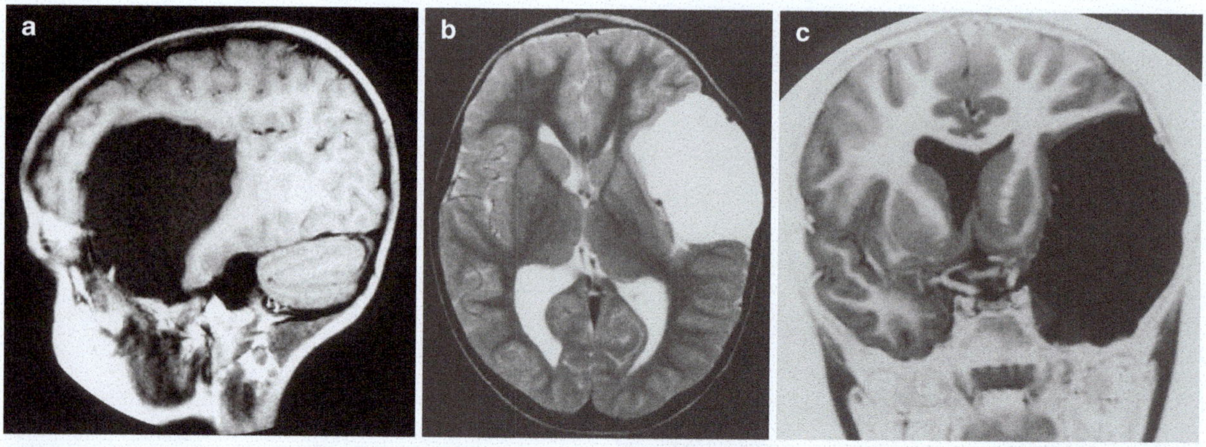

Fig. 2.13 Arachnoid cyst. (**a**) Sagittal SE T1-WI. (**b**) Axial TSE T2-WI. (**c**) Coronal TIR image. These images illustrate the typical appearance of a middle cranial fossa arachnoid cyst. Cyst contents are isointense to CSF. Branches of the middle cerebral artery, seen as small areas of flow void, are displaced medially. Note that there is some outward bulging of the skull overlying the cyst (this 5-year-old boy presented with a growing "bump" on the head). The cyst is lined by displaced cortical gray matter (coronal image)

gradient echo sequence (GRE) with magnetization preparation, such as MP-RAGE, 3D-FSPGR, or 3D-TFE. On these MR scans, gray matter appears "gray" and white matter appears "white." These images are well-suited for the detection of cortical lesions and neuronal migrational disorders. Embryologically, these conditions result from the abnormal migration of neurons from the germinal matrix to the brain surface. The spectrum of these disorders is wide and varied and includes lissencephaly, cortical dysplasias, heterotopias, schizencephaly, megalencephaly, etc.; these conditions are discussed in greater detail in Chap. 13.

When evaluating complex malformations of the brain or cystic lesions (Fig. 2.13), imaging should be performed in the three orthogonal planes to show the extent and anatomic relationships of the lesion accurately. Alternatively, a 3D sequence can be employed. IR images are also of value in following the process of myelination and in the diagnosis of myelin disorders. Fast FLAIR images are an alternative for the detection of white-matter diseases.

2.3 Mass Lesions

2.3.1 Introduction

One of the most common indications for MRI of the brain is to rule out an intracranial mass lesion, especially in patients presenting with focal neurological deficits (e.g., hemiparesis, hemianopia, etc.) and seizures. Clinical symptoms depend on the location of the lesion. Some of these patients have had a prior computed tomography (CT) scan of the brain. If the CT scan shows a mass lesion, MRI should be performed to look for additional lesions, to characterize the mass, and to plan the treatment. If the CT scan is negative but there is strong clinical suspicion of an intracranial mass, MRI should also be performed. Administration of contrast material is essential. MRI is the method of choice for virtually all types of intracranial mass lesions.

When confronted with an intracranial lesion, the radiologist should be able to answer the following questions:

1. Is the lesion a tumor?
2. What is the location of the lesion? (supra- or infratentorial? intra-axial or extra-axial?)
3. What is the amount of mass effect and edema?
4. What is the most likely diagnosis, keeping in mind the location of the lesion, the clinical history, and the patient's age?

2.3.2 Tumor or Not?

The clinical and MRI diagnosis of an intracranial mass lesion can be challenging. In most cases, the initial clinical symptoms are nonspecific and result only from mass effect, local pressure, and distortion of adjacent structures. Not all mass lesions are tumors. Tumors are usually characterized by a gradual onset of symptoms, preferential involvement of white matter with sparing of cortical gray matter, round or infiltrating shape, and are not confined to a specific vascular distribution. Some of the major differential diagnostic considerations include: recent infarct, abscess, resolving hematoma, encephalitis, and developmental anomaly. The use of intravenously injected contrast agents does not always solve the issue. Some tumors do not enhance (e.g., low-grade astrocytoma), whereas intense enhancement is sometimes observed in nontumoral conditions (e.g., enhancement in recent stroke due to blood–brain barrier (BBB) breakdown, ring-like enhancement of an abscess). It is important to remember that in tumors, the amount of enhancement is not directly related to the degree of malignancy.

2.3.3 Lesion Location

Intracranial lesions can be classified as *supra- or infratentorial*, depending on their position relative to the tentorium cerebelli. Infratentorial tumors are more frequent in the pediatric age group. Some tumors occur in different topographical compartments, depending on the patient's age. A typical example are choroid plexus papillomas; in infants, they tend to occur supratentorially (lateral ventricles), whereas in adults they are more common infratentorially (fourth ventricle). Other tumors preferentially occur in one compartment, e.g., hemangioblastoma is almost exclusively an infratentorial tumor.

Perhaps, even more important for the differential diagnosis is to determine whether the site of origin of the lesion is *intra-axial or extra-axial*, depending on whether the neoplasm originates in the brain parenchyma or from the coverings of the brain. The prognosis and surgical approach for the two types differ. ***Extra-axial tumors*** can be of meningeal origin (meningioma, leptomeningeal seeding, lymphoma), nerve-sheath origin (schwannoma of N. VIII, V, VII), or osseous origin (chordoma, eosinophilic granuloma). In the broad sense of the definition, extra-axial tumors also include maldevelopmental cysts and tumors (arachnoid cyst, (epi)dermoid cyst, lipoma). The cardinal feature of extra-axial tumors is that they are separated from the brain surface. The diagnosis depends primarily on the identification of anatomical boundary layers, which are interposed between the brain surface and the extra-axial tumor, e.g., CSF cleft, vascular cleft, and dural cleft. Most extra-axial tumors are benign. Because they are located outside of the brain, they do not possess a BBB. When an extra-axial tumor enhances after intravenous injection of a contrast agent, it is because of its intrinsic tumor vascularity. Enhancement often helps to define the anatomic compartmentalization of extra-axial tumors. Contrast enhancement is highly characteristic of some extra-axial tumors (meningioma, schwannoma), whereas others almost never enhance (epidermoid, dermoid).

The most common supratentorial extra-axial tumors are meningiomas and metastases. Meningioma is the most common primary nonglial intracranial tumor (13–19% of all operated brain tumors). Small meningiomas may be difficult to detect because they are almost isointense to cortical gray matter on T1- and T2-WI, and may be overlooked on noncontrast imaging studies (Fig. 2.14). Since meningioma capillaries lack a BBB, these tumors enhance strongly with Gd. Invasion of the skull bones is common (Fig. 2.3); another typical finding is the so-called "enostotic spur" (Fig. 2.15). Some meningiomas are intraventricular. Extra-axial metastases are most commonly caused by breast carcinoma (most common primary tumor). Metastases may involve the skull, pachymeninges (dura mater), and leptomeninges (arachnoid-subarachnoid metastases, pial metastases). Other supratentorial extra-axial tumors include lymphoma, sarcoidosis, and chordoma.

Infratentorially, extra-axial tumors occur predominantly in the cerebellopontine angle (CPA). In decreasing order of frequency, they include acoustic schwannoma (80%), meningioma (13–18%), epidermoid tumor (5%), and other lesions (schwannoma of N. V, VII, foramen jugulare tumors, chordoma, arachnoid cyst, aneurysm of basilar artery, and exophytic glioma).

Intra-axial tumors originate within the substance of the brain. They can be subdivided into primary and secondary tumors. The most common primary brain tumors are of glial cell origin. Gliomas account for 40–50% of

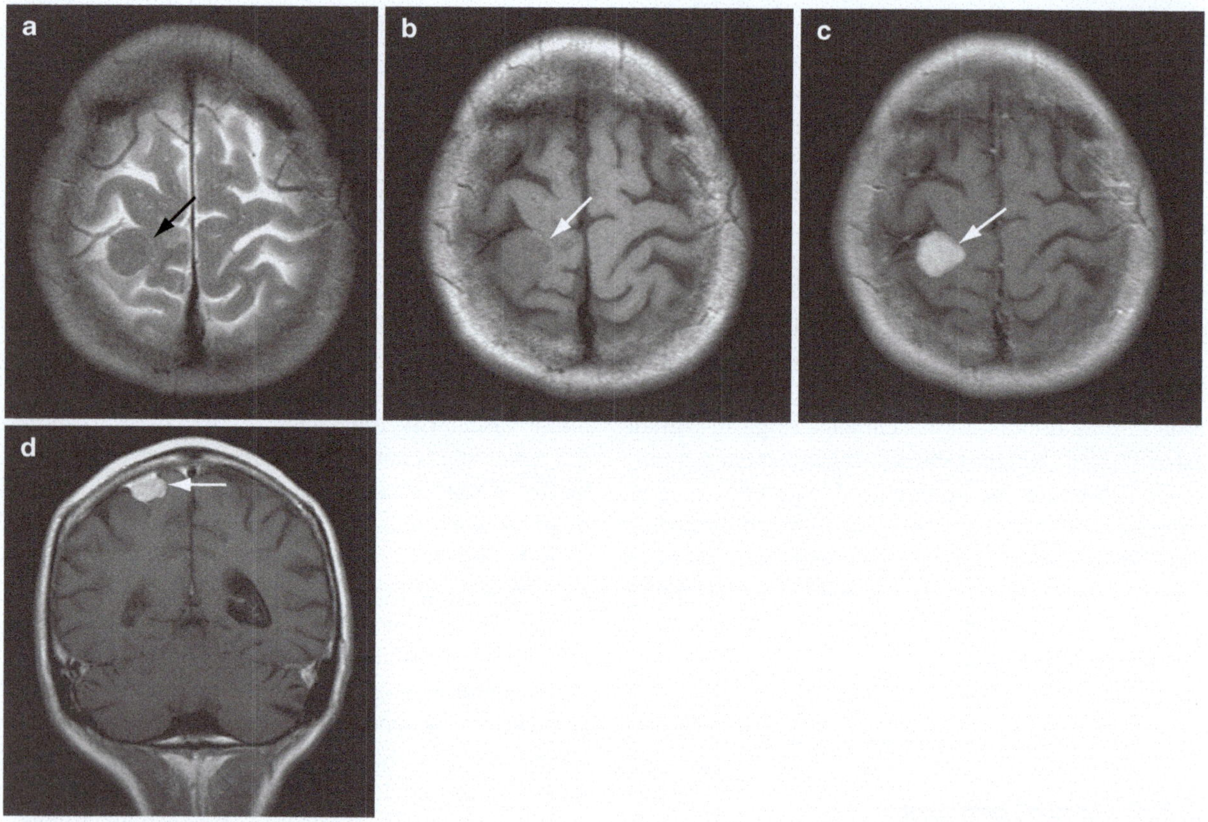

Fig. 2.14 Right parietal convexity meningioma (in a 65-year-old woman). (**a**) Axial TSE T2-WI. (**b**) Axial TSE T1-WI. Gd-enhanced axial (**c**) and coronal (**d**) TSE T1-WI. On T2- and T1-WI, this meningioma is almost isointense to hypointense compared to the adjacent cortical gray matter in the central sulcus. Small meningiomas can be easily overlooked on precontrast images. After Gd injection, there is homogeneous enhancement, and the broad dural base of the lesion is well seen on the coronal scan (*arrows*)

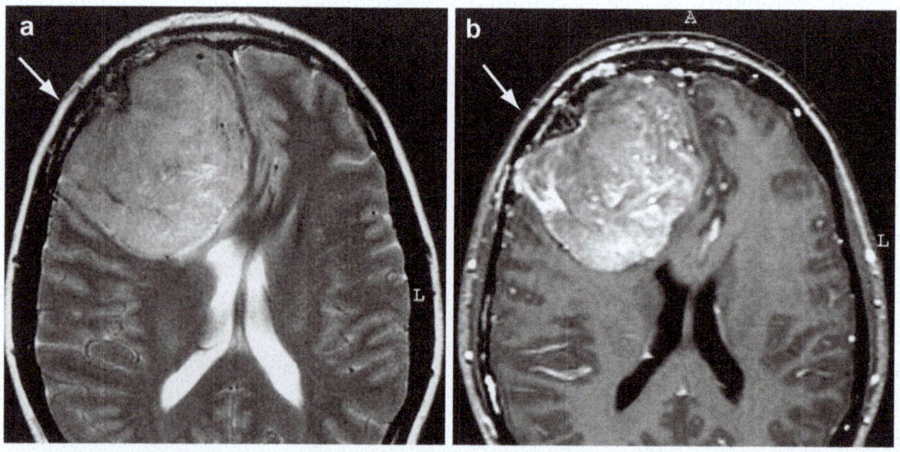

Fig. 2.15 Frontal convexity meningioma. (**a**) Axial TSE T2-WI. (**b**) Axial gadolinium-enhanced gradient-echo 3D FT T1-WI. The T2-WI reveals a large tumor which is isointense to cortical gray matter. The lesion is well demarcated. Displaced vessels and CSF clefts are visible in the brain-tumor interface, indicating the extra-axial nature of the tumor. There is no perifocal edema. The tumor enhances inhomogeneously. Numerous intratumoral vessels are present. Note the pathognomonic enostotic spur and the accordeon sign at the posterior margin of the lesion (*arrows*)

Table 2.2 Topography of intracranial tumors

	Intra-axial	Extra-axial
Supratentorial	Primary: glioma (astrocytoma, GBM, oligodendroglioma, ependymoma, DNET/ PNET, lymphoma)	Primary: meningioma, pituitary adenoma, epidermoid, dermoid, bone tumors
	Secondary: intraparenchymal metastases	Secondary: leptomeningeal metastases
Infratentorial	Primary: astrocytoma, medulloblastoma(PNET), ependymoma, brainstem glioma, hemangioblastoma	Primary: schwannoma, meningioma, (epi)dermoid, chordoma
	Secondary: intraparenchymal metastases	Secondary: leptomeningeal metastases

all primary intracranial tumors. Examples of intra-axial tumors include astrocytoma (low-grade, anaplastic, glioblastoma multiforme (GBM)), oligodendroglioma, ependymoma, dysembryoplastic neuroectodermal tumor (DNET), and lymphoma. However, metastases are still the most frequent intra-axial tumors in the supratentorial compartment. Intra-axial tumors can enhance because of the BBB breakdown (e.g., high-grade astrocytoma) or because of their intrinsic tumor vascularity (hemangioblastoma). The degree of enhancement may play a role in differentiating high-grade from low-grade gliomas. Table 2.2 provides an overview of intracranial tumors depending on their location.

Some tumors are located in the ventricles. Table 2.3 provides a differential diagnostic list for intraventricular mass lesions.

2.3.4 Edema and Mass Effect

MRI is more sensitive than CT in detecting intracranial mass lesions because of the intrinsically higher soft tissue contrast resolution and because the associated edema is easily observed on FLAIR and T2-WI. In many instances, peritumoral edema is more conspicuous than the tumor itself. Three types of edema can be discerned.

Table 2.3 Intraventricular tumors (listed alphabetically)

Astrocytoma, Glioblastoma
Choroid plexus papilloma/carcinoma
Colloid cyst (third ventricle) Craniopharyngioma
Ependymoma
Epidermoid/dermoid Medulloblastoma (PNET)
Meningioma Metastases (CSF seeding)
Neurocytoma (or neuroepithelioma, usually centered around the septum pellucidum)

Vasogenic edema is caused by a breakdown of the BBB, which allows excessive fluid to pass from the capillaries into the extracellular space. Vasogenic edema extends along white-matter tracts and generally spares the cortical gray matter (Fig. 2.16). Vasogenic edema is associated with primary and metastatic tumors, contusion, inflammation, hemorrhage, and the subacute stage of cerebral infarcts.

Cytotoxic edema is most often due to ischemia. When the blood supply to brain cells is decreased below a certain threshold (approximately 15 mL/min/100 g of tissue), the production of adenosine triphosphate (ATP) is reduced, and the Na/K pump fails. This results in cellular swelling and a decrease in the volume of the extracellular spaces. Cytotoxic edema is typically seen in (hyper)acute ischemic arterial infarction (Fig. 2.17) and can involve both gray and white matter. If damage to the BBB follows, vasogenic edema may ensue in addition to the cytotoxic edema.

Interstitial edema occurs around the ventricles and is induced by acute hydrocephalus. It results from transependymal migration of CSF into the periventricular white matter, due to a pressure gradient.

All types of edema result in an increased water content of the tissues and are therefore hyperintense on FLAIR and T2-WI. Interstitial edema results in diffuse periventricular hyperintensity along the lateral ventricles. Diffusion-weighted MRI is the technique of choice for early detection of cytotoxic edema, which may be detected within minutes after an acute cerebral infarct.

Intracranial mass effect is determined not only by the tumor volume, but also by the amount of edema that is present. Mass effect can lead to displacement of brain tissue, a process that is known as "cerebral herniation." This is important to recognize, because it can lead to severe neurological dysfunction and is more commonly the cause of death than the tumor itself. Four types of internal *brain herniation* are distinguishable.

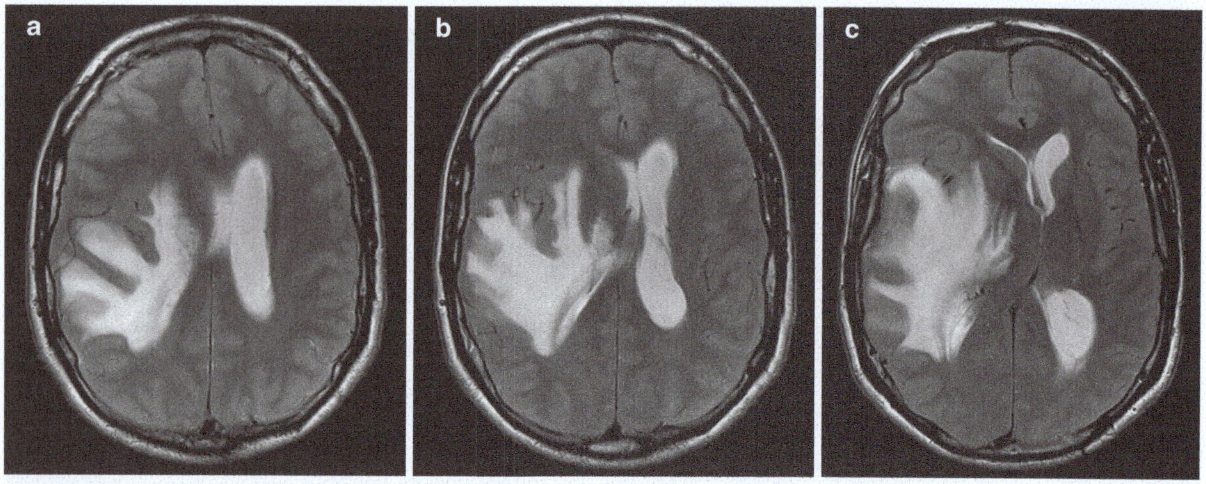

Fig. 2.16 Vasogenic edema, associated with anaplastic astrocytoma (WHO grade III). (**a–c**) Axial TSE T2-WI. "Fingers of edema" extend along white-matter tracts, into the subcortical white matter (**a**). The claustrum is outlined by vasogenic edema in the capsula externa and extrema (**b**). Edema also extends into the posterior limb of the internal capsule and surrounds the different layers of the lentiform nucleus. Vasogenic edema is due to increased vascular permeability with accumulation of fluid in the intercellular spaces

1. Subfalcine herniation: Brain tissue is displaced horizontally from left to right or vice versa, and the cingulate gyrus is pushed under the falx. This process is best seen on coronal MR images, though it should also be recognized on axial scans.
2. Descending transtentorial herniation (uncal herniation, hippocampal herniation): The uncus and/or hippocampal gyrus of the temporal lobe are pushed medially and downward into the tentorial incisura, thereby compressing the mesencephalon and upper pons. Displacement of the medial temporal lobe is best seen on coronal images, but the compression of the brainstem is best observed on axial T2-WI.
3. Ascending transtentorial herniation: Upward displacement of the vermis and cerebellum through the incisura due to an infratentorial mass. The sagittal imaging plane is preferred.
4. Cerebellar tonsillar herniation: Downward displacement of the cerebellar tonsils and hemispheres through the foramen magnum behind the cervical spinal cord. Sagittal and coronal imaging planes are preferred.

2.3.5 Lesion Characterization

2.3.5.1 Signal Intensity

Most tumors appear hyperintense on FLAIR and T2-WI, and are iso- to hypointense on precontrast T1-WI. These MR findings are not helpful in characterizing the lesion. Some mass lesions display unusual signal features, which may narrow the differential diagnosis. Table 2.4 lists a differential diagnosis for lesions that are hypointense on T2-WI. Table 2.5 provides a differential diagnostic list for lesions that are hyperintense on T1-WI. Cystic lesions are relatively rare, and their differential diagnosis is listed in Table 2.6.

Enhancement Pattern and Perfusion

Presence of contrast enhancement does not necessarily differentiate a tumor from a nontumoral lesion, since many nonneoplastic conditions also enhance. Moreover, the boundary of the enhancing area does not always delimit the tumor extent. This is especially true for gliomatous tumors, which project areas of infiltrating tumor cells beyond the margin of enhancement. Moreover, the intensity of contrast enhancement is not always correlated with the degree of malignancy of the lesion (e.g., pilocytic astrocytomas demonstrate marked enhancement, despite their relatively benign nature). Some specific types of enhancement provide interesting diagnostic gamuts, e.g., ring-like enhancement which may be encountered in a wide variety of lesions including GBM, metastasis, abscess, areas of demyelination, and others (Table 2.7).

The use of perfusion imaging has opened up new horizons in tumor imaging (see below).

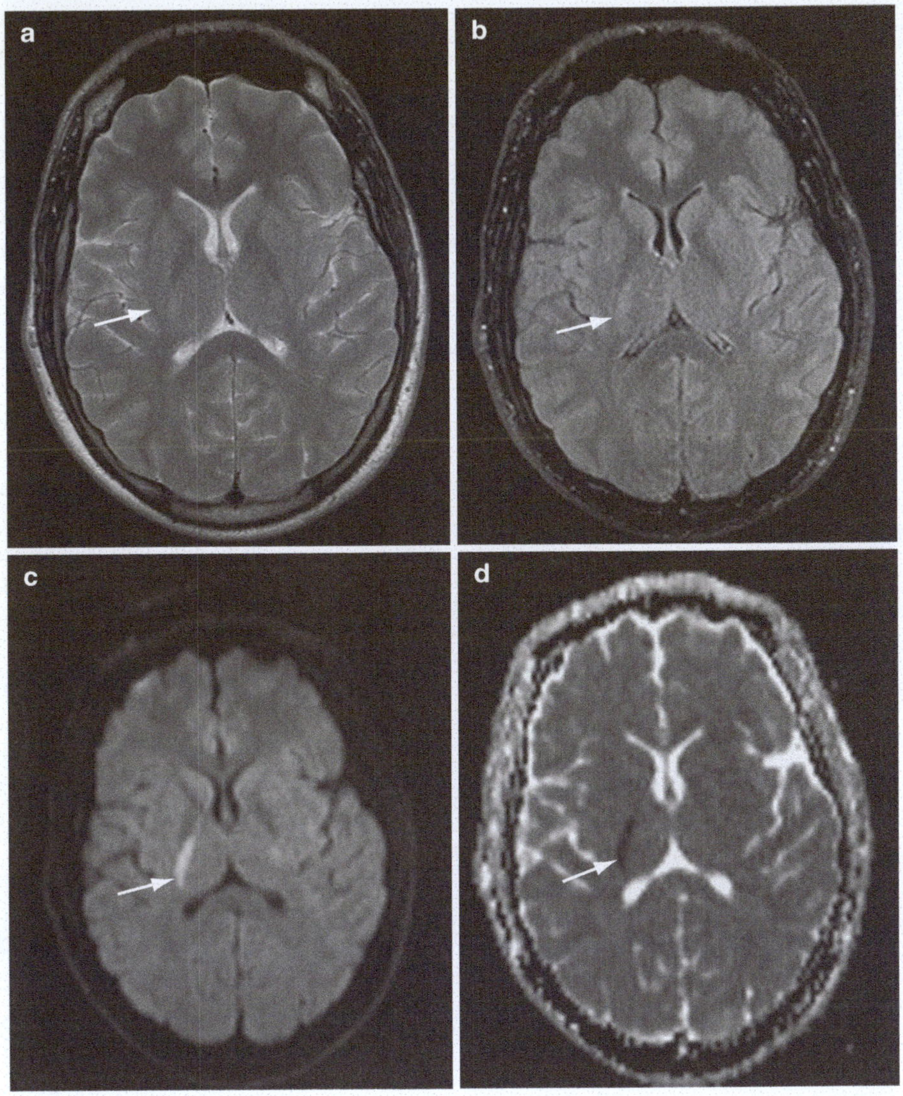

Fig. 2.17 Cytotoxic edema in hyperacute infarction (*arrows*). (**a**) Axial TSE T2-WI. (**b**) Axial fat-sat turbo FLAIR. (**c**) Axial EPI diffusion-weighted "trace" image (DWI). (**d**) Apparent diffusion coefficient (ADC) map. The patient is a previously healthy 38-year-old man who presented with sudden onset of left hemiparesis, left hemianesthesia, left homonymous quadranopia No signal abnormality is seen on T2 (**a**) or FLAIR (**b**) images. Conversely, diffusion-weighted trace images show a focal area of high signal intensity (**c**) with lowered ADC values (**d**) in the posterior limb of the right internal capsule. These findings are consistent with a hyperacute infarction of the right anterior choroidal artery. This case illustrates the importance of DWI and ADC maps for early detection of cytotoxic edema, at a time when other imaging sequences are negative

Table 2.4 Differential diagnosis of lesions with low signal intensity on T2-W images

Paramagnetic effects	• Iron in dystrophic calcification • Old hemorrhage (ferritin, hemosiderin) • Acute hemorrhage (deoxyHb) • Subacute hemorrhage (intracellular metHb) • Melanin (free radicals)
Low proton density	• Calcification • High nucleus/cytoplasm ratio • Dense cellularity
Macromolecule content	• Very high protein concentration • Fibrocollagenous stroma • Caseating granuloma (e.g., tuberculoma)
Intratumoral vessels	• Rapid blood flow (flow voids)

Table 2.5 Differential diagnosis of lesions with high signal intensity on T1-W images

Paramagnetic effects from hemorrhage	• Subacute-chronic blood, e.g., methemoglobin
Paramagnetic effects without hemorrhage	• Melanin • Ions associated with necrosis or calcification: Mn, Fe, Cu
Nonparamagnetic effects	• Very high protein concentration • Fat • Flow-related enhancement in vessels

Table 2.6 Differential diagnosis of cystic lesions

True cyst	• Sharply demarcated, ovoid or round
Signal intensity	• Isointense with CSF on all pulse sequences (e.g., arachnoid cyst, cysts associated with extra-axial masses) • Slightly higher SI than CSF on T1-WI and PD-WI (proteinaceous debris and/or small concentrations of paramagnetic substances
Diffusion	• No diffusion restriction (e.g., arachnoid cyst, necrotic tumor, …) • Diffusion restriction (e.g., bacterial abscess, epidermoid, mucinous metastasis, …)
Enhancement	• Ring enhancement • Mural nodule (e.g., hemangioblastoma)

Table 2.7 Differential diagnosis of ring-enhancing brain lesions

Neoplasm	• Primary neoplasm (high-grade glioma, meningioma, lymphoma, acoustic schwannoma, cranio-pharyngioma) • Metastatic tumor
Abscess	• Bacterial, fungal, parasitic abscess • Empyema (epidural, subdural, or intraventricular)
Hemorrhagic-ischemic lesion	• Resolving infarction • Aging hematoma • Operative bed following resection
Demyelinating disorder	
Radiation necrosis	

2.4 Supratentorial Brain Tumors

2.4.1 Introduction

Traditionally, MR examinations for supratentorial brain tumors have provided anatomic and structural data: location and margins of the tumor in various imaging planes, SI behavior, pattern of contrast enhancement, etc. Recently, MR has evolved toward a "multimodal" or "multi-parametric imaging platform" which incorporates perfusion and diffusion imaging, spectroscopy, tensor imaging, etc.

The axial plane is the plane of first choice for the supratentorial compartment; the coronal plane is the second best. In cases of midline lesions, such as pineal region tumors, the sagittal plane must be used.

Intravenous (i.v.) contrast agents, such as Gd-chelates are frequently necessary for the detection and improved delineation and characterization of the tumor. Without i.v. contrast, it is not possible to differentiate nonspecific high-intensity foci attributed to aging or ischemia from metastasis or lymphoma. Small lesions, such as metastases can be invisible without Gd. The pattern of contrast enhancement yields important information about the differential diagnosis and the degree of malignancy.

The questions to be answered are: what is the exact location of the tumor, and what is the probable histologic type and degree of malignancy? The radiologist must be aware of other factors of clinical importance: the mechanical effects such as obstructive hydrocephalus and descending transtentorial herniation.

Although intrinsically superior to CT, MRI also has its limitations! Neuroradiological examinations do not show the true neuropathological extent of many intra-axial brain tumors. MRI is a highly sensitive technique, but there is still a lack of specificity. On T2-WI, high SI lesions from a MS plaque and a metastasis can be very similar. MRI is not as sensitive for intratumoral calcifications as CT. Necrosis, a prognostically important factor in brain tumor diagnosis is not reliably detected by MRI.

2.4.2 Basic Neuroradiological Features

2.4.2.1 Description of the Lesion

In an MRI report, the following basic neuroradiological characteristics of an intracranial tumor should appear: location (intra-axial or extra-axial, supratentorial or infratentorial, frontal or temporal, etc.), SI, degree of perifocal edema, space-occupying characteristics, what happens after i.v. contrast, solitary or multiple lesions. Together with other factors, such as the clinical information, the speed of evolution, the age of the patient, and the relative frequency of certain tumors in certain locations, these neuroradiological features should lead to a probable neuropathological diagnosis or differential diagnosis.

2.4.2.2 Intra-Axial or Extra-Axial Location

The most important question for the radiologist when confronted with an intracranial mass lesion is whether it is located in the intra-axial or extra-axial compartment. This is of great clinical importance. The location affects the operative planning and prognosis. Extra-axial tumors are located outside the brain parenchyma and are mostly benign. There are several signs of an extra-axial location (Table 2.8).

2.4.2.3 Signal Intensity

Because of their high water content, most brain tumors are hypointense on T1-WI and hyperintense on T2-W images. However, there are many exceptions to this rule. The signal behavior of a tumor can be homogeneous or heterogeneous. There are many causes of heterogeneous SI (Table 2.9).

Tumors with a dense cellularity have a relatively low SI on T2-WI. This is a characteristic MR feature of medulloblastoma, pinealoblastoma, neuroblastoma, lymphoma, and mucinous adenocarcinoma metastasis (Table 2.4).

Some tumors exhibit high SI on T1-WI. This characteristic is mainly found in tumors containing fat (lipoma, dermoid), melanin (metastatic melanoma), methemoglobin (hemorrhagic tumors), or high protein concentrations (craniopharyngioma) (Table 2.5).

Table 2.8 MR signs of extra-axial tumor location

Difference in signal intensity between the tumor surface and the cortex	Arterial encasement; dural sinus invasion
Elements of a brain-tumor interface	Dural-tail sign
White-matter buckling	Gyral compression: the accordeon sign
Osseous changes	Paradoxical cisternal widening
Vascular pedicle	Broad-based dural contact

Table 2.9 Causes of heterogeneous signal intensity

Hemorrhage
Necrosis
Calcification
Cyst
Blood vessels
Inhomogeneous enhancement
Fat
Melanin

2.4.2.4 Patterns of Contrast Enhancement in Brain Tumors

The pattern of contrast enhancement supplies important information about the possible histological type of the tumor (Tables 2.7, 2.10, and 2.11).

2.4.2.5 MR Perfusion Imaging of Brain Tumors

Brain tumors are known for their capacity to induce the formation of new blood vessels, a process which is known as angiogenesis. When a brain tumor starts to outgrow its blood supply, it produces angiogenic cytokines, which are the driving force behind angiogenesis. The blood vessels which are produced in this way are histologically abnormal, tortuous, irregular, and disorganized. They do not possess a BBB and are more permeable than normal capillaries. When tumors enhance after injection of a gadolinium-chelate, it is because the contrast agent leaks out of the abnormal blood vessels, and through these fenestrations, enters the interstitial space. The vascular abnormalities and changed flow dynamics in tumor blood vessels can be used in MR perfusion imaging. The most frequently used parameter in neuro-oncology is regional cerebral blood volume (rCBV). It is expressed in mL/100 g of brain tissue, and is a good indicator of the blood passing through the tumor or

Table 2.10 Superficial tumor with homogeneous enhancement

Meningioma
Lymphoma
Anaplastic astrocytoma
Metastasis

Table 2.11 Cyst with enhancing mural nodule

Pilocytic astrocytoma
Hemangioblastoma
Pleomorphic xanthoastrocytoma
Ganglioglioma

normal brain tissue. High-grade glial brain tumors have greater rCBV than their low-grade counterparts, reflecting their greater angiogenetic activity. In patients with brain tumors, MR perfusion imaging is helpful:

- To identify high-grade tumor components, and thus to guide stereotactic biopsy (and avoid areas of necrosis)
- To better delineate and define the true extent of glial tumors (since the hyperintense areas on FLAIR or T2-WI do not always correspond to the true tumor margins)
- To assist in surgical planning or radiation therapy, by outlining the tumor boundaries
- To differentiate tumor recurrence (increased rCBV) from radiation-induced necrosis (diminished rCBV)

2.4.3 Extra-Axial Supratentorial Tumors

Extra-axial tumors, are by definition, located outside the brain parenchyma. Meningioma is the most common tumor in this category. Other extra-axial tumors include schwannoma, arachnoid cyst, epidermoid-dermoid, lipoma, extra-axial metastasis, etc.

Meningiomas arise from meningothelial (arachnoidal) cells along the inner surface of the dura mater. They have a distinct predilection for specific locations: convexity (Fig. 2.15), parasagittal, sphenoidal ridge (Fig. 2.3), anterior skull base, cavernous sinus, CPA, etc. Most meningiomas demonstrate a heterogeneous SI pattern. They are typically isointense with gray matter on most sequences and may, therefore, be missed unless contrast is administered (Fig. 2.14). On T1-WI, meningiomas are almost always hypo- to isointense compared with brain tissue. On PD-WI and T2-WI, meningiomas tend to be iso- to hyperintense compared with the adjacent brain parenchyma. The identification of an anatomic brain-tumor interface is pathognomonic for the extra-axial localization. Three different anatomic interfaces may be identified with MRI: pial vascular structures, CSF clefts, and dural margins.

Following Gd administration, meningiomas generally display intense and homogeneous enhancement. Even heavily calcified meningiomas tend to enhance. Multiplanar imaging is useful for the preoperative delineation of the extent of the meningioma. Dural enhancement adjacent to the tumor is a striking finding in contrast-enhanced MRI. It is referred to as the "dural-tail sign." It is not specific for meningiomas; it indicates dural involvement by an adjacent mass.

2.4.4 Intra-Axial Supratentorial Tumors

2.4.4.1 Neuroepithelial Tumors

Tumors of neuroepithelial tissue, also known as glial tumors or "gliomas," account for 40–45% of all primary intracranial tumors. They arise from the glial cells, which have a great propensity to malignant transformation. The three most common groups of gliomas, which correspond to the three histologic subgroups of glial cells, are: astrocytoma, oligodendroglioma, and ependymoma. Neoplasms arising from the choroid plexus can also be considered as neuroepithelial tissue tumors, because the choroid plexus contains modified ependymal cells. Gliomas occur predominantly in the cerebral hemispheres, but the brain stem and cerebellum are frequent locations in children, and they can also be found in the spinal cord. In 2007, the World Health Organization (WHO) published a new classification of tumors of the CNS, which lists several new entities.

Astrocytic Tumors

Astrocytic brain tumors can be divided into two major groups: the fibrillary (also known as infiltrative or diffuse) astrocytoma and the circumscribed (localized or noninfiltrative) astrocytoma (Table 2.12).

Well-differentiated (diffuse) low-grade *astrocytomas* (WHO grade II) are the low-grade member of the fibrillary or diffuse astrocytomas (Fig. 2.18). Well-differentiated low-grade astrocytomas are relatively rare, affect younger patients, and have a better prognosis than their more aggressive counterparts. On MRI, a low-grade astrocytoma is seen as a homogeneous mass lesion, involving gray and white matter. The lesion is typically hypo- or isointense on T1-WI and hyperintense on FLAIR and T2-WI. The tumor causes local mass effect with gyral swelling, though perifocal edema is usually absent or slight. MRI misleadingly displays these lesions as clearly defined, especially on T2-WI. However, it should be remembered that they belong to the group of diffuse astrocytoma, and tumor cells extend beyond the MRI

Table 2.12 Classification of astrocytic brain tumors

Name	Fibrillary (diffuse or infiltrative) astrocytoma	Circumscribed (localized or noninfiltrative) astrocytoma	Glioblastoma multiforme	Pilocytic astrocytoma	Giant-cell astrocytoma	Pleomorphic xanthoastrocytoma
	Low-grade astrocytoma	Anaplastic astrocytoma				
Common locations	Cerebral hemispheres, pons (in children)	Cerebral hemispheres, brainstem	Cerebral hemispheres	Cerebellum, diencephalon	Subependymal in lateral ventricle (at the foramen of Monro)	Cerebral hemispheres, superficially located, often temporal lobe
Demographics	4th and 5th decades	Variable	Peak 50–65 years	5–15 years (peak around 10 years)	Children, young adults	Young adults with a history of seizures
Imaging findings	Expansion, no enhancement (intact BBB), follows white matter tracts	Variable appearance, enhancement, no necrosis or cyst formation	Grossly heterogeneous (necrosis, ring enhancement, vasogenic edema, hemorrhage)	Cyst with enhancing nodule	Variable enhancement, associated with other features of tuberous sclerosis	Heterogeneous (cyst with enhancing mural nodule, dural tail due to superficial location)
Malignancy grading (WHO)	Grade II	Grade III	Grade IV	Grade I	Benign	Benign (10% may have malignant degeneration)
Enhancement	Enhancement with Gd-chelates increases with degree of malignancy (breakdown of blood-brain barrier)	Enhancement is not related to degree of malignancy				

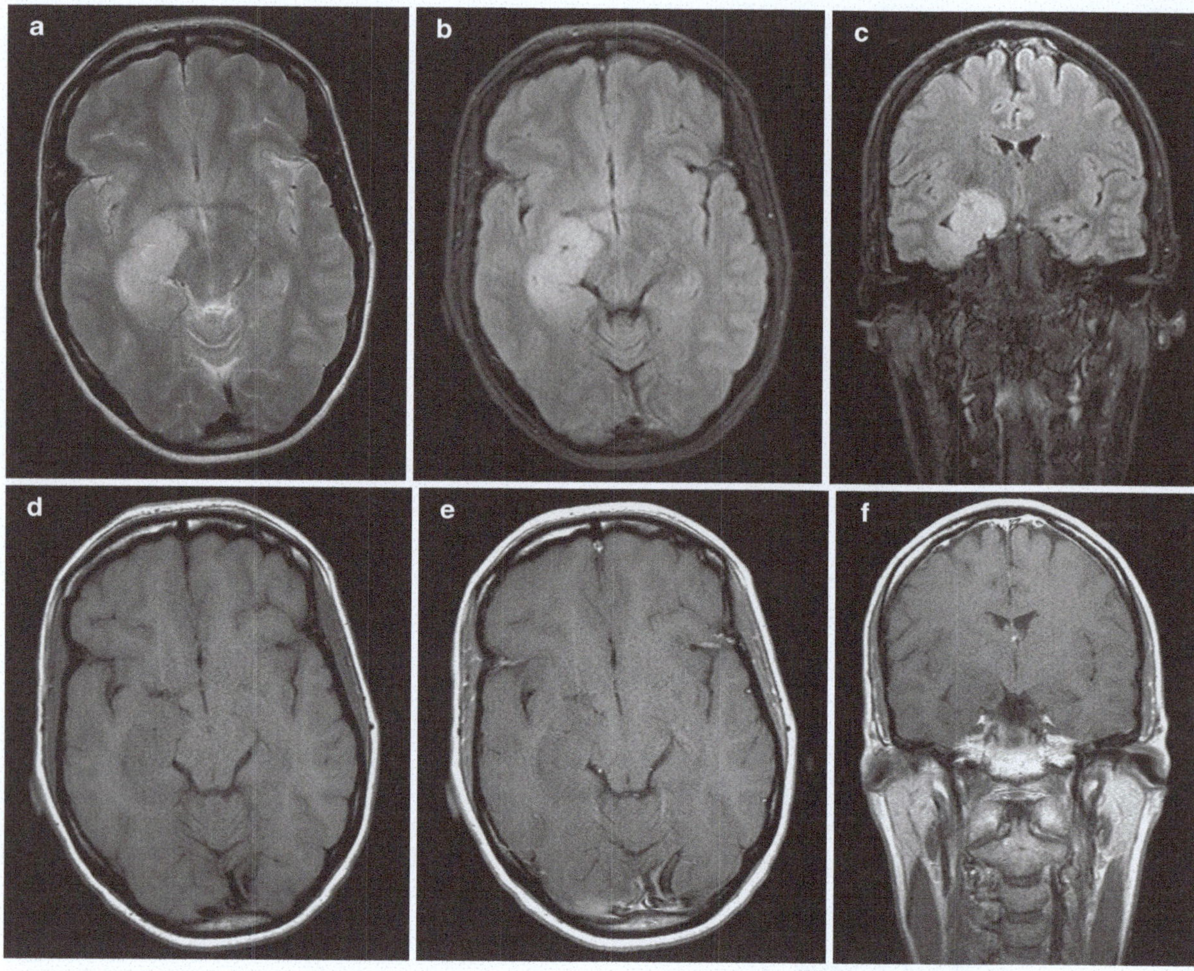

Fig. 2.18 Low-grade diffuse astrocytoma (WHO grade II). (**a**) Axial TSE T2-WI. (**b**) Axial fat-sat turbo FLAIR. (**c**) Coronal fat-sat turbo FLAIR. (**d**) Axial TSE T1-WI. (**e**) Gd-enhanced axial T1-WI. (**f**) Gd-enhanced coronal T1-WI. This 44-year-old woman presented with an epileptic seizure. MRI of the brain reveals a tumor in the medial part of the right temporal lobe. The tumor is hyperintense on T2 and FLAIR images (**a–c**) and hypointense on T1 images (**d**). There is no enhancement (**e, f**). Stereotactic biopsy revealed a low-grade diffuse astrocytoma (WHO grade II)

visible margins of the tumor! Typically, a low-grade astrocytoma shows no contrast enhancement. Moreover, though initially benign, a low-grade astrocytoma can evolve into a higher grade tumor over time. Different parts of the tumor can exhibit varying degrees of malignancy; this makes histological grading from biopsies difficult. MRI perfusion imaging and/or magnetic resonance spectroscopy (MRS) may be helpful in identifying a suitable stereotactic biopsy site.

Anaplastic astrocytomas (WHO grade III) are more common than their low-grade counterparts. These malignant, aggressive tumors infiltrate adjacent brain structures, and have a poor prognosis. On MRI, anaplastic astrocytomas present a more heterogeneous appearance, both on T1-WI and FLAIR or T2-WI. They exhibit marked mass effect and perifocal vasogenic edema, which spreads with fingerlike projections along white-matter tracts. The tumor may contain hemorrhagic foci. Marked but irregular enhancement is usually present, indicating breakdown of the BBB (Fig. 2.19). MRS shows increased choline (Cho), decreased *N*-acetylaspartate (NAA), and may show lactate (indicating necrosis, even though the tumor does not contain macroscopically visible cysts or areas of necrosis) (Fig. 2.20). MRS can be useful to differentiate recurrent tumor from radiation necrosis.

Glioblastoma multiforme (GBM) is the most malignant neuroglial tumor (WHO grade IV). In the older adult (>45 years), high-grade GBM is the most common primary intra-axial supratentorial neoplasm. The imaging

Fig. 2.19 Anaplastic astrocytoma. (**a**) Axial TSE T1-WI. (**b**) Axial TSE T2 WI. (**c**) Axial FLAIR TSE. (**d**) Gd-enhanced axial T1-WI. This 17-year-old young woman presented with a right frontal headache. MRI of the brain reveals a large tumor in the frontal right lobe with partial extension to the left side. The tumor consists of solid and cystic components extending from the right frontal lobe to the contralateral side with some vasogenic edema. The solid component shows mixed and inhomogeneous contrast enhancement. Stereotactic biopsy followed by tumor resection revealed an anaplastic pilocytic astrocytoma

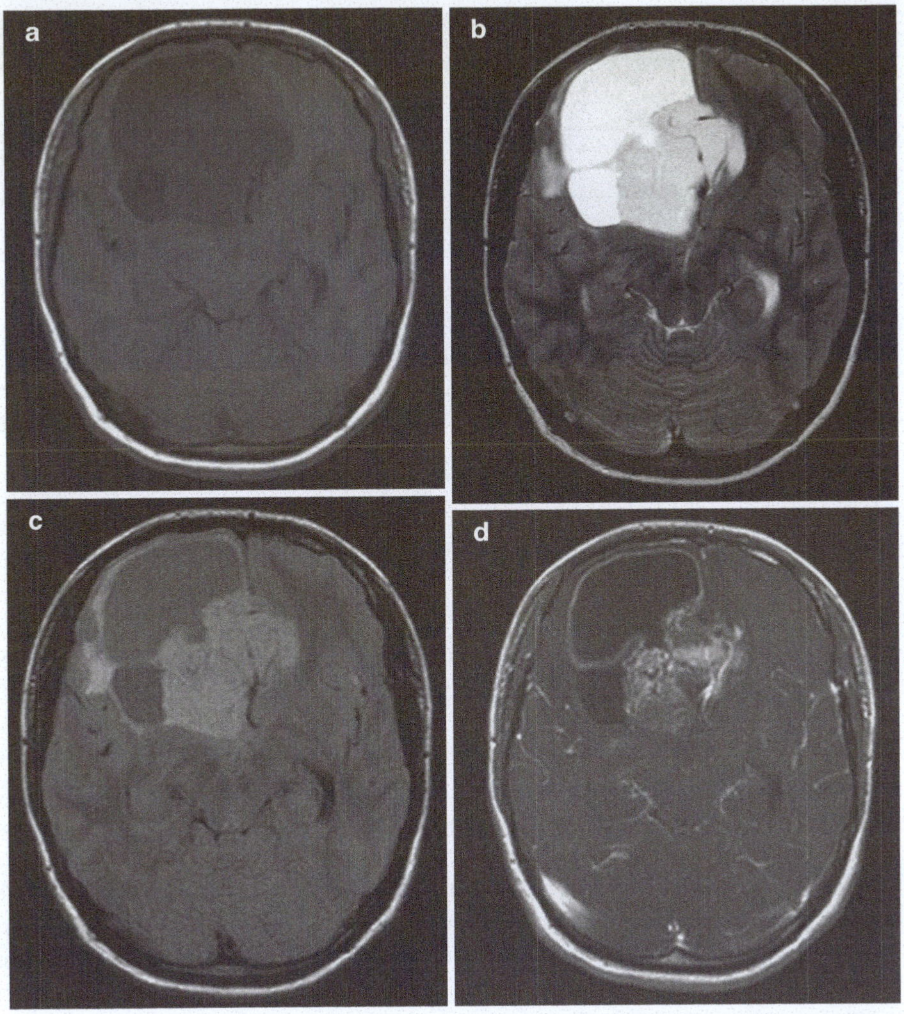

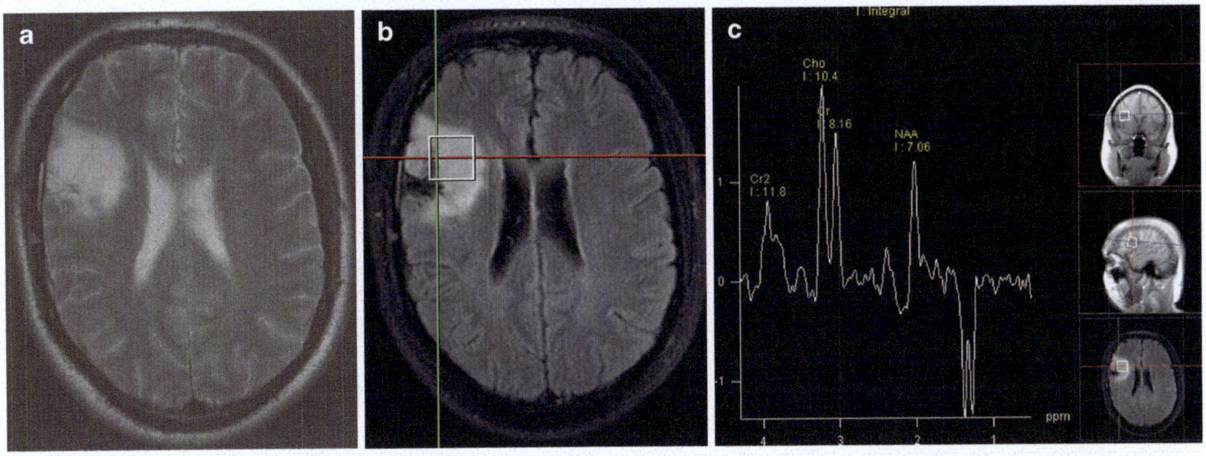

Fig. 2.20 Recurrent anaplastic astrocytoma (WHO grade III) in a 36-year-old man. (**a**) Axial TSE T2-WI. (**b**) Axial fat-sat turbo FLAIR. (**c**) Single voxel proton MR spectroscopy (MRS) (TE: 135 ms). The tumor recurrence is located in the right operculo-frontal region, and is hyperintense both on T2 and FLAIR images. Single voxel proton MRS shows moderate increase in choline (Cho), decrease in *N*-acetyl-aspartate (NAA), and an inverted doublet of lactate (indicating necrosis, even though the tumor does not contain macroscopically visible cysts or areas of necrosis)

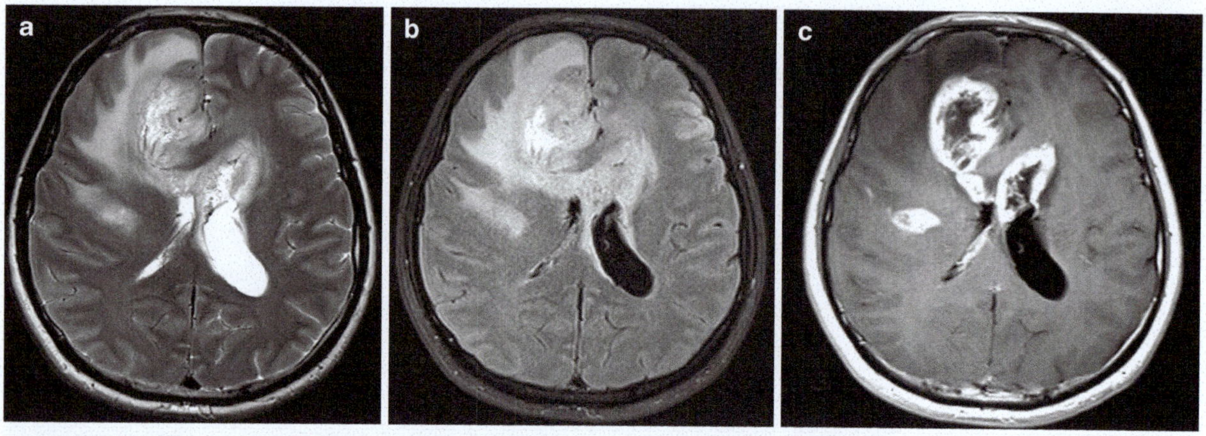

Fig. 2.21 Glioblastoma multiforme. (**a**) Axial TSE T2-WI. (**b**) Axial fat-sat turbo FLAIR. (**c**) Gd-enhanced axial T1-WI. Glioblastoma is an aggressive tumor, surrounded by vasogenic edema, with strong contrast enhancement (reflecting tumor angiogenesis), and areas of necrosis or cyst formation. The tumor has spread from the right frontal lobe across the corpus callosum to the left hemisphere, along the ventricular surface, and there is a satellite nodule in the right fronto-parietal region

findings can be predicted from the neuropathologic key features: cell heterogeneity, vascular cell proliferation (angiogenesis), necrosis, and infiltration. On MR images, these properties are translated into: heterogeneous signal intensities, cystic or necrotic areas, perifocal edema (with tumor inside and outside), intratumoral signal void of vessels, extensive mass effect, and inhomogeneous contrast enhancement (Fig. 2.21). Sometimes, these highly vascular tumors can even mimic arteriovenous malformations (AVMs). They often contain intratumoral hemorrhages. Enhancement with contrast is intense and heterogeneous.

Gliomatosis cerebri is an unusual condition in which multiple lobes of the brain are diffusely invaded by contiguous extension of glial tumor cells. It may represent the extreme form of diffusely infiltrating glioma.

The group of circumscribed (localized or noninfiltrative) astrocytomas includes pilocytic astrocytoma, pleomorphic xanthoastrocytoma (PXA), and subependymal giant cell astrocytoma (SCGA).

Pilocytic astrocytomas occur predominantly in children and adolescents. They are also known as "juvenile pilocytic astrocytomas" (JPA). The most common location for pilocytic astrocytomas is infratentorial (Fig. 13.46), but the tumor can be encountered supratentorially in the optic chiasm or hypothalamus or, less commonly, in the cerebral hemispheres (Fig. 2.22). Optochiasmatic-hypothalamic pilocytic astrocytomas are usually solid tumors, with moderate or even strong enhancement. When large, these tumors may contain cysts or trapped CSF, and should be differentiated from craniopharyngioma. There is an association with neurofibromatosis type 1.

Subependymal giant cell astrocytoma (SGCA) is a slow-growing, indolent, benign tumor, and is typically found in a subependymal location at the foramen of Monro. It occurs most commonly in children and young adults. Symptoms are usually secondary to obstructive hydrocephalus. SCGA shows intense and heterogeneous enhancement. The tumor occurs with tuberous sclerosis.

Pleiomorphic xanthoastrocytoma (PXA) is a rare and generally benign tumor. It is found predominantly in young adults, who often present with a history of seizures. PXA occurs in the cerebral hemispheres and is often located superficially, with the temporal lobes most commonly affected. On MRI, PXA presents as a superficial, partially cystic mass, with an enhancing mural nodule.

In the revised and updated WHO classification of tumors of the CNS, many other tumors are listed. A full discussion of these entities, many of which are very rare, is beyond the scope of this chapter.

Oligodendroglial and Oligoastrocytic Tumors

Oligodendrogliomas arise from oligodendrocytes. They are less common than astrocytic tumors, and constitute 2–5% of all primary brain tumors. They tend to occur in adults between the ages of 25 and 50 years, with a peak

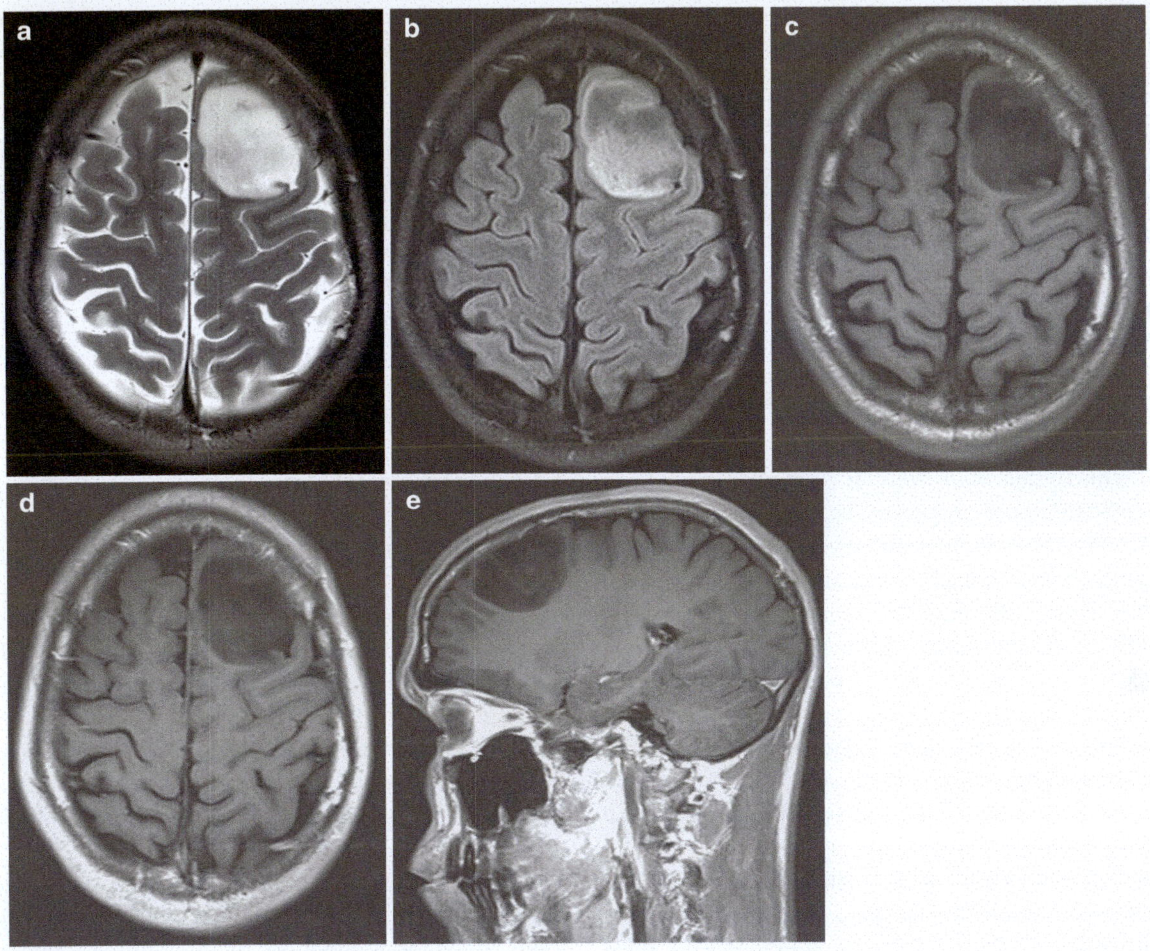

Fig. 2.22 Low grade astrocytoma (WHO grade I). (**a**) Axial TSE T2-WI. (**b**) Axial fat-sat turbo FLAIR. (**c**) Axial TSE T1-WI. (**d**) Gd-enhanced axial T1-WI. (**e**) Gd-enhanced sagittal T1-WI. This 26-year-old man presented with an epileptic seizure. The tumor in the left frontal lobe is inhomogeneously hyperintense on T2 and FLAIR, hypointense on T1, and does not enhance (no signs of angiogenesis, no blood-brain barrier breakdown). The tumor was surgically resected and neuropathological examination revealed pilocytic astrocytoma. Differential diagnosis for such a lesion should include low grade astrocytoma (WHO grade II), dysembryoplastic neuroepithelial tumor (DNET), ganglioglioma or oligodendroglioma

incidence around 35–45 years. Oligodendrogliomas are the most benign of the gliomas. They are slow-growing and are found predominantly in the frontal lobes and tend to infiltrate the cortex. MRI is less sensitive than CT in detecting calcifications, which occur in >70% of cases.

Oligoastrocytomas are brain tumors of mixed glial cell origin, containing elements from both astrocytoma and oligodendroglioma. They are also known as "mixed gliomas," and represent approximately 2% of all primary brain tumors. Oligoastrocytomas can be further subdivided into low-grade and anaplastic types.

Ependymal Tumors

Ependymomas are slow-growing neoplasms arising from cells of the ependymal lineage. They comprise 4–8% of primary brain tumors and are most commonly found in children. Two-thirds of ependymomas occur infratentorially (especially in the fourth ventricle), and one-third are found supratentorially. Of supratentorial ependymomas, more than half are extraventricular, presumably arising from ependymal cell nests in the cerebral parenchyma. On MRI, ependymomas present as a heterogeneous tumor of mixed signal intensities.

Calcifications, present in 50% of cases, may be difficult to detect on routine MRI sequences, and the use of a gradient-echo T2*-weighted sequence or susceptibility-weighted imaging (SWI) sequence can be helpful. After contrast injection, the enhancement is moderate to intense, depending on the vascularization of the tumor.

2.4.4.2 Intracranial Lymphoma

Intracranial lymphoma may be primary or secondary. Primary CNS lymphoma is usually non-Hodgkin's lymphoma (NHL), B-cell type and there is a strong association with Epstein-Barr virus. It is an aggressive brain tumor with a poor prognosis. Typically, primary CNS lymphoma shows multicentric involvement of the deepest parts of the hemispheres, around the ventricles and in the corpus callosum. The tumor tends to disappear rapidly with corticosteroids and/or radiation therapy; hence the name "ghost tumor." The risk of primary CNS lymphoma dramatically increases in immunocompromised patients (AIDS, after renal transplantation, immunoglobulin deficiency syndromes, etc.). Secondary CNS lymphoma is a complication of systemic lymphoma. It shows a tendency to invade the dura mater and leptomeninges; common clinical presentations include cranial nerve palsies and hydrocephalus.

Imaging studies reveal a well-demarcated mass lesion (Fig. 2.23), which is typically found supratentorially in the paramedian structures, including the deep white matter and corpus callosum, as well as the deep central gray matter (basal ganglia, thalamus, hypothalamus). Contact with an ependymal surface is a characteristic feature. Involvement of the posterior fossa occurs, but is not as common as in the supratentorial compartment. Up to half of all cases are multicentric.

On noncontrast CT, lymphoma is hyperdense relative to the surrounding brain tissue, because of the cell density. On MRI, primary CNS lymphoma tends to be iso- to hypointense to brain on both T1-WI and FLAIR or T2-WI (in contradistinction to glioma). The diminished signal on FLAIR and T2-WI may reflect the dense cellularity and relatively decreased water content (high nucleus-to-cytoplasmic ratio) of these tumors. The SI is of course altered in the presence of necrosis, which is a feature frequently found in AIDS patients. There is relatively little mass effect for the size of the tumor. After intravenous injection of Gd-chelates, CNS lymphoma typically enhances intensely (Fig. 2.23), but the pattern of enhancement is variable. Solid homogeneous enhancement is usually observed in immunocompetent patients. Conversely, in immunocompromised patients, the enhancement pattern tends to be irregular, heterogenous, or ring-like. Periventricular enhancement is highly specific (though not pathognomonic) for CNS lymphoma.

The differential diagnosis of CNS lymphoma includes tumors (glioma, metastases, primitive neuroectodermal tumor (PNET), …), infectious diseases (toxoplasmosis, tuberculosis, ependymitis,…), and demyelinating disorders (MS, PML).

2.4.4.3 Intracranial Metastasis

Intracranial metastases are the most common intracranial neoplasms. They account for 15–40% of all clinically detected brain tumors. Metastases can be located in the skull, epidural space, meninges, and subarachnoid space (meningeal carcinomatosis), but they occur most frequently in the brain parenchyma. The most common primary tumors to metastasize to the adult brain are, in order of decreasing frequency, bronchial carcinoma, breast carcinoma, gastrointestinal tract tumors (colon, rectum), renal cell carcinoma, melanoma, and choriocarcinoma. Together, these six primary tumors account for 95% of all brain metastases in adults. In children, the most common primary tumors are leukemia, lymphoma, and neuroblastoma.

Cerebral metastases can occur anywhere in the brain, but they occur most frequently in the cortex or at the corticomedullary junction (hematogenous spread). Intraparenchymal metastases are most common in the cerebral hemispheres, but they also occur in the cerebellum and brainstem. At the time of diagnosis, multiple lesions are found in 2/3 of cases, and a single metastasis is found in 1/3. Metastatic cells can also spread via the CSF, a condition known as carcinomatous meningitis. Subependymal spread is encountered, for example, in metastatic breast carcinoma. Nodular metastatic deposits in the dura mater are not uncommon, and this is known as dural carcinomatosis.

On MRI, cerebral metastases are hypointense on T1-WI and present a variable SI on FLAIR and T2-WI (due to hemorrhage, melanin, necrosis, cyst formation, etc.). They are generally round and better circumscribed than primary tumors. Cerebral metastases from a "mucinous" adenocarcinoma may appear hypointense on

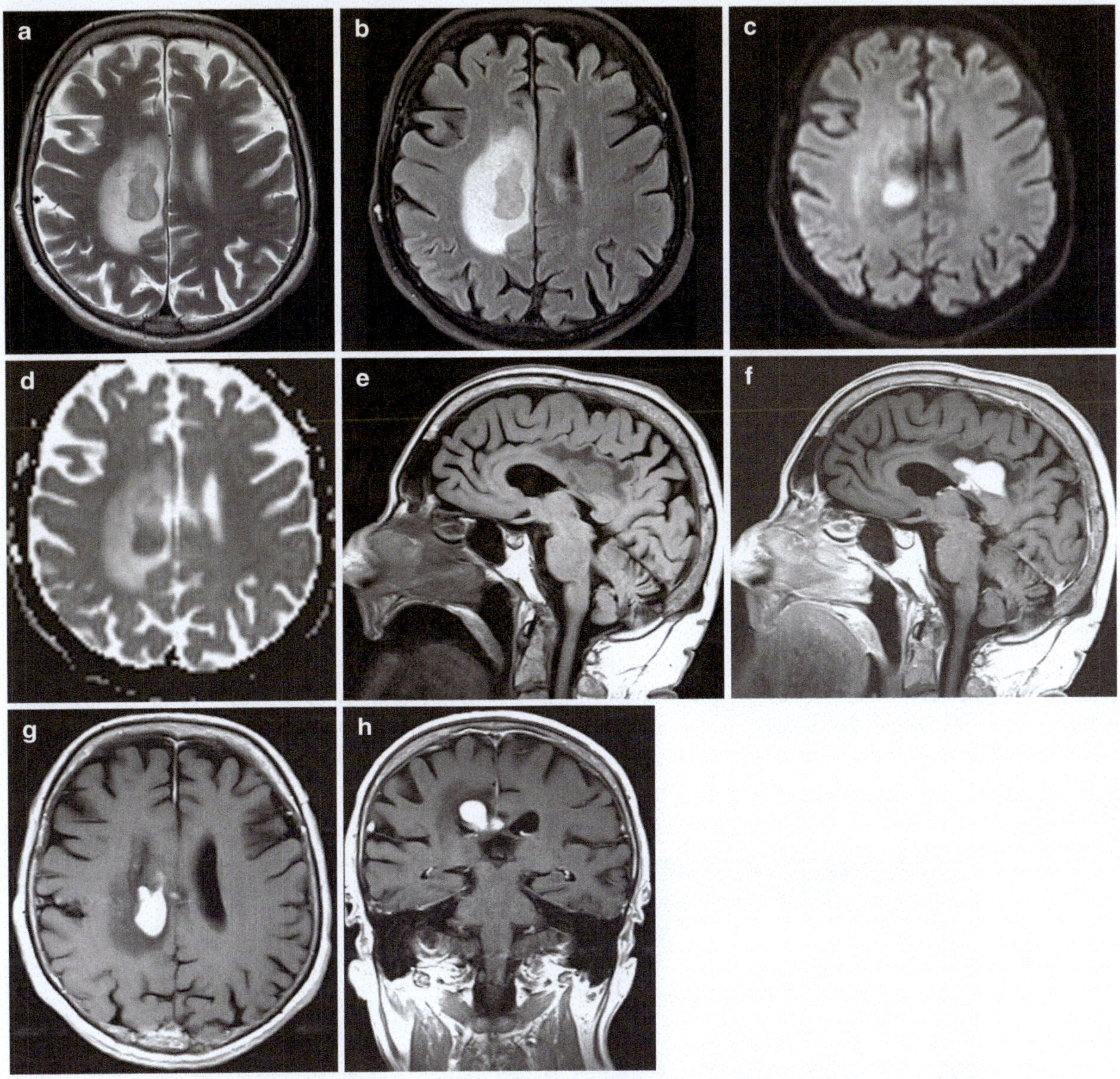

Fig. 2.23 Non-Hodgkin's lymphoma. (**a**) Axial TSE T2-WI. (**b**) Axial fat-sat turbo FLAIR. (**c**) Axial EPI diffusion-weighted 'trace' image. (**d**) Apparent diffusion coefficient (ADC) map. (**e**) Sagittal TSE T1-WI. (**f–h**) Gd-enhanced sagittal (**f**), axial (**g**) and coronal (**h**) TSE T1-WI. This 73-year-old man has a history of Wegener's disease, and was treated with steroids and cyclophosphamide. He presented with sudden onset of gait instability and falling to the left side. The tumor is located above the right lateral ventricle, extends into the corpus callosum, and is surrounded by a large rim of vasogenic edema. The tumor is relatively hypointense on T2-WI (**a**), hyperintense on diffusion-weighted trace images (**b**), with lowered ADC values (**c**); these findings reflect a high cell density and/or high nucleus/cytoplasm ratio, with little mobile water. After Gd injection, there is intense and homogeneous enhancement of the tumor

T2-WI and show diffusion restriction (their viscous content lowers apparent diffusion coefficient (ADC) values). When metastases are hyperintense on T1-WI, this can be due to the presence of hemorrhage or melanin (paramagnetic effect). The amount of peritumoral edema is variable. In small cortical lesions, edema may be absent, but in general, the degree of edema is greater with metastatic lesions than with primary neoplasms (Fig. 2.24).

By far, the most sensitive examination for the detection of intracerebral metastases is gadolinium-enhanced MRI, especially for detecting small metastatic lesions. Gd-enhanced MRI is far superior to contrast-enhanced

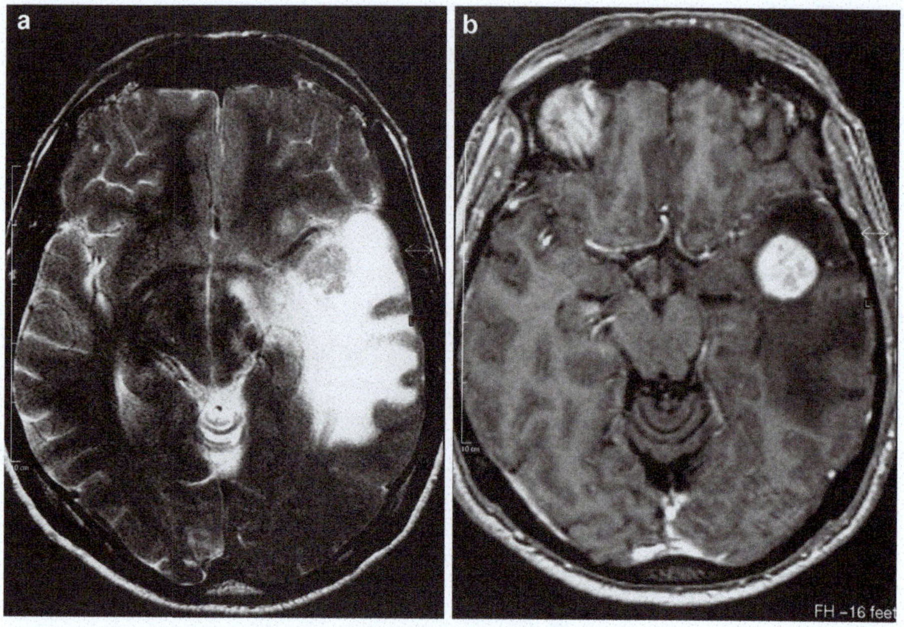

Fig. 2.24 Solitary brain metastasis. (**a**) Axial TSE T2-WI. (**b**) Axial Gd-enhanced GRE 3D FT T1-WI. A nodular mass lesion is observed in the anterior part of the left temporal lobe. On T2-WI, the tumor is isointense with gray matter. Relative to the size of the tumor, there is a disproportionately large amount of perilesional vasogenic edema. After Gd injection, there is intense enhancement. The enhancing tumor can be sharply separated from the surrounding vasogenic edema

CT in the detection of cerebral metastases. On postcontrast T1-WI, cerebral metastases present strong enhancement, which can either be homogeneous, nodular, inhomogeneous, or ring-like (see Table 2.7) (Figs. 2.25 and 2.26). Some authors have shown that a high-dose (0.3 mmol/kg) immediate study is superior to a normal-dose or delayed study in detecting small lesions. With the arrival of newer contrast agents with higher relaxivity there is less need for high-dose imaging. The use of magnetization transfer improves the contrast between

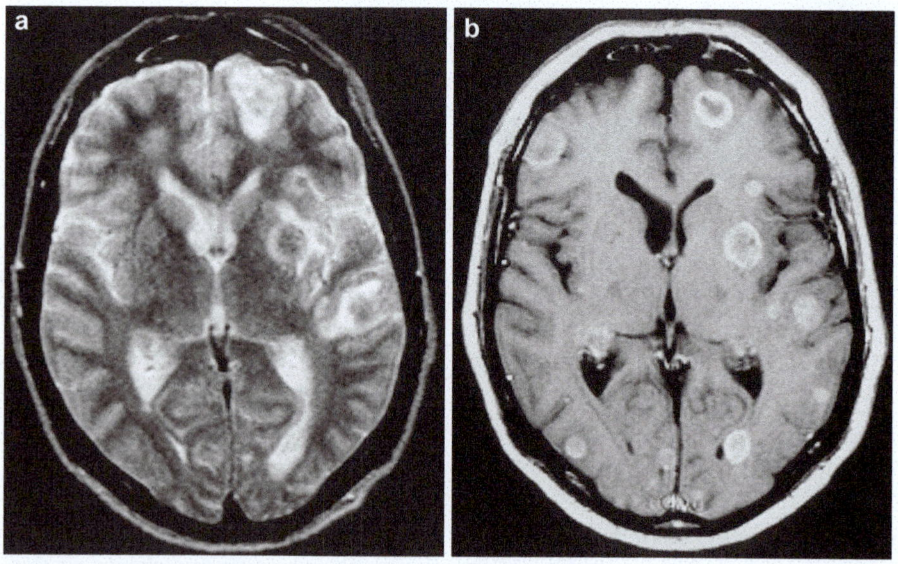

Fig. 2.25 Multiple metastases. (**a**) Axial TSE T2-WI. (**b**) Axial gadolinium-enhanced SE T1-WI. The precontrast T2-WI shows only a few lesions compared with the postcontrast T1-WI. The enhancement characteristics of the different metastatic tumors are not uniform; some enhance homogeneously, while other lesions display a ring-shaped enhancement pattern. Also the amount of perilesional edema is variable. Notice the characteristic location of many of the metastatic lesions at the corticomedullary junction

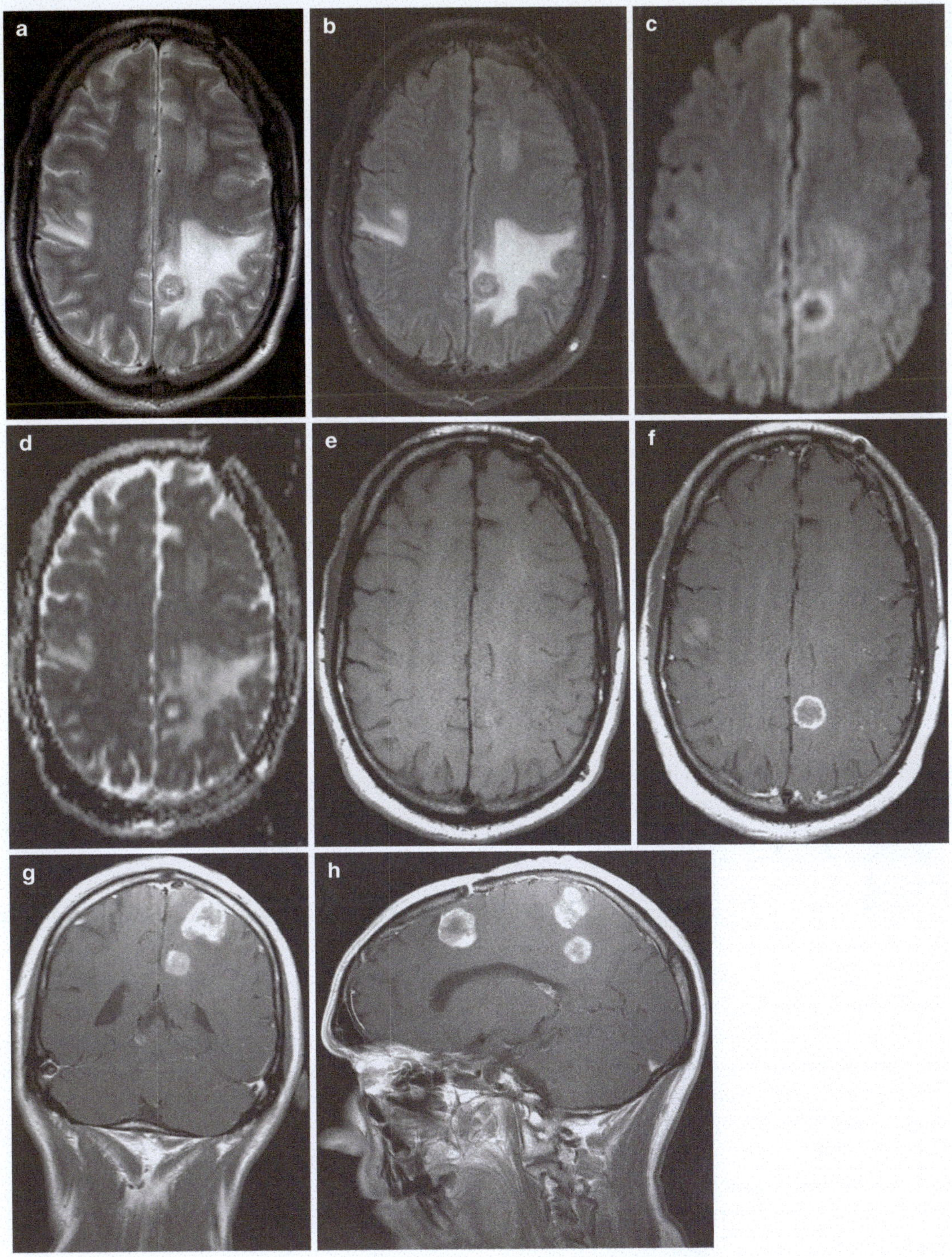

Fig. 2.26 Multiple cerebral metastases. (**a**) Axial TSE T2-WI. (**b**) Axial fat-sat turbo FLAIR. (**c**) Axial EPI diffusion-weighted "trace" image. (**d**) Apparent diffusion coefficient (ADC) map. (**e**) Axial TSE T1-WI. (**f–h**) Gd-enhanced axial (**f**), coronal (**g**) and sagittal (**h**) TSE T1-WI. The primary tumor of this 43-year-old man is a poorly differentiated pulmonary adenocarcinoma. A solitary left frontal lobe metastasis had been resected the previous year. He now presents with multiple metastases, with solid or ring-like enhancement pattern. The metastasis in the medial part of the left parietal lobe has a thick hypointense wall with a hyperintense center, consistent with necrosis. Dense ring enhancement is noted on the Gd-enhanced T1-WI. The diffusion-weighted image (**c**) and the ADC map (**d**) do not show restricted diffusion (DDx with cerebral abscess)

the enhancing lesion and the background. Enhancement and thickening (often asymmetric) of the dura mater suggests dural carcinomatosis (but beware of dural enhancement after recent lumbar puncture or intracranial hypotension syndrome). Leptomeningeal enhancement indicates carcinomatous meningitis.

Although there are no pathognomonic MRI features of cerebral metastases, the following findings are highly suggestive:

- One or more intracranial, enhancing tumor(s) in a patient with a known primary extracranial neoplasm
- A small lesion with a disproportionate amount of peritumoral edema
- Multiple enhancing lesions (Figs. 2.25 and 2.26)
- A solitary, thick-walled, ring-enhancing lesion (Ddx abscess)

2.5 Infratentorial Tumors

2.5.1 Anatomy and Technique

The posterior fossa is bordered anteriorly in the midline by the dorsum sellae and the clivus (body of sphenoid bone, basilar part of occipital bone, separated by the spheno-occipital synchondrosis). The posterior aspect of the petrous bone constitutes the anterior lateral border, while the lateral and posterior borders are formed by the occipital bone, parietal bone, sigmoid, and transverse sinus. The tentorium cerebelli and straight sinus compose the roof of the posterior fossa; the foramen magnum and jugular foramen are found in the floor of the posterior fossa.

The posterior fossa contains the brainstem (mesencephalon, pons, and medulla oblongata), cranial nerves III-XII, cerebellum (vermis, hemispheres, and tonsils), CSF spaces (fourth ventricle, cisterna magna, prepontine cistern, and CPA cisterns), arteries [vertebrobasilar artery and branches: posterior-inferior cerebellar artery (PICA), anterior-inferior cerebellar artery (AICA), superior cerebellar artery (SCA)], veins, and dural sinuses.

For the evaluation of posterior fossa lesions, axial and coronal imaging planes are preferred. Sagittal imaging is useful in fourth-ventricle mass lesions and CCJ abnormalities. When studying cranial nerve lesions, thin slices (<1 mm) should be obtained. T2-WI are useful for demonstrating edema, cysts, areas of necrosis, and the presence of a CSF cleft in extra-axial tumors. Ultra-thin T2-WI (3D TSE with flip back pulse, e.g., RESTORE, FRFSE or DRIVE sequences) or T2*-WI constructive interference in the steady state (CISS, FIESTA, FFE) are useful for visualizing the CSF within the internal auditory canal and the fluid within the inner ear structures (cochlea, vestibule, and semicircular canals). When a tumor is suspected clinically, pre- and postcontrast T1-WI must be obtained.

2.5.2 Age-Related Frequency of Posterior Fossa Tumors

In children, posterior fossa tumors constitute the largest group of solid neoplasms. Posterior fossa tumors are second only to leukemia in overall frequency during childhood. They remain associated with a high mortality rate, despite recent therapeutic advances. In children over the age of 1 year, 50% of brain tumors occur infratentorially. Conversely, in infants (<1 year old), supratentorial tumors are more frequent [PNET, low-grade gliomas, and choroid plexus tumors]. Topographically, posterior fossa tumors can be subdivided into extra- and intra-axial tumors. The latter group can be further split into brainstem, cerebellar, and fourth-ventricle tumors.

2.5.3 Extra-Axial Posterior Fossa Tumors

In adults, the most common posterior fossa tumors are extra-axial in nature. The site of predilection is the CPA cistern, which is located between the anterolateral surface of the pons and cerebellum and the posterior surface of the petrous temporal bone. The following imaging signs may be helpful to determine the extra-axial nature of a mass lesion:

- Widening of the ipsilateral CPA cistern
- Presence of a CSF cleft between the tumor and the cerebellum
- Rotation of the brainstem away from the lesion
- Displacement of the gray matter–white matter interface around the mass

Mass lesions in the CPA in decreasing order of frequency are: acoustic schwannoma (80%), meningioma

Table 2.13 Mass lesions in the cerebellopontine angle cistern

Common	• Acoustic schwannoma (80%) • Meningioma (13–18%) • Epidermoid (5%)
Less common	• Other schwannomas: facial nerve, trigeminal nerve • Vascular: vertebrobasilar dolichoectasia, aneurysm of basilar artery, AVM • Metastases • Paraganglioma • Arachnoid cyst • Lipoma • Foramen jugulare tumors • Chordoma

(15%), epidermoid (5%), other schwannomas (facial nerve, trigeminal nerve), vascular lesions (vertebrobasilar dolicho-ectasia, aneurysm of basilar artery, AVM), metastases, paraganglioma, arachnoid cyst, lipoma, foramen jugulare tumors, and chordoma (Table 2.13). Some intra-axial tumors may secondarily extend into the CPA cistern, e.g., exophytic glioma, metastasis, hemangioblastoma, and ependymoma.

Acoustic nerve schwannoma is the most common CPA tumor (80%). Clinically, this tumor presents with sensorineural hearing loss, dizziness, and gait disturbance. Many acoustic schwannomas have both an intracanalicular and a CPA component. They may be solid or cystic (in large tumors necrosis occurs secondary to hemorrhage) (Fig. 2.27). In less than 5% of cases, there is an associated CPA arachnoid cyst. The hallmark of acoustic schwannomas on MRI, except for their typical location, is the intense, often heterogeneous, enhancement. Small, purely intracanalicular schwannomas can be detected with thin (submillimeter), heavily T2-WI (e.g., 3D CISS), and their presence can be confirmed on Gd-enhanced T1-WI (Fig. 2.28). On these thin-section T2-W scans, there is often a decreased SI of the labyrinthine fluid on the affected side. This finding should be mentioned in the report, since it is associated with poor outcome.

Bilateral acoustic schwannomas occur in the setting of neurofibromatosis type 2 (Fig. 2.29). This is a neurocutaneous disorder with autosomal dominant inheritance (with high penetrance, linkage to chromosome 22). The occurrence frequency is ±1/40,000. The condition is characterized by bilateral acoustic schwannomas, intracranial meningiomas (convexity, falx), schwannomas of cranial nerves V, VII, IX, and X, spinal cord ependymoma, and astrocytoma. Neurofibromatosis type 2 is sometimes described by the acronym "MISME" (multiple inherited schwannomas, meningiomas, and ependymomas). Cutaneous lesions are less frequent than in neurofibromatosis type 1. Symptoms usually develop in the second decade (adolescents and young adults).

Meningioma is the second most common CPA tumor (<10%). Meningiomas show a broad-based dural attachment at the posterior surface of the petrous pyramid. A "dural-tail" sign is a frequent finding and is an important element in the differential diagnosis

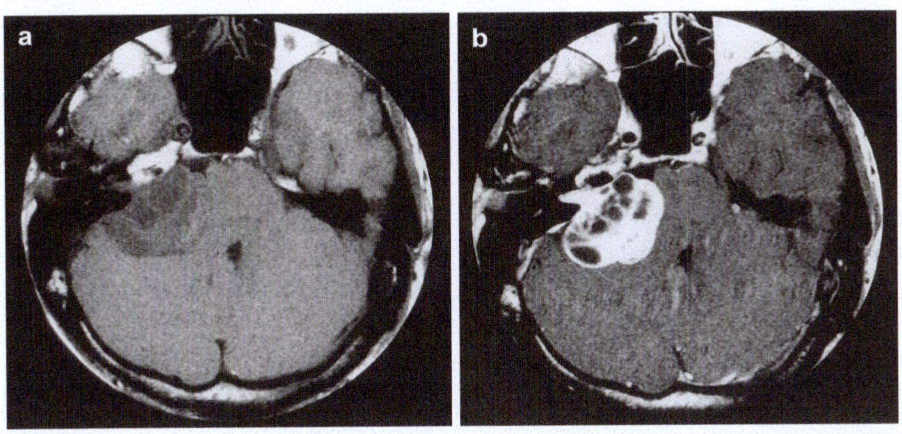

Fig. 2.27 Acoustic schwannoma. (**a**) Axial SE T1-WI. (**b**) Gd-enhanced axial SE T1-WI. A large tumor extends from the right internal auditory canal to the cerebellopontine angle cistern. The enhancement pattern is inhomogeneous. The tumor contains numerous cystic areas. The brainstem is displaced, and the fourth ventricle is flattened, due to mass effect. Note that there is some enhancement of the meninges lining the posterior surface of the petrous bone

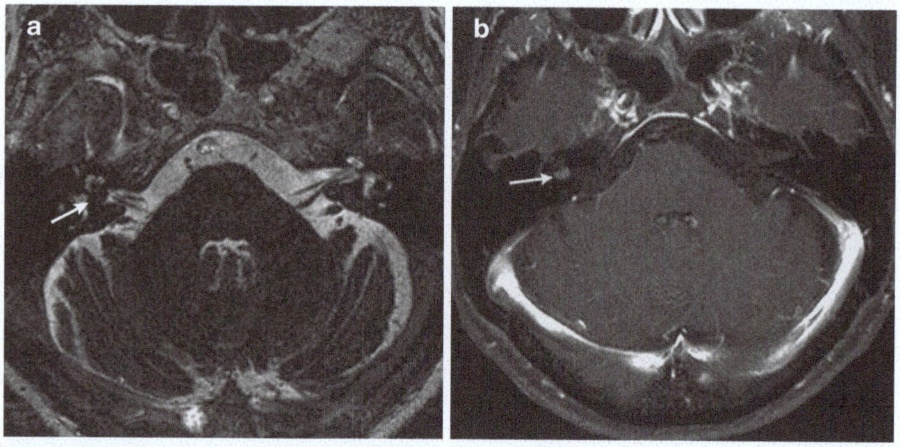

Fig. 2.28 Intracanalicular acoustic schwannoma. (**a**) Axial CISS T2-WI. (**b**) Gadolinium-enhanced axial SE T1-WI with fat saturation. On the heavily T2-W CISS image, the intracanalicular acoustic schwannoma appears as a "filling defect," outlined by bright CSF (*arrow*). Enhancement is intense and homogeneous (*arrow*). Fat saturation can be of use to distinguish the enhancing tumor from the bright fatty bone marrow signal of the petrous apex or the walls of the IAC

with acoustic schwannomas. Meningiomas tend to be eccentric from the internal auditory canal. These tumors may contain (extensive) calcifications, which may be overlooked on MRI. After Gd-injection, enhancement can be heterogeneous or homogeneous, depending on the composition and size of the tumor.

Epidermoid tumor is the third most common CPA tumor. This benign, slow-growing cystic lesion results from an "inclusion" of epithelium during neural tube closure (third to fifth week of gestation). The wall of an epidermoid is composed of a connective tissue capsule (stratified squamous epithelium); the cyst contains desquamative epithelial debris (keratin products) and cholesterol crystals. On MRI, SI can be highly variable, but most often the cyst is isointense to CSF and the lesion is hyperintense on T2-WI and heterogeneously hypointense on T1-WI; this appearance is sometimes referred to as a "black epidermoid," and is due to the presence of cholesterol crystals, keratin, and CSF in the interstices of the tumor. Conversely, a "white epidermoid" is hyperintense on T1-WI due to the presence of triglyderides and polyunsaturated fatty acids which cause shortening of the T1 relaxation time. Epidermoids do not enhance; they are avascular in nature. Diffusion-weighted imaging (DWI) typically shows diffusion restriction (high SI on diffusion trace images, and lowered ADC values). This is an important differential diagnostic feature, since arachnoid cysts and other cystic/necrotic tumors show no diffusion restriction. Though the CPA cistern is the site of predilection, epidermoids can also occur in the middle cranial fossa in the parasellar-paracavernous region. Moreover, epidermoids can also be extradural, located within the calvarium, producing well-defined bone erosion.

Other schwannomas include facial nerve schwannoma, trigeminal nerve schwannoma (also known as gasserian ganglion schwannoma), and jugular fossa schwannomas arising from the glossopharyngeal (IX), vagus (X), accessory (XI) nerves. Less common CPA lesions are listed in Table 2.13.

2.5.4 Intra-Axial Posterior Fossa Tumors

2.5.4.1 Brainstem

Brainstem gliomas represent 25% of intracranial gliomas in children and young adults compared with only 2.5% in adults. Patients usually present with cranial nerve symptoms; hydrocephalus is uncommon at the time of initial presentation. The fourth ventricle is displaced backwards, and its width may be increased (stretching). The cardinal imaging feature is the characteristic location of the tumor (Fig. 2.30). Brainstem gliomas can present two different growth patterns: diffusely infiltrating growth with symmetric expansion, or focally exophytic growth in the adjacent cisterns. Regardless of their growth pattern, brainstem gliomas are not resectable. On MRI, they

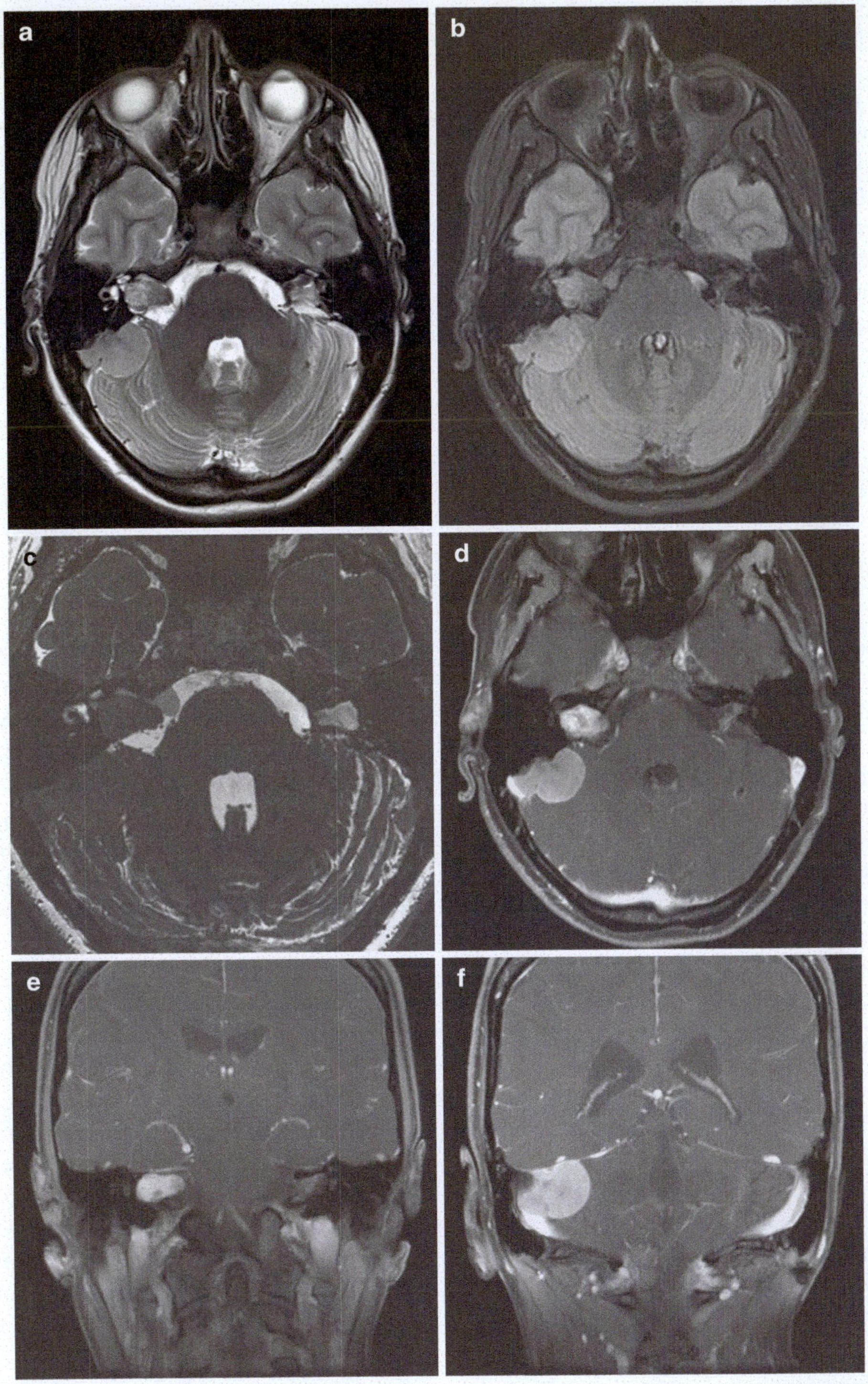

Fig. 2.29 Neurofibromatosis type II. (**a**) Axial TSE T2-WI. (**b**) Axial fat-sat turbo FLAIR. (**c**) Axial high-resolution CISS image. (**d**) Gd-enhanced fat-saturated axial TSE T1-WI. (**e, f**) Gd-enhanced coronal fat-saturated TSE T1-WI. There is an acoustic schwannoma on the *right*, which expands the internal auditory canal and extends into the *right* cerebellopontine angle cistern. On the *left*, there is a postoperative status after resection of an acoustic schwannoma, with enhancing scar tissue (**d**). There is a large meningioma on the posterior wall of the right petrous bone (**a**, **b**, **d**), growing into the sigmoid sinus (**e**). A smaller meningioma sits on the anterior lip of the right internal auditory meatus (**c**)

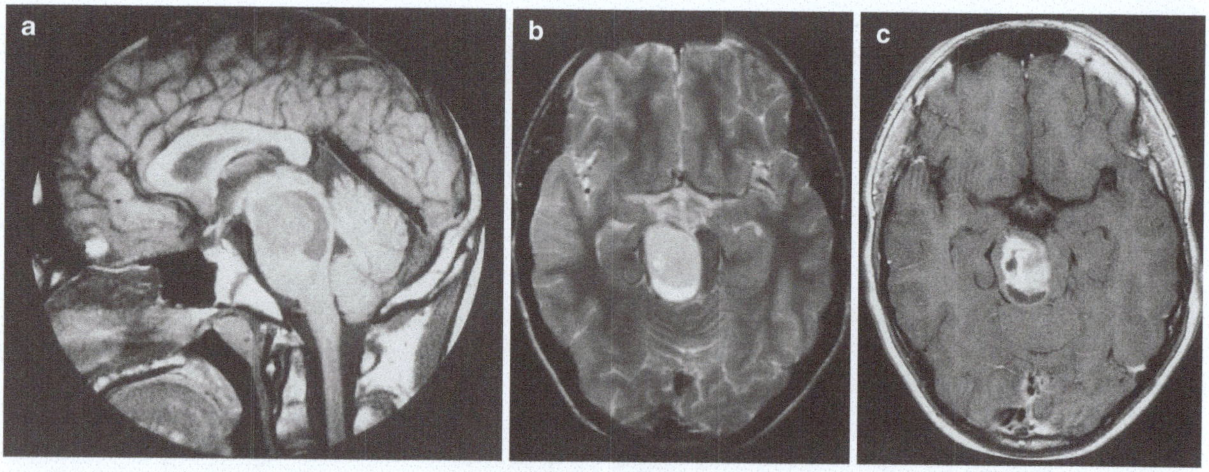

Fig. 2.30 Brainstem glioma. (**a**) Sagittal SE T1-WI. (**b**) Axial TSE T2-WI. (**c**) Gd-enhanced axial SE T1-WI. In this 16-year-old boy with a brainstem glioma, the tumor consists of an anterior solid component and a posterior cystic component. The signal intensity within the cyst is higher that that of CSF, reflecting a higher protein content. Within the solid portion of the tumor, a necrotic area can be discerned. The necrotic portion does not enhance. There is linear enhancement along the walls of the cyst, confirming that this is an intrinsic part of the tumor

are hypointense on T1-WI and hyperintense on T2-WI, and may exhibit subtle enhancement indicating BBB breakdown. The expanding tumor enlarges the brainstem (usually the pons) and may engulf the basilar artery, which becomes trapped between the tumor and the clivus. MRS provides information regarding the biochemical signature of the tumor; high concentration of choline indicates increased cell membrane turnover, and is consistent with a more malignant tumor (Fig. 2.31).

Although 90% of cavernous malformations (syn. cavernous angioma) occur supratentorially, they can also be encountered in the brainstem. Clinical symptoms of brain-stem cavernous malformations include focal motor or sensory changes and are related to the exact location of the lesion. Imaging characteristics are discussed in Chap. 2.7.4.4.

2.5.4.2 Tumors in or Around the Fourth Ventricle

PNET constitute the second most common group of CNS tumors in children. *Medulloblastoma* is the most common representative of this group in the posterior fossa. The peak age range is 5–10 years, with a second, lesser peak between 20 and 30 years. In children, medulloblastoma typically arises in the midline in the posterior vermis (Fig. 13.45). Due to its origin in the roof of the fourth ventricle, obstructive hydrocephalus is common. The presenting symptoms are related to increased intracranial pressure (headache, vomiting). On MRI examinations, these tumors are hypointense on T1-WI and hyperintense on T2-WI. They enhance with Gd-chelates. They have a propensity to leptomeningeal dissemination (metastatic seeding in the subarachnoid space). Therefore, during follow-up examinations, not only the posterior fossa, but the entire neuraxis should be examined. In adults, medulloblastoma typically arises in a cerebellar hemisphere.

Ependymoma represents 10% of childhood brain tumors. There appears to be a bimodal age peak at the age of 5 and 34 years. Two-thirds of intracranial ependymomas are located in the infratentorial compartment, especially in children. Ependymomas are often situated in the floor of the fourth ventricle (Fig. 13.47). They have a propensity to extend through the foramina of Magendie or Luschka, and grow into the CPA cistern or cisterna magna. As in medulloblastomas, the presenting symptoms are related to increased intracranial pressure (obstructive hydrocephalus). On noncontrast CT images, calcifications are present in 50% of cases. The MRI appearance of ependymomas is markedly inhomogeneous, due to the presence of calcifications, necrosis, and hemorrhage (hemosiderin deposits). Ependymomas

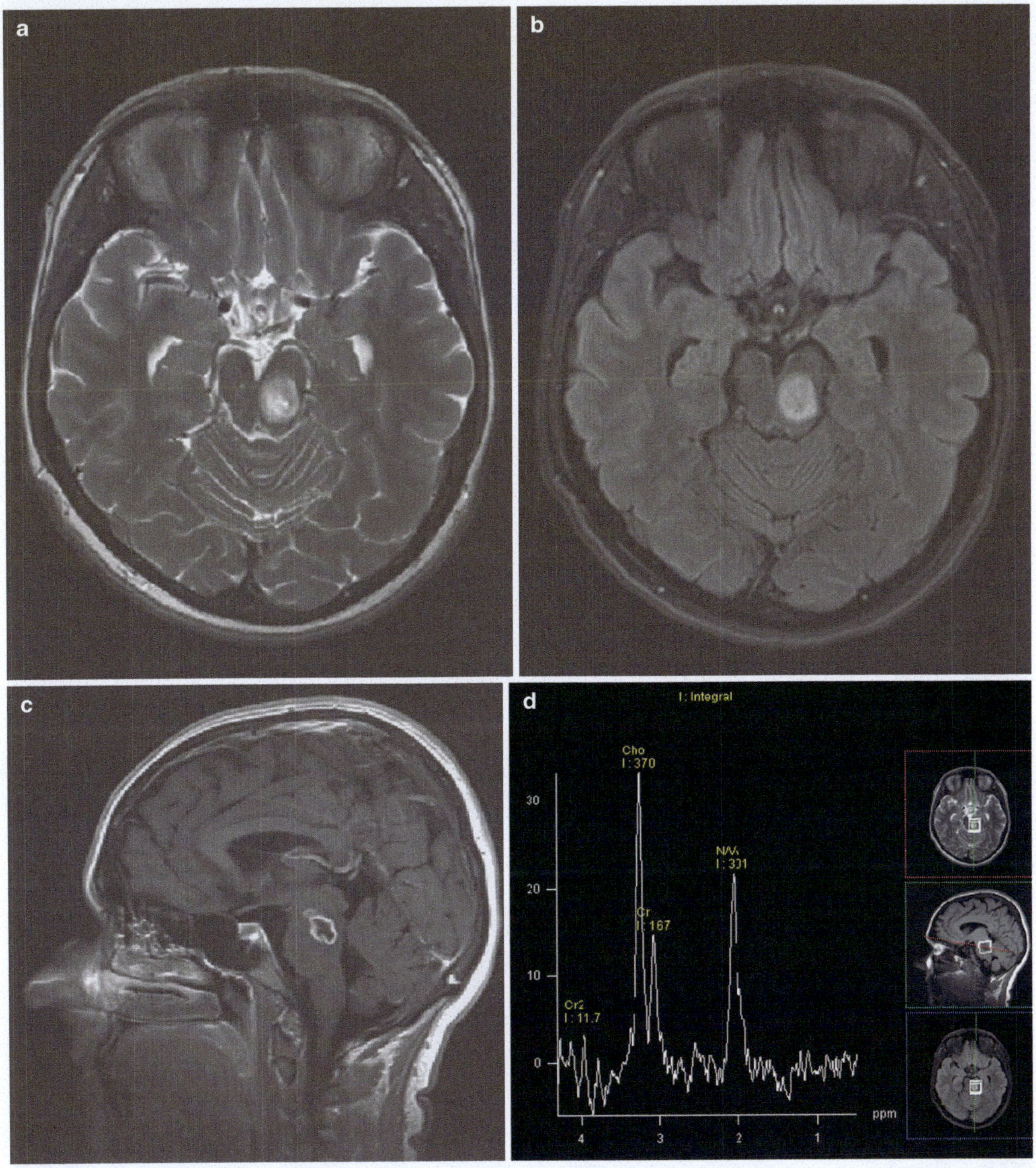

Fig. 2.31 Brainstem glioma in a 40-year-old woman. (**a**) Axial TSE T2-WI. (**b**) Axial fat-sat turbo FLAIR. (**c**) Gd-enhanced sagittal TSE T1. (**d**) Single voxel proton MR spectroscopy (MRS). The tumor extends from the left side of the pons to the mesencephalon and left cerebral peduncle. The mass appears homogeneously hyperintense on T2 and FLAIR, but after Gd administration, there is ring-enhancement, with a central nonenhancing area. MRS shows a markedly increased choline peak, indicating high cell-membrane turnover. Stereotactic biopsy of the lesion revealed astrocytoma grade III

are vascular in nature and enhance moderately or intensely with Gd.

Lesions of the choroid plexus can be cysts, papillomas, or carcinomas. *Choroid plexus cysts* are most often discovered in the lateral ventricles and are infrequent in the fourth ventricle. The MRI appearance is that of a small cystic lesion that is hypointense on T1-WI; there is no enhancement of the cyst contents. On DWI, plexus cysts may show restricted diffusion because of the high viscosity of their gelatinous content. The location of *choroid plexus papilloma* is age-related. In adults, choroid plexus papilloma is found in the fourth ventricle and CPA. In infants, it is found in the trigone of the lateral ventricle. On MRI, choroid plexus papilloma is iso-hypointense on T1-WI and slightly hypointense on T2-WI. The papilloma enhances markedly with Gd. Ventricular dilatation is a frequently associated finding; this can be due to overproduction of CSF by the papilloma and also due to the obstruction of CSF pathways by tumor and by repeated episodes of occult hemorrhage.

2.5.4.3 Primary Cerebellar Tumors

Cerebellar astrocytoma is the most common CNS tumor in children and the second most common posterior fossa tumor (PNET is slightly more frequent) (Chap. 13.2.6.1); it is much less frequent in adults. Histologically, most cerebellar astrocytomas are low-grade and slow growing. They are typically large at diagnosis. Cerebellar astrocytomas arise in the cerebellar hemisphere or vermis. The fourth ventricle is displaced forward and often obliterated; obstructive hydrocephalus is common. The prepontine cistern is narrowed, due to mass effect. Many cerebellar astrocytomas are cystic, often with an enhancing mural nodule (Fig. 2.32). They can be indistinguishable from hemangioblastoma on MRI.

A special type of astrocytoma is the *juvenile pilocytic astrocytoma* (Fig. 13.46). It is the most benign histologic subtype of astrocytoma and predominantly affects children and young adults (Table 2.12). The typical appearance on the MRI is that of a cyst with an enhancing mural nodule (Table 2.11). The SI of the cyst is higher than CSF on T1-WI and T2-WI due to an increased protein content. However, solid forms are not unusual. On the MRI, they are characterized by a heterogeneously increased SI on early Gd-enhanced T1-WI, representing an enhancing matrix; homogeneous enhancement is observed on delayed images.

Hemangioblastoma is the most common primary intra-axial tumor of the adult posterior fossa. It is a benign tumor arising along a pial surface of the

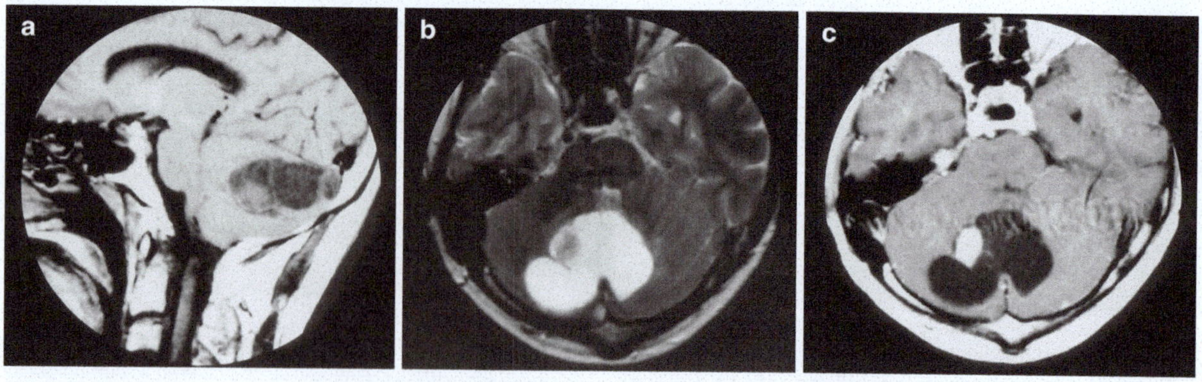

Fig. 2.32 Cystic cerebellar astrocytoma. (**a**) Sagittal SE T1-WI. (**b**) Axial TSE T2-WI. (**c**) Gd-enhanced axial SE T1-WI. There is a cystic-appearing cerebellar mass with a mural nodule. The fourth ventricle is flattened and displaced anteriorly. The cyst contents are of higher signal intensity than CSF, both on the T1-WI and T2-WI, presumably indicating higher protein content. After contrast injection, the mural nodule enhances strongly and uniformly. The principal differential diagnosis involves hemangioblastoma, a tumor which can exhibit similar imaging characteristics

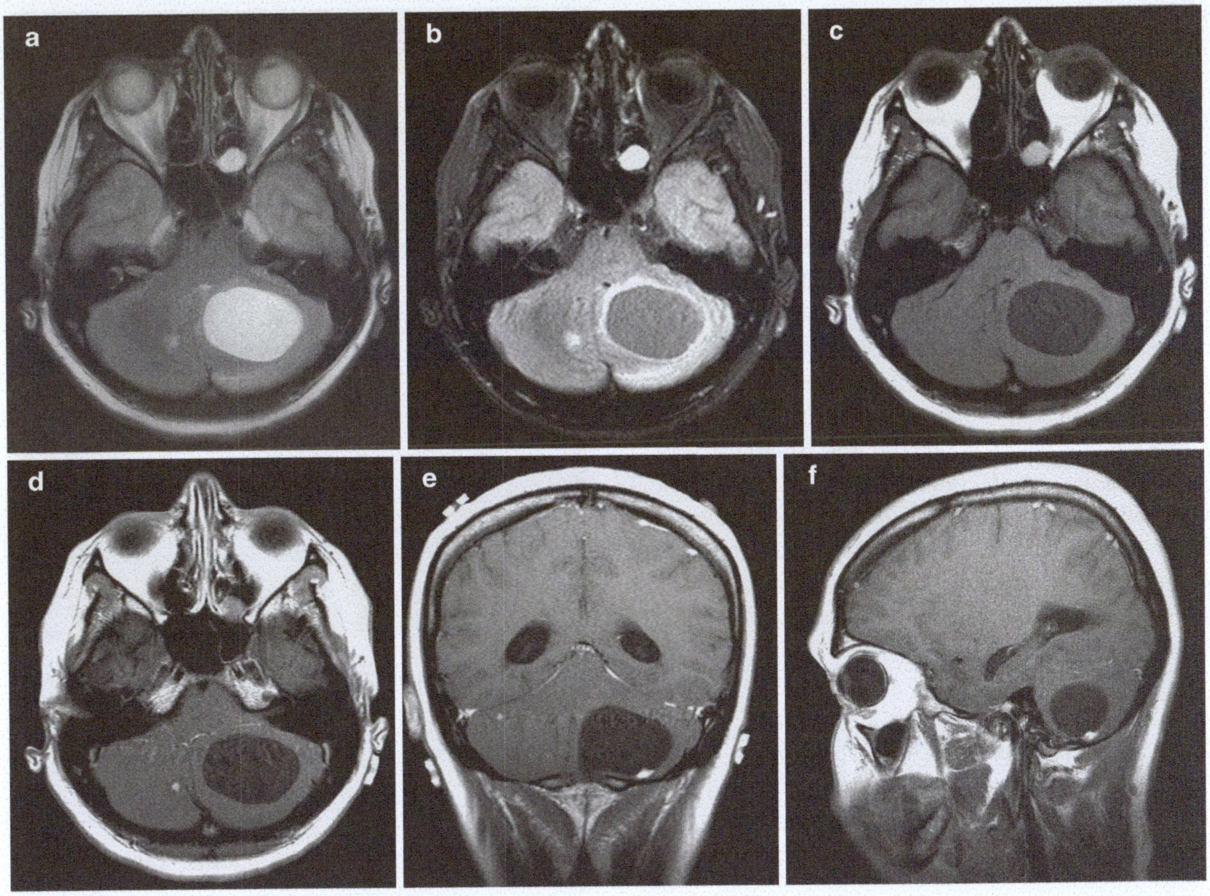

Fig. 2.33 Multiple cerebellar hemangioblastomas. (**a**) Axial TSE T2-WI. (**b**) Axial fat-sat turbo FLAIR. (**c**) Axial TSE T1-WI. Gd-enhanced axial (**d**), coronal (**e**) and sagittal (**f**) TSE T1-WI. The patient is a 25-year-old woman with von Hippel-Lindau syndrome, who presented with headaches, nausea, and vomiting. The largest tumor in the left cerebellar hemisphere presents the classic appearance of a cystic mass, with a small enhancing mural nodule inferiorly. In addition, there are several other small, solidly enhancing hemangioblastomas in the right cerebellar hemisphere

cerebellum, brainstem, or spinal cord. The MRI appearance is characterized by a combination of cysts containing proteinaceous fluid and solid mass lesions (Fig. 2.33). A typical appearance is that of a sharply demarcated cyst with an enhancing mural nodule (Table 2.11). Hemangioblastomas can be sporadic or inherited, solitary or multiple (von Hippel-Lindau). Between 4 and 40% of patients with hemangioblastoma match criteria for *von Hippel-Lindau syndrome*. This syndrome is a neurocutaneous disorder. It is defined by the association of two or more CNS hemangioblastomas (cerebellar hemangioblastoma, retinal angiomatosis, spinal cord, cauda equina hemangioblastoma) with multiple visceral organ cysts or neoplasms (kidney, liver, pancreas, epididymis, pheochromocytoma) and a family history of von Hippel-Lindau disease.

2.5.4.4 Secondary Tumors (Metastasis)

Although 85% of metastatic lesions are supratentorial, metastasis is still the most common intra-axial neoplasm of the adult posterior fossa; 15–20% of all intracranial metastases occur in the posterior fossa. Multiple lesions are the hallmark, but in the posterior fossa, there is a relatively high incidence of solitary lesions (25–50%). Metastases typically are found at gray–white matter interfaces; presumably because tumoral micro-emboli become stuck in the small capillaries. The MR SI of metastases can be altered by the presence of hemorrhage (methemoglobin, hemosiderin), mucin content (hypointense appearance on T2), melanin (paramagnetic effect), and necrosis (high SI on T2-WI, no enhancement in the necrotic areas). Diffusion restriction occurs in metastases from mucinous tumors; conversely there is no diffusion restriction in necrotic areas of cystic metastatic lesions. Abscess, primary glial tumor, and radiation necrosis should be considered in the differential diagnosis. The origin of metastases is in decreasing order of frequency: lung > breast > skin (melanoma) > GIT & GUT. Lung cancer remains the most common source of brain metastases; 50% of lung tumor patients have CNS metastases. Breast carcinoma is the second most common source of intracranial tumors; 30% of breast carcinomas have associated CNS metastases. Malignant melanoma is the third most common tumor to involve the brain secondarily. Other primary tumors arise from the GIT and GUT.

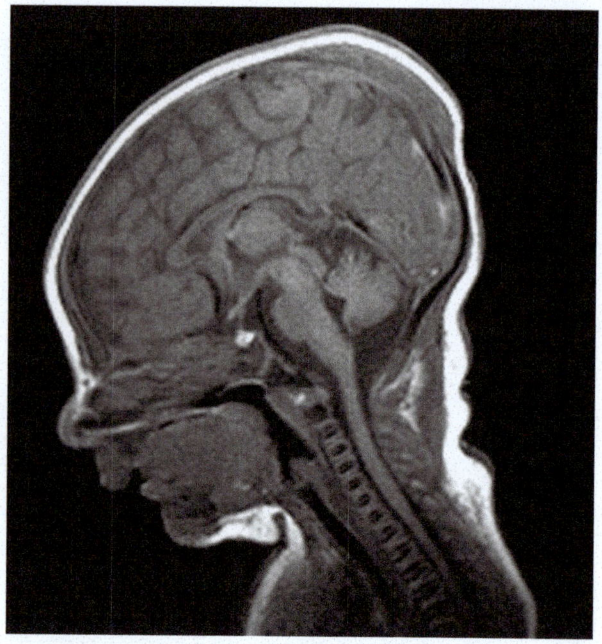

Fig. 2.34 In newborns, the pituitary gland is hyperintense on sagittal T1-WI. This is a normal finding up to the age of 2 months. The subcutaneous swelling in the parietal region represents a caput succedaneum

2.6 Sella Turcica and Hypophysis

2.6.1 Introduction

The pituitary gland consists of two lobes that are physiologically and anatomically distinct: the anterior lobe (adenohypophysis) and the posterior lobe (neurohypophysis). Both are contained within the sella turcica.

The appearance of the pituitary gland depends on the age and the gender of the subject. In neonates (up to 2 months of age), the pituitary gland is normally very hyperintense on T1-WI (Fig. 2.34). It also appears larger than later in life. In adults, the adenohypophysis is isointense to cerebral white matter, whereas the neurohypophysis is hyperintense on sagittal T1-WI. The higher signal of the posterior lobe is believed to be caused by the presence of neurosecretory granules containing vasopressin. Absence of high signal can be associated with diabetes insipidus, but can also occur as a normal finding.

In men, the hypophysis is generally smaller than in women, with a maximum height of 6–8 mm. The pituitary gland decreases in size with aging. In pregnant women, the pituitary gland is spherical or upwardly convex. The anterior pituitary is enlarged, and the height may reach up to 12 mm. It may be hyperintense on precontrast T1-WI. Pituitary lesions associated with pregnancy are lymphocytic adenohypophysitis and Sheehan's syndrome.

2.6.2 MRI Technique

The examination of the sella turcica and hypophysis places high demands on the MRI equipment and sequences. Because of the small volume of the pituitary gland, thin slices must be obtained (1–3 mm). In order to improve in-plane spatial resolution, a small FoV (<20 cm) and appropriate matrix (256 or higher) are recommended.

The close proximity of the air-filled sphenoid sinus constitutes an additional difficulty, because susceptibility artifacts may occur. Therefore, SE sequences are preferred; GRE sequences are generally avoided, except when operating at lower field strengths.

Presaturation pulses can be applied to eliminate phase-shift artifacts from the pulsatile arterial flow in the internal carotid arteries or venous flow in the superior sagittal sinus. For sagittal postgadoinium T1-WI, we routinely place an oblique coronal presaturation pulse on the superior sagittal sinus to eliminate flow artifacts, which are more pronounced after contrast administration due to T1 shortening of the venous blood.

To improve the intrinsically lower SNR in mid- and low-field MRI units, SE sequences with a narrow bandwidth are often used. These sequences have a longer minimal TE value, and therefore, the number of slices (coverage) is lower. However, this is not a problem in pituitary imaging, since only a limited number of slices are needed to cover the area of interest. Another disadvantage is that sequences with narrow bandwidth increase chemical-shift artifacts. This may cause the fatty marrow of the dorsum sellae to overlap the high signal of the posterior pituitary on sagittal T1-WI; this artifact can be avoided by setting the read-out gradient in the anteroposterior direction, so that fat is shifted posteriorly. Similarly, on coronal images, the read-out gradient should be adjusted so that the fatty marrow of the sellar floor is shifted inferiorly. This technique ensures adequate visualization of the inferior part of the pituitary gland. Our standard imaging protocol is given in Table 2.14.

Following i.v. injection of Gd contrast agents, there is an immediate and intense enhancement of the pituitary stalk, adenohypophysis, and cavernous sinus. Enhancement is maximal after 1–3 min. The dynamic process of progressive enhancement of the pituitary gland can be visualized by using sequential T1-WI. In many institutions, dynamic imaging in the coronal plane has become part of the standard imaging protocol for pituitary adenoma. It is generally performed with a TSE T1-sequence, which is repeated every 20 s. Ideally, multiple slice locations should be imaged to completely cover the anterior pituitary lobe. GRE sequences are to be avoided because of the magnetic susceptibility artifacts caused by the air-containing sphenoid sinus.

Literature data suggest that for dynamic postcontrast pituitary imaging, a half dose of Gd may be sufficient (0.05 mmol/kg body weight). Moreover, a half dose of Gd improves contrast between the pituitary gland and the cavernous sinuses. However, when performing MRI of the pituitary at lower field strengths, we recommend a standard dose of Gd (0.1 mmol/kg body weight), because the T1-shortening effect of Gd is less pronounced.

For postcontrast images, magnetization transfer should not be used, because it further reduces the SNR of the thin-section, small-FoV images.

The protocol, as suggested in Table 2.14, should be adapted to the clinical demand. In children with growth-hormone-deficient dwarfism, the imaging protocol can be limited to precontrast sagittal and coronal SE T1-W sequences, which show an ectopic posterior pituitary lobe and absence of the stalk (Fig. 2.35). In patients with central diabetes insipidus, precontrast T1-WI demonstrates the absence of the posterior pituitary lobe high signal.

Table 2.14 Protocol for MRI of the pituitary gland

Sequence	Rationale
Coronal T1-WI	Baseline sequence
Sagittal T1-WI	Look for the signal intensity difference between adenohypophysis (isointense to white matter) and neurohypophysis (hyperintense)
Coronal T2-WI	Look for high signal abnormalities in the pituitary gland or adjacent structures (cavernous sinus, sphenoid sinus, …)
Coronal DWI (trace images and ADC maps) (optional)	Useful in the preoperative evaluation of macroadenomas to assess the viscosity of the lesion
Intravenous contrast injection (half dose)	
Dynamic coronal T1-WI sequence	To assess the progressive enhancement which starts at the pituitary tuft and moves outward to the pituitary lobes
Coronal T1-WI	Look for adenomas, which in the early phase, enhance less intensely than normal pituitary tissue
Sagittal T1-WI	Look for thickening of the pituitary stalk, extension of lesion into the suprasellar cistern or sphenoid sinus

For pituitary gland imaging, high spatial resolution is required. This implies use of a small FoV (≤200 mm) with a 256 matrix. Alternatively, when a 512 matrix is used, the FoV can be somewhat larger. The key issue is pixel size. For the dynamic sequence, the FoV may need to be increased some what, to improve SNR. A limited number of slices is sufficient for a non-enlarged pituitary gland. In cases of pituitary macroadenoma, more slices should be obtained to cover the tumor. Slice thickness for the dynamic study may need to be increased to cover the whole mass. For the dynamic TSE coronal T1-W images, a high ETL increases the speed of the sequence, but also increases T2-W of the image, which is an unwanted effect. Therefore, a balance must be found between a short acquisition time (which requires a high ETL) and a sufficient number of T1-W images (which requires a shorter ETL)

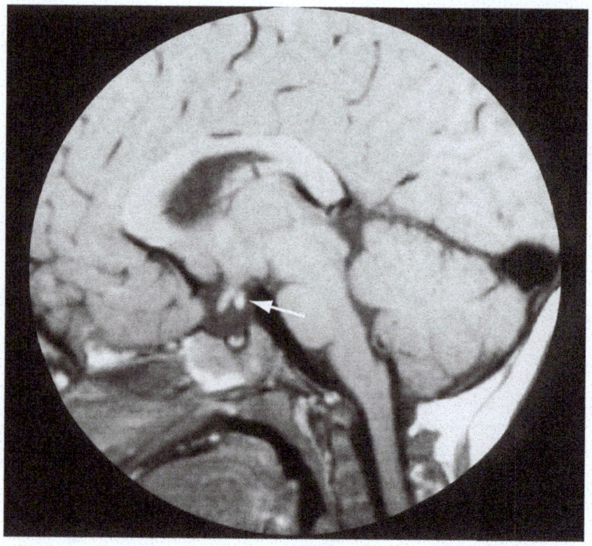

Fig. 2.35 Growth-hormone-deficient dwarfism. In this 3-year-old child with growth-hormone-deficient dwarfism, the sagittal SE T1-WI shows the ectopic posterior pituitary lobe as a focal area of high signal intensity at the proximal infundibulum (*arrow*). The pituitary stalk is absent. This example illustrates that precontrast sagittal SE T1-WI constitute an important part of the examination, especially in children and patients with diabetes insipidus

2.6.3 Pituitary Adenoma

Pituitary adenomas are benign, slow-growing neoplasms arising from the adenohypophysis. They represent 10–15% of all intracranial neoplasms and are the most frequent indication for pituitary MRI. On the basis of histology, pituitary adenomas are subdivided into chromophobe (80%), acidophilic or eosinophilic (15%), and basophilic (5%) types. Alternatively, pituitary adenomas can be classified into functioning (prolactinoma, corticotrophic,and somatotrophic adenoma) or nonfunctioning lesions. An "incidentaloma" is defined as a nonfunctioning pituitary adenoma or pituitary cyst. However, there are no imaging features to distinguish between different types of adenomas. For medical imaging purposes, the most useful classification is to categorize pituitary adenomas by size into microadenoma (≤10 mm) or macroadenoma (>10 mm).

Microadenomas are by definition no larger than 10 mm in diameter. In many cases, MRI provides direct visualization of the adenoma. Typically, on precontrast or (early) postcontrast scans, the adenoma is seen as a small lesion of low SI relative to the normally enhancing pituitary gland (Fig. 2.36). This is due to the greater relative enhancement of normal pituitary tissue vs. adenoma. Adenomas display a later peak of enhancement, with slower washout. This implies that early postcontrast scans are required for lesion identification. On later postcontrast T1-WI, the adenoma may become isointense to normal pituitary tissue and may even become slightly hyperintense. Indirect signs of the presence of a pituitary adenoma include: focal depression or erosion of the sellar floor, displacement of the pituitary stalk, asymmetrical, focal upward convexity of the hypophysis, and invasion of the cavernous sinus.

By definition, *macroadenomas* are 10 mm or greater in size. Frequently, macroadenomas are nonsecretory. Clinical symptoms are caused by pressure on adjacent structures, especially the optic chiasm (Fig. 2.37). This

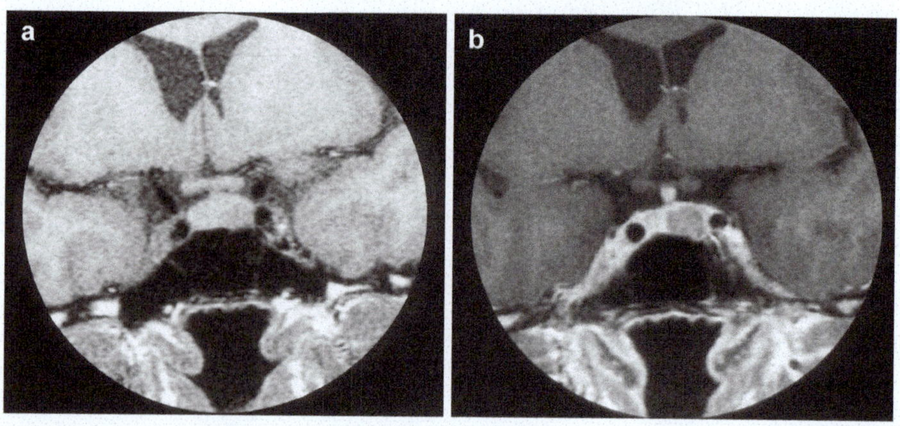

Fig. 2.36 Pituitary microadenoma. (**a**) Coronal SE T1-WI. (**b**) Coronal Gd-enhanced SE T1-WI. This 38-year-old woman had elevated serum prolactin levels. The precontrast image shows an asymmetry between the right and left pituitary lobes. On the postcontrast image, the adenoma in the left pituitary lobe is outlined by the normally enhancing pituitary tissue. Thin slices with high spatial resolution are required

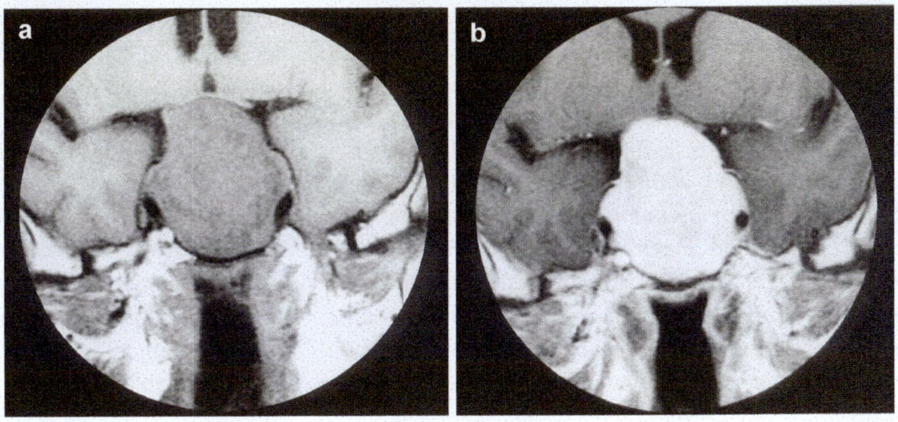

Fig. 2.37 Pituitary macroadenoma. (**a**) Coronal SE T1-WI. (**b**) Coronal Gd-enhanced SE T1-WI. This 45-year-old woman presented with progressive visual loss. The images show a typical pituitary macroadenoma. Note the upward displacement of the optic chiasm, which is draped over the top of the tumor. After Gd, the tumor enhances strongly but inhomogeneously

may lead to visual loss, most commonly bitemporal hemianopia. Compression of normal pituitary tissue may lead to hypopituitarism. The MRI technique is essentially the same, although more (or thicker) slices should be obtained to cover the tumor completely. On T1-WI and T2-WI, macroadenomas are usually isointense to brain tissue. They enhance with contrast; intratumoral cysts or areas of necrosis do not enhance and are hypointense on T1-WI and hyperintense on T2-WI. The use of Gd improves delineation of the mass, especially from the cavernous sinus. Many macroadenomas display enlargement and erosion of the sella, as well as extension into the suprasellar cistern, cavernous sinus, sphenoid sinus, and even the nasopharynx. On sagittal and coronal images, macroadenomas often display a dumbbell configuration, the "waistline" being caused by a constriction of the diaphragma sellae. Cavernous sinus invasion is common but difficult to ascertain on MRI. The most reliable sign is encasement of the internal carotid artery. The differential diagnosis includes suprasellar meningioma, pituitary metastasis, and craniopharyngioma. MRI allows reliable differentiation from an aneurysm. A recent development is the use of DWI in the preoperative assessment of macroadenomas. Signal intensities on DWI and ADC values provide an idea of the consistency of macroadenomas and are correlated with the percentage of collagen content at histologic examination. This is an important information for the neurosurgeon, when planning a transsphenoidal resection, to decide whether the tumor is "suckable" or not.

The appearance of a pituitary adenoma changes after treatment. Imaging findings after medical treatment (bromocriptine, cabergoline) include a decrease in the size of the adenoma, hemorrhage, and low SI on T2-WI. After transsphenoidal surgery, the following can be observed: a defect in the anterior floor of the sella, fat and/or muscle plug, secondary empty sella, and herniation of the optic chiasm. After surgery via craniotomy, the FoV should be enlarged to study potential brain damage along the surgical approach route.

2.6.4 Other Intra-, Supra-, and Parasellar Lesions

Empty sella is defined as an extension of the subarachnoid space into the sella turcica. *Primary empty sella* can be due to a defect in the diaphragma sellae, involution of a pituitary tumor, or regression of the pituitary gland after pregnancy. *Secondary empty sella* is postsurgical in origin, presumably secondary to disruption of the diaphragma sellae. MRI shows an enlarged sella turcica, filled with CSF. The position of the optic chiasm is important to note; visual symptoms may occur if there is downward herniation of the optic chiasm.

Empty sella should be differentiated from a *suprasellar arachnoid cyst*, which is developmental in origin, due to an imperforate membrane of Lillequist. On MRI, a suprasellar arachnoid cyst appears as a well-marginated, homogeneous lesion, which is isointense to CSF on all pulse sequences. In the differential diagnosis, epidermoid and craniopharyngioma should be considered.

Enlargement of the pituitary stalk, best seen on the coronal and sagittal postcontrast T1-WI, is a nonspecific finding. The differential diagnosis includes histiocytosis X, leptomeningeal carcinomatosis, metastasis, and granulomatous disorders (sarcoidosis, giant cell granuloma, tuberculosis, syphilis).

Craniopharyngiomas are slowly growing, benign tumors arising from epithelial remnants of Rathke's pouch. They represent 3–4% of all intracranial neoplasms and are the most common suprasellar mass lesions; 70% are both intra- and suprasellar, whereas 20% are entirely suprasellar. The age distribution is bimodal: the *adamantinomatous type* is encountered in children (first and second decades), whereas the *papillary type* occurs in adults (fourth and fifth decades). The pediatric craniopharyngioma (adamantinomatous type) is the most frequently occurring form. It typically contains cystic and solid components, and calcifications are frequent. It often invades the adjacent brain, leading to dense gliosis. Recurrence after surgery is common. The adult variety (papillary craniopharyngioma) is generally solid and often extends into the third ventricle.

Clinical symptoms are related to compression of the optic chiasm (bitemporal hemianopsia), hypothalamus, and pituitary gland (hypopituitarism, diabetes insipidus, and growth failure in children). Headaches may be secondary to hydrocephalus and increased intracranial pressure.

MRI typically shows a heterogeneous tumor with cystic and solid components. The cysts display variable SI on T1-WI, depending on their contents (cholesterol, protein, hemorrhage). Most frequently, the cysts are of higher SI than CSF on both T1-WI and T2-WI (Fig. 13.52). The solid components and the rim of cysts display enhancement with Gd. This is helpful in defining the extent of the lesion. Though essentially benign in nature, craniopharyngiomas have a tendency to recur after surgery, and Gd is useful in defining recurrent or residual tumor in the postoperative patient.

Calcifications, which occur in up to 80% of craniopharyngiomas in children (30–40% in adults) and are the hallmark of the lesion on plain skull films and CT, are difficult to detect on MR images. In theory, it would be useful to add a spoiled GRE T2*-WI sequence [fast low-angle shot sequence (FLASH), spoiled gradient recalled acquisition into steady state (GRASS), and fast-field echo sequence (FFE)] to the imaging protocol, to detect susceptibility effects from calcifications. Unfortunately, this sequence also brings out susceptibility artifacts due to air in the sphenoid sinus, and therefore, is of limited use.

Meningiomas occur in the suprasellar and parasellar region (sphenoid wing and cavernous sinus meningioma). They are usually slow growing but may compress vital structures. Meningiomas are isointense relative to gray matter on T1-WI. On precontrast T1-WI, the sole clue to the diagnosis may be the presence of a dural or CSF cleft. Therefore, postGd images should always be obtained: meningiomas enhance intensely and homogeneously with Gd. A dural-tail sign is frequent: extension along the anterior margin/floor of the middle cranial fossa or along the tentorium. A meningioma arising from the planum sphenoidale may cause progressive expansion of the sphenoid sinus, a condition known as pneumosinus dilatans.

Optochiasmatic and hypothalamic gliomas are discussed together because the point of origin is often undeterminable. They account for 10–15% of all supratentorial tumors in childhood, with 75% occurring in the first decade (peak age 2–4 years). Histologically, most optochiasmatic-hypothalamic astrocytomas are of the pilocytic type. There is a strong association with neurofibromatosis type 1 in 20–50% of cases. Symptoms include vision loss, diencephalic syndrome, obesity, sexual precocity, and diabetes insipidus. MRI shows a suprasellar, lobulated mass with intense, but heterogeneous contrast enhancement. The presence of intratumoral cysts and areas of necrosis, as well as calcifications render the tumor inhomogeneous. Hydrocephalus is common, due to obstruction of the foramen of Monro by large tumors.

Germinoma is a highly malignant tumor with a predilection for the suprasellar and pineal region. If, in a child, an enhancing suprasellar lesion is discovered in conjunction with a pineal tumor, germinoma should be the primary diagnosis (Fig. 13.51). Germinoma is histologically similar to seminoma and is characterized by a rapid clinical evolution. It is also called "ectopic pinealoma." Germinoma enhances strongly with Gd, because of its highly vascular nature. CSF spread is common, and therefore, the entire neuraxis should be examined for staging and follow-up.

Tuber cinereum hamartoma is not a true neoplasm. It can be sessile or pedunculated and is attached to the hypothalamus between the pituitary stalk and the mammillary bodies. It typically causes precocious puberty. On MRI, the hamartoma is isointense to gray matter on all pulse sequences (Fig. 13.53). It does not enhance because it contains an intact BBB.

An *aneurysm* of the cavernous segment of ICA (extradural portion) must not be missed and should not be mistaken for a solid tumor. Cavernous sinus aneurysm may cause progressive visual impairment and cavernous sinus syndrome (trigeminal nerve pain and oculomotor nerve paralysis). MRI is helpful in showing flow artifacts along the phase-encoding direction. The aneurysm is often of mixed SI and contains different stages of hemorrhage, thrombus, and calcifications.

An infrequent parasellar tumor is *trigeminal schwannoma*, arising from the Gasserian ganglion, in Meckel's cave. It is located in the middle cranial fossa, posterior cranial fossa, or both. On MRI, a dumbbell- or saddle-shaped mass of variable SI is seen. Enhancement is inhomogeneous due to necrosis and cyst formation in large tumors. The tumor may erode the petrous tip. Thin slices should be obtained to look for enlargement of contiguous fissures, foramina, and canals (extension into the infratemporal fossa through an enlarged foramen ovale).

2.7 Cerebrovascular Disease

2.7.1 Stroke

The term *stroke* refers to a sudden or rapid onset of a neurologic deficit (in a vascular territory) due to a cerebrovascular disease. If the neurologic dysfunction lasts for less than 24 h, the term *transient ischemic attack* (TIA) is used. A cerebral infarct that lasts longer than 24 h, but less than 72 h, is called a reversible ischemic neurologic deficit (RIND). Two major types of stroke can be discerned: ischemic and hemorrhagic stroke (Table 2.15). In this section, we shall focus on the role of MRI in ischemic stroke. Hemorrhage is covered in Chap. 1.2.8 and shall not be discussed here.

Stroke is a medical emergency and can cause permanent neurological damage, complications, and even death. The arrival of promising new aggressive therapies aimed at reestablishing the blood flow, reducing the size of the infarction, and protecting the surrounding brain at risk (penumbra) has changed the traditional role of neuroimaging. CT and MRI play a crucial role in the diagnosis, clinical management, and treatment monitoring of stroke. The narrow time window for thrombolytic therapy (up to 6 h after the onset of symptoms) necessitates a rapid and accurate diagnosis.

In a patient with acute stroke, the imaging protocol should be able to (Table 2.16):

- Rule out intracranial hemorrhage. Traditionally, CT has been the gold standard for detecting intracranial blood, but there is growing evidence that MRI with susceptibility imaging (e.g., gradient-echo T2* or SWI) may be equally valid, for example, in ruling out hemorrhagic infarction. FLAIR sequences have been shown to be highly sensitive and specific for the detection of acute subarachnoid and intraventricular blood. The role of MRI as compared to CT remains a matter of discussion.
- Show parenchymal injury. DWI can reveal regions of acute cerebral infarction within minutes after onset of symptoms.
- Provide information on tissue blood flow. Perfusion-weighted imaging (PWI) can identify areas of brain with decreased perfusion.
- Indicate areas of potentially salvageable brain tissue. It is generally accepted that, if the PWI deficit is larger than the DWI abnormality (diffusion-perfusion mismatch), there is brain tissue to be saved (penumbra), though there are exceptions to this theory.
- Assess vessel patency. Magnetic resonance angiography (MRA) can reveal vessel occlusion, narrowing, or intracranial stenoses.

Table 2.15 Classification of stroke types

1. **Ischemic stroke**
1.1 Thrombotic stroke
1.1.1 Internal carotid artery disease
1.1.2 Vertebrobasilar disease
1.1.3 Lacunar infarcts
1.2 Embolic stroke (from cardiac or arterial source)
1.2.1 Middle cerebral artery and branches
1.2.2 Anterior cerebral artery
1.2.3 Posterior cerebral artery
1.2.4 Vertebrobasilar distribution
1.3 Hypercoagulable states (including veno-occlusive disease)
1.3.1 Primary (e.g., protein S/protein C deficiency, antithrombin III deficiency)
1.3.2 Secondary (e.g., antiphospholipid antibody syndrome, paraneoplastic)
2. **Hemorrhagic stroke**
2.1 Intracerebral hemorrhage (e.g., due to hypertension or amyloid angiopathy)
2.2 Subarachnoid hemorrhage
2.2.1 Aneurysm rupture
2.2.2 Arteriovenous malformation

Table 2.16 Protocol for MRI of acute stroke

Sequence	Rationale
Axial DWI (trace images and ADC maps)	to detect foci of diffusion restriction (cytotoxic edema)
Axial turbo FLAIR	to detect other signs of recent stroke (e.g., hyperintense vessel sign, subarachnoid or intraventricular hemorrhage) and to detect signs of preexisting cerebrovascular disease
MRA 3D-TOF through base of skull and circle of Willis	to detect occlusion of a major blood vessel
Axial T2-W sequence (single echo)	to assess white-matter hyperintensities in the brain, including the posterior fossa (where FLAIR is less sensitive)
Axial gradient echo T2* or SWI	to look for hemorrhage and blood breakdown products
EPI MR perfusion with bolus injection of contrast	to reveal CBF and CBV, and mismatch with DWI
Contrast-enhanced MR angiography	to look for occlusion of a major blood vessel

The diffusion-weighted EPI sequences are motion sensitive; therefore the patient should be instructed to keep perfectly still. It is important to immobilize the patient's head as much as possible. Scan time for these sequences is <30 s. The sequence parameters depend on the equipment used. For MR perfusion imaging, contrast medium should be injected as a very tight bolus, about 10 s after the start of the EPI sequence. A MR-compatible power injector is useful. When evaluating for hemorrhagic stroke, add a partial flip angle spoiled GRE sequence, because of its increased sensitivity in detecting susceptibility artifacts. To evaluate internal carotid artery dissection, add an axial SE T1-W sequence which includes the upper neck and the skull base

2.7.1.1 Large Vessel Infarction

Imaging manifestations of cerebral infarction caused by large vessel occlusion vary over time. We can consider four stages: hyperacute (0–6 h after symptom onset), acute (first 4 days), subacute (between 4 days and 8 weeks), and chronic (after 8 weeks).

Hyperacute and Acute Infarction

The pathophysiological changes induced by acute stroke should be understood to interpret the MRI findings. In normal circumstances, cerebral blood flow (CBF) is approximately 50 mL/100 g/min; blood flow is higher in gray matter than in white matter. When CBF starts to decrease, vasodilatation occurs, and the brain attempts to compensate for the diminished blood supply by increasing the oxygen and glucose extraction fractions. A mild decrease in CBF interferes with protein synthesis. A moderate decrease in CBF causes glycolysis, with lactate accumulation and acidosis. With a more severe decrease in CBF (10–20 mL/100 g/min), the metabolic pathway of oxydative phosphorylation becomes compromised and the cellular energy supply starts to fail. Brain cells are no longer able to produce sufficient quantities of ATP to fuel the Na^+/K^+ -ATPase sodium-potassium pump. Active membrane transport becomes impaired, and failure of the sodium-potassium pump causes irreversible ion fluxes across the cell membrane. The loss of membrane integrity, and the ensuing ion fluxes, causes rapid swelling of cells; this is known as *cytotoxic edema*. The process of cytotoxic edema, once started, is irreversible and ultimately leads to cell death. The cascade of events leading to cytotoxic edema starts within minutes after the onset of an arterial stroke, and causes neurological dysfunction.

Vasogenic edema starts to occur several hours (2–6 h) after the onset of ischemia and is caused by injury to endothelial cells and disruption of the capillary tight junctions, with the breakdown of BBB. This results in an accumulation of plasma proteins and water in the extracellular space from the intravascular space. Vasogenic edema usually peaks around 3–4 days after the onset of infarction.

Conventional MRI techniques are of limited use in demonstrating hyperacute stroke (<12 h). On the other hand, diffusion-weighted MRI and perfusion MRI are very useful, and compete with CT for a role in the management of the patient presenting with an acute stroke.

DWI is an echo-planar imaging (EPI)-based technique that measures the random motion of water molecules (i.e., diffusion) in biological tissues during the application of strong magnetic field gradients. The sensitivity to diffusion is expressed by the "*b* value" of the sequence (in s/mm^2). The higher the *b* value, the more dephasing occurs, and the more heavily the signal reflects areas of restricted diffusion. In clinical practice, *b* values around 1,000 s/mm^2 are most commonly used.

Diffusion gradients are applied in (at least) three orthogonal directions. These images can be combined in a so-called "trace" image, which represents the sum of the elements along the main diagonal of the 3 by 3 matrix, which is formed by applying individual diffusion gradients to the slice, read, and phase directions. In practice, the trace image represents a sort of mean of the individual images. In clinical practice, we obtain three images per anatomic slice position (Fig. 2.38):

- $b = 0$ image. This is merely a heavily T2-W EPI image, with the diffusion gradients switched off.
- $b = 1{,}000$ trace image. In regions of acute cerebral infarction (cytotoxic edema), diffusion of water is restricted, causing the lesion to appear bright on DWI.
- ADC maps. ADC maps are parametric images in which each pixel reflects the "ADC" at that location. Tissues in which water mobility is restricted appear dark on ADC maps (the ADC is lower in the infarcted lesion).

In case of a complete arterial occlusion, DWI can depict the lesion within minutes, due to the rapid onset of cytotoxic edema. The DWI lesion volume progressively increases up to day 3 or 4; this enlargement presumably reflects progressive infarction of the ischemic penumbra, as well as increasing edema. After 1 week, the volume of

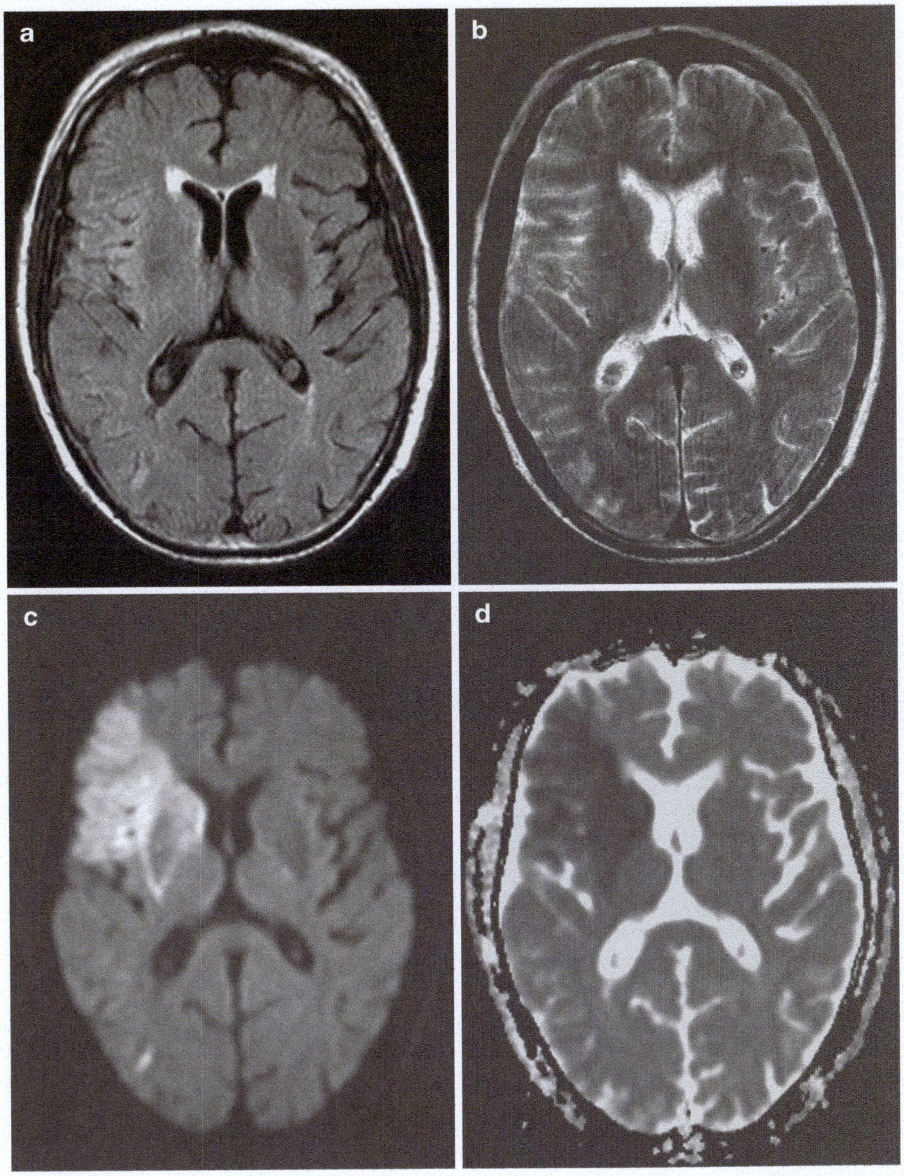

Fig. 2.38 Diffusion-weighted MRI in hyperacute infarction. The patient is a 71-year-old man examined within 2 h after acute onset of left hemiplegia and left facial nerve paralysis. (**a**) Axial turbo FLAIR image. (**b**) Axial TSE T2-WI. (**c**) Axial diffusion-weighted image (DWI), trace image. (**d**) Axial apparent diffusion coefficient map (ADC). The axial FLAIR and TSE T2-WI are within normal limits. Image quality is somewhat degraded by motion artifacts. The DWI shows a focal area of bright signal intensity in the right operculofrontal and sylvian region. On the ADC map, the area of restricted diffusion is confirmed as a hypointense lesion (decreased ADC). Signal abnormalities in the DWI and ADC maps indicate cytotoxic edema. The findings are consistent with hyperacute infarction of the right middle cerebral artery

the DWI abnormality starts to decrease to a level approaching the T2-defined lesion on day 30. This is explained by the fact that, as cells die, cell membranes and other microstructures restricting diffusion disappear.

PWI can be performed using two basic approaches. In arterial spin labeling (ASL), hydrogen protons are labeled outside the head, and the flow of this *endogenous* contrast agent (i.e., tagged spins) through the brain is observed. There are two main approaches: continuous ASL and pulsed ASL. Despite recent technical advances and promising results, ASL is not yet widely used in clinical practice, because it suffers from poor SNR, requires longer imaging times, and can only be applied at higher field strengths (3 T or higher). The currently more widespread approach uses injection of an *exogenous* contrast agent (Gd-based chelate) to act as a T2* contrast agent during its first pass through the cerebral vasculature. The contrast agent causes a transient decrease in SI (T2*-shortening susceptibility effect), proportional to the concentration in a given region (Fig. 2.39). The technique is known as *dynamic susceptibility contrast (DSC) imaging*. Using a rapid imaging sequence (typically EPI), as many as 50 sequential images can be obtained during bolus injection of contrast, covering a time interval of roughly 70 s. Bolus injection of contrast is performed 5–10 s after

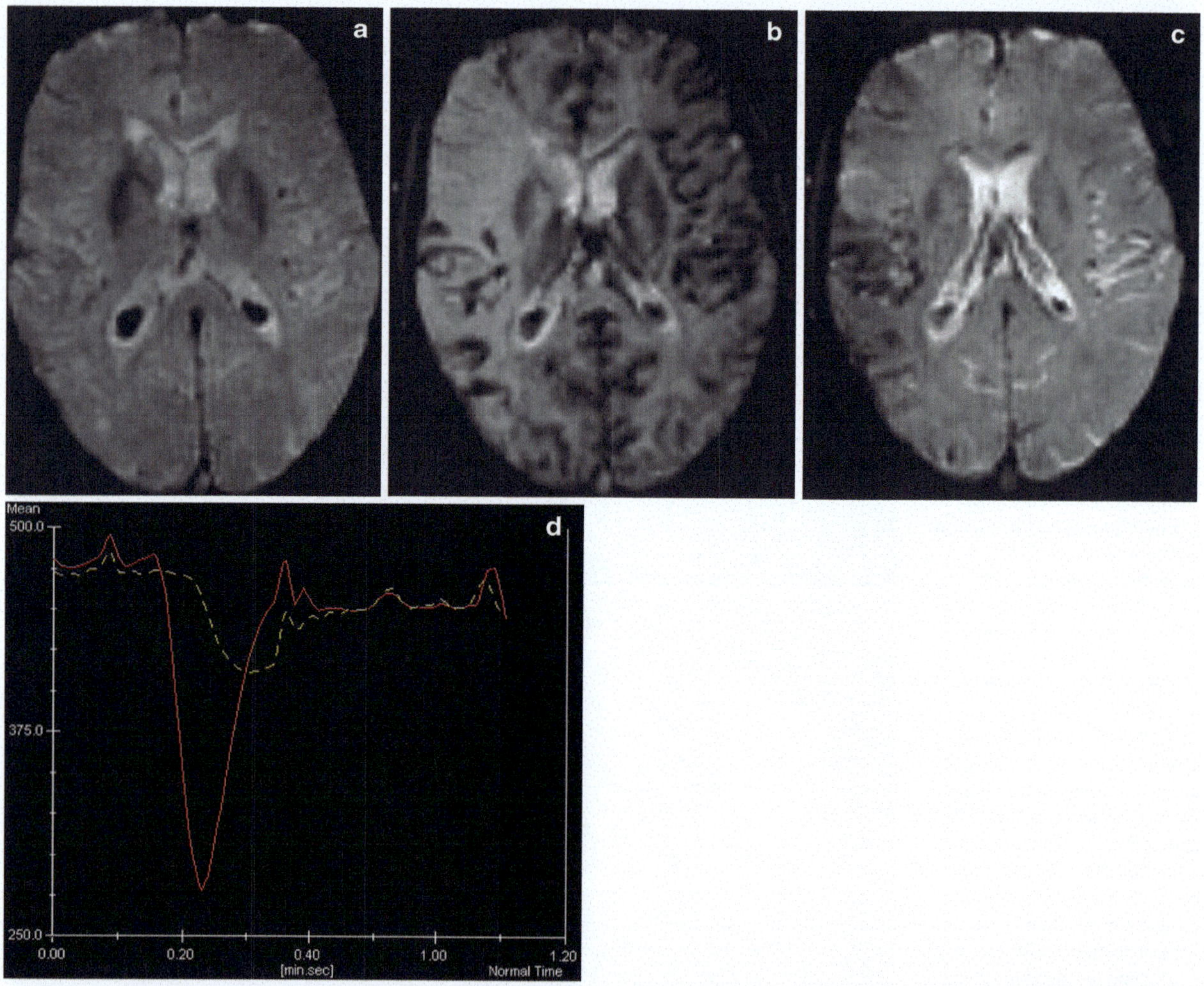

Fig. 2.39 Technique of perfusion-weighted imaging in a patient with hyperacute right middle cerebral artery stroke (same patient as Fig. 2.38). Fast EPI images are obtained during rapid intravenous injection of a contrast bolus (5 mL/s, antecubital vein, 18-gauge IV catheter). (**a**) Baseline image before arrival of the bolus. (**b**) Image during first pass of the contrast bolus. (**c**) Image after passage of the bolus. (**d**) Time-intensity plot, covering 70 s. The first pass of the contrast agent through the cerebral vasculature causes a rapid and sharp decrease in signal intensity, which is due to a T2-shortening susceptibility effect. Specific regions-of-interest can be placed on the image to assess local differences in the bolus arrival time

the start of the imaging sequence, to ensure that an adequate number of baseline images are obtained. We inject a contrast volume of 0.2 mmol/kg body weight (i.e., 30 mL for a 75 kg person) at an injection rate of 5 mL/s (antecubital vein, 18-gauge i.v. catheter). This is followed by injection of 20–30 mL of saline, to flush the gadolinium out of the tubing, arm vein, and lung vasculature. When available, a power injector should be used, although with some experience, adequate results can be obtained also with hand injection (two syringes, containing contrast and saline flush, connected to a bifurcated "Y" check valve system). Sequential images are acquired simultaneously in multiple slice positions. The EPI sequence that we currently use performs 50 chronological images in 12 slice positions, yielding to a total dataset of 600 images. If more slice positions are required, a slightly longer TR is needed, and this would negatively influence the quality of the sequence.

These images must then be processed in parameter maps such as Fig. 2.40:

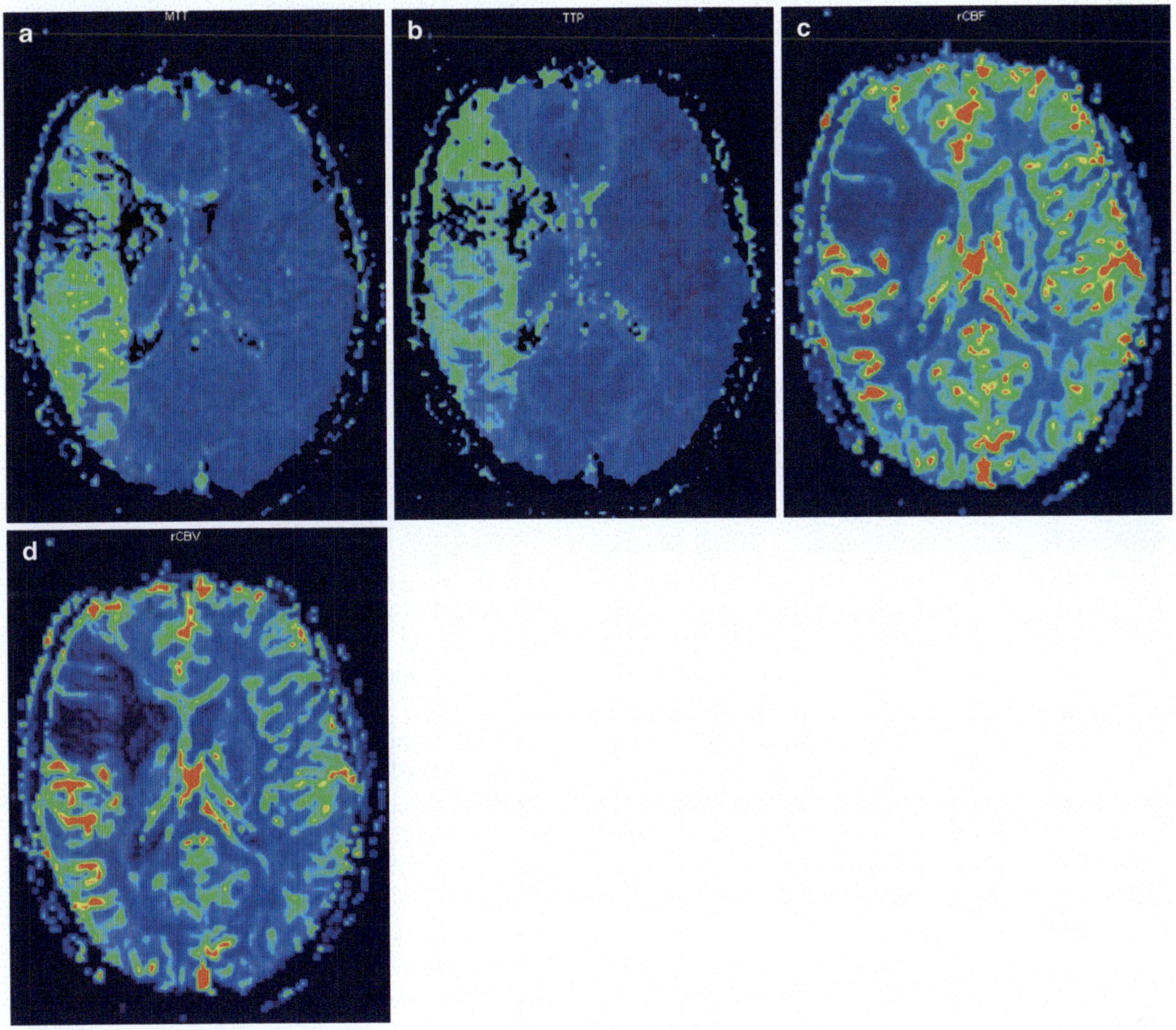

Fig. 2.40 Parametric maps generated by perfusion-weighted imaging (PWI) in a patient with hyperacute right middle cerebral artery stroke (same patient as Fig. 2.38 and 2.39). (**a**) Mean transit time (MTT) map. (**b**) Time to peak (TTP) map. (**c**) Regional cerebral blood flow (rCBF) map. (**d**) Regional cerebral blood volume (rCBV) map. The hypoperfused area corresponds to the distribution territory of the right middle cerebral artery. The perfusion deficit is much larger than the diffusion abnormality (compare with Fig. 2.38c, d). This represents a diffusion-perfusion mismatch, and indicates potentially salvageable brain tissue (see text)

- Time to peak (TTP)
- Mean transit time (MTT)
- Cerebral blood volume (CBV)
- CBF, which can be calculated using the formula: CBF = CBV/MTT

Perfusion MRI has been widely used in the setting of (hyper)acute (and subacute) stroke. However, with the arrival of multi-detector computed tomography (MDCT) scans, CT perfusion has become a valuable alternative to MR perfusion. In the diagnostic work-up of an acute stroke patient, many stroke centers start with a noncontrast CT (to rule out intracranial hemorrhage), followed by CT perfusion (to show the ischemic tissue and penumbra), and CT angiography (to reveal occlusion of a major blood vessel).

DWI/PWI Mismatch. In patients with (hyper)acute stroke, the volume of ischemic tissue documented by PWI is often greater than the region of parenchymal injury shown by DWI. In these patients, intravenous thrombolysis with recombinant tissue plasminogen activator (r-TPA) is of proven benefit within 3 h of symptom onset, and intra-arterial thrombolytic therapy shows promise within a 6-h window of therapeutic opportunity. The DWI/PWI mismatch has been considered as a possible correlate of the ischemic penumbra (i.e., tissue at greatest risk for infarct progression). The DWI abnormality reflects the area of brain tissue that is irretrievably lost (cytotoxic edema with cell death). The penumbra region indicates an area of decreased CBF, but the threshold for irreversible cell death has not yet been reached. Table 2.17 provides an overview of the theoretical possibilities and clinical implications of comparing PWI and DWI abnormalities.

Even without the use of such advanced techniques as diffusion and perfusion imaging, MRI is more sensitive than noncontrast CT in the detection of acute stroke. In the hyperacute and acute stages of a stroke, in addition to DWI, FLAIR is the most sensitive "conventional" imaging sequence. MRI findings of acute ischemic infarction include:

- Blurring of the gray–white matter interface on long TR images.
- Hyperintense swollen cortical gyri. These gyriform areas of increased SI on FLAIR images indicate cytotoxic edema of brain parenchyma, which occurs more rapidly in gray matter than in white matter, due to its higher metabolic activity.

Table 2.17 Clinical implications of comparing perfusion-weighted imaging (PWI) and diffusion-weighted imaging (DWI) abnormalities

PWI and DWI findings	Clinical implication
Normal PWI and normal DWI	No stroke
Normal PWI and abnormal DWI	Early reperfusion (the DWI abnormality indicates some cytotoxic edema, but vessel patency has been restored, and PWI is normal)
Abnormal PWI and normal DWI	This situation can be found in chronic vessel stenosis. Alternatively, this could reflect a false-negative DWI
Abnormal DWI = abnormal PWI	Constituted stroke. The nonperfused brain has evolved to infarction with cytotoxic edema. The involved brain tissue is irretrievably lost, and there is no indication for thrombolysis
Abnormal PWI > abnormal DWI	Mismatch. The DWI abnormality (core infarct) surrounds the PWI deficit, reflecting the penumbra. In this case, there is a potential role for thrombolytic therapy to prevent the penumbra region from evolving to infarction

- Low-SI on T1-WI and high-SI on FLAIR images. The cortical hyperintensity of gyral infarcts may be masked on T2-WI due to the high signal of CSF in the cortical sulci.
- Hyperintense vessel sign. Arterial hyperintensity, most commonly observed in the middle cerebral artery on FLAIR, may reflect slow moving or stationary blood or intraluminal thrombus. The presence of the hyperintense vessel sign, together with abnormal findings on DWI, should prompt consideration of revascularization and flow augmentation strategies.
- Absence of normal signal void. MRI can detect the alteration in blood flow during acute ischemia immediately. High velocity blood flow is normally seen on MRI as an absence of signal. Absence of flow void indicates a significant compromise of arterial blood flow.
- Intravascular contrast enhancement. Enhancement of cortical arteries is often observed 1 or 3 days after the infarct, and most likely represents slow blood flow in collateral arteries, via leptomeningeal anastomoses.

- Meningeal enhancement, adjacent to the infarcted brain tissue, is a sign of meningeal inflammation. It usually appears in the subacute stage, after 1 to 7 days.
- Hyperintense intracranial hemorrhage or hemorrhagic transformation of an infarct (Fig. 2.41). FLAIR images are also useful in detecting hyperacute hemorrhagic lesions, including subarachnoid and intraventricular hemorrhage.
- MRA shows an occluded vessel.

Other later acute (1–3 days) findings include (Fig. 2.42):

- Sulcal effacement, gyral swelling, insular ribbon sign.
- Loss of gray-white matter distinction. The SI changes in infarction involve both white and gray matter. This is an important element in differentiating infarct from tumor. The vasogenic edema associated with a brain tumor involves the white matter and tends to spare the gray matter.
- Increased SI of the brain parenchyma on FLAIR and T2-WI (due to increased water content), in a typical vascular distribution pattern.
- Mass effect (maximal 1–5 days after the event).
- Meningeal enhancement adjacent to the infarct.

In addition to the diffusion (and perfusion)-weighted sequences, the MRI protocol for a stroke patient should include a T1-WI sequence, a FLAIR sequence and/or a dual echo TSE sequence with PD-W and T2-W images, as well as an MRA sequence. Pay particular attention to the presence of normal signal void in all the *major* arteries, especially at the skull base. Use of i.v. contrast

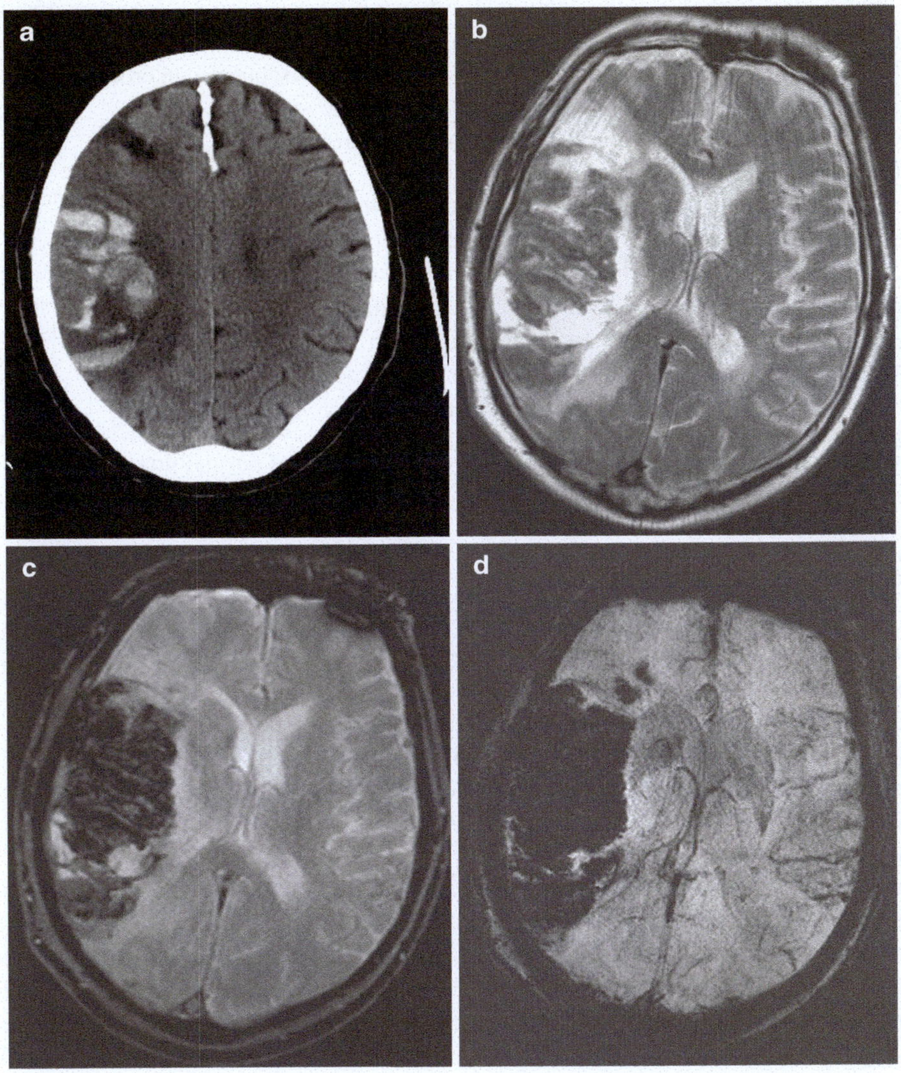

Fig. 2.41 Hemorrhagic transformation of right middle cerebral artery infarct. (**a**) Axial noncontrast CT scan. (**b**) Axial TSE T2-WI. (**c**) Axial gradient echo FLASH T2*-weighted image. (**d**) Axial susceptibility-weighted image (SWI). This 65-year-old man suffered a stroke involving the right middle cerebral artery distribution 4 days before. Noncontrast CT shows hemorrhagic transformation of the infarct (**a**). On T2-WI, the hemorrhagic infarct is hypointense, surrounded by a hyperintense halo of nonhemorrhagic infarction and edema (**b**). On T2* (**c**) and SWI (**d**), the involved area is markedly hypointense, due to susceptibility effects caused by blood breakdown products

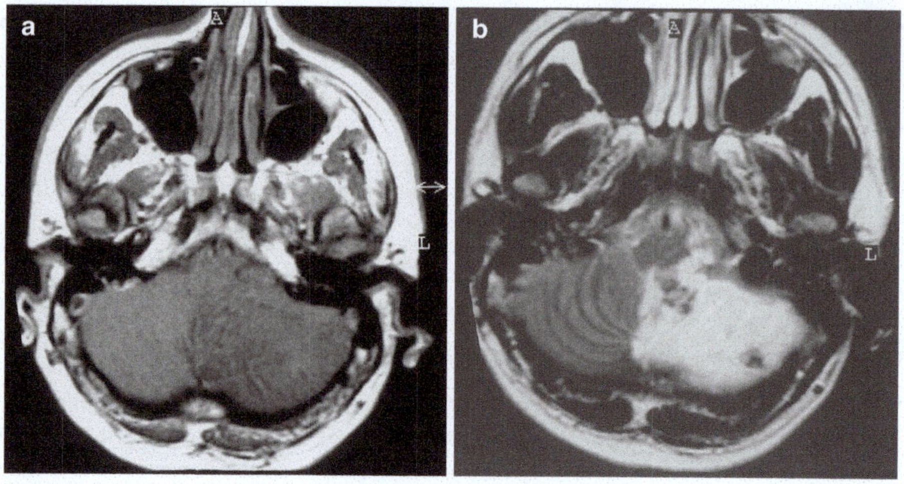

Fig. 2.42 Cerebellar infarct in the distribution of the posterior inferior cerebellar artery (PICA). (**a**) Axial SE T1-WI. (**b**) Axial TSE T2-WI. The signal abnormality involves both gray and white matter in the distribution of the left PICA. The mass effect is limited compared with the size of the lesion. There are a few hemorrhagic components, which are isointense on T1-WI and hypointense on T2-WI (deoxyhemoglobin)

allows identification of the abnormal intravascular enhancement. Use of two different imaging planes facilitates identification of other acute findings. The sagittal plane is more useful as a second plane than the coronal plane for vertebrobasilar stroke. An MRI protocol for acute stroke is given in Table 2.16.

Accurate determination of the patency of the internal carotid artery can be difficult with conventional MRI. The presence of normal signal void in the carotid siphon does not exclude significant stenosis in the extracranial carotid artery. Isointense signal in the lumen may be due to either occlusion or high-grade stenosis with slow flow. With MRA, we can investigate both the carotid bifurcation and the intracranial circulation. This topic is covered elsewhere.

Subacute Infarction (Days to Weeks)

In the early subacute stage, the vasogenic edema becomes more prominent. The infarct is hyperintense on T2-WI and FLAIR, and hypointense on T1-WI. The high SI on diffusion-weighted "trace" images remains for 10–14 days, but the ADC values start to normalize a few days earlier (Fig. 2.43). The mass effect initially increases and then gradually diminishes. Although experimentally disruption of the BBB occurs 6 h after the onset of ischemia, parenchymal enhancement becomes visible only in subacute infarctions, because it requires reestablishment of a certain amount of blood supply. The parenchymal enhancement tends to follow a gyriform pattern (Fig. 2.44). Hemorrhagic changes are more frequently observed (25%) than with CT. Therefore, it is useful to add a partial flip-angle gradient echo T2* or a SWI sequence, in order to detect hemorrhagic changes.

Chronic Infarction (Months to Years)

Prolonged ischemia causes irreversible brain damage. Tissue loss (negative mass effect), encephalomalacia, and replacement of tissue by CSF and/or gliosis are the causes of the SI abnormalities in this stage. Dilatation of the ipsilateral ventricle is common. The encephalomalacic area is sharply demarcated. Absence of normal flow void in major vessels in this stage indicates permanent vascular thrombosis. Wallerian degeneration of the corticospinal tracts can lead to volume loss of the ipsilateral cerebral peduncle and pons, and is due to antegrade degeneration of axons secondary to neural injury. Wallerian degeneration usually occurs as a late finding in old, large infarcts that involve the motor cortex (e.g., middle cerebral artery infarctions).

2.7.1.2 Small-Vessel Disease

Lacunar Infarct

The occlusion of small, penetrating end arteries arising from major cerebral arteries causes deep cerebral "lacunar" infarcts. The term "lacune" refers to a small area of cystic encephalomalacia. Lacunar infarcts account for 15–25% of all strokes, are most frequently

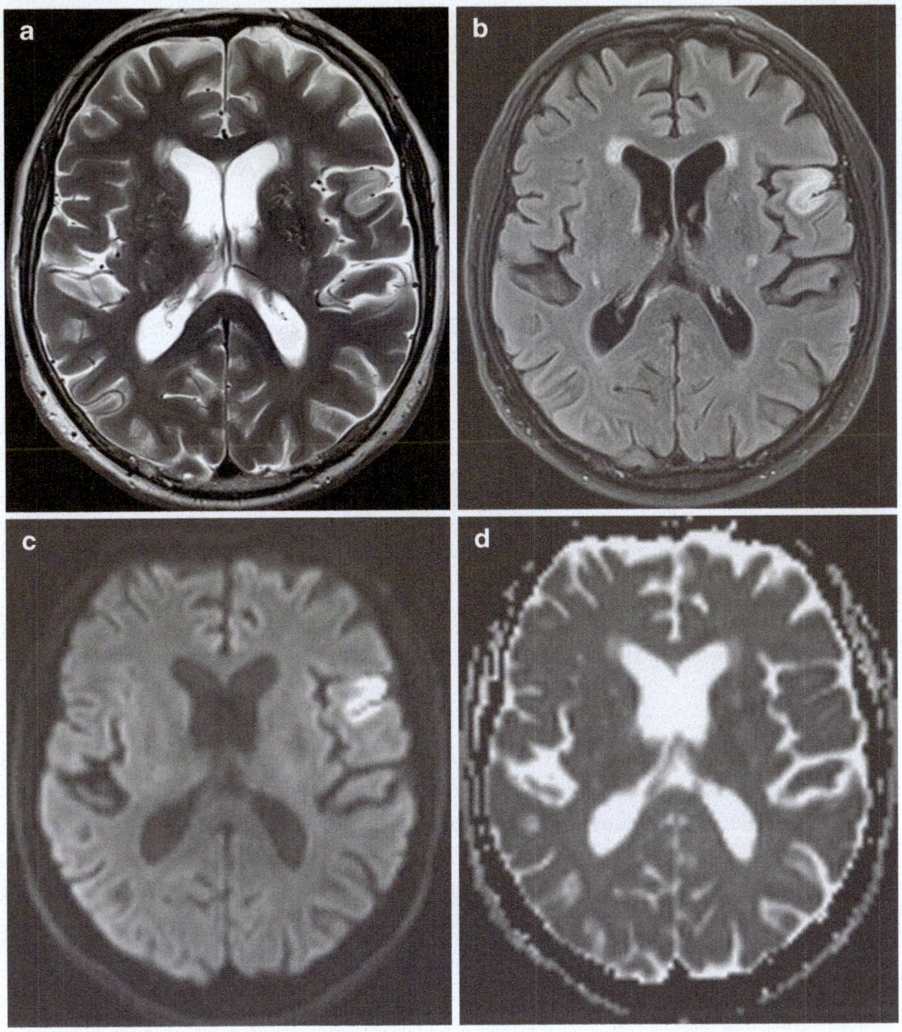

Fig. 2.43 Subacute infarction. (**a**) Axial TSE T2-WI. (**b**) Axial fat-sat turbo FLAIR. (**c**) Axial EPI diffusion-weighted "trace" image. (**d**) Apparent diffusion coefficient (ADC) map. This 70-year-old man presented 9 days before with acute motor aphasia. There is a cortical infarct involving the left inferior frontal gyrus, pars opercularis (Broca's area). The infarction of the cortical gray matter is hyperintense on T2-WI (**a**) and FLAIR images (**b**). There is marked hyperintensity on the diffusion-weighted scan (**c**) but ADC values have started to normalize, a normal finding after 9 days

associated with hypertension, and usually occur in late middle-aged or elderly individuals (>55 years of age). The most commonly involved locations are the basal ganglia (putamen, caudate), thalamus, internal capsule, and pons. This is because lacunar infarcts occur in the distal distribution of small penetrating vessels, such as the lenticulostriate arteries, recurrent artery of Heubner, thalamoperforating arteries, and pontine perforating arteries. If multiple lacunes are present, which is often the case, this is referred to as a lacunar state or "état lacunaire."

In the acute stage, lacunar infarcts may be difficult to detect on standard MRI sequences, although DWI may show focal areas of diffusion restriction. Later, when they become associated with edema, they may be seen as hyperintense, small, rounded lesions on FLAIR and T2-WI. In the acute and subacute phase, they may enhance following Gd-chelate administration, indicating disruption of the BBB. Older lacunar infarcts are isointense to CSF on all sequences, but they may be surrounded by hyperintense rim due to marginal gliosis (formation of scar tissue).

Subcortical Arteriosclerotic Leukoencephalopathy

Subcortical arteriosclerotic (leuko) encephalopathy (SAE) (also known as "leukoaraiosis" or "Binswanger's disease") is characterized by ischemia in the distribution territories of the poorly collateralized distal penetrating arteries. Hyperintense lesions are found on PD-WI, T2-WI, and FLAIR (Fig. 2.45). These signal

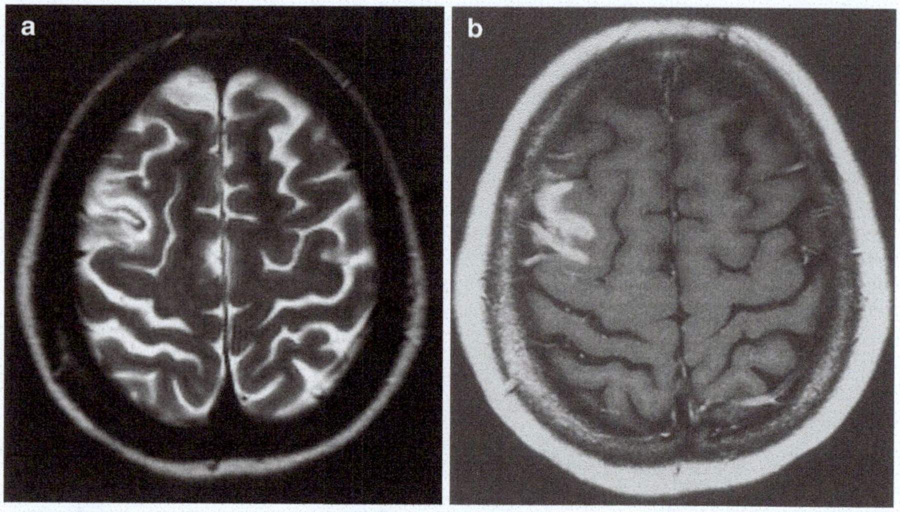

Fig. 2.44 Gyral enhancement in subacute right middle cerebral artery infarction. (**a**) Axial TSE T2-WI. (**b**) Gd-enhanced axial SE T1-WI. Two weeks prior to the present MRI examination, this 49-year-old woman suffered a stroke in the anterior part of the right middle cerebral artery distribution. The T2-WI shows mildly increased signal intensity in the cortical-subcortical region of the right frontal lobe. After Gd injection, the typical gyriform enhancement is seen. This parenchymal enhancement denotes breakdown of the BBB

abnormalities occur in the periventricular white matter, centrum semiovale, basal ganglia, and subcortical "U"-fibers. The lesions may be focal, multifocal, or confluent and extend from the periventricular white matter to the subcortical region. The corpus callosum is usually spared (in contradistinction to MS, which typically involves the corpus callosum). The signal abnormalities of SAE reflect focal areas of demyelination and infarcts, as a result of microvascular arteriolar disease. SAE is a frequent finding in routine MRI, particularly in elderly people. There is a strong association with hypertension. No mass effect is present, and little or no abnormality is seen in the T1-WI. On the Fazekas Scale for scoring periventricular and deep white matter hyperintensities, SAE corresponds to grade 3 lesions: large confluent hyperintense areas in the deep white matter and irregular hyperintensities in the periventricular region.

In patients with chronic cerebrovascular disease, it is useful to add a T2*-WI and/or susceptibility-weighted sequence to the imaging protocol to look for punctuate hemosiderin deposits or so-called "micro-bleeds." They are commonly found in patients with hypertension or amyloid angiopathy. SWI is the preferred technique for the detection of micro-bleeds, since it shows more lesions than T2*-WI (Fig. 2.46).

Normal Hyperintense Areas in the T2-WI

Lacunar infarcts and SAE must be distinguished from normal and age-related areas of hyperintense signal on FLAIR and T2-WI. They include:

- Areas of late myelination in the deep parieto-occipital white matter, adjacent to the ventricular trigone
- Focal breakdown of the ependymal lining with periventricular hyperintense signal anterolateral to the frontal horns ("ependymitis granularis")
- Decreased myelination in posterior internal capsule
- Perivascular spaces of Virchow-Robin

2.7.1.3 Acute Hypertensive Encephalopathy

Acute hypertensive encephalopathy, perhaps more commonly known as posterior reversible encephalopathy syndrome (PRES) is a disorder of cerebrovascular autoregulation associated with hypertension. Patients usually present with headache, seizures, visual field deficits, and altered mental status. There are many precipitating factors including, abrupt elevation of blood pressure, (pre)eclampsia, renal decompensation, fluid retention, and immunosuppressive drug toxicity

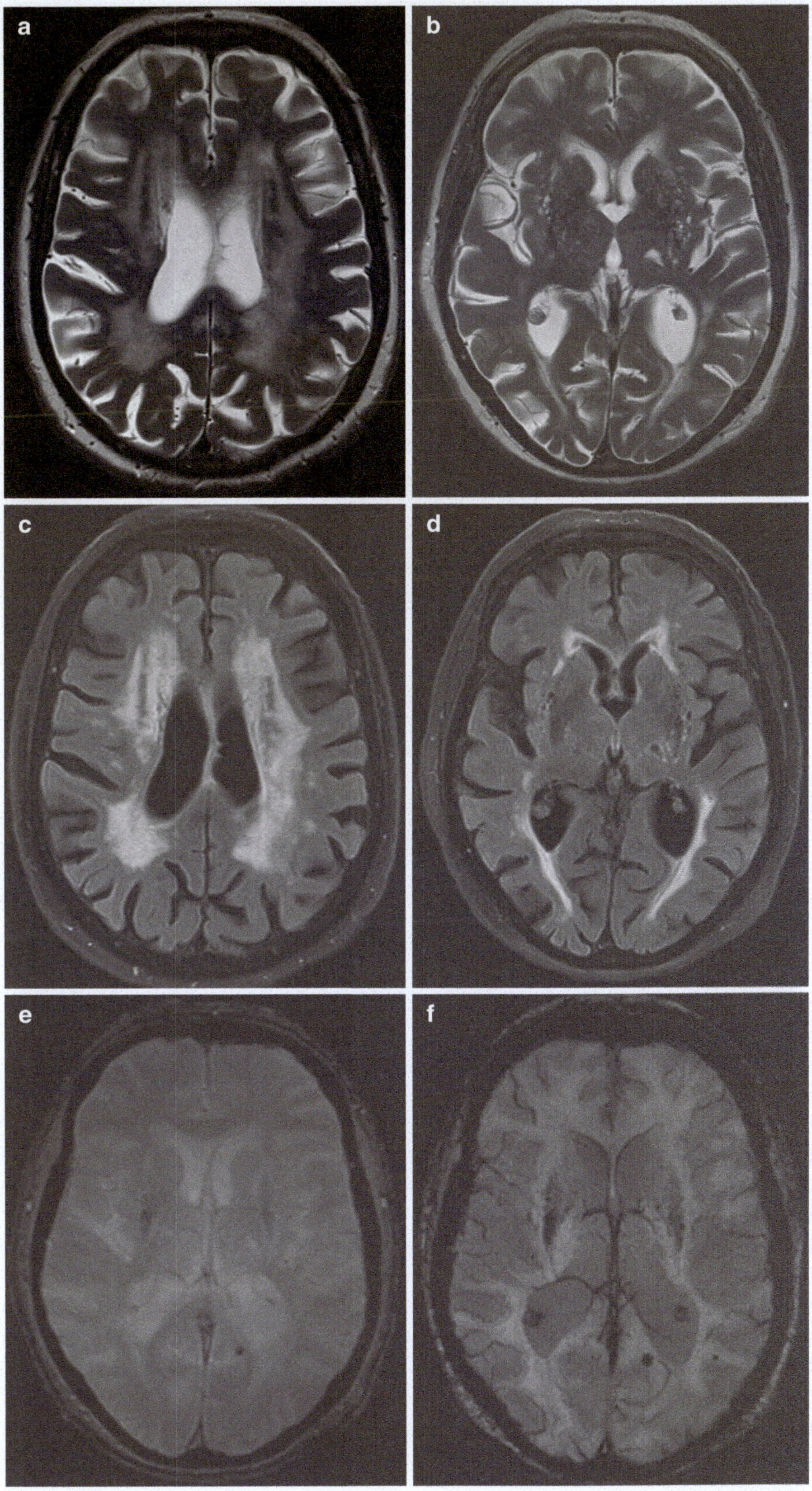

Fig. 2.45 Subcortical arteriosclerotic leukoencephalopathy and micro-bleeds. (**a, b**) Axial TSE T2-WI. (**c, d**) Axial fat-sat turbo FLAIR. (**e**) Axial gradient-echo FLASH T2*-WI. (**f**) Axial susceptibility-weighted image (SWI). The patient is a 76-year-old man with hypertension. In both cerebral hemispheres, there are confluent hyperintense areas in the deep white matter and centrum semiovale and irregular multifocal hyperintensities in the basal ganglia. These signal abnormalities reflect focal areas of demyelination and infarcts, as a result of microvascular arteriolar disease. The T2* and SWI images show micro-bleeds, which are not visible on the other sequences

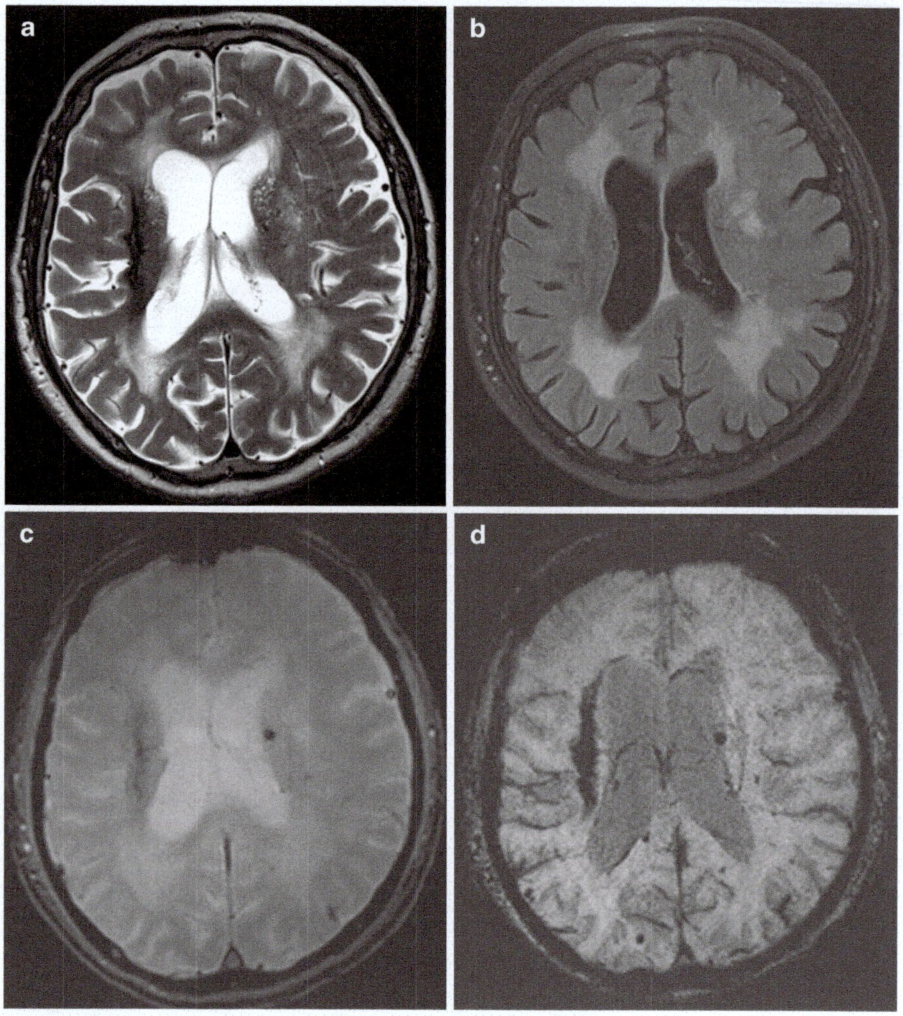

Fig. 2.46 SWI is superior to T2* in the detection of microbleeds. (**a**) Axial TSE T2-WI. (**b**) Axial fat-sat turbo FLAIR. (**c**) Axial gradient-echo FLASH T2*-WI. (**d**) Axial susceptibility-weighted image (SWI). This 73-year-old man has a history of long-standing arterial hypertension. Axial TSE-T2 (**a**) and FLAIR (**b**) show patchy hyperintensities involving the deep white matter in a pattern consistent with subcortical arteriosclerotic leukoencephalopathy. On T2*-WI (C) and SWI, multiple punctate hyperintensities are seen, consistent with microbleeds in the setting of amyloid angiopathy, as well as a large area of hemosiderin deposition in the right putamen (the patient had suffered a putaminal hemorrhage several years earlier). SWI shows more microbleeds than T2*-WI

(especially cyclosporin). Hypertension is a common component and causes disruption of the BBB in the posterior circulation.

On MRI, the most typical findings are patchy, cortical and subcortical hyperintensities on T2 and FLAIR images in the posterior cerebral artery distribution territory (Fig. 2.47). The cerebellum may also be involved. There is no diffusion restriction, because the hyperintense signal abnormalities in PRES are caused by vasogenic (not cytotoxic) edema (due to damage of the vascular endothelium by hypertension) and are not due to cytotoxic edema (as in acute arterial infarction). PRES is a "must-not-miss" diagnosis because the condition is potentially life threatening; most cases resolve with aggressive therapy to normalize blood pressure and withdrawal of the drug producing the symptoms.

2.7.2 Subarachnoid Hemorrhage

CT remains the preferred imaging method for the detection of acute subarachnoid hemorrhage (SAH). On MRI, the diagnosis of subarachnoid and intraventricular hemorrhage relies on FLAIR imaging; in FLAIR, the SI of CSF is suppressed, and blood is seen as hyperintense. There is good evidence that FLAIR imaging is equally sensitive as CT for detection of SAH; other reports indicate that small amounts of SAH may be missed on MRI. The higher oxygen tension of the CSF in the subarachnoid space slows the transformation of oxyhemoglobin to paramagnetic breakdown products such as deoxyhemoglobin and methemoglobin. Additionally, pulsatile CSF flow tends to dilute and disperse the red blood cells.

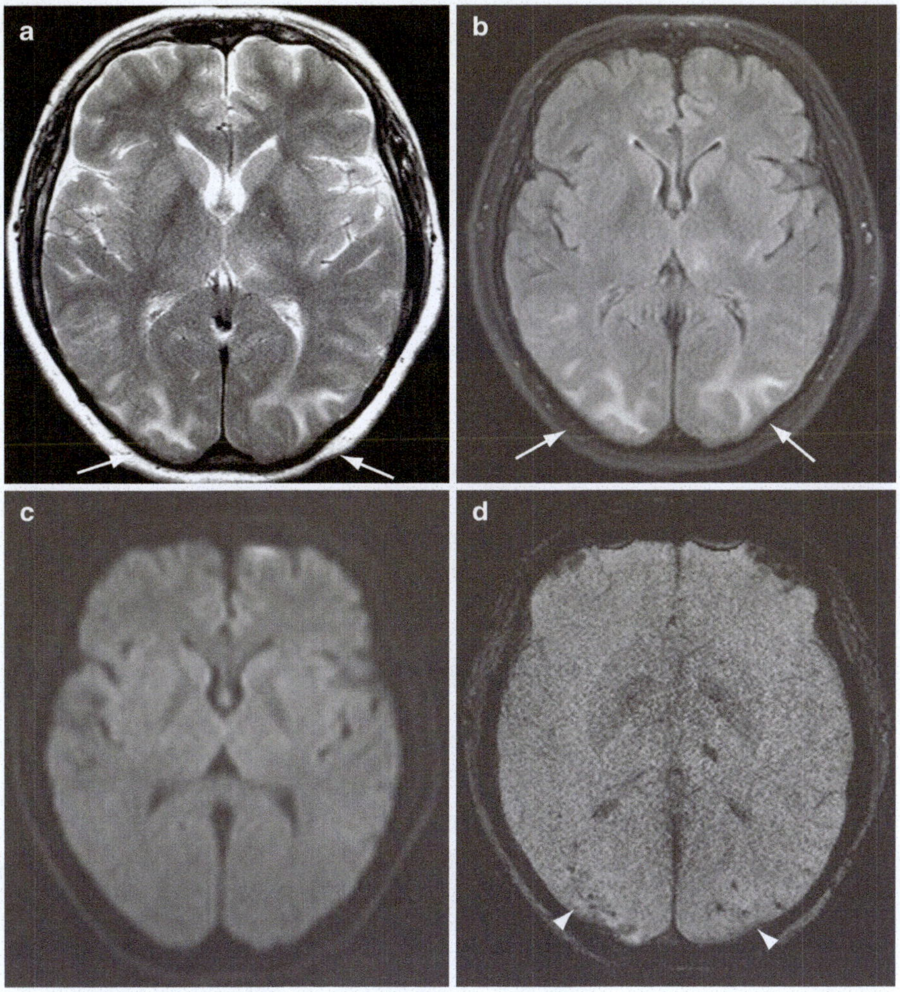

Fig. 2.47 Posterior reversible encephalopathy syndrome (PRES) (*arrows*). (**a**) Axial TSE T2-WI. (**b**) Axial fat-sat turbo FLAIR. (**c**) Axial EPI diffusion-weighted "trace" image (DWI). (**d**) Axial susceptibility-weighted image (SWI). This 62-year-old woman was admitted with headache, vomiting, and visual field disturbances, associated with an acute hypertensive attack. Axial T2 (**a**) and FLAIR (**b**) images show foci of high signal intensity involving the cortex and subcortical white matter of both occipital lobes. There is no diffusion restriction (**c**), since PRES is associated with vasogenic edema and not cytotoxic edema. The SWI (**d**) shows hypointense punctate hemorrhagic foci. The patient recovered after aggressive antihypertensive therapy (*arrowheads*)

Repeated episodes of SAH may cause ferritin and hemosiderin deposition on the leptomeninges covering the brain. This condition is known as superficial siderosis. On T2-WI or T2*-WI MRI, superficial siderosis is seen as a hypointense line along the surface of the brain, especially the pons, mesencephalon, and cerebellar vermis.

In the postoperative follow-up of a patient after aneurysm clipping or after endovascular coiling, MRI is useful because the clip/coil causes fewer artifacts on MRI than on CT. Most aneurysm clips currently used are composed of nonferromagnetic material. However, in the past, many patients have undergone aneurysm clipping with ferromagnetic clips. There is a danger of fatal intracranial hemorrhage after movement of a ferromagnetic aneurysm clip in a MRI unit. Never scan a patient with an aneurysm clip without identifying the exact type of the clip! Contrast-enhanced MRA is the preferred imaging technique in the follow-up of patients after endovascular coiling or clipping of aneurysms.

2.7.3 Dural Sinus and Cerebal Vein Thrombosis

Thrombosis of a dural sinus (or cerebral vein) is a serious, and in some cases, potentially lethal condition. The clinical presentation is often confusing and nonspecific, and the radiologist may be the first to suggest the diagnosis to the clinicians. The goal of neuroradiologic examination is twofold: (1) to prove the existence of a thrombosis and (2) to evaluate the intracranial damage caused by the thrombosis. MRI is the method of choice for both of these tasks.

2.7.3.1 Identification of a Thrombosed Sinus or Vein by MRI

The superior sagittal sinus is the most common site of dural sinus thrombosis, followed by the transverse sinus, sigmoid sinus, and cavernous sinus. Deep cerebral vein thrombosis is less common, but even more dangerous. Cortical vein occlusion usually occurs in association with dural sinus thrombosis, though it can occur as an isolated finding.

There are several methods of identifying an occlusion of a dural sinus by MRI:

1. Conventional MRI: careful interpretation of the SI within the lumen of the venous sinus may indicate whether it corresponds to flow or thrombosis. Thrombosis of a dural venous sinus can be detected as an intravascular area of high SI on T1-WI (Fig. 2.48) or FLAIR.
2. MR venography which can either be performed with a phase-contrast technique (Fig. 2.49) or time-of-flight (TOF) MRA ("slow flow" technique or magnetic resonance "venography").

Conventional MRI is unreliable. In practice, it is sometimes difficult to decide whether the intraluminal signal within a dural sinus or cerebral vein corresponds to flow or to thrombosis. The SI of a clot varies with its age. An acute clot is isointense to gray matter on T1-WI (and therefore easily missed) and hypointense on T2-WI. A subacute clot becomes hyperintense on both T1-WI and T2-WI; this corresponds to the formation of extracellular methemoglobin. However, in the intermediate stage, the clot can be hypointense on T2-WI (due to intracellular methemoglobin) and thus mimic normal flow void in a patent dural sinus. The SI of normal flow in a sinus is also variable. Instead of flow void, a high signal may be observed on T1-WI because of an entry

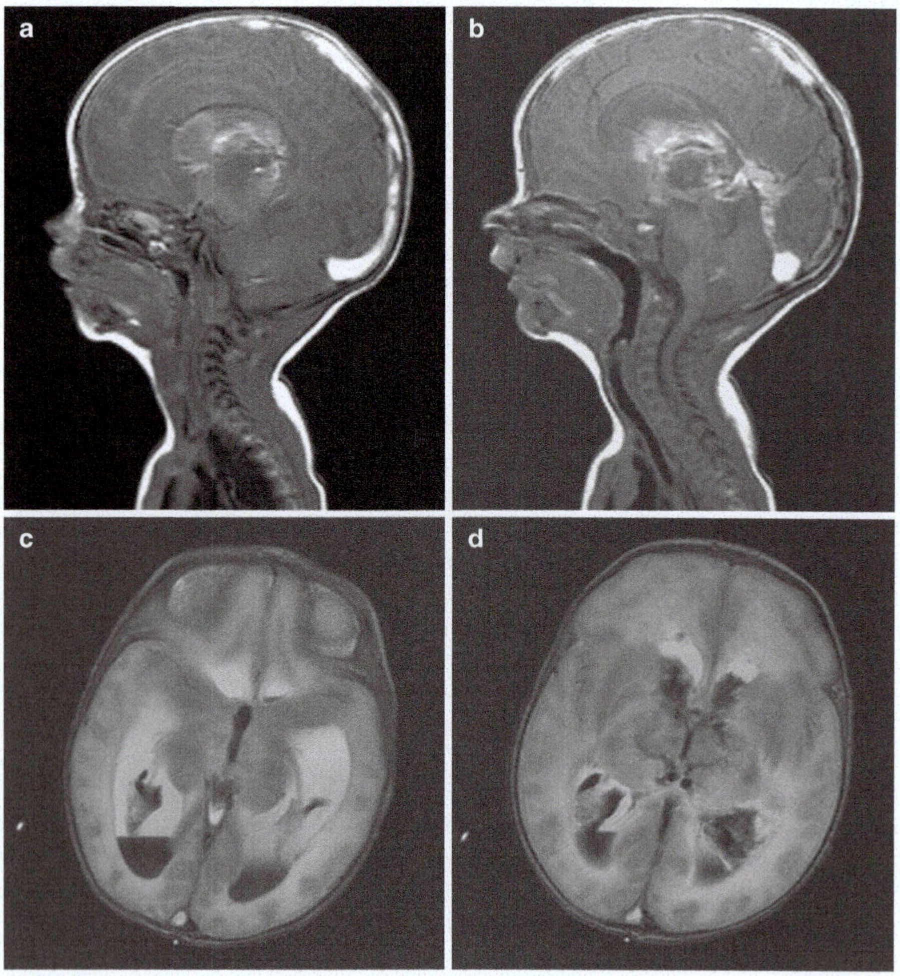

Fig. 2.48 Thrombosis of the cerebral veins and sinuses. (**a**, **b**) Sagittal TSE T1-WI. (**c**, **d**) Axial TSE T2-WI. This newborn baby boy presented with seizures and neurologic deficits. Sagittal T1-WI show complete sinovenous thrombosis involving the dural sinuses (superior sagittal sinus, torcular, transverse, and sigmoid sinus), but also the deep venous system (sinus rectus, great cerebral vein, internal cerebral veins). Axial T2-WI reveal venous infarctions in the thalami and diencephalic structures. There is intraventricular blood (with hemorrhagic sedimentation layers). The child expired after a few days

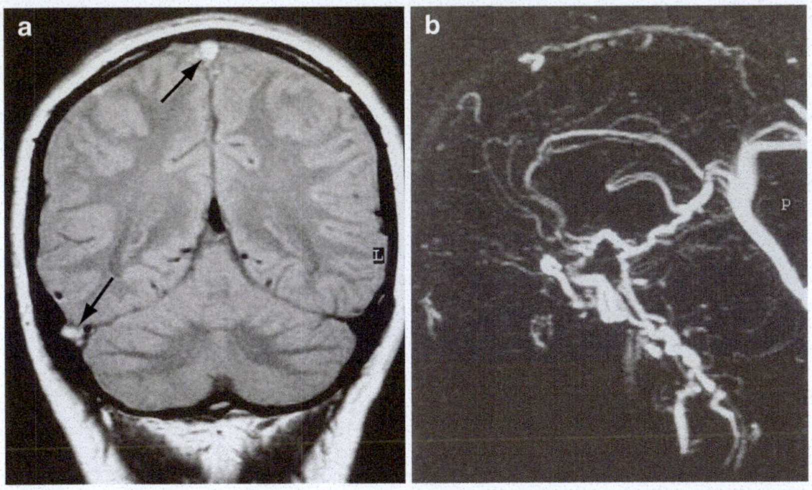

Fig. 2.49 Thrombosis of the superior sagittal and right transverse sinus. (**a**) Coronal SE PD-WI. (**b**) MIP reconstruction of a phase-contrast MR angiography (MRA) (sagittal view). On the coronal PD-WI, the signal within the lumen of the superior sagittal and right transverse sinus is hyperintense (*arrows*). The intraluminal signal intensity was also high on the T1-WI and T2-WI (not shown). This signal-intensity behavior is consistent with a blood clot (extracellular methemoglobin). The phase-contrast MRA image reveals an absence of flow within the superior sagittal sinus, thereby confirming the diagnosis of thrombosis

slice phenomenon, in-plane flow, or slow flow. In T2-WI, the luminal signal can be high because of even-echo rephasing or slow in-plane flow, accentuated by flow compensation techniques. Wall enhancement of the thrombosed sinus or enhancement of the intraluminal thrombus may further confound the issue.

MR venography is the preferred technique for the detection of dural sinus or cerebral vein thrombosis. MR venography can be performed with slow flow TOF MRA, (e.g., oblique coronal 2D TOF (2D FLASH) with saturation of arterial inflow) or with phase-contrast MRA (e.g., single-slab phase-contrast angiography). A more detailed discussion of MRA techniques can be found in Chap. 1. Yet, even these techniques are not fool-proof, since a hyperintense thrombus on T1-WI can simulate flow-related enhancement on a slow-flow TOF (due to the T1-shortening effect).

2.7.3.2 Evaluation of the Intracranial Damage

Dural sinus and cerebral vein thrombosis can cause intracranial hypertension, hydrocephalus, venous infarction, and hemorrhage. MRI may show swelling of the brain with mass effect and sulcal effacement. On T2-WI, hyperintense lesions, not corresponding to an arterial territory may be found; they are frequently bilateral or involve more than one vascular distribution. Hemorrhagic transformation of these venous infarcts is common. Parasagittal hemorrhages are highly specific for superior sinus thrombosis, and are secondary to cortical venous infarction. As a general rule, venous infarctions do not exhibit diffusion restriction; this is because, in the early phase, venous occlusion causes vasogenic edema unlike an arterial infarction which causes cytotoxic edema. After contrast injection, prominent venous enhancement in dilated cortical veins and collaterals is observed.

2.7.4 Vascular Malformations

2.7.4.1 Classification

The four archetypal vascular malformations are (1) AVM, (2) capillary telangiectasia, (3) cavernous angioma, and (4) developmental venous anomaly (venous angioma). The latter is considered an anatomic variant and not a true malformation.

2.7.4.2 Arteriovenous Malformation

AVMs are congenital disorders. The angioarchitecture of an AVM consists of one or more enlarged feeding arteries, a tangled collection of blood vessels (the nidus), and a tortuous assortment of dilated draining veins. AVMs are a cause of intracerebral hemorrhage; they are also associated with headaches, ischemic or hemorrhagic infarctions, or SAH. The MRI examination is complementary to cerebral angiography for treatment planning. It must identify:

- Number, location, and course of the feeding arteries
- Exact delineation of the nidus
- Location of the draining veins
- Aneurysms or dilated blood vessels
- Parenchymal damage, atrophy
- Presence of hemorrhage and its relationship to the nidus

An important target of the MRI protocol is the accurate anatomic definition of the nidus and its relationship to vital cerebral structures. Therefore, the MRI examination has to include images in three imaging planes (axial, coronal, and sagittal), eventually supplemented by MRA. In at least one imaging plane, T1-WI and T2-WI should be performed. MRI findings in the typical case are:

- Multiple round, linear, or serpiginous areas of signal void (Fig. 2.50)
- Little or no mass effect in the absence of recent bleeding
- Atrophy of the surrounding brain, gliosis
- Absence of brain tissue inside the nidus

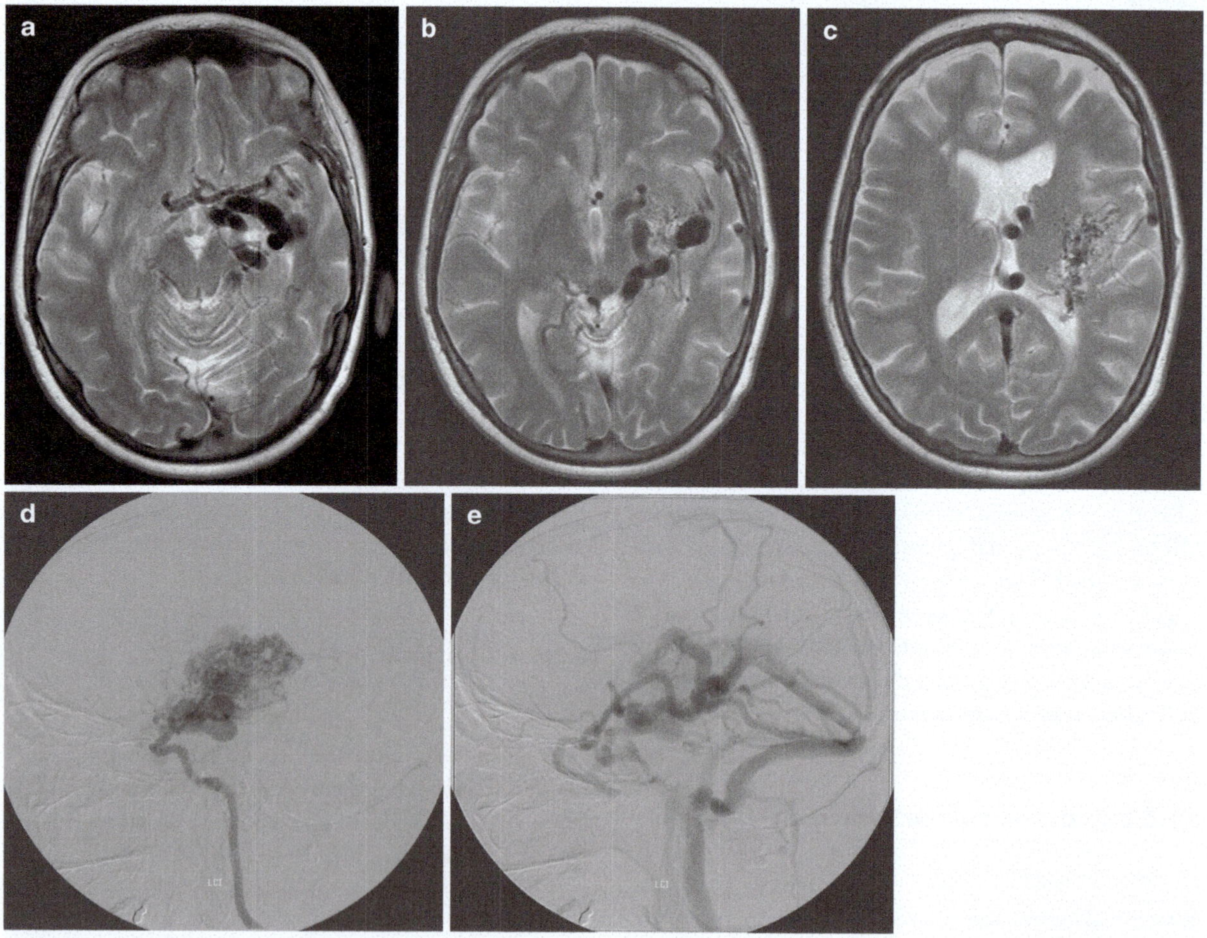

Fig. 2.50 Arterio-venous malformation. (**a–c**) Axial TSE T2-WI. (**c, d**) Cerebral angiography, left internal carotid artery injection, lateral view, late arterial phase (**d**) and venous phase (**e**). This 50-year-old woman has a high-flow arteriovenous malformation in the left subinsular/basal ganglia region. The draining veins are hypointense on the axial T2-WI (**a–c**), reflecting their high flow speed. Despite the size of the malformation and the large caliber of the draining veins, there is no mass effect, nor perilesional edema (and this is a typical feature of AVMs, unless there has been a hemorrhagic episode)

2.7.4.3 Capillary Telangiectasia

Capillary telangiectasias are vascular malformations which are composed of dilated capillaries with interposed normal brain parenchyma. They are the second most common vascular malformation (second only to venous developmental anomalies). At autopsy, they are frequently found as multiple lesions. The brainstem, especially the pons, is the most typical location, but capillary teleangiectasias can also be found in the cerebellum, spinal cord, and supratentorially. Most of these lesions are clinically silent and are incidentally discovered on imaging studies. Capillary telangiectasias are invisible on cerebral angiography. On Gd-enhanced MR images, the so-called "racemose" type of capillary teleangiectasia may be seen as a region of mild, stippled contrast enhancement. The "cavernous" type presents as hypointense lesions on SWI or T2*-WI, indicating evidence of old hemorrhage with hemosiderin deposition.

2.7.4.4 Cavernous Malformation (Syn. Cavernous Hemangioma)

Cavernous malformations occur in the brain and the spinal cord. The most frequent location is in the cerebral hemispheres, though they also occur in the brainstem. Sporadic and familial forms are possible. Lesions are frequently multiple (20–30%), with a familial pattern in 10–15% of the patients. Cavernous malformations may be asymptomatic. When symptomatic, their clinical presentation consists of seizures, headache, hemorrhage, and progressive neurological deficit.

Histopathologically, a cavernous malformation has three components: sinusoidal vascular spaces lined by a single layer of endothelial cells, fibrous septa with calcifications, and a peripheral component of gliotic hemosiderin-laden tissue. There is no brain parenchyma within the lesion. The flow is very slow or absent, with frequent intravascular thrombosis.

Noncontrast CT demonstrates cavernous angiomas as small, rounded, dense foci, often with associated calcification. However, MRI is more sensitive and more specific, due to its sensitivity to old blood–breakdown products.

In a typical cavernous angioma, MRI findings are:

- A well-delineated lesion, often with a high SI on T1-W images
- Reticulated "pop-corn" appearance; heterogeneous SI represents blood products of different age; hypointense signal areas (due to blood-breakdown products such as hemosiderin) are more prominent on T2-W and GRE images (Fig. 2.2)
- Peripheral closed rim of hemosiderin
- No flow; no arterial feeders, no draining veins
- No mass effect and no perifocal edema, unless a recent episode of bleeding has occurred

The MRI protocol should contain pulse sequences sensitive for old blood products (hemosiderin). The TSE sequence is insensitive and may miss the lesions. Susceptibility-weighted imaging (SWI) is the most sensitive sequence for detection of small, punctate cavernous malformations. The second choice is a spoiled partial flip-angle T2*-weighted GRE (Fig. 2.51).

2.7.4.5 Developmental Venous Anomaly

Developmental venous anomalies (DVAs; also known as "venous malformation" or "venous angioma") are believed to represent an anatomic variant of the normal venous drainage pattern, and not a true malformation. Most often, they are discovered as an incidental finding. DVAs do not contain an arterial or capillary component. They consist of small tributary veins that drain into an enlarged venous channel. On T1-WI, they are seen as linear or curvilinear flow voids, often perpendicular to the cortex or the ventricular wall. On T2-WI, their SI is variable, depending on the direction and speed of flow, as well as technical factors, such as the entry phenomenon. After Gd injection, the small tributary veins enhance in a stellate fashion, often presenting the shape of a caput medusae (Fig. 2.52). Developmental venous anomalies are difficult to detect on precontrast images, and up to one-third are discovered only after an injection of Gd. Alternatively, susceptibility-weighted images (SWI) can be used to detect abnormalities of venous drainage, for example in Sturge–Weber syndrome (Fig. 2.53). The SWI sequence is very sensitive to veins because they contain paramagnetic deoxyhemoglobin. Therefore, SWI should constitute an important part of any neuroimaging protocol to reveal microarchitecture of neurovascular diseases.

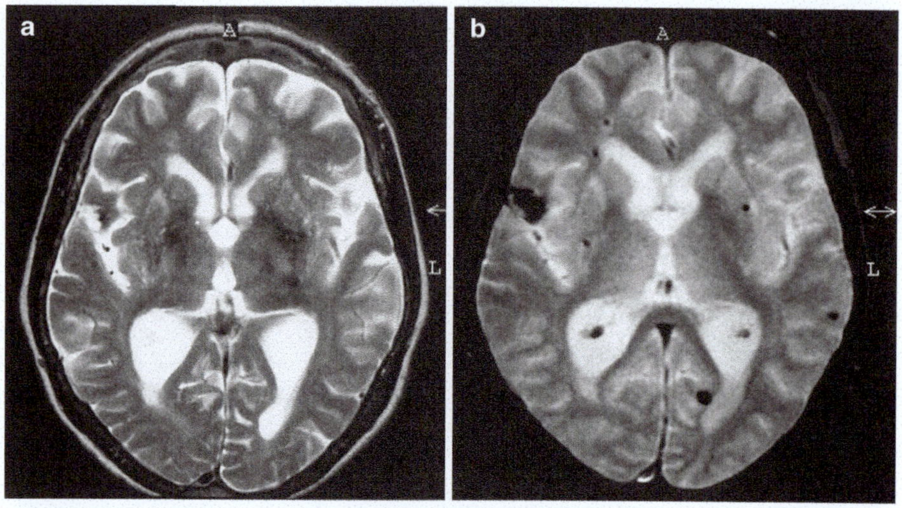

Fig. 2.51 Multiple cavernous hemangiomas. (**a**) Axial TSE T2-WI. (**b**) Axial GRE image. In this patient with multiple cavernous malformations, note the striking difference in the number of lesions detected by the partial flip-angle T2*-weighted GRE compared with the TSE T2-W sequence. This is due to the insensitivity of the TSE sequence for blood degradation products, such as hemosiderin

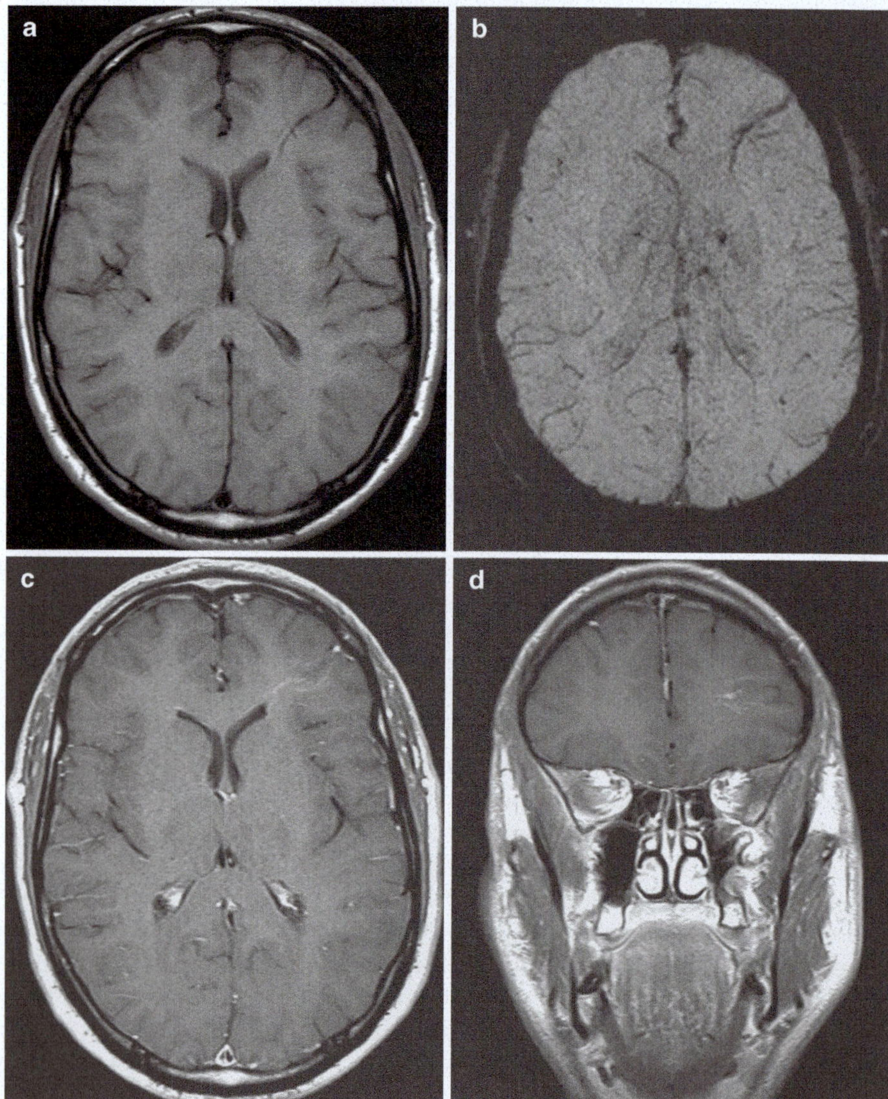

Fig. 2.52 Developmental venous anomaly ("venous angioma"). (**a**) Axial TSE T1-WI. (**b**) Axial susceptibility-weighted image (SWI). Gd-enhanced axial (**c**) and coronal (**d**) TSE T1-WI. The tubular structure in the left frontal lobe represents a large draining vein. Since this vein contains deoxygenated blood, it appears dark on the SWI (as all venous structures). After Gd injection, a cluster of small tributary veins enhance in a stellate fashion, (the so-called "caput medusae"), and they converge toward the large draining vein

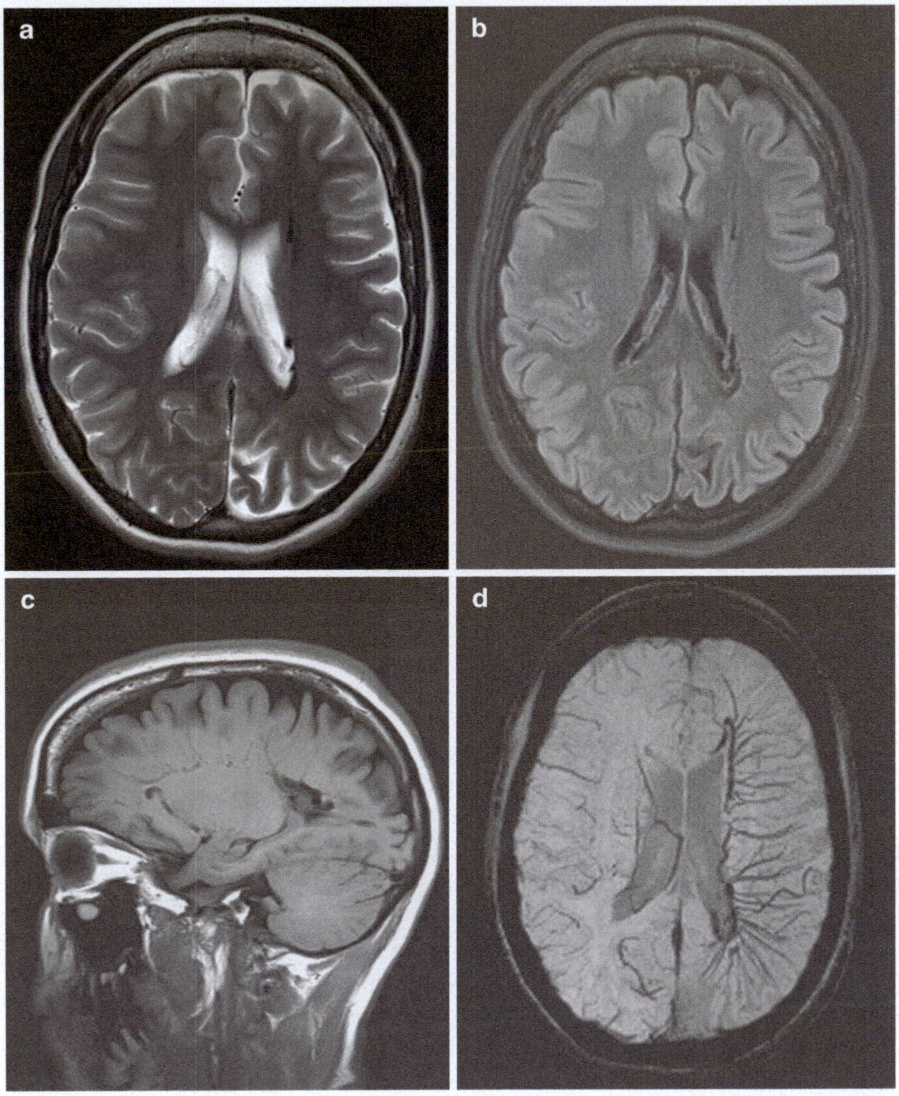

Fig. 2.53 Sturge-Weber syndrome with complex collateral venous drainage. (**a**) Axial TSE T2-WI. (**b**) Axial fat-sat turbo FLAIR. (**c**) Sagittal TSE T1-WI. (**d**), Axial susceptibility-weighted image (SWI). The axial T2 and FLAIR images show mild cortical atrophy of the left cerebral hemisphere (**a**, **b**). There are prominent vascular structures along the left lateral ventricle (**a–c**). The SWI shows extensive medullary collateral venous drainage (**d**). SWI is very sensitive to veins because of their deoxyhemoglobin content, and SWI should constitute an important part of any neuroimaging protocol to reveal micro-architecture of neurovascular diseases

2.8 White Matter Lesions

2.8.1 Introduction

In the neuroradiological assessment of white-matter disease, it is important to consider both the patient's age and the clinical presentation. Most white-matter diseases present with similar findings on MRI, with hyperintense lesions on T2-WI and hypointense lesions on T1-WI. Contrast enhancement occasionally occurs, and indicates breakdown of the BBB. Subtle differences in the pattern of white matter changes may direct us to the correct diagnosis.

Imaging strategy should be directed by the expected pathology, which depends on the age of the patient. In the first year of life, periventricular leucomalacia and delayed myelination are frequent findings. In the first decade, the leukodystrophies can be the cause of white matter changes. In the adult population, MS is the most common white-matter disease, with an increasing incidence of nonspecific and vascular-related white matter changes with aging. Within certain patient groups, other diseases are more frequent (toxic demyelination, radiation necrosis).

2.8.2 Normal Development

Myelination of the CNS starts in the fifth fetal month. At the age of 2 years, 90% of myelination is complete. The remainder of the process continues to early adulthood. The progression of myelination can be studied with MRI, and the visualization of this process depends on the pulse sequence and field strength. T2 Early changes (≤6–8 months) are best studied with a T1-W sequence; at a later age (6–18 months), changes are best depicted on T2-WI. The process of myelination follows a distinct pattern. In broad terms, myelination progresses from caudad to craniad, and from posterior to anterior. The myelination process is discussed in greater depth in Chap. 13.2.3.

The posterior limb of the internal capsule contains an area with different SI than the anterior limb. On T2-WI, this is seen as a focal symmetric area of high SI. Proton density and T1-WI show no difference between the anterior and posterior limb of the internal capsule. These regions probably represent a portion of the pyramid tract (parieto-pontine bundles). This normal finding should not be mistaken for lesions in the internal capsule.

2.8.3 T2-W and FLAIR

Myelinated structures are hypointense on T2- and FLAIR images. At birth, the dorsal white-matter tracts of the brainstem, the superior and inferior cerebellar peduncles, and the medio-dorsal tracts in the diencephalon are myelinated. Supratentorially, only the posterior limb of the internal capsule and the white matter in the postcentral gyrus are myelinated. As the process continues, more cerebral structures become myelinated. At the age of 6 months, the brainstem presents a mature myelination pattern, and the cerebellar hemispheres show central myelination. The optic radiation is fully myelinated, while the internal capsule and the corpus callosum are partially myelinated. The occipital and parietal lobes and the motor areas myelinate earlier than the frontal and temporal lobes. This is also reflected in the myelination of the internal capsule and the corpus callosum. The anterior limb of the internal capsule and the genu of the corpus callosum myelinate 4 months later than the posterior limb and the splenium. The occipital and parietal lobes reach a mature myelination between 6 and 18 months; the frontal and temporal lobes reach this point between 21 and 27 months.

2.8.4 T1-W Sequence

Myelinated structures are hyperintense on T1-WI. The myelination process as seen on IR T1-WI proceeds parallel to that seen on T2-and FLAIR. However, myelination is seen earlier on T1-WI than on T2-WI. At birth, all three cerebellar peduncles are myelinated, and the optic pathways also show a high SI due to myelination. Not only the postcentral, but also the precentral gyrus is myelinated at birth on IR-SE T1-WI. At the age of 6 months, most of the brain reaches a mature myelination on the IR-SE T1-WI, and the frontal and temporal poles are fully myelinated on IR-SE T1-WI after 10 months.

2.8.5 Delayed Myelination

There is a close correlation between myelination and psychomotor development, both in normal and delayed myelination. In infants with a developmental delay of unknown cause, delayed myelination is present in 10% of cases. The most common causes of delayed myelination are malnutrition, hypoxia-ischemia, infections, congenital heart failure, hydrocephalus, and chromosomal abnormalities (Down's syndrome).

2.8.6 Leukodystrophy

Leukodystrophies constitute a group of disorders that are characterized by abnormal formation, turnover, or destruction of myelin. The underlying cause is an enzyme deficiency. Most of these disorders are encountered in the pediatric population. White matter changes on MRI are often nonspecific, though some are suggestive of certain diseases.

Canavan disease (see Chap. 13.2.4.8, Fig. 13.31) is rare and results in a diffuse, symmetric, low SI of the white matter on T1-WI. On T2-WI, the supratentorial white matter has a uniformly high SI. In *Alexander disease* (see Chap. 13.2.4.9, Fig. 13.32), the abnormal SI is initially located in the frontal lobes. Enhancement after contrast-medium administration of the basal ganglia and periventricular white matter has been reported. *Adrenoleukodystrophy* (see Chap. 13.2.4.3, Fig. 13.27) affects only boys and results in high SI in the occipital lobes on T2-WI; in due course, these abnormalities advance anteriorly. The anterior rim of the lesion may enhance after contrast-medium administration. An almost complete lack of myelination is seen in the *Pelizaeus–Merzbacher disease* (Fig. 2.54). Hyperintense lesions on T2-WI are found in the basal ganglia or

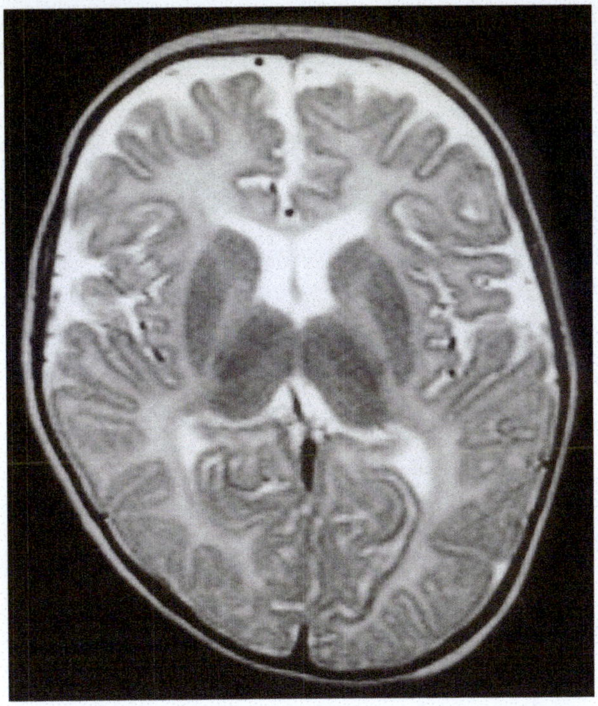

Fig. 2.54 Pelizaeus-Merzbacher disease. This axial TSE T2-WI shows abnormally high signal intensities throughout the white matter in both hemispheres. This finding is consistent with an almost complete lack of normal myelination

thalamus in *Krabbe disease, Leigh disease* (see Chap. 13.2.4.4, Fig. 13.28), and *methylmalonic acidemia.* A more exhaustive discussion of leukodystrophies is presented.

2.8.7 Multiple Sclerosis

MS is an inflammatory demyelinating disease of the CNS. It is the most common demyelinating disease after vascular- and age-related demyelination. MS is characterized by multiple "plaques" of demyelination in the white matter of the brain and spinal cord. The primary lesions are found in the perivascular spaces along penetrating veins. Though the etiology of MS is not fully understood, the destruction of myelin is most likely caused by an autoimmune process. Initial symptoms can sometimes be triggered by trauma or a viral infection, but a convincing link to the disease has not been made.

The clinical course of MS is highly variable. The age of symptom onset in MS is usually between 18 and 40 years; onset is uncommon in childhood and after the age of 50 years. Initial symptoms may include numbness, dysesthesia, double vision, or problems with balance and coordination. Loss of motor function is also a frequent initial presentation. Less commonly, spinal-cord-related symptoms constitute the initial presentation of MS. There is a female:male ratio of 3:2.

The most common clinical presentation is *"relapsing-remitting"* MS (70% of cases). Patients experience symptomatic episodes (known as "attack" or "Schub" in German), which can last from 24 h to several weeks, followed by complete or partial disappearance of symptoms (remission). The interval between relapses may be weeks to years (and even decades). As white-matter lesions increase over time, and neurologic disabilities increase, the disease frequently becomes *"secondary progressive."* Accumulating neurological deficits eventually lead to permanent disability. The evolution from relapsing-remitting to secondary-progressive MS occurs in approximately half of patients within 10 years after onset. Alternatively, in 10–20% of cases, MS can follow a *"primary progressive"* course; in this type of disease, there is a continuous, gradual evolution from the beginning, rather than relapses.

2.8.7.1 Diagnostic Criteria

No single clinical or laboratory test is pathognomonic for MS. For this reason, diagnostic criteria have been developed to assess the relative probability of MS. In 2001, an international panel convened by the National Multiple Sclerosis Society of North America and chaired by Ian McDonald recommended revised diagnostic criteria for MS. They replace the older Poser Criteria and have become known as the "McDonald criteria," after their lead author (Table 2.18). These new criteria integrate MRI image assessment with clinical and other paraclinical methods in drawing diagnostic conclusions. The McDonald criteria take into account the high sensitivity of MRI in detecting lesions. In 2005, a revision to the "McDonald criteria" was proposed to clarify the exact definition of terms such as "attack," "dissemination," a "positive MRI" etc. It is now widely accepted that MRI plays an important role as a noninvasive diagnostic test to establish the diagnosis of MS lesions, showing demyelinating lesions in the brain and spinal cord. Because of its greater sensitivity, compared with clinical measures, MRI can be used to measure subclinical disease. Moreover, MRI outcome measures are routinely used in clinical trials of MS patients, and MRI has become the method of choice for patient follow-up and treatment monitoring.

Table 2.18 McDonald criteria for the diagnosis of Multiple Sclerosis

Clinical presentation	Additional data needed
Two or more attacks (relapses) Two or more objective clinical lesions	None; clinical evidence will suffice (additional evidence desirable but must be consistent with MS)
Two or more attacks One objective clinical lesion	Dissemination in space, demonstrated by: MRI A positive CSF and two or more MRI lesions consistent with MS Further clinical attack involving different site
One attack Two or more objective clinical lesions	Dissemination in time, demonstrated by: MRI Or second clinical attack
One attack One objective clinical lesion (monosymptomatic presentation)	Dissemination in space demonstrated by: MRI Or positive CSF and two or more MRI lesions consistent with MS and Dissemination in time demonstrated by: MRI Or second clinical attack
Insidious neurological progression suggestive of MS (primary progressive MS)	One year of disease progression (retrospectively or prospectively determined) and Two of the following: Positive brain MRI (nine T2 lesions or four or more T2 lesions with positive VEP) Positive spinal cord MRI (two focal T2 lesions) Positive CSF

2.8.7.2 MRI Appearance of MS

The characteristic abnormalities of MS in the brain consist of multiple white-matter lesions with a high SI on FLAIR, PD-WI, and T2-WI and low SI on T1-WI. Lesions are found predominantly in a periventricular distribution, centrum semiovale, and the callososeptal interface (Fig. 2.55). Additional sites of involvement include other parts of the cerebral white matter such as the subcortical white matter, optic nerves, corpus callosum, internal capsule, cerebellar peduncles, brainstem, and spinal cord.

Demyelinating lesions appear smaller on T1-WI than on T2-WI. Occasionally, they show a hyperintense border on T1-WI. Lesions in MS can be small, large, or confluent. The typical configuration is that of an ovoid lesion extending perpendicularly from the ventricular surface (Dawson's finger) (Fig. 2.55). This probably reflects the perivascular inflammation along

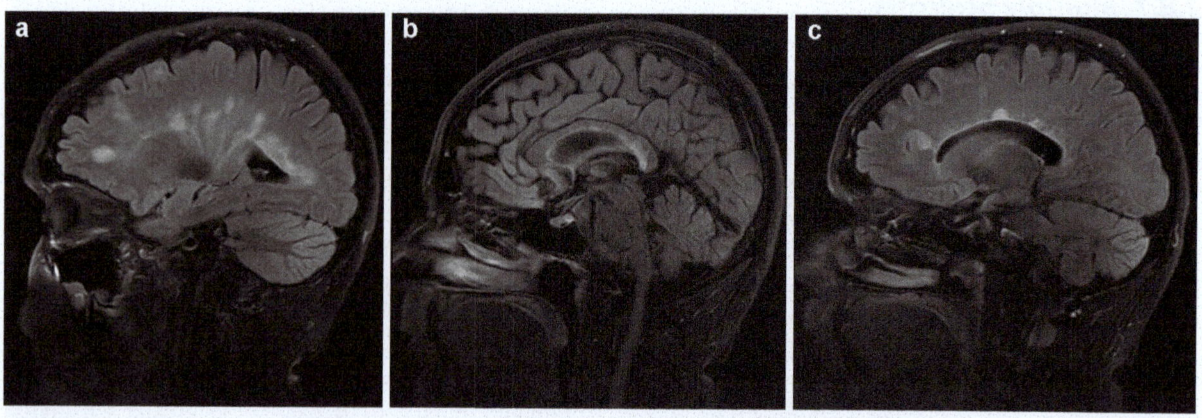

Fig. 2.55 Multiple sclerosis: value of sagittal FLAIR images. (**a–c**) Sagittal fat-sat turbo FLAIR images. These images, obtained in a 27-year-old woman with multiple sclerosis, show multiple demyelinating lesions in the periventricular white matter and corpus callosum. The periventricular lesions characteristically extend perpendicularly from the ventricular surface (Dawson's finger). There is extensive involvement of the corpus callosum, which is a hallmark of MS

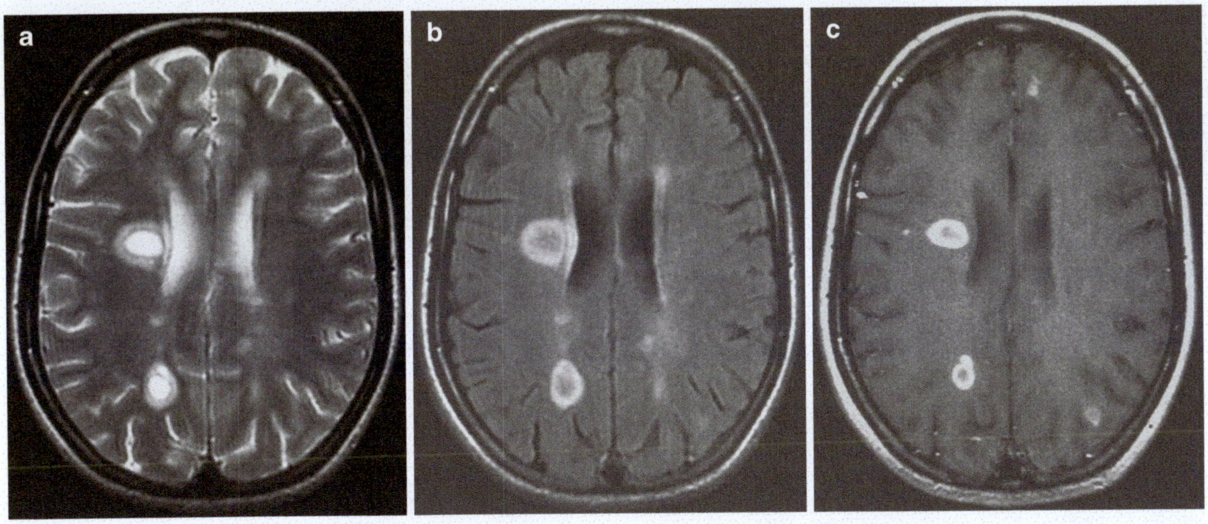

Fig. 2.56 Multiple sclerosis: role of gadolinium. (**a**) Axial TSE T2-WI and (**b**) axial TSE Flair through the centrum semiovale. (**c**) Gd-enhanced axial SE T1-WI through the centrum semiovale. On the T2-WI, all white-matter lesions are hyperintense. Active lesions have basically the same imaging appearance as older lesions. After Gd injection, only a few lesions enhance, indicating disruption of the BBB. The pattern of enhancement can be solid (presumably indicating a fresh lesion) or ring-like (believed to represent an older or reactivated lesion)

a penetrating medullary vein. Atypical lesions and mass-like lesions occur with sufficient frequency to cause diagnostic errors.

MS lesions may enhance after contrast administration on T1-WI, depending on the age and activity of the lesion. New and active lesions commonly show contrast enhancement, due to BBB breakdown. New lesions tend to show solid enhancement, whereas reactivated lesions enhance in a ring-like fashion (Fig. 2.56). After 2 months, the integrity of the BBB is restored, and the majority of lesions no longer show contrast enhancement.

As with unenhanced lesions, the contrast-enhancing lesions are smaller than the corresponding lesions on the T2-W scan. The discrepancy between the size of the lesion on T1-WI and T2-WI reflects the different components of the local process: edema, inflammation, and demyelination.

The poor correlation between the MRI findings and the clinical events is demonstrated by the frequent finding of enhancing lesions in clinically stable patients.

2.8.7.3 Lesion Distribution

White-matter lesions are abundant in the centrum semiovale, corpus callosum, optic chiasm, and optic nerves. Hyperintense lesions on T2-WI are commonly found in the corpus callosum. Typically, these lesions occur along the inner callosal-ventricular margin, creating an irregular ventricular surface of the corpus callosum. This aspect can be differentiated from callosal atrophy due to the lobar white-matter lesions. The existence of callosal lesions improves both the sensitivity and the specificity of MRI for the diagnosis of MS. The absence of callosal lesions renders the diagnosis of MS less likely, but does not exclude it.

A frequent initial presentation of MS is optic neuritis, although there is controversy regarding the likelihood of definitive MS developing in patients who have had an optic neuritis. Brainstem lesions are common, and a lesion in the medial longitudinal bundle affects approximately one-third of MS patients. In patients with clinically possible MS and a normal MRI study of the brain, a spinal MRI study should be performed.

2.8.7.4 Imaging Strategies in MS

Initial and Baseline MRI Evaluation

Many patients are referred for an “initial evalution” standardized MRI scan of the brain after an episode of neurological symptoms which is known as a “clinically isolated syndrome” or a “monosymptomatic

Table 2.19 Brain imaging protocols in multiple sclerosis in patients presenting with a clinically isolated syndrome and as a baseline or follow-up scan

Sequence	Diagnostic scan in a patient presenting with a clinically isolated syndrome	MS baseline or follow-up scan	Remarks
Scout (three-plane or other)	Yes	Yes	Use scouts to align axial scans according to protocol (e.g., parallel with the subcallosal or intercommissural line)
Sagittal Turbo FLAIR	Yes	Optional	Sensitive to show early MS lesions within the corpus callosum and at the callososeptal interface, as well as lesions perpendicular to the ventricular surface
Axial TSE PD/T2	Yes	Yes	TE1≤30 ms and TE2≥80 ms
Axial Turbo FLAIR	Yes	Yes	Sensitive to white-matter lesions including subcortical and cortical lesions
Axial T1 pregadolinium	Optional	Optional	Routine part of most neuroimaging protocols
3D T1	Optional	Optional	Can be used for volumetric assessment (e.g., atrophy measures)
Coronal fat-sat T2 or STIR	Optional	Optional	Indicated in cases of optic neuritis; slices to be positioned from the eye globe to the optic chiasm
Intravenous contrast injection (0.1 mmol/kg body weight)			
Five minutes delay			This delay can be filled by performing the axial turbo FLAIR after injection of contrast medium
Axial and/or T1 postgadolinium	Yes	Optional	It is advised to perform more than one postgadolinium T1-W sequence, because enhancement tends to increase with time after injection

attack," or with a past history that is suspicious for MS. Alternatively, for patients with an established diagnosis of MS, it is recommended that the "baseline evaluation" should include an MRI of the brain that meets the standardized protocol (in addition to a complete neurologic history and examination). Imaging protocols for the initial and baseline MRI evaluation are based on the consensus statement representing the consortium of MS centers consensus guidelines, published in 2006 by Simon et al. (Table 2.19).

In order to detect demyelinating lesions in white matter, the optimal MRI sequence should provide: (1) high contrast between lesions and CSF and (2) high contrast between lesions and normal white matter.

Traditionally, these dual goals have been achieved by a double-echo SE sequence, which provides PD-WI (first echo, TE ≤ 30 ms) and T2-WI (second echo, TE ≥ 80 ms). On PD-WI, the SI of CSF is almost equal to that of periventricular white matter; this allows excellent detection of periventricular lesions which stand out as high-signal areas. On T2-WI, lesions are markedly hyperintense relative to the cerebral white matter. However, small periventricular lesions may be difficult to separate from the high SI CSF in the ventricles.

The combination of high-lesion CSF and high-lesion white-matter contrast can also be achieved by the turbo FLAIR sequence. FLAIR is an IR technique and typically uses a long inversion time of ±2,000 ms (2 s) to suppress the signal of CSF in combination with a long TR/long TE sequence. Turbo FLAIR possesses a superior sensitivity for focal white matter changes in the supratentorial brain, but lesions can be missed in the posterior fossa (Fig. 2.57).

Sagittal turbo FLAIR images are particularly useful for the detection of MS plaques in the corpus callosum and at the callosal-septal interface. Moreover, sagittal images demonstrate the radial orientation of plaques, perpendicular to the ventricular margins (Dawson's fingers). This characteristic finding reflects the perivenular inflammation of MS.

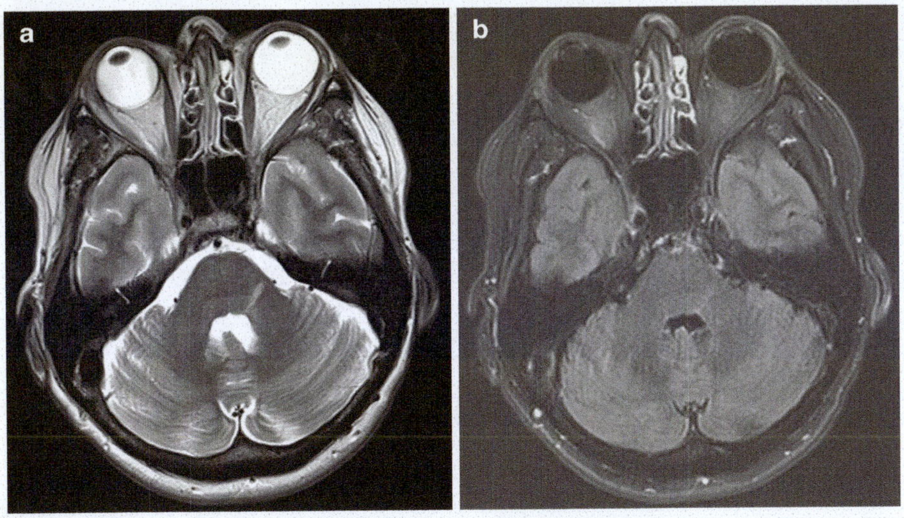

Fig. 2.57 T2-WI are superior to FLAIR images for the detection of posterior fossa lesions. (**a**) Axial TSE T2-WI. (**b**) Axial fat-sat turbo FLAIR. The demyelinating lesion in the left brachium pontis (middle cerebellar peduncle) is better seen on T2-WI than on FLAIR. In the posterior fossa, T2-WI provide better lesion-to-background contrast; FLAIR images are less sensitive in the depiction of demyelinating lesions involving the brainstem and cerebellum. In patients with multiple sclerosis, on FLAIR images, the lesion load in the posterior fossa may be underestimated

Follow-Up MRI Scans

Follow-up MRI scans of the brain (and/or spine) are indicated if a patient's clinical condition is worsening unexpectedly, to reassess the disease burden for patients enrolled in therapeutic trials, or to rule out a secondary diagnosis. However, in the absence of these conditions, routine follow-up MRI scans are generally not recommended.

When follow-up MRI scans are obtained in MS patients, they should be performed in accordance with the standardized imaging protocol. The follow-up scans must be compared with previous studies. The radiologist should pay attention to the appearance of new lesions or enlarging T2-hyperintense lesions as well as to the number of contrast-enhancing lesions. Follow-up scans should also report on the presence or appearance of so-called "black holes." These are lesions that are markedly hypointense on T1-WI, indicating severe tissue injury (including axonal damage, matrix destruction, and myelin loss). Black holes cannot be ascertained on a single MRI scan, since, by definition, these chronic T1 hypointensities should persist for at least 6 months. Black holes should be differentiated from acute MS lesions, which may also appear hypointense on T1-WI due to transient vasogenic edema, which usually disappears after a few weeks. In clinical practice, T1 black holes are lesions that remain hypointense on postgadolinium T1-W scans, indicating a focal area of tissue loss (Fig. 2.58).

Follow-up MRI scans are of great value to count new or enlarging lesions over time, to register changes in enhancement, and to perform quantitative analysis of the T2-lesion volume (the so-called "burden of disease"). Standardized MRI protocols have proven to be useful to correlate imaging findings with clinical outcomes for patients enrolled in therapeutic trials. Cerebral atrophy, which can be assessed from the size of the ventricles and width of the cortical sulci, indicates overall volume loss of brain tissue and is mildly correlated with disabiltiy in MS patients. The use of 3D scans allows volumetric measurements of white-matter lesions and brain tissue.

Gd-Enhanced MRI in Patients with MS

Gd-enhanced MRI of the brain is recommended in patients with (suspected) MS for diagnosis and initial diagnostic evaluation. New and active demyelinating lesions are associated with BBB breakdown and may therefore enhance after contrast administration. The identification of enhancing white-matter lesions is an important component of the

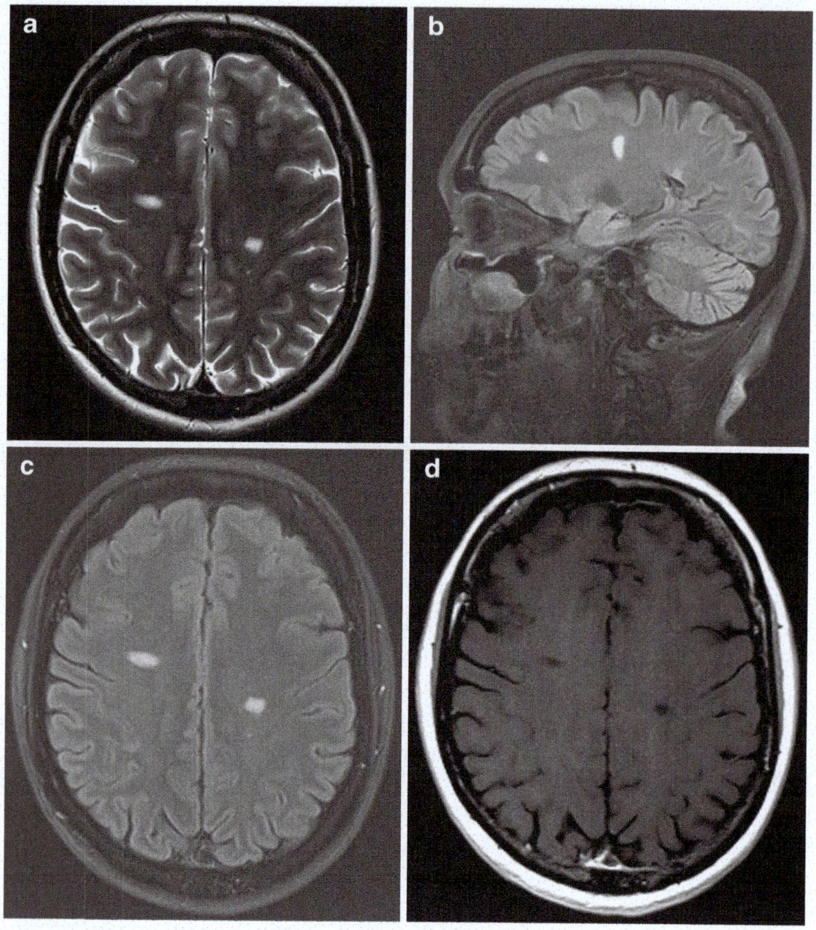

Fig. 2.58 Black holes in multiple sclerosis. (**a**) Axial TSE T2-WI. (**b**) Sagittal fat-sat turbo FLAIR. (**c**) Axial fat-sat turbo FLAIR. (**d**) Gd-enhanced axial TSE T1-WI after a 5-min delay. There are several demyelinating plaques in the subependymal white matter and centrum semiovale; they are hyperintense on FLAIR and T2-WI. On contrast-enhanced T1-WI, the lesions remain hypointense and there is no enhancement. Black holes are defined as lesions that remain hypointense on postgadolinium T1-W scans, indicating a focal area of neural tissue loss

criteria providing evidence for dissemination in time and space. Enhancing white-matter plaques, at the time of the initial diagnostic evaluation, is a strong predictor of future clinical attacks and a diagnosis of MS. Enhancement tends to be solid with fresh lesions and becomes ring-like when the lesion is several weeks old (Fig. 2.56). In addition to showing enhancing MS lesions, the use of gadolinium-enhanced sequences is also very useful to rule out confounding diagnoses, which could otherwise be missed (e.g., leptomeningeal disease, meningioma, tumors, vascular malformations, etc.).

A 5-min delay is suggested between the start of the contrast injection and the postcontrast T1-W sequence. This delay is necessary to provide sufficient time for Gd to leak through the BBB. Some authors have suggested filling up the delay by obtaining the axial turbo FLAIR sequence postgadolinium. Although it is not recommended in the consensus guidelines (Table 2.19), we routinely obtain at least axial and coronal postgadolinium T1-WI. The conspicuity and number of enhancing white-matter lesions can be increased by use of double-dose contrast or by increasing the delay after injection. However, there is no convincing evidence that supports higher doses at this time. We routinely use a standard dose of gadolinium-chelate (0.1 mmol/kg body weight, 20 mL maximum) with a 5-min delay. Application of a MTC (magnetization transfer contrast) prepulse renders the T1-W sequence more sensitive for contrast enhancement (Fig. 2.59). To avoid confusion between enhancement and an MTC effect, the precontrast T1-W sequence should also be performed with a MTC prepulse.

It is well-known that anti-inflammatory medications (e.g., corticosteroids) restore the BBB. Therefore, it is important to perform the MRI examination before

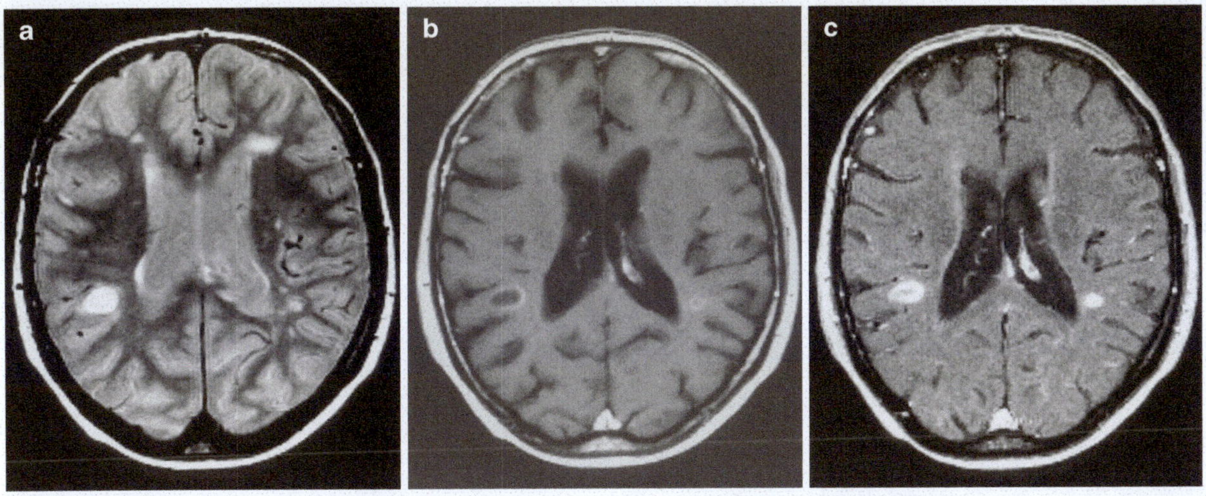

Fig. 2.59 Multiple sclerosis: value of magnetization transfer contrast. (**a**) Axial TSE PD-WI through the lateral ventricles. (**b**) Gd-enhanced axial SE T1-WI (same level). (**c**) Gd-enhanced axial SE T1-WI with MTC (same level). PD-WI shows multiple white-matter lesions in both hemispheres. The distribution pattern is consistent with MS. After Gd injection, ring-like enhancement is observed in two lesions. The Gd-enhanced image with MTC shows more intense enhancement. The signal-to-noise ratio is poorer due to background suppression

medical treatment is instituted. If not, the activity of the disease may be underestimated.

Patients Presenting with Optic Neuritis

In patients presenting with a clinically isolated syndrome with visual disturbances, e.g., optic neuritis, the imaging protocol should include sequences that depict the optic nerve, optic chiasm, and visual pathways. Imaging of the optic nerve is best performed with thin coronal images with fat-suppression (STIR or T2-WI with spectral fat saturation) (Fig. 2.60). Coronal images should cover the orbit and include the optic chiasm and optic tracts. On T2-WI, high SI indicating edema of the optic nerve can be seen. Due to the swelling of the nerve, the CSF-filled perioptic sheath is compressed, and the normal "target" configuration of the optic nerve surrounded by CSF disappears. T1-W sequences after contrast administration may show enhancement of the optic nerve.

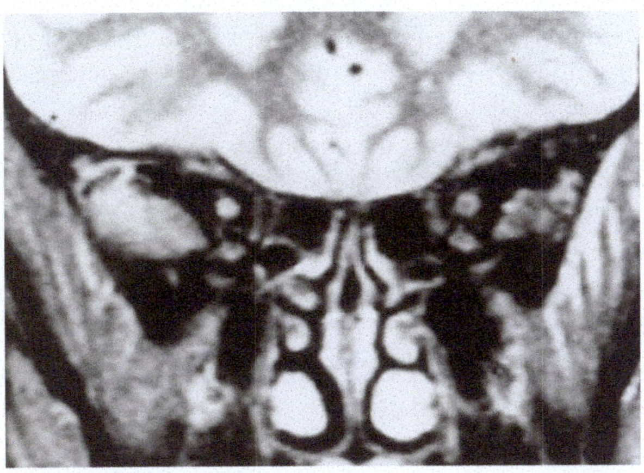

Fig. 2.60 Optic neuritis. This coronal STIR image with fat suppression shows abnormally high signal intensity in the right optic nerve. Note normal "target" appearance of the left optic nerve, which is outlined by the CSF space surrounding it

2.8.7.5 Differential Diagnosis

A diagnosis of MS should not only be made on the basis of MRI findings, but should take into account the patient's history, clinical signs and symptoms, as well as the appropriate laboratory tests. Because of improved MRI techniques, it is relatively easy to rule out obvious MS mimickers such as tumors or vascular malformations. However, it remains difficult to differentiate MS lesions from other diseases involving white matter such as: neurosarcoidosis, Sjögren syndrome,

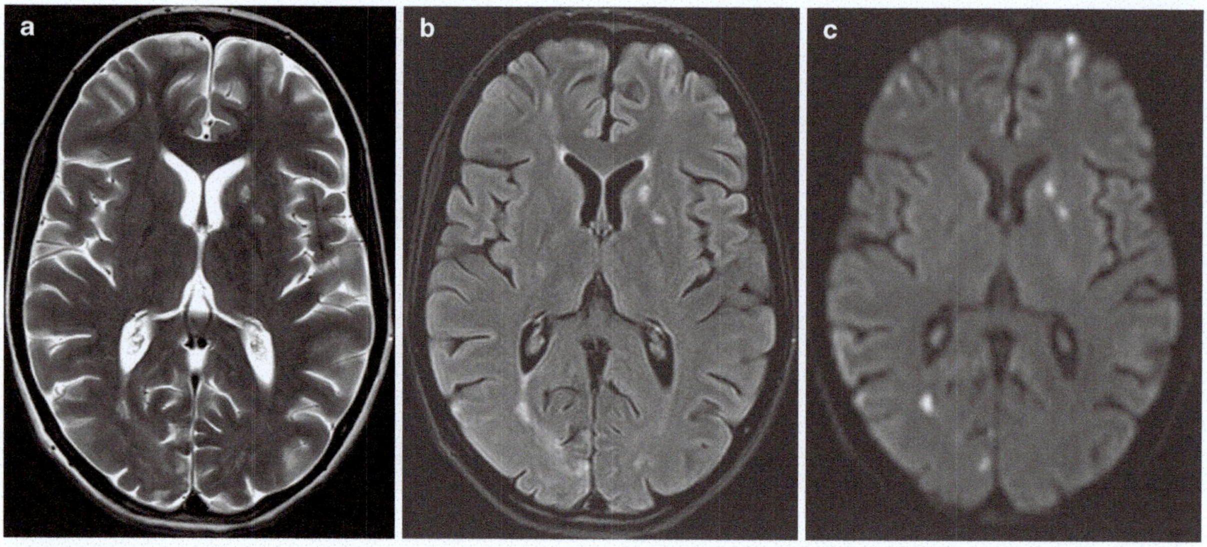

Fig. 2.61 Vasculitis. (**a**) Axial TSE T2-WI. (**b**) Axial fat-sat turbo FLAIR. (**c**) Axial EPI diffusion-weighted "trace" image (DWI). This 22-year-old woman with neuropsychiatric systemic lupus erythematosus and antiphospholipid syndrome was admitted with coordination difficulties, drowsiness, and confusion. T2 (**a**) and FLAIR (**b**) images show scattered, punctate hyperintensities throughout both hemispheres. These lesions exhibit restricted diffusion (**c**), indicating recent infarctions. Vasculitis should be considered in the differential diagnosis of multiple sclerosis, even though in this case, the topography and distribution pattern of the lesions is suggestive of vascular rather than demyelinating etiology

vasculitis (e.g., systemic lupus erythematosus, Behçet disease, …), Lyme disease, acute disseminated encephalomyelitis (ADEM), etc. These conditions may present clinical and MRI findings remarkably similar to MS. Lyme disease can mimic MS on an MRI study, and in endemic regions, this treatable disease should be considered in the differential diagnosis. Vasculitis is associated with multifocal T2-hyperintense lesions, representing micro-infarctions, sometimes with diffusion restriction (Fig. 2.61). Vasculitis preferentially involves the peripheral, subcortical white matter and gray matter, with focal gray matter atrophy. ADEM is a monophasic disease with an MRI appearance which is often indistinguishable from MS.

In the elderly population, the main differential diagnosis is with nonspecific ischemic white-matter lesions associated with microvascular disease or systemic hypertension (subcortical arteriosclerotic leukoencephalopathy).

On MRI studies, overdiagnosis of MS should be avoided and the radiologist should be aware of pitfalls and differential diagnoses. A short list of multifocal white-matter lesions is provided in Table 2.20.

Table 2.20 Differential diagnosis of multifocal white-matter lesions

Aging
Multiple sclerosis
ADEM
Lyme disease
PML
Metastasis
Trauma
Vasculitis
Hypertension
Migraine

2.8.8 Toxic and Degenerative Demyelination

Radiation therapy and chemotherapy may lead to degeneration of cerebral white matter. T2-WI shows focal or diffusely confluent lesions in the lobar white matter. Local mass effect can be present due to focal necrosis. Peripheral enhancement is often seen after

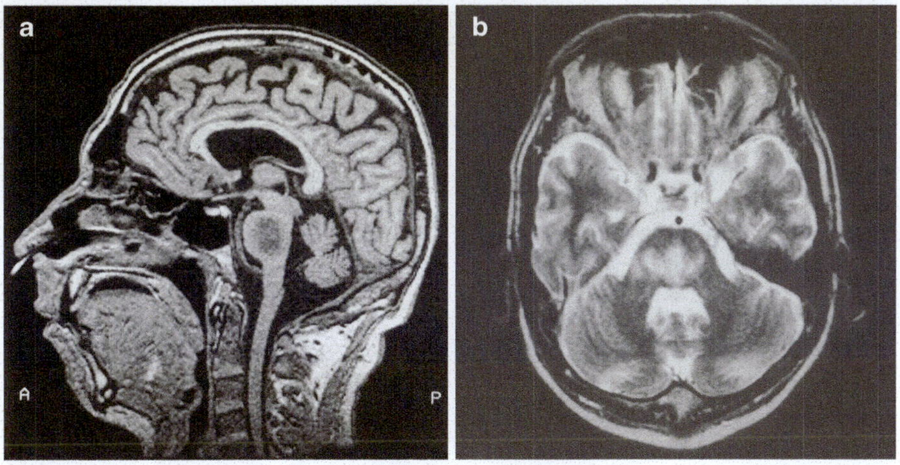

Fig. 2.62 Central pontine myelinolysis. (**a**) Sagittal SE T1-WI. (**b**) Axial TSE T2-WI. Within the pons, there is a lesion which is hypointense on the T1-WI and hyperintense on the T2-WI. There is a surrounding rim of normal-appearing pontine parenchyma. On the axial image, the "trident" shape reflects the position of the corticospinal tracts in the anterior lateral part of the pons

contrast administration. Radiation-induced contrast-enhancing lesions may develop in patients after treatment for brain tumors, and these lesions can mimic recurrent or residual tumor. MRS can be used to differentiate recurrent tumor (increased choline/creatine ratio and decreased *N*-acetylaspartate) from radiation necrosis (elevated lactate). Alternatively, dynamic susceptibility-weighted contrast-enhanced perfusion MRI can be used, since recurrent tumor shows elevated CBV (presumably reflecting tumor angiogenesis), whereas CBV is decreased in areas of radiation-induced necrosis (indicating that radiation necrosis is ischemic in nature and due to an insufficient blood supply).

Alcohol is another cause of toxic demyelination. Osmotic myelinolysis is an acute neurologic condition, which may occur as a complication of severe and prolonged hyponatremia, particularly when corrected too rapidly. This condition is most frequently found in alcoholics, but other risk factors include malnutrition, liver transplant surgery, burn patients, etc. The most common site of involvement is the central pons, and this condition is known as central pontine myelinolysis (Fig. 2.62). On MRI, an area of prolonged T1- and T2- relaxation times is observed in the pons. On axial T2-WI, the hyperintense signal abnormality presents a characteristic "trident"-shape in the central pons, with sparing of the pontine tegmentum and ventrolateral pons (corticospinal tracts). Extrapontine osmotic myelinolysis can also be found in the basal ganglia and the thalamus. Peripheral enhancement may be observed after contrast administration. Chronic alcoholism can also cause nonspecific deep white-matter lesions and periventricular demyelination.

2.9 Intracranial Infection

2.9.1 Imaging Strategy

MRI is superior to CT for the detection of intracranial infections. The pulse-sequences used for the evaluation of intracranial infections are straightforward. Use of a paramagnetic contrast agent is crucial. In most cases, we use the same protocol as proposed for intracranial mass lesions.

2.9.2 Meningitis

Meningitis is the most common presentation of CNS infection. It can be caused by bacterial, viral, or fungal agents. Clinically, meningitis presents as an acute febrile illness with severe headache, stiffness of the neck, photophobia, and vomiting. Imaging does not contribute to the diagnosis, but can be used to exclude parenchymal abscess or localized empyema, to look for a source of infection (paranasal sinuses, petrous bones), to monitor the complications of meningeal infections (hydrocephalus, subdural effusion, infarction), and to rule out confounding diagnoses when the clinical presentation is atypical.

In most cases of meningitis, no abnormality is seen on unenhanced MRI scans; in some cases, obliteration of the basal cisterns is observed, with hyperintense signal on proton-density and FLAIR images. After contrast-medium administration, leptomeningeal

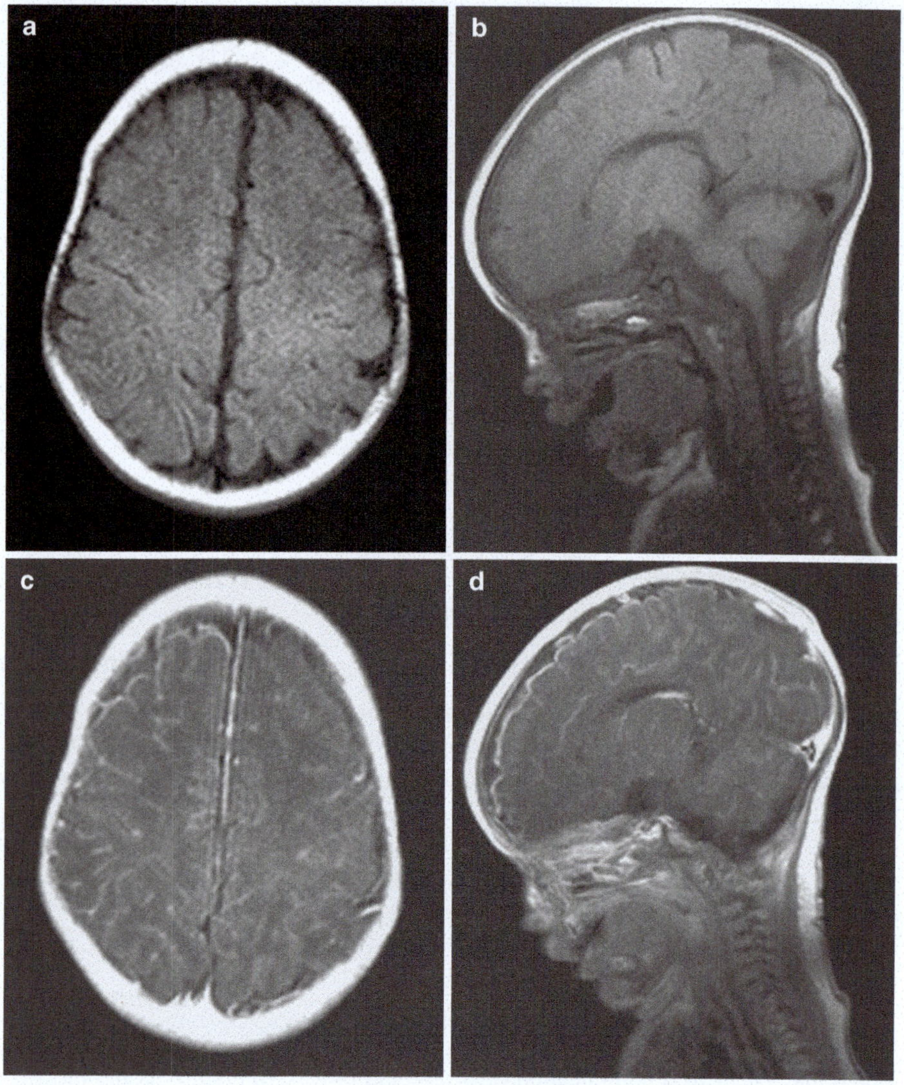

Fig. 2.63 Acute bacterial meningitis. (**a**, **b**) Precontrast axial and sagittal SE T1-WI. (**c**, **d**) Gd-enhanced axial and sagittal SE T1-WI (identical slice positions). Precontrast T1-WI is unremarkable because the thickened leptomeninges are isointense to CSF. T2-WI were normal (not shown). After Gd-administration, there is extensive enhancement of the leptomeningeal bacterial exudate involving the subarachnoid spaces and cortical sulci. Lumbar puncture confirmed meningococcal meningitis

thickening and enhancement is observed, especially in patients with chronic bacterial infection (Fig. 2.63).

In adults, 50% of patients with bacterial meningitis develop complications, which include:

- *Hydrocephalus*, due to fibropurulent infectious exudate and cellular debris, which obstructs the CSF flow at the foramina of Monro, aqueduct, fourth ventricle outlet foramina, and subarachnoid spaces.
- The infection can spread to the ventricular system, resulting in *ventriculitis* (also known as ependymitis) and *choroid plexitis*, both showing ependymal enhancement after contrast administration.
- *Subdural effusions* are a common complication of meningitis. They are seen as extra-axial fluid collections with smooth contours that displace the cortical veins medially and do not extend into the sulci. They should be differentiated from widened subarachnoidal spaces, where the extra-axial fluid extends into the sulci and does not displace the cortical veins.
- *Subdural empyema* (a collection of pus and fluid from infected tissue) can be caused by meningitis, but the most common cause is sinusitis. Empyema is recognized on MRI as a lentiform or crescentic extra-axial fluid collection, adjacent to the inner table, overlying the cerebral convexities, or extending into the interhemispheric fissure along the falx, or into the posterior fossa with strong enhancement of the surrounding pseudomembrane (Fig. 2.64). Most subdural empyemas are found in close proximity to the

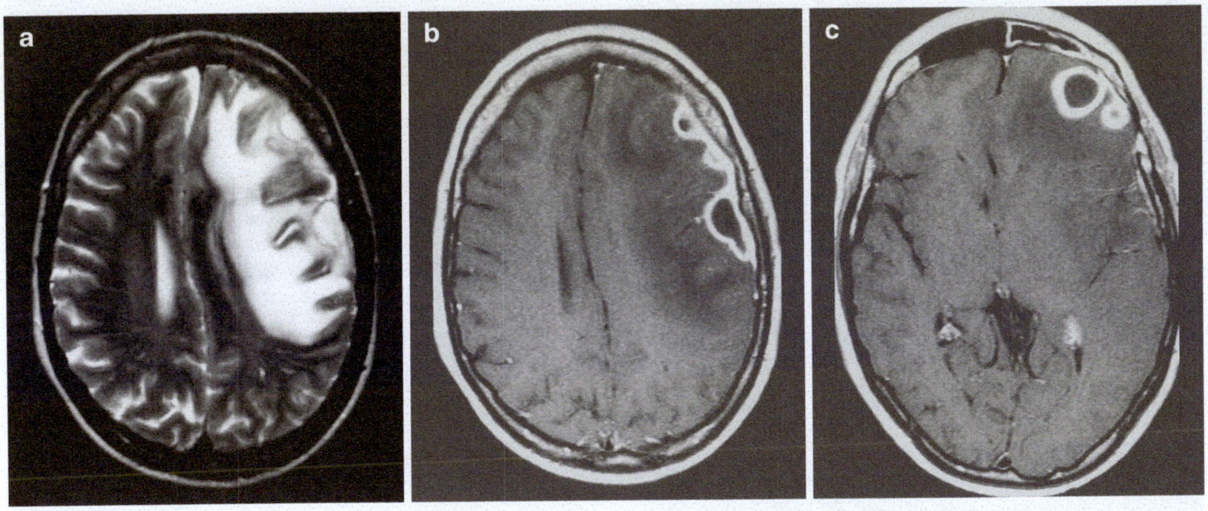

Fig. 2.64 Subdural empyema and intracerebral abscess. (**a**) Axial TSE T2-WI through the centrum semiovale. (**b**) Axial Gd-enhanced SE T1-WI (same level as **a**). (**c**) Axial Gd-enhanced SE T1-WI through the lower frontal lobes. The axial T2-WI shows nodular meningeal thickening over the left frontal convexity; there is extensive vasogenic edema in the white matter of the left cerebral hemisphere. After Gd injection, extra-axial fluid collections are observed. There is strong enhancement of the meninges and surrounding pseudomembranes. In the lower frontal lobe, the pyogenic empyema has spread into the cerebral parenchyma with the formation of an intracerebral abscess, which enhances in a ring-like pattern

paranasal sinuses (anterior cranial fossa, frontal region) or the temporal bones (bases of the skull, middle and posterior cranial fossa).

- Pyogenic meningitis can spread into the cerebral parenchyma causing *cerebritis*. Hematogenous spread, however, is the most common cause of a cerebritis. MRI shows an ill-defined region of low signal on T1-WI and high signal on T2-WI. Patchy enhancement can be seen after contrast-medium administration.

The appearance of an intraparenchymal area of ring enhancement indicates formation of a *cerebral abscess* (Fig. 2.65). This process of encapsulation may take weeks depending on the organism, immune response, and therapy. An abscess has a thick enhancing wall and is surrounded by vasogenic white-matter edema. Because most abscesses result from hematogenous spread of microorganisms, the preferred location is the corticomedullary junction. On T2-WI, the wall of the abscess is hypointense (dark rim). After Gd-injection, there is thick-walled ring-enhancement. Characteristically, a bacterial abscess exhibits restricted diffusion on DWI trace images (hyperintense), and lowered ADC values (hypointense). This is due to the high cellular content and increased viscosity of the pus (decreased motion of water). This is a useful differentiating feature from a necrotic tumor, which does not show diffusion restriction. However, some metastases, especially from mucinous primary tumors, may also exhibit diffusion restriction. Table 2.7 provides a differential diagnosis for ring-enhancing lesions in the brain.

Cranial nerve dysfunction is a common complication of bacterial or tuberculous meningitis.

Cerebral infarcts can occur as a complication of meningitis, due to arteritis, vascular compression, or dural sinus or cerebral vein thrombosis.

2.9.3 Encephalitis

The term encephalitis refers to a diffuse, nonfocal, inflammatory process of the brain parenchyma, usually of viral origin. The most common causative agents are: herpes simplex virus (HSV), cytomegalovirus, and, in patients with AIDS, the papovaviruses. Most of the encephalitides resemble each other and have few identifying imaging characteristics. Areas of involvement are characterized by mass effect, edema, hyperintensity on T2-WI, and, less frequently, small infarctions or petechial hemorrhages. A common nonviral cause of encephalitis is toxoplasmosis, especially in immunocompromised patients. ADEM is an autoimmune allergic encephalitis.

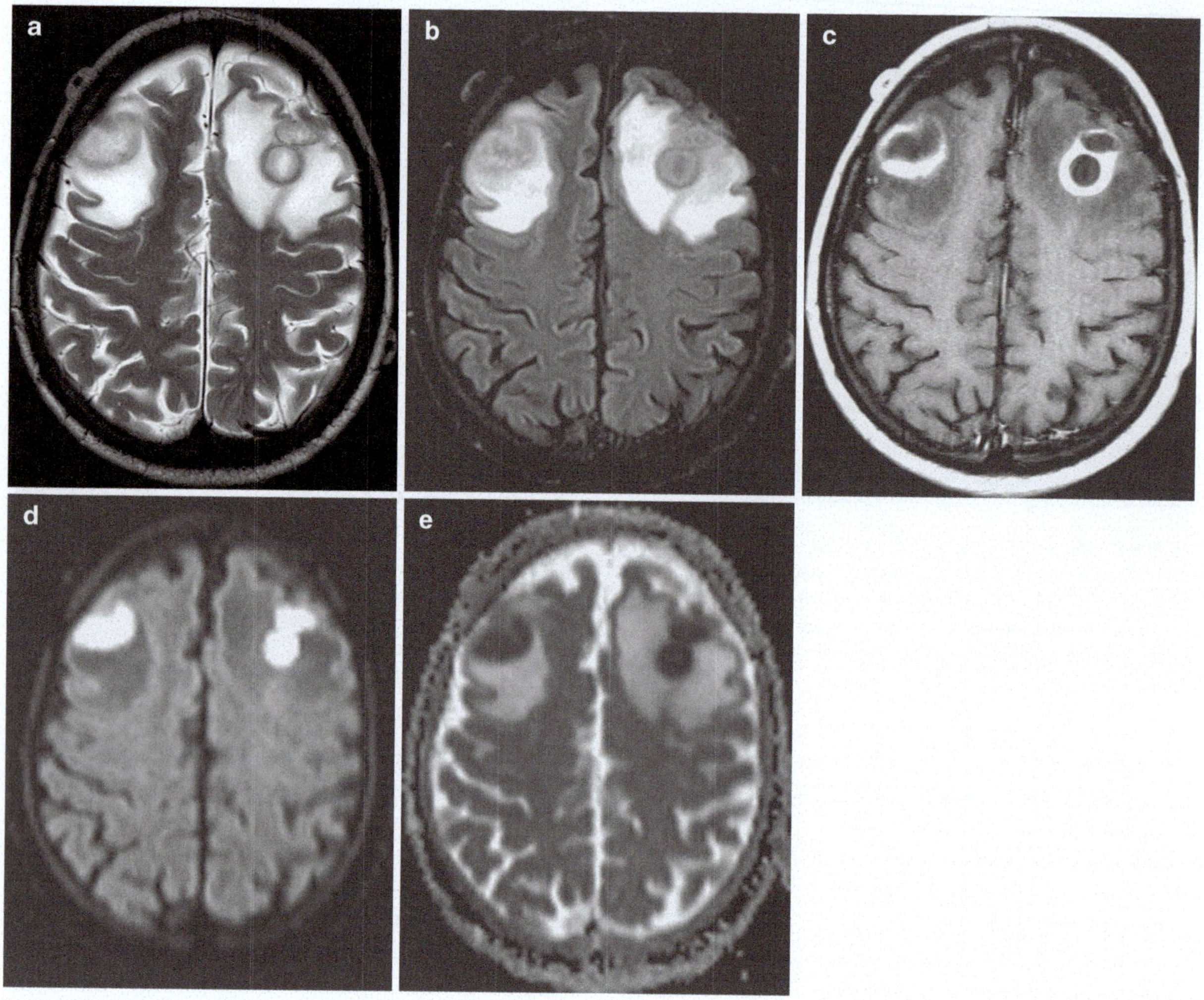

Fig. 2.65 Bacterial cerebral brain abscesses. (**a**) Axial TSE T2-WI. (**b**) Axial fat-sat turbo FLAIR. (**c**) Gd-enhanced axial T1-WI. (**d**) Axial EPI diffusion-weighted "trace" image. (**e**) Apparent diffusion coefficient (ADC) map. The patient is a 43-year-old man with alcoholic liver cirrhosis, chronic pancreatitis, portal vein thrombosis, and septicemia. There are pyogenic abscesses in both frontal lobes, surrounded by a large area of vasogenic edema. On T2-WI the abscess capsule is hypointense (*dark rim*). After Gd-injection, there is bilateral ring-enhancement. The lesions show markedly restricted diffusion on the trace images (hyperintense), and lowered ADC values (hypointense). Diffusion restriction in pyogenic abscesses is due to the high cellular content and increased viscosity of the pus (decreased motion of water)

2.9.3.1 Herpes Encephalitis

There are two types of HSV encephalitis, type I (in adults) and type II (in neonates).

HSV type 1 (oral herpes) is the most common cause of sporadic viral encephalitis. It has a predilection for the subfrontal and medial temporal lobes. Although initially unilateral, most patients develop lesions in both hemispheres. The temporal lobe, insular cortex, subfrontal area, and cingulate gyrus are affected. Early MRI changes are: gyral effacement due to edema on T1-WI and high signal of the temporal lobe and cingulate gyrus on T2-WI (Fig. 2.66). Bilateral temporal lobe involvement is considered nearly pathognomonic of HSV encephalitis. Later in the course of the disease, T1-WI may demonstrate gray matter hyperintensities in a gyriform pattern (indicating petechial hemorrhages). After contrast administration, gyral enhancement may be observed. HSV encephalitis has a high mortality rate (50–70%), and those who survive show marked atrophy and encephalomalacia of the temporal and frontal lobes.

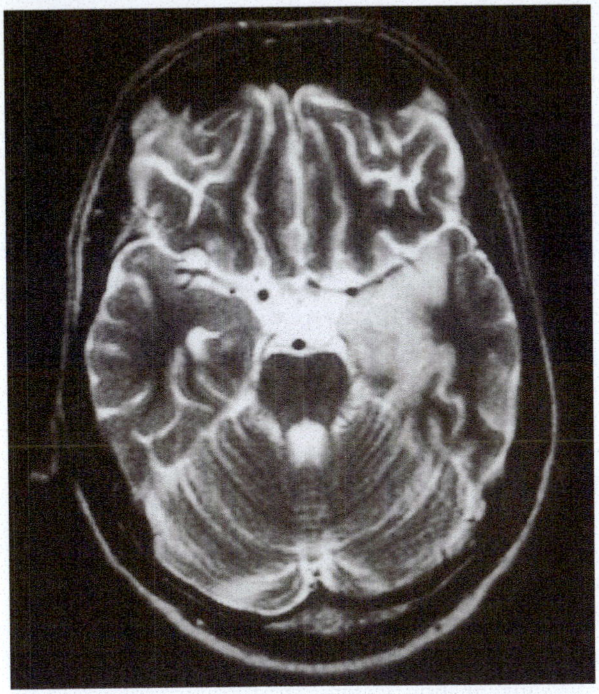

Fig. 2.66 Herpes simplex virus encephalitis. This axial TSE T2-WI was obtained in a patient with Herpes type 1 encephalitis. Note the increased signal intensity of the medial part of the left temporal lobe. There is some mass effect due to edema

The neonatal HSV type 2 (genital herpes) is a diffuse nonfocal encephalitis, known as panencephalitis. Because the neonatal brain is largely unmyelinated, diffuse edema is difficult to detect with MRI. Diffusion-weighted images may show increased signal intensities, consistent with cytotoxic edema. Patchy meningeal or parenchymal enhancement can be seen.

2.9.3.2 HIV and AIDS-Related CNS Diseases

The retrovirus that causes AIDS is neurotropic and directly invades the peripheral nervous system and CNS. This virus is the most common pathogen in AIDS patients. Other AIDS-related CNS infections are opportunistic and are caused by *Toxoplasma gondii*, *Cryptococcus neoformans*, and papovaviruses.

HIV Encephalitis

The HIV virus causes a variety of neurological disorders, including encephalopathy (AIDS dementia complex), myelopathy, and peripheral neuropathy. HIV encephalitis is often found in combination with CMV encephalitis. The predominant imaging characteristic of HIV encephalitis is marked cerebral atrophy (Fig. 2.67). On T2-WI, confluent or patchy areas of increased signal are observed in the periventricular and deep white matter, most commonly in the frontal lobes There is no enhancement after contrast injection.

Progressive Multifocal Leukoencephalopathy

Progressive multifocal leukoencephalopathy (PML) is a CNS infection caused by reactivation of the JC

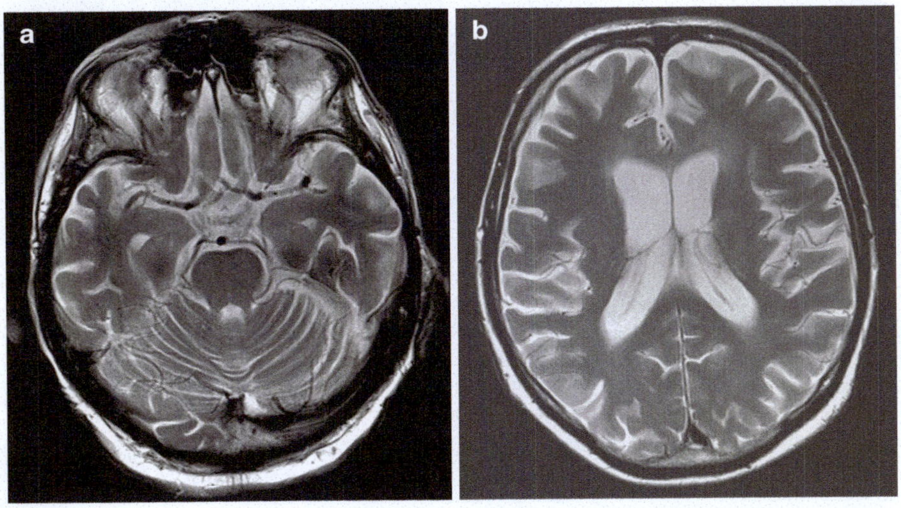

Fig. 2.67 HIV-encephalitis (AIDS dementia complex). (**a**, **b**) Axial TSE T2-WI. The patient is a 51-year-old man with AIDS, presenting with memory loss and confusion. The most striking finding of AIDS dementia complex is marked cerebral atrophy. In addition, there may be confluent areas of increased signal in the periventricular and deep white matter, most commonly in the frontal lobes

papovavirus. This viral infection causes destruction of oligodendrocytes, which results in extensive demyelination. Initial FLAIR and T2-WI show multifocal, subcortical, high-signal lesions, especially in the fronto-parietal and temporo-occipital white matter. In due course, these lesions become confluent and show central cavitation. Contrast enhancement is uncommon. Although PML can be unilateral, an asymmetric distribution in the white matter of both cerebral hemispheres is more common. Signal abnormalities can also be seen in the gray matter of the thalamus and basal ganglia (presumably secondary to involvement of traversing white-matter fibers). In many cases, the posterior fossa is also affected with areas of demyelination involving white-matter tracts in the brainstem and cerebellum.

Toxoplasmosis

Toxoplasmosis is the most common opportunistic CNS infection in AIDS patients. The infection is caused by toxoplasma gondii. Cerebral toxoplasmosis causes multiple mass lesions in brain parenchyma, which are found near the corticomedullary junction and in the basal ganglia (Fig. 2.68). The lesions are difficult to see on unenhanced T1-WI; T2-WI are more sensitive in localizing multifocal lesions. After gadolinium-chelate administration, most lesions show ring-shaped or nodular enhancement. It is important to look for multiple lesions, because multifocality helps to differentiate a toxoplasmosis infection from a primary CNS lymphoma.

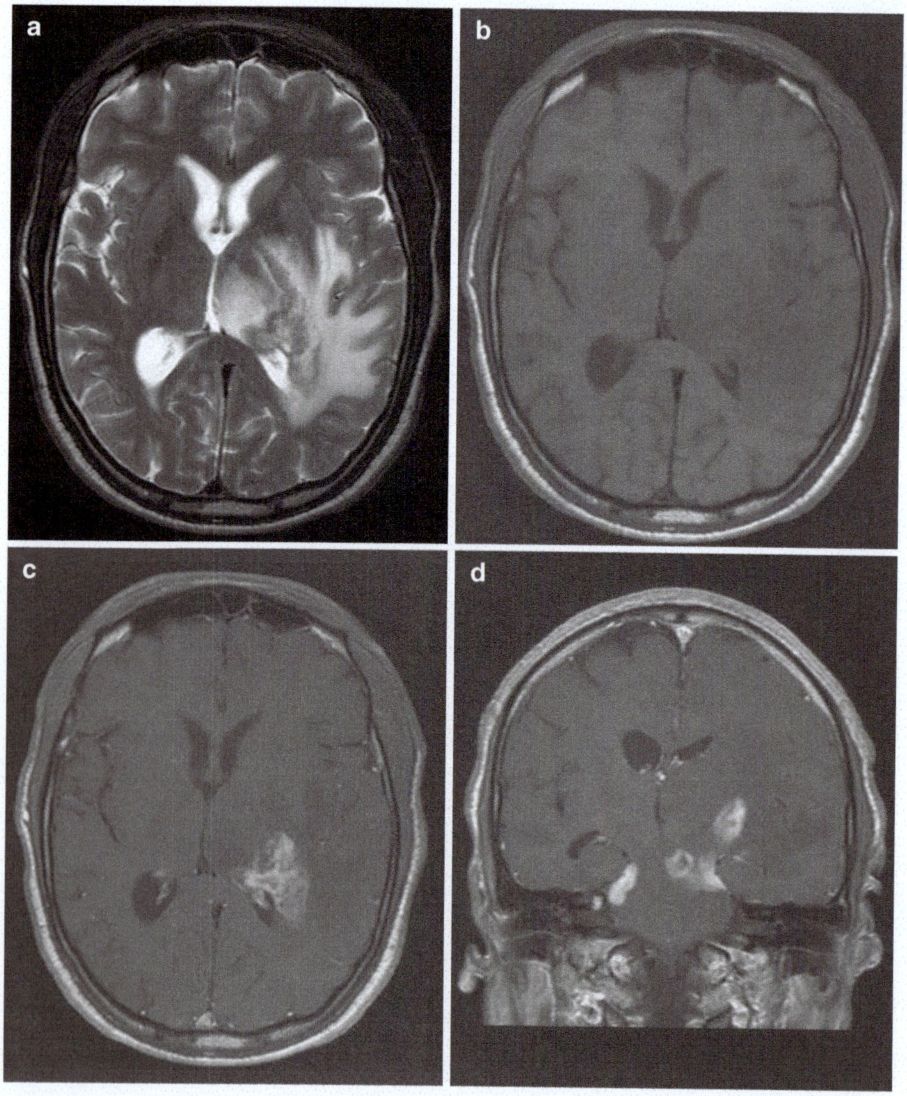

Fig. 2.68 Cerebral toxoplasmosis. (**a**) Axial TSE T2-WI. (**b**) Axial TSE T1-WI. Gd-enhanced axial (**c**) and coronal (**d**) TSE T1-WI. This 47-year-old man with AIDS developed cerebral toxoplasmosis. On TSE T2-WI, lesions present a mixed appearance with extensive white-matter edema. The abscesses are isointense with the surrounding edema on T1-WI. After Gd-injection, multiple enhancing lesions of varying size are seen; they represent parenchymal toxoplasma abscesses with necrosis and surrounding inflammation. Differential diagnosis should include cerebral lymphoma and other infectious diseases

Primary CNS Lymphoma

Lymphoma is the second most common cause of a CNS mass lesion in AIDS patients (preceded only by toxoplasmosis). Primary CNS lymphoma in AIDS patients is typically a high-grade B-cell non-Hodgkin lymphoma, with strong association with the Epstein-Barr virus infection. Lymphomas can occur anywhere in the brain, but they are most commonly found in periventricular region and the corpus callosum. On T1-WI, lymphoma is iso-to hypointense to the surrounding brain tissue. The SI on FLAIR and T2-WI is variable, but frequently lymphoma is hypointense, reflecting its high-cell density. After gadolinium-chelate administration, primary CNS lymphoma enhances intensely and homogenously (Fig. 2.23). Ring enhancement is also a frequent finding and reflects central necrosis. It is important to remember that steroids may inhibit contrast enhancement, and may confound the diagnosis.

Cryptococcosis

Cryptococcosis is the most common cause of fungus infection in AIDS patients. Cryptococcus is a common soil fungus, which may infect the lungs and spread hematogenously to the CNS in patients with immunodeficiency. In the brain, cryptococcosis causes choroid plexitis, meningitis, and encephalitis. The fungus spreads along the perivascular Virchow–Robin spaces (VRS). It causes an enhancing granulomatous meningitis (if the immune response is still sufficient); otherwise, hydrocephalus and generalized brain atrophy are found (if the immune response is inadequate). On MRI, signal abnormalities (hypointense on T1-WI and hyperintense on FLAIR and T2-WI) can be observed in the lenticulostriate region; these lesions reflect gelatinous pseudocysts. After administration of gadolinium-chelates, leptomeningeal enhancement may be observed.

2.9.4 Acute Disseminated Encephalomyelitis

ADEM, also known as postviral leukoencephalopathy, is a type of postinfectious encephalomyelitis, following a viral illness (e.g., measles, chickenpox, rubella, mumps, varicella, pertussis, Epstein-Barr, and viral upper airway infections). ADEM can also be triggered by a vaccination.

ADEM should be regarded as an autoimmune response against the patient's white matter resulting in demyelination. ADEM is usually a self-limiting disease, and as opposed to relapsing-remitting MS, is a monophasic disease. It is mostly found in children and young adults, but can be seen in all ages. FLAIR or T2-WI show multifocal subcortical areas of increased SI, with or without the involvement of posterior fossa. Lesions are widely distributed in both hemispheres, usually asymmetrically. After contrast injection, some lesions will enhance on a T1-W sequence. Although most patients recover completely without residual lesions, 10–20% of patients develop permanent sequelae. The main differential diagnosis is with MS (which usually occurs as a recurrent disease), autoimmune vasculitis, and even aging brain.

2.9.5 Tuberculosis

Tuberculosis remains a major public health problem, not only in developing countries, but also in industrialized nations. CNS tuberculosis results from hematogenous dissemination. Tuberculosis can affect the CNS in several ways (Fig. 2.69):

- *Tuberculous meningitis* is presumed to occur after rupture of an initial subependymal or subpial focus tuberculosis (a so-called Rich focus). Tuberculous meningitis in the brain typically involves the basal cisterns, interhemispheric fissure, Sylvian fissure, and the cerebral convexities. It causes meningeal thickening ("pachymeningitis") and marked enhancement of the basal cisterns, corresponding on pathology to a gelatinous exudate. Hydrocephalus is a common complication, due to obstruction of the subarachnoid spaces and CSF drainage pathways. Ischemic infarctions of the basal ganglia, internal capsule, and thalami occur due to vascular compression of the lenticulostriate and thalamoperforating arteries. T1-WI after contrast administration show thickening and intense enhancement of the meninges in the basal cisterns.
- *Tuberculomas* occur in the brain as a result of granuloma formation within the brain parenchyma. Tuberculomas are most commonly found in the posterior

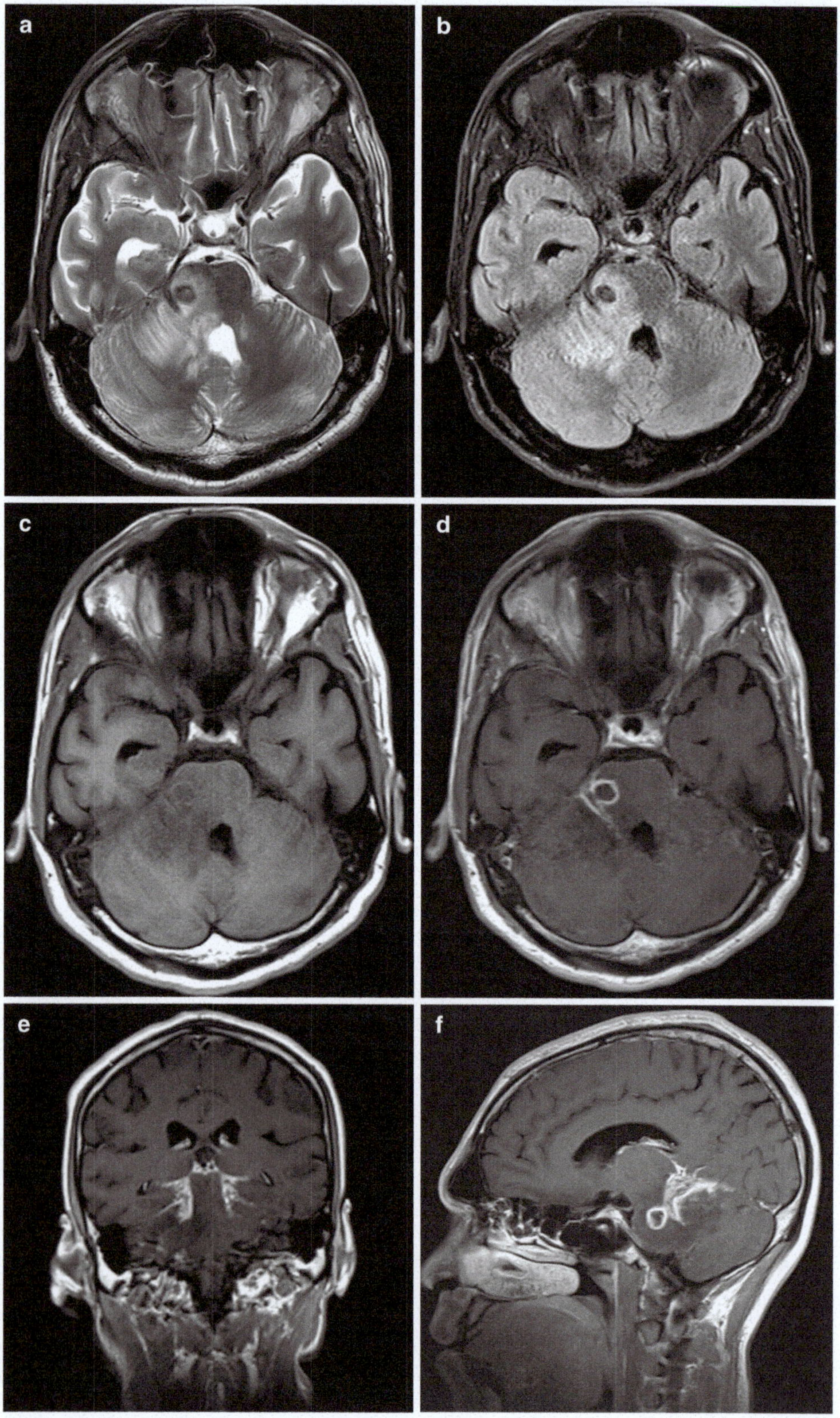

Fig. 2.69 Tuberculous pachymeningitis and tuberculoma in the brainstem. (**a**) Axial TSE T2-WI. (**b**) Axial fat-sat turbo FLAIR. (**c**) Axial TSE T1-WI. Gd-enhanced axial (**d**), coronal (**e**) and sagittal (**f**) TSE T1-WI. This 32-year-old man, with pulmonary tuberculosis was admitted with chronic bifrontal headaches, papilledema, nuchal rigidity, and worsening general condition. On the right side of the pons, there is a tuberculoma. This lesion is hypointense on T2-WI, is surrounded by vasogenic edema, and show rim enhancement. These characterictics indicate a caseating tuberculoma. In addition, there is severe pachymeningitis around the upper brainstem (pons and mesencephalon), with extension into the ambient and pontocerebellar cisterns. This combination of tuberculous pachymeningitis with (multiple) tuberculous brain abscesses has been compared to a "soap-bubble" appearance on gadolinium-enhanced MRI scans

fossa, and in the cortical and subcortical regions near the gray–white matter junction of the frontal and parietal lobes. More than two-third of tuberculomas are found as a solitary lesion, which poses a differential diagnostic problem. The MRI appearance depends on the maturity of the tuberculoma. A non-caseating tuberculoma is hypointense relative to brain tissue on T1-WI, hyperintense on T2-WI, and shows homogeneous, solid enhancement. A caseating tuberculoma with a solid center is isointense or even markedly hypointense on T2-WI, is surrounded by an area of vasogenic edema, and tends to show rim enhancement. When the caseating tuberculoma has developed a necrotic center, the core becomes hyperintense on T2-WI, the perilesional edema disappears, though ring enhancement may persist. Tuberculous meningitis with formation of multiple tuberculous brain abscesses can present a so-called "soap-bubble" appearance on gadolinium-enhanced MRI scans (Fig. 2.69).

2.10 Normal and Abnormal Aging of the Brain

The morphologic appearance of the brain changes with aging. These changes start to occur in adults, but become more pronounced in elderly individuals. In addition to an irreversible loss of brain substance (a process known as cerebral atrophy), specific age-related changes occur in the cerebral white matter, CSF spaces, and gray matter. These findings should be considered as normal aging phenomena, and should not be mistaken for disease.

2.10.1 White Matter Changes in Aging

2.10.1.1 Periventricular Hyperintensities: "Caps" and "Bands"

In almost all adult and elderly individuals, one finds so-called "caps" and "bands" around the lateral ventricles. The periventricular caps, which are hyperintense on FLAIR images, are found predominantly around the frontal horns of the lateral ventricles. They are usually small, although larger, often symmetric foci can also be found in normal individuals. High-signal rims (bands), contiguous with the margins of the lateral ventricles on FLAIR images, are also a frequent normal finding. These periventricular hyperintensities (PVH) correspond to areas of mild demyelination, associated with subependymal gliosis, discontinuity of the ependymal lining, and widening of the extracellular spaces (known as "ependymitis granularis"). The ependymal lining of the ventricles is regular and thin in the younger population, but becomes thicker and irregular, with extensions into the white matter, in the elderly population. Larger lesions cannot reliably be differentiated from demyelinating disease and infarcts; the MRI appearance can be indistinguishable. Extensive, confluent T2-hyperintense periventricular signal abnormalities are also found in hydrocephalus as a result of intraparenchymal leakage of CSF ("interstitial edema").

2.10.1.2 Deep White-Matter Hyperintensities

With increasing age, focal T2-hyperintense regions are found in the deep white matter of normal individuals. With the exception of the subcortical U-fibers, they can be located anywhere in the cerebral white matter. Minor perivascular damage (but not infarction) is the most likely substrate of punctate MR white-matter hyperintensities in elderly brains. These foci show high SI on both echoes of a long TR sequence, are best seen as hyperintense foci on FLAIR images, show low SI on T1-WI, and there is no contrast enhancement or mass effect. There is a correlation between the incidence of these nonspecific white-matter lesions and cerebrovascular disease and hypertension. On MRI alone, it is often impossible to distinguish these age-related lesions from multifocal disease, although the MRI characteristics together with the clinical data usually lead to correct interpretation.

In 1987, a scoring system was proposed, which subsequently became known as the "Fazekas scale," after the first author. The Fazekas scale rates periventricular and deep white-matter hyperintensities (PVH and DWMH) on a four grade scale (Table 2.21).

Table 2.21 The Fazekas Scale for scoring periventricular and deep white-matter hyperintensities (1987)

Periventricular hyperintensities (PVH)	Deep white-matter hyperintensities (DWMH)
(0) Absence	(0) Absence
(1) "Caps" or pencil-thin lining	(1) Punctate foci
(2) Smooth "halo"	(2) Beginning confluence of foci
(3) Irregular PVH extending into the deep white matter	(3) Large confluent areas

2.10.1.3 Perivascular Hyperintensities

Perivascular spaces or VRS surround penetrating arteries for a short distance as they enter the cerebral parenchyma. They are lined by pia mater and contain interstitial fluid. They are in continuity with the subpial space, and are separated from the subarachnoid space by a single layer of pia mater. VRS are found predominantly in the basal ganglia (in the lower putamen, around the anterior commissure) and in the centrum semiovale (Fig. 2.70). However, VRS can also occur in other parts of the brain, such as the mesencephalon and cerebral peduncles On T1-WI, they are hypointense, and on T2-WI they appear as punctate or linear hyperintensities. Since they are filled with interstitial fluid, their signal is suppressed on FLAIR images, unlike nonspecific age-related white-matter lesions which appear bright on FLAIR images. Most VRS are small and punctuate, or linear, larger, and more confluent perivascular spaces can occur in the basal ganglia. The occurrence of VRS is age related. VRS are an almost constant finding in adults, and a frequent finding in children.

2.10.2 Age-Related Changes in the CSF Spaces and Cortical Gray Matter

Volume loss of the cerebral parenchyma and subsequent widening of the CSF-containing spaces (ventricles, sulci, and cisterns) is a normal effect of aging. There is, however, a large overlap with neurodegenerative diseases such as Alzheimer's disease, frontotemporal dementia, or dementia with Lewy bodies. Prominent sulci are also seen in young children up to the age of 1 year. The interhemispheric distance can be as wide as 6 mm in normal neonates.

Widening of the ventricles in elderly patients can be due to atrophy, reflecting central volume loss of the brain; this is known as ventriculomegaly (we try to avoid the older term "hydrocephalus ex vacuo"). However, ventricular enlargement due to central atrophy may be impossible to differentiate from certain types of hydrocephalus, such as normal pressure hydrocephalus.

2.10.3 Age-Related Changes in Brain Iron

Iron metabolism in the brain is independent of the iron metabolism and storage in the rest of the body. It is an

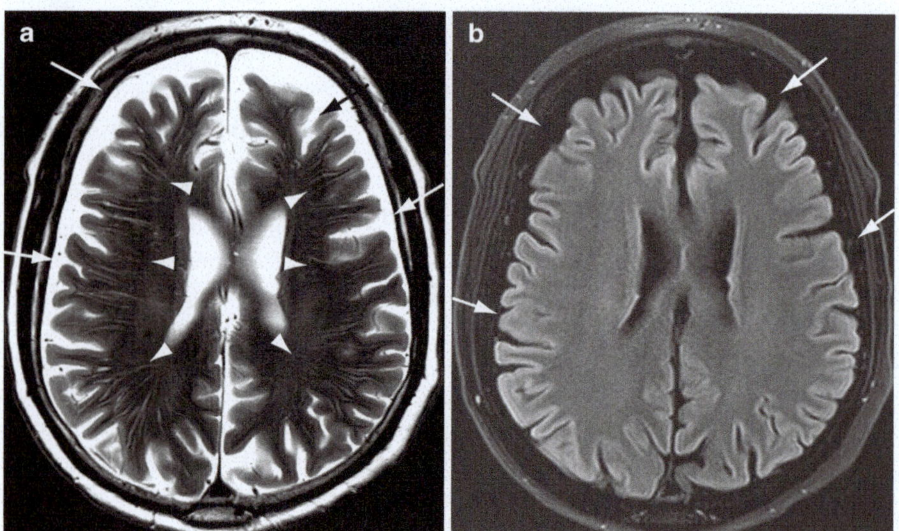

Fig. 2.70 Perivascular Virchow-Robin spaces. (**a**) Axial TSE T2-WI. (**b**) Axial fat-sat turbo FLAIR. The T2-WI (**a**) shows prominent perivascular Virchow-Robin (VRS) spaces throughout the white matter of a 65-year-old man with diffuse atrophy (*arrows*) and widening of the extracerebral CSF spaces. The VRS, which contain interstitial fluid, are seen as linear hyperintensities. On the FLAIR image, the VRS spaces are not visible, because the fluid signal is suppressed (*arrowheads*)

essential element for the maturation and function of the brain. Iron depositions can be detected on MRI because of the susceptibility effect. On T2*-W scans, or susceptibility-weighted imaging (SWI), foci of iron deposition are seen as hypointense areas. In the first year of life, iron deposition becomes visible in the basal ganglia, substantia nigra red nucleus. In childhood, the dentate nucleus also becomes hypointense on T2-WI and T2*-WI. The iron content of the basal ganglia increases with age; the globus pallidus becomes hypointense on T2-WI in the middle-aged and elderly population, and the putamen is hypointense only in the elderly population.

2.10.4 MRI in Abnormal Aging and Dementia

The boundary between "normal" and "abnormal" aging is not clearly defined. In patients with clinical signs and symptoms of dementia, MRI is useful, though imaging findings are often nonspecific and there is considerable overlap with physiologic changes of the brain of the aging patient.

Alzheimer's disease is the most common of all dementing disorders in the elderly. It is a disease of gray matter, with loss of cells from the cerebral cortex. On MRI, the brain presents a "cracked walnut" appearance, with symmetrical enlargement of the sulci in the high-convexity regions. Focal atrophy is most obvious in the medial temporal lobes, with volume loss of the hippocampus and parahippocampal gyrus. Frequently, a smooth periventricular halo of T2-hyperintensity is also present.

Other types of dementia include frontotemporal lobar degeneration, dementia with Lewy bodies, Vascular dementia, Creutzfeld-Jacob disease or variant Creutzfeld-Jacob disease, and HIV-related dementia.

As a general rule, in patients with dementia, MRI is preferred over CT. Common imaging findings include atrophy of the medial temporal lobes and white matter damage. The imaging protocol to evaluate patients with dementia should include a FLAIR sequence, because of its high sensitivity to periventricular and DWMH, and its ability to differentiate lacunes (hypontense) from areas of demyelination or gliosis (hyperintense). As an alternative, a long TR dual-echo TSE (providing proton-density and T2-WI) sequence can be employed; this sequence is not as good as FLAIR to characterize ischemic lesions, but has the advantage of a higher sensitivity for posterior fossa lesions. The MRI protocol should also include at least one sequence to detect intracerebral deposits of iron, calcium, and hemosiderin. This can be achieved either with a gradient echo T2*-W sequence or with a susceptibility-weighted sequence (SWI). It is important to look for "microbleeds" (punctate hemosiderin deposits), which have a much higher prevalence in subjects with dementia than those without dementia (Fig. 2.46). Microbleeds occur in patients with amyloid angiopathy, and it has been shown that SWI is more sensitive than gradient echo T2*-imaging in the detection of these small hemosiderin deposits. Finally, it is recommended that the imaging protocol for patients with dementia should also include a 3D volumetric sequence, e.g., a 3D MP-RAGE.

2.11 Craniocerebral Trauma

Traumatic injury of the brain and spinal cord is a leading cause of death and permanent disability. Clinical management of patients with craniocerebral trauma requires an assessment of the degree of patient risk according to the symptoms of intracranial injury. However, the severity of brain injury cannot be evaluated exclusively by the extent of impairment as determined by clinical examination. Modern imaging techniques play an important role in the management of the patient with craniocerebral trauma, and should be used to detect anatomic and physiologic abnormalities.

Multidetector computed tomography (MDCT) is the initial imaging modality of choice in severe acute craniocerebral trauma. MDCT is used for the detection of intracranial hemorrhage, mass effect and edema (including brain herniation), skull fractures, displaced bone fragments, foreign bodies, intracranial air, etc. New generation MDCT scanners (with 64, 128 or more detector rows) provide isotropic data sets, which can be used for high-resolution three-dimensional postprocessing, to show fractures of the skull vault, maxillofacial region, and even the petrous bones and skull base.

2.11.1 MRI in Acute and Subacute Trauma

MRI is generally not the preferred technique in acute trauma. There are significant logistic difficulties in installing a traumatized patient in the MR unit. Appropriate MRI-compatible monitoring and life-support equipment should be available. All staff involved in the procedure should be aware of the dangers and necessary precautions for working near an MRI scanner. MRI is contraindicated if there is any suspicion that the patient might harbor an intracranial or intraorbital metallic foreign object, implant or incompatible device (e.g., penetrating injury, bullet fragment, shrapnel, stainless steel aneurysm clip, etc.). MRI is relatively insensitive for the detection of skull fractures and small bone fragments. Long acquisition times cause problems with regard to patient motion. The availability of the MR scanner on a stand-by basis may be problematic and interferes with normal patient flow. For all of these reasons, in most hospitals, MDCT scanning remains the preferred technique in acute trauma patients.

However, thanks to recent technological developments, the role of MRI is growing in the assessment of acute and subacute craniocerebral injury. MRI provides superior contrast resolution and has the highest sensitivity for parenchymal lesion detection. MRI has the potential to reveal nonhemorrhagic (and hemorrhagic) white-matter shearing injuries, even in patients with normal CT examinations.

Phased-array head coils, in combination with PAT such as SENSE and GRAPPA have significantly shortened MRI scan times. This has led to decreased motion artifacts and improved image quality, even in poorly cooperative head-injured patients. In the acute stage, FLAIR sequences are used for the detection of diffuse axonal injury (DAI), edema, and hemorrhage. Moreover, FLAIR has a high sensitivity for the detection of intracranial hemorrhage, including subarachnoid and intraventricular hemorrhage. Gradient echo T2* and SWI sequences are valuable for detection of intracranial hemorrhage and blood degradation products. DWI has been shown to be useful in the evaluation of craniocerebral trauma, and especially DAI (Fig. 2.71). Decreased ADC values can be demonstrated in patients with DAI in the acute setting and may persist into the subacute period (up to 18 days after the initial event), beyond that described for cytotoxic edema in ischemia. DWI is able to identify traumatic shearing injuries which are not visible on routine pulse sequences. Moreover, DWI can show hypoxic-ischemic brain damage, for example in cases of nonaccidental head injury (e.g., shaken baby syndrome) or vascular damage (e.g., carotid or vertebral artery dissection).

As a general rule, MRI is indicated in stable patients in whom there is a discrepancy between clinical symptoms and CT findings. Patients with DAI and nonaccidental head trauma (child abuse) should be examined with MRI. There is growing evidence that DWI serves as a valuable biomarker for the severity of tissue injury and as a predictor for outcome.

2.11.2 MRI in Chronic Trauma

MRI is of great use in the evaluation of trauma patients in the chronic phase, due to its superior contrast resolution. MRI is superior to CT for the detection of chronic subdural hematomas, which are often isodense to CSF on noncontrast CT scans, but can be seen on MRI, because they contain blood degradation products (methemoglobin) and high concentrations of protein. Fat-saturated FLAIR sequences are superior to T2-WI in the detection of small subdural hematomas (Fig. 2.72). When a subdural hematoma contains blood of varying ages, due to repeated episodes of bleeding, MRI may show layers of different SI, reflecting varying phases of the blood-breakdown process.

FLAIR sequences are used mainly for the detection of gliosis and cystic encephalomalacia. Gradient echo T2* or SWI sequences allow visualization of hypointense hemosiderin deposits after DAI. These punctate hemosiderin deposits are the result of shearing injuries due to rotational acceleration and deceleration forces, commonly encountered in motor vehicle accidents and blunt trauma to the head. DAI lesions occur in the cerebral hemispheres (subcortical brain parenchyma, gray–white matter junction, centrum semiovale), corpus callosum, basal ganglia, brainstem, and cerebellum. In every patient with a history of previous head trauma, a T2* or SWI sequence, which is highly sensitive to blood-breakdown products such as hemosiderin and ferritin, should be routinely added to the MRI scanning protocol. DAI lesions are seen as punctate hypointense foci; multiple lesions are frequent.

Posttraumatic encephalomalacia is much better appreciated with MRI than with CT, because of the absence of bone artifacts and the multiplanar imaging capabilities of MR. Foci of encephalomalacia often result from cortical contusions and should be looked

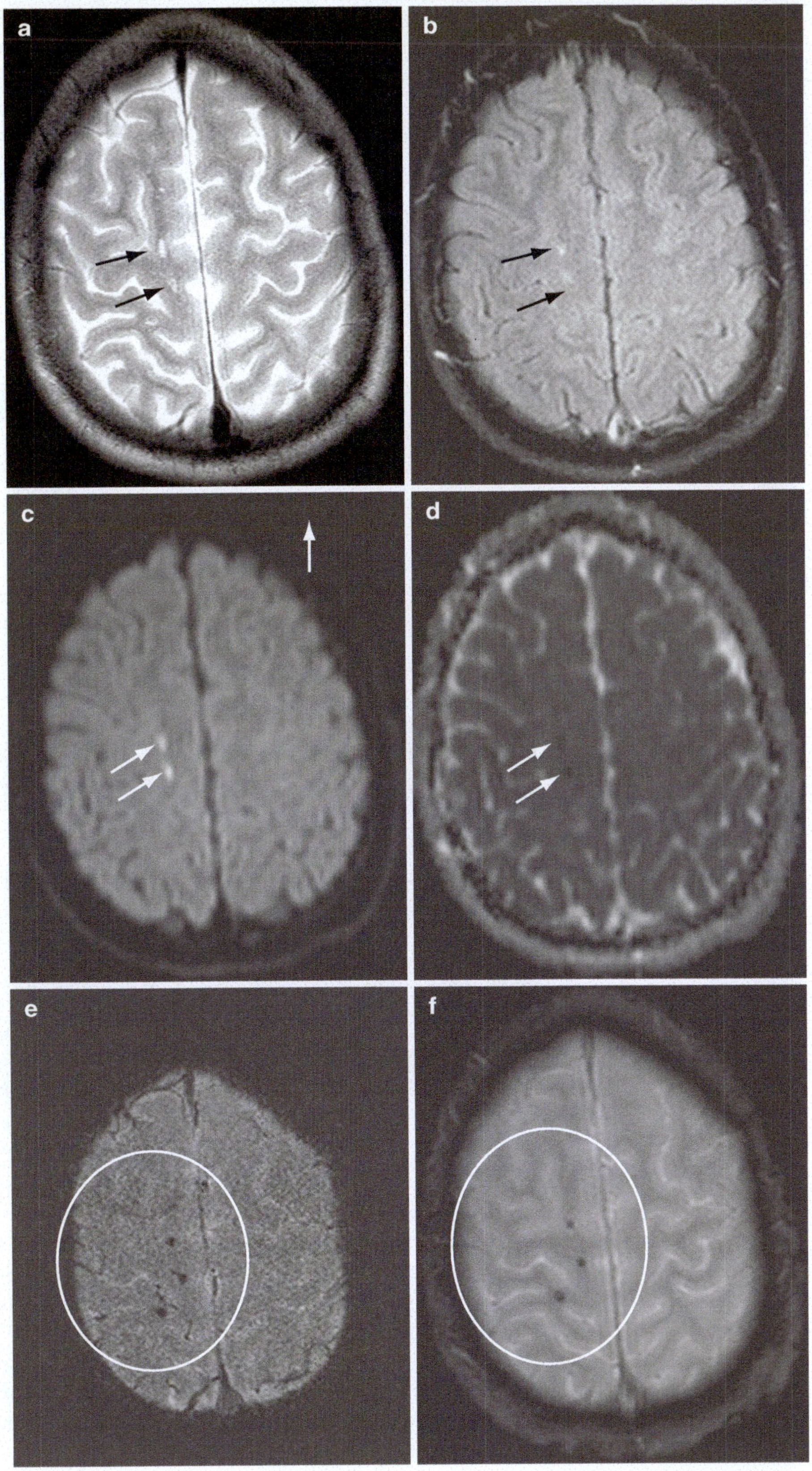

Fig. 2.71 Diffuse axonal injury (DAI). (**a**) Axial TSE T2-WI. (**b**) Axial fat-sat turbo FLAIR. (**c**) Axial EPI diffusion-weighted "trace" image. (**d**) Apparent diffusion coefficient (ADC) map (*arrows*). (**e**) Axial susceptibility-weighted image (SWI). Axial and coronal gradient echo FLASH T2*-WI.
This 17-year-old boy suffered a high-velocity deceleration trauma when his motorcycle struck a parked truck at high-speed. Upon admission, GCS was 9/15. Noncontrast CT scan of the brain was unremarkable. Because of the discrepancy between the patient's clinical status and the normal CT findings, MRI of the brain was performed on the same day. Diffuse axonal injuries (DAI) are scattered throughout both cerebral hemispheres, mainly involving the hemispheric gray-white matter interfaces, centrum semiovale, and corpus callosum.
The DAI lesions are hyperintense on T2 (**a**) and FLAIR (**b**). They exhibit diffusion restriction (**c**) with lowered ADC values (**d**). On axial SWI (**e**) and axial (**f**) and coronal (**g**, **h**) gradient echo T2* images, multiple, punctate, hypointense lesions (*circles*) are seen in the centrum semiovale, at the corticomedullary junctions, and in the subcortical white matter (corresponding to areas of shearing stress). The pattern of distribution and signal intensity behavior is typical for DAI with petechial hemorrhages

(*continued*)

Fig. 2.71 (continued)

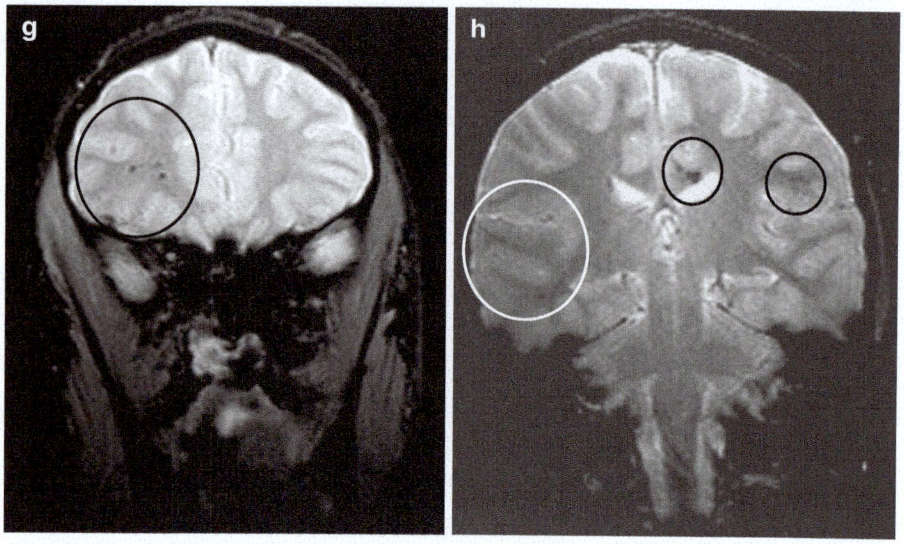

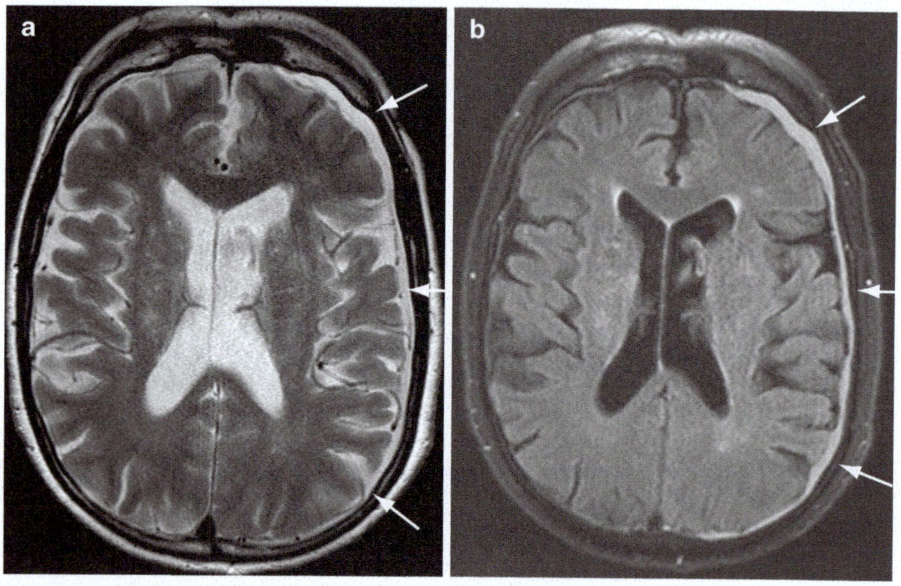

Fig. 2.72 Chronic subdural hematoma (*arrows*). (**a**) Axial TSE T2-WI. (**b**) Axial fat-saturated FLAIR. There is a thin subdural hematoma overlying the left cerebral hemisphere (missed on a noncontrast CT scan performed 2 days earlier). The hyperintense subdural hematoma is much better seen on the FLAIR image, due to the suppression of fluid and fat

for in the basal, frontal, and anterior temporal lobes. These regions are vulnerable to deceleration injury. They are seen as areas of tissue loss, which are hyperintense on T2-WI. On PD or FLAIR images, the area of tissue loss is isointense to CSF and is surrounded by a hyperintense rim of gliosis.

Diffusion tensor imaging (DTI) with fractional anisotropy (FA) maps is used to evaluate white-matter tracts, by measuring the degree and spatial distribution of anisotropic diffusion within the brain. FA maps and DTI reveal changes in the white matter that are correlated with both acute Glasgow Coma Scale and Rankin scores at discharge. Because FA and DTI changes are present at both early and late time points following injury, they are valuable biomarkers and could be used as an early indicator for the severity of tissue injury and as a prognostic measure of subsequent brain damage.

2.12 Seizures

The primary goal of MRI in the evaluation of epilepsy is to identify and localize the neuropathologic substrate of a partial onset seizure. The diagnosis and localization of the lesion determines the therapeutic possibilities. Many different abnormalities can cause epilepsy (Table 2.22). Most of these abnormalities are dealt with in other sections; in this section, we will discuss mesial temporal sclerosis (MTS) and a general imaging strategy for epilepsy.

Table 2.22 Causes of partial-onset epileptic seizures

Tumors	Astrocytoma Oligodendrogioma Ganglioma DNET Metastasis
Migration disorders	Tuberous sclerosis Focal cortical dysplasia Schizencephaly Nodular heterotopia Laminar heterotopia Lissencephaly Hemimegaloencephaly
Vascular malformations	Cavernous angioma AVM Sturge-Weber
Mesial temporal sclerosis	
Brain injury	Ischemia Trauma

2.12.1 Mesial Temporal Sclerosis

MTS is the most common cause of intractable temporal lobe epilepsy. The condition is characterized histopathologically by marked neuronal loss in the hippocampus (with relative sparing of the CA2 subfield), amygdala, parahippocampal gyrus, mesial temporal cortex, and entorhinal cortex. The terms MTS, hippocampal sclerosis, and Ammon's horn sclerosis are used interchangeably, but the extent of the lesion differs for each term.

On T2-WI and FLAIR images, the main MRI findings are increased SI and decreased volume of the hippocampus (Fig. 2.73), compared to the contralateral side. These abnormalities are best seen on coronal slices, preferably orientated perpendicular to the long axis of the temporal lobe. T1-WI shows hippocampal atrophy and dilatation of the temporal horn (Fig. 2.73). FLAIR sequences are more sensitive to the signal changes than (fast) SE sequences. There is no enhancement of the hippocampal sclerosis after contrast-medium administration. In the majority of cases, the abnormality is bilateral but asymmetric, and the most affected side is presumed to be the origin of the seizures.

MTS is frequently associated with abnormalities of the limbic system, including atrophy of the ipsilateral fornix and ipsilateral mammillary body. Patients with MTS may show hyperintensity of the cerebral cortex in the anterior temporal lobe; rarely cerebral hemiatrophy is found.

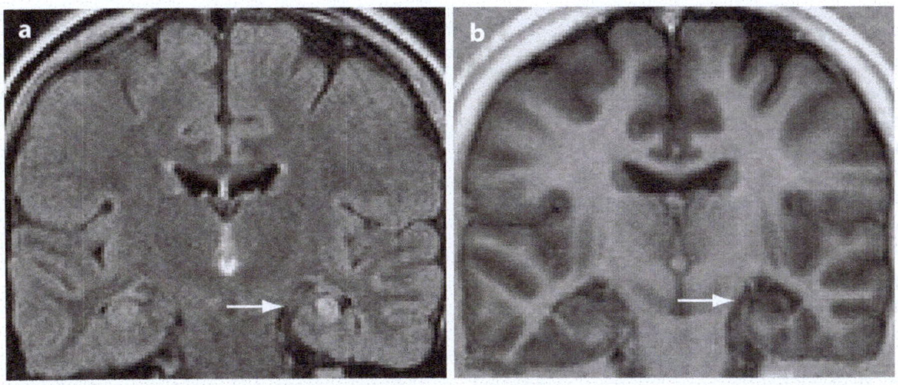

Fig. 2.73 Mesial temporal sclerosis (*arrows*). (**a**) Coronal FLAIR T2-WI through the hippocampus. (**b**) Coronal IR-T1-WI (same slice position). On the FLAIR T2-W sequence, there is an area of abnormally increased signal intensity in the left hippocampus. IR T1-WI shows focal tissue loss with widening of the left temporal horn. T1-WI shows hippocampal atrophy and dilatation of the temporal horn. T2-WI shows an increased signal intensity of the hippocampus

2.12.2 MRI Strategy for Epilepsy

Imaging protocols for the diagnosis of hippocampal sclerosis vary widely from center to center. An imaging protocol for epilepsy should be guided by the location of the epileptogenic focus as provided by the clinical presentation and the electroencephalogram (EEG). For general screening, one can substitute axial turbo FLAIR and TSE T2-W sequences for the traditional double-echo long TR sequence. The imaging protocol should include most cerebral pathologies associated with seizures, including cortical development disorders. Therefore, a coronal T1-W sequence with thin slices should be added, e.g., an MP-RAGE sequence. Cortical alterations, e.g., migration disorders, can be detected on this high-resolution scan, and side-to-side comparison of the hippocampus can be made. A coronal turbo-FLAIR sequence will show signal changes in the hippocampus more clearly than the conventional T2-WI. In patients with seizures, it is always wise to include a gradient echo T2*-sequence or a susceptibility-weighted imaging (SWI) sequence to detect old hemorrhagic foci or cavernous malformations. Finally, the imaging protocol must be adapted to the equipment that is available (field strength, gradient performance, available sequences, etc.).

Further Reading

Armed Forces Institute of Pathology (1994) Tumors of the central nervous system. Armed Forces Institute of Pathology, Washington DC

Atlas SW (1996) Magnetic resonance imaging of the brain and spine. Lippincott-Raven, Philadelphia

Atlas SW (2002) Magnetic resonance imaging of the brain and spine, 3rd edn. Lippincott Williams & Wilkins, Philadelphia

Barkovich JA (2000) Pediatric neuroimaging, 3rd edn. Lippincott Williams & Wilkins, Philadelphia

Barkovich JA (2005) Pediatric neuroimaging, 4th edn. Lippincott Williams & Wilkins, Philadelphia

Byrd SE, Darling CF, Wilczynski MA (1993) White matter of the brain: maturation and myelination magnetic resonance in infants and children. Neuroimaging Clin North Am 3: 247–266

Castillo M (1997) Prethrombolysis brain imaging: trends and controversies. AJNR Am J Neuroradiol 18:1830–1833

Castillo M (guest ed) (1998) New techniques in MR neuroimaging. Magnetic resonance imaging clinics of North America 1998, vol 6. Saunders, Philadelphia

Castillo M (1998) New techniques in MR neuroimaging. In: Magnetic resonance imaging clinics of North America, vol 6. Saunders, Philadelphia

Fazekas F, Ropele S, Enzinger C, Gorani F, Seewann A, Petrovic K, Schmidt R (2005) MTI of white matter hyperintensities. Brain 128:2926–2932

Finelli DA, Hurst GC, Gullapalli RP (1998) T1-W three dimensional magnetisation transfer MR of the brain: improved lesion contrast enhancement. AJNR Am J Neuroradiol 19: 59–64

Forsting M, Wanke I (2008) Intracranial vascular malformations and aneurysms, from diagnostic work-up to endovascular therapy (2nd revised edition). Springer, New York

Gillard JH, Waldman AD, Barker PB (2005) Clinical MR neuroimaging. Cambridge University Press, New York

Gilman S (1998) Imaging the brain (first of two parts). N Engl J Med 338:812–820

Gilman S (1998) Imaging the brain (second of two parts). N Engl J Med 338:889–896

Hergan K, Schaefer PW, Sorensen AG, Gonzalez RG, Huisman TA (2002) Diffusion-weighted MRI in diffuse axonal injury of the brain. Eur Radiol 12:2536–2541

Hartmann M, Jansen O, Heiland S, Sommer C, Münkel K, Sartor K (2001) Restricted diffusion within ring enhancement is not pathognomonic for brain abscess. AJNR Am J Neuroradiol 22:1738–1742

Hoang TA, Hasso AN (1994) Intracranial vascular malformations. Neuroimaging Clin North Am 4:823–847

Jack CR (1995) Magnetic resonance imaging: neuroimaging and anatomy. Neuroimaging Clin North Am 5:597–622

Lacerda S, Law M (2009) Magnetic resonance perfusion and permeability imaging in brain tumors. Neuroimaging Clin N Am 19:527–557

Law M (2009) Advanced imaging techniques in brain tumors. Cancer Imaging 9(special issue A):S4–S9

Law M, Young RJ, Babb JS, Peccerelli N, Chheang S, Gruber ML, Miller DC, Golfinos JG, Zagzag D, Johnson G (2008) Gliomas: predicting time to progression or survival with cerebral blood volume measurements at dynamic susceptibility-weighted contrast-enhanced perfusion MR imaging. Radiology 247:490–498

Lee SH, Rao KCVG, Zimmerman RA (1992) Cranial MRI and CT, 3rd edn. McGraw-Hill, New York

Lee SH, Rao KCVG, Zimmerman RA (2004) Cranial MRI and CT, 4th edn. McGraw-Hil, New York

Louis DN, Ohgaki H, Wiestler OD, Cavenee WK (eds) (2007) WHO classification of tumours of the central nervous system. IARC, Lyon

Louis DN, Ohgaki H, Wiestler OD et al (2007) The 2007 WHO classification of tumours of the central nervous system. Acta Neuropathol 114:97–109

Lufkin RB (1998) The MRI manual, 2nd edn. Mosby-Year Book, St Louis

McDonald WI, Compston A, Edan G et al (2001) Recommended diagnostic criteria for multiple sclerosis: guidelines from the International Panel on the diagnosis of multiple sclerosis. Ann Neurol 50:121–127

Osborn AG (1994) Diagnostic neuroradiology. Mosby-Year Book, St Louis

Osborn AG (2004) Diagnostic imaging – brain. Amirsys, Salt Lake City

Parizel PM, Van Goethem JW, Özsarlak Ö, Maes M, Philips CD (2005) New developments in the neuroradiological diagnosis of craniocerebral trauma. Eur Radiol 15:569–581

Pierallini A, Caramia F, Falcone C, Tinelli E, Paonessa A, Ciddio AB, Fiorelli M, Bianco F, Natalizi S, Ferrante L, Bozzao L (2006) Pituitary macroadenomas: preoperative evaluation of consistency with diffusion-weighted MR imaging – initial experience. Radiology 239:223–231

Polman CH, Reingold SC, Edan G (2005) Diagnostic criteria for multiple sclerosis: 2005 revisions to the "McDonald Criteria". Ann Neurol 58:840–846

Provenzale JM, Mukundan S, Barboriak DP (2006) Diffusion-weighted and perfusion MR imaging for brain tumor characterization and assessment of treatment response. Radiology 239:632–649

Sahraian MA, Radue E-W (2007) MRI atlas of MS lesions. Springer, Berlin

Simon JH, Li D, Traboulsee A, Coyle PK, Arnold DL, Barkhof F, Frank JA, Grossman R, Paty DW, Radue EW, Wolinsky JS (2006) Standardized MR imaging protocol for multiple sclerosis: Consortium of MS Centers consensus guidelines. AJNR Am J Neuroradiol 27:455–461

Sorensen AG, Reimer P (2000) Cerebral MR perfusion imaging: principles and current applications. Thieme, Stuttgart

van der Knaap MS, Valk J (1995) Magnetic resonance of myelin; myelination and myelin disorders. Springer, Berlin

van der Knaap MS, Valk J (2005) Magnetic resonance of myelin; myelination and myelin disorders, 3rd edn. Springer, Berlin

Magnetic Resonance Imaging of the Spine

3

Johan W. M. Van Goethem

Contents

J. W. M. Van Goethem
Department of Radiology, Universitair Ziekenhuis Antwerpen, Wilrijkstraat 10, 2650 Edegem, Belgium
e-mail: johan.vangoethem@ua.ac.be

3.1 Patient Positioning and Coils

3.1.1 Positioning of the Patient

Depending on the type and manufacturer of your magnet, and the type of examination you are going to perform, patients can be positioned either head first or feet first. The main advantage of positioning patients feet first is the diminution of claustrophobic feelings. Many magnet systems, however, obligate you to position patients for cervical spine (CS) examinations head first the fixed location of the head and/or the CS coil. If you have the choice, patients, especially anxious ones and children, should be positioned feet first whenever possible. We use a knee support for patient comfort in examinations of the cervical and thoracic spine; this, in turn, is favorable for the image quality as patients are less likely to move during the examination. In lumbar spine examinations, however, a lumbar support diminishes lumbar lordosis, and therefore, may diminish the amount of disc protrusion. Only when patients are unable to remain motionless without the support of the legs, e.g., patients with substantial back pain, should a knee support be used in lumbar spine examinations. In any case, the patient should be positioned as comfortably as possible to minimize movement artifacts. On high field magnets and/or magnets with strong gradients, earplugs or a headphone should be provided to the patient.

3.1.2 Coils

In general, two types of coils are used in spine imaging: linearly polarized and circularly polarized (CP) coils. CP coils are constructed to generate more signal and,

P. Reimer et al. (eds.), *Clinical MR Imaging*,
DOI: 10.1007/978-3-540-74504-4_3, © Springer-Verlag Berlin Heidelberg 2010

hence, provide images with a higher signal-to-noise ratio (SNR). Therefore, CP coils are preferred and are standard today.

Although all coils are designed to receive the signal generated by the patient during imaging, only certain coils are also used to transmit the radiofrequency (RF) pulses used in magnetic resonance imaging (MRI). These so-called send-receive coils tend to produce better images, as the RF transmission is performed closer to the region of interest.

Usually, one type of coil is used for imaging the thoracic and lumbar spine. It consists of a flat box incorporated in a lumbar (or thoracic) support or directly into the patient's table. Depending on the type of coil and the manufacturer, these coils generate a maximum field of view (FoV) of 25–40 cm.

A CS coil is usually more raised so that it provides better support for the patient's neck. In general, it is made of a lower and an upper part, the latter being fixed in position after the patient is placed on the lower part. The maximum FoV of these coils usually covers the craniocervical junction, the CS, and the cervicothoracic junction. Depending on the coil design and the patient's stature, imaging down from the first to the sixth thoracic vertebra may be possible. Some manufacturers also provide circular solenoid coils, which can be placed around the neck. These coils tend to generate a smaller FoV. Flexible coils can be used in patients who cannot be positioned in the normal cervical coil, e.g., patients with large neck collars or extreme thoracic kyphosis.

If the magnet is equipped with phased-array spine coils, they should be used as they make coil selection and patient positioning in relation to the coil less critical. The use of several phased-array coils simultaneously allows for a larger FoV. Moreover, parallel acquisition technique (PAT) and sensitivity encoding (SENSE) permit a considerable reduction in acquisition time and/or better SNR using phased-array coils in spine imaging with a large FoV. If phased-array spine coils are not available and a very large section of the spine, or even the entire spine, needs to be imaged, the built-in body coil should be used. Depending on the homogeneity of the magnetic field outside the magnet center and the length of the gradient coils, 45–50 cm of the spine may be visualized (which is the complete spine in children or small individuals). Indications for imaging the entire spine without the use of phased-array coils should be carefully monitored. If the body coil is used, image quality and, in particular, contrast and spatial resolution are not up to par with images generated with local coils. Therefore, subtle lesions may be missed, e.g., smaller disc herniations or intramedullary lesions as in multiple sclerosis (MS). It is, therefore, preferable to perform separate examinations of the cervical, thoracic, and/or lumbosacral segments of the spine in such cases.

3.1.3 Positioning of the Coil in Relation to the Patient

When imaging the thoracic spine, it can be useful to attach one or more markers on the skin of the patient's back prior to starting the examination. These markers simplify the problem of determining the examined levels afterward, especially in a system in which it is not possible to obtain large FoV (50 cm) localizer images with the body coil when the surface coil is already in place. The use of a console-operated table movement, if available, also simplifies this problem.

When positioning patients in the cervical coil, one must try to place the coil relatively low down so that cervicothoracic junction is included in the images. To minimize movement, a cervical collar can be used for cervical magnetic resonance (MR) examinations. In patients with a very pronounced thoracic kyphosis and/or stiff CS, normal positioning in the cervical coil may be impossible. Some coils allow imaging without the upper part attached, but one still has to ensure that the distance between the coil and the neck is not too large. It sometimes helps when cushions are placed under the patient's buttocks and/or legs. In extreme cases, it may be necessary to allow the patient to lay his or her head on a pillow. In these cases, one can use a flexible or collar-like coil or, if this is not available, the body coil. This may also be the case in patients with dyspnea, who are unable to lie completely flat.

For MRI of the lumbar spine without phased-array coils, the center of the coil should be positioned about 5 cm above the iliac crest (which is usually at the L4-L5 level). The conus medullaris and the sacrum should be included in the FoV. For all examinations, one should try to match the center of the region of interest to the center of the bore of the magnet. In some magnets, this is done automatically.

3.1.4 Patient Information

Patients should be cleared for any MRI contraindications before they enter the magnet room. They should also be informed of the benefits and potential risks of MRI before the examination is performed. In particular, before administering intravenous contrast products, informed consent (written or oral) should be obtained.

The scenario and length of the examination should be explained in understandable terms. It is helpful to keep the patient informed during the examination about the length of each sequence. This way, swallowing and movement can be minimized as patients will have a better idea about the time they must keep still.

As with all MR examinations, the patient should be instructed to lie as motionless as possible. Excessive thoracic or abdominal breathing movements should be avoided when imaging that region. In imaging the CS, the patient must be cautioned against swallowing or instructed to at least minimize swallowing during the measurements. Since this is very hard for some patients, it may be useful to leave enough time between measurements (more than 15 s) to allow the patient to swallow or cough.

When examining children, we allow a parent(s) to be present in the magnet room. With young children (<6 years), parents are sometimes placed together with their child inside the magnet, lying in prone position, head to head with the child. With anxious patients, it can be helpful to leave a member of the nursing staff inside the magnet room to calm the patient down when necessary. Anxiolytic medication can be beneficial in claustrophobic patients.

MRI in patients with metallic or electronic implants is discussed further below (see Sect. 3.2.3.2 The Postoperative Lumbar Spine).

3.2 Sequence Protocol

3.2.1 General Guidelines

In general, both sagittal and axial images are obtained in spine imaging.

T1- and T2-weighted images (WI) offer different and complementary information.

On T2-WI, normal intervertebral discs are bright. With aging, water loss occurs, the T2 relaxation time shortens, and the discs gradually become darker (degenerative disc disease or "black disc disease"). However, with longer echo train length (ETL) (more echoes sampled after each 90° pulse), normal discs also become darker due to certain physical effects (Fig. 3.1). Therefore, in order to diagnose degenerative disc disease, sagittal T2-WIs with

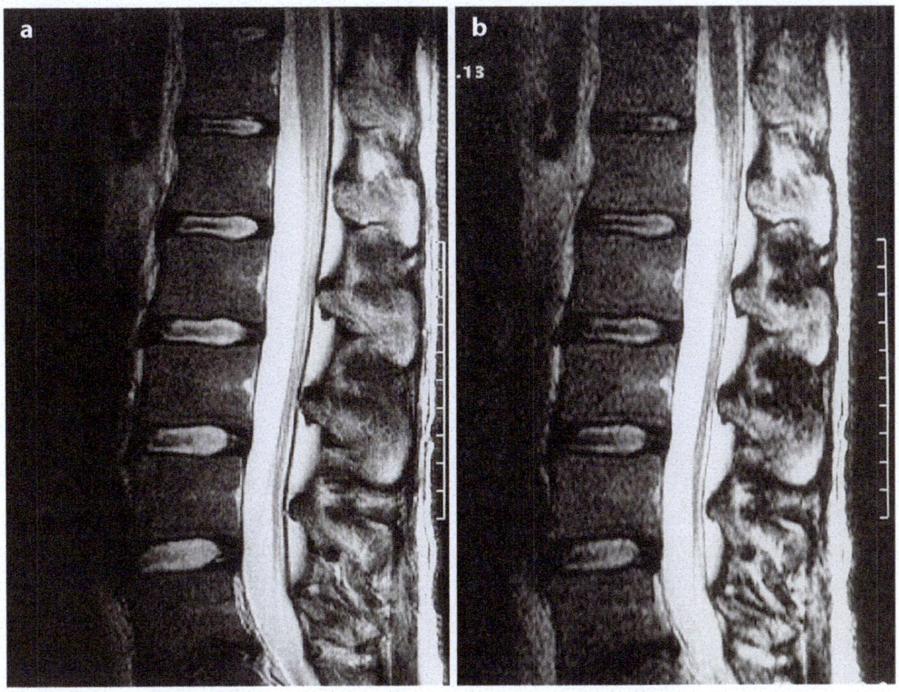

Fig. 3.1 Normal and ultrafast T2-weighted images from the same volunteer. (**a**) The routine turbo spin-echo sequence. (**b**) The ultrafast sequence (see Tables 3.1 and 3.2 for the complete sequence parameters). Notice the excellent spatial resolution of both images (both obtained with a 512 matrix). The ultrafast sequence is noisier and darker in most areas except cerebrospinal fluid, due to lengthening of the echo train. This may cause problems in accurately diagnosing degenerative disc disease

Table 3.1 Overview of some commonly used MRI sequences for the *lumbar* spine

T1	• typically TSE 2D sequence, can be replaced by T1 FLAIR on 3.0T imagers (superior contrast) • sagittal and axial for evaluation of the anatomy, especially foraminal stenosis • evaluation of endplate changes (Modic changes) • no fat saturation
T2	• typically TSE 2D sequence • *sagittal*, especially for evaluation of the discs, including degenerative changes, tears and disc herniation, but also medullary lesions • *axial*, especially for (1) evaluation of the location and extent of disc herniation and its relation to the dural sac and nerve roots, (2) evaluation of spinal stenosis and (3) evaluation of degenerative facet joint disease
T2 fatsat	• indicated in all patients • typically sagittal, STIR because of superior fat suppression but can be replaced by TSE T2 fatsat • evaluation of 'inflammatory' changes in endplates, soft tissue and especially facet joints • evaluation of endplate changes (Modic changes)
T1 +/– Gd	• axial, to be done in majority of post-herniectomy patients to distinguish fibrosis for recurrent herniation • no need for fat saturation • infectious or tumoral pathology
MR-myelogram	• can be either T2 TSE 3D sequence with postprocessing or multiple singleshot sequences, typically HASTE • mainly to evaluate spinal stenosis
Diffusion	• no routine use

Table 3.2 Overview of some commonly used MRI sequences for the *cervical* spine

T1	• typically TSE 2D sequence, can be replaced by T1 FLAIR on 3.0T imagers (superior contrast) • sagittal for evaluation of the anatomy • no fat saturation
T2 - sagittal	• typically TSE 2D sequence • especially for evaluation of the discs, including degenerative changes, tears and disc herniation, but also medullary lesions
T2 - axial	• typically GRE 2D sequence but should be replaced by TSE 2D sequence in the patient with metal spinal implants • especially for (1) evaluation of the location and extent of disc herniation and its relation to the spinal cord, (2) evaluation of spinal stenosis, (3) evaluation of degenerative facet joint disease and especially (4) evaluation of foraminal narrowing (due to uncarthrosis and facetarthrosis)
T2 fatsat	• indicated in all patients • typically sagittal, STIR because of superior fat suppression but can be replaced by TSE T2 fatsat • evaluation of 'inflammatory' changes in endplates, soft tissue and facet joints
T1 +/– Gd	• no routine use in the postop patient, only in infectious or tumoral pathology
MR-myelogram	• can be either T2 TSE 3D sequence with postprocessing or multiple singleshot sequences, typically HASTE • mainly to evaluate spinal stenosis
Diffusion	• no routine use

a relatively short ETL are preferable (e.g., 15 or less). Sagittal T2-WIs are also excellent to visualize the spinal cord and cauda equina nerve roots. Finally, spinal canal stenosis and impressions on the thecal sac are most easily recognized on sagittal T2-WI. One should be aware of the fact that turbo spin-echo (TSE) or fast spin-echo (FSE) T2-W sequences are not effective in diagnosing marrow-infiltrating disease, unless fat-suppression techniques are used. Fat-suppression techniques are also very valuable in detecting degenerative changes in and around facet joints and posterior elements in general. We have included a sagittal short T1 inversion recovery (STIR) sequence in our standard imaging algorithm of the cervical, thoracic, and lumbar spine.

Sagittal T1-WIs are more sensitive than conventional nonfat-suppression TSE/FSE T2-WI in detecting bone-marrow disease, e.g., degenerative endplate changes or vertebral metastases, but STIR or other fat-suppression T2-WIs are also able to increase the detection of certain bone-marrow diseases. Also, the difference between osteophytes and disc material (with or without posterior disc protrusion) is usually better appreciated on T1-WI, especially in the CS. This contrast is somewhat less on 3T imaging because of T1-lenghtening effects. Therefore, SE T1-W imaging is sometimes replaced by fluid-attenuated inversion recovery (FLAIR) T1 or gradient echo (GRE) sequence T1 on 3T machines.

The epidural fat tissue in the lumbar (and thoracic) spine is very bright on T1-WI and contrasts well with the dural sac and the intervertebral disc. This is why axial T1-WIs are preferred in the (thoraco-)lumbar region. Since acquisition times are substantially shortened with the newer techniques, we also use axial T2-WIs in our standard imaging protocol of the (thoraco-)lumbar spine. This sequence allows excellent visualization of the nerve roots in relation to other structures, especially the intervertebral disc.

In the CS, there is no epidural fat tissue, but an epidural venous plexus. To optimize contrast between the dural sac and the intervertebral discs, axial T2-WIs are preferred. These images are also useful in detecting medullary disease. On conventional spin-echo (SE) and TSE T2-WI sequences, it is difficult to differentiate osteophytes from disc material. On GRE images, these can usually be differentiated because bone is markedly hypointense whereas disc is hyperintense. Moreover, the shorter echo time (TE) of GRE T2-W sequences in comparison to SE sequences reduces cerebrospinal fluid (CSF)-induced pulsation artifacts.

3.2.2 Localizer Images

After positioning the patient, midsagittal and coronal localizer images (syn. scout images, survey images) are obtained. The type of sequences used for this purpose is of little importance and depends on the manufacturer of the system. The FoV of the localizers should be larger than the FoV of the images desired. The same coil (surface or body) as the one to be used during the actual examination should be used. The coronal localizers are positioned so that they intersect the spine.

When imaging the thoracic spine, extra-large FoV sagittal localizers using the body coil (or phased-array coils) are useful to determine the exact levels to be imaged. Sagittal sequences are positioned parallel to the spine on coronal localizers. Axial images are positioned on sagittal localizers, perpendicular to the spinal canal, rather than parallel to the intervertebral disc space.

3.2.3 Specific Types of Sequences

The sequences used in MRI of the spine depend on the kind of pathology (expected to be) found.

3.2.3.1 Degenerative Disc Disease

In imaging patients with degenerative spinal disease, sagittal T1, T2-W SE or TSE and T2-fatsat sequences are used for all spine examinations. In the CS, axial T2-W GRE sequences are added, while in the thoracic and lumbosacral region, axial T1-W and T2-W TSE images are applied. In axial T2-WI of the CS, GRE sequences are preferable over SE sequences since SE sequences, and especially TSE sequences, tend to be severely degraded by CSF-flow artifacts. Also, as mentioned before, GRE sequences are of value in differentiating between disc and bone, e.g., soft disc herniation vs. osteophytic spur formation.

For all axial and sagittal T1-WI, TSE is preferable over SE imaging since the imaging time is considerably shorter, except in imaging on 3T. The slight blurring or loss in spatial resolution is an acceptable penalty to pay for the shorter imaging time (Fig. 3.2). In choosing a TSE T2-W sequence for sagittal imaging, one should experiment with different ETLs. If a long ETL is chosen (>10), the discs become darker, the contrast with the vertebrae decreases, and only the bright CSF stands out. An ETL should be chosen that is long, but with an acceptable remaining signal of the intervertebral discs to be able to differentiate between normal and degenerative discs (Fig. 3.1). Some sagittal T2-W sequences are flow compensated; this means they are specifically designed for imaging the (cervical and thoracic) spine by minimizing flow artifacts caused by the craniocaudal CSF pulsations. If these sequences are available, they should be used (Fig. 3.3).

In the CS, axial images are usually positioned from C2 down to T1. Since the cervical neural foramina are not visible on sagittal images, axial images should be obtained even if no pathology is discernible on the sagittal images. No examination of the CS is complete

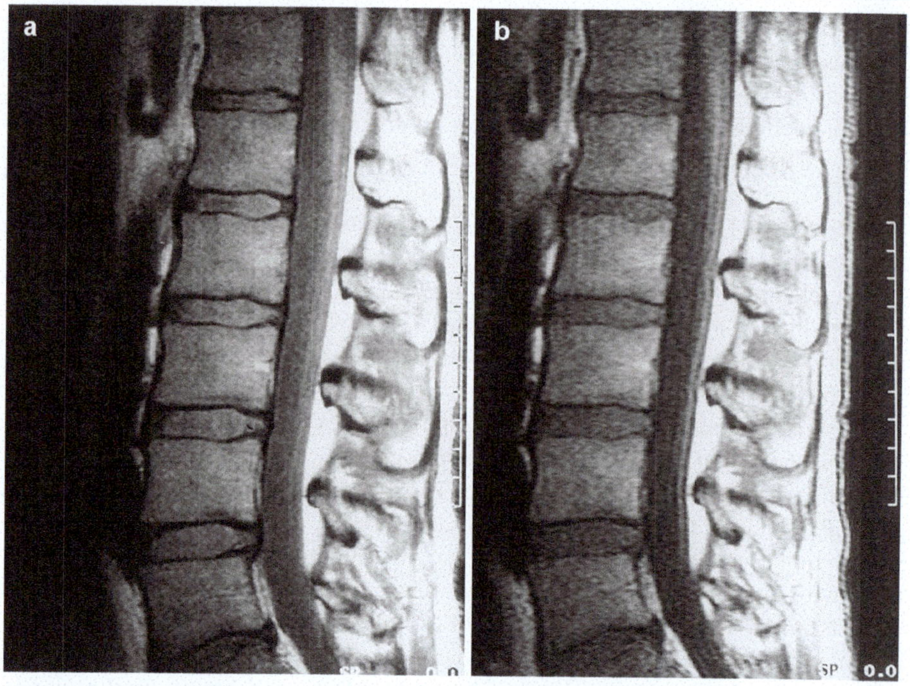

Fig. 3.2 Turbo spin-echo (TSE) and spin-echo (SE) T1-weighted images (WI). Sagittal T1-WI from the same volunteer. (**a**) The routine TSE sequence (see Table 3.1 for the complete sequence parameters). (**b**) The SE sequence (TR 500, TE 15, 256 x 512, TA 4′19″). The SE sequence has a lower resolution in the phase direction (anteroposterior) to partially compensate for the longer acquisition time. Image contrast is very similar, but signal-to-noise ratio is clearly superior in the TSE image. Therefore, there is no reason for using SE T1-W sequences in normal spine imaging

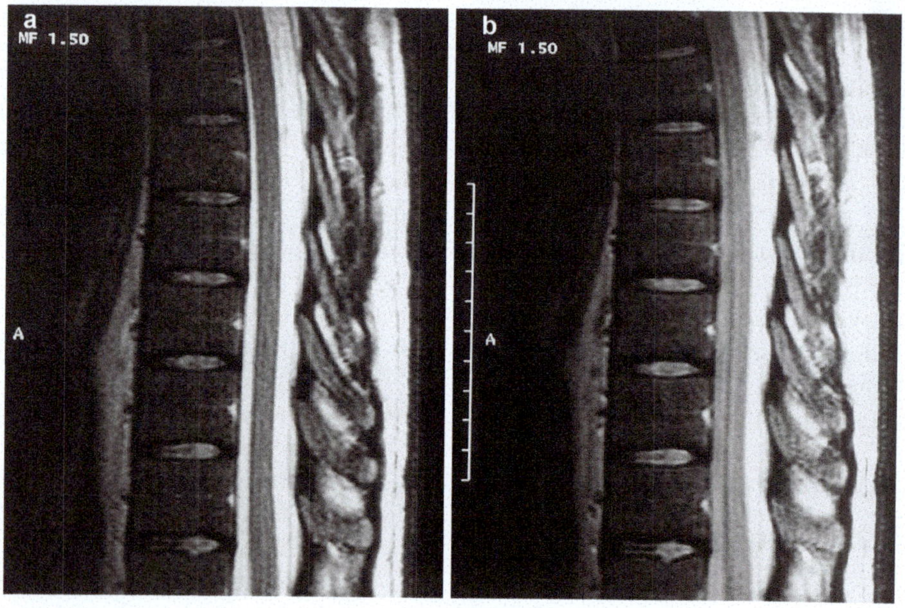

Fig. 3.3 Cerebrospinal fluid (CSF) flow compensation. Sagittal T2-weighted images of the midthoracic spine from the same volunteer. (**a**) The routine TSE sequence for the thoracic spine. (**b**) The sequence without CSF-flow compensation (actually the sequence used in the lumbar spine) (see Table 3.1 for the complete sequence parameters). The latter (**b**) is slightly blurred, especially at the level of the thoracic medulla, due to the noncompensated up and downward movement of the CSF (pulsating CSF in the read direction)

without axial images. In the lumbosacral or thoracic spine, axial images are usually to be obtained only at the level(s) of the (most) affected discs (as seen on the sagittal T2-WI). The thoracolumbar neural foramina are much more accurately displayed on sagittal images than on axial images (Fig. 3.4). Alternatively, 3D T2-W TSE sequences allow image reconstruction in all directions. They are a viable alternative on 3T machines where the imaging time of these sequences is reasonable.

3.2.3.2 Postoperative Lumbar Spine

Additional axial SE T1-WI after intravenous gadolinium injection should be obtained in patients after lumbar disc surgery. The postcontrast images should be obtained as quickly as possible after gadolinium injection (sequence completed within 5–8 min after injection). The most important use of gadolinium is in differentiating scar tissue from (recurrent or residual)

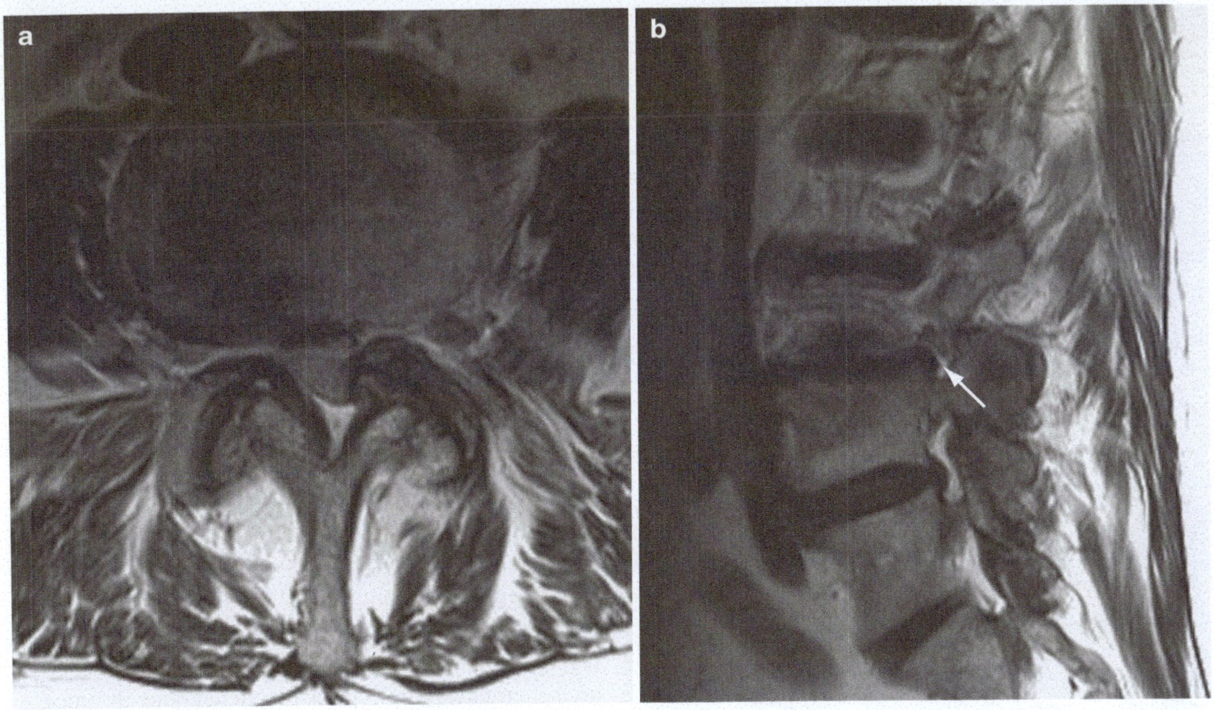

Fig. 3.4 Foraminal stenosis. Foraminal stenosis can be underestimated on axial images. The axial image (**a**) shows severe degenerative facet disease and disc bulging with a spinal stenosis and foraminal narrowing. It is however very hard to evaluate possible foraminal nerve root compression. This is clearly depicted on the sagittal image (**b**) where one can see compression of the L3 nerve root between the bulging disc and the hypertrophic degenerative facet joint (*arrow*)

disc herniation, since the latter is generally accepted to be a possible indication for reintervention. Also, the evaluation of enhancement of nerves, meninges, posterior spinal facet joints (i.e., zygapophyseal joints), and perispinal soft tissues is important in some patients. Some authors also stress the usefulness of (T)SE T2-WI or FLAIR T2-WI in addition to or instead of T1-WI after gadolinium in the differentiation of recurrent disc herniation and epidural fibrosis. If you routinely use FLAIR T1 on a 3T machine, you might consider switching to (T)SE T1 for pre- and postgadolinium imaging since contrast enhancement is less marked on FLAIR T1 imaging sequence.

Fat suppression can be used to differentiate enhancing scar tissue from epidural fatty tissue in i.v. gadolinium-enhanced T1-WI of the postoperative spine. However, the detection of abnormal postoperative nerve root enhancement may be more difficult to differentiate from the normal small amount of enhancement usually seen on fat-suppression images. In some rare cases, fat suppression can be helpful in the differentiation between postoperative blood and normal epidural fat.

Metallic implants used for spinal fusion are not a contraindication for MRI. However, superparamagnetic materials, e.g., some sorts of steel, will create severe susceptibility artifacts (Fig. 3.5). TSE sequences are less susceptible than SE sequences, which in turn are less susceptible than GRE sequences (Fig. 3.5). Also, shortening the TE and increasing the bandwidth of the sequence lessens artifacts. If a particular region is not interpretable due to artifacts, it may be worthwhile trying to swap read- and phase-encoding directions. Nonsuperparamagnetic metals, e.g., tantalum or titanium, only produce RF artifacts, which are smaller in size.

Spinal stimulators and other electronic implant devices in principle constitute an absolute contraindication for MRI. Some types of electronic implants, however, are "MR-compatible." This should be checked with the manufacturer and the surgeon or clinician who implanted the device before the patient is brought into the magnet room. In any case, these devices have to be switched off before the MR examination. Patients have to be carefully instructed to signal during the examination when they have the impression

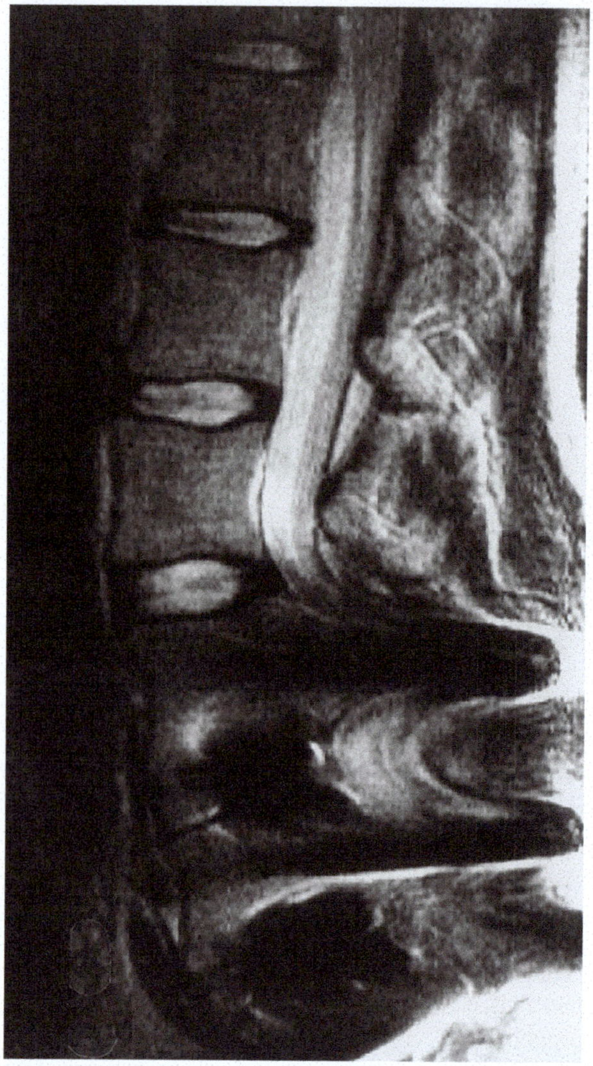

Fig. 3.5 Susceptibility artifacts. Superparamagnetic metal implants (e.g., some sorts of stainless steel) cause severe susceptibility artifacts. Although these spinal orthopedic implants are not a contraindication for MR imaging in general, they almost always exclude imaging of the involved region. Note, however, that the disc spaces above the fusion are not affected

the device is turned on again, or in any case when they sense something unusual.

3.2.3.3 Postoperative Cervical Spine

No additional sequences are necessary since the problem of epidural fibrosis is nonexistent in the CS. As in the lumbar spine, one should be aware of the susceptibility artifacts on GRE sequences that may be caused by metallic implants (Fig. 3.6). In these cases, SE or, better, TSE sequences are preferred.

3.2.3.4 Nontumoral Medullary Lesions

When looking for inflammatory (MS) or infectious medullary lesions, one should perform axial GRE T2-WI (instead of T1-WI) in the thoracic spine. In addition, the routine sagittal T1-W and T2-W sequences are performed. Also, sagittal STIR imaging might be more sensitive for detecting medullary lesions than TSE-sequences. Gadolinium-enhanced images may be useful in suspected inflammatory and infectious lesions, especially in nonviral myelomeningitis.

For suspected ischemic medullary lesions, diffusion-weighted imaging (DWI) is very useful, both in the detection and the differential diagnosis. Moreover, DWI allows us to make an assumption about the age of an ischemic lesion (hyperacute, acute, and chronic).

3.2.3.5 Intraspinal Tumoral Lesions

In addition to the normal imaging protocol, one should perform axial and sagittal TSE T1-WI after gadolinium injection.

3.2.3.6 Vertebral Metastases

In screening for vertebral metastases, one should perform sagittal TSE T1- and T2-WI. In addition, a sagittal GRE so-called out-of-phase sequence can be used. This is a sequence with a specific TE corresponding to the time it takes for water and fat protons to move exactly 180° out of phase. This time depends on the field strength of the magnet and is approximately 7 ms for a 1.5-T imager, and 11 ms for a 1.0-T machine. In the normal adult human, the medullary bone of the vertebral bodies contains approximately equal amounts of water and fat protons. In out-of-phase conditions, the signal of both will cancel out, leaving the vertebrae completely black. In the case of vertebral pathology, however, the signal will increase, and as such, vertebral metastases (or other lesions) will clearly stand out (Fig. 3.7).

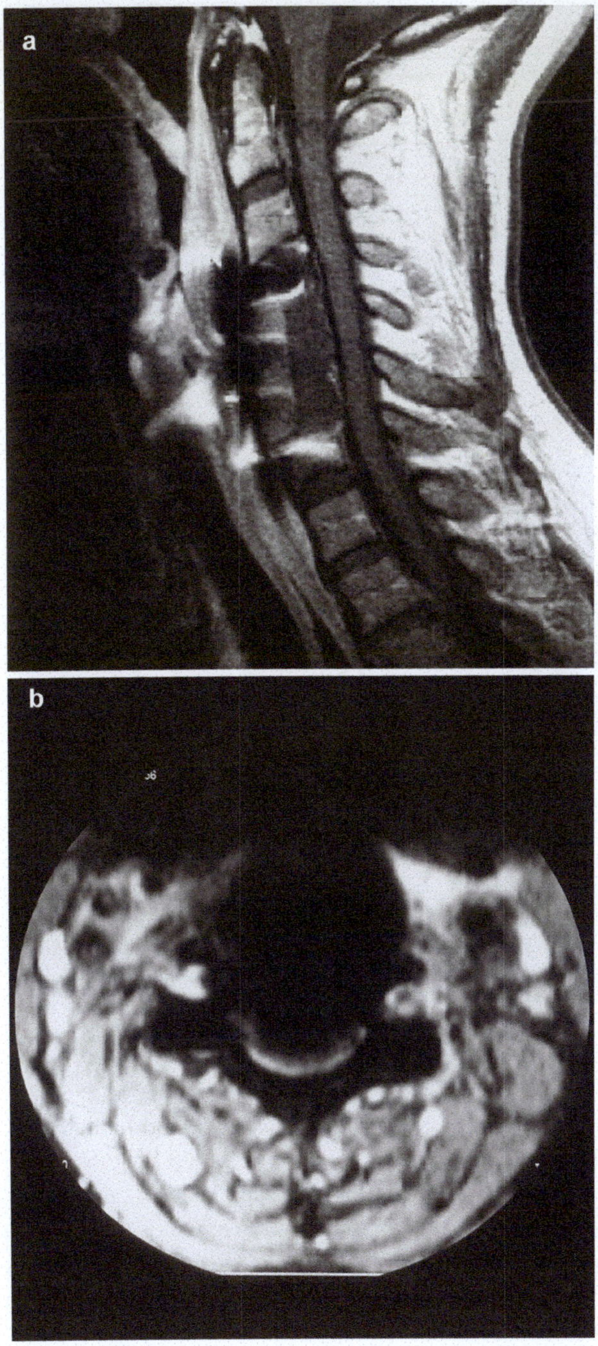

Fig. 3.6 Radiofrequency (RF) artifacts. Nonsuperparamagnetic metals (e.g., titanium) do allow imaging of the region of the implants, since they only cause RF artifacts, which are smaller than susceptibility artifacts. However, note that SE and especially TSE sequences are preferred over gradient-recalled echo (GRE) sequences; compare the sagittal TSE T1-W sequence (**a**) with the axial GRE T2-W sequence (**b**). Therefore, in these cases, GRE sequences should be replaced by (T)SE sequences, also in the axial plane

If a metastasis extends into the spinal canal or neural foramen, additional axial T1-WI after gadolinium injection should be performed.

3.2.4 Sequence Parameters

Table 3.1 lists the standard sequence parameters for MRI of the CS, thoracic, or lumbar spine. All matrices of images with a large FoV (lumbar spine) should be at least 512. On some newer machines, even 1,024 matrices are possible.

Rectangular field of views (RFoV) can be used to shorten the imaging time. However, this can also be achieved by decreasing the number of acquisitions, e.g., a sequence with two acquisitions and 50% RFoV is identical in imaging time and SNR to the same sequence with one acquisition and no RFoV (100%). RFoV, however, may cause infolding (or wraparound) artifacts. To avoid infolding artifacts in general, oversampling can be used. In the read direction, this can be achieved without lengthening the acquisition. In the phase direction, oversampling linearly increases the imaging time, but SNR also increases. For this reason, 100% oversampling and one acquisition is equal to no oversampling and two acquisitions, both in imaging time and SNR. Therefore, we can state:

4 acquisitions with 50% RFoV
= 2 acquisitions with 100% RFoV
= 1 acquisition with 200% RFoV
(also called 100% phase oversampling)

This occurs in both imaging time and SNR, but the latter solution prevents infolding artifacts. There may, however, be an advantage in obtaining more acquisitions with RFoV, since image degradation by motion artifacts decreases when more averages are obtained.

Since motion (respiration, movement, pulsatile blood flow, CSF flow, etc.) usually causes artifacts in the phase-encoding direction, it can be useful to swap the read-out and phase-encoding directions. In the lumbar spine, choosing phase encoding in the craniocaudad direction diminishes artifacts due to CSF pulsations (Fig. 3.8).

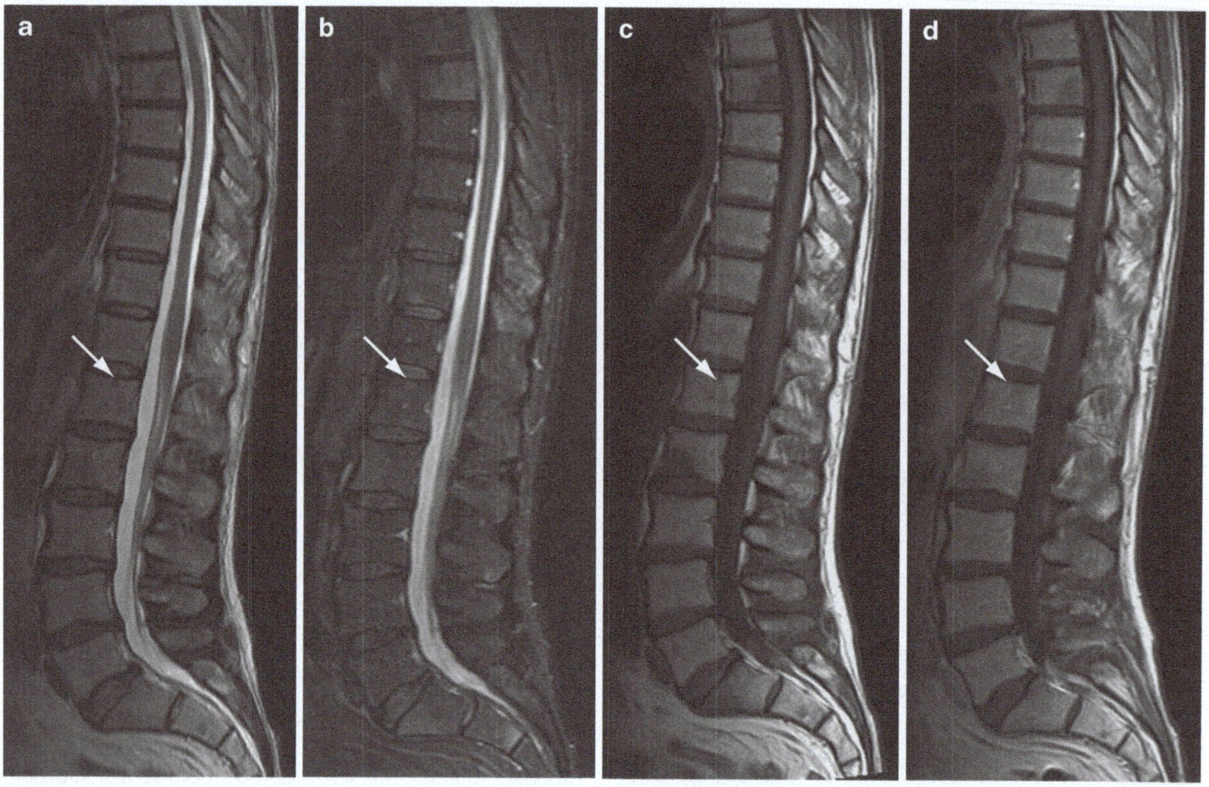

Fig. 3.7 Vertebral metastases. Sagittal TSE T2-weighted image (**a**), STIR image (**b**), and unenhanced (**c**), and gadolinium-enhanced (**d**) TSE T1-weighted images (WI). This is a patient with vertebral metastases of an epiglottic carcinoma. Since the metatstatic tissue that replaces fatty bone marrow is usually hypointense on T1 and can be either hypo-, iso-, or hyperintense on T2, the T1-weighted sequence without gadolinium most clearly depicts the lesions. In this case, lesions are seen in the vertebral bodies of Th7, L1, L2, L5, S1, and S2 as well as in the spinous process of Th8 (**c**). Note that hypointense bone-marrow lesions on the T1-WI (**c**) (such as most metastases) become less conspicuous after administration of gadolinium, since enhancement of the lesions renders them less hypointense or even isointense to normal bone marrow (**d**). Also, T2-weighted images (**a**), even with fat suppression (**b**), show the lesions not as clearly (**a**, **b**). The small lesion in L1 for example is hardly visible on any sequence except the T1-WI before gadolinium (**c**) (*arrows*)

3.2.5 Slice Thickness and Orientation

Standard slice thickness for sagittal sequences in the spine is 3–4 mm. One should use an uneven number of slices so that the middle slice is precisely centered on the midpoint of the spinal cord. For axial slices, one can use 3–4 mm slices in the neck and 4–5 mm slices in the lumbar region, since lumbar disc spaces are relatively thick and the foramina are large. Thicker slices, although generating a significantly better SNR, are unsatisfactory in depicting small disc herniations due to partial volume effects.

These axial slices should be oriented perpendicular to the spinal canal rather than parallel to the intervertebral disc. Usually, this does not make much difference except in the CS when the discs are angulated downward.

Coverage on the sagittal images should include the neural foramina on either side. At least part of the adjacent anatomic region should be imaged, e.g., the conus medullaris in imaging the lumbar spine or the craniocervical junction in imaging the CS. It is not unusual for a conus medullaris tumor to present clinically as a radiculopathy or low-back pain.

3.2.6 Saturation Zones

Saturation techniques use a selective pulse that is applied to tissues either inside or outside the FoV. Their purpose is to excite (or saturate) moving spins that lie outside the region of interest. They are extremely

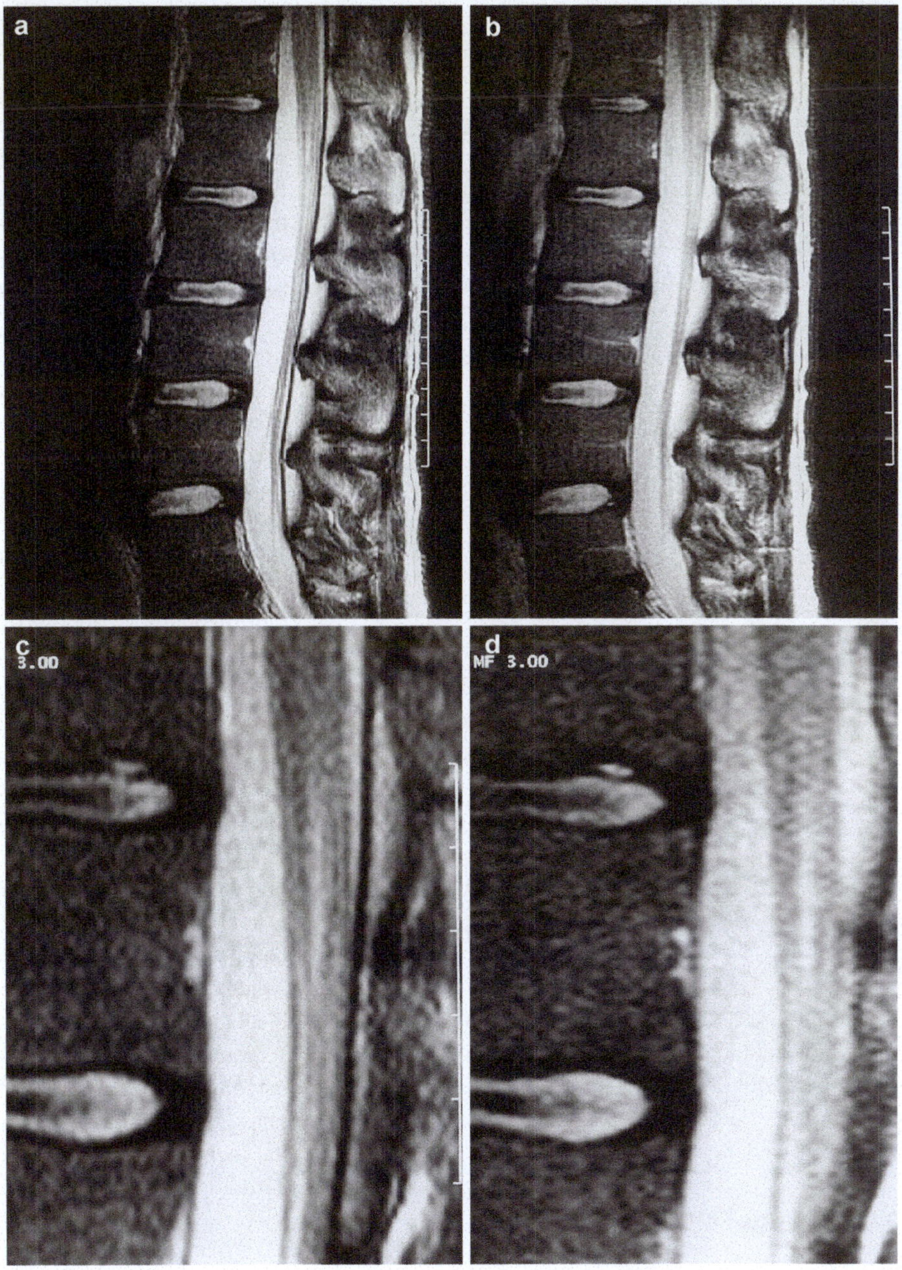

Fig. 3.8 Sagittal T2-WI from the same volunteer. (**a**) The sequence with swapped phase and read directions (phase direction craniocaudal). (**b**) The nonswapped sequence. Swapping reduces blurring due to artifacts from the pulsating cerebrospinal fluid. Magnified views (**c**, **d**) of the same anatomic region clearly show blurring of the conus medullaris and the nerve roots on the nonswapped image (**d**). Do not use rectangular field-of-views in combination with swapped images since this will create infolding artifacts

useful to eliminate motion-induced artifacts arising outside the spine. If possible, all tissues in front of the spine should be saturated. This diminishes the phase-encoding artifacts caused by moving tissues in this region, e.g., breathing, swallowing, cardiac motion, pulsating blood flow, etc. If the saturation is not effective enough, two smaller bands instead of one larger band can be used.

3.2.7 Special Sequences

3.2.7.1 Coronal Images

Coronal images can be useful in evaluating spinal scoliosis. Also, paraspinal extension of processes such as foraminal neurinomas are more clearly depicted. Finally, developmental anomalies, such as lumbosacral

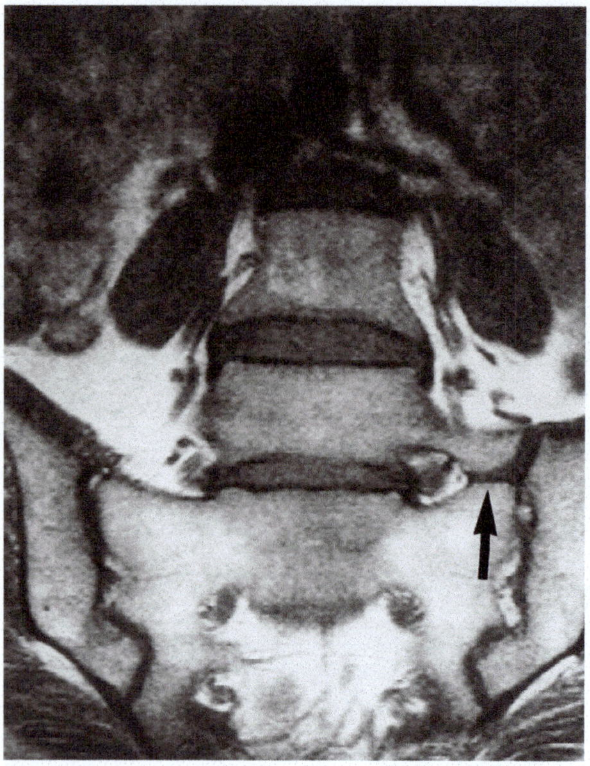

Fig. 3.9 Transitional vertebra. A lumbosacral transitional vertebra can be difficult to detect if only axial and sagittal images are acquired. This (para)coronal image clearly depicts the abnormal articulation of the left L5 transverse process with the sacrum and the ilium, with formation of a pseudarthrosis (*arrow*)

transitional vertebrae (Fig. 3.9), craniocervical junction abnormalities, or failures of segmentation and fusion of vertebrae, are more readily assessed on coronal images.

3.2.7.2 Large FoV

In some cases, the use of a large FoV can be helpful. In particular, when screening or staging a patient with vertebral metastases, an overview of the spine is sensible. When phased-array coils are available, large segments of the spine can be portrayed with excellent image quality. However, when phased-array coils are not available, the body coil must be used, and the image quality will be suboptimal. For vertebral metastases, this should not pose a major problem, but in screening for more subtle lesions, such as intramedullary lesions in MS, these large FoV images may give false-negative results.

3.2.7.3 Sequences with Fat Suppression

In the lumbar spine, fat suppression can be used to differentiate enhancing scar tissue from epidural fat tissue in gadolinium-enhanced T1-WI of the postoperative spine. Nevertheless, the same result can be obtained by subtracting pre- and postcontrast images without fat suppression. In some rare cases, fat-suppression techniques can be helpful in the differentiation between blood and fat.

Fat-suppression techniques are also very useful in imaging degenerative pathology of the facet joints and posterior elements in general. Intraarticular fluid, facet joint cysts, ganglionic cysts, yellow ligament cysts, and bone edema are all clearly depicted.

3.2.7.4 Out-of-Phase Imaging

Out-of-phase or opposed-phase images occur in GRE sequences when the TE equals the time needed for water and fat protons to progress 180° out of phase. In these circumstances, objects consisting of equal amounts of water and fat protons are hypointense (black) on MR images, since the contributions of water and fat protons to the overall signal intensity effectively cancel each other out. During adult life, vertebral bodies consist more or less of equal amounts of water and fat. When a pathologic process disturbs this equilibrium, the vertebrae will show areas of higher signal, which clearly stand out in relation to the normal black background. A frequently used indication involves screening for vertebral metastases. One exception is osteoblastic metastases, which remain dark on out-of-phase images since they are already hypointense due to the lack of mobile protons (Fig. 3.7). Therefore, standard T1-WI should always also be obtained.

3.2.7.5 Ultrafast Imaging

In some patients, it can be useful to shorten the imaging time in order to decrease motion artifacts (children, uncooperative patients, etc.) or to decrease the overall examination time (claustrophobic patients, monitored patients, etc.). In these cases, the sequence parameters listed in Table 3.2 can be used. Although the acquisition time is reduced to 1 min or less, these ultrafast sequences still produce high-quality images or even better images with patient movement (Fig. 3.10).

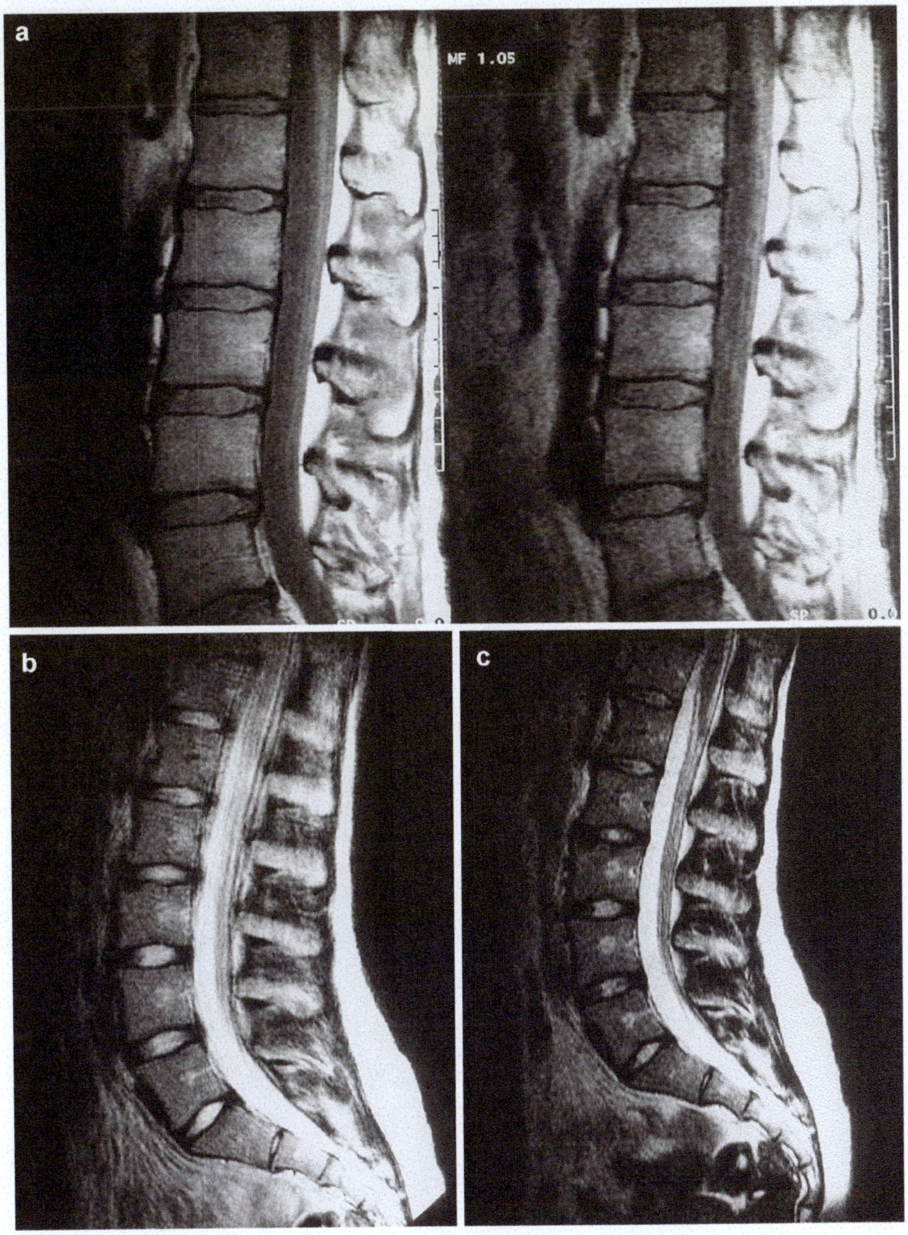

Fig. 3.10 Ultrafast imaging. (**a**) Sagittal TSE T1-WI from the same volunteer. On the *left* is the routine sequence (repetition time (TR) 1,350, echo time (TE) 15, echo train length (ETL) 7, acquisition time (TA) 2 min 28 s), on the right, the ultrafast sequence (TR 1270, TE 15, ETL 7, TA 53 s', see also Tables 3.1 and 3.2 for complete sequence parameters). Notice the comparable spatial resolution of both images (both 512 matrix), but the higher SNR of the routine sequence on the *left*. (**b**) Routine sagittal TSE T2-W sequence (TR 3000, TE 96, ETL 7, TA 4 min 19 s) in a patient with considerable low-back pain. The image is degraded by motion artifacts, and the quality is unsatisfactory. (**c**) Ultrafast sequence (TR 3200, TE 128, ETL 23, TA 1 min 7 s; see Tables 3.1 and 3.2 for the complete sequence parameters) in the same patient. Owing to the shorter imaging time, the quality of the ultrafast sequence is clearly better

Imaging time is (or can be) further decreased by eliminating saturation zones. SNRs are substantially lower but still sufficient.

3.2.7.6 MR Myelography

MR myelography can be helpful in addition to the normal imaging sequences. Although three-dimensional (3D)-TSE sequences have been proposed, they significantly add to the total imaging time of the examination. Therefore, I prefer single-shot wide-slab T2-W sequences with a very long echo train (Fig. 3.11). Although these allow only one view of the thecal sac at a time, their imaging time is very short, making it possible to obtain different views by running the sequence in different orientations (one frontal view, one sagittal view, and two obliques). This sequence has the added advantage of eliminating postprocessing (no maximal intensity projection is necessary).

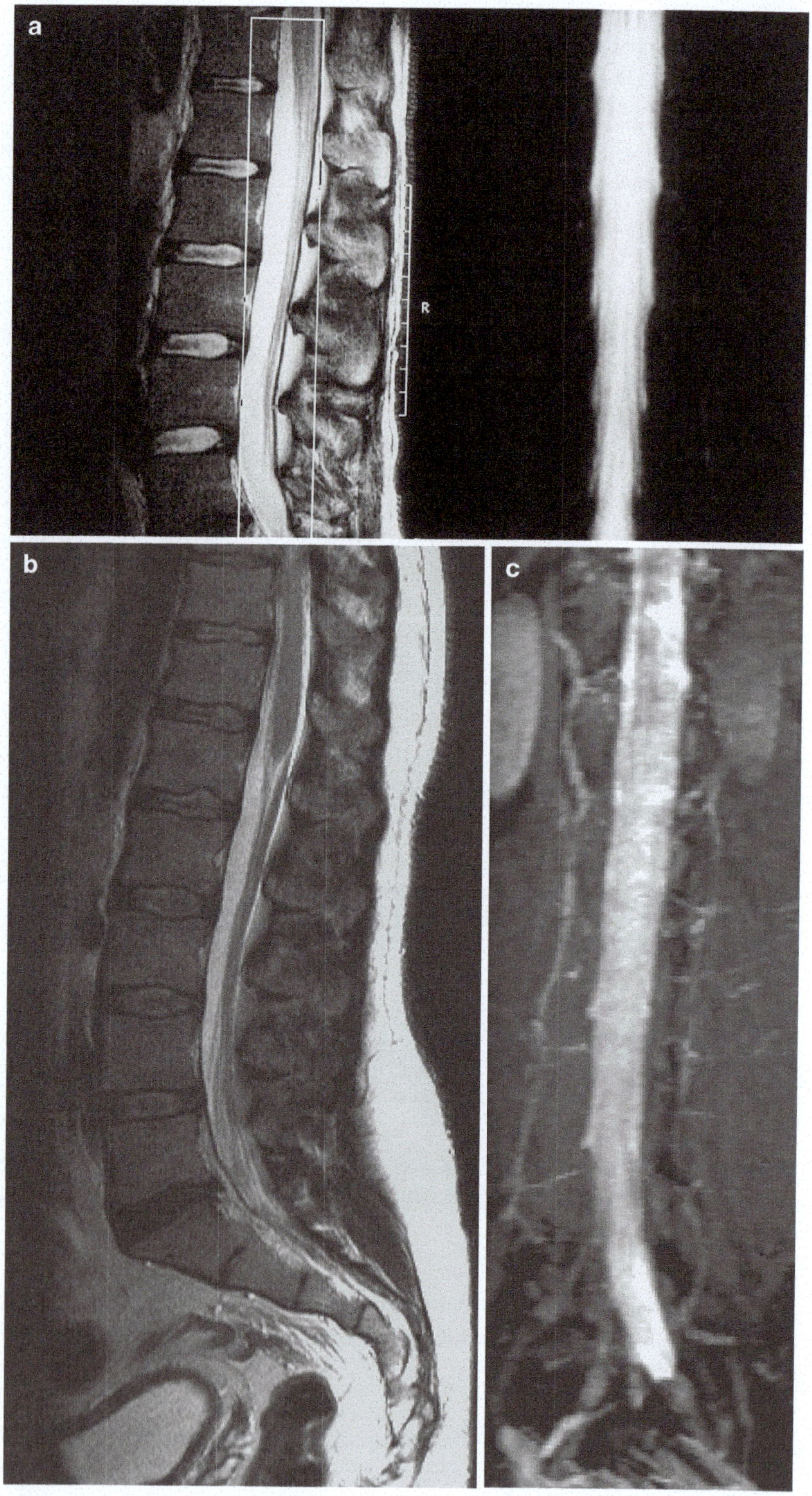

Fig. 3.11 MR myelogram. (**a**) Routine MR myelogram in a normal volunteer (repetition time (TR) 2,800, echo time (TE) 1,100, echo train length 240, TA 7 s). In this example, a frontal view MR myelogram (*right*) is obtained by placing the slice on a sagittal image (*left*). Slice thickness should be adjusted to include the complete dural sac and nerve sheaths. Excellent detail with symmetric nerve roots and sheaths. The sequence can be run in different directions to obtain frontal, lateral, or oblique-view myelograms. (**b**, **c**) For comparison, a 3D TSE T2-W sequence. This sequence has a markedly longer acquisition time but has the advantage of producing multiple views

3.2.7.7 MR Angiography

Magnetic resonance angiography (MRA) has limited use in spinal imaging. Even arteriovenous malformations or fistulae are hard to image with MRA. Normally, postcontrast T1-W sequences are sufficient (Fig. 3.12).

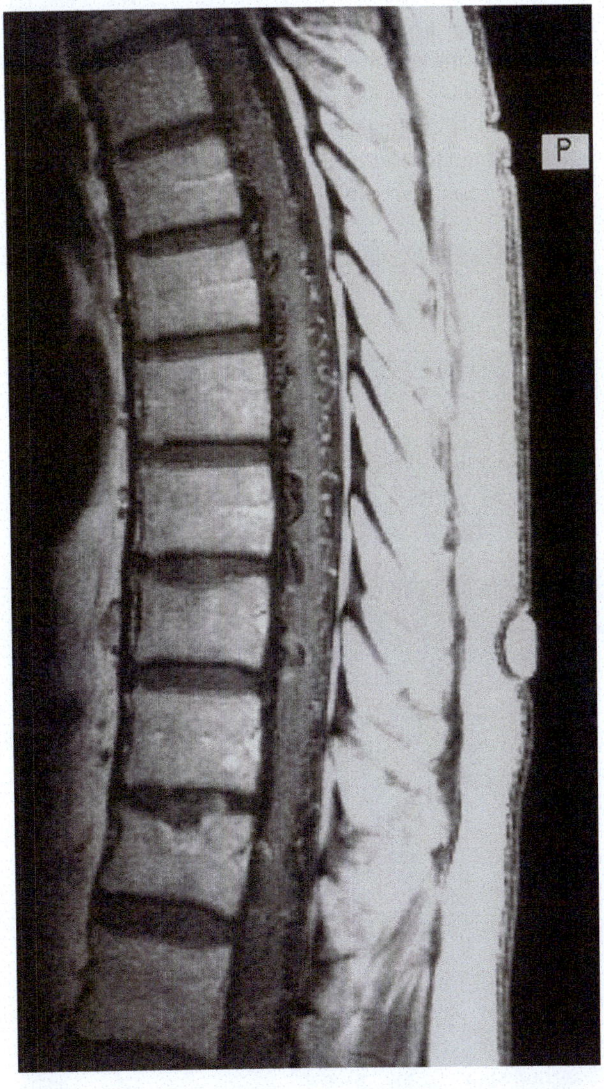

Fig. 3.12 Spinal AV malformation, gadolinium-enhanced T1-WI. Notice the presence of multiple serpiginous blood vessels on the surface of the thoracic cord in this typical example. The small blood vessels with slow flow enhance with gadolinium, and the medium-sized vessels with higher flow do not enhance and are seen as areas of flow void. These gadolinium-enhanced images are typical and sufficient for making the diagnosis. High-quality MR angiography images are difficult to obtain due to the small size and tortuous course of these blood vessels

3.2.7.8 Diffusion-Weighted Imaging

DWI is a special technique using very strong magnetic gradients, effectively canceling signal from protons in free moving water, e.g., CSF. Protons that are more restricted in movement, e.g., in intracellular water, still produce a measurable MR signal. The spontaneous movement of protons is known as "Brownian motion" and results among others in diffusion, hence the term DWI.

This technique is especially useful in detecting cytotoxic edema, where there is cell swelling effectively increasing the amount of intracellular over extracellular water and thereby reducing water diffusion. Since ischemia produces cytotoxic edema very early on (after 1 h), DWI is capable of the early detection of ischemic lesions.

Newer applications of DWI, such as in MS, are emerging but not ready for daily clinical practice.

3.2.7.9 Functional Imaging

Functional imaging of the spine consists mainly of semidynamic imaging. Flexion/extension imaging of the CS is relatively easy to perform with fast sequences. The first images are made with the head flexed forward. This can be readily achieved by placing an inflated balloon under the patient's head. By letting air out of the balloon in small amounts, imaging can be performed in different positions between flexion and extension. This way, dynamic relationships between anatomic structures and pathology, e.g., herniated disc, can be assessed. Depending on the coil design, it can be necessary to switch the normal neck coil for a flexible coil or to use the body coil.

Dynamic imaging of the lumbar spine is more difficult because of the limited space available in the magnet; this problem can be solved in two ways. The most simple solution is to image the patient supine and prone, thus simulating extension and flexion. Another possibility is to use specially designed devices and/or balloons or to image the patient in lateral decubitus. These techniques are relatively cumbersome. Flexion-extension views of the spine have also been obtained with the patient in sitting position with a special type of open interventional MR system ("double-donut" design). Newer machines allow standing weight-bearing MR of the spine. These have the advantage of imaging the spine under physiological loading, and during bending and rotation.

The term functional magnetic resonance imaging (fMRI) is also used for the detection of neuronal activity. Usually, a special MR technique, called blood oxygen level-dependent imaging, is used to detect minute changes in the blood level of deoxyhemoglobin due to neuronal activity and secondary autonomous blood flow adaptation. The technique is mostly used in the brain, since susceptibility artifacts make it very hard to obtain useful images of the spinal cord. Another technique, based on proton density changes during neuronal activity, SEEP, is also used experimentally in fMRI of the spinal cord.

3.2.8 Contrast Media

The use of contrast agents has been discussed in previous sections of this chapter. The most common indications for the use of intravenous gadolinium in the spine are:

1. The postoperative lumbar spine, especially after discectomy (use of gadolinium obligatory)
2. Detection of small tumors, especially neurinomas
3. Imaging of tumors in general
4. MS and other inflammatory diseases

3.3 Clinical Examples

The MRI findings in some typical examples of spinal pathology are demonstrated in Figs. 3.13–3.26.

3.3.1 Degenerative Disease

The most frequently encountered pathology in the spine is degenerative disease. Degenerative disc disease is typified by dehydration of the intervertebral disc. This phenomenon is easily recognized on T2-W sequences as black or dark discs. Secondary changes, such as reduced intervertebral space, osteophytic reactions, and bulging disc, are also easily recognized. Sometimes tears of the annulus fibrosus can be detected on T2-WI as a region of high signal intensity near the posterior margin of the disc (Fig. 3.13). These annular tears typically enhance after intravenous gadolinium injection.

Other characteristic findings in degenerative disc disease are alterations in the adjacent vertebral body endplates (Table 3.3). These endplate changes were first categorized by Modic (Fig. 3.14). Type I endplate changes represent vascularized bone marrow and/or edema and are seen as low-SI changes on T1-WI and high-SI areas on T2-WI. Type II changes represent more chronic alterations with proliferation of fatty tissue and are bright both on T1-WI and T2-WI. Type III changes, also seen on conventional radiographs and computed tomography (CT) images, represent dense, sclerotic bone and are dark on T1-WI and T2-WI. Type I and II changes may enhance with gadolinium, but should not be confused with inflammatory enhancement commonly seen with disc infection.

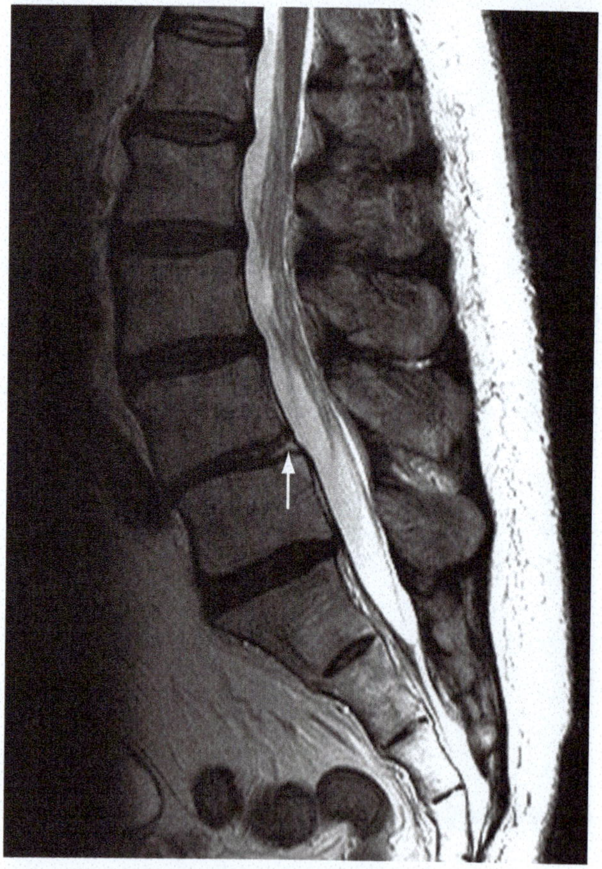

Fig. 3.13 Degenerative disc disease is characterized by T2-shortening of the disc and decreased intervertebral height, degenerative vertebral endplate changes, bulging disc, and/or osteophytes. A radial tear of the annulus (*arrow*), which is found consistently with the other degenerative changes in the intervertebral disc, involves all layers of the annulus fibrosus. It may be detected by MR imaging as a band of high signal intensity on T2-WI (L4-L5 disc in this case)

Table 3.3 Modic type changes of vertebral endplates in degenerative disease (Modic et al. 1988)

Modic classification	T1-SI changes	T2-SI changes	Represents
I marrow and/or edema	–	+	Vascularized bone
II tissue	+	+	Proliferation of fatty
III	–	–	Sclerotic bone

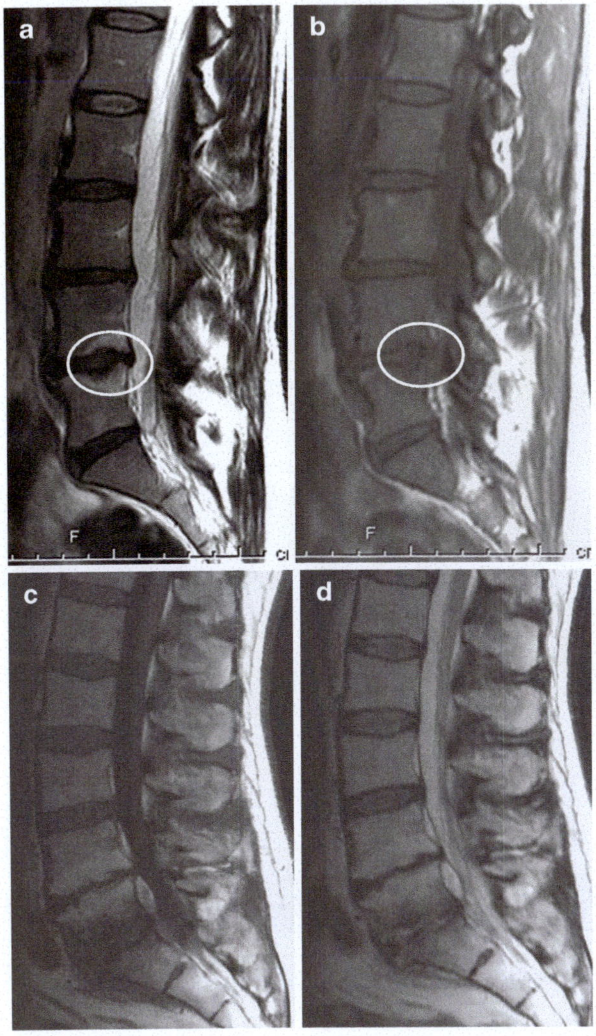

Fig. 3.14 Modic type endplate changes. (**a**, **b**) T2, respectively. T1-WI signal intensities of endplates in Modic I changes at the L4-L5 level (*oval*). These changes correspond to bone edema and may represent "active" degeneration. (**c**) T2 and (**d**) T1 on the other hand show chronic changes with high signal intensities in the endplates at the L4-L5 level and low signal intensities at the L5-S1 level, representing lipomatous (Modic type II), respectively. sclerotic changes (Modic type III)

Degenerative changes of the facet joints may play an important role in low-back pain, but may also cause irradiating leg pain due to secondary foraminal stenosis (Fig. 3.4). Foraminal narrowing, or foraminal pathology in general, is more accurately assessed on sagittal images than on axial images (CT or MRI) (Fig. 3.4).

In the CS, uncovertebral degenerative disease may play an important role in irradiating shoulder or arm pain due to secondary foraminal narrowing. In assessing the cervical neural foramen, one should be aware of the underestimation of the diameter (up to 10%) on MRI because of chemical shift artifacts.

3.3.2 Herniated Disc

Herniated discs are more easily detected with MRI than with CT. First, MRI allows visualization of the complete lumbar (or cervical or thoracic) spine in one examination. Second, sagittal images also depict the spinal canal in between intervertebral disc spaces. It is not unusual for a disc fragment to migrate (or extend) into the area behind the vertebral body (Fig. 3.15). Some of these migrated discs can be missed on CT if axial slices are limited to the intervertebral disc spaces examined. Third, the intrinsic tissue contrast is usually better on MR. Especially, the cervicothoracic and/or lumbosacral region can be hard to assess on CT due to beam hardening, especially in larger patients.

The terms used to describe or classify bulging or herniated discs are somewhat ambiguous and sometimes misused. Recently, a nomenclature project initiated by the American Society of Spine Radiology has found wide acceptance among radiologists, clinicians, and surgeons (Table 3.4). In this nomenclature, herniation is defined as a localized displacement of disc material beyond the limits of the intervertebral disc space. The disc material may be nucleus, cartilage, fragmented apophyseal bone, anular tissue, or any combination thereof. The term "localized" contrasts to "generalized," the latter being arbitrarily defined as greater than 50% (180°) of the periphery of the disc.

Localized displacement in the axial (horizontal) plane can be "focal," signifying less than 25% of the disc circumference, or "broad-based," meaning between 25 and 50% of the disc circumference. The presence of disc tissue "circumferentially" (50–100%) beyond the edges of the ring apophyses may be called

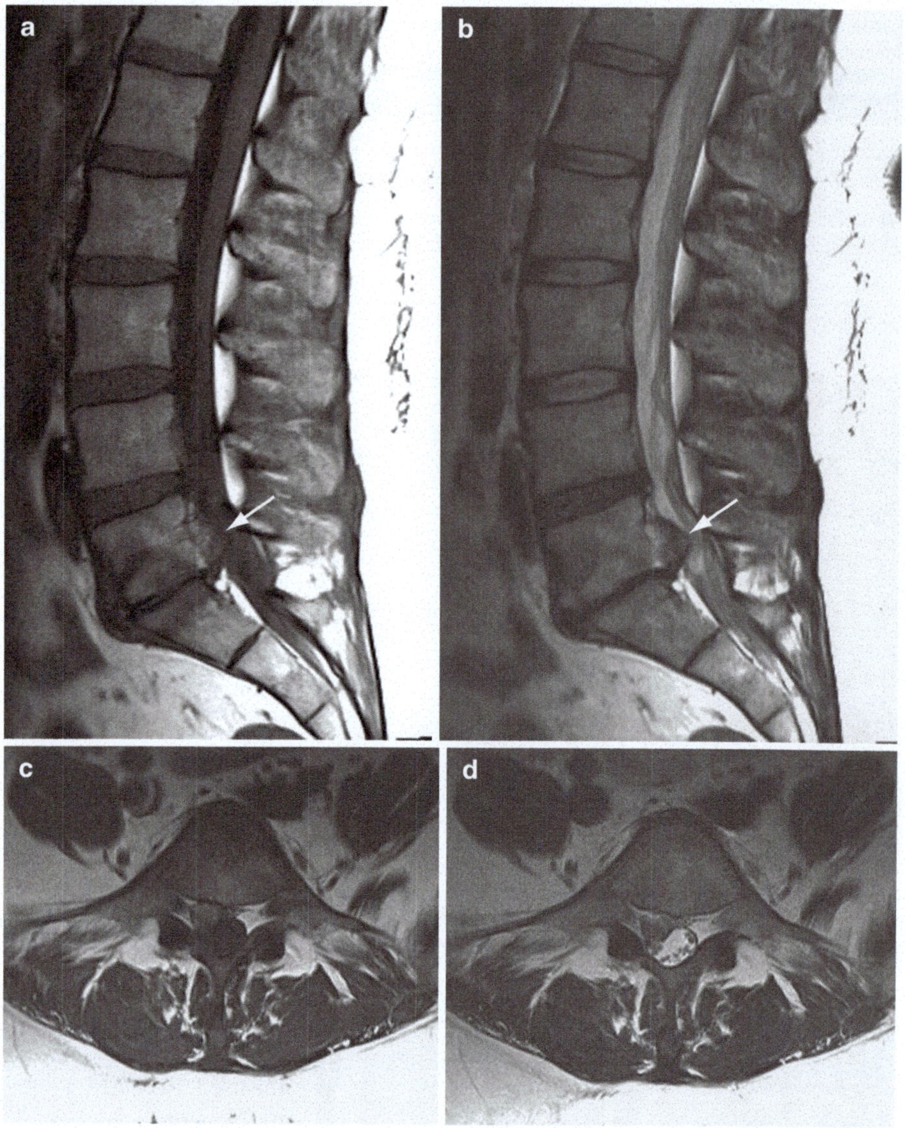

Fig. 3.15 Sequestered disc. Sequestered disc fragments can migrate upward (or less frequently downward) behind the vertebral bodies, all the way up to the next intervertebral space (*arrows*). As such, they may be missed on axial computed tomography. Therefore, sagittal imaging is an important advantage of MR imaging (**a**, **b**). Sequestered disc fragments tend to be hyperintense on T2-WI when they are relatively young. Older disc fragments dehydrate and become dark on all sequences. In this case, the disc fragment is still relatively bright, both on T1 and T2-WI. The contrast between the extruded disc fragment and the surrounding epidural fat tissue is slightly better seen on T1-WI (**c**) than on T2-WI (**d**)

Table 3.4 Nomenclature of disc herniation

General terminology	Definition	Specification I	Specification II	Definition
Bulging	Displacement over >50% of the periphery of the disc			
Herniation	Localized displacement (<50% of the periphery of the disc)	Focal (<25%) OR broad-based (25 … 50%)	Protrusion	No extrusion
			Extrusion	Distance of the edge of the herniated material > disc height or hernia base
			Sequestration (= special form of extrusion)	No continuity with parent disc

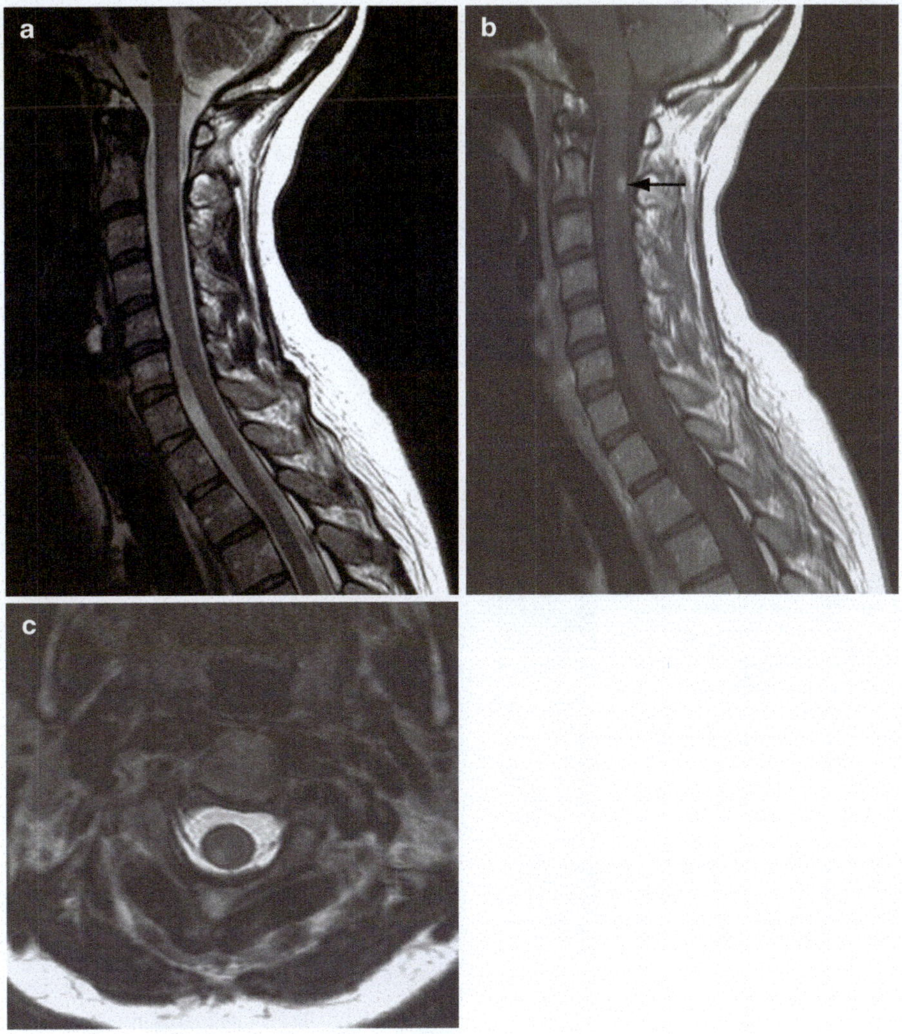

Fig. 3.16 Multiple sclerosis. In this young woman with multiple sclerosis, sagittal TSE T2-weighted images (WI) (**a**), axial gradient echo T2-WI (**c**), and sagittal unenhanced (not shown) and gadolinium-enhanced TSE T1-WIs (**b**) were obtained. The signal changes observed with intramedullary multiple sclerosis lesions are comparable to those in the brain. The sagittal T2-WI shows an unsharply demarcated hyperintense lesion posterior and paramedial in the cord (**c**) that manifests enhancement (**b**) (*arrow*). Note that multiple sclerosis can be seen on magnetic resonance (MR) imaging with lesions in the brain and/or the spine. Therefore, when a presumptive diagnosis of spinal multiple sclerosis plaques is made, MR examination of the brain should be performed to confirm the diagnosis, by demonstrating typical brain lesions

"bulging" and is not considered a form of herniation, nor are diffuse adaptive alterations of the disc contour secondary to adjacent deformity as may be present in severe scoliosis or spondylolisthesis.

Herniated discs may take the form of protrusion or extrusion, based on the shape of the displaced material. Protrusion is present if the greatest distance, in any plane, between the edges of the disc material beyond the disc space is less than the distance between the edges of the base in the same plane. The base is defined as the cross-sectional area of disc material at the outer margin of the disc space of origin, where disc material displaced beyond the disc space is continuous with disc material within the disc space. In the craniocaudal direction, the length of the base cannot exceed, by definition, the height of the intervertebral space. Extrusion is present when, in at least one plane, any one distance between the edges of the disc material beyond the disc space is greater than the distance between the edges of the base in the same plane, or when no continuity exists between the disc material beyond the disc space and that within the disc space. Extrusion may be further specified as sequestration, if the displaced disc material has completely lost all continuity with the parent disc (Fig. 3.15). The term migration may be used to signify displacement of disc material away from the site of extrusion, regardless of whether it is sequestrated

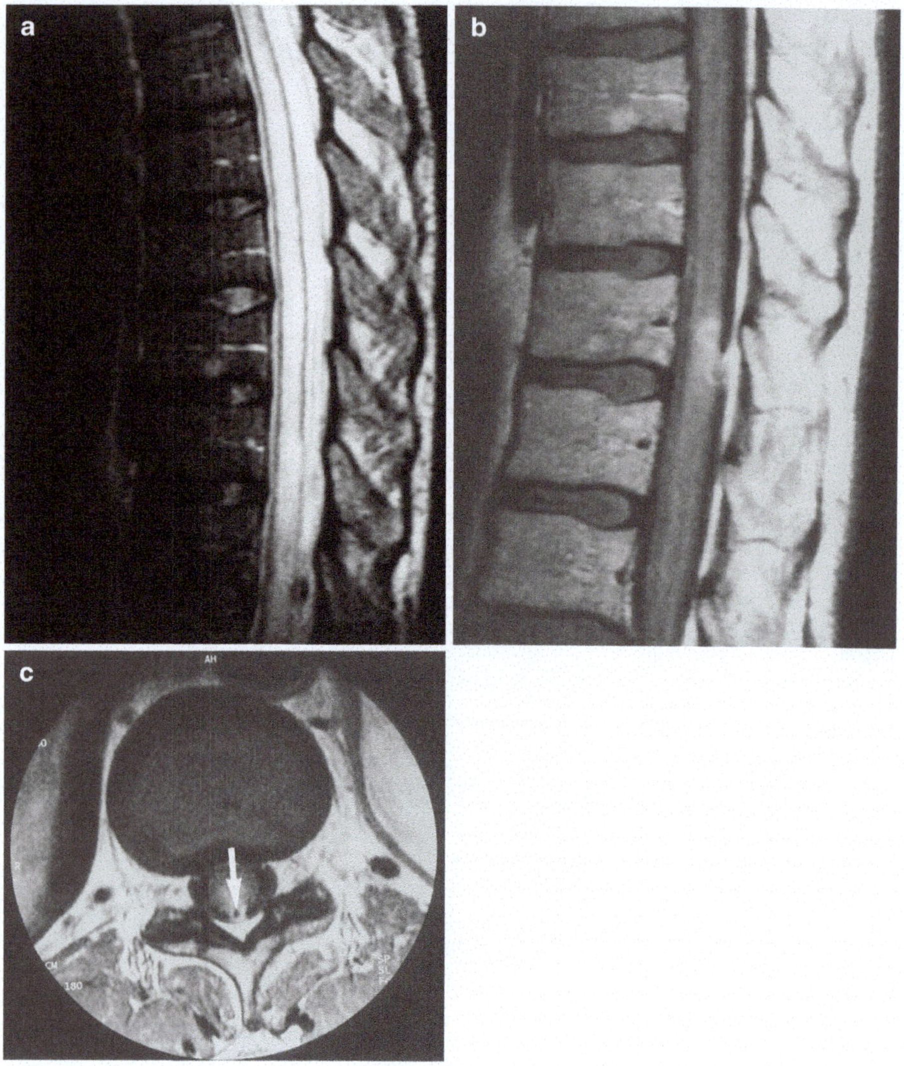

Fig. 3.17 Tuberculous myelomeningitis. Tuberculous myelomeningitis in a patient with an epidural morphine catheter for pain release in case of incurable pancreatic carcinoma. The sagittal TSE T2-weighted image (WI) shows extensive medullary edema (**a**). The sagittal (**b**) and axial (**c**) T1-WI after gadolinium enhancement shows a much smaller nidus of active inflammation in the medulla and in the subdural space around the tip of the catheter (*arrow*). Granulomatous changes in cases of tuberculous or bacterial meningitis show marked enhancement after gadolinium injection. Conversely, in patients with viral meningitis, magnetic resonance imaging findings are often normal. Myelitis can be either infectious as in this case, with extensive medullary edema, or inflammatory, as for example in multiple sclerosis

or not. Because posteriorly displaced disc material is often constrained by the posterior longitudinal ligament, images may portray a disc displacement as a protrusion on axial sections and an extrusion on sagittal sections, in which cases the displacement should be considered an extrusion. Herniated discs in the craniocaudal (vertical) direction through a break in the vertebral body endplate are referred to as intravertebral herniations.

Disc herniations may be further specifically described as contained, if the displaced portion is covered by the outer anulus, or uncontained when any such covering is absent. Displaced disc tissues may also be described by location, volume, and content.

3.3.3 Inflammatory and Infectious Lesions

The most common inflammatory intramedullary lesions are seen in patients with MS. Most of these lesions are hard to detect on precontrast T1-WI, as are MS lesions of the brain. On T2-WI, lesions are hyperintense (Fig. 3.16) and can be quite large in the acute phase. Sometimes, they also exhibit uptake of gadolinium contrast, which is believed to be a sign of an active lesion. An MRI examination of the brain and the complete spinal cord should be performed to search for other lesions. Clinically, one-third of MS patients exhibit spinal symptoms only.

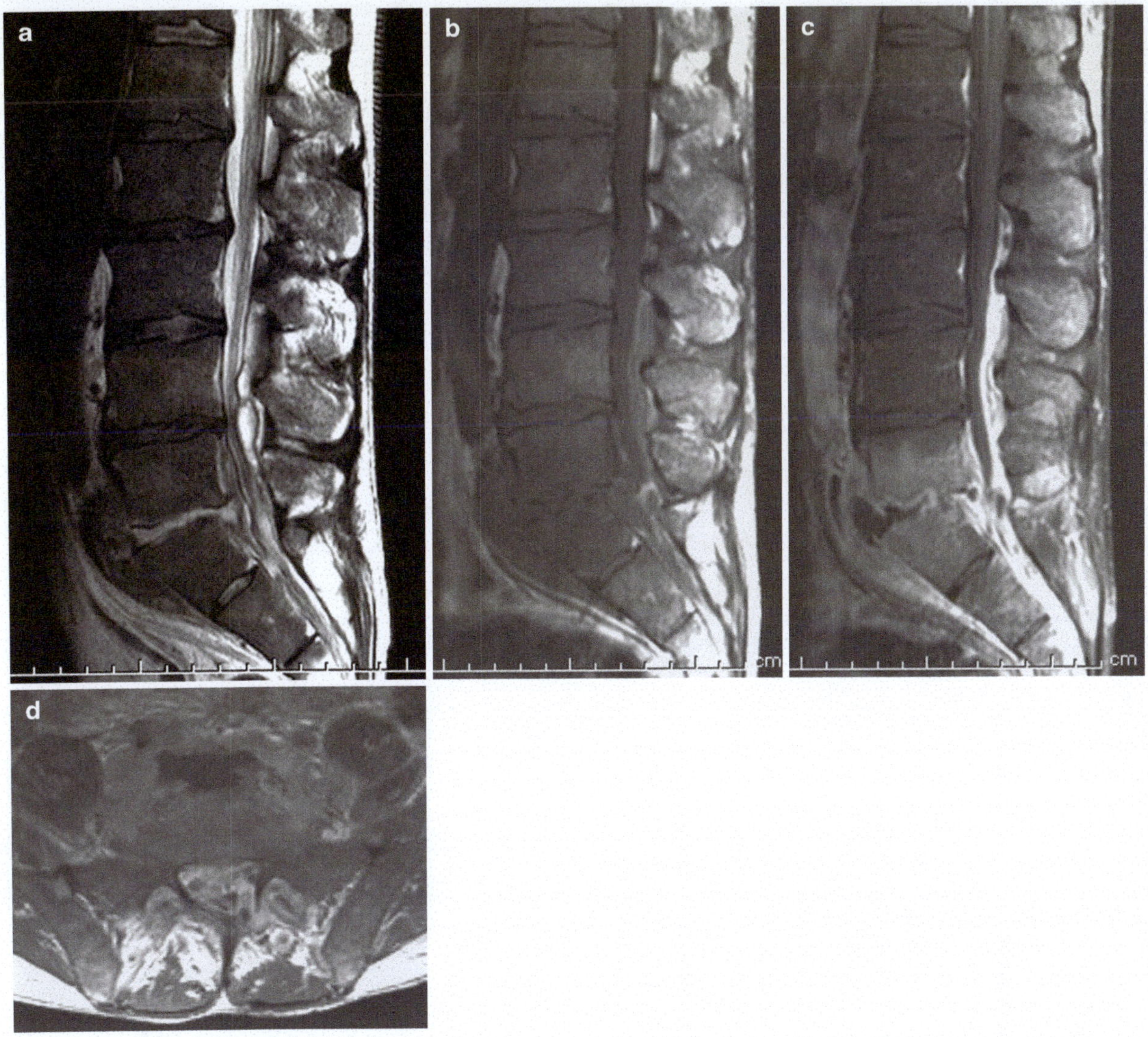

Fig. 3.18 Spondylodiscitis. Spondylodiscitis or disc space infection with osteomyelitis. Note the substantial signal changes both in the vertebral bodies and in the intervertebral disc space. The blurry margins of the vertebral endplates on the T1-WI (**b**) and the high SI of the disc space on the T2-WI (**a**) allow differentiation with degenerative or postoperative changes. Also, the important enhancement, especially of the peripheral disc space and less so of the vertebral bodies is typical for an infectious spondylodiscitis (**c**). In this case, there is also an extensive involvement of the paraspinal soft tissues and the epidural space (**c**, **d**) with phlegmona

The cervical cord is twice as likely to be involved as the lower levels.

Spinal infections can be (intra-)medullary (Fig. 3.17), intraspinal or, more frequently, vertebral and/or discal in location. Spondylodiscitis is frequently caused by bacteria or tuberculosis (Fig. 3.18). Postoperative spondylodiscitis can be difficult to diagnose in the early postoperative phase, since normal (inflammatory) postoperative changes may resemble infectious pathology.

3.3.4 The Postoperative Lumbar Spine

As mentioned earlier, MRI is capable of differentiating postoperative epidural fibrosis and recurrent disc herniation. This is important since the latter can be an indication for reintervention. On postcontrast T1-WI, herniated disc material shows no or minor enhancement (Fig. 3.19), while epidural fibrosis enhances intensely, especially in the first years after surgery (Fig. 3.20). However, smaller disc fragments or "older" recurrent

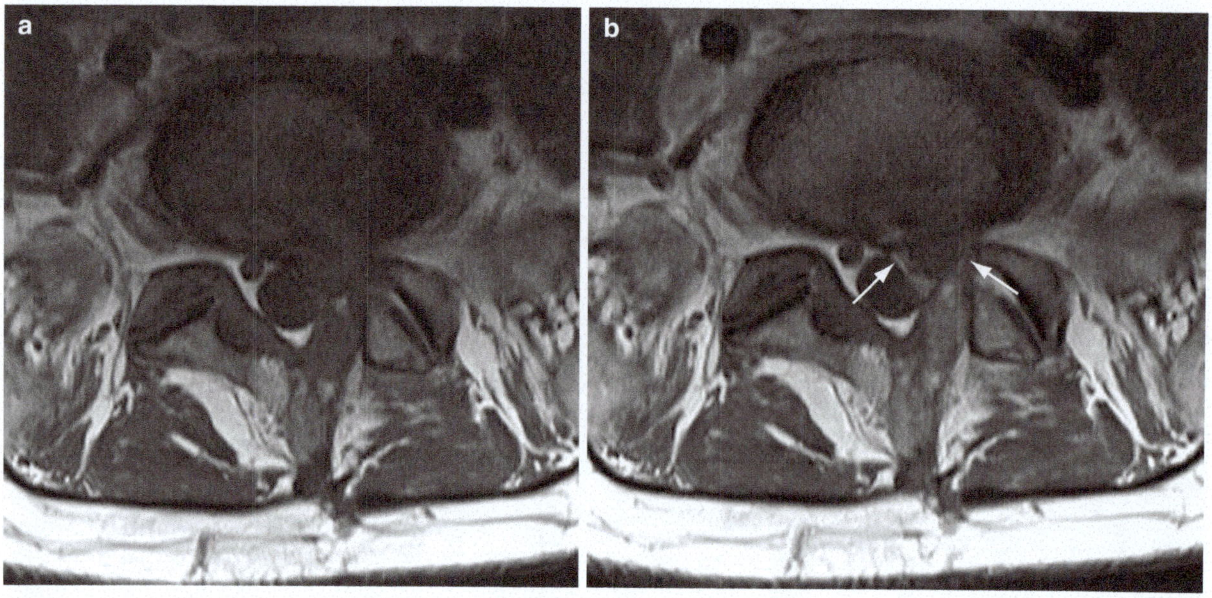

Fig. 3.19 Recurrent disc herniation. Axial T1-WI before (**a**) and after (**b**) gadolinium enhancement in a patient with a large recurrent disc herniation. Differentiating postoperative recurrent disc herniation from epidural fibrosis is important, since the latter is no indication for surgical reintervention. When imaging is performed directly after gadolinium injection, disc material only shows peripheral enhancement (*arrows*), which represents inflammatory tissue

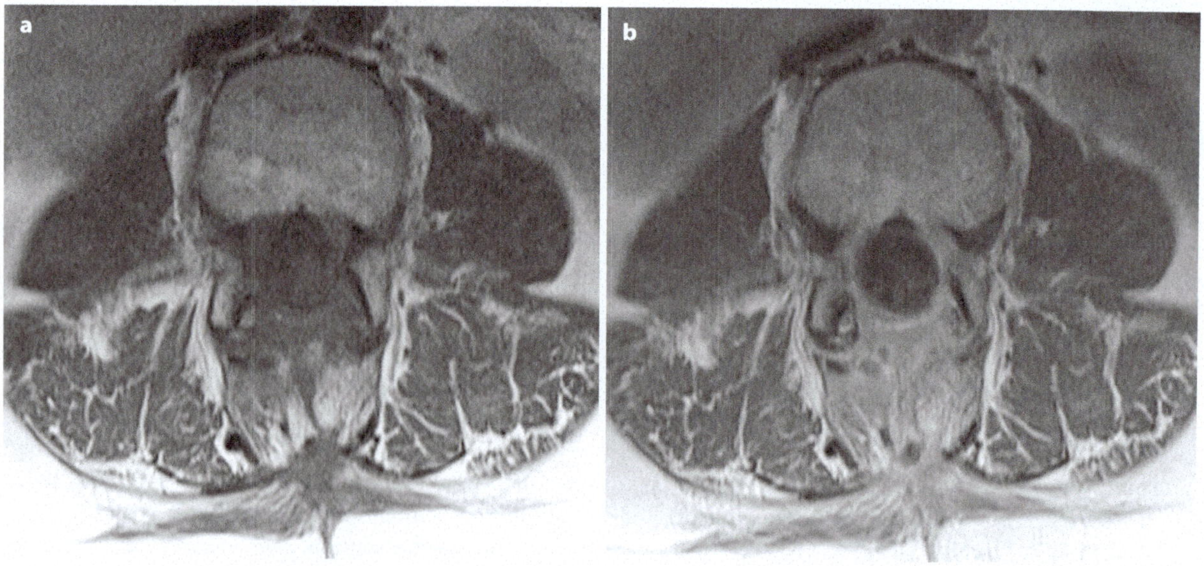

Fig. 3.20 Postoperative epidural fibrosis. Axial T1-WI before (**a**) and after (**b**) gadolinium enhancement in a patient with postoperative epidural fibrosis. Compare with Fig. 3.18; epidural fibrosis shows complete enhancement after contrast administration. In this case, both left and right epidural space enhances. The location of enhancement depends on the surgical route and can be unilateral or bilateral depending on the surgery that was performed

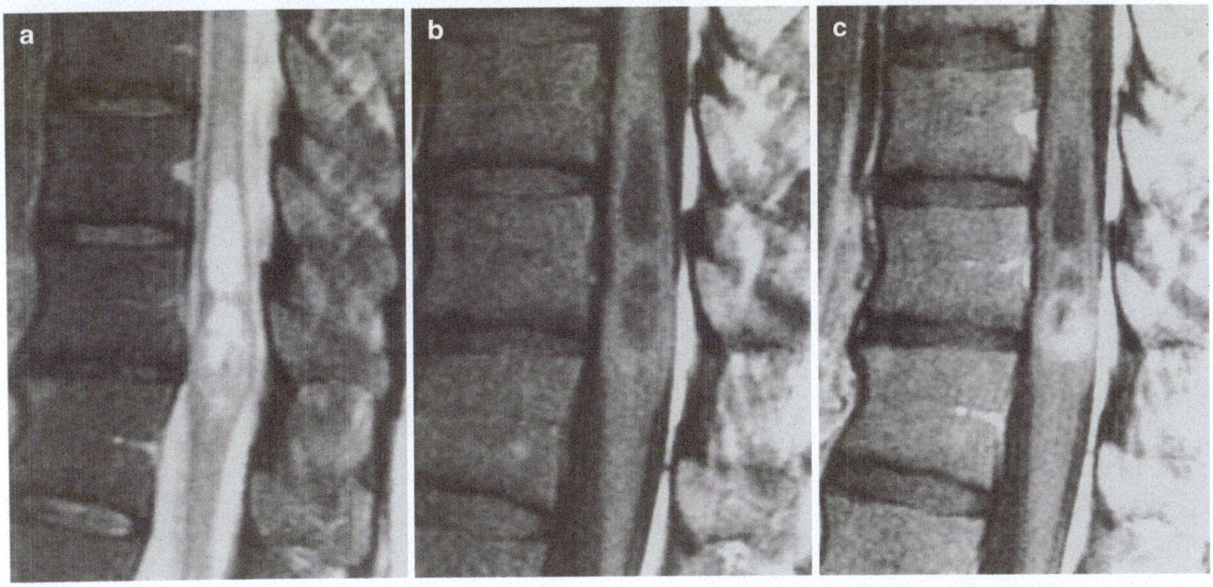

Fig. 3.21 Spinal cord astrocytoma. Astrocytoma of the thoracic spinal cord: sagittal T2-WI (**a**), unenhanced T1-WI (**b**), and gadolinium-enhanced T1-WI (**c**). Because of their infiltrative nature, intramedullary astrocytomas nearly always enhance. Often, there are associated cysts, but the cysts are usually not lined by tumor and do not require excision

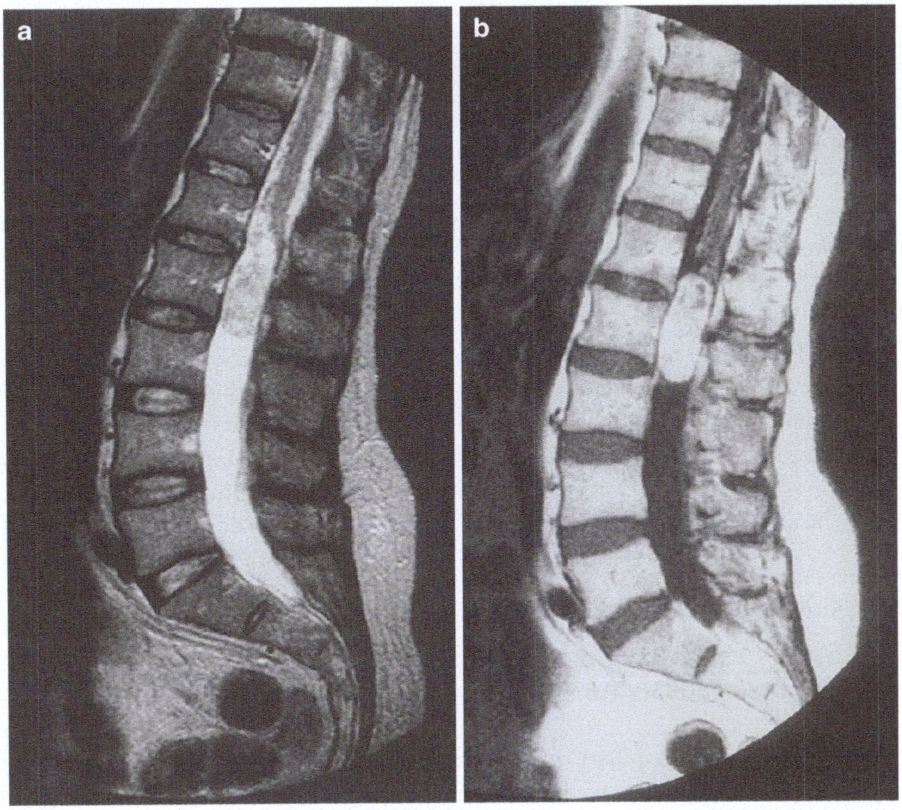

Fig. 3.22 Ependymoma of the conus medullaris. In this patient, with an ependymoma of the conus medullaris (myxopapillary type), sagittal T2-WI (**a**) and gadolinium-enhanced T1-WI (**b**) were performed. Ependymomas are usually better delineated than astrocytomas. On histopathologic examination, they are often surrounded by a capsule. Ependymomas usually show intense and homogeneous enhancement. Ependymomas tend to be central and are more frequently hemorrhagic than astrocytomas

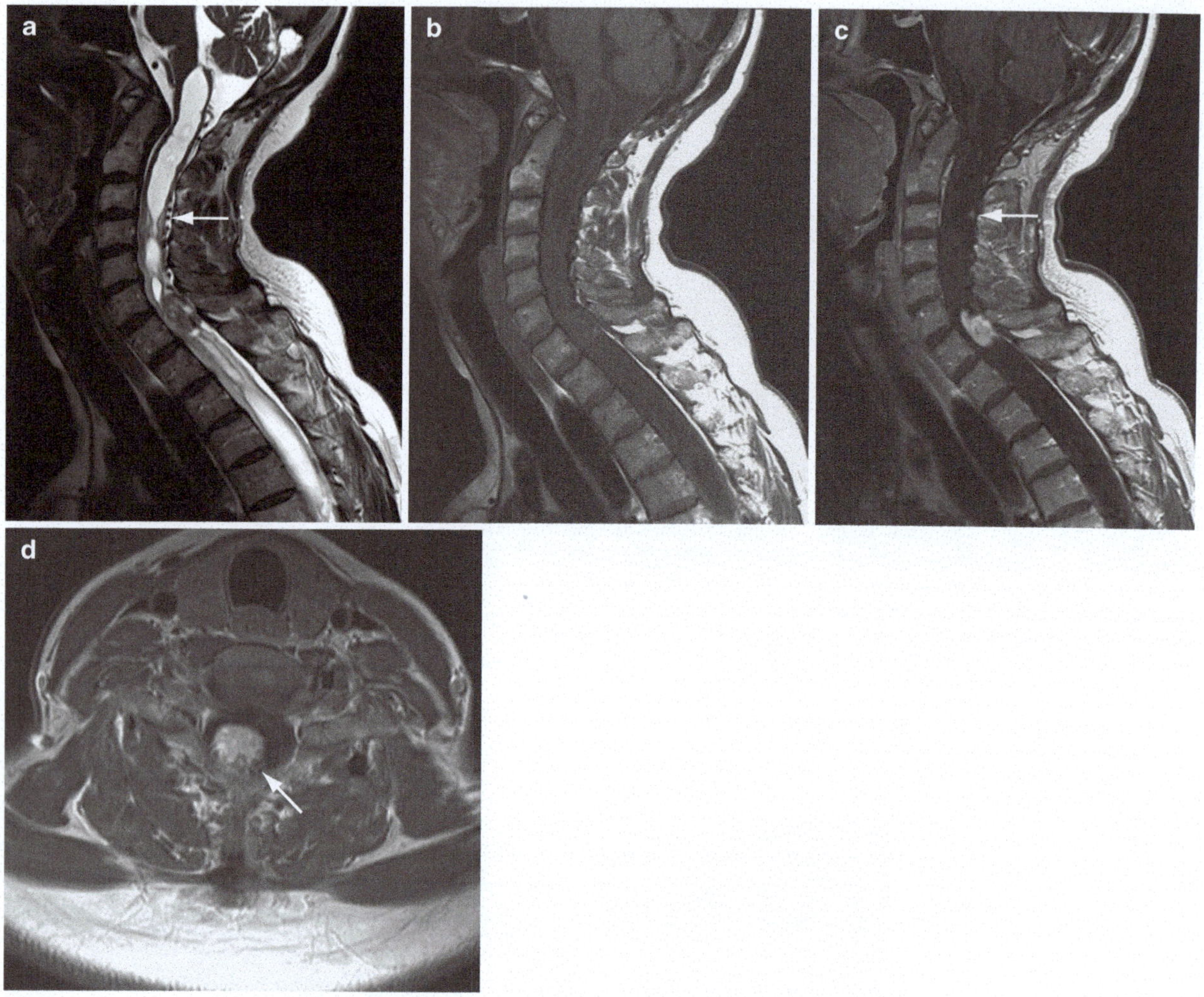

Fig. 3.23 Spinal hemangioblastoma. In this patient, with a spinal hemangioblastoma, sagittal T2-WI (**a**), sagittal T1-WI (**b**), and gadolinium-enhanced sagittal (**c**) and axial T1-WI (**d**) were performed. The typical pattern of this tumor is a strongly enhancing nodule with a large accompanying cystic lesion and edema. There is marked swelling of the cord, and the lesion is very extensive, especially compared to the enhancing tumor nodule. Also, note the prominent vessels (flow voids) in and around this highly vascular tumor (*arrows*)

herniated discs may progressively show more enhancement due to secondary inflammatory changes.

It is important to note that when the intervertebral disc space narrows after discectomy, secondary foraminal stenosis may occur, causing irradiating pain without recurrent herniation.

3.3.5 Spinal Tumors

3.3.5.1 Intramedullary Tumors

Three primary intramedullary tumors are frequently encountered: astrocytoma, ependymoma, and hemangioblastoma.

The peak incidence of spinal astrocytomas is around the third and fourth decade, and they are most often found in the thoracic cord. Clinical symptoms vary and are sometimes very minor. Most often, patients have motor changes with gait difficulties, but pain and bladder disturbances are also possible. In children, sometimes a secondary scoliosis is found. The cord is often enlarged, and most cord astrocytomas are low signal on T1, high signal on T2, and, contrary to brain astrocytomas, show enhancement after gadolinium injection (Fig. 3.21). After gadolinium injection, the delineation of potential cysts is usually more apparent.

Cord ependymomas are usually found in older patients, with a peak incidence around the fourth and fifth decade. It is the most frequent tumor of the lower

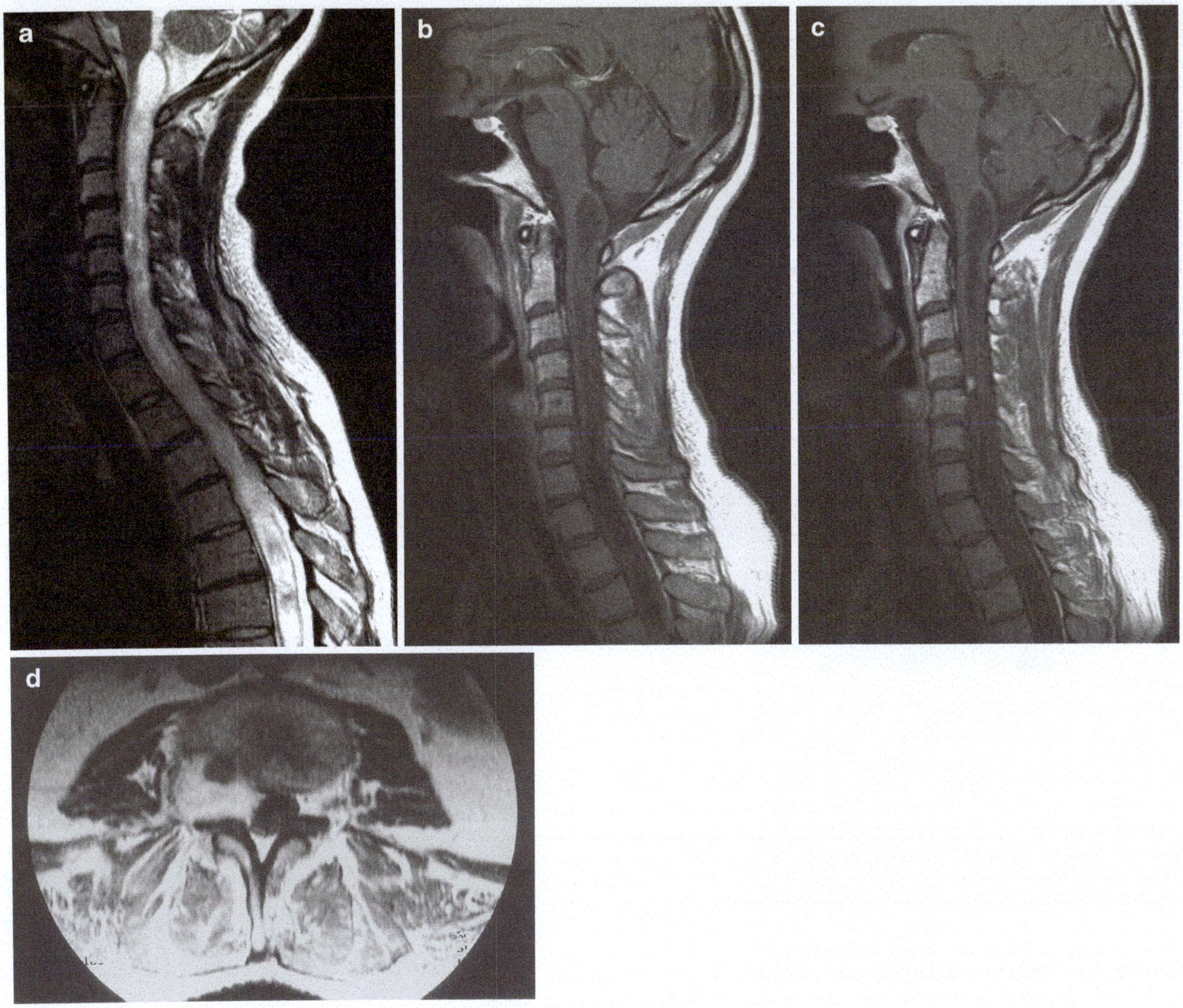

Fig. 3.24 Neurofibroma. In this patient with a neurofibroma in the lumbar region, sagittal T2-WI (**a**), sagittal T1-WI (**b**), and gadolinium-enhanced sagittal (**c**) and axial (**d**) T1-WI were performed. Scalloping of the vertebral bodies and widening of the neural foramen are typical in nerve sheath tumors. The high signal on T2-WI reflects the high water content of the tumor. Enhancement is usually homogeneous, although central fibrous portions may enhance less intensely. Tumors extending through the neural foramen are typically dumbbell-shaped, as in this case (**d**)

thoracic cord and conus medullaris, where they are usually of the myxopapillary type. Clinically, patients with ependymomas more often present with back or neck pain and sometimes radicular pain, but bladder dysfunction and gait problems are also encountered. These lesions also show cord enlargement and tend to be more centrally located than cord astrocytomas. Cord ependymomas are usually hypointense on T1 and hyperintense on T2, but can be more heterogeneous than astrocytomas due to areas of hemorrhage. Ependymomas show strong enhancement after gadolinium injection (Fig. 3.22).

Finally, spinal hemangioblastomas are less common than the two other types of intramedullary tumors. One out of three patients with spinal hemangioblastomas have von Hippel-Lindau syndrome. Spinal hemangioblastomas typically have associated cyst formation and substantial cord edema. Strong enhancement of the tumor nidus after gadolinium injection is always seen in these tumors (Fig. 3.23).

3.3.5.2 Intraspinal Extramedullary Tumors

Two types of tumors are frequently encountered: neurinoma (Figs. 3.24 and, 3.25) and meningioma (Fig. 3.26).

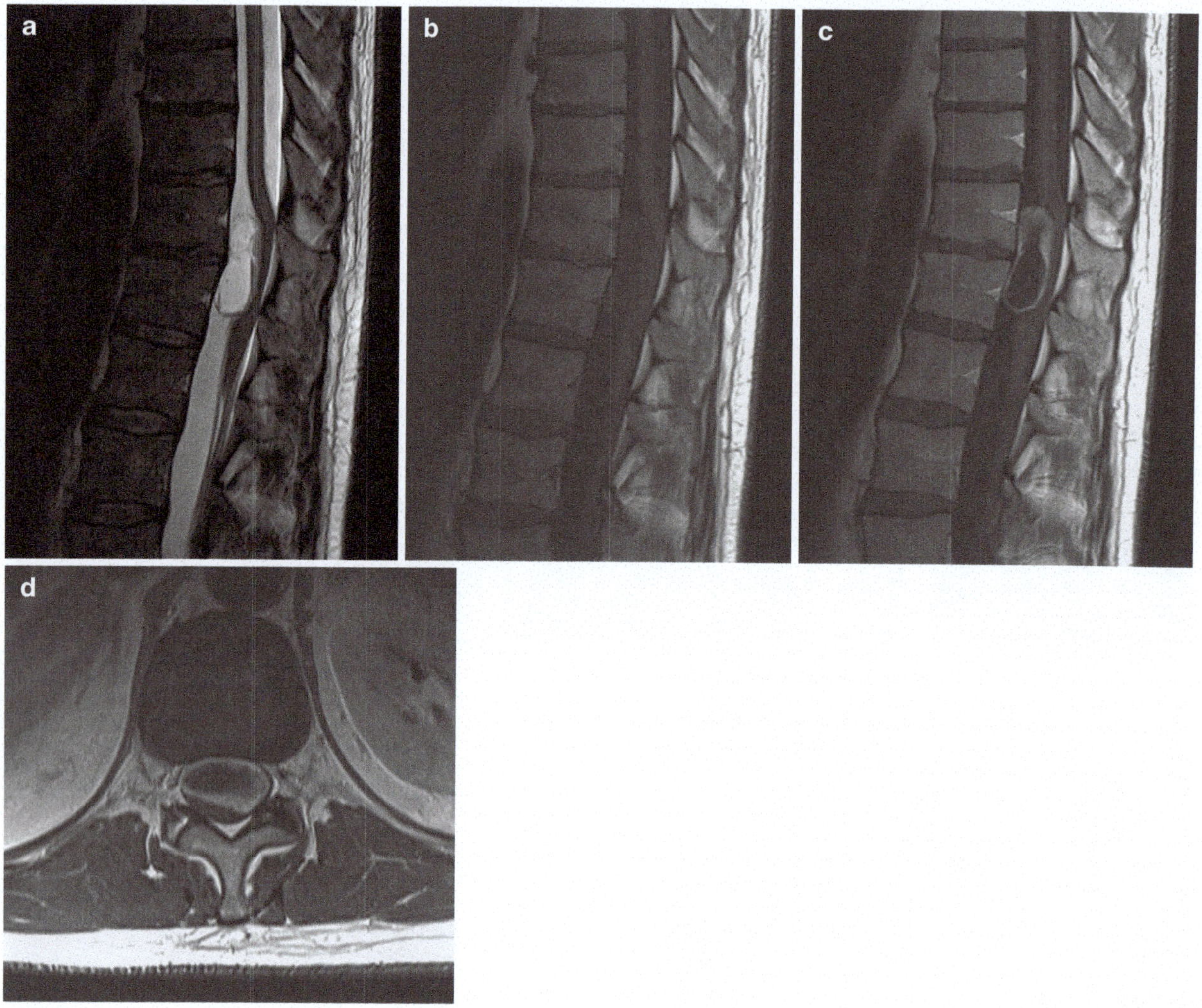

Fig. 3.25 Intradural schwannoma (neurinoma). In this patient with a large schwannoma at the lower thoracic cord, sagittal T2-WI (**a**), sagittal T1-WI (**b**) and both sagittal (**c**) and axial T1-WI (**d**) with gadolinium enhancement were obtained. Schwannomas cannot reliably be distinguished from neurofibromas on imaging findings alone. Therefore, it is sometimes more appropriate to call these nerve sheath tumors before final pathological diagnosis

Neurinoma, neurofibroma, neurolemmoma, and schwannoma are various names for tumors that arise from Schwann cells or nerve sheaths. Schwannoma, neurinoma, and neurolemmoma are synonyms. Usually, neurinomas (Fig. 3.25) do not envelop the adjacent, dorsal sensory root, while neurofibromas (Fig. 3.24) surround the nerve and are mostly associated with neurofibromatosis, even when single. Nerve sheath tumors are the most frequent intraspinal tumors, and they have a peak incidence around the fourth decade. Patients usually present with radicular pain. These lesions are most often markedly hyperintense on T2-WI, and iso- to hyperintense on T1-WI. After gadolinium injection, there is homogeneous tumor enhancement.

Spinal meningiomas tend to be encapsulated and are attached to the dura. They do not invade the spinal cord, but displace it. They are usually anterior in the cervical region and posterolateral in the thoracic region. Only 3% of spinal meningiomas occur in the lumbar region. Most patients are women, with a peak incidence in the sixth decade. Generally, patients

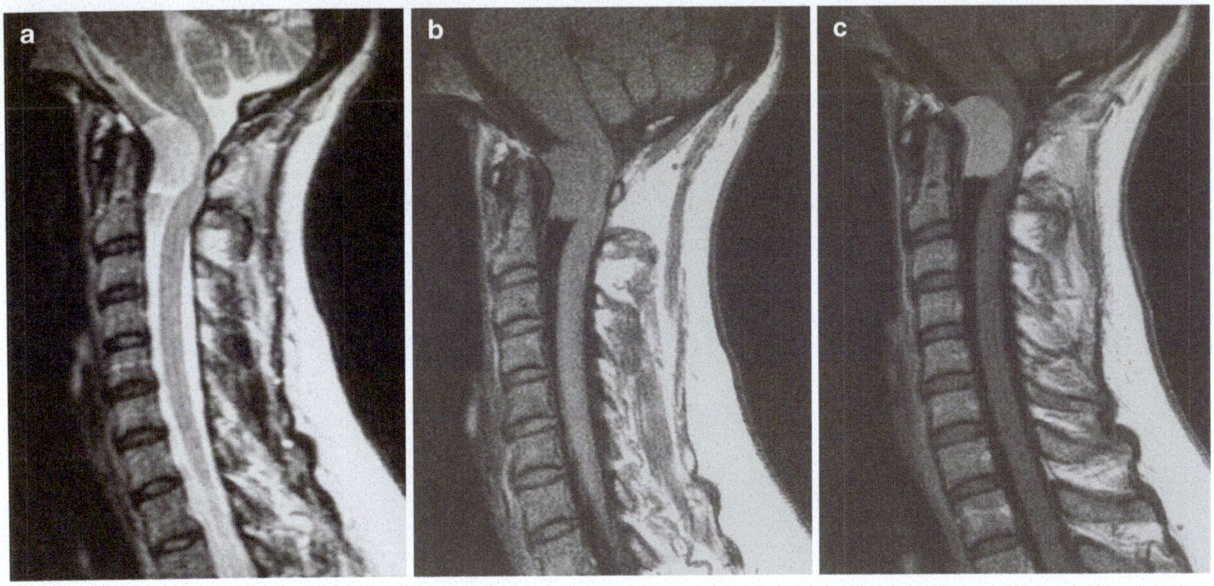

Fig. 3.26 Intradural extramedullary meningioma. In this 65-year-old woman with a meningioma near the craniocervical junction, the following imaging sequences are shown: sagittal T2-WI (**a**), sagittal T1-WI (**b**), and gadolinium-enhanced sagittal T1-WI (**c**). From 60 to 80% of meningiomas are seen in middle-aged to elderly women. The average age at presentation is in the fifth and sixth decades. The lesions are hypo- to isointense to the spinal cord on T1-WI (**b**) and slightly hyperintense on T2-WI (**a**). Intense and homogeneous enhancement is typical (**c**), and the presence of a dural tail indicates the dural-based nature of the tumor

present with radicular, neck, or back pain. Meningiomas are hypo- to isointense on T1-WI, iso- to hyperintense on T2-WI, and show intense, homogeneous contrast enhancement.

Acknowledgments I would like to thank Bavo Van Riet, Paul Parizel, Geert Van Hoorde, and Chris Goris for their collaboration.

Further Reading

Modic MT, Steirnberg PM, Ross JS et al (1988) Degenerative disk disease: assessment of changes in vertebral body marrow with MR imaging. Radiology 166:193–199

Osborn AG, Ross J, Crim J (2008) Expert Differential Diagnoses: Brain and Spine. Amirsys, p 1000, ISBN 1931884021/9781931884020

Ross J, Brant-Zawadzki M, Chen M, Moore K, Salzman K (2004) Diagnostic imaging: spine. Amirsys, Salt Lake City, p 992. ISBN 978-0721628806

Van Goethem JWM, van den Hauwe L, Parizel PM (eds) (2007) Spinal imaging: diagnostic imaging of the spine and spinal cord. Springer, Berlin, p 602. ISBN 978-3-540-21344-4

Magnetic Resonance Imaging of the Head and Neck

4

Bert De Foer, Bernard Pilet, Jan W. Casselman, and Luc van den Hauwe

Contents

B. De Foer (✉)
Department of Radiology, AZ Sint–Augustinus Hospital, Oosterveldlaan 24, 2610 Wilrijk, Belgium
e-mail: bert.defoer@GZA.be

4.1 General Imaging Principles

In order to detect pathology in the head and neck region, one should always try to achieve imaging with the highest possible detail. For this, imaging with a high matrix of up to 512 × 512 is necessary. This can however be very time consuming and may result in images with an insufficient signal-to-noise ratio (SNR). There are several methods to overcome these drawbacks.

The use of small phased-array surface coils inside the head or neck coil is one of them. These surface coils can be placed on the region of interest and will provide a much better SNR. Usually commercially available surface coils of 7 or 8 cm diameter are used. A drawback of these small surface coils is that, on the midline, one is often confronted with a reduced signal due to the limited depth of penetration of the signal of these coils. This is a relative drawback, however, as the SNR in the small structures of larynx and neck will still be sufficiently high. In temporal bone imaging, signal in the temporal bones located off centre will also be highly accurate for a detailed temporal bone examination.

The evaluation of the brain and/or neck can be performed using a multi-channel head and/or neck coil.

Moreover, the use of phased-array coils also makes the use of parallel imaging techniques possible. The use of a two element phased-array coil will enable us to reduce the imaging time by 50%, using a parallel imaging factor, *R*, of maximum 2. The maximum imaging factor is equal to the number of coil elements.

Precautions should be taken when using these small surface coils. There must always be an isolating material covering the coil. The coils must never touch each other, and connection cables must be placed parallel to the long axis of the tunnel.

P. Reimer et al. (eds.), *Clinical MR Imaging*,
DOI: 10.1007/978-3-540-74504-4_ 4, © Springer-Verlag Berlin Heidelberg 2010

4.1.1 Temporal Bone

4.1.1.1 Introduction

The external and middle ear are best examined with computed tomography (CT). There are, however, a growing number of indications for the evaluation of the middle ear using magnetic resonance imaging (MRI). One of the most important indications for MR examination of the middle ear is acquired middle ear and/or congenital cholesteatoma. MR clearly has an additional value in complicated acquired middle ear cholesteatoma with suspicion of complications, such as infection, fistulisation through the lateral semicircular canal and disruption of the tegmen. MR and more specific non-echo planar imaging (non-EPI)-based diffusion-weighted imaging (DWI) is far superior to CT for the evaluation of the post-operative ear to exclude residual or recurrent cholesteatoma.

In patients presenting with sensorineural hearing loss (SNHL), vertigo and tinnitus, one must evaluate the inner ear, the internal auditory canal (IAC), the cerebellopontine angle (CPA) and the auditory/vestibular pathways in the brain and brainstem. Only MRI is able to visualise all these structures and detect a sufficient amount of pathology in these patients. MRI has also become the method of choice in the detection and characterisation of lesions of the petrous apex (cholesterol granuloma, congenital cholesteatoma) and in the diagnosis of meningo(encephalo)celes in case of defects in the tegmen of the middle ear.

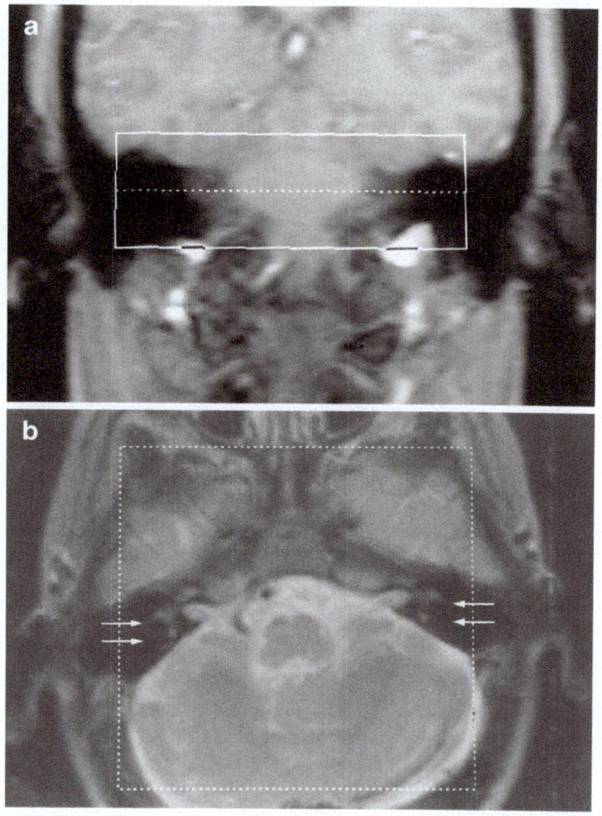

Fig. 4.1 Positioning and orientation of the T2-weighted (T2-W) gradient echo (GRE) or turbo spin-echo (TSE) slab on the coronal scout view (**a**) and a transverse spin-echo T2-weighted image (T2-WI) (**b**). The internal auditory canal is not always easy to visualise on the thick and blurred coronal scout views. However, the complete inner ear is included in the study if the slab covers the inferior border of the temporal lobes and reaches the level of the jugular foramen and hypo-glossal canal inferiorly. The slab can be angulated to correct for skull or positioning asymmetries (**a**). Transverse T2-WI or T1-WI can be used to verify whether the small field of view (FoV) TSE/GRE slab is correctly positioned so that both lateral semicircular canals (*arrows*) are included in the study (**b**)

4.1.1.2 Coils and Patient Positioning

Patients are examined in the supine position with the head firmly fixed in the head coil. Axial images should be centred on the superior border of the external auditory canal. Multiple coronal localisers may be required to correct for imperfect positioning (head tilting) or intrinsic asymmetries of the skull (Fig. 4.1). We prefer the use of a multi-channel head coil together with two small surface coils inside the multi-channel head coil. By doing so, the membranous labyrinth and IAC can be evaluated using the small coils, and the evaluation of midline structures and the brain can be done using the multi-channel head coil. Evaluation of the entire brain is mandatory when performing MRI in patients presenting with SNHL, vertigo and tinnitus. The use of small surface coils inside the head coil averts the need for changing coils during the examination. Precautions should be taken while using these small coils inside the head coil (cfr supra).

Before positioning the patient in the magnet, hearing aids should be removed. Most cochlear implants are incompatible with MRI. In general, modern prostheses used for ossiculoplasty are not a contraindication for MRI.

4.1.1.3 Sequence Protocol

1. In almost all indications for a temporal bone MRI, a routine T2-weighted (T2-W) brain study, with axial scans from the base of the skull to the vertex, should be performed in order to exclude a central cause of SNHL or vertigo (Fig. 4.2).
2. Axial un-enhanced spin-echo (SE) T1-weighted images (T1-WI) are needed to detect intrinsically hyper-intense lesions, such as schwannoma, lipoma, blood (trauma), cholesterol granuloma or fluid with a high protein concentration. Without these images, it becomes impossible to differentiate enhancement from spontaneous hyper-intensities on the gadolinium (Gd)-enhanced T1-WI. An alternative solution is to not acquire un-enhanced images routinely to save time and to re-examine the patient the next day, whenever intra-labyrinthine enhancement or high signal is found (about 2% of all cases).
3. A Gd-enhanced T1-W sequence provides the most sensitive images for detecting pathology in the membranous labyrinth, IAC and CPA (Figs. 4.3–4.5). It is, therefore, obligatory to obtain this sequence. Intravenous (i.v.) administration of 0.1 mmol/kg of Gd is sufficient. The axial Gd-enhanced images must be obtained in the same positions (table positions) as the pre-contrast images so that comparison is possible. Slice thickness of the pre- and post-contrast T1-WI should not exceed 3 mm; 2-mm thin slices are considered state of the art. Slices should be contiguous, i.e. there should be no interslice gap. The same technique should be applied for coronal images, which can be helpful to confirm doubtful or subtle pathology. As an alternative, a 3D gradient echo (GRE) T1-W sequence with a thickness of 1 mm or less can be used. By doing so, a maximum number of slices through the IAC and membranous labyrinth can be acquired. When searching for a cholesteatoma, a late (45 min) post-gadolinium T1-W sequence can be helpful for detection of the cholesteatoma (Fig. 4.6).
4. T1-WI with fat suppression are particularly useful in the post-operative patient to separate residual/recurrent schwannoma from high signal fatty material used by the surgeon to fill up the created defect in case of a translabyrinthine approach. On Gd-enhanced T1-WI, both have a high signal intensity and can be difficult to differentiate.
5. Heavily T2-WI, usually turbo spin-echo (TSE) T2-WI or GRE T2-WI are required to evaluate the very small structures of the CPA, the four nerve branches in the IAC and the fluid inside the membranous labyrinth (Figs. 4.4 and 4.7). It is important to obtain the GRE images prior to the administration of Gd to avoid Gd-intensified flow artefacts. When possible, 0.4–0.7-mm thick slices should be used; slice thickness should not exceed 1 mm. The slab becomes thinner when sub-millimetric images are used, and hence, positioning becomes critical in the coronal plane. High-resolution imaging can be achieved with a 512 × 512 matrix at the expense of increasing the acquisition time and decreasing the SNR. Alternatively, we prefer to use a very small field of view (FoV) of 10 cm with a 256 matrix, which provides a similar in-plane spatial resolution, but without increasing the acquisition time. In most patients, both inner ears will just fit in a FoV of 10 cm, but accurate positioning is crucial, and it is best to use the thin-section axial un-enhanced T1-WI or T2-WI to check whether the TSE/GRE slab also covers the outer borders of the lateral semicircular canals. Only these heavily T2-WI can discriminate high signal intra-labyrinthine fluid from low signal intra-labyrinthine fibrosis or tumour.

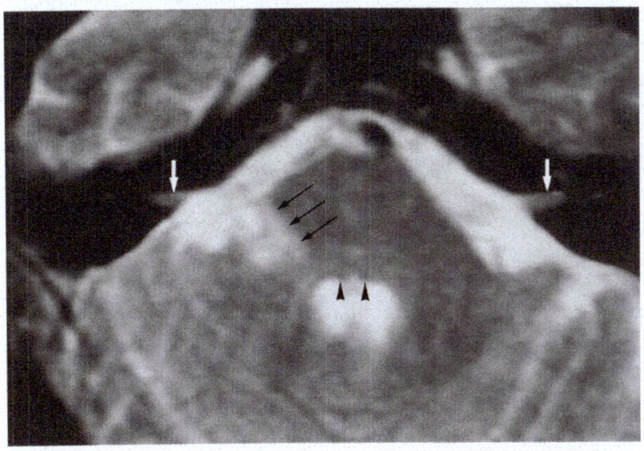

Fig. 4.2 Brainstem infarction. Thin SE T2-WI of the brainstem in a patient with acute SNHL on the right side. A high signal intensity (SI) infarction (*black arrows*) can be seen at the level of the right cochlear nucleus in the lower pons. Notice also the low SI of the myelinated medial longitudinal fasciculus on both sides (*arrowheads*). The IAC is also recognizable (*white arrows*)

In acoustic neuroma surgery, these T2-WI will allow us to determine the type of surgery to be performed. If fluid is still present between the schwannoma and the fundus

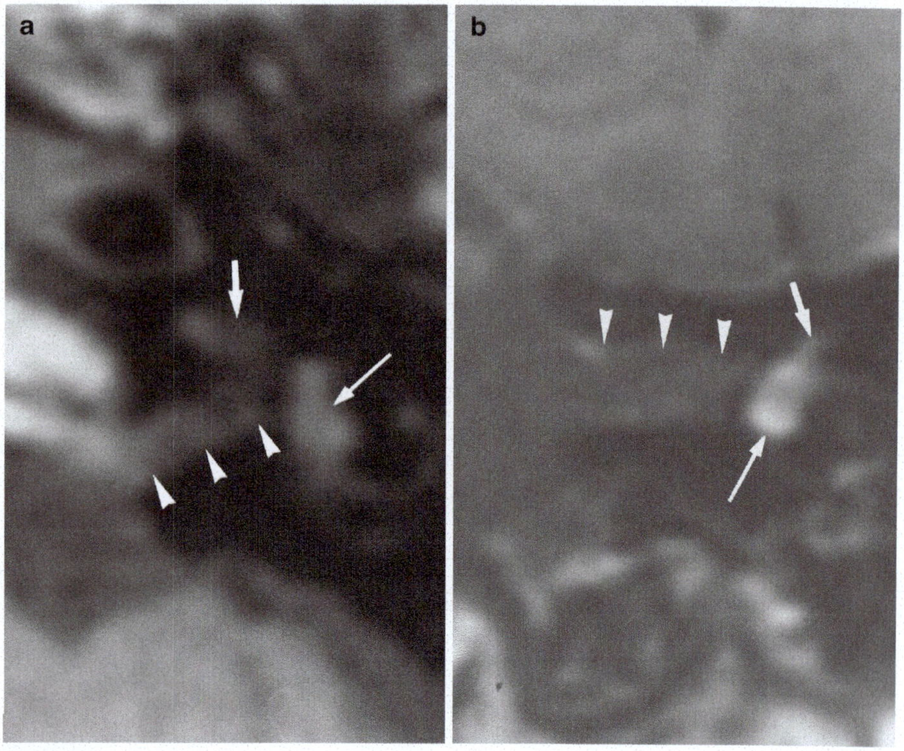

Fig. 4.3 Labyrinthitis. Transverse un-enhanced (**a**) and coronal gadolinium (Gd)-enhanced (**b**) SE T1-WI through the left membranous labyrinth in a patient with labyrinthitis. A spontaneous high SI is seen in the vestibule (*long white arrow*) and represents intra-labyrinthine fluid with a high protein concentration or fluid mixed with blood (**a**). The posterior wall of the IAC (*arrowheads*) and the cochlea (*small white arrow*) are seen. On the Gd-enhanced image (**b**), enhancement is observed in the vestibule (*long white arrow*) and superior semicircular canal (*small white arrow*). The roof of the IAC is indicated by *arrowheads*. The GRE T2-WI (not shown) demonstrated the presence of fluid throughout the left membranous labyrinth

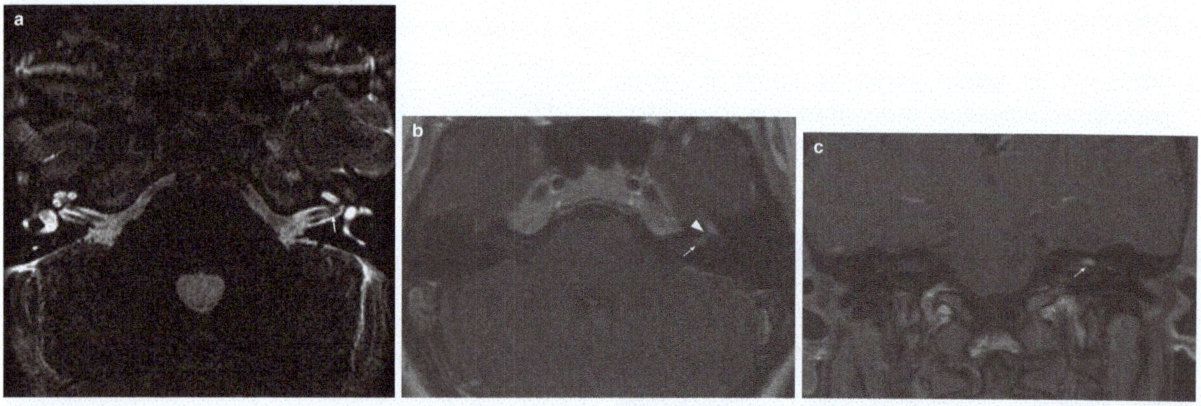

Fig. 4.4 Facial nerve neuritis in a patient with sudden onset of facial nerve palsy. Axial 0.8 mm 3D TSE T2-W (**a**), axial (**b**) and coronal (**c**) 2-mm thick T1-W MR images. All images were acquired through the IAC. On the axial 0.8-mm thick 3D TSE T2-WI (**a**) the right IAC shows a slice at the level of the cochlear nerve and the inferior vestibular nerve. Due to a slight asymmetric position of the head of the patient, the level of the slice at the left IAC is situated higher than on the right side. On the left side, the facial nerve can be seen anteriorly in the IAC and the superior vestibular branch posteriorly in the IAC. Note that there is a nodular thickening anteriorly in the left IAC situated at the level of the fundus of the IAC (*arrow*) (**a**). This corresponds to a nodular enhancing lesion in the fundus of the IAC on the axial post-gadolinium T1-WI (*small arrow*) (**b**). The labyrinthine segment of the facial nerve also enhances on the left side (*arrowhead*) (**b**) and the geniculate ganglion also enhances strongly compared to the right side. Enhancement of the facial nerve in the fundus of the IAC and/or enhancement of its labyrinthine segment is always to be considered as pathological. Enhancement of the tympanic segment is considered normal due to the surrounding venous plexus. The coronal T1-W post-gadolinium image (**c**) demonstrates the nodular enhancing lesion located superiorly in the IAC (*arrow*). The fact that the enhancement is situated superiorly and anteriorly in the IAC confirms that pathology is situated in the facial nerve. The nodular aspect of the lesion is explained by the fact that the narrowest segment of the entire course of the facial nerve is situated in the fundus of the IAC, before entering the temporal bone with the labyrinthine segment. The facial nerve neuritis causes oedema and a retrograde swelling of the nerve just before this most narrow segment, causing the swelling of the nerve in the IAC, as well on the 3D TSE T2-W sequence as on the post-gadolinium T1-WI. A control examination performed 6 months later (not shown) demonstrated a normal sized nerve without any enhancement. This case demonstrates that facial neuritis can appear as a pseudo-tumoral thickening of the nerve. Tumoural thickening of the nerve due to a schwannoma will persist over time

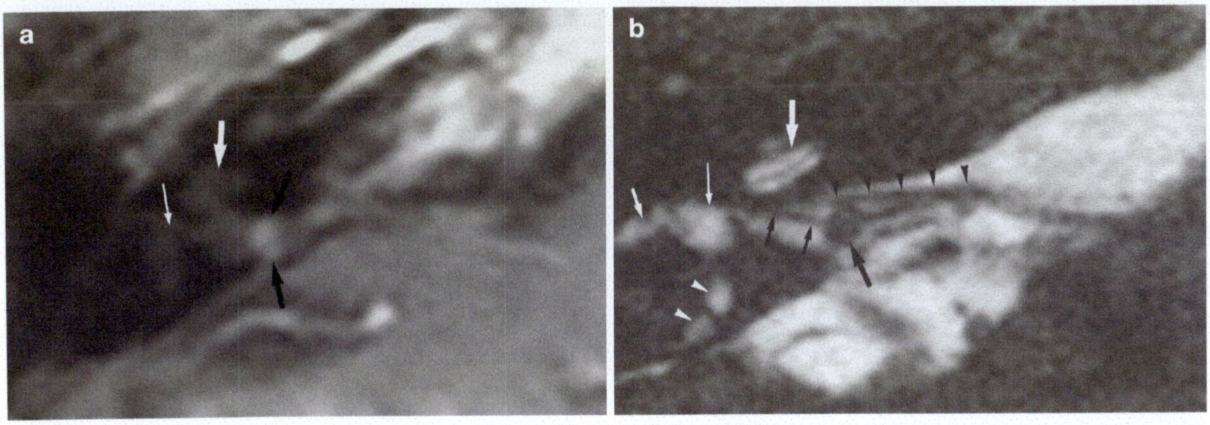

Fig. 4.5 Acoustic schwannoma. Transverse 2-mm thick Gd-enhanced T1-WI (**a**) and 0.7-mm thick GRE T2-WI (**b**) in a patient with a schwannoma of the superior vestibular branch of the vestibulo-cochlear nerve. A nodular enhancing lesion (*black arrows*) can be seen in the IAC, but it is impossible to further define the exact position of the lesion on this image (**a**). The cochlea (*thick white arrow*) and vestibule (*thin white arrow*) are noticed. On the thin-section GRE T2-WI (**b**), the facial nerve (*black arrowheads*) can be recognised anteriorly in the IAC. A nodular lesion (*large black arrow*) can be seen in the course of the vestibular branch of the vestibulo-cochlear nerve (*small black arrows*). Notice the cochlea with separate visualisation of the scala tympani and scala vestibuli (*large white arrow*), the vestibule (*long white arrow*), the lateral (*small white arrow*) and posterior (*white arrowheads*) semicircular canals

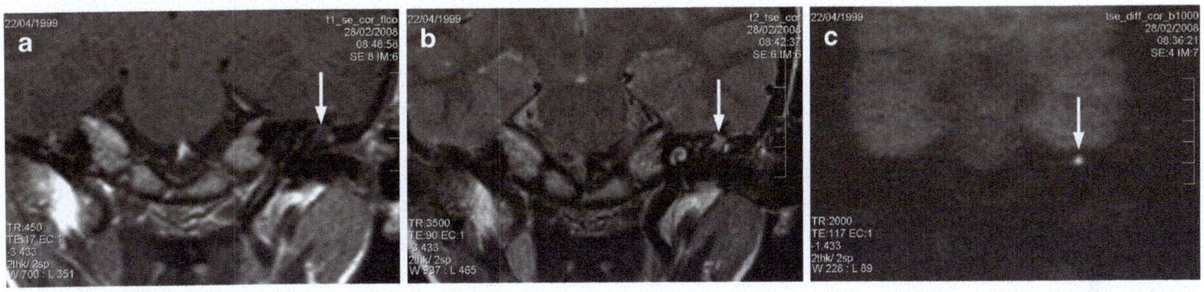

Fig. 4.6 5 year-old boy evaluated prior to second look surgery looking for residual cholesteatoma. Coronal (**a**) late (45 min) post-gadolinium SE T1-WI, coronal TSE T2-WI (**b**) and coronal single-shot TSE DWI (**c**). The cholesteatoma is seen on this image, acquired through the cochlea, as a moderately intense nodular lesion in the epitympanum, underneath the tegmen (*arrow*) (**b**). Note that the SI of the cholesteatoma is comparable to the SI of the grey matter in the adjacent temporal lobe. On late post-gadolinium SE T1-WIs (**a**), the cholesteatoma is seen as a hypo-intense nodular lesion with peripheral enhancement (*arrow*). The non-EPI (single-shot TSE) DWI clearly shows the cholesteatoma as a nodular high SI lesion (*arrow*) in the signal void of the left temporal bone (**c**). MR demonstration of a small residual epitympanal cholesteatoma prior to second look surgery. Residual cholesteatoma was confirmed at surgery

of the ICA, hearing preservation surgery (middle cranial fossa or retrosigmoid approach) is possible. If no fluid is observed, the surgeon has to remove all the tissue up to the base of the cochlea, leaving the patient deaf. In these patients, a less invasive translabyrinthine approach is performed. An even more important sign is the signal intensity of the cerebrospinal fluid (CSF) between the schwannoma and the fundus of the ICA and the signal intensity of the intra-labyrinthine fluid. Hearing preservation is achieved four times more often when a normal signal intensity of these fluids is observed (Fig. 4.8).

6. To detect vascular malformations and neurovascular conflicts, 1-mm (or submillimetre) thick, high-resolution, 3D time of flight (ToF) MR angiography (MRA) images should be used, with and without i.v. gadolinium administration. This sequence should be routinely added to the imaging protocol in patients with pulsatile tinnitus as a major complaint (Figs. 4.9 and 4.10).
7. Selective, 4-mm thick, SE T2-WI of the brainstem (axial) and auditory cortex (coronal) are used when more subtle pathology along the auditory/vestibular pathway is suspected (Fig. 4.2). They should always be added in case of vertigo.
8. DWI has gained growing importance for the detection and diagnosis of acquired or congenital middle ear

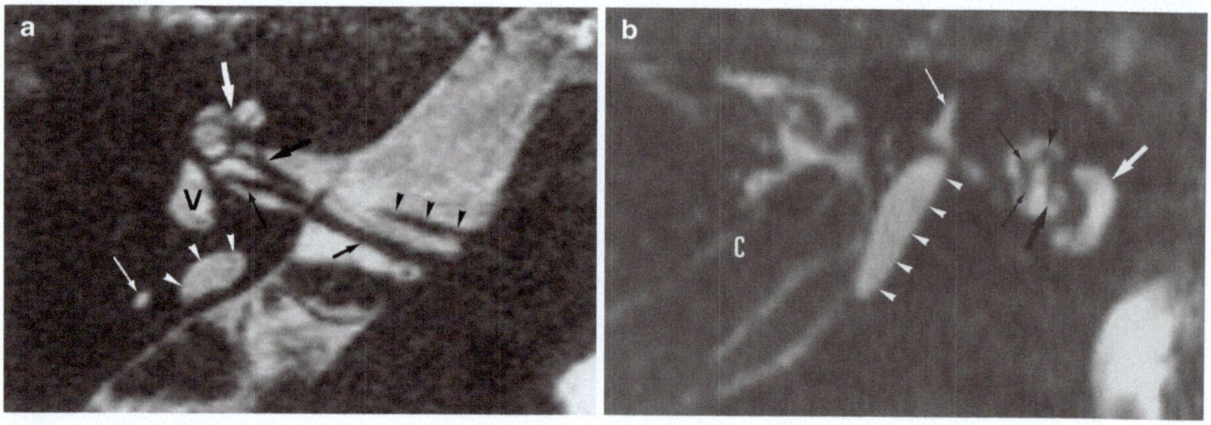

Fig. 4.7 Large vestibular aqueduct syndrome. Transverse 0.7-mm thick GRE T2-WI (**a**) and a parasagittal reconstruction (**b**) of the right membranous labyrinth, made from these transverse 0.7-mm thick images, in a patient with a large endolymphatic duct and sac (large vestibular aqueduct syndrome). The patient was referred for MR evaluation of SNHL. An enlarged, fluid-filled endolymphatic sac can be recognised (*white arrowheads*). The sac is abnormal when its diameter is larger than the diameter of the fluid-filled posterior semicircular canal (*long white arrow*). Fluid-filled vestibule (*V*) and cochlea with separate visualisation of the two scalas (*large white arrow*). Facial nerve (*black arrowheads*), common trunk of the vestibulo-cochlear nerve (*small black arrow*) and its more peripheral cochlear (*large black arrow*) and inferior vestibular (*long black arrow*) branches (**a**). The enlarged, fluid-filled endolymphatic sac (*white arrowheads*) can be followed from the labyrinth to the anterior border of the cerebellum (*C*). Fluid-filled superior semicircular canal (*long white arrow*) and cochlea (*large white arrow*). Facial nerve (*black arrowhead*), cochlear branch (*large black arrow*) and vestibular branches (*long black arrows*) of the vestibulo-cochlear nerve, surrounded by CSF in the fundus of the IAC (**b**)

cholesteatoma. Non-EPI DWI sequences should be preferred over EPI DWI because of their higher spatial resolution, slightly thinner slices and a lower susceptibility to artefacts. Non-EPI DWI sequences are usually single-shot or multi-shot TSE sequences. 2-mm thick (matrix 134 × 192) non-EPI DWI sequences should be performed in the coronal plane (Fig. 4.6).

For an overview of the imaging protocols, see Tables 4.1–4.3.

4.1.1.4 Pathology

The most frequent pathology of the inner ear is the schwannoma. These tumours can be found in the labyrinth, IAC (Figs. 4.5, 4.8 and 4.11) and CPA (Figs. 4.8 and 4.11). The second most frequent pathology in the membranous labyrinth is acute/chronic labyrinthitis (Fig. 4.3). Other frequently found lesions causing SNHL, vertigo, tinnitus or a combination of these clinical signs include labyrinthine malformations (Fig. 4.7) and other types of CPA tumours such as meningiomas or epidermoids (Fig. 4.12), neurovascular conflicts (Fig. 4.9), brainstem infarctions (Fig. 4.2) or demyelination, vascular tumours (Fig. 4.13), and vascular malformations (Fig. 4.10), etc.

MRI has become indispensable in the workup of these patients. MRI has also become indispensable in patients who are candidates for cochlear implant surgery, as only the heavily T2-WI can inform the surgeon whether the cochlea is filled with fluid and a normal cochlear branch of the vestibulo-cochlear nerve is present. Other associated pathologies can be excluded.

MRI is also the method of choice for the detection of post-operative meningo(encephalo)coeles in patients with defects of the tegmen (Fig. 4.14).

MRI - including late post-gadolinium T1-WI and non-EPI DWI - is gaining importance in the evaluation of (chronic) middle ear pathology, as well as for acquired middle ear cholesteatoma, the congenital cholesteatoma and the evaluation of the pre-second look residual cholesteatoma (Fig. 4.6). Especially in the evaluation of post-operative cholesteatoma, MRI, including late post-gadolinium T1-WI and non-EPI DWI, is highly superior to CT and even EPI DWI for the detection of the post-operative residual or recurrent cholesteatoma. Non-EPI DWI should be the examination of choice in the evaluation of pre-second look residual cholesteatomas.

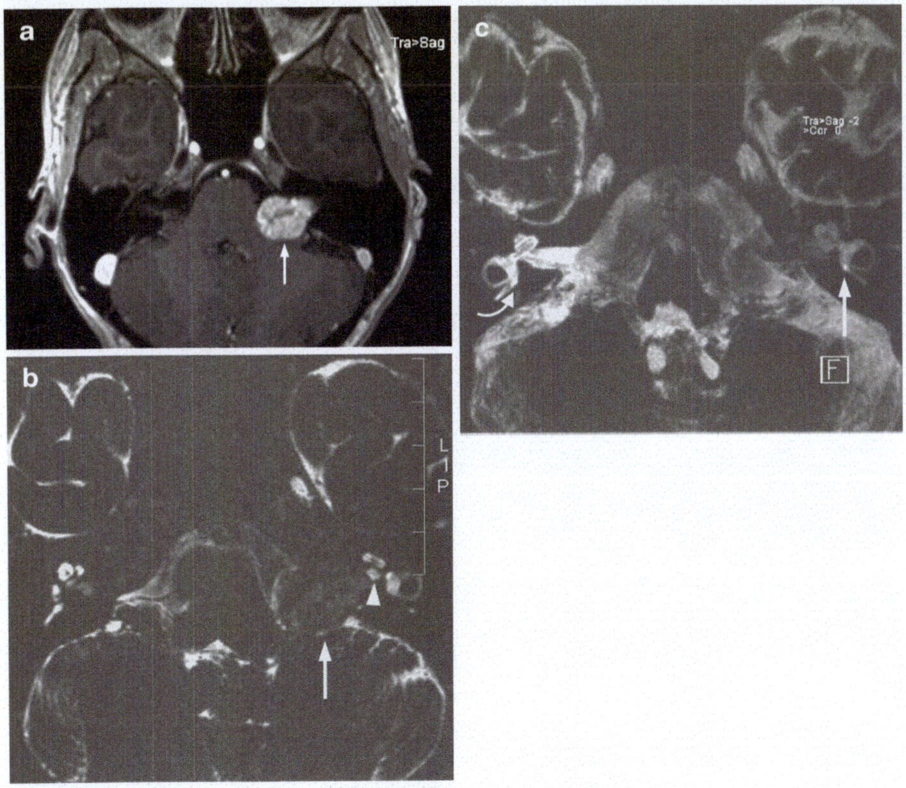

Fig. 4.8 Large vestibulo-cochlear schwannoma in the IAC and CPA. Axial reformation of a 1-mm thick 3D GRE T1-W sequence (**a**), axial 0.4 mm 3D TSE T2-W sequence (**b**) and MIP reconstruction of the 3D thin slice T2-W sequence (**c**). The schwannoma is seen as a large nodular enhancing mass lesion (*arrow*) in the IAC, protruding in the CPA, with compression of the left middle cerebellar peduncle (**a**). On the axial 3D TSE T2-W sequence (**b**) the tumour replaces the signal of CSF in the CPA and IAC (*arrow*). Note that there is still a little amount of fluid in the fundus of the IAC (*arrowhead*): this is considered a positive predictive sign for hearing preservation surgery. The MIP reconstruction (**c**) of the 0.4 mm 3D TSE T2-W dataset clearly demonstrates a signal drop in the membranous labyrinth on the left side (*arrow*) compared to the normal right side (*curved arrow*). This is considered a negative predictive sign for hearing preservation surgery

4.1.2 Eye and Orbit

4.1.2.1 Introduction

CT scanning still plays an important role in the diagnosis of orbital pathology. The differences in attenuation values of the orbital contents (retrobulbar fat, extrinsic muscles, globe, bone, air and vessels) provide an excellent natural tissue contrast. However, MRI is the modality of choice when available. The major advantage of MRI over CT is that the entire visual pathway can be examined in one go with higher sensitivity and specificity. In this manner, MRI not only detects orbital lesions, but is also able to demonstrate a wide range of intra-cranial pathology associated with visual impairment [parasellar lesions, multiple sclerosis (MS) plaques]. At present, CT still remains the imaging modality of choice in the following circumstances: detection of calcifications, traumatic lesions, primary lesions arising from the bony orbit, or non-availability of MRI. Fat-suppressed images allow better discrimination between enhancing structures located within the retrobulbar fat (Fig. 4.15).

4.1.2.2 Coils and Patient Positioning

Prior to performing MRI of the eye and orbit, patients must be screened in order to rule out the presence of

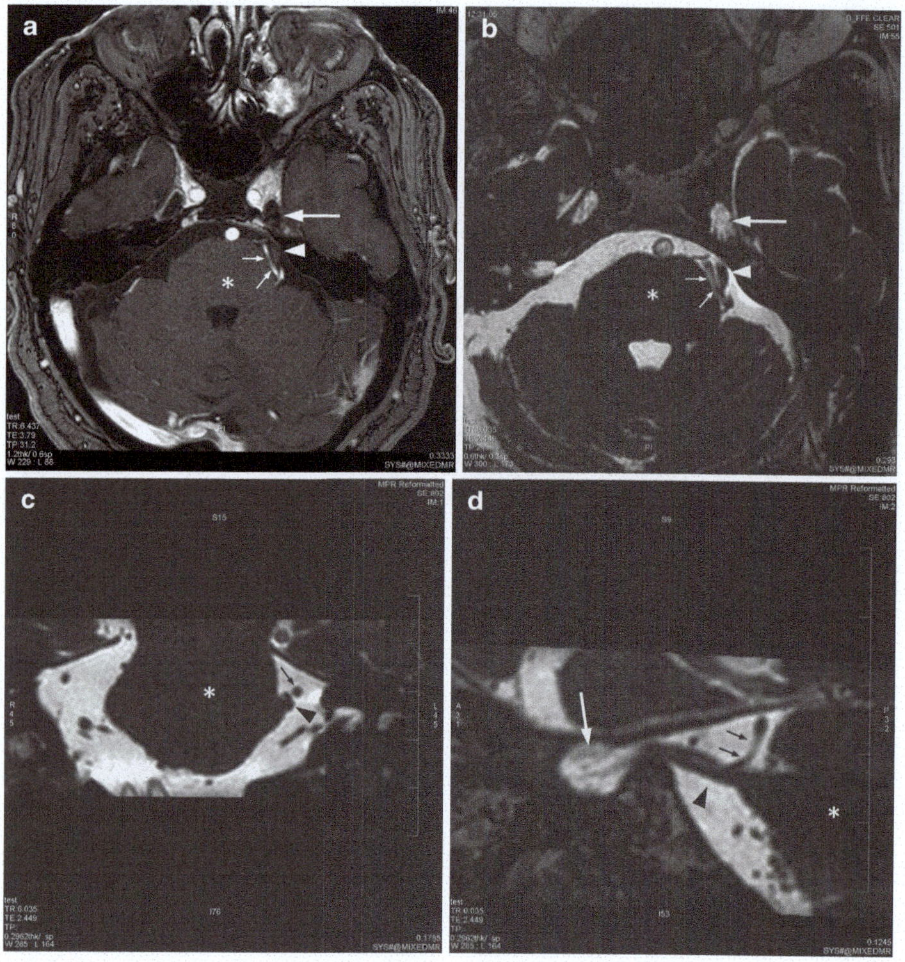

Fig. 4.9 Neurovascular compression syndrome. Neurovascular conflict of the left superior cerebellar artery with the left trigeminal nerve. Axial 1.2-mm thick 3D T1-WI (**a**), axial (**b**), coronal (**c**) and sagittal (**d**) 3D T2-W sequence at the level of the left trigeminal nerve. The axial very thin T1-W sequence (**a**) after i.v. injection of gadolinium demonstrates the superior cerebellar artery (*small arrows*) crossing the nerve root entry zone (*arrowhead*) of the left trigeminal nerve, coming from the brainstem (*asterisk*) and running towards Meckel's cave. The corresponding thin heavily T2-WI (**b**) shows the hypo-intense vascular structure of the left superior cerebellar artery (*small white arrows*) crossing the nerve root entry zone of the left trigeminal nerve (*arrowhead*). Note the fluid in Meckel's cave (*arrow*). On the coronal T2-WI (**c**), the superior cerebellar artery (*small black arrow*) approaching the nerve root entry zone (*arrowhead*) of the left trigeminal nerve, near its origin at the brain stem (*asterisk*) can be seen. The sagittal plane of the T2-W sequence (**d**) clearly shows the superior cerebellar artery (*small black arrows*) making a loop towards the left trigeminal nerve (*arrowhead*) causing a slight depression of the left trigeminal nerve. Note the branches of the trigeminal nerve in Meckel's cave (*arrow*) and the posteriorly located brain stem

metallic foreign bodies in or near the orbit, e.g. metallic slivers, fragments, or iron dust in industrial workers. These objects can move under the influence of the magnetic field, with blindness as a possible consequence. Therefore, thorough questioning of the patient is necessary. When in doubt, conventional X-rays should be obtained before placing patients in the magnet. Patients are asked to remove their mascara since it may contain ferromagnetic components, causing image degradation due to susceptibility artefacts. It is important to encourage the patient to fix his or her gaze on one point during the examination to avoid motion artefacts, which might arise during blinking.

The MR examination of the orbit can best be performed using the combination of a multi-channel head coil and small binocular surface coils. Ultrathin slices with a high spatial resolution can thus be obtained. This is useful to examine the globe for the presence of tumours (Fig. 4.16). A disadvantage of surface coils is that only the anterior portion of the

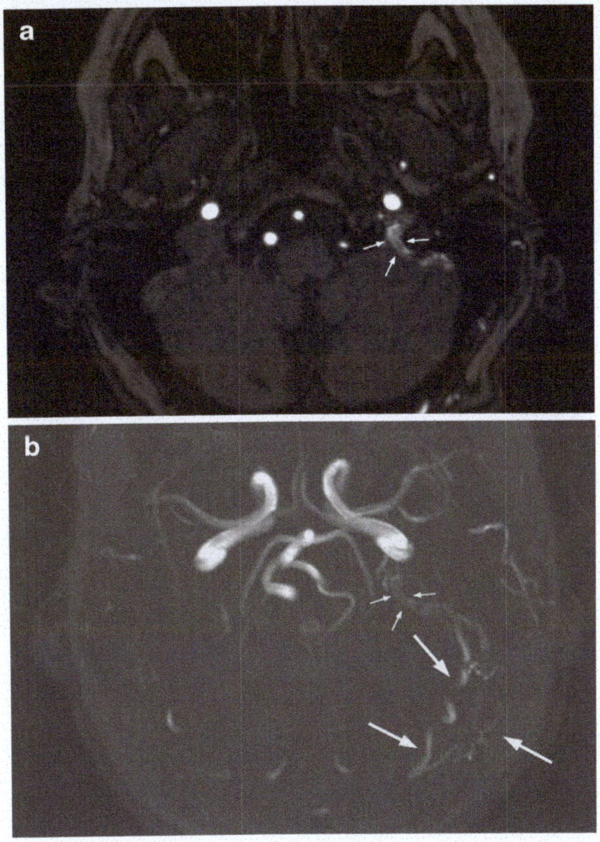

Fig. 4.10 Dural arterio-venous (AV) fistula in a patient with acute onset of a left sided pulsatile tinnitus. There was no prior trauma reported. Axial image of a 0.6 mm 512 matrix 3D ToF MRA (**a**) and subsequent MIP reconstruction (**b**). Un-enhanced 3D ToF MRA demonstrates high signal in high velocity vessels or arteries at the skull base (**a**). In this patient, the 3D ToF MRA shows a normal carotid and vertebro-basilar circulation, best seen on the MIP reconstruction (**b**). However, serpiginous high signals can be found in the left sigmoid sinus and jugular bulb (*arrows*) (**a**). This high signal demonstrates a high flow status in the left sigmoid sinus and jugular bulb caused by a transcranial dural AV-fistula (*arrows*), best seen on MIP reconstruction (**b**). The MIP reconstruction not only shows the high flow in the jugular bulb on the left side (*small arrows*), but also the serpiginous transcranial vessels coming from the external carotid artery, causing the AV-fistula (*large arrows*)

orbit is depicted (the globe), leaving the remainder of the orbit and the optic pathway un-examined. The deeper parts of the orbit and the optic pathway can be evaluated using the multi-channel head coil.

4.1.2.3 Sequence Protocol

To reduce motion artefacts, the scanning time should be kept as short as possible. This can be achieved by reducing the repetition time (TR) and/or the number of excitations (NEX). Thin slices (maximum thickness of 3 mm) and a small FoV are combined to optimise spatial resolution. For the MR protocol for imaging of the orbit and visual pathway, see Table 4.4.

1. High-resolution SE T1-W semi-axial or coronal imaging sequences are performed as the initial screening sequence. Both slice orientations allow comparison of both orbits. The semi-axial slices are oriented along the course of the optic nerve.
2. TSE T2-W and fat-suppressed sequences are added when a lesion is seen, and further characterisation is required. Fat suppression is necessary to subdue the bright signal arising from the retrobulbar fat. This causes chemical-shift misregistration artefacts at fat-water interfaces (the margins of the globe), and furthermore, the bright signal of the retrobulbar fat may overwhelm small structures of intermediate to low signal intensity (the use of fat suppression is mandatory for lesion demonstration in the optic nerve, e.g. optic neuritis). Fat suppression can be obtained by frequency-selective spectral pre-saturation or short tau inversion recovery (STIR) techniques.
3. Gd-enhanced SE T1-WI with fat suppression may be required for further differentiation of tumours, optic nerve lesions and orbital masses. After intravenous injection of Gd, spectral fat saturation is the technique of choice (Fig. 4.15). STIR sequences should be avoided for post-contrast MRI, because the fat signal as well as the signal arising from enhancing structures will be suppressed. This phenomenon is known as negative enhancement.
4. GRE sequences are of limited use, but may detect changes in susceptibility in the presence of calcifications (retinoblastoma) or haemorrhage.

4.1.2.4 Pathology

Major indications for MRI of the eye and orbit include tumours (Tables 4.5 and 4.6) such as uveal melanoma (Fig. 4.16), retinoblastoma, optic nerve glioma, optic nerve sheath meningioma (Fig. 4.17), haemangioma (Fig. 4.18) and metastases (Fig. 4.19). Also, inflammatory lesions of the orbit, e.g. idiopathic inflammatory pseudo-tumour (Fig. 4.15) and inflammatory lesions of the optic nerve (Fig. 4.20), may be demonstrated. Lesions that arise outside the orbit and interfere with

Table 4.1 Magnetic resonance imaging protocol recommendations for temporal bone examinations

Pulse sequence	WI	Plane	No. of sections	TR (ms)	TE (ms)	Flip angle	Echo train length	Section thickness (mm)	Matrix	FoV	recFoV	BW	No. of acq.	Acq. time (min:s)
TSE T2 cholestea-toma	T2	Cor	12	3,500	90	180	20	2	256 × 256	200	75	129	2	2:25
3D GRE T1	T1	Tra	160	1,900	3.37	15	–	1	180 × 256	256	75	130	1	3.55
3D TSE T2	T2	Tra	48	1,500	302	170	9	0.4	448 × 448	200	50	189	1	6.21
SE T1 cholestea-toma	T1	Tra/cor	12	400	17	90	–	2	256 × 256	200	75	130	2	3:24
3D ToF MOTSA	–	Tra	44	39	7	25	–	0.6	256 × 256	180	100	100	1	5:12
SS TSE DWI ($b = 0$, 1,000)	DWI	Cor	12	2,000	117	180	–	2	134 × 192	220	100	401	10	4:02
TSE T2 (brain)	T2	Tra	20	4,710	108	180	24	5	403 × 448	230	75	130	2	3:52
TSE T2 (brainstem)	T2/PD	Tra	16	3,000	14/81	180	48	4	256 × 256	230	56.3	130	3	7:17

WI weighted image; *TR* repetition time (ms); *TI* inversion time (ms); *TE* echo time (ms); matrix (phase × frequency matrix); *FoV* field of view (mm); *recFoV%* rectangular field of view; *BW* bandwidth (Hz)

Table 4.2 Overview of imaging protocols for sensorineural hearing loss, vertigo and tinnitus

SNHL	Vertigo	Tinnitus
Axial T2-W brain	Axial T2-W brain	Axial T2-W brain
Axial un-enhanced T1-WIs	T2-W brain stem sequence	*Axial un-enhanced T1-WIs*
Thin 3D T2-W TSE sequence	Thin 3D T2-W TSE sequence	Thin 3D T2-W TSE sequence
Axial + coronal Gd-enhanced T1-W or Gd-enhanced 3D GRE T1-W sequence	Axial + coronal Gd-enhanced T1-W or Gd-enhanced 3D GRE T1-W sequence	Un-enhanced and Gd-enhanced 3D ToF MOTSA MRA
		Axial + coronal Gd-enhanced T1-W or Gd-enhanced 3D GRE T1-W sequence

Italics: optional sequence, can be omitted. *Gd* gadolinium; *GRE* gradient echo; *TSE* turbo spin echo

Table 4.3 Imaging protocol for cholesteatoma evaluation. All sequences are centred over both temporal bones. Entire examination is performed 45 min after Gd administration

Cholesteatoma
Coronal TSE T2-W
Axial SE T1-W
Coronal SE T1-W
Thin 3D T2-W TSE sequence
SS TSE DWI sequence

Gd gadolinium; *TSE* turbo spin echo; *SS* single shot; *DWI* diffusion-weighted imaging; *SE* spin echo

the function of the optic pathways can be seen, e.g. pituitary macro-adenoma (Fig. 4.21).

4.1.3 Paranasal Sinuses

4.1.3.1 Introduction

CT and MRI are complementary techniques in imaging of the paranasal sinuses. The bony structures surrounding the air-filled sinus cavities are better seen on CT. Therefore, CT is the preferred imaging modality in trauma patients. Moreover, CT is superior in demonstrating the ostiomeatal complex, which occupies a key position in inflammatory/infectious disease, especially when functional endoscopic sinus surgery (FESS) is planned. The use of MRI is advocated in patients with complicated inflammatory sinus disease and in those with suspected tumoural pathology in this region.

4.1.3.2 Coils and Patient Positioning

The patient is placed in a supine position in the multichannel head coil with the head firmly fixed.

4.1.3.3 Sequence Protocol

1. The MR examination of the paranasal sinuses starts with coronal un-enhanced SE T1-WI and TSE T2-WI. The purpose of these sequences is to discriminate between different soft-tissue structures and retention of serous and mucinous fluid.
2. Contrast-enhanced, high-resolution, axial and coronal SE T1-WI are obtained to further differentiate soft-tissue structures, thereby allowing discrimination between tumoural components from normally enhancing mucosa or polyps (Fig. 4.22). Also, intra-cranial and/or intra-orbital extension of pathology can be better demonstrated (Fig. 4.23).

For the MRI protocol for sinonasal examinations, see Table 4.7.

4.1.3.4 Pathology

Complications of inflammatory sinus diseases, such as mucocoele (Fig. 4.24), brain abscess or sub-dural empyema, cavernous sinus thrombosis, meningitis, etc., are much better demonstrated on MRI than on CT. MRI is indicated to demonstrate the exact extent of tumoural lesions and discriminate them from normal mucosa and secondary retention of fluid, whereas on CT, only opacification of the sinuses will be seen. Tumoural lesions (Table 4.8) include both benign (inverted papilloma, juvenile angiofibroma, fibro-osseous lesions, etc.) (Fig. 4.22) and malignant lesions [squamous cell carcinoma (SCCA), adenocarcinoma,

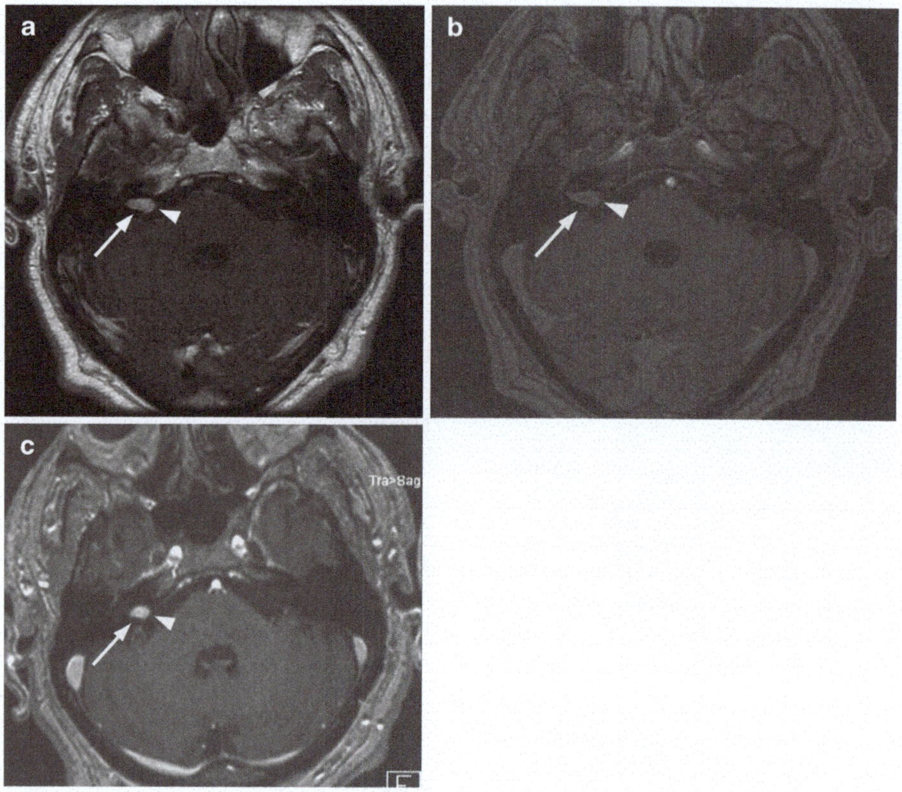

Fig. 4.11 Vestibulo-cochlear schwannoma in the IAC with volume loss over several years. Axial reformation of a 1-mm thick 3D GRE T1-W sequence (**a**), axial reformation of a 3D ToF MRA after gadolinium administration (**b**) and axial 2-mm thick T1-W MR image (**c**). Images acquired in the same patient in 2003 (**a**), 2004 (**b**) and 2005 (**c**). About 50–60% of all vestibulocochlear schwannomas in the IAC and CPA show no growth at all. About 40–50% of schwannomas demonstrate growth over time. It is extremely rare to have a schwannoma showing a loss of volume over time, as demonstrated in this patient, best seen at the component of the tumour protruding in the CPA (*arrowheads*)

adenoid cystic carcinoma, lymphoma, esthesioneuroblastoma, etc.] (Fig. 4.23). Aspergillus infection of the maxillary sinuses gives a very peculiar signal intensity (Fig. 4.25). It presents with a characteristic low signal on T2-WI. Interpretation based on T2-WI alone can therefore lead to a misdiagnosis of air in the sinus.

4.1.4 Skull Base

4.1.4.1 Introduction

The bony structures of the skull base are easier to recognise on CT. However, lesions of the skull base can also involve the extra-cranial and intra-cranial soft tissues, the nerves and vessels in the skull base foramina and the bone marrow. MRI provides adequate contrast and spatial resolution to distinguish all these structures, and has therefore become the method of choice to study skull-base lesions and cranial nerve involvement. CT is however complementary since the technique provides a better idea of the type of bone lysis or erosion.

4.1.4.2 Coils and Patient Positioning

A multi-channel head coil provides the best images of the skull base. Patients are examined in the supine position, and their head is placed as high as possible in the multi-channel head coil. The closer the skull base is to the centre of the head coil, the better the image quality. Images are made parallel and/or perpendicular to the part of the skull base to be examined.

4.1.4.3 Sequence Protocol

The MR technique will depend on the structures surrounding the region of interest.

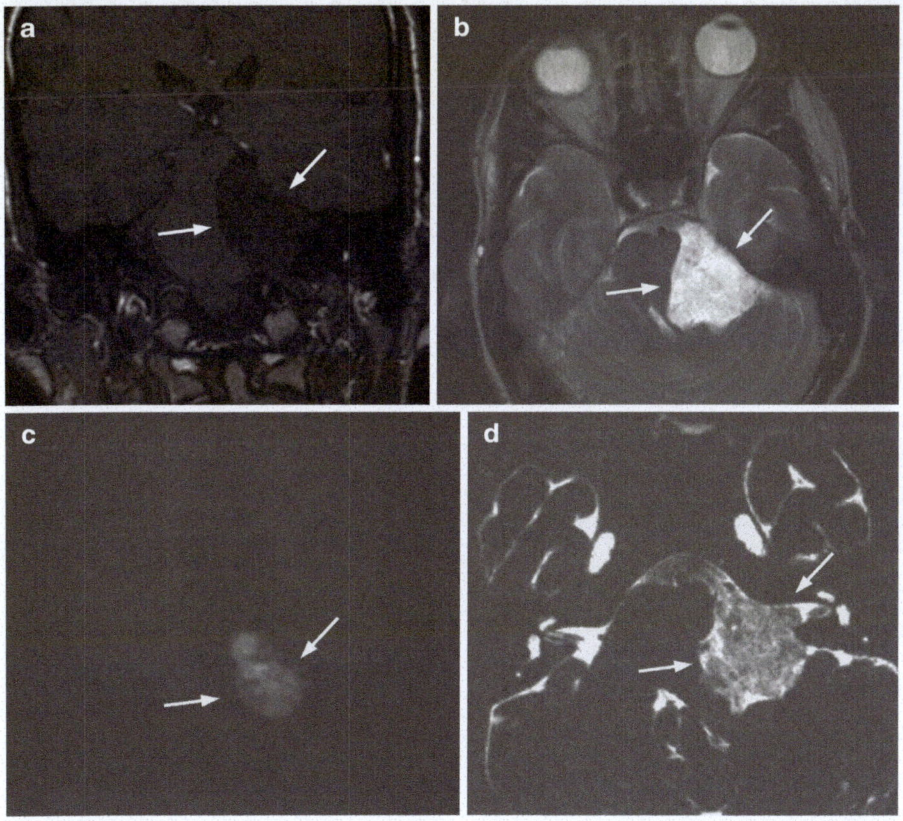

Fig. 4.12 Epidermoid tumour in a young patient with epilepsy. Coronal T1-W sequence (**a**), axial TSE T2-W sequence (**b**), coronal single-shot TSE DWI sequence (**c**), axial 0.4 mm 3D TSE T2-W sequence (**d**). On un-enhanced coronal T1-WI, a nearly iso-intense mass lesion is found in the left CPA compressing the brain stem (*arrows*) (**a**). Note that the SI of the lesion is slightly higher than the signal of CSF in the ventricles. On the corresponding axial T2-WI (**b**), the mass lesion compressing the brain stem and fourth ventricle has a slight hyper-intense aspect compared to the SI of CSF in the fourth ventricle (*arrows*). On non-EPI DWI, the lesion displays high SI (*arrows*) (**c**) without any lesion distortion or artefact as usually seen on the more frequently used EPI DWI sequences. On the axial 0.4-mm thick 3D TSE T2-WI, the lesion demonstrates an inhomogeneous moderate hyper-intensity (*arrows*). The moderate high SI of the lesion in the left CPA has an intensity that is clearly lower than the intensity of the CSF in the right CPA. Characteristic appearance on all sequences of a large epidermoid tumour

1. High-resolution SE or TSE T1-WI are used when cortical bone, soft tissues and nerves surrounded by bone or soft tissues must be visualised. Un-enhanced and enhanced images should be used. On the un-enhanced images, the fatty bone marrow signal should be carefully evaluated (Fig. 4.26).
2. In the central skull base and especially in the posterior skull base, nerves and vessels approach the skull base surrounded by CSF. In these regions, normal nerves and tumour extension along nerves are best seen on transverse GRE or TSE T2-WI. On these images, the tumour/nerves are seen as intermediate to low signal-intensity structures, outlined by high signal-intensity CSF. High resolution and sub-millimetre images are required.
3. Within the skull-base foramina, the nerves, vessels and surrounding bone are best distinguished from one another when high-resolution 3D ToF MRA images are used. These images should be un-enhanced and enhanced so that the venous lakes become hyper-intense and provide a different signal intensity from the nerves and surrounding bone (Fig. 4.27). On the un-enhanced images, the flow status of a tumour lesion can be evaluated. They are of particular use in the case of a suspected glomus tumour, as they nicely demonstrate the high flow in the tumour vessels.
4. Lesion characterisation and screening of the skull base can be performed using high-resolution transverse TSE T2-WI (Fig. 4.27). This sequence can also be used as the first screening sequence in severe pathology.

The parameters of these four routine skull-base sequences are shown in Table 4.9.

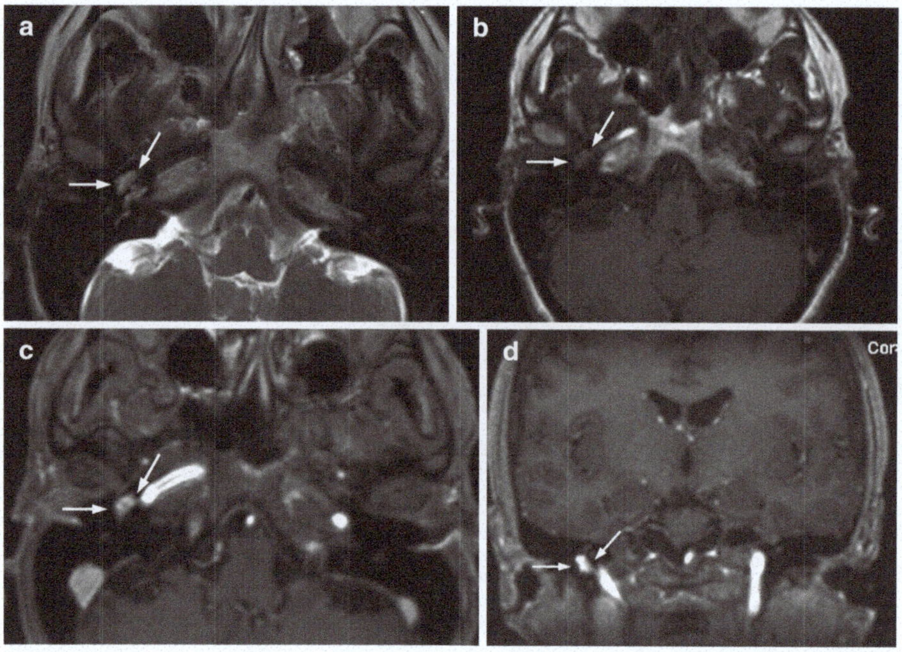

Fig. 4.13 Glomus tympanicum tumour located in the anterior hypo-tympanum, on its characteristic location adjacent to the promontory of the middle ear. Axial T2-WI (**a**), axial un-enhanced T1-WI (**b**), axial and coronal reformation of a gadolinium-enhanced GRE T1-W sequence (**c, d**). A small hyper-intense mass lesion located anterior to the cochlea, located in the anterior part of the hypo-tympanum is noticed (*arrows*) (**a**). The lesion is located adjacent to the promontory, which is the characteristic location of a small glomus tympanicum tumour, originating from the glomus bodies against the promontory. On un-enhanced T1-WI (**b**) it is slightly hyper-intense (*arrows*). The lesion shows very strong enhancement on the post-gadolinium T1-W GRE sequence (*arrows*) (**c, d**). It enhances almost as strong as the adjacent horizontal intra-petrosal segment of the carotid artery. Location, aspect and enhancement pattern are characteristic for a glomus tympanicum tumour

A routine TSE T2-W sequence of the brain should be added in order to exclude central pathology.

Contrast-enhanced, high-resolution T1-WI with fat suppression can be used to detect bone-marrow invasion, and they are sometimes better at distinguishing tumour from normal fat. Un-enhanced SE T1-WI remain the most sensitive images to detect bone-marrow invasion.

4.1.4.4 Pathology

MRI is used in the skull base mainly to evaluate tumour extension (especially along nerves and vessels), detect bone invasion and achieve better tumour characterisation. Tumours can originate intra-cranially in the marrow/cortical bone of the skull base or in the extra-cranial soft tissues. All possible extension routes through neuroforamina should be checked. Inflammatory lesions, congenital malformations, traumatic lesions and all types of cranial nerve pathology may also involve the skull base and be studied by MRI. However, congenital malformations and traumatic lesions are best studied with CT, with some exceptions. The anterior skull base is best studied in the coronal and sagittal planes. Un-enhanced and Gd-enhanced high-resolution SE T1-WI are best suited to study the olfactory bulbs and tracts (trauma patients, congenital anosmia, etc.) and tumours originating in the sinuses or intra-cranially (meningiomas, esthesioneuroblastomas, etc.). Coronal, thin TSE/GRE T2-WI are only required when a CSF leak or meningo(encephalo)coele is suspected. The central skull base, and especially the parasellar region and neuroforamina are best studied in the coronal and transverse planes with high-resolution SE T1-WI. Most of the tumoural lesions and cranial nerve lesions may be studied this way, and when necessary, be further characterised using TSE T2-WI. Transverse MRA images are only used when aneurysms or other vascular pathology is suspected (Fig. 4.27). Transverse TSE/GRE T2-WI are used when posterior extension into the pre-pontine cistern or CPA is present. In the posterior skull base, axial and coronal images perform best. The sagittal plane is only used to study midline lesions of

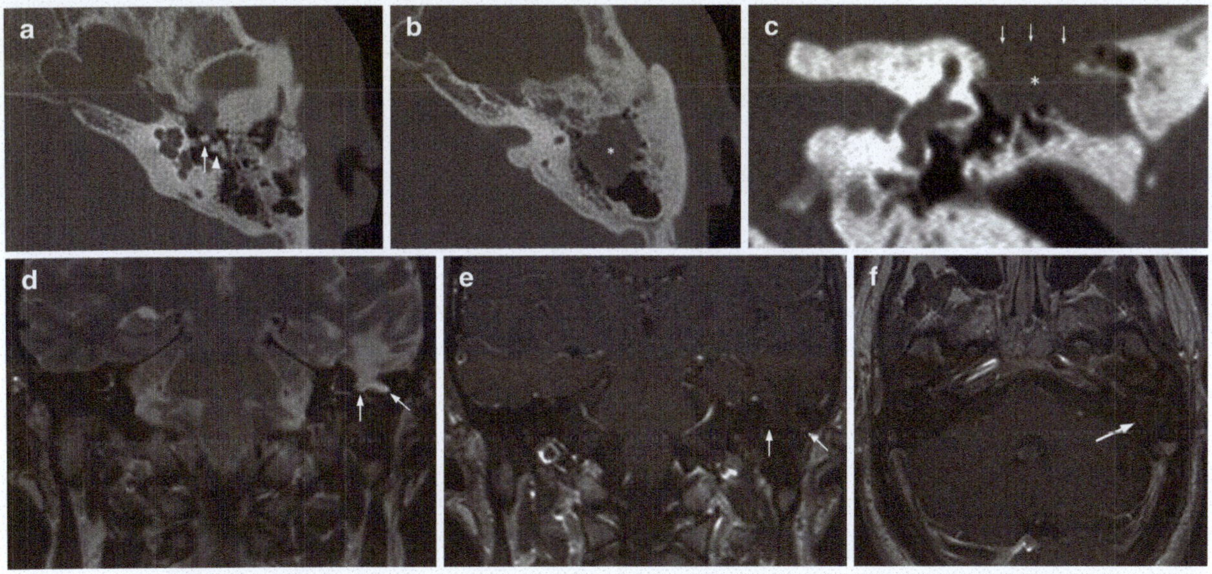

Fig. 4.14 Post-traumatic herniation of a meningocoele through a large defect in the tegmen on the left side. Associated loss of brain tissue in the left temporal lobe. Axial CT image at the level of the incudostapedial joint on the left side (**a**) and at the level of the antrum (**b**). Coronal reformation of a helical CT dataset (**c**). Coronal T2-WI (**d**), coronal (**e**) and axial T1-WI (**f**) after i.v. injection of gadolinium. On the axial CT image at the level of the incudostapedial joint, the separation of the head of the maleus (*small arrow*) from the corpus of the incus (*arrowhead*) is clearly seen (**a**). On an axial slice through the antrum at the level of the superior semicircular canal, a large nodular soft tissue mass lesion can be seen (*asterisk*) (**b**). The coronal reformation clearly demonstrates the loss of delineation of the tegmen (*arrows*) and the protruding soft tissues in the middle ear (*asterisk*) (**c**). The coronal T2-WI (**d**) nicely demonstrates the post-traumatic loss of brain tissue in the left temporal lobe. Note the herniation of the meninges and residual brain tissue (*arrows*) into the signal void of the temporal bone on the left side. The corresponding coronal post-gadolinium T1-WI shows the hypo-intense signal of the CSF herniating through the defect into the middle ear (*arrows*) (**e**). The axial T1-WI through the left middle ear shows the hypo-intense CSF in the middle ear surrounded by the enhancing meninges (*arrows*) (**f**)

the clivus and craniocervical junction (Fig. 4.28). High-resolution T1-WI are used to study tumours and look for enhancing tumoural and inflammatory lesions. Thin, transverse TSE/GRE T2-WI are often used to study the relationship of the lesions to the cranial nerves VI to XII in the cisterns surrounding the lower brainstem. Finally, transverse, high-resolution, Gd-enhanced MRA images are needed when a lesion involves or grows through the jugular foramen (e.g. glomus jugulare tumour) (Fig. 4.27).

4.1.5 Nasopharynx and Surrounding Deep Spaces and Parotid Glands

4.1.5.1 Introduction

The nasopharynx is an anatomic area in the head and neck region, which is difficult to visualise clinically. Moreover, the surrounding deep spaces cannot be examined clinically, and lesions in these spaces become visible only when they become sufficiently large or start to involve surrounding structures, such as nerves, blood vessels, etc. Therefore, high-quality imaging is needed in these anatomical regions. Only MRI is able to consistently provide images with sufficient tissue-contrast resolution and spatial resolution in these regions, and therefore, is the imaging modality of choice.

4.1.5.2 Coils and Patient Positioning

A selective examination of the nasopharynx and surrounding spaces is best performed with a multi-channel head coil. Patients are examined in the supine position with the head positioned as high as possible in the head coil. To obtain high-quality images, the patients should be instructed to avoid motion, swallowing and talking, because it degrades image quality. Breathing through the nose with the mouth closed also reduces motion artefacts.

A dedicated neck coil is used when the complete oral cavity or complete oropharynx must be included,

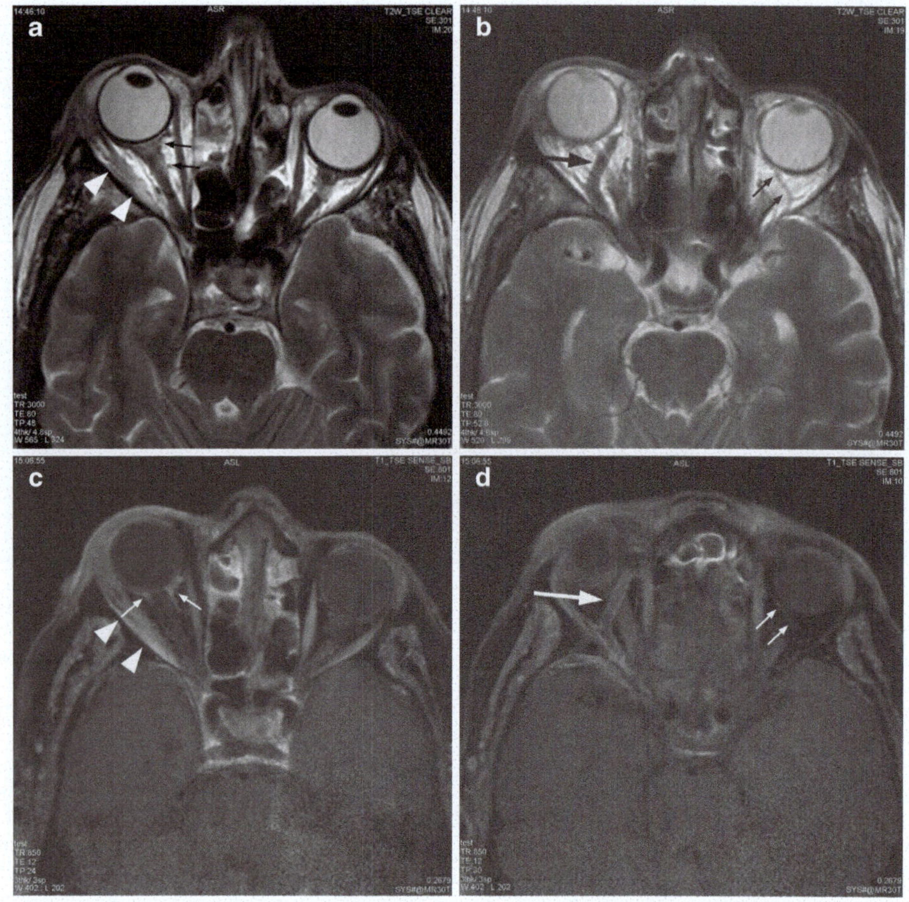

Fig. 4.15 Idiopathic inflammatory pseudo-tumour. Patient with painful proptosis of the right eye caused by an inflammatory pseudo-tumour of the right orbit. There is associated thrombosis of the left superior ophthalmic vein. Axial T2-WI at the level of the optic nerve (**a**) and at the level of the superior ophthalmic vein (**b**). Axial T1-WI with fat suppression after i.v. injection of gadolinium at the level of the optic nerve (**c**) and at the level of the superior ophthalmic vein (**d**). On the axial T2-WI at the level of the optic nerve, there is a marked proptosis of the right eye. There is also thickening of the lateral rectus muscle (*arrowheads*) with also a hyper-intense thickening of the optic nerve sheath (*black arrows*) (**a**). The MR image a few slices higher, at the level of the superior ophthalmic vein, demonstrates a clear asymmetry between both sides. The right superior ophthalmic vein (*black arrow*) is thickened compared to the contralateral superior ophthalmic vein (*small black arrows*) (**b**). There is enhancement of the thickened right lateral rectus muscle (*arrowheads*) on a post-gadolinium T1-WI with fat suppression (**c**). Note also the enhancement of the thickened optic nerve sheath (*arrows*). The thickened and thrombosed superior ophthalmic vein can be noted on the right side (*large arrows*); compare to the normal sized superior ophalmic vein on the left side (*small arrows*) (**d**)

or when a complete staging of the neck lymph nodes is required.

The parotid glands can be examined with surface coils. With these coils, higher spatial resolution can be achieved, but there is a drop in signal intensity from the superficial to the deep part of the gland, and this may result in insufficient visualisation of the deep lobe. Therefore, we prefer a head coil for imaging the parotid glands. In order to increase the spatial resolution, a 512 × 512 matrix is used. Another advantage is that the patient is better fixed in a head coil, and this will result in less motion artefacts. Again, the patient must be positioned as high as possible in the head coil so that the inferior part of the parotid gland can be included in the imaging FoV (Fig. 4.29). The preferred slice orientation for the above-mentioned studies is the axial plane, parallel to the hard palate. A nasopharynx study should start at the superior border of the pituitary fossa in order to exclude intra-cranial extension. The inferior landmark is the inferior border of the mandible; however, the signal is often already insufficient

Table 4.4 Magnetic resonance protocol recommendations for imaging of the orbit and visual pathway

Pulse sequence	WI	Plane	No. of sections	TR (ms)	TE (ms)	Flip angle	TI (ms)	Echo train length	Section thickness (mm)	Matrix	FoV	rec-FoV	BW	No. of acq.	Acq. time (min:s)
SE T1	T1	Tra/cor	16	350	17	90	–	–	2	256 × 512	200	75	130	1	2:47
STIR	T2	Cor/tra	20	9,000	123	180	2,500	–	3	256 × 256	230	75	130	1	3:20
TSE T2	T2	Tra/cor	20	4,710	100	180	–	36	3	288 × 320	160	80	130	1	2:56
SE T1 FS	T1	Tra/cor	16	500	17	90	–	–	3	192 × 192	113	75	130	1	2:30

WI weighted image; *TR* repetition time (ms); *TI* inversion time (ms); *TE* echo time (ms); *TD* time delay (sec); *No of acq* number of acquisition or partitions; matrix (phase × frequency matrix); *FoV* field of view (mm); *recFoV%* rectangular field of view; *BW* bandwidth (Hz)

at this level when a head coil is used. A parotid-gland study starts at the superior border of the external auditory canal and ends at the inferior border of the mandible. When additional coronal slices are used, they are made in a plane perpendicular to the hard palate.

4.1.5.3 Sequence Protocol

The nasopharynx, surrounding deep spaces and parotid glands are best examined in the transverse plane; the MRI protocol for examinations of these regions is shown in Table 4.10.

1. Transverse high-resolution TSE T2-WI can be used as the first sequence. These images have a high contrast and spatial resolution, making them very sensitive for the detection of parotid lesions. Moreover, these images are needed when further tissue characterisation is necessary (Figs. 4.29–4.31). Malignant tumours usually display a lower signal intensity on TSE T2-WI than benign lesions, such as pleomorphic adenomas (compare Figs. 4.29–4.31)
2. The MR examination continues with transverse un-enhanced and Gd-enhanced high-resolution TSE or SE T1-WI. The un-enhanced images are the most sensitive images in the detection of bone marrow involvement, and therefore, can detect early skull-base or mandible invasion. Moreover, they prevent confusion of areas with high signal intensity on T1 images (blood, fat, proteinaceous fluid, etc.) with areas of enhancement. Gd-enhanced T1-WI have a better SNR than the un-enhanced images, and this results in better tumour delineation. The solid and cystic parts of a tumour are also better distinguished on the Gd-enhanced images.
3. Additional coronal and/or sagittal Gd-enhanced T1-WI of a nasopharynx lesion or a lesion of the surrounding spaces or the parotid gland often provide important information about the exact location and extension of the tumour. These are mandatory when the skull base is invaded.
4. Finally, the transverse and coronal Gd-enhanced images can be replaced by similar images with spectral fat suppression. On these images, tumour enhancement can be better distinguished from the surrounding fat. The drawback of fat suppression is that fewer slices are available when the same acquisition time is used. Therefore, the slice thickness should be increased if the complete region must be imaged, or the total acquisition time must be increased. Also, the signal-to-noise ratio is inferior on images with fat suppression.
5. In the evaluation of tumoural pathology, a dynamic 3D GRE T1-W sequence during i.v. gadolinium administration can be used, as tumoural lesions enhance earlier and stronger than normal tissue. This often makes the delineation of the tumour easier, as moreover, these sequences are less prone to motion artefacts which are frequently encountered in patients with head and neck cancer.
6. In the assessment of tumoural pathology, an EPI DWI sequence can be added. In tumoural pathology of the parotid gland, this sequence enables differentiation between malignant and benign tumoural lesions. In patients treated by radio- and chemotherapy, EPI DWI sequences are able to make the differentiation between residual and/or recurrent tumour vs. scar tissue, inflammation and fibrosis. A major drawback of DWI (especially EPI DWI) is its sensitivity to susceptibility artefacts, frequently found in the head and neck region at the various interfaces between air and soft tissues.

Table 4.5 Ocular tumours

Uveal melanoma
Metastasis
Choroidal haemangioma
Retinoblastoma
Astrocytic hamartoma (tuberous sclerosis, neurofibromatosis)
Intra-ocular calcifications

Table 4.6 Orbital tumours

Optic nerve glioma
Optic nerve sheath meningioma
Plexiform neurofibroma
Haemangioma (capillary, cavernous)
Lymphangioma
Lymphoma – pseudo-tumour
Rhabdomyosarcoma
Metastases

4.1.5.4 Pathology

Nasopharynx

About 70% of nasopharynx tumours are SCCAs, while lymphomas account for approximately 20% of lesions. Hence, the differential diagnosis is not the major problem. Rather than differentiating between these two tumours, the main role of MRI in these patients is to delineate the exact extent of the tumour, and this is possible only when 512 × 512 matrix images are used (Fig. 4.32).

Surrounding Spaces

These spaces (pre- and post-styloid parapharyngeal space, retropharyngeal space, pre-vertebral space, masticator space, etc.) contain different anatomical structures and can give rise to different kinds of tumours. The list of possible tumours is long but can be reduced considerably if one can recognise in which space the tumour originates. This is easier when high-resolution images are available because they better show anatomical landmarks of the different spaces, as well as the displacement of the fat of the pre-styloid parapharyngeal space (Fig. 4.30). Lesions originating in different spaces (medial, lateral, posterior to the pre-styloid parapharyngeal space) displace the fat in different directions. The direction of fat displacement indicates the space in which the lesion originates.

Parotid Gland

Most parotid-gland tumours are benign, and up to 80% of the benign tumours are pleomorphic adenomas (Fig. 4.29). The role of MRI is to demonstrate whether the deep lobe is involved and whether the tumour is located near the known course of the main branch of the facial nerve. Aggressive characteristics, suggesting malignant degeneration or the presence of a malignant tumour, can sometimes be seen, but are not always present in the case of malignant tumours.

A frequently encountered malignant tumour is the adenoid cystic carcinoma (Fig. 4.31) which typically has a tendancy of perineural spread along the facial nerve.

One can attempt to visualise the intra-parotid course of the different branches of the facial nerve using surface coils. EPI DWI sequences using ADC maps may be able to differentiate a benign from a malignant parotid-gland lesion (Figs. 4.29 and 4.30).

4.1.6 Oropharynx and Oral Cavity

4.1.6.1 Introduction

CT is frequently used in the staging of oropharynx and oral cavity tumours. Both the local and nodal staging can be performed easily with CT. MRI can also be used as the initial technique, but today MRI is most often performed when additional information concerning local tumour extension or tumour characterisation is required.

4.1.6.2 Coils and Patient Positioning

Dedicated neck coils are necessary when the complete oropharynx and oral cavity must be covered. Images with sufficient SNR at the level of the mandible and under the mandible can be obtained only when such

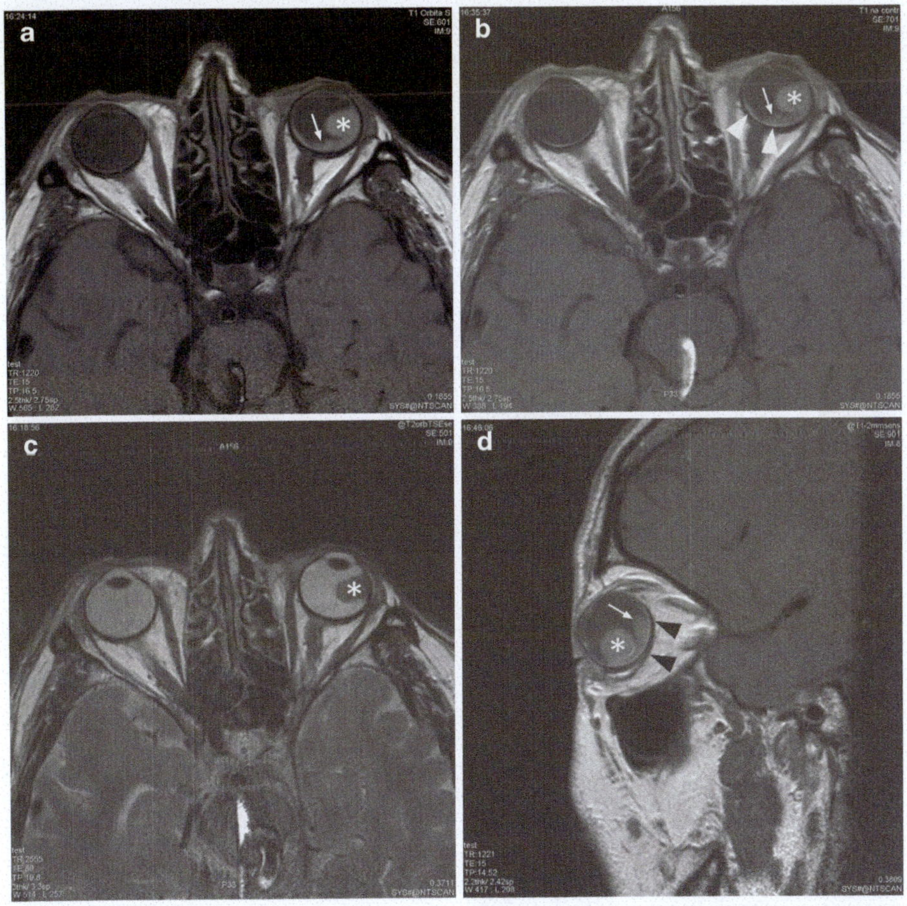

Fig. 4.16 Uveal melanoma. Patient with a malignant melanoma in the left eye with associated sub-retinal haemorrhage. Axial SE T1-WI before (**a**) and after gadolinium administration (**b**). Axial TSE T2-WI (**c**) and sagittal SE T1-WI (**d**) after gadolinium administration. On the axial un-enhanced T1-WI (**a**), there is a nodular tumoural component situated in the temporal side of the left globe (*asterisk*). The spontaneous hyper-intensity is caused by the melanin in the malignant melanoma. The curvilinear spontaneous hyper-intensity posterior in the globe is compatible with associated sub-retinal haemorrhage (*arrow*). On the axial post-gadolinium T1-WI (**b**), the tumour does not seem to enhance due to its already high SI on un-enhanced images (*asterisk*). Note that there is a fine curvilinear enhancement (*arrowheads*) underneath the blood (*arrow*) caused by the enhancing choroidea. On the axial TSE T2-WI (**c**), only the nodular hypo-intense melanoma (caused by the melanin) can be seen (*asterisk*). The sub-retinal haemmorhage cannot be seen as it displays the same SI as the fluid in the globe. The sagittal post-gadolinium T1-WI image (**d**) shows the same three components as the axial image: the nodular melanoma (*asterisk*), the associated sub-retinal haemorrhage (*arrow*) and the enhancing choroidea (*arrowheads*)

dedicated coils are used (Fig. 4.33). Moreover, dedicated neck coils also allow imaging of the lower neck, which is mandatory if simultaneous MR assessment of the lymph nodes is required. On MRI, lymph node staging is much easier in the coronal plane; this is possible with a dedicated neck coil as these coils easily cover the region from the skull base to the upper mediastinum. Patients are examined in the supine position. They are instructed not to move, swallow or talk during the examination, and they are also asked to close their mouths and breathe quietly through their noses. Images are made parallel and/or perpendicular to the floor of the mouth or inferior border of the mandible. In the oropharynx, images are made in the axial plane; coronal images are optional. In the oral cavity, at least one sequence should be made in the coronal plane, preferably a fat-suppressed, high-resolution, Gd-enhanced SE T1-W sequence.

4.1.6.3 Sequence Protocol

1. The examination starts with a transverse TSE T2-WI sequence, covering the complete region of interest. These images are very sensitive in the detection of

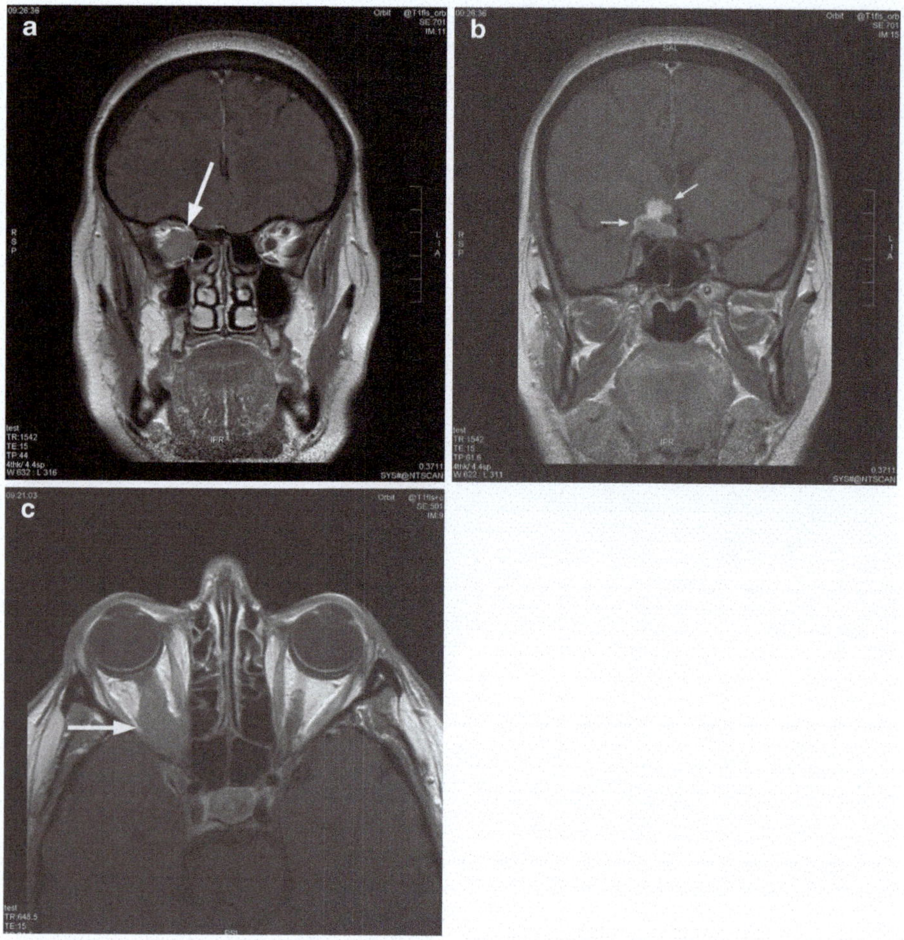

Fig. 4.17 Optic nerve sheath meningeoma. Patient with progressive loss of vision on the right side and a slight proptosis. Coronal post-gadolinium T1-WI at the level of the optic nerve (**a**) and at the level of the clinoid process (**b**). Axial gadolinium-enhanced T1-WI (**c**). There is a diffuse thickening of the optic nerve caused by a large optic nerve sheath meningeoma (*arrows*) (**a**, **c**). There is extension of the meningeoma to the parasellar region with a mass lesion surmounting the anterior clinoid process (*arrow*) (**b**)

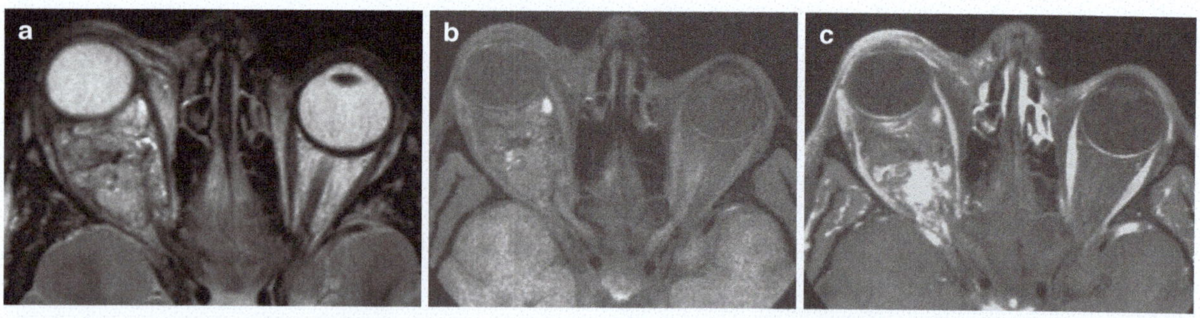

Fig. 4.18 Intra-conal cavernous haemangioma of the right orbit. Transverse turbo TSE T2-WI (**a**), transverse SE T1-WI with spectral fat saturation before (**b**) and after (**c**) Gd injection in a 27-year-old man presenting with proptosis of the right eye. A heterogeneous, lobulated, retrobulbar mass of the right orbit is observed. On T2-WI, the lesion is markedly hyperintense (**a**). The lesion contains areas of high signal intensity on T1-WI (**b**) that may represent areas of thrombosed vascular spaces. Cavernous haemangiomas always enhance after Gd injection (**c**)

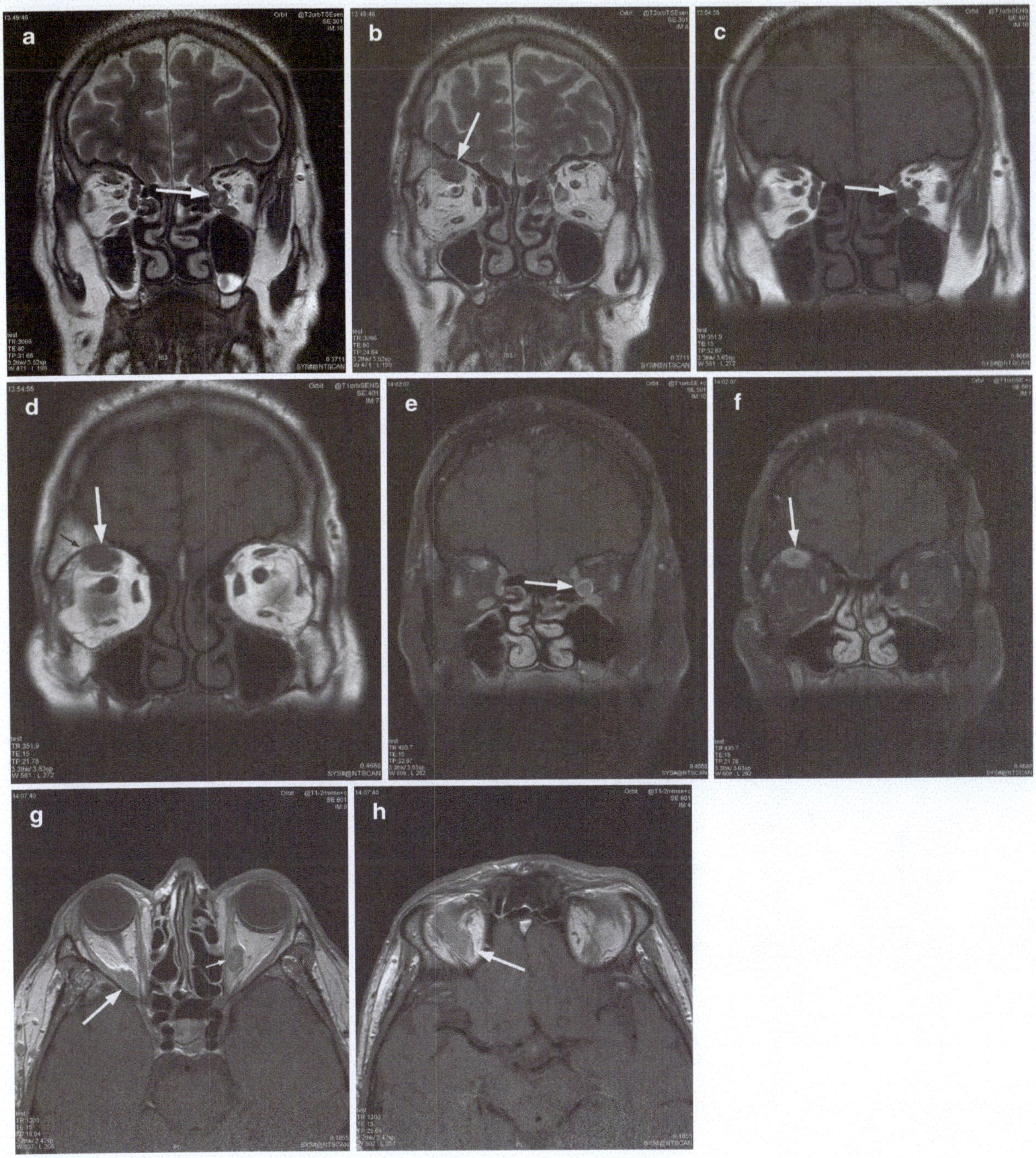

Fig. 4.19 Bilateral rectus muscle metastases. Patient presenting with diplopia and with a previous medical history of adenocarcinoma of the parotid gland. TSE T2-WI (**a**, **b**), un-enhanced SE T1-WI (**c**, **d**), and gadolinium-enhanced SE T1-WI image with fat suppresion (**e**, **f**), all in the coronal plane, and axial gadolinium-enhanced T1-WI (**g**, **h**). On the coronal TSE T2-WI (**a**, **b**) a nodular hypo-intense thickening of the left medial rectus muscle (*arrow*) (**a**) and the right superior rectus muscle (*arrow*) (**b**) is noted. The mass lesions display an iso-intensity to muscle on the un-enhanced T1-WI (*arrows*) (**c**, **d**). On the right side, there is loss of delineation of the superior orbital cortex, suggestive of tumoural invasion (*small black arrow*) (**d**). The mass lesions show moderate enhancement, more pronounced on the right side on the post-gadolinium T1-WI with fat suppression (*arrows*) (**c**, **d**). Corresponding axial T1-WI (**g**, **h**) show the nodular enhancing lesions in the medial rectus muscle on the left side (*small arrow*) (**g**) and the superior rectus muscle on the right side (*arrow*) (**h**). There is an additional lesion in the right orbital apex invading the right lateral rectus muscle (*large arrow*) (**g**). Biopsy of the superior rectal muscle lesion on the right side showed a metastasis of the parotid-gland adenocarcinoma

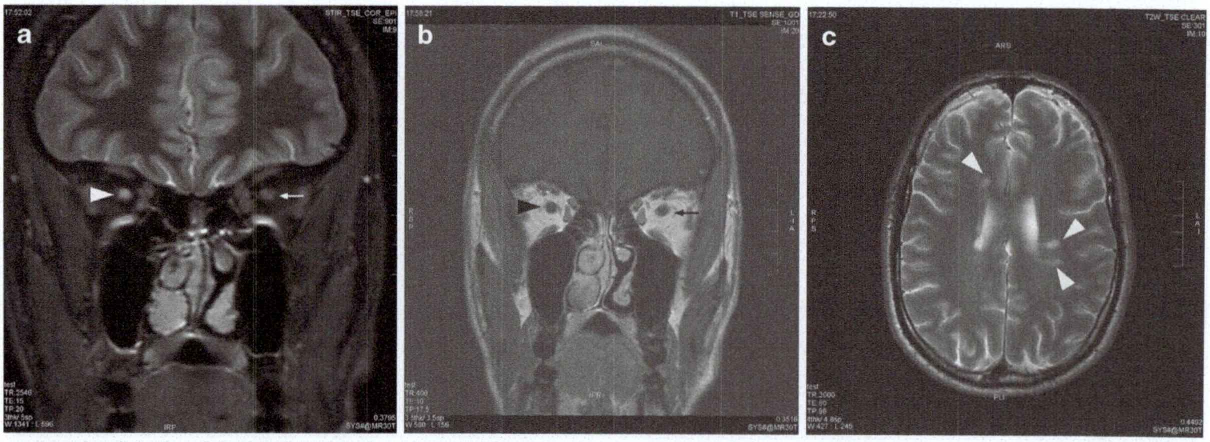

Fig. 4.20 Optic neuritis. Patient clinically presenting with visual disturbance of the right eye. Final diagnosis based upon MRI was optic neuritis in a patient with multiple sclerosis. Coronal STIR image through the optic nerves (**a**). Coronal post-gadolinium T1-WI image (**b**). Axial TSE T2-WI of the brain (**c**). On the coronal STIR image (**a**), the hyper-signal of the right optic nerve (*arrowhead*) is clearly seen compared to the contralateral normal side (*arrow*): imaging findings compatible with optic neuritis. Note that there are no abnormalities visible on the post-gadolinium T1-WI (**b**). SI and enhancement pattern is identical on both sides (*arrow and arrowhead*). The post-gadolinium T1-W sequence is not suited to demonstrate optic neuritis. STIR images are considered most sensitive in demonstrating optic neuritis. Axial TSE T2-WI (**c**) shows the characteristic ovoid hyper-intense lesions periventricular compatible with demyelinated plaques (*arrow heads*)

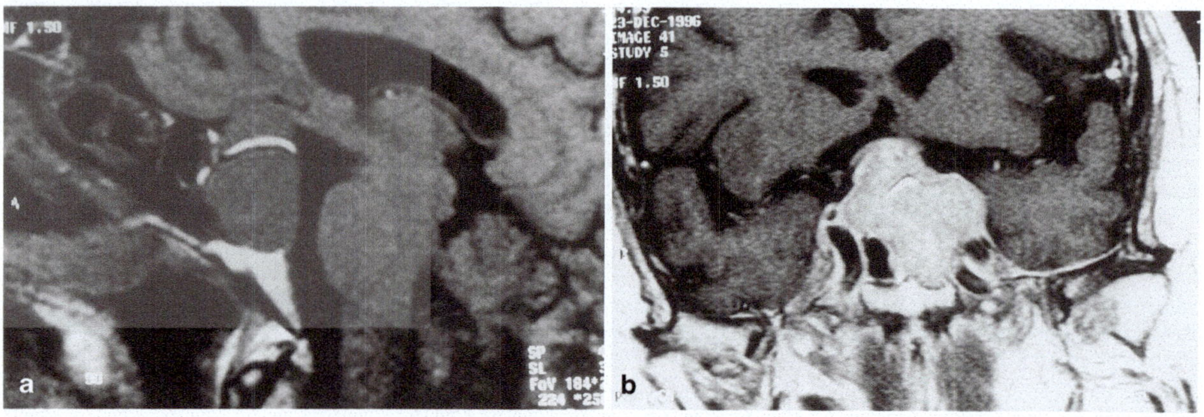

Fig. 4.21 Pituitary macro-adenoma. Sagittal SE T1-WI (**a**) and coronal Gd-enhanced SE T1-WI (**b**) through the pituitary gland and parasellar region. The suprasellar component of the pituitary macro-adenoma displaces and compresses the optic chiasm. The lesion arises from the left lobe of the pituitary gland and invades the left cavernous sinus. There is also extension into the sphenoid sinus

lesions, and therefore, well suited as an initial sequence (Fig. 4.34).

2. Transverse high-resolution, un-enhanced and Gd-enhanced SE T1-WI are then performed. The un-enhanced images are needed as they are the most sensitive images to detect early bone marrow involvement (Fig. 4.35). Moreover, spontaneous hyper-intensities (fat = dermoid cyst, blood = haemangioma or vascular malformations, etc.) can be detected on these images. Gd-enhanced T1-WI are used to evaluate the extent of the lesions. Solid lesions can sometimes become iso-intense with the surrounding soft tissues or fat on these images (Figs. 4.36–4.38). Therefore, fat-suppressed images are often more sensitive, especially in the oral cavity.
3. In case of the evaluation of tumoural pathology, dynamic GRE T1-W sequence during i.v. gadolinium administration can be used as tumoural lesions enhance earlier and stronger than normal tissue. This often makes the delineation of the tumour easier since these sequences are less prone to motion artefacts, frequently encountered in patients with head and neck cancer (Figs. 4.36–4.38). Moreover,

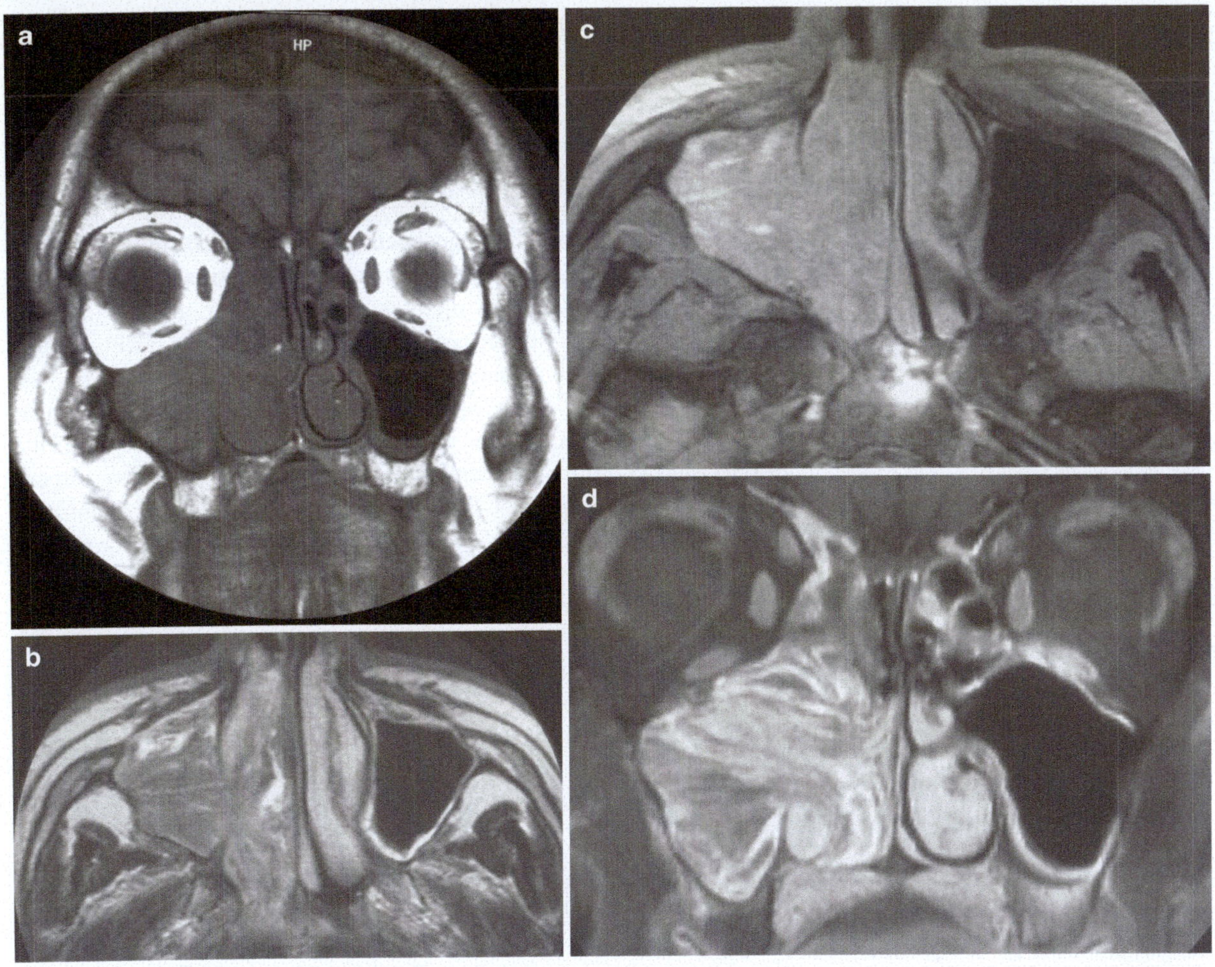

Fig. 4.22 Inverted papilloma. Coronal SE T1-WI (**a**), transverse TSE T2-WI (**b**) and Gd-enhanced SE T1-WI with spectral fat saturation in the transverse (**d**) and coronal planes (**c**) in a 60-year-old man with complaints of nasal obstruction and epistaxis. The lesion appears to arise from the lateral nasal wall near the middle turbinate and extends into the left maxillary sinus (**a**). There is remodelling of the medial wall of the maxillary sinus, without frank bone destruction. Complete opacification of the maxillary sinus is noticed. No differentiation can be made between tumoural tissue, normal mucosa and retention of mucus on the pre-contrast T1-WI (**a**). After Gd injection (**c**, **d**), there is enhancement of the normal mucosa with heterogeneous enhancement of the tumour. No enhancement is noticed in the retained secretions. Biopsy of the lesion demonstrated inverted papilloma

the fat suppression of these sequences makes the tumour delineation more clear.

4. In case of evaluation of tumoural pathology an echo planar diffusion-weighted sequence can be added. In patients treated by radio- and chemotherapy, EPI DWI sequences are able to make the differentiation between residual and/or recurrent tumour vs. scar tissue, inflammation and fibrosis. A major drawback of DWI is its sensitivity to susceptibility artefacts, frequently found in the head and neck region at the various interfaces between air and soft tissues (Figs. 4.36 and 4.38).

The longest diameter of the oropharynx and oral cavity is anteroposterior; hence, when a rectangular FoV is used in the transverse plane, phase encoding should be chosen in the left-right direction. In the infra-hyoid neck, the phase encoding should be chosen in the anteroposterior direction in order to avoid infolding of the shoulders.

For the MRI protocol for examinations of the oropharynx and oral cavity, see Table 4.11.

4.1.6.4 Pathology

The majority of tumours involving the oropharynx are SCCAs (Figs. 4.35–4.38). Again, the cardinal role of MRI is the precise evaluation of tumour extent. The

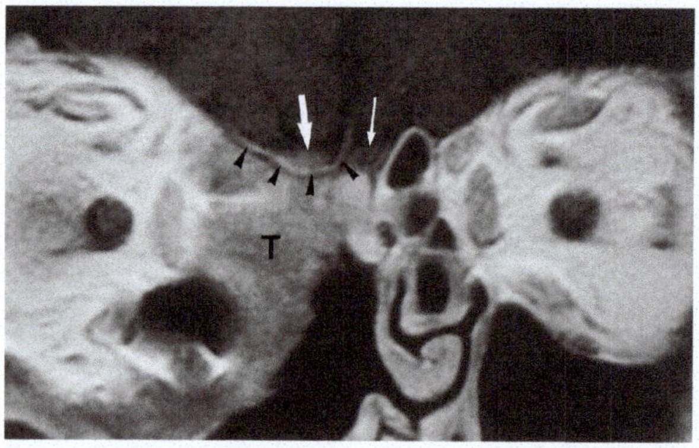

Fig. 4.23 Recurrent ethmoid adenocarcinoma. Coronal Gd-enhanced, high-resolution SE T1-WI through the anterior skull base. Tumour recurrence (*T*) can be seen in the right ethmoid region. Enhancement of the meninges can be appreciated above the right cribriform plate (*arrowheads*), and enhancement of the olfactory bulb (*large white arrow*), representing tumour invasion, can also be recognised. Compare with the normal low signal intensity of the left olfactory bulb (*long white arrow*)

preferred imaging direction is the axial plane, because it allows comparison of both sides. Coronal images are only of benefit when the lateral walls of the oropharynx are involved and for the evaluation of tumoural extension in the floor of the mouth.

In the oral cavity, SCCA is again the most frequently encountered pathology. However, congenital malformations (Fig. 4.34), inflammatory lesions and benign tumours also occur in this anatomical region. Therefore, un-enhanced T1-WI should be used to detect the presence of fat, blood or proteinaceous fluid in these lesions, and TSE T2-WI can be used to further characterise the lesions. Moreover, un-enhanced T1-WI are extremely important to evaluate the often very subtle fat planes. Careful evaluation of these fat planes might demonstrate tumoural invasion.

Malignant tumours in the oropharynx are situated close to the mandible and maxilla and often invade these bony structures. Early involvement can be recognised as loss of the high signal-intensity bone marrow on the un-enhanced T1-WI (Fig. 4.35). The loss of high signal marrow, is however not specific for tumoural invasion; it also occurs in cases of inflammation. At least one sequence in the coronal plane should be performed in order to avert partial volume problems in the region between the floor of the mouth and the tongue, and at the superior and inferior borders of the mandible.

4.1.7 Larynx and Hypo-Pharynx

4.1.7.1 Introduction

The major indication for MRI is to demonstrate the exact extent of the tumour in patients with laryngeal-hypo-pharyngeal cancer. The piriform sinus and retro-cricoid hypo-pharynx are located so close to the laryngeal structures that a tumour arising in these regions necessitates total laryngectomy, as in patients with advanced laryngeal cancer. Today, however, partial (voice-sparing) laryngectomy can be performed successfully, depending on the extent of depth of the tumour. Therefore, landmarks for conservative surgery should be carefully checked. Anterior commissure extension, spread in the pre-epiglottic fat space and the perilaryngeal fat, and cartilage invasion are important signs to look for in patients with laryngeal cancer. Both CT and MRI can detect tumoural spread beneath the mucosa. Moreover, sub-mucosal lesions, tumours arising at the sub-glottic level or at the apex of the piriform sinus can be visualised, where endoscopic techniques fail (so-called blind mucosal areas). The advantage of MRI over CT is that this region can be better evaluated because of its high soft-tissue contrast, high spatial resolution and the multi-planar approach without ionising radiation. These factors contribute to the higher sensitivity and accuracy of MRI in detecting early cartilage invasion. The disadvantage of MRI is the longer examination time, resulting in more artefacts due to swallowing, respiration and blood flow. With the advent of multi-detector spiral CT, detailed examinations with multi-planar reconstructions can be made. The advantage of CT over MRI is that its speed of acquistion is not disturbed by motion artefact. Moreover, CT has the capability of performing dynamic examinations such as the modified Valsalva manoeuvre to expand the piriform sinus. The choice between CT and MRI should be made based upon the availability of both techniques and the expertise of the radiologist performing the examination.

4.1.7.2 Coils and Patient Positioning

The patient is placed in the standard supine position. It is important to explain to the patient the importance of the

Table 4.7 Magnetic resonance imaging protocol recommendations for sinonasal examinations

Pulse sequence	WI	Plane	No. of sections	TR (ms)	TE (ms)	Flip angle	Echo train length	Section thick-ness (mm)	Matrix	FoV	rec-FoV	BW	No. of acq.	Acq. time (min:s)
SE T1	T1	Cor/tra	20	500	11	70	–	3	307 × 512	210	75	89	2	3:55
TSE T2	T2	Cor/tra	16	5,000	112	150	56	3	307 × 512	200	–	130	2	4:47

WI weighted image; *TR* repetition time (ms); *TI* inversion time (ms); *TE* echo time (ms); matrix (phase × frequency matrix); *FoV* field of view (mm); *recFoV%* rectangular field of view; *BW* bandwidth (Hz)

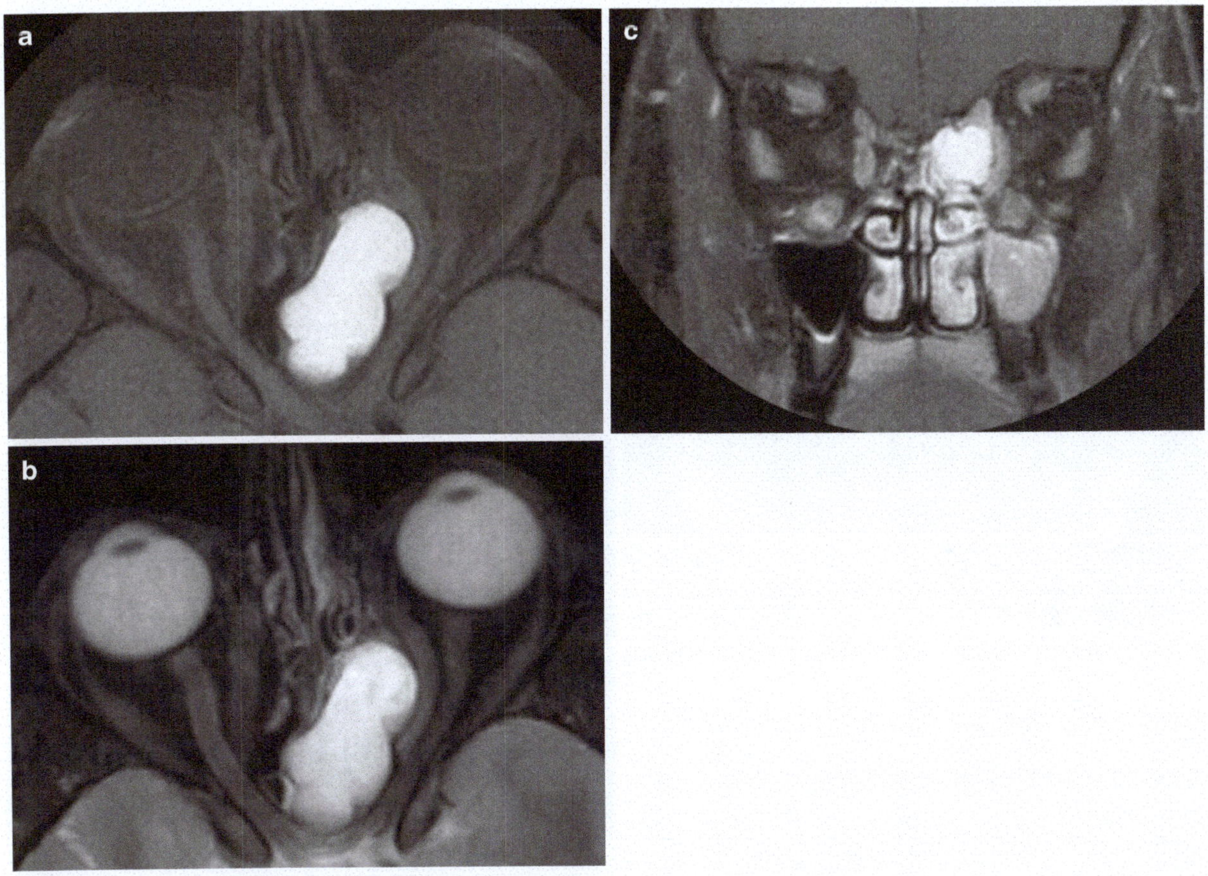

Fig. 4.24 Mucocoele. Transverse SE T1-WI (**a**) and transverse (**b**) and coronal (**c**) TSE T2-WI at the level of the sphenoid sinus in a patient who complained of progressive diplopia. Spectral fat saturation was applied in all sequences. An expansile lesion with high signal intensity is noticed at the sphenoid sinus. There is clear expansion of the sinus cavity with intra-orbital extension of the mucocoele and displacement of the medial rectus muscle. The signal intensity of a mucocoele depends on the viscosity of the secretions

examination to achieve maximum cooperation during the examination (quiet breathing through the nose, avoiding swallowing and coughing). Special surface coils dedicated for imaging of the neck and cervical spine can be used to obtain the best results. The coils are centred at the level of the thyroid prominence (Fig. 4.39).

Table 4.8 Paranasal sinus masses

Mucocoele
Mucus retention cyst
Polyp
Antrochoanal polyp
Inverted papilloma
Sinusitis
Carcinoma

4.1.7.3 Sequence Protocol

1. The MR study starts with semi-axial high-resolution un-enhanced SE T1-WI and TSE T2-WI, parallel to the true vocal cords.
2. After Gd injection, high-resolution SE T1-WI are obtained in the axial and coronal planes. To demonstrate tumoural extension in the base of the tongue, sagittal images are used instead of (or in addition to) coronal slices.
3. Fat-suppressed images after Gd injection can demonstrate enhancing tumour tissue in the paralaryngeal fat space even better.

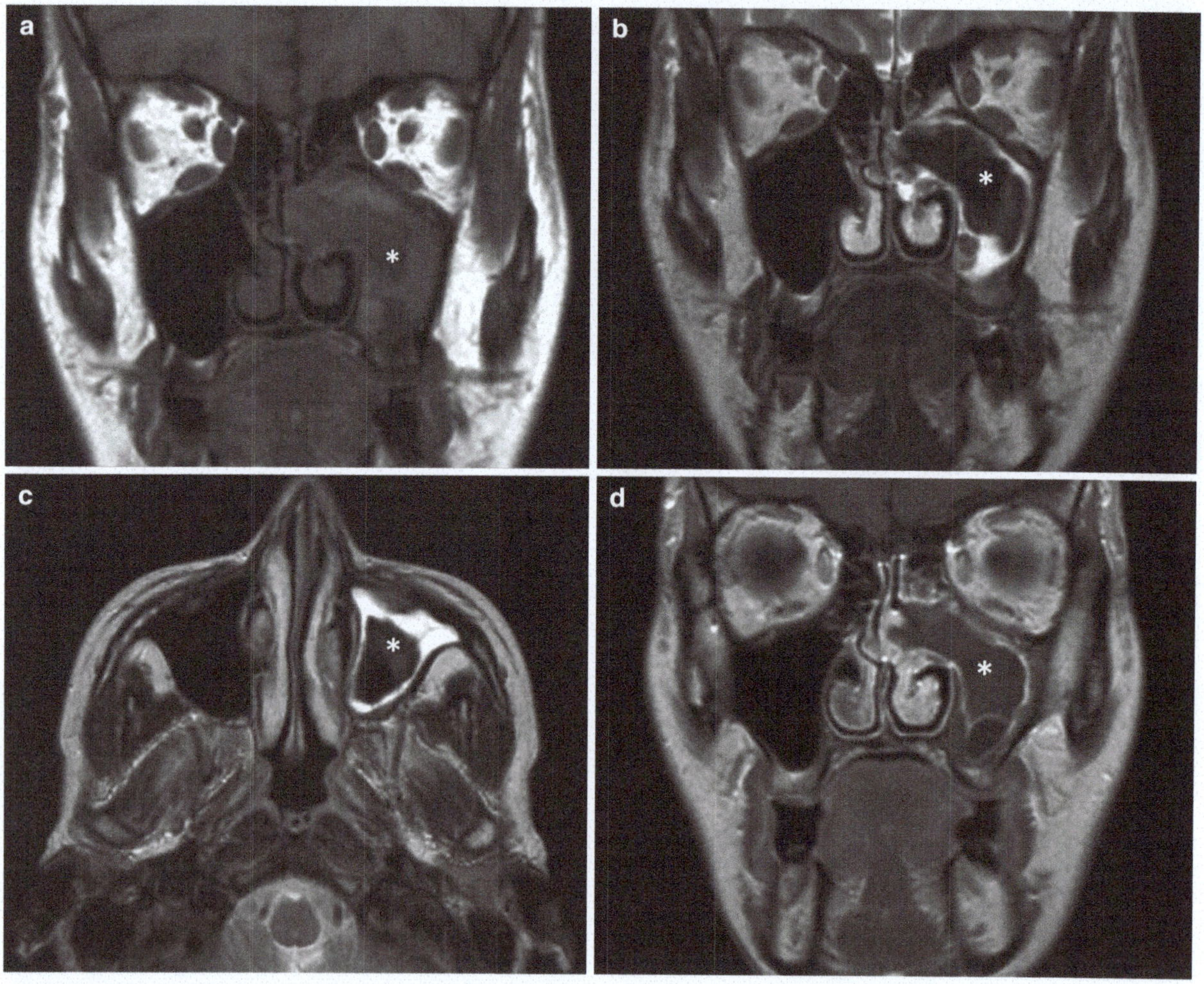

Fig. 4.25 Aspergillus infection in the left maxillary sinus presenting with a characteristic low signal on T2-WI. Coronal T1-WI (**a**), coronal and axial T2-WI (**b**, **c**) and coronal post-gadolinium T1-WI (**d**). On all sequences, the entire maxillary sinus is filled with a lesion (*asterisk*) protruding into the middle nasal meatus. The lesion has mixed SI on un-enhanced T1-WI (**a**). On T2-WI (**b**, **c**), the lesion has a very characteristic central hypo-intense appearance (*asterisk*), caused by the paramagnetic effect of the mycelia of the aspergillus. This characteristic hypo-intense appearance can be misinterpreted as air in the sinus when evaluating the T2-WI alone. On coronal post-gadolinium T1-WI, the lesion enhances peripherally (*asterisk*). The characteristic appearance of the lesion on T1- and T2-W sequences gives the diagnosis of aspergillus infection

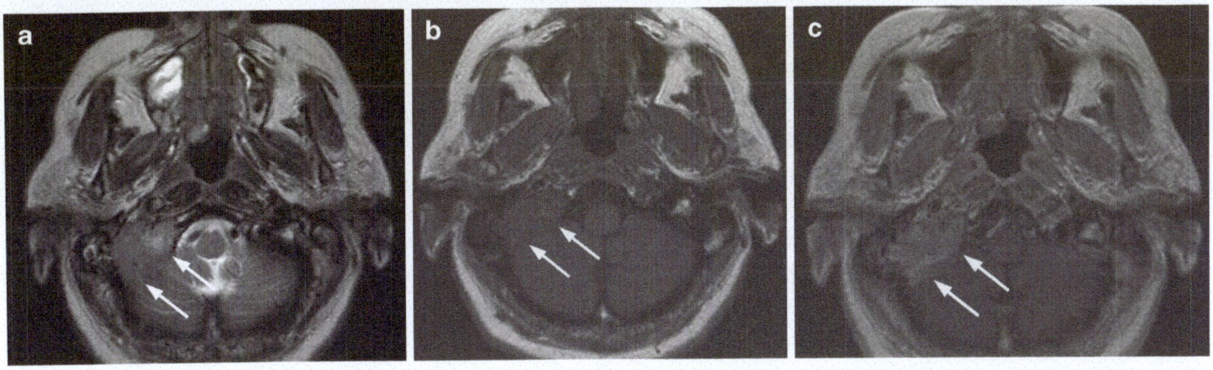

Fig. 4.26 Metastatic lesion in the right skull base, from a bronchial carcinoma. The bronchial carcinoma was detected based upon the detection of the skull base metastasis. Patient complained of right sided headache and tinnitus. The tinnitus can probably be explained by the high vascular flow status of the metastatic lesion. Axial T2-WI (**a**), axial un-enhanced (**b**) and gadolinium-enhanced (**c**) T1-WI. Axial T2-WI (**a**) shows a moderately intense mass lesion (*arrows*) in the right skull base invading also the region of the hypo-glossal canal. The mass lesion has an iso-intense aspect on T1-WI (**b**) (*arrows*) with strong enhancement (*arrows*) on post-gadolinium T1-WI (**c**)

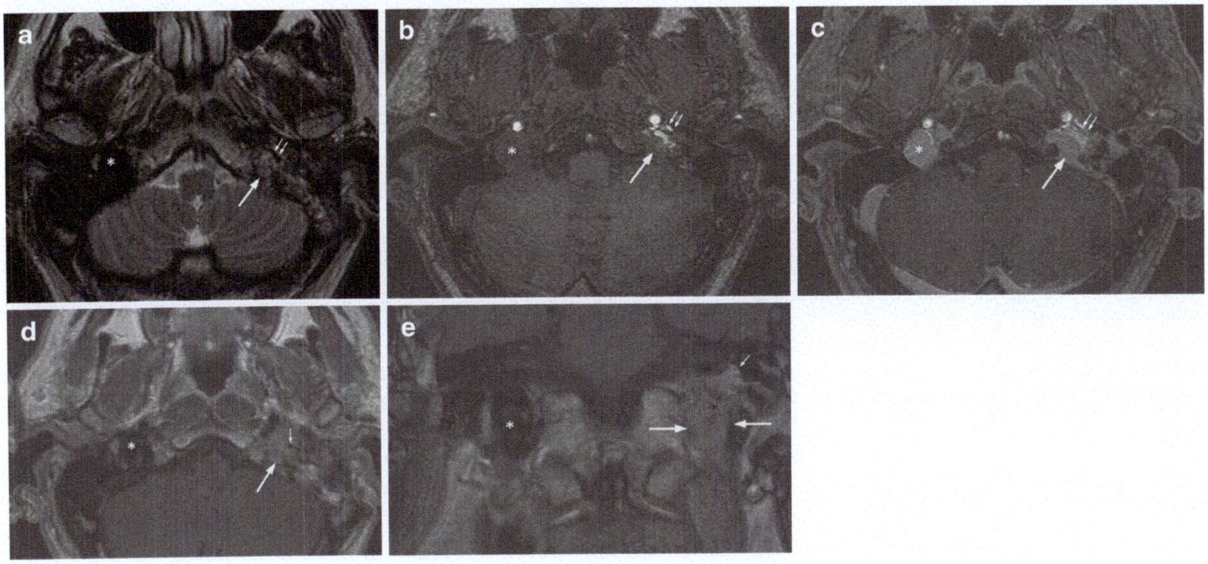

Fig. 4.27 Large glomus jugulare tumour located in the left jugular foramen. The glomus jugulare tumour is a highly vascular tumour originating from the glomus bodies in the jugular foramen. This particular glomus jugulare tumour demonstrates extension towards the middle ear cavity. Axial T2-WI (**a**), axial 3D ToF MRA before (**b**) and after i.v. gadolinium administration (**c**). Axial (**d**) and coronal (**e**) T1-WI after i.v. gadolinium administration. Axial T2-WI (**a**) demonstrates the loss of signal void of the left jugular foramen by an iso- to slightly hyperintense lesion (*large arrow*); some punctate areas of signal void caused by high velocity vessels in the lesion (*small arrows*) can be discerned. Compare to the normal flow void in the right jugular bulb (*asterisk*). Axial un-enhanced 3D ToF MRA (**b**) at the level of the skull base shows the high flow status of the common carotid artery bilaterally. In the left jugular bulb, some serpiginous high signal intensities (*small arrows*) can be seen caused by the high flow in the vessels of the tumour (*large arrow*). Note again the lack of high signal in the normal jugular bulb on the right side (*asterisk*). On the enhanced 3D ToF MRA (**c**) the enhancing vessels (*small arrows*) can still be seen in the enhancing tumour (*large arrow*). The normal jugular bulb on the right side (*asterisk*) is also enhancing. On the axial post-gadolinium T1-WI (**d**), the enhancing mass lesion can be seen filling up the entire jugular foramen on the left side (*large arrow*). Note the flow voids of the high velocity vessels in the tumoural lesion (*small arrow*) and the complete signal void in the normal right jugular foramen (*asterisk*). Coronal post-gadolinium T1-WI (**e**) demonstrates the enhancing mass lesion in the left jugular foramen (*large arrows*). Note the component of the tumour protruding into the middle ear (*small arrow*): glomus jugulo-tympanicum. Note again the flow void in the normal jugular bulb on the right side

Table 4.9 Magnetic resonance imaging protocol recommendations for examinations of the skull base

Pulse sequence	WI	Plane	No. of sections	TR (ms)	TE (ms)	Flip angle	Echo train length	Section thickness (mm)	Matrix	FoV	rec-FoV	BW	No. of acq.	Acq. time (min:s)
TSE T2 skull	T2	Tra	20	4,710	108	180	24	5	403 × 448	230	75	130	2	3:52
TSE T1 ± Gd skull base	T1	Tra/cor/sag	20	570	14	180	77	3	512 × 512	220	75	130	2	4:27
TSE T2 skull base	T2	Tra	14	4,710	100	180	20	3	403 × 448	240	62.9	130	4	6:23
3D ToF MOTSA ± Gd	–	Tra	44	30	4.04	25	–	0.6	394 × 512	240	62.5	130	1	6:32
3D TSE T2	T2	Tra	48	1,500	297	170	9	0.5	448 × 448	240	50	189	1	6.21

WI weighted image; *TR* repetition time (ms); *TI* inversion time (ms); *TE* echo time (ms); matrix (phase × frequency matrix); *FoV* field of view (mm); *recFoV%* rectangular field of view; *BW* bandwidth (Hz)

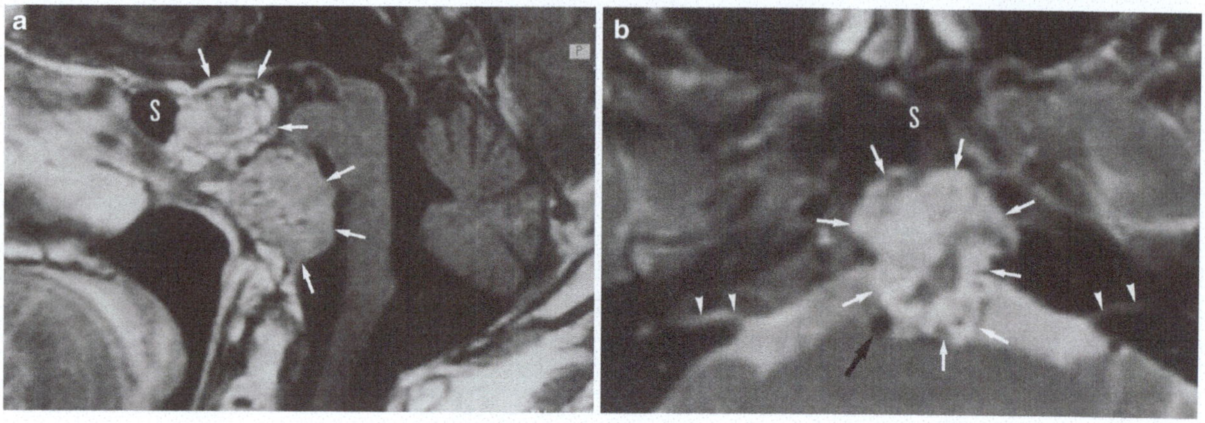

Fig. 4.28 Clival chordoma. Sagittal Gd-enhanced T1-WI (**a**) and axial T2-WI (**b**) through the clivus. A bilobular enhancing mass can be seen behind the sphenoid sinus (*S*) and in the clivus (*white arrows*). The sagittal plane is best suited to image these midline lesions and to demonstrate the displacement of the brainstem. On the T2-WI (**b**) through the level of the IAC (*arrowheads*), the mixed signal intensities inside the tumour (*white arrows*), the multiple convex peripheral protrusions and the midline location help to further establish the diagnosis of a chordoma. The basilar artery (*black arrow*) is compressed between the chordoma and the brainstem

4. In the evaluation of tumoural pathology, dynamic GRE T1-W sequence during i.v. gadolinium administration can be used as tumoural lesions enhance earlier and stronger than normal tissue. This often makes the delineation of the tumour easier, as moreover these sequences are less prone to motion artefacts which are frequently encountered in patients with head and neck cancer.
5. In the evaluation of tumoural pathology an EPI DWI sequence can be added. In patients treated with radio- and chemotherapy, echo planar diffusion-weighted sequences are able to make the differentiation between residual and/or recurrent tumour vs. scar tissue, inflammation and fibrosis. A major drawback of DWI is its sensitivity to susceptibility artefacts, frequently found in the head and neck region at the various interfaces between air and soft tissues.

For MRI protocol for examinations of the larynx and hypopharynx, see Table 4.12.

4.1.7.4 Pathology

Most frequently, MRI is performed to delineate the exact extent of the tumour in patients with SCCA (Fig. 4.40). Other tumours include adenoid cystic carcinoma, lymphoma, plasmocytoma, chondrosarcoma and melanoma. Pseudo-tumoural lesions can also be encountered (laryngocoele, haematoma, etc.).

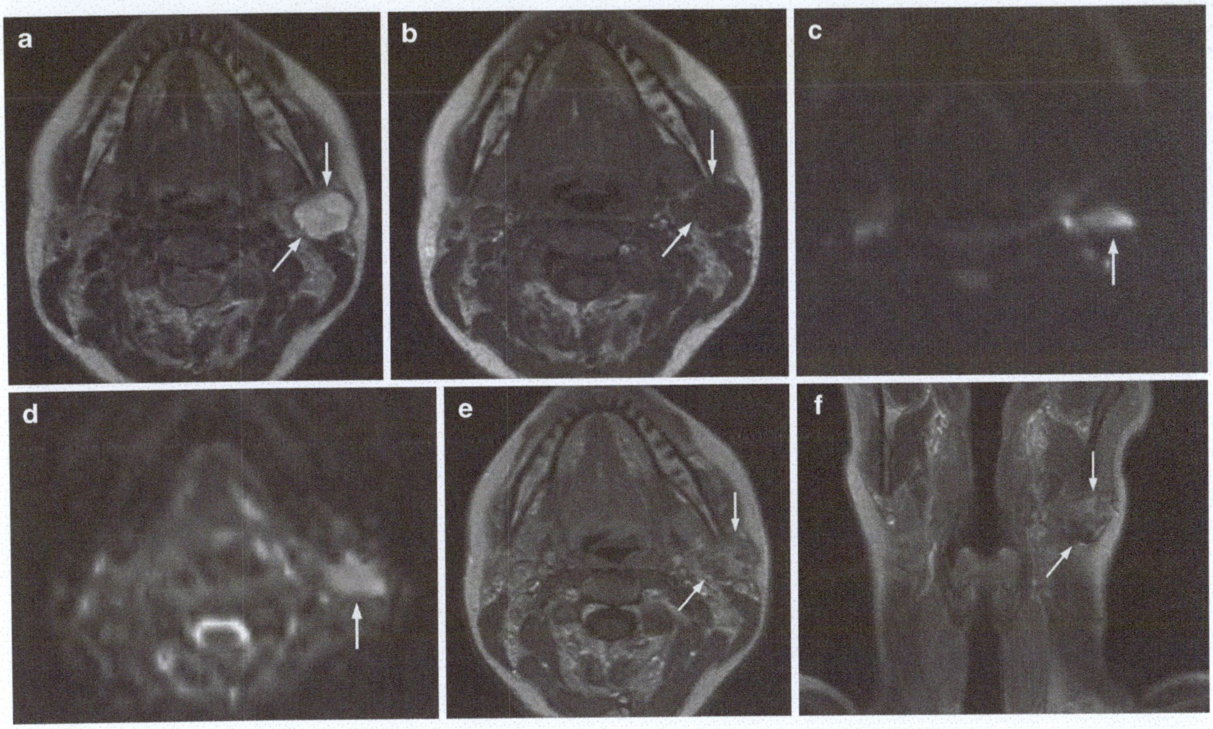

Fig. 4.29 Pleomorphic adenoma in the lower pole of the left parotid gland. Axial T2-WI (**a**), axial un-enhanced T1-WI (**b**), axial EPI diffusion-weighted image (b = 1,000) (**c**) with corresponding ADC map (**d**). Axial post-gadolinium T1-WI (**e**). A nodular lesion (*arrows*) in the lower pole of the superficial lobe of the left parotid gland can be found. The lesion is clearly hyperintense on T2-WI (**a**). This hyper-intensity is already very suggestive of pleomorphic adenoma. The lesion is hypo-intense to the surrounding glandular tissue of the parotid gland on T1-WI (*arrows*) (**b**). Note the very high SI of the lesion on the EPI DWI (*arrows*) (**c**). The high SI on ADC maps (*arrows*) indicates a high ADC value, consistent with a lack of diffusion restriction and highly suggestive of a benign lesion in the parotid gland (**d**). On post-gadolinium T1-WI (**e**), the lesion demonstrates inhomogeneous enhancement (*arrows*). The coronal image (**f**) shows the location of the lesion in the lower pole of the parotid gland and its inhomogeneous enhancement (*arrows*). Surgery revealed a pleomorphic adenoma of the left parotid gland

Table 4.10 Magnetic resonance imaging protocol recommendations for nasopharynx, surrounding deep spaces and parotid-gland examinations

Pulse sequence	WI	Plane	No. of sections	TR (ms)	TE (ms)	Flip angle	Echo train length	Section thickness (mm)	Matrix	FoV	recFoV	BW	No. of acq.	Acq. time (min:s)
TSE T2	T2	Tra	26	6,130	111	180	24	4	403 × 448	230	75	130	2	5:02
TSE T1 ± Gd	T1	Tra/cor/sag	20	570	14	180	77	4	512 × 512	229	76.6	130	3	6:38
EP *b*0-b750	DWI	Tra	30	15,500	91	–	–	4	128 × 128	250	81.3	1,502	3	3:53
3D GRE T1 + Gd	T1	Tra	64	5.12	2.14	12	–	1.6	205 × 256	220	100	400	1	1:11

WI weighted image; *TR* repetition time (ms); *TI* inversion time (ms); *TE* echo time (ms); matrix (phase × frequency matrix); *FoV* field of view (mm); *recFOV%* rectangular field of view; *BW* bandwidth (Hz); *EP* echo planar; *DWI* diffusion-weighted imaging

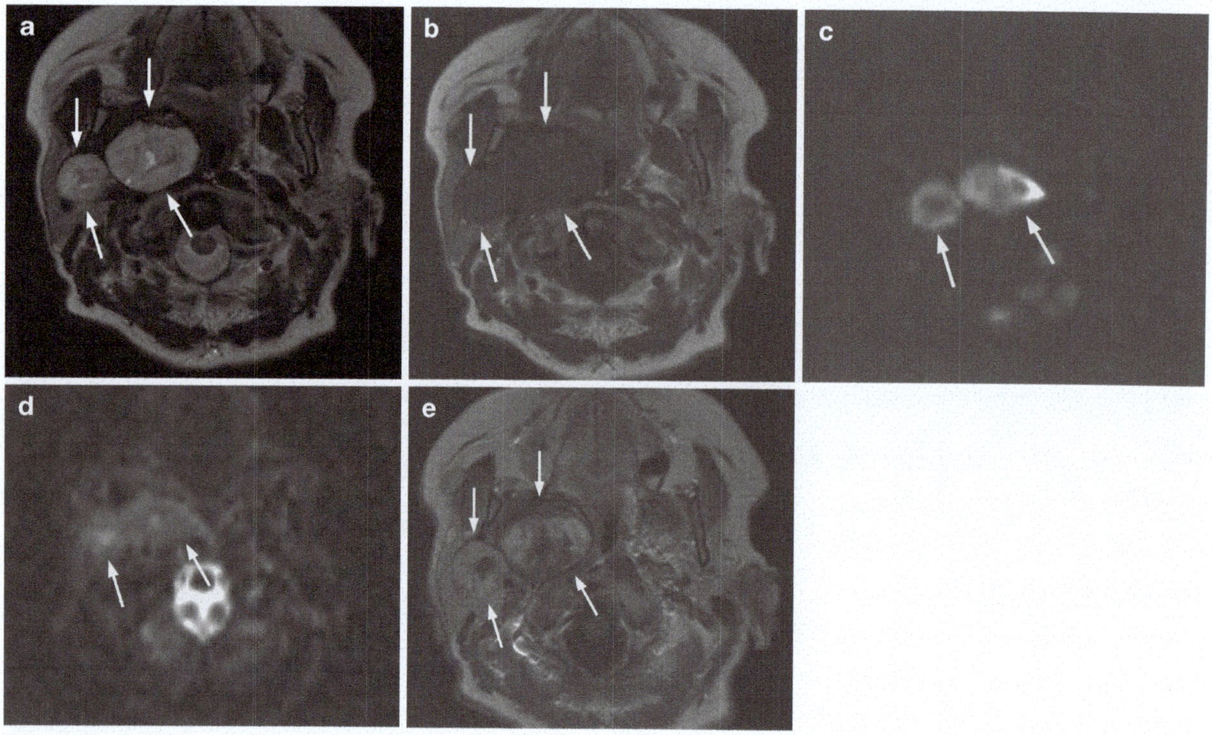

Fig. 4.30 Very large pleomorphic adenoma in the left parapharyngeal space. This lesion originates either from the deep lobe of the parotid gland or from small salivary glands in the parapharyngeal fat space. The enlargement of the left stylomandibular tunnel suggests an origin in the deep lobe of the right parotid gland. Due to the large volume of the lesion, a "carcinoma ex pleomorphic adenoma" (originating in a pre-existing pleomorphic adenoma) cannot be excluded. Axial T2-WI (**a**), axial unenhanced T1-WI (**b**), axial EPI DWI (b = 1,000) (**c**) with corresponding ADC map (**d**). Axial enhanced T1-WI (**e**). The large lesion has a bilobular shape, compressing the left pharyngeal wall. The lesion has a hyper-intense aspect on T2-WI (*arrows*) (**a**), an iso-intense aspect on T1-WI (*arrows*) (**b**) and a clear hyper-intense aspect on DWI (*arrows*) (**c**). The high SI on ADC maps (*arrows*) (**d**) corresponds to a high ADC value, measured in several parts of the lesion: this indicates the benign nature of the lesion. There is an inhomogeneous diffuse enhancement of the lesion (**e**). At surgery, a pleomorphic adenoma was found. At pathology, there were no arguments for a malignant degeneration

4.1.8 Temporomandibular Joint

4.1.8.1 Introduction

Clinically, it is almost impossible to differentiate patients with internal derangement of the temporomandibular joint (TMJ) from patients with myofascial pain dysfunction syndrome. The latter is a stress-related psychophysiological disorder, whereas the former is caused by an asynchrony of the various anatomic subunits of the joint. Today, MRI provides direct visualisation of these different components, and therefore, has surpassed techniques such as CT and arthrography. The most important structure within this joint is the articular disc, a biconcave dense fibrocartilaginous plate, which separates the mandibular condyle from the mandibular fossa. The role of MRI is to demonstrate the position and morphology of the disc and its relationship to the mandibular condyle during motion. The presence of bony abnormalities should also be looked for.

4.1.8.2 Coils and Patient Positioning

As in most examinations, the patient is placed in a supine position. Examination of the TMJ can be best performed using a surface coil. A surface coil diameter between 8 and 12 cm provides an optimal SNR. Bilateral dedicated surface coils (when available from the manufacturer of your MR system) that are placed symmetrically on both sides of the head and lateral to the joint are preferred, since both TMJs are simultaneously examined. This can be important, since bilateral abnormalities can be noticed in up to 60% of patients, and it allows comparison of both joints.

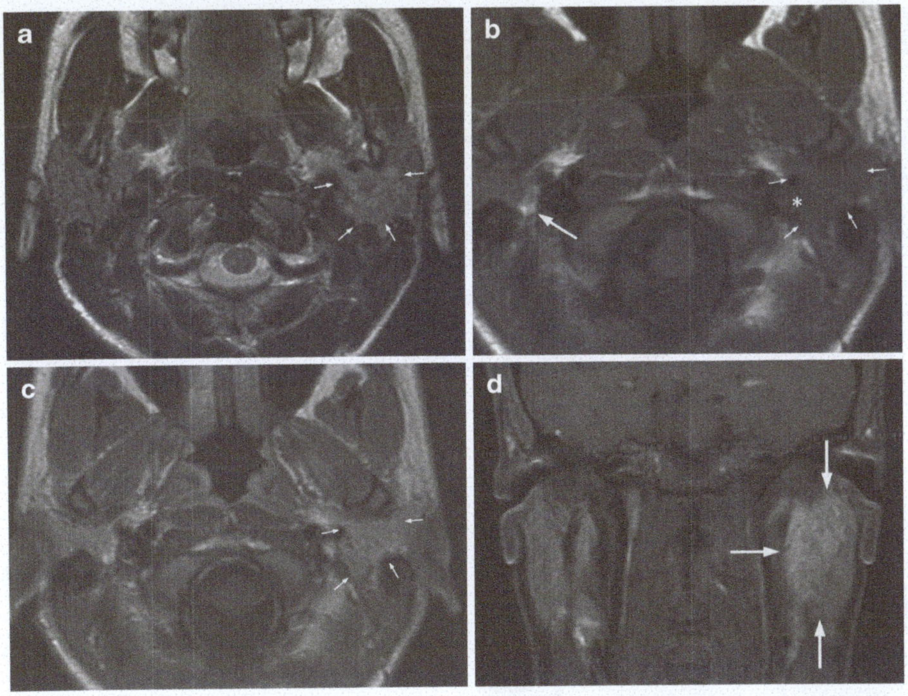

Fig. 4.31 Adenoid cystic carcinoma of the left parotid gland. Patient presenting with a progressive and painful facial nerve palsy on the left side. Axial TSE T2-WI (**a**), axial SE T1-WI before (**b**) and after gadolinium administration (**c**). Coronal gadolinium-enhanced T1-WI with fat suppression (**d**). The T2-WI (**a**) clearly show a diffuse infiltrating mass lesion in the left parotid gland. The lesion has a slightly hyper-intense aspect (*arrows*). On the un-enhanced T1-WI (**b**), the mass lesion presents itself as a hypo-intense mass lesion (*small arrows*) (compare with the slightly higher SI of the normal right parotid gland, caused by fat in the normal parotid gland). More important is the fact that the fat plane in the stylomastoid foramen on the left side has disappeared (*asterisk*) compared to the normal right side (large arrow). This is caused by tumoural infiltration and prompts a very bad prognosis as perineural spread of the tumour is highly probable. The tumour enhances after intra-venous administration of gadolinium and is difficult to discriminate from the surrounding parotid gland (*arrows*) (**c**). On a coronal gadolinium-enhanced T1-WI with fat saturation (**d**) the lesion can be seen as a diffusely enhancing mass lesion in the left parotid gland (*arrows*)

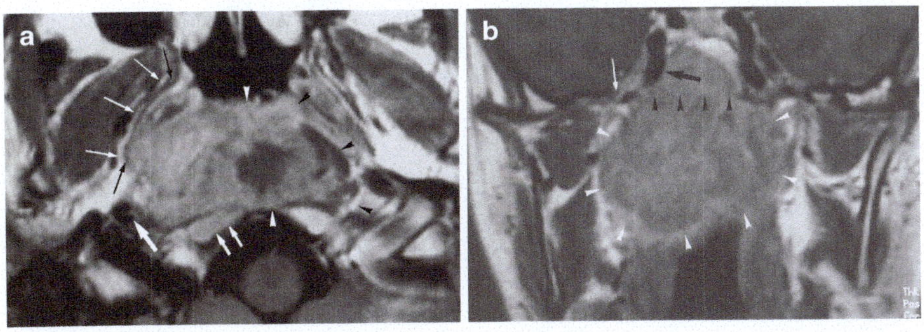

Fig. 4.32 Nasopharyngeal squamous cell carcinoma (SCCA). Transverse (**a**) and coronal (**b**) Gd-enhanced SE T1-WI in a patient with SCCA of the nasopharynx. A large tumour (*arrowheads*) completely fills the nasopharynx lumen and pushes the right tensor veli palatini muscle (*long black arrows*) and pre-styloid parapharyngeal space (*long white arrows*) laterally, but without invading these structures (**a**). The pre-vertebral muscles have been invaded, and signal loss is seen in the marrow of the skull base on the right side (*small white arrows*), indicating bone invasion. The closest and most frequently reached vital structure by nasopharynx tumours is the internal carotid artery; in this patient, the signal void of the internal carotid artery is only 1 mm away from the tumour (*large white arrow*). The destruction of the skull base (*black arrowheads*) by the large nasopharynx tumour (*white arrowheads*) is best seen in the coronal plane (**b**). The sphenoid sinus is completely filled with tumour, and the tumour reaches the medial wall of the internal carotid artery at this level (*black arrow*). The normal mandibular nerve inside the oval foramen (*white arrow*) has not been reached by the tumour

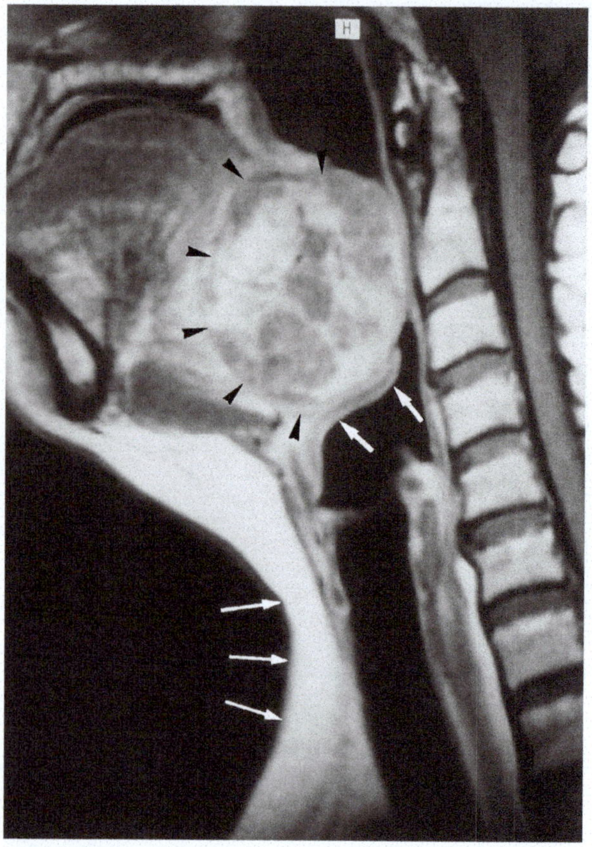

Fig. 4.33 Lingual thyroid. Sagittal Gd-enhanced T1-WI in a patient with a goitre in a lingual thyroid. The complete neck can be studied when a dedicated neck coil is used. Note the absence of a normal thyroid gland in the lower neck (*long white arrows*) and the presence of an inhomogeneously enhancing mass (*arrowheads*) in the base of the tongue, pushing the epiglottis backwards (*small white arrows*)

4.1.8.3 Sequence Protocol

Standard imaging of the TMJ should include oblique, sagittal and coronal images obtained in both the closed- and open-mouth positions. Pseudo-dynamic imaging becomes possible when at least four images at different degrees of opening of the mouth are made (Fig. 4.41). The Burnett bidirectional TMJ device, which is made of plastic, can be used by the patient to control the degree of mouth opening. For the MRI protocol for examinations of the TMJ, see Table 4.13.

1. The basic MR examination, used for screening, consists only of oblique, sagittal and coronal SE T1-WI. The direction of the oblique sagittal scans is parallel to the mandibular ramus.
2. Additional TSE T2-WI in sagittal or coronal planes can be added to look for the presence of joint effusion and inflammatory changes in the joint capsule.
3. GRE T2-WI can also be applied, but these sequences are more vulnerable to artefacts arising from magnetic susceptibility, chemical shift and blood flow.

4.1.8.4 Pathology

Internal derangement (mostly anterior disc displacement) and degenerative joint disease are the most common findings (Fig. 4.42). Other abnormalities include joint effusion (capsulitis), bone marrow oedema (avascular necrosis of the condyle) and tumours (synovial chondromatosis, osteoma, osteochondroma, etc.).

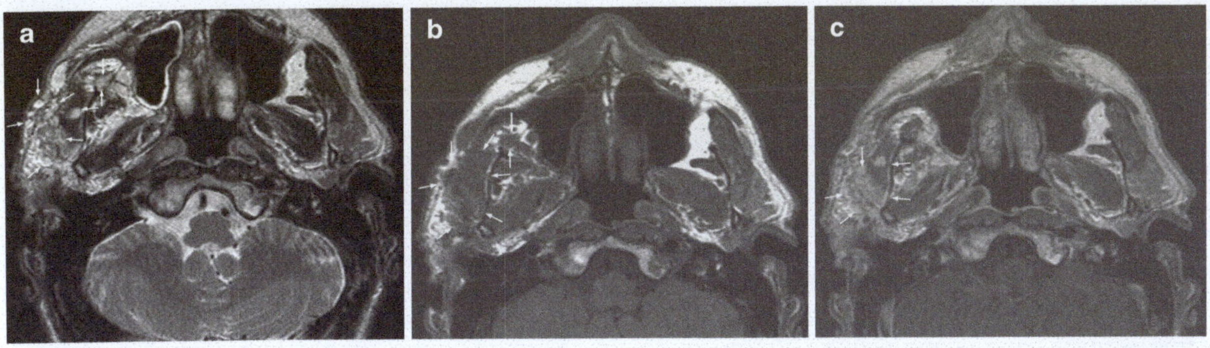

Fig. 4.34 Diffuse infiltrative hemangioma of the masticator space, sub-cutaneous tissues and skin of the right cheek. Axial TSE T2-WI (**a**), un-enhanced (**b**) and Gd-enhanced (**c**) T1-WI at the level of the masticator space. The masticator space on the right side is diffusely infiltrated by multiple nodular mass lesions, with hyper-intense aspect (*arrows*) on T2-WI (**a**). The lesions are situated in the fat planes between the pterygoid muscles and in the pterygoid muscles. The lesions are also situated in the entire masticator muscle, the sub-cutaneous fat planes and skin of the right cheek. On un-enhanced T1-WI (**b**), one can nicely see the diffuse infiltrated aspect of the right masticator space by the multiple nodular iso-intense mass lesions (*arrows*). Although the lesions are infiltrative, they do not look aggressive as they do not displace the normal structures. Note that the sub-cutaneous fat planes and the fat planes in-between the muscles of mastication are also diffusely infiltrated by iso-intense lesions. The lesions enhance after intra-venous gadolinium administration (*arrows*) (**c**). The SI of the lesions on both T1- and T2-WIs, the diffuse infiltrative aspect together with the non-aggressive behaviour of the lesion and their enhancement pattern are highly suggestive of a congenital maxillo-facial hemangioma

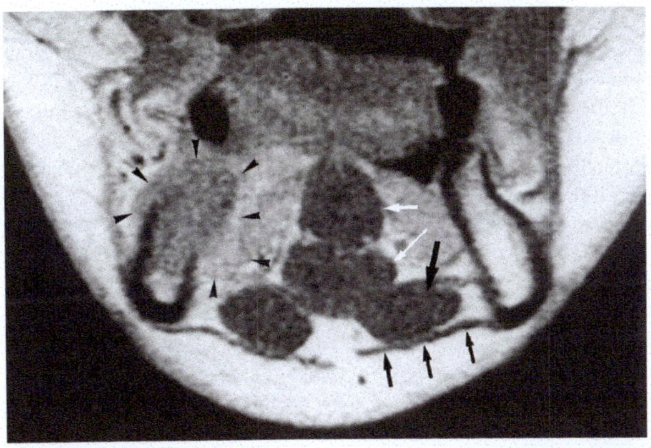

Fig. 4.35 Gingival squamous cell carcinoma (SCCA). Coronal T1-WI through the oral cavity in a patient with SCCA of the gingiva. The tumour can be seen covering the alveolar ridge of the right mandible (*arrowheads*). The cortical bone of the right mandible is destroyed, and the bone marrow is invaded; compare with the normal high signal-intensity bone marrow on the left side. Genioglossus muscle (*small white arrow*), geniohyoid muscle (*long white arrow*), anterior belly of the digastric muscle (*large black arrow*) and platysma (*small black arrows*)

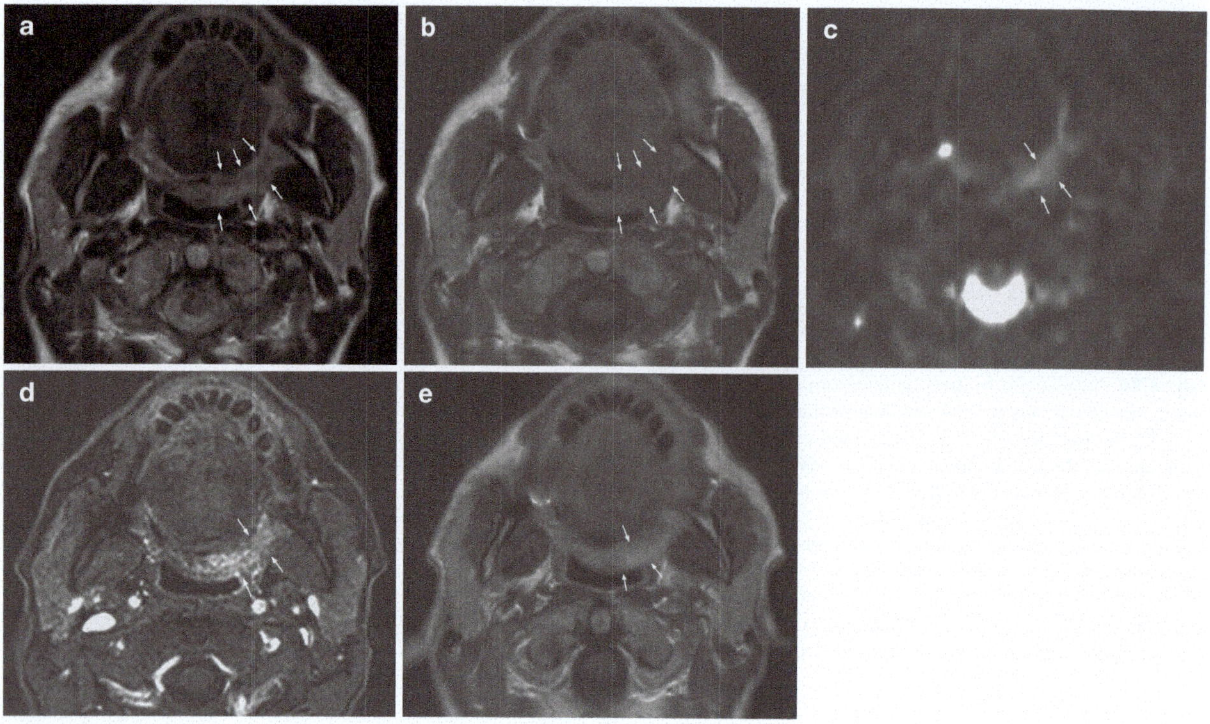

Fig. 4.36 SCCA of the soft palate and anterior tonsillar pillar. Axial TSE T2-WI (**a**), Axial SE un-enhanced (**b**) and Gd-enhanced (**e**) T1-WI. Axial EPI DWI (b = 1,000) (**c**) and axial dynamic GRE T1-WI (**d**). Axial TSE T2-WI (**a**) at the level of the soft palate and uvula shows an asymmetry between both sides of the posterior soft palate. On the left side, a thickening of the soft palate and anterior tonsillar pillar can be noted (*arrows*). The signal is also slightly hyper-intense. The lesion reaches with its lateral margin the medial aspect of the ascending ramus of the left mandible: the hypo-intense cortex has a normal thickness and signal intensity. The medial margin of the lesion is situated at the uvula. On the axial SE T1-WI (**b**), the lesion demonstrates a slightly hypo-intense aspect compared to the contralateral side. There is also a clearly thickened aspect on the left side (*arrows*) compared to the right side. The tumour (*arrows*) displays a hyper-intensity and thickening of the left side of the soft palate on the DWI (**c**). The corresponding ADC map (not shown) demonstrates a hypo-intensity (low ADC value) indicating restricted diffusion, and suggestive of a malignant lesion. On the dynamic GRE T1-WI (**d**), the tumoural lesion enhances strongly. Note again the thickening of the left side of the soft palate (*arrows*). The extension along the anterior tonsillar pillar can clearly be seen (*arrows*). The tumour enhances - in this arterial phase image - very early and strongly. On the post-gadolinium T1-WI (**e**), the thickening of the left side of the posterior soft palate and the anterior tonsillar pillar can be seen (*arrows*). The enhancement is slightly stronger than on the normal right side. The discrimination of the tumour is much more difficult due to the enhancement of the normal structures. Note however the conspicuity of the lesion on the dynamic GRE T1-WI as well as on the DWI

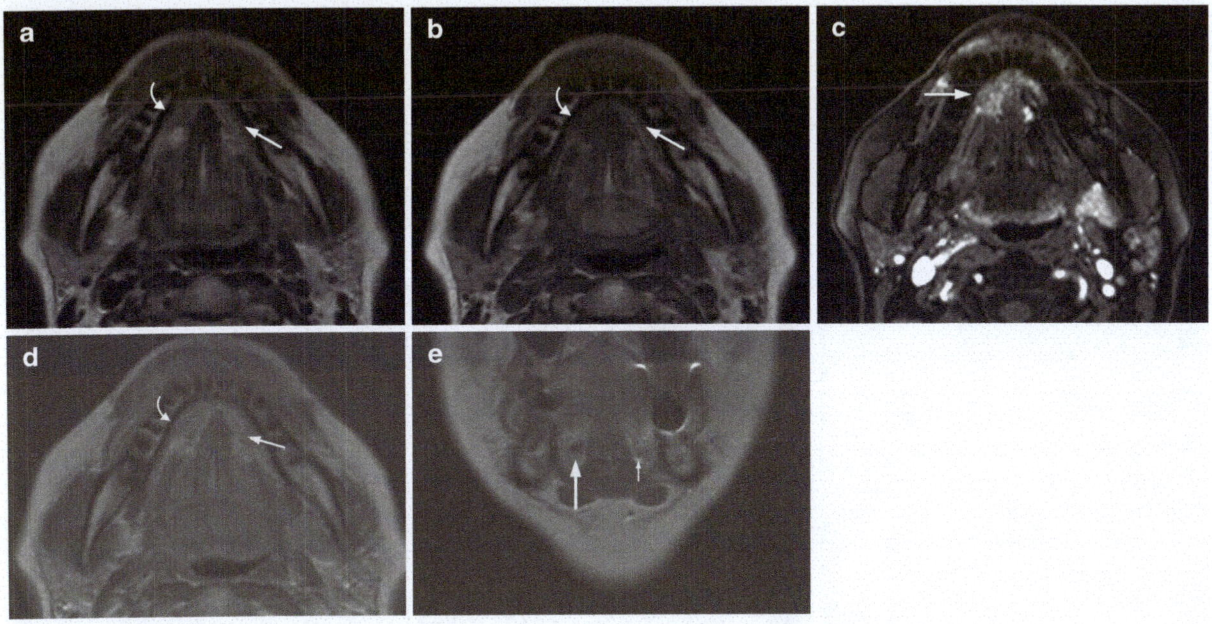

Fig. 4.37 Small SCCA of the anterior floor of the mouth on the right side. Patient presented with complaints of intermittent right sub-mandibular swelling. This swelling was caused by the associated sialadenitis of the right sub-mandibular gland due to the obstruction of the right sub-mandibular gland duct. Axial TSE T2-WI (**a**), axial un-enhanced (**b**) and enhanced (**d**) T1-WI at the level of the floor of the mouth. Axial dynamic contrast enhanced GRE T1-WI (**c**) at the same level. Coronal SE T1-WI (**e**) through the floor of the mouth at a level just posterior to the tumour. On the T2-WI (**a**) there is a slight asymmetry at the anterior aspect of the floor of the mouth. The right sub-lingual space (*curved arrow*) has a slightly lower intensity than the fat containing left sub-lingual space (*arrow*). As fat planes are best evaluated on un-enhanced T1-WI, the lesion (*curved arrow*) can indeed be seen as a hypo-intense mass lesion replacing the fat signal in the right sub-lingual space (**b**). Note the normal hyper-intense fat signal in the left sub-lingual space (*arrow*). On the post-gadolinium T1-WI, discrimination of the tumour becomes much more difficult due to the enhancement of the tumour in the floor of the mouth on the right side (*curved arrow*) and the normally enhancing sub-lingual gland in the left sub-lingual space (*arrow*) (**d**). The only clue to the diagnosis is given by the asymmetry in volume which is more prominent on the right side and caused by the tumour. The dynamic GRE T1-WI however clearly shows the strongly enhancing tumour (*arrow*) in the right floor of the mouth (**c**). The EPI DWI sequence (not shown) could not demonstrate the tumour due to artefacts from dental filling material. A coronal T1-WI (**d**) just posterior to the tumour demonstrates the enlarged sub-mandibular duct on the right side (*large arrow*); compare with the normal left side (*small arrow*)

Table 4.11 Magnetic resonance imaging protocol recommendations for examinations of oropharynx and oral cavity

Pulse sequence	WI	Plane	No. of sections	TR (ms)	TE (ms)	Flip angle	Echo train length	Section thickness (mm)	Matrix	FoV	rec-FoV	BW	No. of acq.	Acq. time (min:s)
TSE-T2	T2	Tra	20	4,030	86	150	45	4	384 × 384	230	75	130	1	3:07
SE T1 ± Gd (with fat suppression)	T1	Tra/cor	20	450	12	90	–	4	384 × 384	230	75	130	1	4:16
EP *b*0-b750	DWI	Tra	20	9,000	71	–	–	4	128 × 128	250	81.3	1,698	1	2:15
3D GRE T1 + Gd	T1	Tra	64	5.12	2.14	12	–	1.6	205 × 256	220	100	400	1	1:11

WI weighted image; *TR* repetition time (ms); *TI* inversion time (ms); *TE* echo time (ms); matrix (phase × frequency matrix); *FoV* field of view (mm); *recFoV%* rectangular field of view; *BW* bandwidth (Hz); *EP* echo planar; *DWI* diffusion-weighted imaging

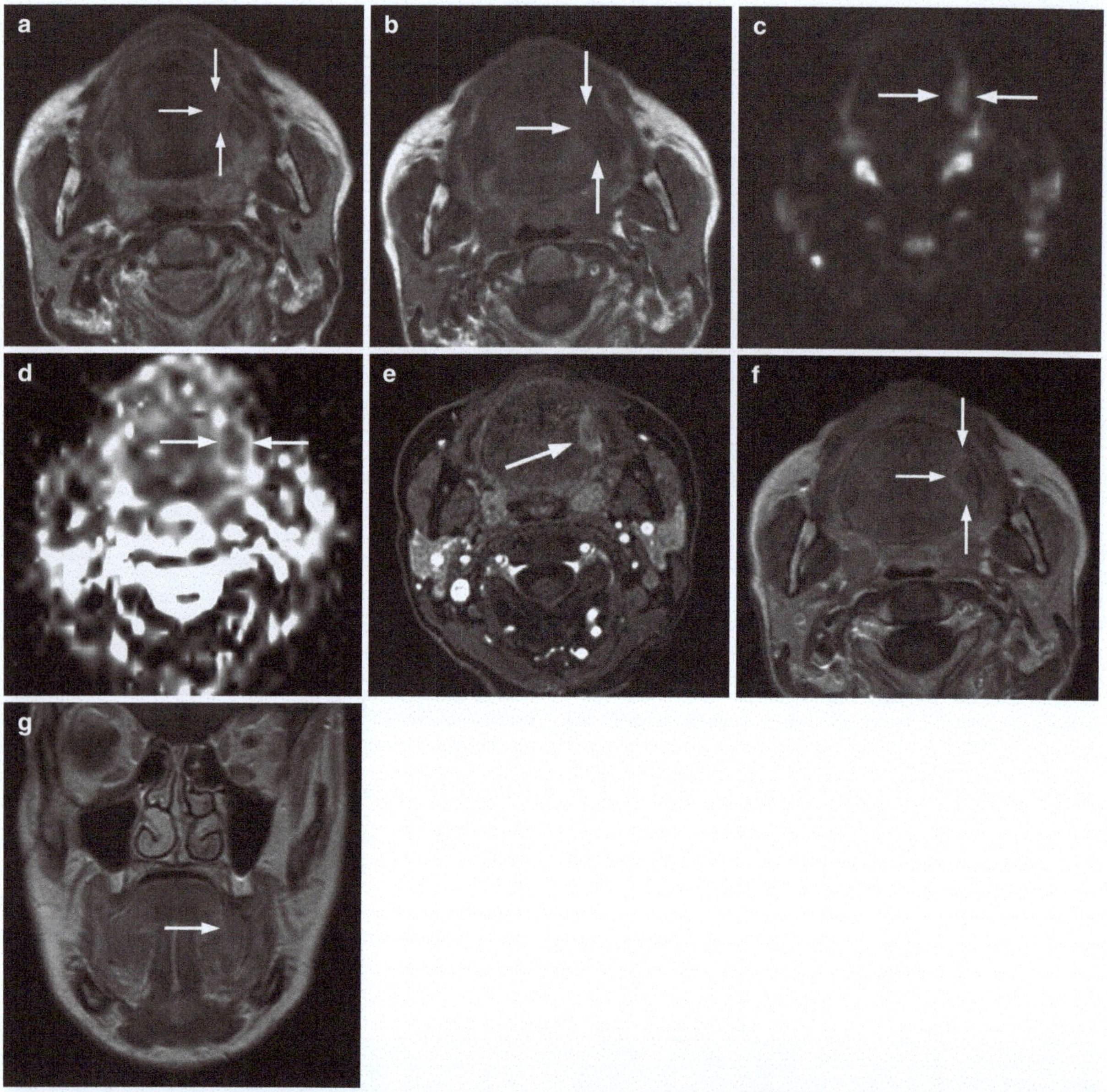

Fig. 4.38 Small SCCA of the left margin of the tongue. Axial TSE T2-WI (**a**), axial un-enhanced (**b**) and Gd-enhanced (**f**) SE T1-WI at the level of the intrinsic muscles of the tongue. Axial EPI DWI ($b = 1{,}000$) (**c**) with corresponding ADC map (**d**) and axial dynamic GRE T1-WI (**e**) at the same level. Coronal (**g**) post-gadolinium SE T1-WI at the level of the tumour. The tumoural lesion (*arrows*) can hardly be discerned on the axial T2-WI (**a**), which is slightly degraded by motion artefacts. Apart from muscular tissue, the tongue also consists of fatty tissue. On an un-enhanced T1-WI (**b**), the tumour can hence be seen as a hypo-intense mass lesion replacing the moderately intense signal of the tongue at the left margin of the tongue (*arrows*). The DWI (**c**) shows the tumour as a small hyper-intense mass lesion at the left lateral margin of the tongue (*arrows*). The corresponding ADC map (**d**) nicely shows the diffusion restriction in the tumour, presenting as a hypo-intense mass lesion (*arrows*). This causes a low ADC value and is highly suggestive of a malignant lesion. Due to the neovascularity, tumoural lesions enhance strongly and early. So, the lesion can nicely be seen as a small enhancing mass lesion (*arrow*) on dynamic GRE T1-WI (**e**) during intra-venous injection of gadolinium. As the lesion enhances, it can be difficult to discriminate the tumour from the fatty tissue containing tongue on post-gadolinium T1-WI. In this case, the mass lesion can be delineated by a small enhancing (*arrows*) line on axial (**f**) and coronal (**g**) post-gadolinium T1-WI. There is no involvement of the extrinsic tongue muscles or the muscles of the floor of the mouth. Pathological lymph nodes cannot be found. Note again that the lesion can be best delineated on the dynamic GRE T1-WI and the DWI

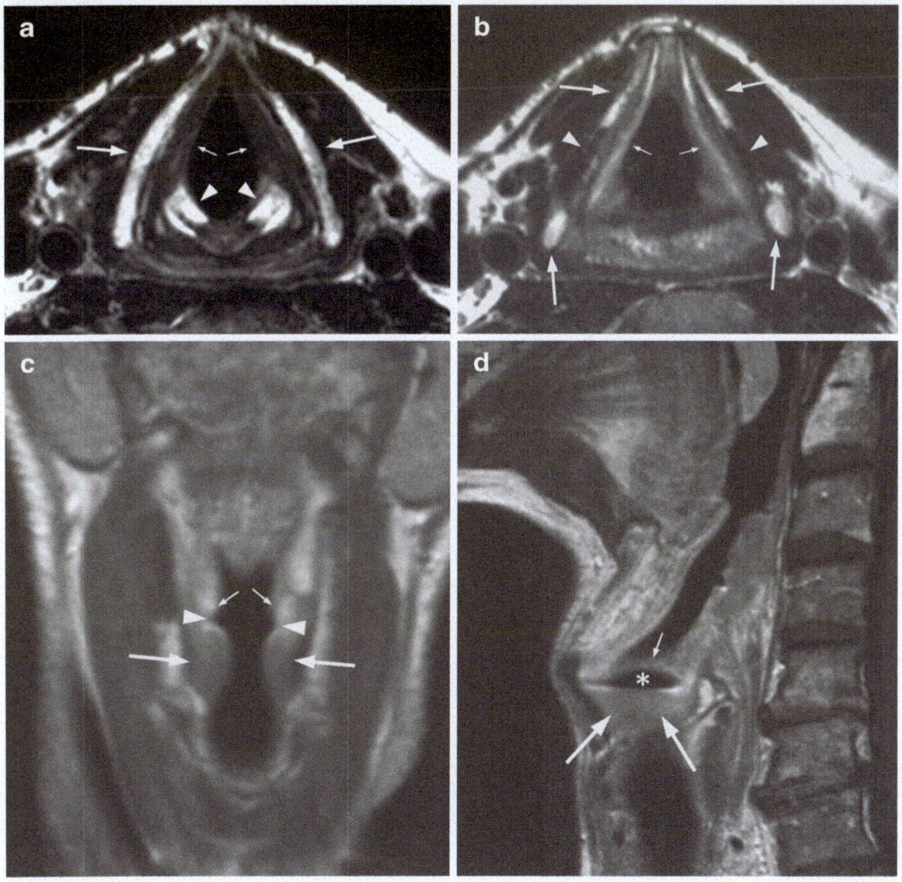

Fig. 4.39 Normal MR anatomy of the larynx. Axial high resolution T1-WI at the level of the true vocal cords (**a**) and at the level of the false vocal cords (**b**), coronal high resolution T1-WI at the level of the true and false vocal cords (**c**), parasagittal high resolution T1-WI through the true and false vocal cords and the laryngeal ventricle (**d**). All images are acquired using small surface coils. On the axial T1-WI at the level of the true vocal cords (**a**), both laminae of the thyroid cartilage (*large arrows*) have a hyper-intense aspect due to the presence of bone marrow in the ossified parts of the laminae. Both true vocal cords have an iso-intense aspect (*small arrows*) which can be explained by the presence of the vocalis muscle which forms the true vocal cord. Both arytenoids cartilages (*arrowheads*) also display a bone marrow signal, due to ossification. On the axial T1-WI at the level of the false vocal cords (**b**), both thyroid laminae display a hyperintense signal in their anterior and posterior aspects (*arrows*). In-between, the thyroid laminae are clearly hypo-intense (*arrowheads*) due to the fact that this part of the lamina is not ossified and contain no fatty bone marrow. Both false vocal cords display a hyper-intense signal due to the fact that the false vocal cords contain only fat (*small arrows*). On the coronal T1-WI (**c**), the relation between true and false vocal cords can nicely be demonstrated. The muscular true vocal cords display an iso-intense signal (*large arrows*), whereas the higher situated false vocal cords display a hyper-intense signal (*small arrows*). In-between, the orificium of the laryngeal ventricle (ventricle of Morgagni) can be seen (*arrowheads*). The parasagittal T1-WI (**d**) shows the relation between true (*large arrows*) and false vocal cords (*small arrow*) as well as the air-filled laryngeal ventricle (*asterisk*). The laryngeal ventricle can not only be filled with air – as in this case – but can also be collapsed or even be filled with some fluid in the case of a laryngocoele

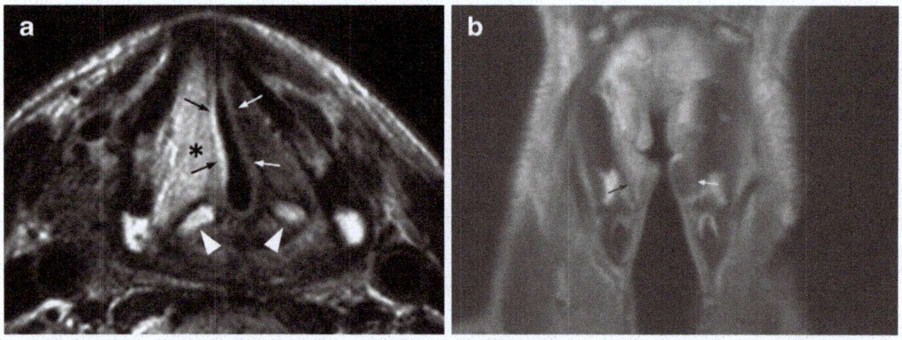

Fig. 4.40 Laryngeal carcinoma of the right vocal cord. Axial high resolution T1-WI (**a**) at the level of the true vocal cords and coronal high resolution T1-WI (**b**) in a different patient with SCCA of the right vocal cord. Both images are acquired after intra-venous administration of gadolinium. On the axial T1-WI, there is a clear asymmetry between both vocal cords. The right vocal cord is thickened and diffusely enhancing (*asterisk*). The overlying mucosa (*black arrows*) seems to be normal but enhances. Endoscopy revealed a normal looking mucosa with normal findings at biopsy. The enhancement is caused by some oedema. Compare to the SI and delineation of the normal left sided mucosa over the left true vocal cord. Note also the normal iso-intense (muscular) aspect of the left true vocal cord. Both arytenoids have a normal hyper-intense aspect (*arrowheads*). This SCCA originated in the right laryngeal ventricle growing into the right true vocal cord underneath an intact mucosa. This pattern of sub-mucosal spread is characteristic of SCCA of the laryngeal ventricle, which can remain occult for a long time. On the coronal T1-WI (**b**) after i.v. gadolinium administration in a different patient with SCCA of the right vocal cord, a clear asymmetry at the level of the vocal cords is noticed. The normal hypo-intense signal, caused by the vocalis muscle (*white arrow*) is replaced by enhancing tumoural tissue (*black arrow*)

Table 4.12 Magnetic resonance imaging protocol recommendations for examinations of the larynx hypo-pharynx

Pulse sequence	WI	Plane	No. of sections	TR (ms)	TE (ms)	Flip angle	TI (ms)	Echo train length	Section thickness (mm)	Matrix	FoV	rec-FoV	BW	No. of acq.	Acq. time (min:s)
SE T1	T1	Tra/cor	19	570	15	90	–	–	3	196 × 512	230	75	130	2	3:44
TSE T2	T2	Tra	19	4,000	19–93	90	–	3	5	192 × 256	230	75	130	1	4:16
EP *b*0-b750	DWI	Tra	20	9,000	71	–	–	–	4	128 × 128	250	81.3	1,698	1	2:15
3D GRE T1 Gd	T1	Tra	64	5.12	2.14	12	–	–	1.6	205 × 256	220	100	400	1	1:11
SE T1 FS	T1	Tra/cor	11	650	15	90	–	–	3	192 × 256	230	75	130	2	4:10

WI weighted image; *TR* repetition time (ms); *TI* inversion time (ms); *TE* echo time (ms); matrix (phase × frequency matrix); *FoV* field of view (mm); *recFoV%* rectangular field of view; *BW* bandwidth (Hz); *EP* echo planar; *DWI* diffusion-weighted imaging

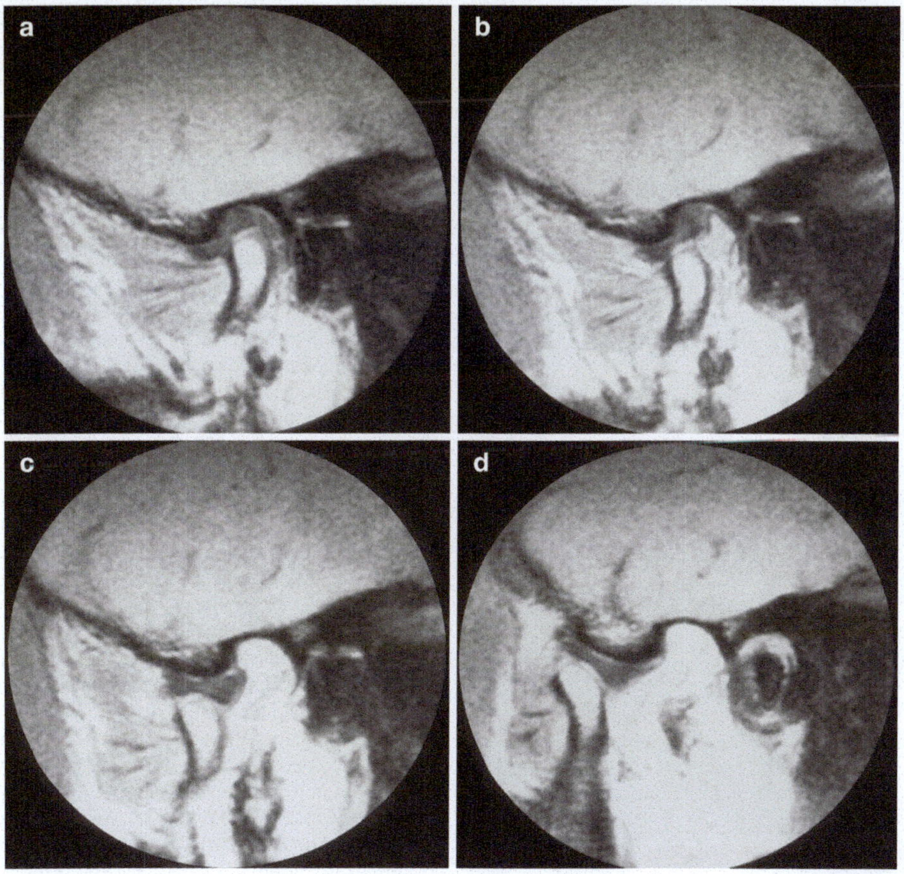

Fig. 4.41 Pseudo-dynamic examination of the normal temporomandibular joint (TMJ). Sequential parasagittal images in a normal volunteer are obtained at various degrees of mouth opening, controlled by the Burnett bidirectional TMJ device. The images with closed mouth show the normal articular disc as a biconcave fibrous structure of low signal intensity (**a**). One can discern three components: the anterior band, the intermediate zone and the posterior band. The posterior band is located above the condyle at the 12 o'clock position. Gradual opening of the mouth is accompanied by anterior translation of the condyle, with movement of the intermediate zone towards the articular tubercle (**b**, **c**). The mandibular condyle lies under the articular tubercle with interposition of the intermediate zone when the mouth is completely opened (**d**)

Table 4.13 Magnetic resonance imaging protocol recommendations or examinations of the temporomandibular joint. All sequences are performed using double loop coils used at the same time

Pulse sequence	WI	Plane	No. of sections	TR (ms)	TE (ms)	Flip angle	Echo train length	Section thickness (mm)	Matrix	FoV	rec-FoV	BW	No. of acq.	Acq. time (min:s)
TSE	T1	Para-sag	2 × 7	768	12	90	109	3	210 × 256	150	100	78	2	2:50
SE	T1	Cor	9	400	20	90	–	3	448 × 512	180	88	78	2	6
TSE	T2	Para-sag	2 × 7	3,000	66	150	33	3	256 × 256	150	100	130	2	3:23

WI weighted image; *TR* repetition time (ms); *TI* inversion time (ms); *TE* echo time (ms); *TD* time delay (s); *No of acq* number of acquisitions or partitions; Matrix (phase × frequency matrix); *FoV* field of view (mm); *recFoV%* rectangular field of view; *BW* bandwidth (Hz)

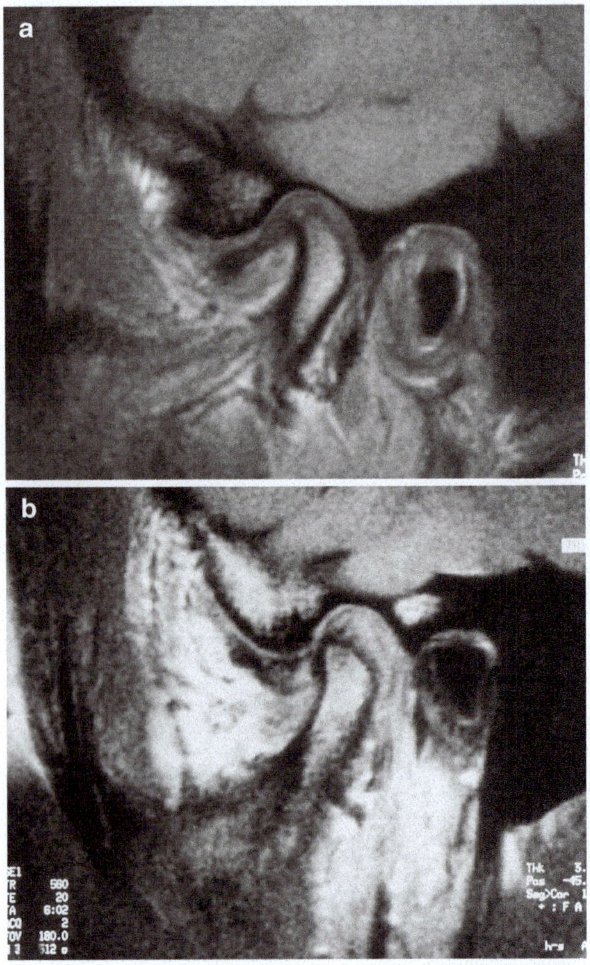

Fig. 4.42 Disc dislocation. Anterior dislocation of the articular disc with the mouth closed (**a**) and mouth opened (**b**) in a patient with a click in the left TMJ. The disc is positioned anteriorly of the condyle with the mouth closed (**a**). Note the disappearance of the biconcave morphology. There is no reduction of the disc on opening of the mouth (**b**)

Further Reading

Armington WG, Bilaniuk LT, Zimmerman RA (1996) Visual pathways. In: Som PM, Curtin HD (eds) Head and neck imaging, 3rd edn. Mosby Year Book, St Louis, pp 1184–1232

Becker M (2000) Oral cavity, oropharynx and hypopharynx. Semin Roentgenol 35(1):21–30

Belden CJ (2004) MRimaging of the globe and optic nerve. Neuroimaging Clin N Am 14:809–825

Castelijns JA, van den Brekel MWM, Hermans R (2000) Imaging of the larynx. Semin Roentgenol 35:31–41

Chong VF, Khoo JB, Fan YF (2002) Imaging of the nasopharynx and skull base. Magn Reson Imaging Clin N Am 10: 547–571

Curtin HD (1996) Larynx. In: Som PM, Curtin HD (eds) Head and neck imaging, 3rd edn. Mosby Year Book, St Louis, pp 612–710

Curtin HD (2002) The skull base. In: Atlas SW (ed) Magnetic resonance imaging of the brain and spine, 3rd edn. Lippincott Williams & Wilkins, Philadelphia, pp 1243–1282

Curtin HD, Hasso AN, Swartz JD, Lo WWM (1996) Temporal bone. In: Som PM, Curtin HD (eds) Head and neck imaging, 3rd edn. Mosby Year Book, St Louis, pp 1233–1535

Davidson HC (2004). Imaging of the temporal bone. Neuroimaging Clin N Am 14:721–760

De Foer B, Vercruysse JP, Offeciers E, Casselman JW (2008) MRI of cholesteatoma. In: Moffat M, Keir J, Sudhoff H (eds) Recent advances in otolaryngology 8. Royal Society of Medicine, London, pp 1–20

Hermans R (2003) Imaging of the larynx. Springer, Berlin

Lemmerling M, Kollias SS (2004) Radiology of the petrous bone. Springer, Berlin

Mafee MF, Atlas SW, Galetta SL (2002) Eye, orbit, and visual system. In: Atlas SW (ed) Magnetic resonance imaging of the brain and spine, 3rd edn. Lippincott Williams & Wilkins, Philadelphia, pp 1433–1526

Mafee MF, Karimi A, Shah JD, Rapoport M, Ansari SA (2006). Anatomy and pathology of the eye: role or MR imaging and CT. Magn Reson Imaging Clin N Am 14:249–270

Mark AS, Casselman JW (2002) Anatomy and disease of the temporal bone. In: Atlas SW (ed) Magnetic resonance imaging of the brain and spine, 3rd edn. Lippincott Williams & Wilkins, Philadelphia, pp 1363–1432

Rao VM, Bacelar MT (2004) MR imaging of the temporomandibular joint. Neuroimaging Clin N Am 14:761–775

Sigal R (1996) Oral cavity, oropharynx, and salivary glands. Neuroimaging Clin North Am 6:379–400

Smoker WRK (1996) Oral cavity. In: Som PM, Curtin HD (eds) Head and neck imaging, 3rd edn. Mosby Year Book, St Louis, pp 488–544

Som PM, Brandwein M (1996) Salivary glands, tumors and tumor-like conditions. In: Som PM, Curtin HD (eds) Head and neck imaging, 3rd edn. Mosby Year Book, St Louis, pp 877–914

Som PM, Brandwein M (1996) Sinonasal cavities: inflammatory diseases, tumours, fractures and postoperative findings. In: Som PM, Curtin HD (eds) Head and neck imaging, 3rd edn. Mosby Year Book, St Louis, pp 126–318

Stambuk HE, Karimi S, Lee N, Patel SG (2007) Oral cavity and oropharynx tumors. Radiol Clin North Am 45:1–20

Vogl TJ, Balzer JO (1996) Base of the skull, nasopharynx, and parapharyngeal space. Neuroimaging Clin North Am 6: 357–378

Weber AL, al-Arayedh S, Rashid A (2003). Nasopharynx: clinical, pathologic, and radiologic assessment. Neuroimaging Clin N Am 13:443–464

5 Musculoskeletal System

Filip M. Vanhoenacker, Pieter Van Dyck, Jan Gielen,
Arthur M. De Schepper, and Paul M. Parizel

Contents

F. M. Vanhoenacker (✉)
Department of Radiology, Universitair Ziekenhuis Antwerpen,
General Hospital Sint-Maarten Duffel-Mechelen,
Wilrijkstraat 10, 2650 Edegem, Belgium
e-mail: filip.vanhoenacker@telenet.be

P. Reimer et al. (eds.), *Clinical MR Imaging*,
DOI: 10.1007/978-3-540-74504-4_5,

5.1 Introduction

The introduction of magnetic resonance (MR) imaging has dramatically changed imaging of the musculoskeletal system. MR examinations of the musculoskeletal system are among the most frequent procedures, performed in most MR units. This chapter will deal with MR of the joints, bone (marrow), and soft tissues. Table 5.1. provides an overview of current MR sequences used in the musculoskeletal system.

Table 5.1 Overview of some commonly used MRI sequences for the MSK system

T1	• SE = basic sequence for assessment of anatomy • TSE/FSE can be used, but less anatomical detail; Large echotrain length should be avoided because of imaging blurring • T1-weighted images (WI) can also be obtained by using T1-weighted gradient echo (GE) or magnetization prepared GE • Routinely without fat saturation, at least one T1-WI without fat saturation should be obtained in every MSK examination • Frequency selective fat saturation before and after IV gadolinium administration is used for assessment of contrast enhancement in MSK infection, inflammation and tumors of the MSK system
PD/T2	• TSE/FSE with or without fat suppression • Selective fat saturation may increase detection of bone marrow edema • Fat suppression may fail due to field inhomogeneity (metallic artifacts or bulk susceptibility). Selective fat saturation should be avoided in postoperative imaging • Long echo for detection of long T2 lesions • Intermediate echo for routine evaluation of joint cartilage
STIR	• Non-selective signal suppression of fat • Screening sequence for detection of bulk water in pathologic processes • Less susceptible to field inhomogeneities than spectral fatsuppression • Lower signal to noise ratio than frequency selective fat saturation • Should not be used in combination with gadolinium contrast administration
Gradient Echo	• Excellent spatial resolution • Relatively poor contrast resolution • 3D T1-spoiled gradient sequences allow thin slice multiplanar reconstructions • Fat saturation or water excitation is added for evaluation of cartilage (e.g. knee and hip) • Gradient echo sequence (T2*) provides information about hemoglobin breakdown products and calcifications (e.g. of muscle hematoma or hemorraghic areas within bone and soft tissue tumors, loose bodies) • Should be avoided in postoperative imaging (increased susceptibility artefacts to metallic artifacts) • Out of phase gradient echo imaging can be used to evaluate bone marrow metastases in the spine • 3D gradient echo with volume interpolation can be used after dynamic gadolinium contrast injection or for MR arthrography in claustrophobic patients (fast sequence)
DWI / ADC	• Sensitive to random water movement • Potential indications: soft tissue tumors (e.g. to differentiate solid from cystic tumor or solid from necrotic tumor), evaluation of osteoporosis, differentiation of benign and malignant vertebral fractures • Use different b values of 50-400-800-1000 s/mm^2
Perfusion imaging	• Depicts blood flow at the microvascular level • Potential indications (follow-up after treatment of MSK tumors, bone marrow disease, assessment of activity of rheumatoid arthritis, viability of vascularized grafts)
T1-WI +/– Gd	• Required in any case where infection, inflammation or tumor is suspected • Imaging planes, depends on the anatomy and location of the lesion • Same imaging plane should be used before and after gadolinium-chelate injection • Subtraction and fatsuppression may enhance lesion conspicuity • For dynamic studies 3D GRE with fat saturation most suited
MR arthro-graphy	• Indicated for pathologic conditions of the joints (particularly useful for evaluation of fibrocartilage of shoulder, hip, other joints…) • Most authors prefer direct MR arthrography with injection of dilute gadolinium contrast within the joint • Combined with T1-WI with selective fat suppression • Indirect MR arthrography (intravenous injection of gadolinium contrast) may be an alternative in postoperative joints
Whole body MRI	• Potential indications: metastases, multiple myeloma, screening malignancies in multiple exostosis syndrome, neurofibromatosis type I, screening early spondylarthropathy,…

Abbreviations: *TSE* Turbo Spin Echo; *FSE* Fast Spin Echo; *STIR* Short Tau Inversion Recovery; *DWI* Diffusion Weighted Imaging; *ADC* Apparent Diffusion Coefficient; *Gd* Gadolinium contrast

5.2 Knee Joint

5.2.1 Anatomy

5.2.1.1 Menisci

The menisci are C-shaped fibrocartilaginous structures, firmly attached to the anterior and posterior aspects of the tibial plateau by the so-called "root ligaments." Conventionally, they are described as having three segments: anterior horn, body, and posterior horn. Each meniscus measures approximately 5 mm in height along its periphery and tapers to a thin inner edge such that it demonstrates a triangular shape in cross section. The outer rims of the menisci are convex and attached to the fibrous joint capsule and through it to the edges of the articular surfaces of the tibia. The inner edges are concave, thin, and free. Their superior surfaces are slightly concave for reception of the femoral condyles, whereas their inferior surfaces that rest on the tibial condyles are flatter (Fig. 5.1).

The *medial meniscus* is C-shaped and occupies 50% of the articular contact area of the medial compartment (Fig. 5.2). Its posterior horn is wider than the anterior horn. Although anatomic variations in meniscal morphology and attachments exist, the anterior horn of the medial meniscus has a firm bony attachment to the tibia anterior to the anterior cruciate ligament (ACL). The posterior horn is attached immediately in front of the attachment of the posterior cruciate ligament (PCL). The outer border of the medial meniscus is firmly attached to the knee joint capsule. The meniscotibial and meniscofemoral ligament attach the meniscus to the tibia and femur, respectively, and is referred to as the deep medial collateral ligament (MCL) (Fig. 5.3).

The *lateral meniscus* is more uniform in width and semicircular, covering 70% of the lateral tibial plateau (Fig. 5.2). The anterior horns of the medial and lateral menisci are attached to each other through the transverse ligament. The posterior horn of the lateral meniscus is attached to the medial femoral condyle through the posterior meniscal-femoral (Wrisberg) and anterior meniscal-femoral (Humphrey) ligament. Therefore, during rotation, the motion of the lateral meniscus is coupled with that of the femoral condyle. The lateral meniscus has loose attachments to the joint capsule and is separated from it by the popliteus tendon posterolaterally where it courses through a meniscocapsular tunnel. In this region, the superior and inferior popliteal meniscal fascicles are seen, running from the peripheral margin of the meniscus, around the popliteus tendon, to the joint capsule (Fig. 5.4). The lateral meniscus is more mobile and is not anchored to the lateral

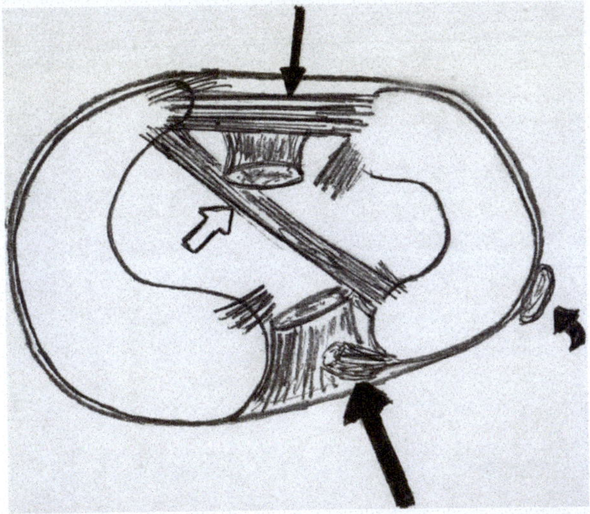

Fig. 5.2 Diagram of the menisci (seen from above). Note the transverse intermeniscal ligament anteriorly (*small arrow*), the meniscofemoral ligament attaching to the posterior horn of the lateral meniscus (*large arrow*), an oblique meniscomeniscal ligament (*open arrow*) and the popliteus tendon (*curved arrow*). (Reprinted with permission from Vanhoenacker et al. 2007)

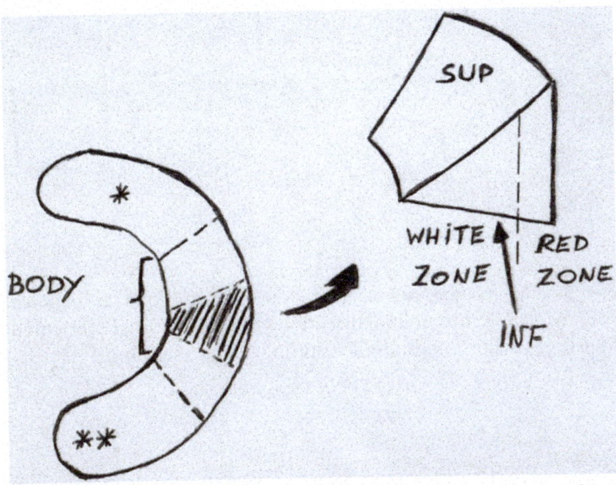

Fig. 5.1 Meniscal anatomy. Each meniscus is arbitrarily divided into anterior horn (*asterisk*), body and posterior horn (*double asterisk*) segments. A cross-section to the body illustrates the superior (*SUP*) and inferior (*INF*) articular surfaces, and the more vascularized periphery of the meniscus (*red zone*), and the relatively avascular inner two thirds of the meniscus (*white zone*). (Reprinted with permission from Vanhoenacker et al. 2007)

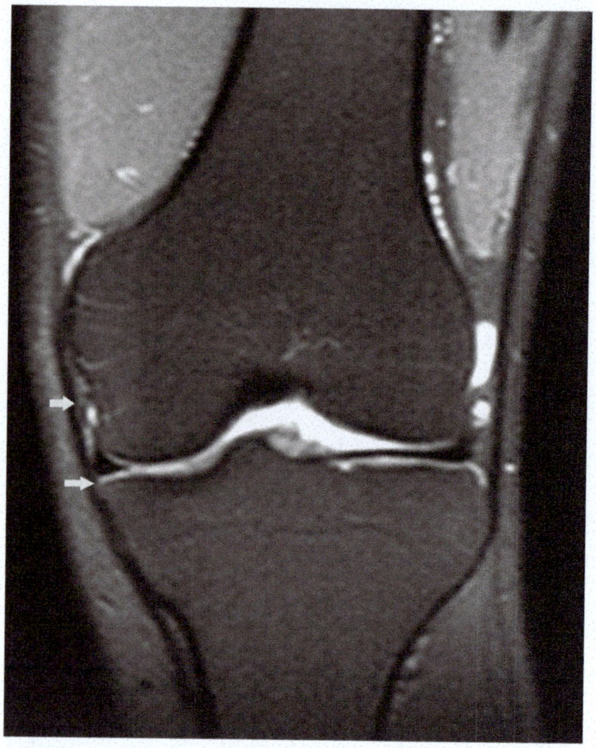

Fig. 5.3 The "deep medial collateral ligament." Coronal fat suppressed – intermediate T2-WI. The meniscofemoral (*thick white arrow*) and meniscotibial (coronary) ligament (*thin white arrow*) attach the meniscus to the femur and tibia, respectively, and is referred to as "the deep medial collateral ligament"

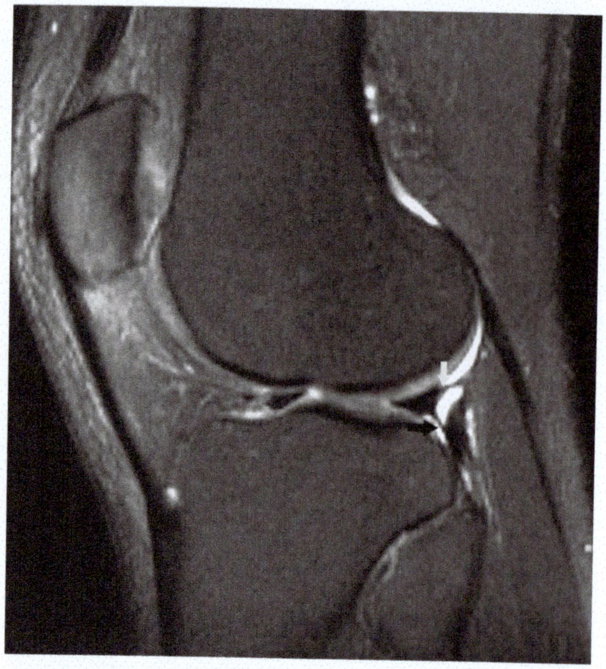

Fig. 5.4 Popliteal meniscal fascicles. Sagittal PD-WI. The superior (*white arrow*) and inferior (*black arrow*) popliteal meniscal fascicles are seen, running from the peripheral margin of the meniscus, around the popliteus tendon, to the joint capsule

collateral ligament. In flexion and internal rotation, the popliteal tendon retracts the posterior horn, thus reducing entrapment of the lateral meniscus between the femur and the tibia. It is therefore less likely to be injured than the relatively immobile medial meniscus.

The *microanatomy of the menisci* may explain injury patterns (Fig. 5.5). A network of type I collagen fibers arranged in a circumferential direction is the dominant morphological pattern, allowing dispersion of compressive loads and the development of "hoop stresses." Radial oriented fibers ("tie fibers") may function to restrain motion between circumferential fibers and resist longitudinal splitting. At the surface of the meniscus, fiber orientation is more of a random configuration.

The *blood supply to the menisci* originates from the lateral and medial superior and inferior genicular arteries. These vessels reach the periphery of the meniscus through the synovial covering of the anterior and posterior horn attachments. Vessels are present throughout the substance of the fetal menisci. Beginning at birth, there is a progressive decrease in vascularity proceeding from the inner to the outer regions of the meniscus. The adult meniscus is avascular in the inner two thirds ("white zone"), and vessels are most prominent in the peripheral one-third of the menisci and in the adjacent coronary and capsular ligaments ("red zone") (Fig. 5.1).

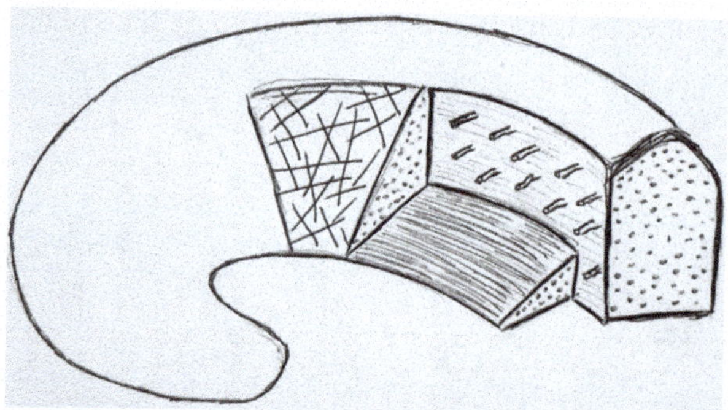

Fig. 5.5 Microanatomy of the meniscus. Most collagen bundles course in a circumferential direction with fewer radially oriented fibers, resisting longitudinal splitting. (Reprinted with permission from Vanhoenacker et al. 2007)

On MR imaging (MRI), the normal menisci demonstrate diffusely low signal intensity on all MRI pulse sequences because of their fibrocartilaginous structure. Menisci must be evaluated on both the sagittal and coronal images. Analysis of axial images – however – is very useful for the detection and characterization of small meniscal tears. Particularly, small peripheral meniscal tears and small radial tears of the free edge of the meniscus are better visualized in the axial plane.

The most peripheral images of the sagittal plane demonstrate a "bow tie" appearance of the meniscus. The normal meniscus should have 1.5–2 bow ties (5–13 mm) on 4–5 mm thick images. Broad and disk shaped menisci (>13 mm) with 3–4 or more bow ties are called "discoid" and are more prone to meniscal tears. The normal meniscus measures 3–5 mm in height. The medial meniscus varies in width from 6 mm at the anterior horn to 12 mm at the posterior horn. The lateral meniscus is approximately 10 mm in width throughout its length.

More centrally, the normal meniscus becomes triangular in appearance. The anterior and posterior horns of the lateral meniscus are nearly equal in size, whereas the posterior horn of the medial meniscus is nearly twice the size of the anterior horn.

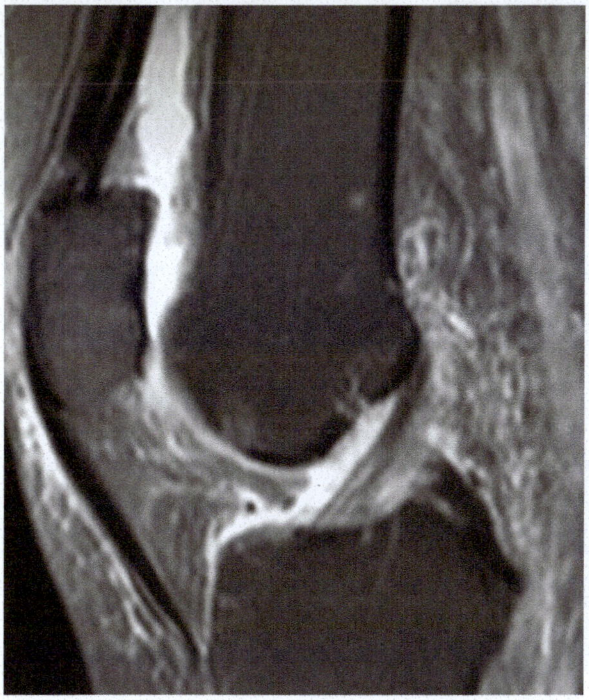

Fig. 5.6 Normal ACL. Sagittal fat-suppressed intermediate T2-W MR image. The anteromedial bundle is represented by a hypointense line. The ACL has a fan-shaped appearance at its distal insertion at the tibia

5.2.1.2 Ligaments

Anterior Cruciate Ligament (ACL)

The ACL runs from the medial aspect of the lateral femoral condyle, forward and laterally to the anterior tibial eminence. In its proximal portion, it runs parallel to the intercondylar roof. It is composed of two principle bundles, the large anteromedial bundle and the more loosely packed posterolateral bundle. The anteromedial band becomes taut in flexion. In extension, the posterolateral portion is under tension.

On MRI, the ACL is of low signal intensity on all pulse sequences (Fig. 5.6). The anteromedial bundle is best depicted on sagittal sections, where the taut ACL shows as a hypointense line. At the tibial insertion, the fibers of the anteromedial bundle spread out, and the space between the fibers is filled with fluid and fibrofatty tissue. This should not be misinterpreted as a tear. The posterolateral bundle is best defined on axial images.

Posterior Cruciate Ligament

The PCL courses from the lateral aspect of the medial femoral condyle to the posterior aspect of the intraarticular tibia. The PCL is stronger than the ACL and is hypointense and more uniform than the ACL on all pulse sequences (Fig. 5.7). Rarely, some internal signal variation can be seen in the proximal third, probably due to a magic angle phenomenon. The PCL consists of two major fiber bundles, an anterolateral (AL) and posteromedial (PM) bundle. These bundles are more difficult to distinguish on routine MR sequences.

Minor Intracapsular Ligaments

Intermeniscal Ligaments

There are three intermeniscal ligaments, anterior, posterior, and oblique. The anterior ligament or transverse geniculate ligament runs between the two anterior meniscal horns. On MRI, a cord-like structure representing the

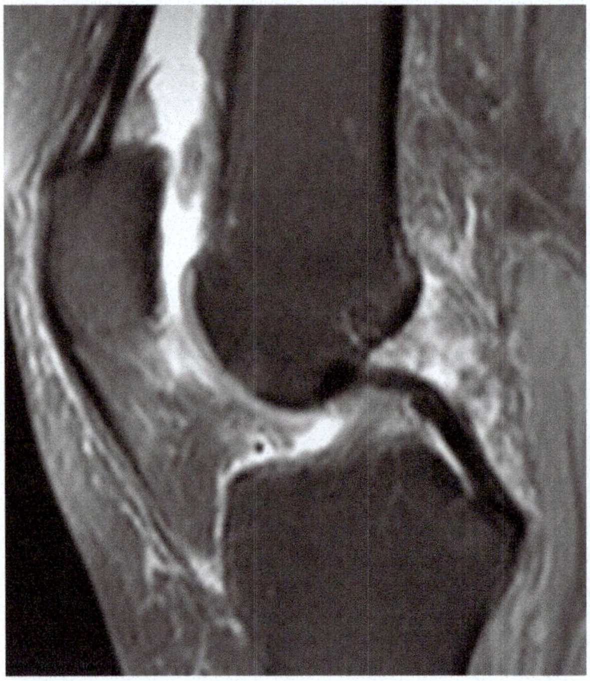

Fig. 5.7 Normal PCL. Sagittal fat-suppressed intermediate T2-W MR image. The ligament is uniform hypointense on all pulse sequences

anterior intermeniscal ligament can be identified. The ligament is generally round or oval shaped (Fig. 5.8). A small layer of fluid between the ligament and the meniscus should not be interpreted as a meniscal tear.

The posterior intermeniscal ligament is less commonly visualized on MR.

The oblique intermeniscal ligament runs in the transverse plane from the posterior horn of the lateral meniscus to the anterior horn of the medial meniscus (Fig. 5.9). It separates the PCL from the ACL. This structure should not be mistaken for an ACL fragment, a displaced meniscal fragment or an osteochondral loose body.

Meniscofemoral Ligaments

The meniscofemoral ligaments run from the posterolateral meniscus obliquely to the lateral aspect of the medial femoral condyle. The posterior meniscofemoral ligament or "ligament of Wrisberg" runs posteriorly to the PCL, whereas the anterior meniscofemoral ligament or "ligament of Humphrey" runs anteriorly to the PCL. The size of the MFL may vary. Fluid between a prominent MFL and the lateral meniscus may mimic a tear (Fig. 5.10).

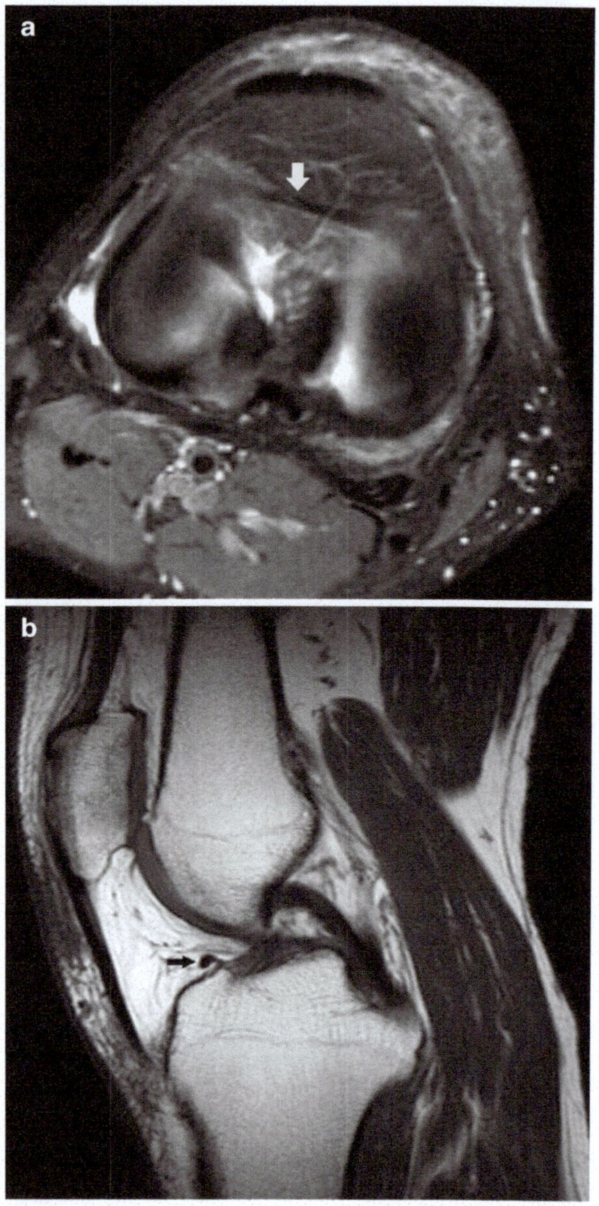

Fig. 5.8 The anterior transverse intermeniscal ligament. Axial fat-suppressed intermediate T2-W MR image (**a**). The ligament runs anteriorly between the two anterior meniscal horns (*white arrow*). Sagittal SE T1-WI (**b**). The ligament is seen as dark oval spot (*black arrow*) at the posterior aspect of Hoffa's fat pad and can be followed on serial images

Ligamentum Mucosum

The infrapatellar plica or ligamentum mucosum has an arcuate course from its posterior femoral attachment just anterior to the ACL, anteriorly and inferiorly to the posteroinferior tip of Hoffa's fat pad, before turning superiorly to the lower pole of the patella (Fig. 5.11).

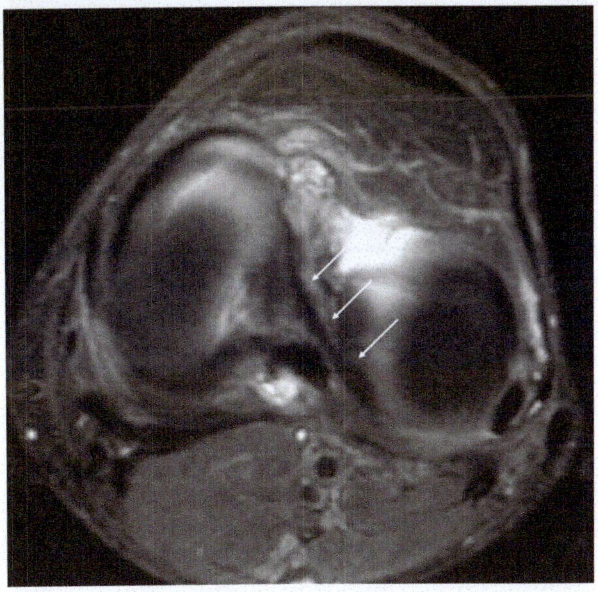

Fig. 5.9 The oblique intermeniscal ligament. Axial fat-suppressed intermediate T2-W MR image. The ligament runs in the transverse plane from the posterior horn of the lateral meniscus to the anterior horn of the medial meniscus (*arrows*)

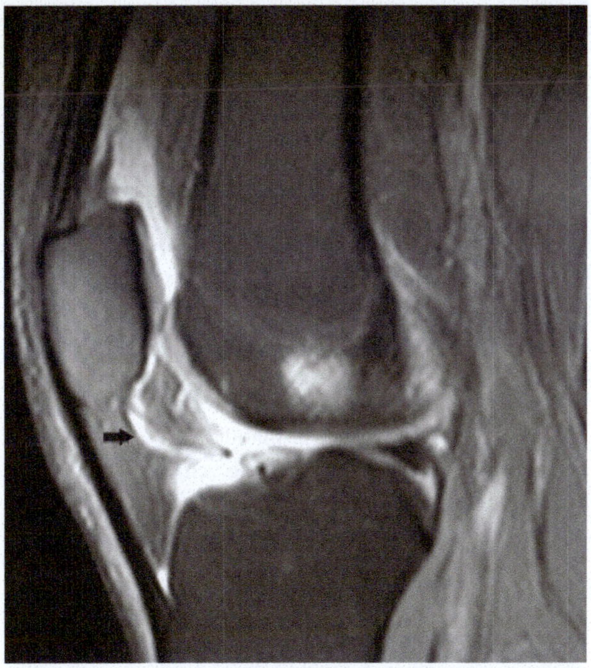

Fig. 5.11 Fluid-filled ligamentum mucosum. Sagittal fat-suppressed intermediate T2-W demonstrates a hyperintense structure that runs from the anterior and inferior aspect of Hoffa's fad pad to the lower pole of the patella (*arrow*)

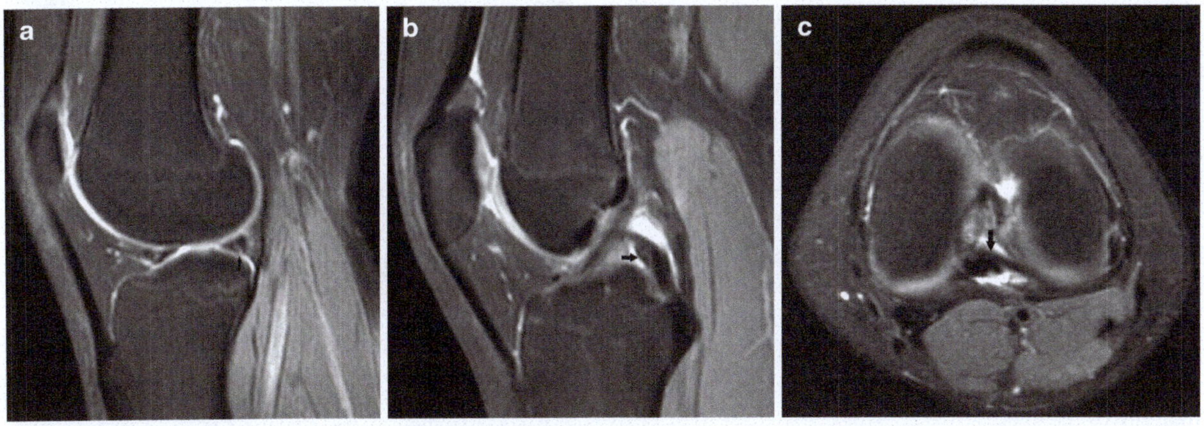

Fig. 5.10 Prominent meniscofemoral ligament of Humphrey mimicking a lateral meniscus tear. Lateral sagittal fat-suppressed intermediate T2-W MR image (**a**). MFL attachment to the posterior third of lateral meniscus simulating a tear (*arrow*). Midsagittal fat-suppressed intermediate T2-W MR image (**b**), demonstrating the course of the anterior MFL (*arrow*), also demonstrated on the axial fat-suppressed intermediate T2-W MR image (*arrow*) (**c**)

Medial Stabilizing Ligaments

The medial knee is stabilized by the deep static components of the MCL and the dynamic PM pes anserine tendons. Anteriorly, the medial retinaculum and fibers of the vastus medialis obliquus provide additional support.

Lateral Stabilizing Ligaments

The lateral collateral ligament consists of two separate ligamentous components: anteriorly the iliotibial band and posteriorly the fibular collateral ligament – biceps – popliteus complex.

Other small structures of the posterolateral corner (PLC) include the arcuate ligament, the popliteofibular ligament, the popliteomeniscal fascicles, the oblique popliteal ligament, and the fabellofibular ligament. Most of these structures can be seen on coronal MR images, although the smaller structures are not always visible in its entire course.

5.2.2 Technique

Equipment and techniques for MRI vary widely. A circumferential surface coil is mandatory to ensure uniform signal-to-noise across the entire image and provide better spatial resolution. Complete assessment of the knee requires that images should be obtained in the sagittal, coronal, and axial planes.

A minimum slice thickness of 4 mm is recommended to ensure that the intraarticular ligaments are properly evaluated. Orientation of images along the axis of the ACL can be helpful, although rarely required. The anterolateral (AL) margin of the lateral femoral condyle can be used as a guide.

Sequences that use a short echo time (TE <20 ms), such as T1, proton-density (PD), and gradient-echo T2*-weighted images (WIs), are most sensitive for identifying meniscal tears. Long echo-time (T2) sequences are less sensitive but more specific. Conventional spin echo (SE) sequences are more sensitive to meniscal pathology than fast spin echo (FSE) sequences. FSE technique offers the advantage of faster data acquisition, but blurring effect inherent to this technique that can obscure a meniscal tear. T2-WIs with spectral fat saturation (FS) (or short inversion time inversion recovery (STIR)) can be performed in conjunction to enhance the detection of bone-marrow edema (BME) or contusion. Table 5.2. summarizes the pulse recommendations for routine imaging of the knee.

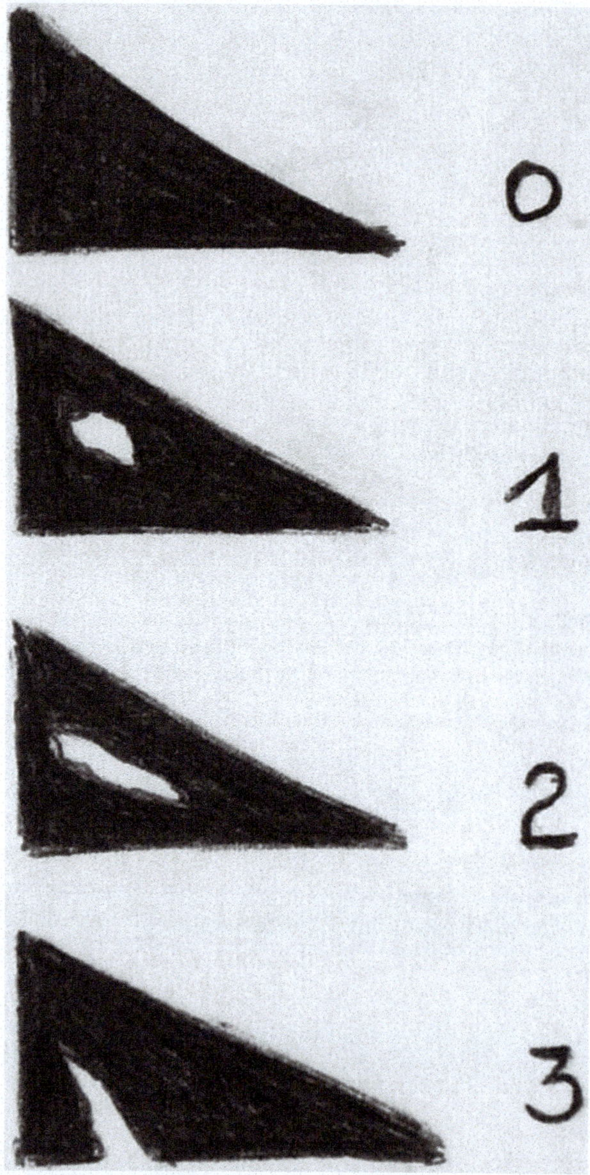

Fig. 5.12 Grading of intrameniscal signal as seen on MRI. *Grade 0*, normal; *grade 1*, intrasubstance globular-appearing signal not extending to the articular surface; *grade 2*, linear increased signal patterns not extending to the articular surface; *grade 3*, the abnormal signal extends to the articular surface. Only grade 3 signal represents meniscal tear. (Reprinted with permission from Vanhoenacker et al. 2007)

5.2.3 Relevant Pathology

5.2.3.1 Meniscal Tears

Classification of Meniscal Tears

To understand the significance of increased signal intensity in meniscal abnormalities, an MR grading system has been developed and correlated with a histopathologic model (Fig. 5.12): *grade 1*, intrasubstance globular-appearing signal not extending to the articular surface; *grade 2*, linear increased signal patterns not extending to the articular surface; and *grade 3*, the abnormal signal extends to the articular surface. The clinical importance of grade 2 signal abnormality in the meniscus, as seen on MRI and not visualized arthroscopically, is still not well

Table 5.2 Pulse recommendations for the knee

Pulse sequence	WI	Plane
SE	T1	Coronal
FS FSE	T2	Coronal
FS FSE	T2	Axial
FSE	PD + T2	Sagittal

understood. Grades 1 and 2 represent intrasubstance mucinous degeneration in an adult or prominent vascularity in a child and have no surgical significance. Grade 3 is visible by arthroscopy and represents a meniscal tear.

In addition to observing increased signal intensity within tears, the morphology of the meniscus should be assessed when evaluating meniscal lesions.

The "direct" signs associated with meniscal tears on MRI (Fig. 5.13) include

1. Unequivocal grade 3 signal: extension of the signal changes should be visible at least two slices to make a confident diagnosis of a meniscustear ("two slice rule").
2. Abnormal meniscal morphology with displaced or missing meniscal tissue: Several signs such as the absent bow tie sign, the double PCL sign ("bucket-handle tear") and the larger anterior horn sign ("flipped meniscus") are indicative of displaced meniscus fragments.
3. Meniscocapsular separation.

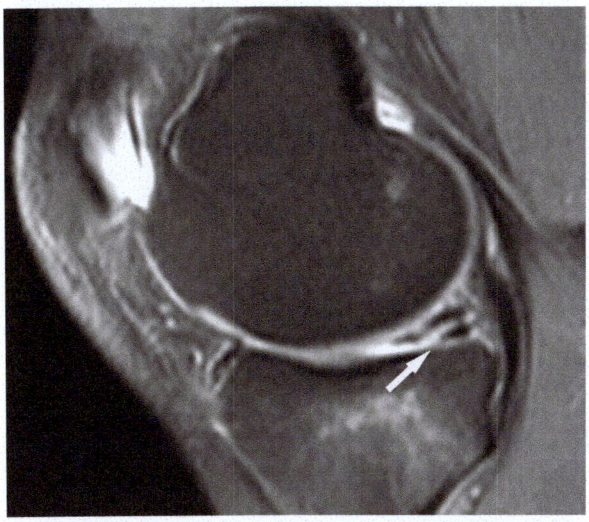

Fig. 5.13 Direct sign of meniscal tear. Sagittal PD-WI demonstrates grade 3 signal intersecting the inferior articular surface of the meniscus, representing oblique meniscal tear (*arrow*)

The "indirect" signs associated with meniscal tears on MRI include

1. Abnormal superior popliteomeniscal fascicle and posterior pericapsular edema: lateral meniscal tear, most commonly posterior horn.
2. Posterior bone bruise of the medial tibial plateau: peripheral tears of the posterior horn of the medial meniscus or tears of the posterior root ligament of the medial meniscus. Tears of this ligament can be associated with ganglioncysts at the posterior aspect of the tibia as well.
3. Extrusion (>3 mm) of the medial meniscus: degeneration, complex, or large radial tear, tear involving the meniscal root.

Meniscal tears can be classified into two primary tear planes: vertical and horizontal (Fig. 5.14). Vertical tears are often of a traumatic origin and occur in younger individuals, whereas horizontal tears are usually secondary to meniscal (mucoid) degeneration and occur at later age.

Vertical tears are further subdivided into radial (perpendicular to the surface of the meniscus) and longitudinal (parallel to the long axis of the meniscus) varieties. An oblique vertical ("flap") tear is the most common meniscal tear type and demonstrates both radial and longitudinal components, as it courses obliquely across the meniscus, resulting in a flap of unstable meniscus. They most commonly affect the posterior horn and are seen as predominantly horizontal on sagittal MR images originating along the inferior surface at the free edge.

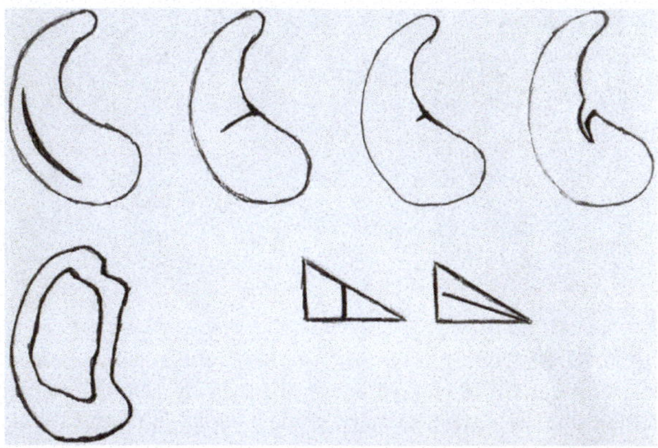

Fig. 5.14 Classification of meniscal tears (*left to right*): peripheral, longitudinal tear; large and small radial tear; oblique parrot-beak tear; bucket-handle tear; vertical tear; horizontal tear. (Reprinted with permission from Vanhoenacker et al. 2007)

Radial tears are relatively uncommon meniscal tears and most commonly occur at the junction of the anterior horn and body of the lateral meniscus and at the meniscotibial attachment of the posterior horn of the medial meniscus. They are often seen as blunting of the free edge on coronal (MR) images. On sagittal images, the only evidence of a radial tear may be increased signal intensity on one or two peripheral sections (Fig. 5.15).

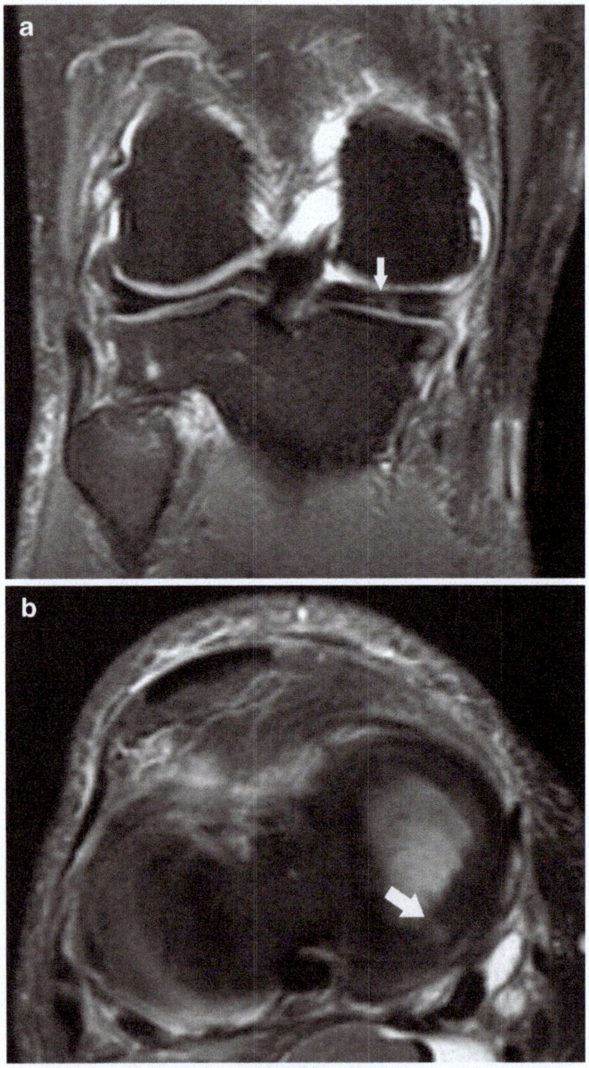

Fig. 5.15 Radial tear of the posterior horn of the medial meniscus. Coronal fat-suppressed intermediate T2-W MR image (**a**) demonstrates a vertical oriented grade 3 signal in the posterior horn of the medial meniscus (*arrow*). On the axial fat-suppressed intermediate T2-W MR image (**b**), the radial orientation of the tear is confirmed (*arrow*). Note also the ill delineation of the free edge of the posterior horn of the medial meniscus

A bucket-handle tear is an important and not infrequent type of meniscal injury, occurring in about 10% of meniscal tears in most series. It typically consists of a vertical or oblique tear in the posterior horn that extends longitudinally through the body segment and anterior horn, usually occurring acutely with a sudden impact, splitting the meniscus longitudinally. Coronal and sagittal MR images demonstrate blunting of the meniscus donor with the remaining meniscus being smaller than normal. The inner meniscal fragment is often displaced in the intercondylar notch, creating a "handle." Reported MRI signs for bucket-handle tears include absent bow tie sign, the double PCL sign, the disproportional posterior horn sign, the anterior flipped fragment sign, and double anterior horn sign (Fig. 5.16).

Horizontal tears extend through the meniscus along a plane parallel to the tibial plateau, dividing the meniscus in inferior and superior segments. A horizontal cleavage tear is the most common type of tear to be associated with a meniscal cyst (Fig. 5.17). These cysts occur as a result of fluid extruding through the tear by a ball valve effect, and collecting either in the meniscus (intrameniscal cyst) or at the meniscocapsular junction (parameniscal cyst). These cysts tend to recur after resection if the underlying meniscal cyst is not repaired. With a horizontal tear, a portion of the meniscus may flip into the adjacent synovial gutter along the margin of the joint. These fragments may be missed easily at arthroscopy, when they are not identified on MRI.

Complex meniscal tears display combinations of vertical and horizontal tear patterns (Fig. 5.18).

Meniscocapsular separation is a subtype of meniscal tear, occurring most commonly along the medial meniscus, but the lateral meniscus may be affected also. Typically, the posterior meniscal horn is separated from the capsule with displacement of the posterior meniscal margin from the posterior tibial border by more than 8–10 mm.

Postoperative Meniscus

For the radiologist, imaging the postoperative meniscus remains a challenge. As in preoperative patients, MRI is the most valuable imaging method for postoperative evaluation of the knee.

Standard MRI protocols are less reliable in imaging postoperative knees than in unoperated knees, especially for the diagnosis of meniscal tears, with accuracies

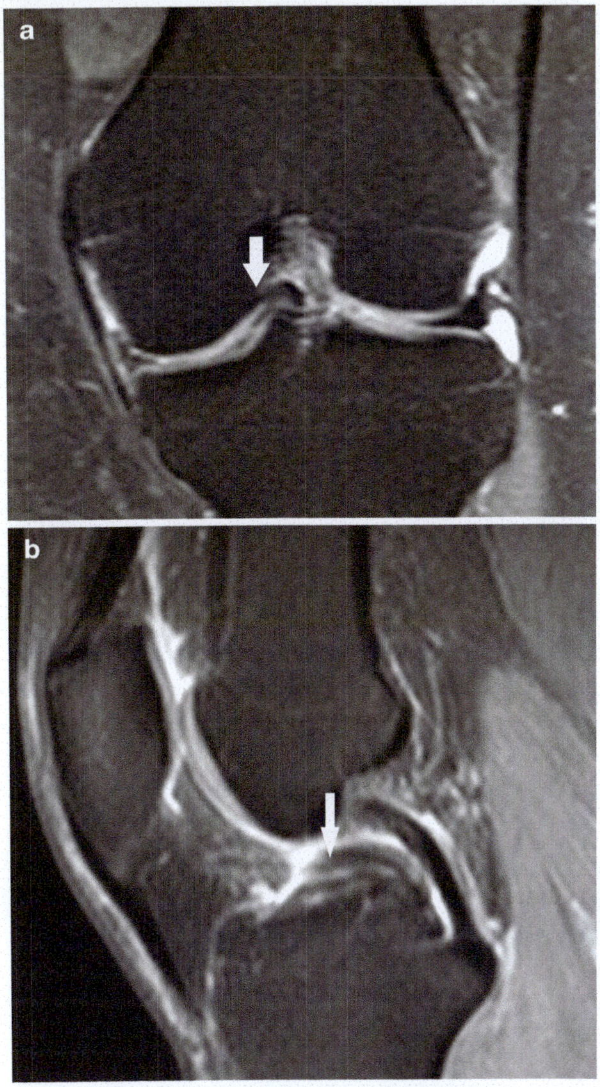

Fig. 5.16 Bucket-handle tear of the medial meniscus. Coronal fat-suppressed PD-WI (**a**) displays abnormal morphology and grade 3 signal in the medial meniscus with internally displaced meniscal fragment (*arrow*). Sagittal fat-suppressed PD-WI (**b**) demonstrates the meniscal fragment (*arrow*) in front of the PCL ("double PCL sign")

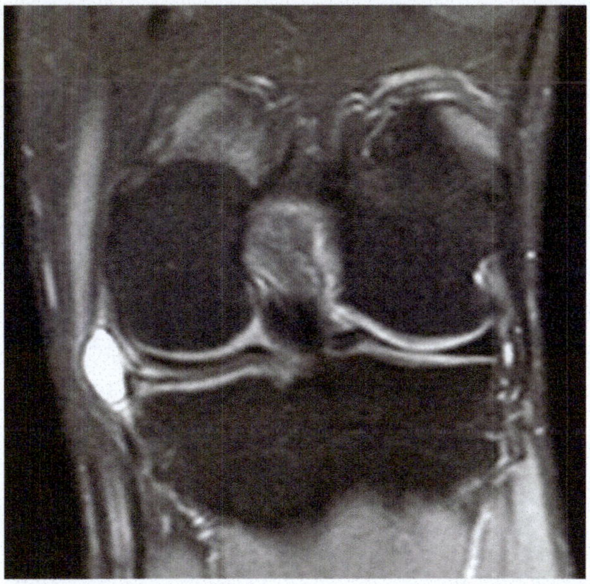

Fig. 5.17 Meniscal cyst. Coronal fat-suppressed PD-WI shows a large horizontal tear in the medial meniscus with parameniscal cyst

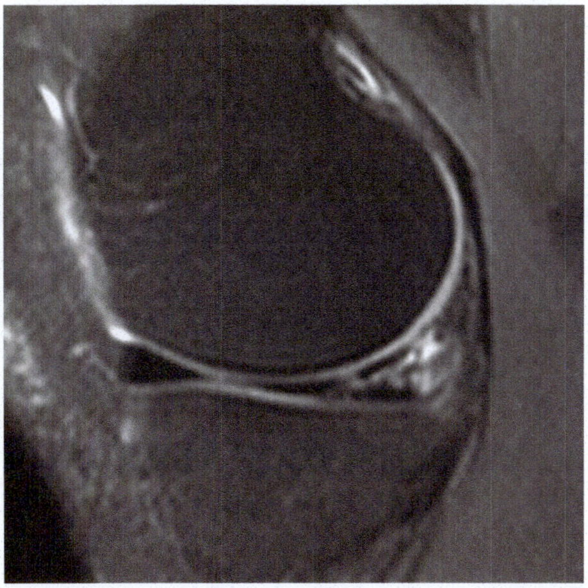

Fig. 5.18 Complex meniscal tear. Sagittal fat-suppressed PD-WI shows a medial meniscus tear with a combined vertical and horizontal tear pattern

ranging from less than 50–80%. Contour abnormalities and diffuse signal changes may be present in both normal postoperative menisci and in recurrent meniscal tears. The basic criteria for identifying a meniscal tear – increased intrameniscal signal on a T1-W or PD-WI extending to the meniscal surface - becomes an unreliable predictor in the postoperative knee. A high-signal line that reaches the articular surface (grade 3) may represent an area of meniscal healing and may be misinterpreted as a new tear. Furthermore, a partial resection could convert a grade 2 intrameniscal signal into a grade 3 signal, extending to the new surface of the partly resected meniscus. Fluid-intensity signal on a T2-WI extending into the meniscus is a stricter criterion for recurrent or residual tear, providing high specificity (92%) but low sensitivity (60%).

In an attempt to increase the diagnostic accuracy, direct MR arthrography (MRA) has been applied to the postoperative meniscus. The criterion for diagnosing a recurrent or residual tear of the meniscus using MRA is seeing extension of the gadolinium into the meniscal fragment or into the site of a meniscal repair.

In general, most patients do not need to undergo MRA, and conventional MRI should be considered as the first line investigation. Of utmost importance in the evaluation of the postoperative meniscus, is the availability of the preoperative images if possible and the operative report with details of the extent of resection.

We look for unequivocal sites of fluid-intensity signal within the meniscal remnant, displaced fragments or tears in a new location, as the only reliable criteria for a recurrent or residual tear. Standard criteria can be used to interpret areas of the menisci known to be separated from the site of prior surgery. Investigation with MRA (or CT arthrography) could then be considered if conventional MRI is normal (no severe degenerative arthrosis, avascular necrosis (AVN), chondral injuries, native joint fluid extending into a meniscus, or a tear in a new area), if the clinical suspicion of recurrent tear is high, or if conventional MRI is inconclusive. In particular, MRA may be useful when there is prior knowledge of significant meniscal resection (more than 25%) or meniscal repair with new symptoms in the same area as the initial symptoms. Furthermore, MRA is of additional value in assessing the articular cartilage, deteriorating more rapidly after meniscectomy.

5.2.3.2 Ligamentous Trauma

Anterior Cruciate Ligament Tears

Injury of the ACL is common and may be due to several mechanisms. Tear can be acute or chronic and complete or partial.

Complete Tears

The diagnosis of an acute complete ACL tear is usually straightforward. The main primary finding on sagittal orientated MR images is failure to identify the normal hypointense low signal line of the anteromedial bundle (Fig. 5.19). The normal linear striated appearance of the ACL is replaced by an amorphous

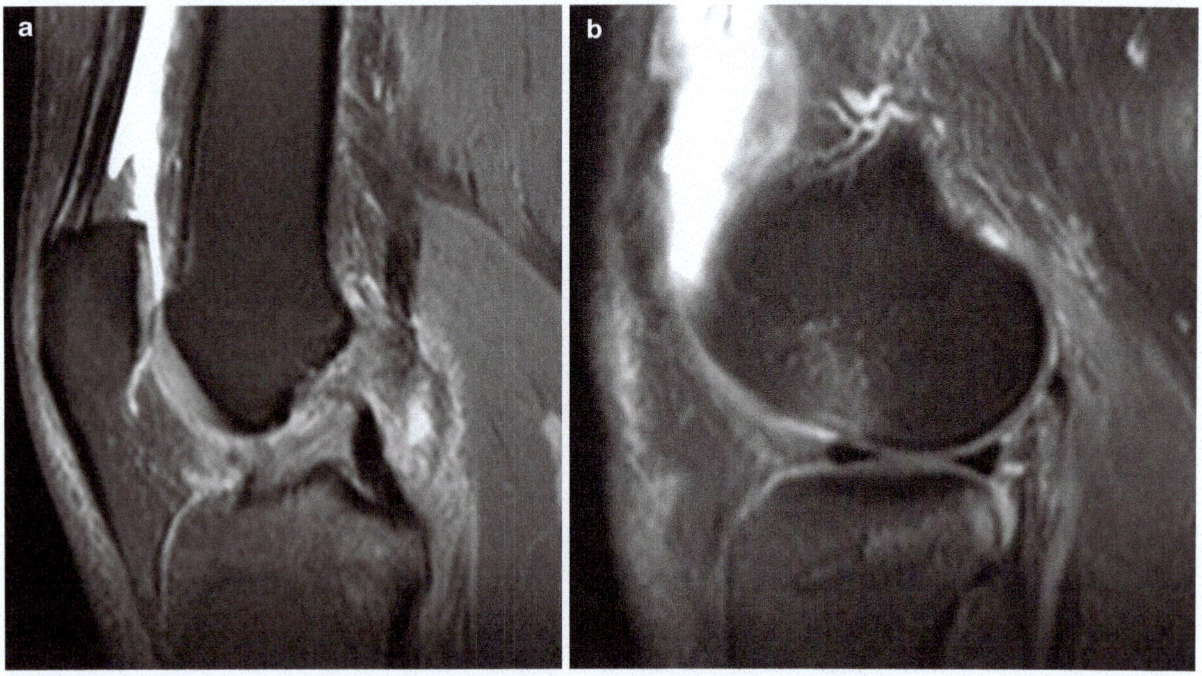

Fig. 5.19 Anterior cruciate ligament tear. Midsagittal fat-suppressed PD-WI (**a**) shows absence of the ACL. Note the presence of bone marrow edema at the posterolateral tibia and the middle third of the lateral femurcondyle (**b**) as a consequence of impaction of the posterior tibia against the lateral femur (secondary signs of ACL tear)

Table 5.3 Secondary signs of ACL tears

Signs of bone injury	Soft tissue signs	Anterior tibial translation
BME posterolateral tibia	ACL angle (between anterior aspect of distal ACL and anterior portion of intercondylar eminence) less than 45°	Buckling of the PCL
BME lateral femoral condyle	Blumensaat angle (between anterior aspect of distal ACL and intercondylar roof) more than 21°	PCL line (drawn along the posterior distal portion of the PCL) not intersecting the femur within 5 cm of the distal aspect of the femur
BME or fracture posteromedial tibia	Horizontal shearing of Hoffa fat pad	Tangent to the lateral femoral condyle passes more than 5 mm from the posterior tibial margin
Deep lateral femoral notch sign (more than 1.5 mm)	Buckling of the patellar tendon	Uncovering of the posterior horn of the lateral meniscus: vertical line along the posterior tibial cortex insects the posterior horn of the lateral meniscus
Associated Segond fracture	Rupture of the iliotibial band	Straight LCL

cloud-like appearance of high or heterogeneous signal intensity on T2-WIs. The rupture is usually located in the proximal or mid-portion of the ligament. Shortly after the injury, the disrupted ligamentous fibers are surrounded by edema and hemorrhage, and therefore it is sometimes difficult to identify the exact location of the tear.

In more chronic stages, the torn ACL can undergo complete atrophy. Remnants of the torn ligament may lie in an abnormal position along the floor of the joint.

Secondary signs of ACL rupture are summarized in Table 5.3. Secondary signs do not significantly improve the diagnostic accuracy compared to the primary signs. Although they are rarely of practical value, they may – however – be helpful in the differential diagnosis of a partial from a complete tear.

Partial Tears

The diagnosis of partial ACL rupture can be more problematic. The reported signs (such as focal areas of loss of signal, thickening or thinning of the ligament, or abnormal orientation) are neither as sensitive nor as specific as those indicating complete rupture.

Posterior Cruciate Ligament Tears

The PCL is a stronger structure than the ACL that rarely ruptures. PCL tear results from a major trauma and occurs usually in combination with other ligamentous trauma. Posterolateral corner injuries are present in approximately half of PCL injuries, resulting in minor edema around the capsule, but fortunately two thirds of these will be clinically stable.

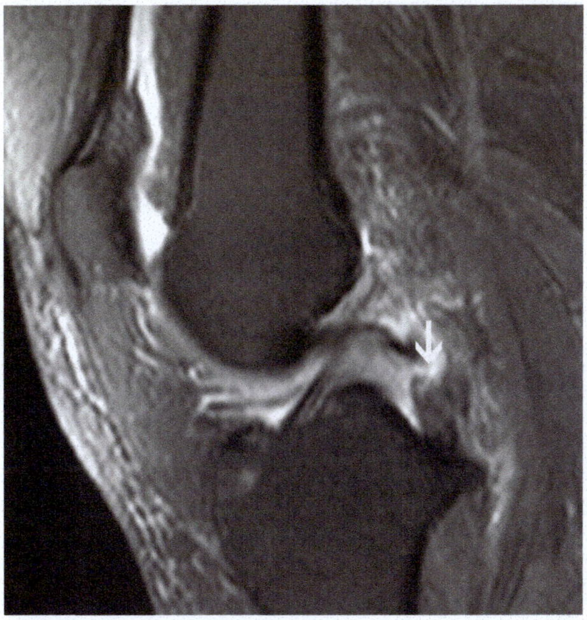

Fig. 5.20 Posterior cruciate ligament tear. Midsagittal fat-suppressed intermediate-WI shows focal discontinuity of the PCL (*arrow*)

MRI plays an important role in the assessment of PCL injuries. Indeed, PCL rupture is difficult to evaluate on clinical examination and at arthroscopy.

Signs of a complete PCL tear include focal discontinuity or nonvisualization of the ligament with or without an hemorrhagic or edematous mass (Fig. 5.20).

Partial intrasubstance tears are identified more commonly than with ACL rupture.

Medial Collateral Ligament Tears

MCL ligament injury results from valgus stress on the knee and is often associated with injury of the menici and ACL. Coronal fat suppressed T2-W MR images are preferred for assessment of the MCL. There is a good correlation between clinical and MRI staging of MCL tears. A grade 1 injury clinically has medial-sided pain, some laxity but with a firm end-point. On MRI, minor edema around the superficial aspect of ligament is seen. A grade 2 injury is a partial tear and has a valgus laxity with a soft but definable end-point. MRI reveals internal signal intensity changes appearing as an onion-skin aspect or partial disruption of MCL (Fig. 5.21). A grade 3 lesion presents clinically as a valgus laxity without a defined end-point and is correlated with complete ligament discontinuity on MRI (Fig. 5.22). Femoral insertion injuries are most common.

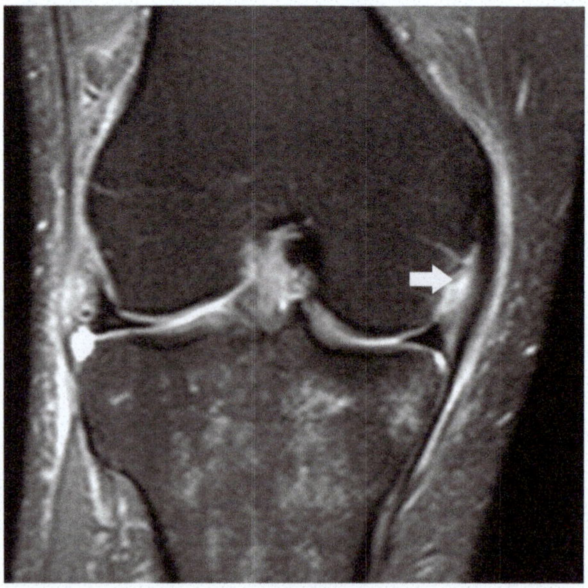

Fig. 5.21 Grade II medial collateral ligament (MCL) tear. Coronal fat-suppressed intermediate-WI shows soft-tissue edema adjacent to the superficial femoral part of the MCL and focal discontinuity of the deep meniscofemoral ligament (*arrow*)

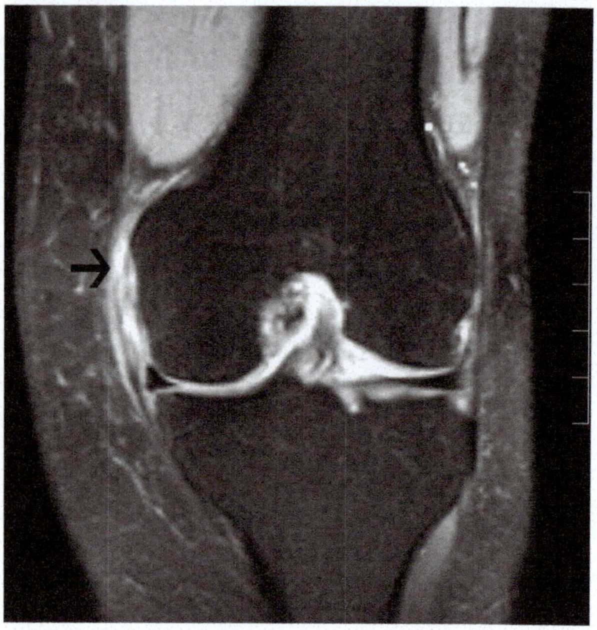

Fig. 5.22 Grade III medial collateral ligament tear. Coronal fat-suppressed intermediate-WI. Focal discontinuity of both the deep and superficial part of the MCL (*arrow*)

Posterolateral Corner Injury

Injuries of the ACL or PCL are often associated with injury of the posterolateral stabilizers of the knee. Unrecognized injury of the PLC can lead to failure of cruciate reconstruction. The different anatomic components of the PLC should be scrutinized for potential lesions. Imaging signs that are associated with significant PLC injury include soft-tissue edema adjacent to the ligamentous components of the PLC and ligamentous discontinuity (Fig. 5.23), and BME at the proximal fibula and at the medial femoral condyle. The latter occurs during varus strain with impaction of the tibial plateau against the medial femoral condyle. Bone avulsion at the insertion of the biceps femoris tendon at the fibula is known at the arcuate sign (Fig. 5.24).

Posteromedial Corner Injury

When MCL or ACL injuries are detected, a careful study of the PMC is warranted, as these may be associated with lesions at the insertion of the semimembranosus tendon.

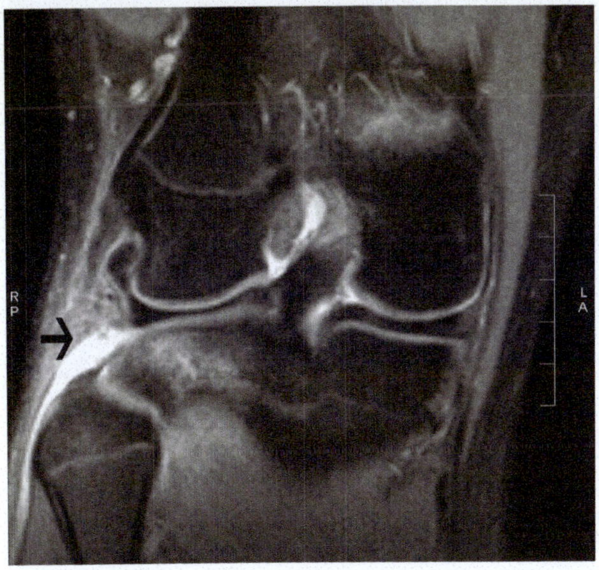

Fig. 5.23 Complete tear at the distal insertion of the fibular collateral ligament. Coronal fat-suppressed intermediate-WI. Focal discontinuity of the ligament at the proximal tibia (*arrow*)

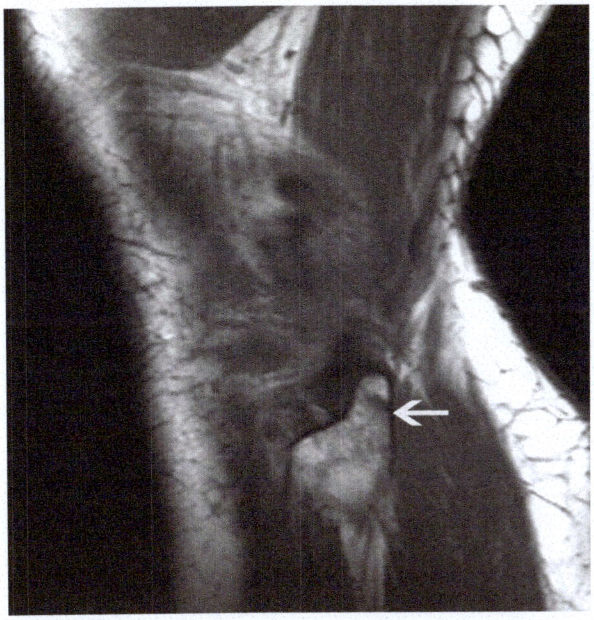

Fig. 5.24 Arcuate sign. Sagittal SE T1-WI. Notice the presence of a fracture at the proximal fibula, indicating a lesion of the conjoint tendon (*arrow*)

5.2.3.3 Bone-Marrow Edema and Osseous Lesions About the Knee

Traumatic BME (bruise) is most frequent and the underlying mechanism may be either acute or chronic.

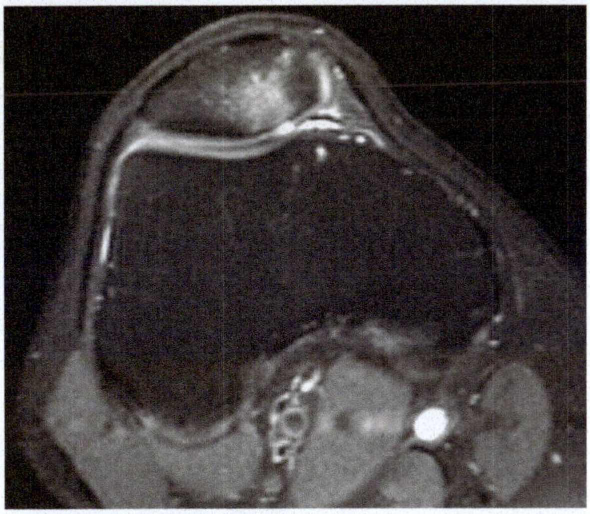

Fig. 5.25 BME due to direct impaction injury. Axial fat-suppressed intermediate-WI. There is extensive BME at the medial aspect of the patella due to a direct blow at the anterior aspect of knee

Variable incidences have been published but edema is often encountered in acute trauma (published incidences vary from 27 to 72%).

A minority of the studies of acute injuries will show bruising only without associated injuries.

Acute Traumatic Lesions

BME is frequently encountered on MRI after an injury to the musculoskeletal system. These osseous injuries may result from several forces acting on the joint. In general, compressive forces vs. traction forces will influence the extent of BME edema around the joint.

Impaction Injuries

Focal bruise may result from direct trauma to the bone (Fig. 5.25), but often a specific pattern of bone marrow changes on adjacent bones occurs due to impaction of one bone on another.

Impaction type of BME is extensive and will involve a broad surface of the involved bony structures.

Avulsive Injuries

Distraction injuries are usually due to valgus, varus or rotational stress on a joint, resulting in a small avulsion fracture related to a tendinous, ligamentous, or capsular attachment on the bone.

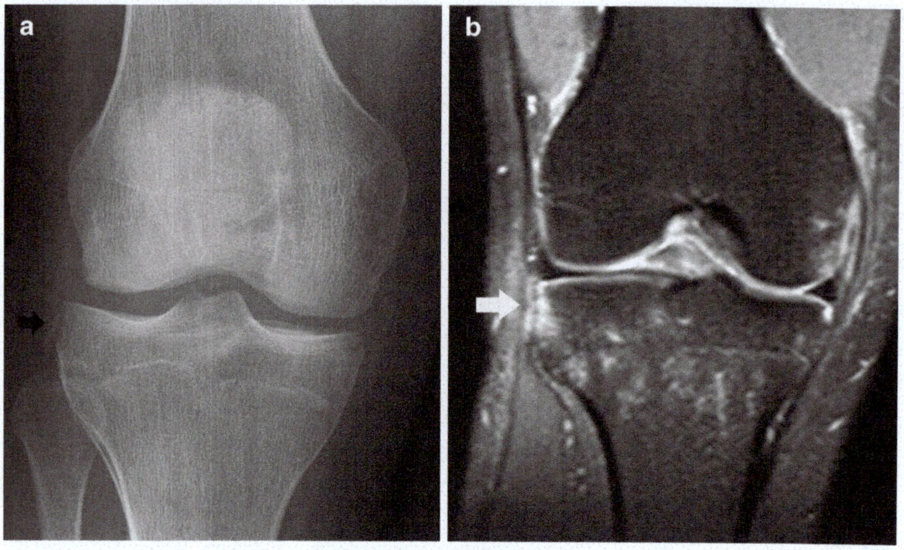

Fig. 5.26 Typical example of an avulsion fracture and associated BME (avulsion type BME). Standard radiograph (**a**) clearly shows an avulsion fracture (Segond fracture). Coronal fat-suppressed intermediate-WI (**b**) of the right knee shows only minor focal BME at the lateral aspect of the tibia

Because the cortical bone is involved rather than the trabecular bone, the resulting "avulsion BME-pattern" is much less extensive than in impaction injuries.

Moreover, the avulsed bone fragment may be very difficult to detect on MRI (Fig. 5.26a). In most instances, a small avulsion is far better demonstrated on conventional radiographs (Fig. 5.26b) or CT.

Complex Patterns

In most clinical situations, this rigorous distinction between *pure impaction type injuries* and *avulsive type injuries* is artificial, because both types will be seen in a single joint after acute traumatic injuries. Generally, the impaction type of BME will be encountered on the *entry site* of the force acting on a joint, whereas a distraction type of BME will be seen on the *exit site* of the force. Although avulsive type BME is less extensive than the impaction type, the former is usually the witness of underlying ligamentous sprain.

These soft-tissue lesions are often less conspicuous than the bruises, though they are more important, at least in the short-term follow-up, for stability reasons.

Indeed, sprain of the supporting structures of the joint may cause instability, if not recognized and appropriately treated.

Moreover, BME around a joint is usually the result of a combination of multiple forces (and not of a single force), which all have a certain amplitude and direction. The impact of these forces may differ with the position of the joint at the moment of the trauma (e.g., degree of flexion, varus, valgus…).

Certain combinations of forces are known to cause a specific injury.

Systematic analysis of the BME-pattern, together with the associated soft tissue changes can often reveal the specific mechanism of injury.

In this regard, the pattern and distribution of BME represents a "footprint" of the mechanism of acute trauma.

In the knee, for example, classic patterns, which are encountered in sports injuries are the pivot shift injury (Fig. 5.27), the hyperextension injury (Fig. 5.28), the clip injury (Fig. 5.29), dashboard injury (Fig. 5.30), and (transient) lateral patellar dislocation (Fig. 5.31).

Pivot shift injury, which occurs when valgus load is applied to the knee in various states of flexion, combined with external rotation of the tibia or internal rotation of the femur, will result in disruption of ACL. Resultant anterior subluxation of the tibia will cause impaction of the lateral femoral condyle against the posterolateral margin of the lateral tibial plateau. Therefore, BME will be present in the posterior aspect of the lateral tibial plateau and the middle portion of the lateral femoral condyle. Associated bone bruising at the posterior lip of the medial tibial plateau may be the result of contrecoup forces due to valgus forces. According to others, this medial-sided bone bruise is attributed to avulsion at the semimembranosus attachment. Concomitant soft-tissue injuries of the pivot shift injury are MCL lesions, lesion of the posterior

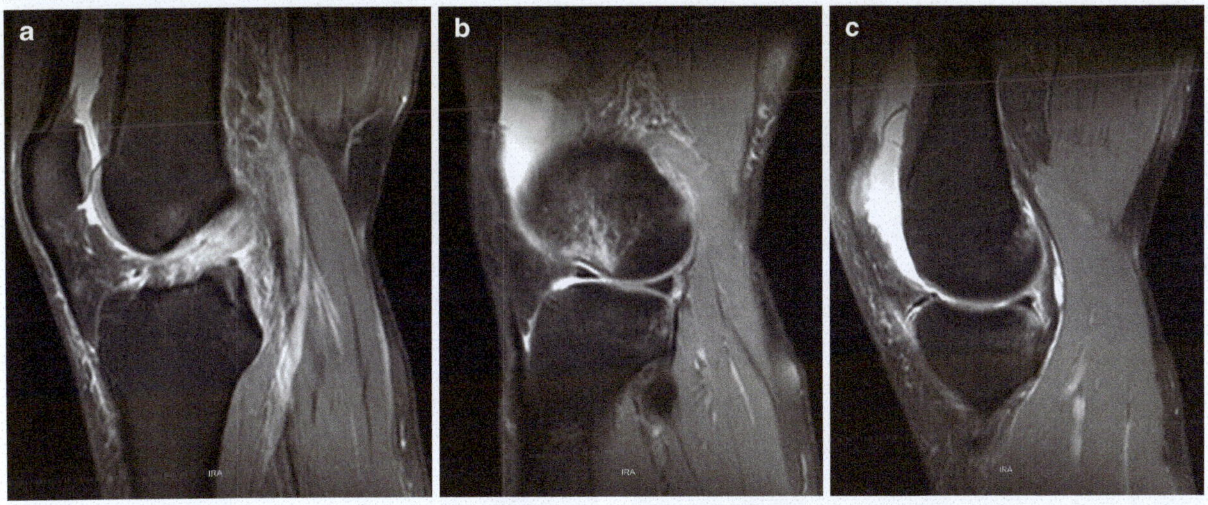

Fig. 5.27 Pivot shift injury in a soccer player with associated BME at the posteromedial corner of the knee. Sagittal fat-suppressed intermediate-WI (**a**) of the lateral aspect of the right knee. BME at the posterolateral aspect of the tibia and corresponding BME at the middle part of the lateral femur-condyle (with associated focal cortical depression). Midsagittal fat-suppressed intermediate-WI of the right knee shows complete disruption of the ACL (**b**). Sagittal fat-suppressed intermediate-WI of the medial aspect of the right knee (**c**). Note also BME at the posteromedial aspect of the tibia near the distal of the semimembranosus tendon. According to some authors, this lesion represents a contre-coup impaction lesion. According to others, however, this lesion represents a traction injury at the posteromedial corner of the knee due to external rotation of the knee. (Reprinted with permission from Vanhoenacker et al. 2007)

Fig. 5.28 Hyperextension trauma. Sagittal fat-suppressed intermediate-WI (**a**) of the right knee at the lateral compartment. Midsagittal fat-suppressed intermediate-WI (**b**) of the right knee. Severe hyperextension of the knee can result in the impaction of the anterior aspect of the femoral condyle against the anterior aspect of the tibial plateau. At the posterior aspect of the knee (distraction site), there is rupture of the posterior cruciate ligament and indistinct outline of the posterior joint capsule

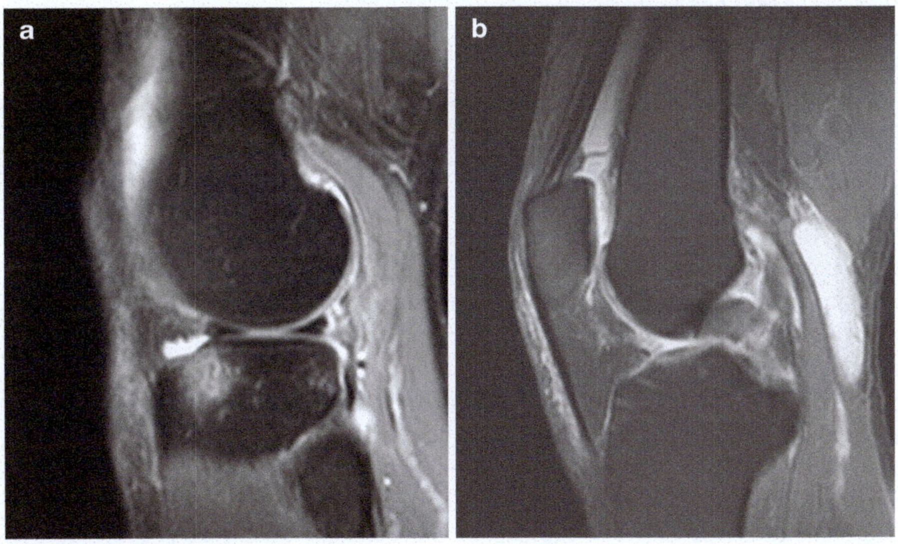

horn of the lateral and medial meniscus or a tear at the posterior joint capsule.

Hyperextension injury results in a kissing contusion pattern in the anterior aspect of the distal femur and proximal tibia. Associated soft-tissue lesions may include ACL or PCL tears or meniscal lesions.

The classic bone contusion pattern seen after lateral patellar dislocation includes involvement of the anterolateral (AL) aspect of the lateral femoral condyle and the inferomedial aspect of the patella.

Associated soft-tissue injuries include sprain or disruption of the medial soft-tissue restraints (medial retinaculum, medial patellofemoral ligament, and the medial patellotibial ligament).

Clip injury occurs when pure valgus stress is applied to the knee while the knee is in mild flexion. BME is

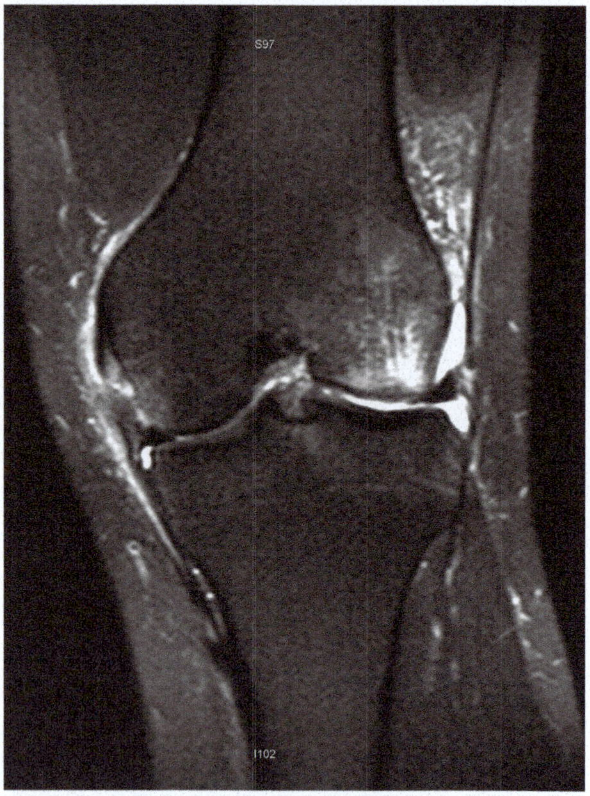

Fig. 5.29 Clip injury. Coronal fat-suppressed FSE T2 W image of the left knee shows a large area of BME involving the lateral femoral condyle. Minimal edema is noted within the medial femoral condyle near the proximal attachment of the MCL. There is partial disruption of the MCL. (Reprinted with permission from Vanhoenacker et al. 2007)

most prominent in the lateral femoral condyle due to impaction forces, whereas a second smaller area of edema may be present in the medial femoral condyle secondary to avulsive forces at the insertion of the MCL.

Dashboard injury occurs when a posteriorly directed force is applied to the anterior aspect of the proximal tibia while the knee is in a flexed position. This will result in BME at the anterior aspect of the tibia and occasionally at the posterior surface of the patella. Associated soft-tissue injuries are disruption of the PCL and posterior joint capsule.

Failure of this pattern approach revealing the underlying mechanism of trauma may be due to several factors, including insufficient trauma, massive injury, or preexisting osteoarthritis associated with BME (usually encountered in older sporters). Moreover, accelerated osteoarthritis is more prevalent in sporters than in the general population, due to previous repetitive trauma.

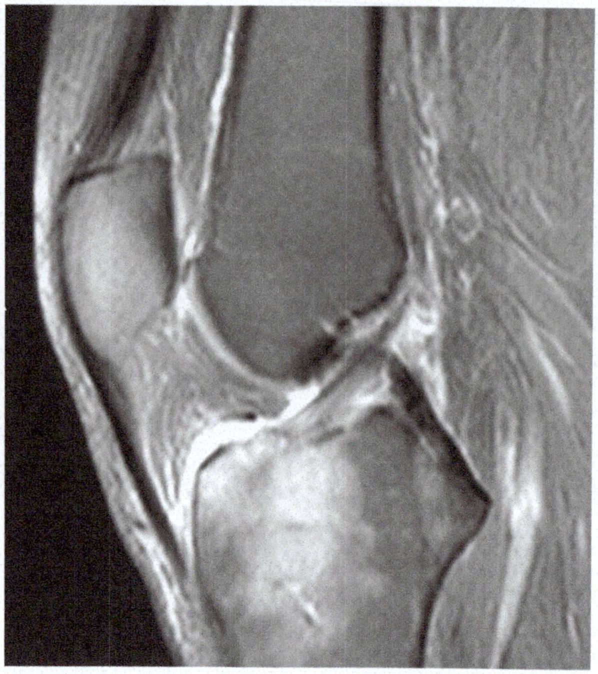

Fig. 5.30 Dashboard injury. Sagittal fat-suppressed intermediate-WI showing BME at the proximal tibia

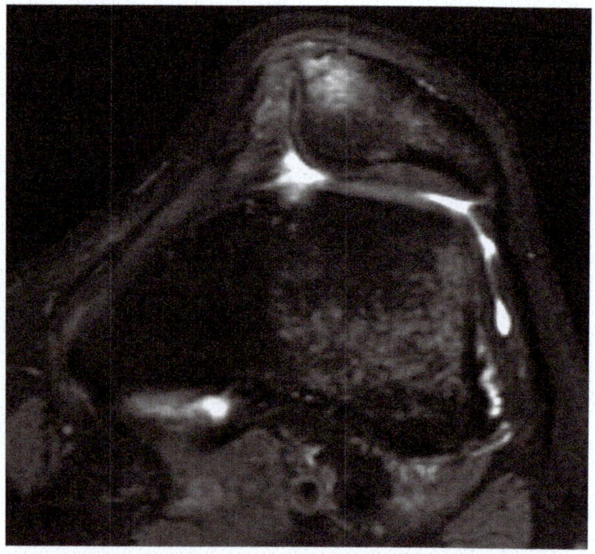

Fig. 5.31 Impaction type bone marrow edema, associated with lateral patellar dislocation. Axial fat-suppressed intermediate-WI of the right knee demonstrates BME involving the medial patellar facet and the anterior aspect of the lateral femoral condyle. Associated distraction at the medial patellar retinaculum will result in thickening and extensive hyperintensity due to partial disruption

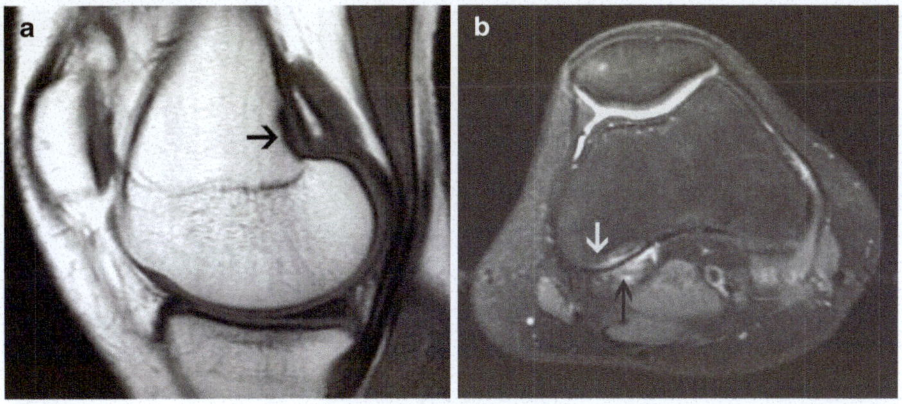

Fig. 5.32 Chronic avulsive irregularity. Sagittal SE T1-WI (**a**). There is a small well-delineated, hypointense lesion at the posteromedial aspect of the femur (*arrow*). Axial fat-suppressed intermediate-WI (**b**) demonstrates BME (*white arrow*) and adjacent soft-tissue edema (*black arrow*) at the proximal insertion of the medial gastrocnemius

Chronic Traumatic Lesions (Repetitive Trauma)

Fatigue and Insufficiency Fractures

This item will be described more in detail in Sect. 5.9.5.

Chronic Avulsive Injuries

Typical examples of chronic avulsive injuries include the chronic avulsive irregularity due to chronic traction at the insertion of the medial gastrocnemius or adductor longus at the posteromedial aspect of the knee. This lesion occurs in active adolescents and was formerly designated as periosteal desmoids or Bufkin lesion. This is – however – a misnomer, because the lesion does not represent a true tumor.

Apart from periosteal edema, MRI may also reveal BME and cortical signal abnormalities (Fig. 5.32).

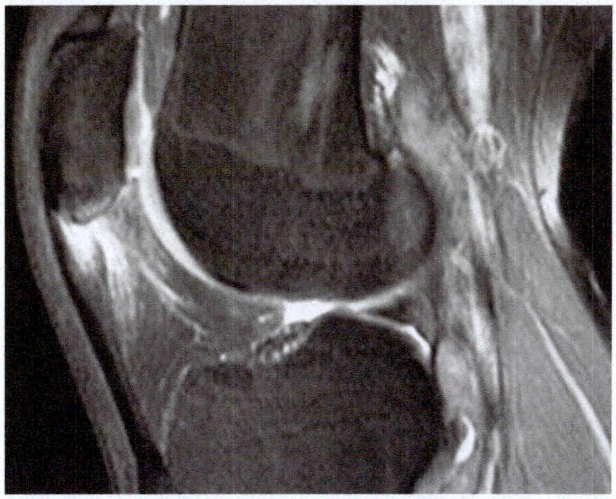

Fig. 5.33 Patellar tendinosis. Sagittal fat-suppressed intermediate-WI showing focal thickening and internal high signal within the proximal patellar tendon. Note also adjacent soft-tissue edema within Hoffa's fat pad and BME at the apex of the patella

5.2.3.4 Tendon Disorders

Generally, tendon disease is characterized by caliber changes, increased signal intensity on T2-WIs, and associated (bone) and soft-tissue edema.

Patellar Tendon Disease

The patellar tendon is vulnerable to overuse type injuries. Jumper's knee (patellar tendinosis) consists of degeneration of the proximal tendon directly adjacent to the inferior pole of the patella. The probable mechanism of injury is impingement of the tendon by the inferior pole of the patella. The abnormality is typically confined to the deep surface of the central portion of the tendon. Ultrasound is the technique of choice to confirm clinical suspected lesions. Plain radiographs may demonstrate calcification. On MRI, the abnormal portion of the tendon is thickened and shows increased signal on all sequences (Fig. 5.33). There may be associated BME at the inferior pole of the patella or fluid in the associated soft tissue. A common finding on MR is impingement of the lateral aspect of the patellar tendon on the anterolateral (AL) articular margin of the lateral femoral condyle (lateral patellar tendon-lateral femoral condyle friction syndrome). Some minor high signal may be detected in the fat that is interposed between the tendon and the condyle. Although this entity may be seen in patients

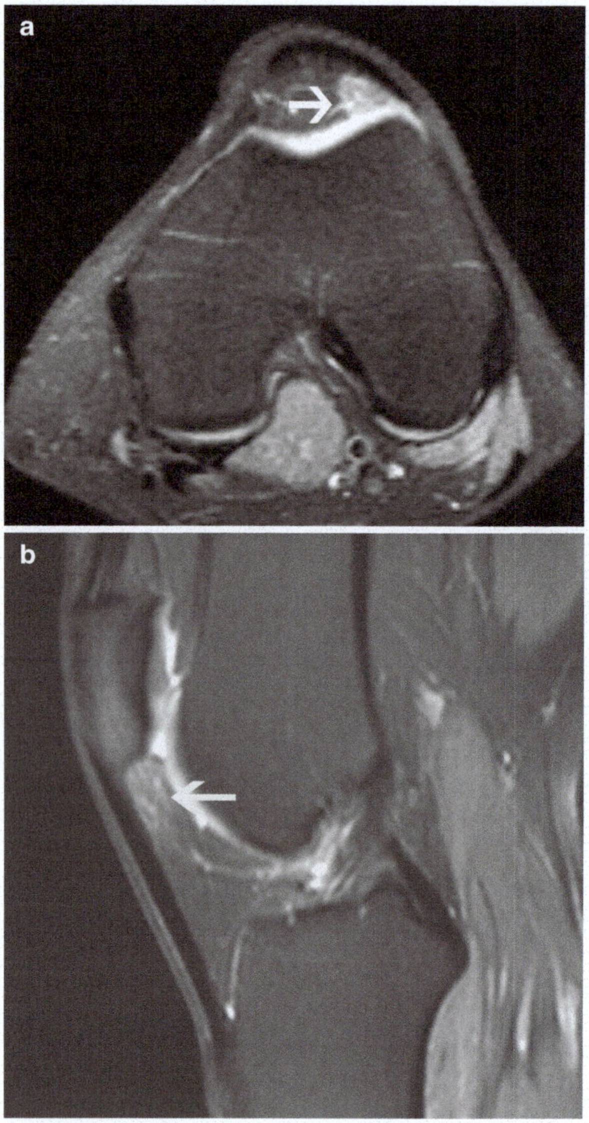

Fig. 5.34 Lateral patellar tendon-lateral femoral condyle friction syndrome. Axial (**a**) and sagittal (**b**) fat-suppressed intermediate-WI demonstrate high signal within Hoffa's fat pad between the lateral femoral condyle and the lateral patellar tendon (*white arrows*)

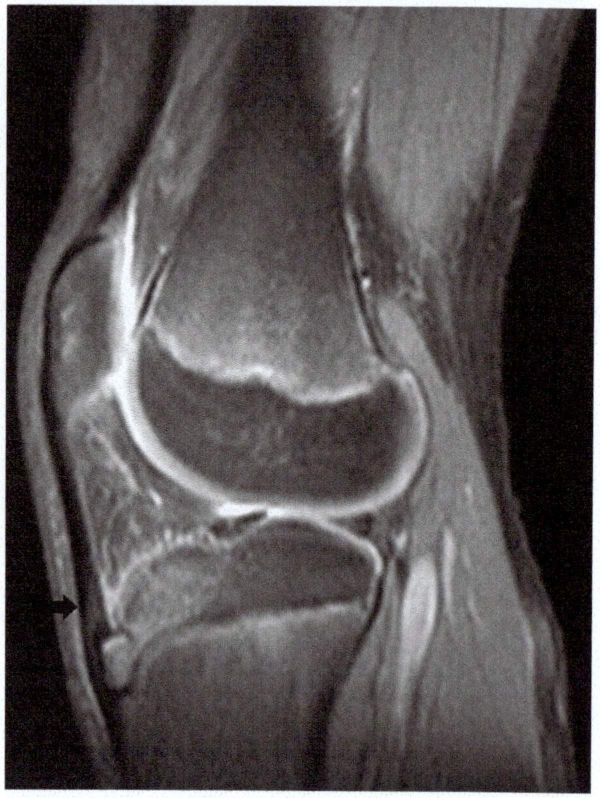

Fig. 5.35 Osgood–Schlatter disease. Sagittal fat-suppressed intermediate-WI reveals a high signal within the distal patellar tendon (*arrow*) and adjacent BME at the tibial tuberosity

with anterolateral pain, it is so common a finding on routine MR that its significance is still a matter of debate (Fig. 5.34).

In the adolescent, the commonest condition is Osgood Schlatter's disease, which is a traction injury of the distal patellar tendon at the tibial tubercle. Sinding–Larsen–Johansson syndrome is a similar traction type injury that occurs at the proximal end of the tendon. In both contions, MR is similar with fragmentation of the tibial tubercle and inferior pole of the patella, respectively and widening of the adjacent tendon with edema (Fig. 5.35). These two conditions have a good prognosis and resolve with conservative management.

Patellar tendon rupture is rare. Predisposing factors are patellar tendinosis, previous steroid injections, previous ACL repair with patellar graft, and certain chronic medical disorders. The tear usually occurs close to the tendon's origin at the inferior pole of the patella. Early surgical repair is indicated, so it is important to make a timely diagnosis. Both ultrasound and MRI may confirm tendon discontinuity and may determine the site and extent of the rupture.

Quadriceps Injuries

Injury to the quadriceps tendon may be the result of acute trauma caused by rapid deceleration, such as running when the foot is planted, or it may be caused

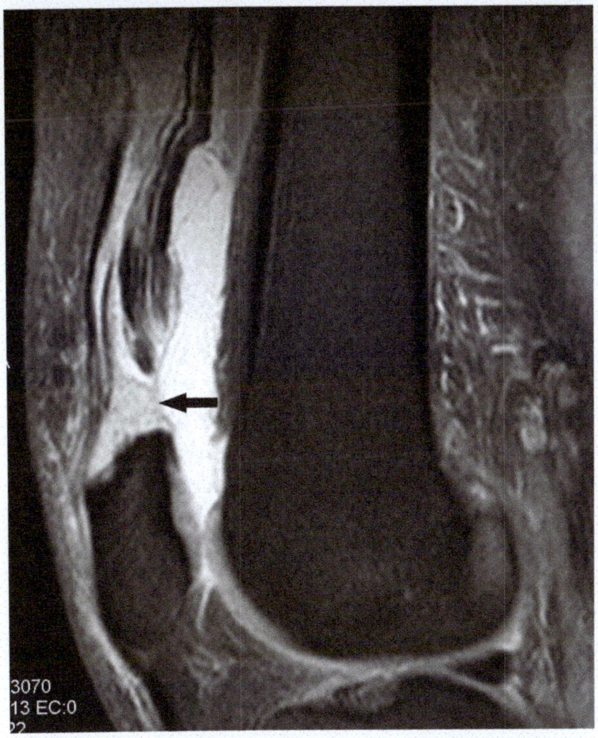

Fig. 5.36 Complete quadriceps tendon rupture. Sagittal fat-suppressed intermediate-WI. There is a fluid-filled gap at the distal insertion of the quadriceps tendon at the patella (*arrow*)

by chronic microtrauma. Predisposing conditions are gout, diabetes, connective tissue disease, and other systemic disorders. Tendon discontinuity is usually seen distally or near the patellar attachment (Fig. 5.36). The rupture may be partial or complete. Complete tears require surgical repair.

5.2.3.5 Cartilage Lesions

Articular cartilage injury is a common finding during arthroscopy. In the knee, most of these injuries are associated with other problems, such as meniscal lesions and ACL injury.

Staging of Cartilage Lesions

The most well-known arthroscopic staging method for articular cartilage is that proposed by Outerbridge in 1961 and modified by Shahriaree (1985).

A practical classification system uses four grades of chondromalacia:

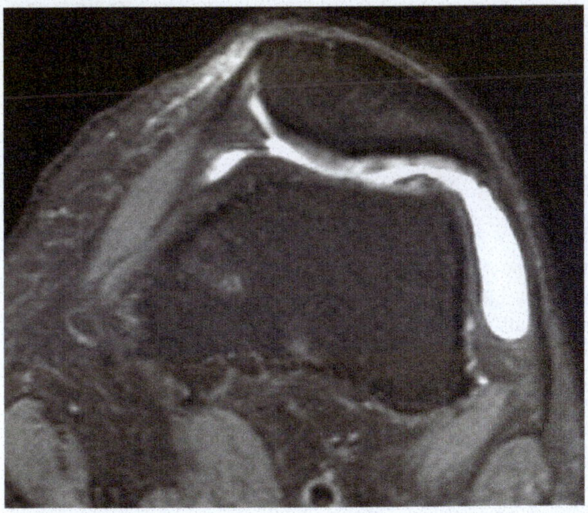

Fig. 5.37 Cartilage lesion grade III. Axial fat-suppressed intermediate-WI demonstrates multiple cartilage defects involving more than 50% but less than 100% cartilage thickness at the lateral facet of the patella

- 0: normal cartilage
- I: slight swelling (not adequately assessable on routine MR and CT imaging)
- II: fissuring or cartilage defects less than 50% of cartilage thickness
- III: fissuring or cartilage defects more than 50% but less than 100% of cartilage thickness (Fig. 5.37)
- IV: cartilage defects and erosion with exposure of subchondral bone

A final grade V could be added to allow for differentiation between full-thickness lesions with intact subchondral bone or with penetration of the bony endplate (Fig. 5.38). These grade V lesions are often associated with focal areas of BME.

Limitations of this classification are the inability MRI to reliably demonstrate early degenerative changes. Moreover, the size of a lesion is not taken into account in this classification as it is difficult to measure the diameter of an irregular lesion.

An ideal MRI study for cartilage should provide accurate assessment of cartilage thickness and volume, demonstrate morphological changes of the cartilage surface, demonstrate internal cartilage signal changes, allow evaluation of subchondral bone, and allow evaluation of the underlying cartilage physiology. Currently, three imaging sequences allow good morphologic evaluation of cartilage and chondral abnormalities. The proton-density and T2-weighted

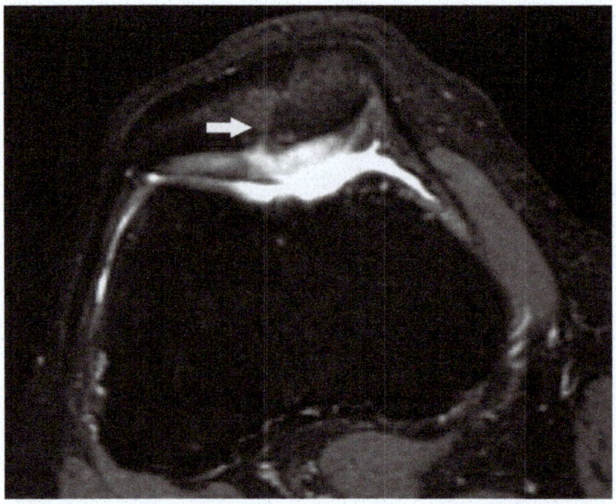

Fig. 5.38 Cartilage lesion grade V. Axial fat-suppressed intermediate-WI. Extensive cartilage lesions at the medial patella, extending down to the bone and adjacent BME (*arrow*)

FSE sequence, fat suppressed T1-weighted 3D spoiled gradient-echo (GRE) sequence and the 3D double echo steady state (3D-DESS) sequence are excellent for detection of grade 2, 3, and 4 chondral lesions. In these sequences, articular cartilage shows an intermediate signal intensity (SI) compared to the high SI of the adjacent joint fluid and the low SI of the subchondral bone.

Even in the absence of fluid, the borders of the cartilage are readily visible. Fatsuppressed intermediate weighted imaging (PD) allows simultaneous evaluation of other structures in the knee, such as menisci, ligaments, and tendons. Therefore, in routine clinical practice, fatsuppressed intermediate weighted imaging (PD) is usually sufficient.

As the deepest cartilage layers are not displayed well, overestimation of the depth of a cartilage lesion may occur. Therefore, more time-consuming high-resolution 3D techniques have to be performed whenever deep cartilage lesions are detected on the FSE images.

Thin-partitioned, fat suppressed 3D-spoiled GRE images, either using selective fat suppression (e.g., fat suppressed 3D-SPGR) or selective water excitation (WE) (e.g., FLASH-3D WE; DESS-3D WE), provide higher spatial and contrast resolution, but require longer acquisition times and are more vulnerable to magnetic susceptibility and metallic artifacts.

Moreover, thin-section volume acquisitions allow segmentation and accurate 3D reconstructions of articular cartilage.

Early cartilage degeneration (grade 1) cannot be reliably demonstrated using any of these sequences, and therefore novel MRI techniques that are sensitive to subtle structural and biochemical changes occurring early in the course of articular cartilage degeneration have been developed (delayed gadolinium-enhanced MRI of cartilage or dGemric and T2 relaxation time mapping of cartilage). These physiological MRI methods of articular cartilage are –however – not used in daily clinical routine.

MR-arthrography (MRA) allows a better delineation of the articular cartilage surface and the detection of small cartilage lesions. In osteochondral lesions, MRA can be performed to differentiate more accurately between stable and unstable lesions.

The outline of a cartilage lesion allows to differentiate between acute and more chronic lesions. In general, if the edges are sharp and the cartilaginous lesion is accompanied by BME in the subjacent bone, an acute lesion must be suspected. A shallow lesion with wide margins, a more gradual slope to its edges and sclerosis of the subchondral bone suggest a chronic, degenerative lesion.

There are many different surgical techniques for cartilage repair. These can be divided into three groups: the palliative (débridement or stabilization of loose articular cartilage), reparative (stimulation of repair from the subchondral bone), and restorative procedures (replacement of damaged cartilage). The palliative procedures are lavage, débridement, and shaving. None of these procedures, induce repair and relief is usually temporary.

Reparative procedures take advantage of the intrinsic repair response. By creating tiny fractures in the subchondral boen, these techniques expose all the vascular-mediated elements necessary for the classic healing response, such as fibrin clot, blood and marrow cells, cytokines, growth factors, and vascular invasion. Microfracturing is the most common used technique. Other reparative procedures are drilling and abrasion arthroplasty.

The restorative procedures include soft-tissue transplants, autologous chondrocyte implantation, allogenic chondrocyte transplantation and auto- or allo-genic stem cell transplantation, and autogenous or allogenous osteochondral transfers.

MRI is a good technique to evaluate cartilage repair by displaying thickness, edge integration, surface, subchondral bone plate, and marrow.

Table 5.4 Criteria of graft failure (modified with permission from Vanhoenacker et al. 2007)

Cartilage	Thickness of repair tissue less than 50% of native cartilage Delamination or dislocation of repair tissue Extensive surface damage with loss of more than 50% of cartilage thickness
Subchondral bone	Persistent bone marrow edema after 8–12 months Subchondral cyst formation Extensive subchondral sclerosis Collapse of the bony endplate

An overview of the most important criteria associated with graft failure is given in Table 5.4.

Osteochondrosis Dissecans (OCD) and Osteochondral Fractures

OCD and osteochondral fractures are mostly caused by shearing forces. While an osteochondral fracture is due to a single traumatic event, OCD is due to repetitive loading on the articular surface. OCD is a disease of childhood and adolescence. In the knee, the lateral aspect of the medial femoral condyle, the weight-bearing portion of the lateral femoral condyle, the patella, and the trochlear groove are typical sites.

MRI manifestations include a crater and a fragment of cartilage and bone, most frequently located at the femoral condyles. The fragment may be in situ or absent, fragmented, or healing in place. MRI assesses important parameters, such as size, location, stability, joint surface congruity, and viability of the fragment. These elements may influence therapeutic planning. Lack of enhancement of the bone fragment after intravenous injection of gadolinium contrast indicates the presence of nonviable bone. Native joint fluid on T2-WI between the fragment and the host bone is seen in unstable nonhealing lesions. Some authors prefer direct MR arthrography for determining surface cartilage irregularities or evaluation of fragment instability (Fig. 5.39).

5.2.3.6 Patellofemoral Disorders Other than Cartilage Lesions

Bipartite Patella

Bipartite patella is a normal variant consisting of a small separate ossification at the superolateral aspect of the patella. A symptomatic bipartite patella is characterized on MRI by BME between the accessory ossification and the main body of the patella (Fig. 5.40).

Patellar Maltracking

Patellofemoral dysplasia present with one or more of the following adverse anatomical features: a high riding patellar (patella alta); a flat trochlear groove; and a laterally positioned tibial tubercle. MRI will identify and quantify the anatomical abnormalities. The degree of patella alta is assessed on sagittal images by calculating the ratio of the minimum length of the posterior surface of the patellar tendon by the maximum length

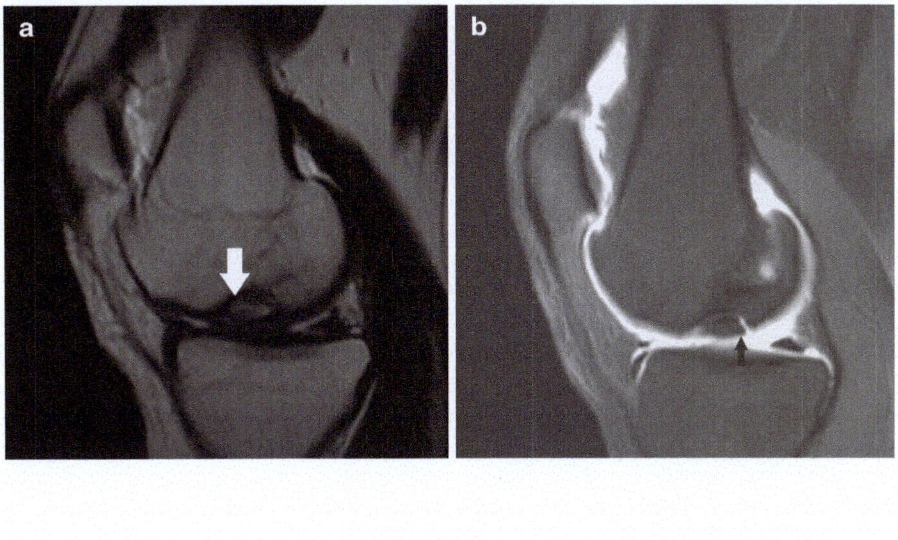

Fig. 5.39 Osteochondrosis dissecans of the medial femoral condyle. Sagittal SE T1-WI (**a**) shows a bony osteocartilaginous lesion at the medial femoral condyle *white arrow*). Sagittal MR arthrogram (**b**) reveals contrast extension between the osteochondral fragment and the underlying host bone (*black arrow*)

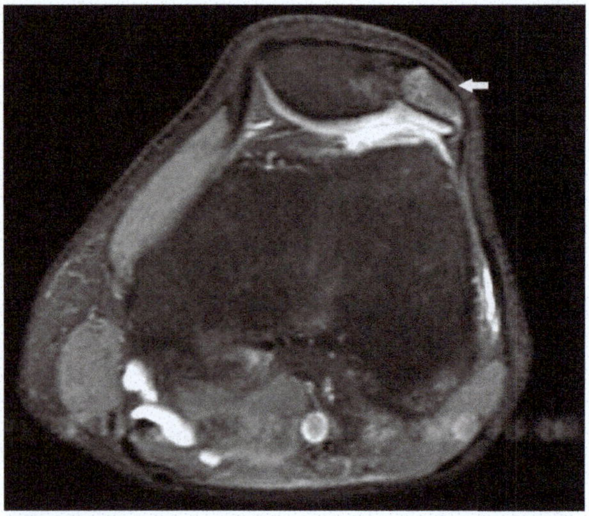

Fig. 5.40 Symptomatic bipartite patella. Axial fat-suppressed intermediate-WI. Notice an accessory bone fragment at the lateral aspect of the patella (*arrow*). There is BME on both sides of the accessory fragment and the patellar bone

of the patella. This ratio should be under 1.3–1.5 (Fig. 5.41). The trochlear groove is best assessed on the axial scans. The groove may be shallow, flat, or even convex. The relative position of the tibial tubercle can be assessed by measuring the tibal tubercle-trochlear groove (TT–TG) distance. This is the distance between the position of the trochlear groove and the tibial tubercle in the sagittal plane. Two slices are selected on an axial scan, one at the level of the trochlear groove and one at the level of the attachment of the patellar tendon at the tubercle. The two slices are superimposed. A baseline is drawn along the back of the femoral condyles. Two lines are drawn perpendicular to this baseline, one through the tibial tubercle and one through the deepest point of the trochlear groove. The TT–TG is the distance between these two lines. The upper limit of normal is about 1.7–1.8 cm.

Although assessment of lateral subluxation may be demonstrated on dynamic MRI, these methods are not often performed in daily clinical routine.

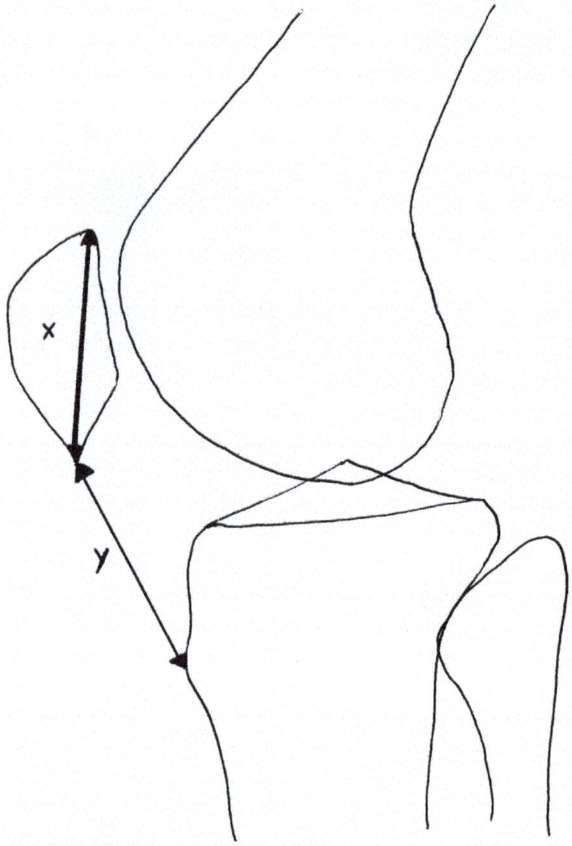

Fig. 5.41 Measurement for evaluation of the position of the patella. X = the maximum length of the patella. Y = the minimum length of the posterior surface of the patellar tendon. This Y/X ratio should be under 1.3–1.5 (Insall–Salvati index)

5.2.3.7 Cystic Lesions About the Knee

Cystic lesions around the knee comprise a diverse group of entities, ranging from benign cysts to complications of underlying diseases such as infection, arthritis, and malignancy. Although the presentation of cystic masses may be similar, their management may differ. Therefore, correct classification is mandatory. Thorough knowledge of the normal anatomy is a prerequisite to diagnose normal and abnormal fluid-filled masses around the knee.

Ultrasound is a quick and cheap imaging method to confirm the cystic nature of the masses and to diagnose superficial cystic structures. MRI may be indicated to demonstrate detailed anatomy, identifies associated intraarticular pathology and is particularly useful in demonstrating deep located cystic masses, such as PCL and ACL cysts.

Not all masses, which display a very high signal intensity on T2-WIs are necessarily fluid filled. A few noncystic masses can mimic cystic structures. Intravenous contrast should be administered whenever there is doubt about the cystic or solid nature of the visualized mass.

Table 5.5 Classification of paraarticular cystic lesions

	Communication with joint	Wall composition	Cell lining	Contents
Recess	Present	Continuous mesothelial lining	"True" synovial cells	Mucinous fluid
(Arthro)synovial cyst	Present	Continuous mesothelial lining	"True" synovial cells	Mucinous fluid
Ganglion(cyst)	Maybe present	Discontinuous mesothelial lining	Flattened pseudo-synovial cells	Mucinous fluid
Bursitis de novo	Absent	Fibrous wall	No mesothelial lining	Fibrinoid necrosis
Bursa (permanent)	Absent	Continuous mesothelial lining	"True" synovial cells	Mucoid fluid

In this paragraph, we will give a brief overview of different cysts and cyst-like lesions of the knee. Table 5.5 summarizes the classification of these lesion based on the combination of topography, the presence or absence of joint communication and the histological composition.

Recesses

Joint recesses are normal extensions or outpouchings of the joint cavity. They may become distented when a joint effusion occurs.

According to their location, the following recesses can be distinguished:

1. Gastrocnemius-semimembranosus recess: posteromedial (Fig. 5.42)
2. Popliteus hiatus: posterolateral
3. Ligamentum mucosum: anterior location within Hoffa's fad pad (Fig. 5.11)
4. Lateral synovial recess: lateral underneath the iliotibial band

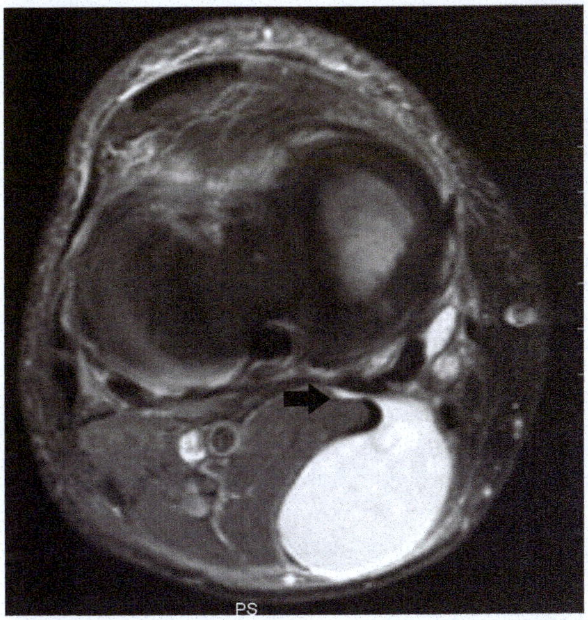

Fig. 5.42 Medial gastrocnemius-semimembranosus recess. Axial fat-suppressed intermediate-WI revealing a fluid-filled structure with the popliteal fossa, with a connecting stalk to the knee joint between the medial gastrocnemius and the semimembranosus tendon (*arrow*)

Bursae

True bursae are synovial-lined structures that act to decrease friction between moving structures. They are found in an anatomically predisposed topography. In normal circumstances, they are not or barely visible, but they may become distented to various pathological conditions, including (repetitive) trauma, inflammatory disease (rheumatoid arthritis, crystal deposition disease, …), synovial proliferative disorders (PVNS, chondromatosis) or infection. Anatomically, the following bursae can be distinguished:

1. Suprapatellar bursa
2. Prepatellar bursa (Fig. 5.43)
3. Superficial infrapatellar bursa
4. Deep infrapatellar bursa
5. Pes anserinus bursa
6. MCL bursa
7. Fibular collateral ligament – biceps femoris bursa (Fig. 5.44)
8. Semimembranosus – tibial collateral ligament bursa (Fig. 5.45)

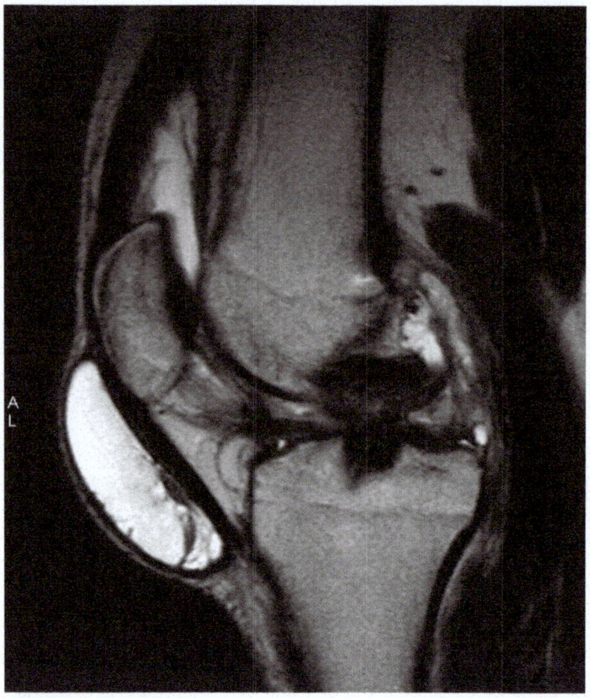

Fig. 5.43 Prepatellar bursitis. Sagittal fat-suppressed intermediate-WI. Large fluid-filled structure in front of the patellar tendon with some internal low signal intensity septa. Note also an excess of fluid within the suprapatellar bursa

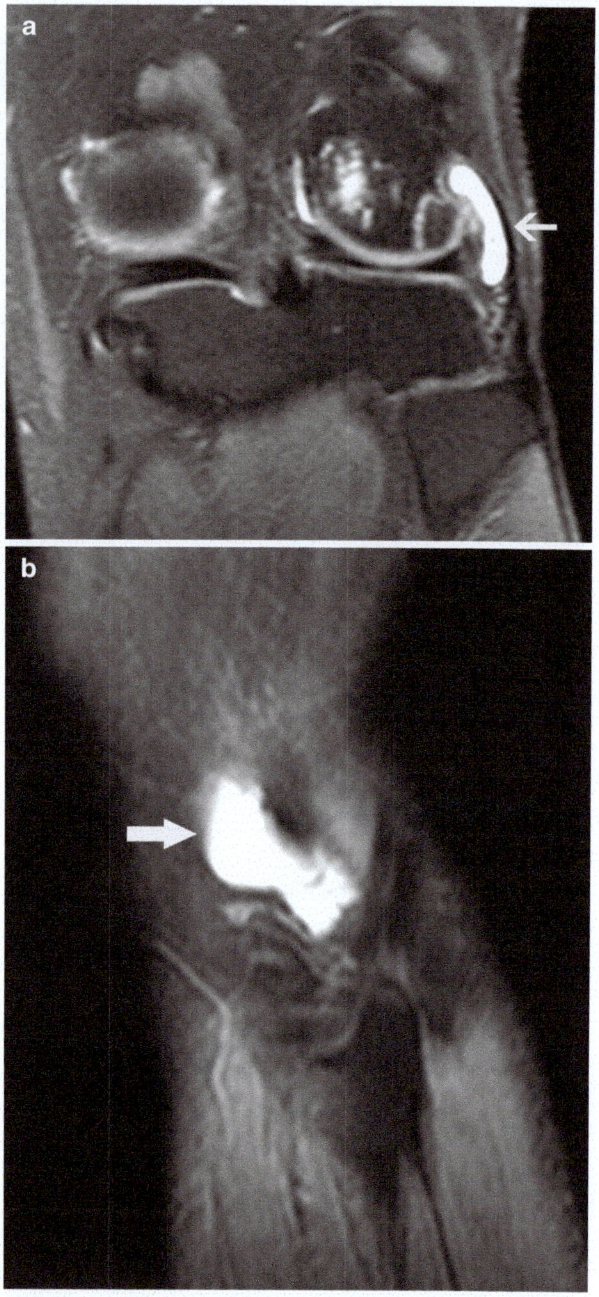

Fig. 5.44 Fibular collateral ligament-biceps femoris bursa. Coronal (**a**) and sagittal (**b**) fat-suppressed intermediate-WI. Well-delineated fluid-filled lesion adjacent to the conjoint tendon (*arrows*)

When these bursae become distended, they can be characterized by its specific location, shape, and extent around the surrounding structures.

"Bursitis de novo," occurring at not anatomically predisposed locations, have no synovial lining, but are the result of fibrinoid necrosis of connective tissue in areas subject to chronic frictional irritation. They are well known around a hallux valgus, but are rarely seen around the knee.

Synovial Cysts

The term synovial cyst describes a continuation or herniation of the synovial membrane through the joint capsule. In the French literature, the term "arthrosynovial" cyst is preferred, which refers to its intimate relationship with the adjacent joint. Indeed, there is always a communication with the adjacent joint, and the histological composition is identical to those of the joint cavity. It consists of a collection of intraarticular fluid, lined by a continous layer of "true" synovial cells. Usually, associated joint diseases are present, like osteoarthrosis, inflammatory, and posttraumatic joint diseases. The elevated intraarticular pressure, due to an accumulation of joint fluid in these diseases, causes herniation of joint fluid and synovium through a "locus minoris resistentiae" within the joint capsule.

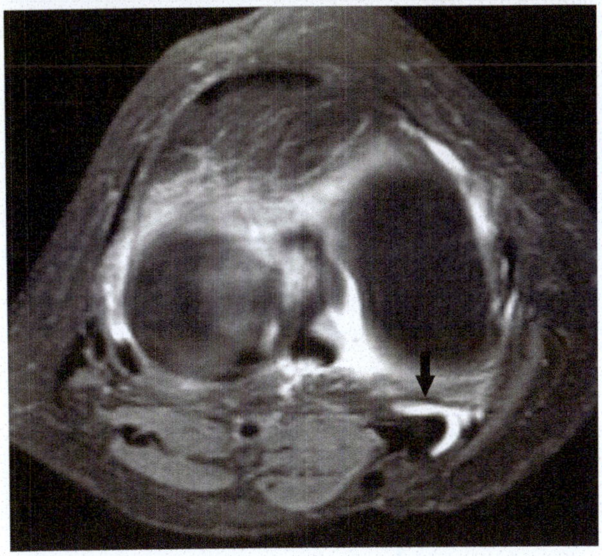

Fig. 5.45 Semimembranosus-tibial collateral ligament bursa. Axial fat-suppressed intermediate-WI shows a typical inverted U-shaped structure around the semimembranosus tendon. The apex of the lesion extends toward the tibial collateral ligament (*arrows*)

Ganglion Cysts and Variants

Ganglia contain also mucinous fluid, but their wall consists of a (discontinous) layer of flattened pseudosynovial cells, surrounded by connective tissue (pseudocapsule).

A communication with the adjacent joint is not always present.

There remains much controversy in the literature, concerning the pathogenesis of ganglion cysts. Several theories have been proposed, including displacement of synovial tissue during embryogenesis, proliferation of pluripotential mesenchymal cells, degeneration of connective tissues after trauma, and migration of synovial fluid into the cyst (synovial herniation theory).

Based upon the similar appearance on imaging, surgery, and similar wall composition of synovial cysts and ganglion cysts, we believe that the synovial herniation hypothesis is the most satisfactory. According to this theory, synovial cysts or ganglion cysts are formed by a herniation of synovium through a breach in the adjacent articulation.

While a synovial cyst has a continuous synovial lining of true synovial cells, the wall composition of a ganglion cyst consists of a discontinuous layer of pseudosynovial cells.

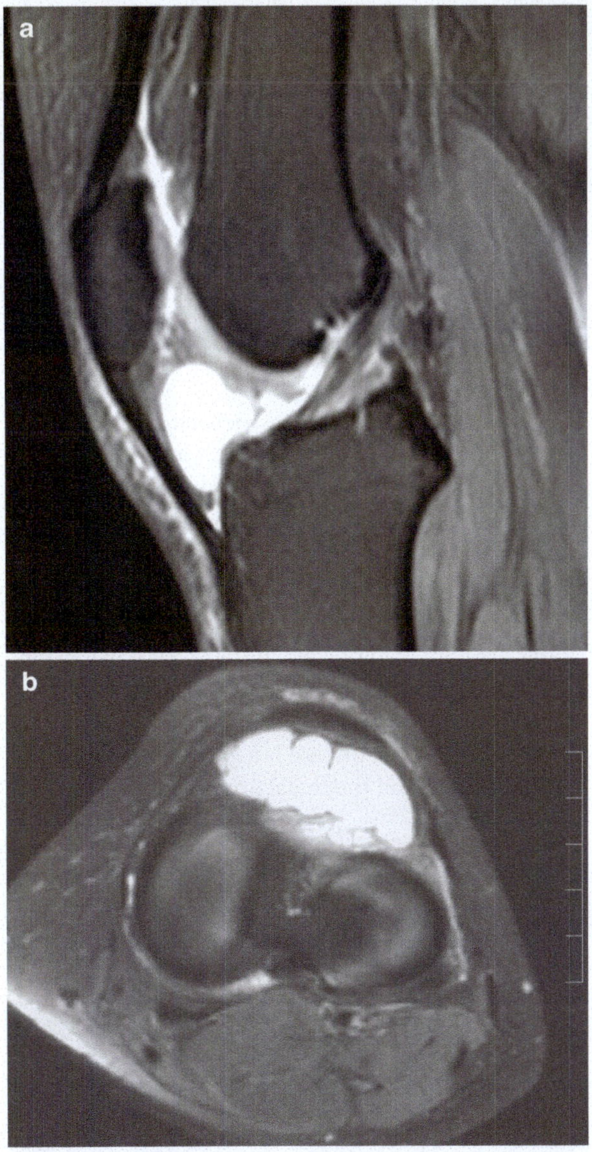

Fig. 5.46 Ganglion cyst within Hoffa's fat pad. Sagittal (**a**) and axial (**b**) fat-suppressed intermediate-WI shows a large hyperintense lesion within Hoffa's fad pad. The axial images show a slight peripheral lobulation of the lesion

A ganglion cyst may represent an advanced stage of a degenerated synovial cyst, in which the continuous synovial lining and the communication with the joint may be lost during the process of degeneration.

Ganglion cysts may be located anywhere around the joints (Fig. 5.46). A paraarticular location in fat layers or muscle is most frequently seen.

Special forms of ganglion cysts include meniscal cysts, cruciate ligament cysts, intraosseous ganglia, cystic adventitial disease and peri- or intra-neural cysts.

A meniscal cyst consists of a collection of synovial fluid, which is extruded through a meniscal tear.

Lateral meniscus cysts are usually located at the periphery of the middle third of the meniscus, whereas medial meniscus cysts may present at a distant location from the joint, because of the firm attachment of the medial meniscus to the joint capsule (Fig. 5.17).

The identification of an associated meniscus tear and the communication of the cyst with the tear is the key to the characterization of a meniscal cyst.

Cruciate ligament cysts occur within the fibers or on the surface of the cruciate ligaments (ACL–PCL), and may be associated with partial tears or healed tears of the ligament (Fig. 5.47).

Intraosseous ganglia are intraosseous extensions from synovial fluid through the subchondral bone (Fig. 5.47).

Cystic adventitial disease is a ganglion cyst, located in the wall of vessel (popliteal artery).

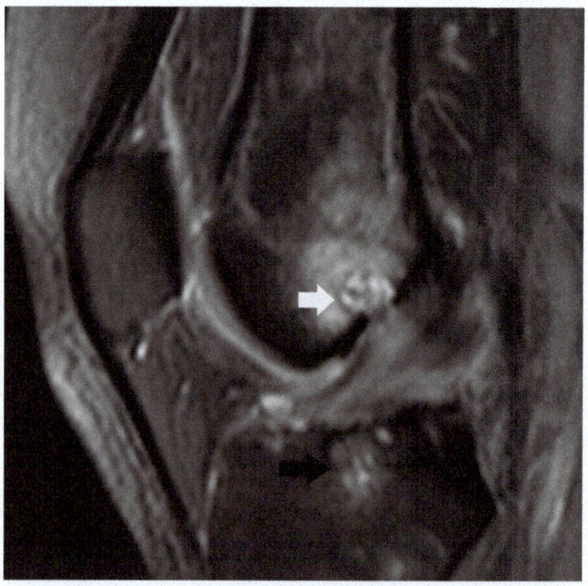

Fig. 5.47 Anterior cruciate ligament ganglion cyst. Sagittal fat-suppressed intermediate-WI. Notice the presence of high signal within the fibers of the ACL (celery stalk appearance). There is also associated intraosseous cyst formation with surrounding BME at the distal femur (*white arrow*) and proximal tibia (*black arrow*)

Mimics of Cystic Lesions

Certain noncystic lesions can mimic cystic lesions, as they are of very high internal signal intensity on T2-WIs.

They include both benign (peripheral nerve sheath tumors and myxomas) and malignant tumors with prominent areas of necrosis or myxoid degeneration (synovial sarcoma, liposarcoma, etc.). Intravenous administration of contrast is mandatory in such cases to distinguish whether the structure is (partially) solid or cystic.

Furthermore, abscesses and vascular masses, such as varices and popliteal artery aneurysms may simulate cystic lesions.

5.3 Ankle and Foot Joints

5.3.1 Anatomy

5.3.1.1 Ankle Anatomy and Related Biomechanics

The complexity of foot and ankle motions during walking is reflected in its anatomy.

Mobility in three directions is a prerequisite to allow stable walking or running, which is achieved by three distinct articulations:

1. The "ankle" or "mortise" joint allowing plantar and dorsal flexion.
2. The three subtalar articulations allowing eversion and inversion.
3. The transverse articulation between the hindfoot and midfoot.

Four major ligamentous complexes act as stabilizers of these joints, including the lateral collateral ligament, the MCL (deltoid ligament), the syndesmotic complex, and the interosseous ligaments in the sinus tarsi.

The Lateral Compartment

The lateral compartment of the ankle consists of the lateral collateral ligament, the peroneal tendons (brevis and longus), and its retinaculum.

The deepest layer is formed by the lateral collateral complex, which consists of three individual ligaments: the anterior and posterior talofibular ligament and the fibulocalcaneal ligament. The latter acts as an important barrier for the peroneal tendons, lying more superficially. In case of rupture of this ligament, fluid will collect around the peroneus tendons.

The peroneus tendons run through a small gutter at the posterior side of the fibular malleolus, acting as a pulley. The brevis tendon lies in the front of the longus tendon.

The tendons are anchored by the extensor retinaculum.

The Medial Compartment

The major part of the medial compartment of the ankle consists of the MCL or deltoid ligament and the flexor tendons, which are contained by a flexor retinaculum.

The deltoid ligament has two distinct layers. The deep layer runs between the tibia and talus and has an anterior and posterior compartment (anterior and posterior tibiotalar ligament).

The superficial part consists of a tibionavicular, tibiospring, and tibiocalcaneal ligament.

The tibiospring and tibiocalcaneal ligaments are continuous, with the latter more posteriorly located than the former. The tibiocalcaneal ligament inserts at the sustentaculum tali and the tibiospring ligament on the spring ligament, which runs between the sustentaculum tali and the navicular bone. The deltoid ligament is a solid complex, which is only injured by severe distortions, invariably associated with disruption of the lateral collateral ligament and/or the syndesmosis and sometimes, fracture of the fibula.

The deltoid ligament is superficially covered by two flexor tendons: the posterior tibialis anteriorly and the flexor digitorum longus tendon just behind it. The third flexor tendon, the flexor hallucis longus lies more posteriorly and runs underneath the sustentaculum tali (mnemonic: Tom, Dick, and Harry).

Syndesmosis

The syndesmosis is the term used to describe the three stabilizing components of the inferior tibiofibular articulation, the anterior and posterior tibiofibular ligaments, and the interosseous membrane. Injury of the syndesmosis is extremely uncommon in the absence of a fracture.

There is an anterior and posterior ligamentous complex. The posterior complex is divided in three parts, including the posterior tibiofibular ligament, the inferior transverse (also referred to as the deep inferior posterior tibiofibular) ligament, and the interosseous tibiofibular ligament.

The posterior ligament is stronger, and therefore, excessive stress results more often in an avulsion fracture at its insertion than soft-tissue injury.

The anterior tibiofibular ligament has an inferior distal fascicle (Bassett's ligament), which may have a role in the pathogenesis of anterolateral (AL) ankle impingement.

Sinus Tarsi

The sinus tarsi is a cone-shaped space interposed between the inferolateral border of the talus and the superolateral surface of the calcaneus.

The sinus tarsi is predominantly filled with fat, allowing the space to narrow slightly on eversion. On inversion, widening of the space and hence stability between the talus and calcaneus is maintained by both the cervical and interosseous ligaments.

At MRI, the sinus tarsi is best visualized on direct coronal images, fat suppressed inversion recovery images facilitating the detection of edema and hemorrhage, whereas SE T1-W or PD images allowing the evaluation of interosseous and cervical ligaments.

The cervical ligament consists of the more lateral and distal structure, whereas the interosseous ligament lies more posteriorly and medially.

Posterior Compartment

Posteriorly, the Achilles tendon, formed by merging of the gastrocnemius and soleus tendon, is the most commonly injured tendon in the ankle.

On axial imaging, the Achilles tendon has a typical semilunar configuration.

A fat-containing structure (Kager's fat pad) lies in front of the tendon.

The retrocalcaneal bursa is a fluid-filled structure between the tendon and the calcaneus at the level of the insertion.

On MRI, the asymptomatic retrocalcaneal bursa normally contains a small high-signal intensity fluid and/or synovium. A bursa larger than 1 mm anteroposteriorly, 11 mm transversely, or 7 mm craniocaudally should be considered abnormal.

Anterior Compartment

Anteriorly, three tendons are found from medially to laterally: the tibialis anterior, extensor hallucis longus, and extensor digitorum longus (mnemonic: Tom Hates Dick).

These tendons are covered by the extensor retinaculum, which has a superior and inferior part.

5.3.1.2 Normal Variants and Pitfalls in MRI of the Ankle and Foot

Multiple normal anatomic variants may erroneously be interpreted as pathologic conditions on MRI of the ankle and foot.

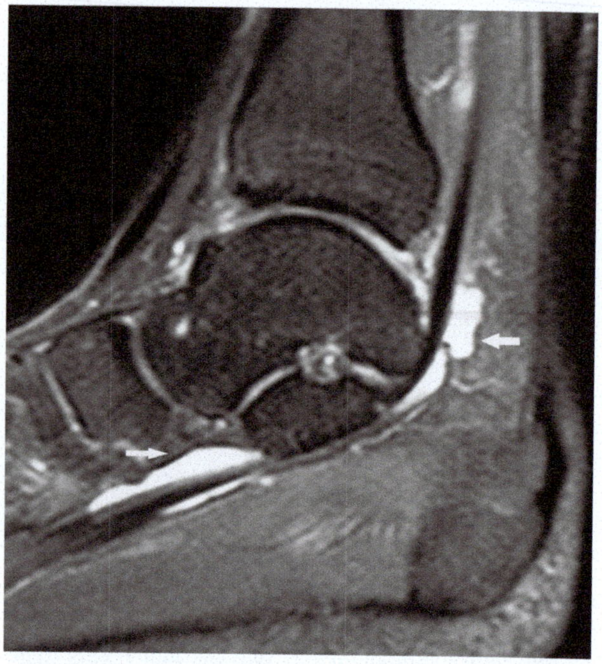

Fig. 5.48 Normal amount of fluid within the flexor hallucis tendon sheath. Sagittal fat-suppressed intermediate-WI shows a normal amount a fluid along the course of the FHL tendon (*arrows*)

Fluid Within Tendon Sheaths

A small amount of tendon sheath fluid is frequently observed in asymptomatic subjects and should not be considered abnormal. Tenosynovial fluid is more common in flexor than extensor tendons. Extensive fluid within tendon sheaths is usually indicative of tenosynovitis; however, communication between the ankle joint and the flexor hallucis longus tendon explains the presence of prominent fluid within this tendon sheath in patients with large joint effusions. Thus, even large amounts of fluid within the tendon sheath of the flexor hallucis longus tendon (Fig. 5.48), particularly in the absence of increased fluid in other flexor tendon sheaths, can be of no clinical significance. A small amount of fluid in the tendon sheath of the posterior tibial tendon, however, should be considered as abnormal.

Heterogeneity of the Ankle Ligaments

Heterogeneity and striation of the ankle ligaments are common findings that are particularly prominent in the posterior talofibular ligament and the posterior talotibial band of the deltoid ligament. The anterior Tibiotalar ligament also can manifest heterogeneity and even apparent fragmentation. These findings are due to fat interposed between the fascicles of the ligaments. The orderly fashion of the striation and the absence of morphological alteration of the ligaments are helpful in the differential diagnosis with a true tear.

Pseudoloose Bodies

The posterior and anterior tibiofibular and talofibular ligaments appear as round low-signal-intensity structures simulating loose bodies on midline sagittal MR images.

Occasionally, the ligaments can even be partly surrounded by fluid owing to their intimate relationship with the joint capsule. Confusing the ligaments with loose bodies can easily be avoided by following the course of the ligaments on sequential parasagittal images.

Cross-sectional imaging of the calcaneofibular ligament on routine coronal images also can manifest as a low signal round structure deep to the peroneal tendons and lateral to the calcaneus.

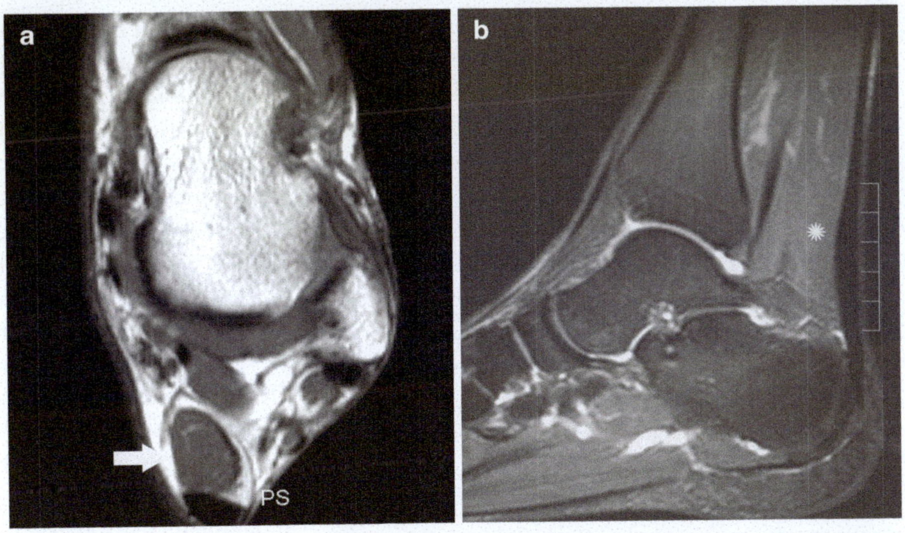

Fig. 5.49 Accessory soleus muscle. Axial SE T1-WI (**a**). There is an abnormal muscle belly lying in front of the distal Achilles tendon (*arrow*). Sagittal fat-suppressed intermediate-WI (**b**) shows obliteration of Kager's fat pad, due to the surnumerary muscle belly (*asterisk*)

Accessory Muscles of the Ankle

Numerous muscle variants are found in the ankle region (Fig. 5.49). Although the presence of these muscles is frequently of no clinical significance, the anomalous muscles can predispose to painful clinical conditions, such as fullness, swelling, and postexercise pain in the involved region. A variety of clinical conditions can develop from impingement of adjacent structures. Sometimes surgical resection of the muscles is required to alleviate the symptomatology.

The four most frequently encountered accessory muscles of the posterior ankle are the accessory soleus (Fig. 5.49), the peroneus quartus, the accessory flexor digitorum longus, and the peroneocalcaneus internus muscles.

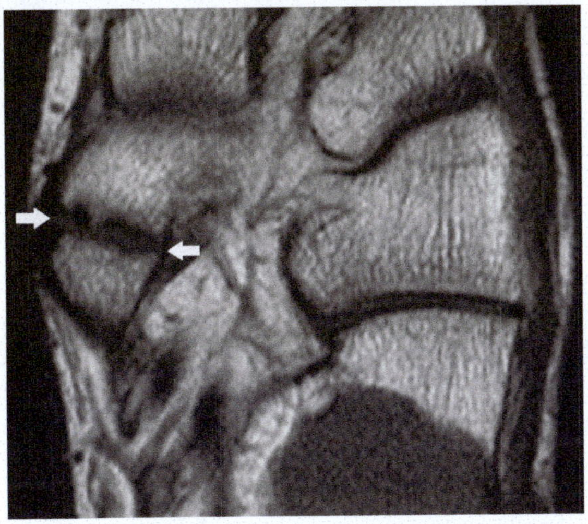

Fig. 5.50 Accessory navicular bone. Axial SE T1-WI showing an accessory bone adjacent to the navicular bone. Note the presence of a syndchondrosis between the two fragments (*arrows*)

Accessory Bones

Multiple accessory bones have been described in the literature. The most frequent among them are the os peroneum, trigonum, supranaviculare, os naviculare accessorium (Fig. 5.50), vesalianum, and intermeta tarsale.

They should not be misinterpreted as fractures.

Pseudocoalition at the Ankle

Pseudocoalition of the medial subtalar joint is depicted on coronal and sometimes axial images as an osseous "bar" between the talus and the calcaneus, which is traversed by a vague, low signal, linear shadow migrating from cranial to caudal location on sequential images.

This appearance reflects partial volume averaging generated by the obliquity of the medial subtalar joint relative to the orthogonal coronal or axial planes. The presence of a medial subtalar joint and morphologically normal sustentaculum tali on sagittal MR images aids in distinguishing pseudocoalition from true coalition.

A bony coalition between the calcaneus and the navicular bone is often simulated on sagittal T1-WIs of the hindfoot. This pitfall can be avoided easily by noting a normal relationship between the two bones on axial and coronal images. Also, in the absence of a true coalition, gradient-echo or STIR sagittal images demonstrate bright signal between the calcaneus and navicular bone, precluding the existence of a calcaneonavicular bar.

5.3.2 Imaging Technique

Currently, 8-channel ankle coils are currently used. Routine MR of the ankle is performed in supine position with the foot in 20° of plantar flexion to decrease the magic angle and for better visualization of the calcaneofibular ligament. Some authors recommend additional prone positioning with plantar flexion of the foot to reduce the magic angle effect. Table 5.6. summarizes the pulse recommendations for routine imaging of the ankle joint.

5.3.3 Pathology

5.3.3.1 Ligamentous Disorders

Ankle sprains are among the most common musculoskeletal disorders, of which 85% are inversions sprains of the lateral ligaments. The anterior talofibular ligament is always affected. Involvement of the calcaneofibular ligament and posterior talofibular ligament occurs in more severe trauma. The anterior talofibular ligament is best evaluated on axial MR images.

Syndesmotic injuries and medial ligament sprains are less common than lateral ligament injuries. Although these lesions may occur in isolation (e.g., due to eversion in case of deltoid rupture), involvement of these ligamentous structures are usually associated with severe lateral eversion sprains.

Acute ligamentous injury is characterized by focal discontinuity or absence of the ligament in most severe cases, whereas milder injuries show adjacent soft-tissue edema around the ligament. Fluid around the peroneal tendons indicates discontinuity of the calcanofibular ligament. Signal intensity changes are best assessed on fluid-sensitive sequences (Fig. 5.51).

Chronic injury appears as thickening or thinning of the ligament.

Associated BME may occur due to similar mechanisms as described in the knee. The compression side will reveal extensive *impaction type* BME, whereas tension side demonstrates minor bone *avulsive type* BME.

Repetitive ankle sprains may be accompanied with OCD (see Sect. 5.3.3.3) and sinus tarsi syndrome.

Sinus tarsi syndrome refers to a clinical entity consisting of pain and instability. Trauma is the causative agent in 70%, whereas other causes include underlying inflammatory disorders, foot deformities, or synovial or ganglion cysts extending into the sinus tarsi.

Table 5.6 Pulse recommendations for the ankle joint

Pulse sequence	WI	Plane
FS FSE	PD	Oblique coronal
FS FSE	T2	Oblique coronal
FSE	T2	Oblique axial
FS FSE	PD	Sagittal

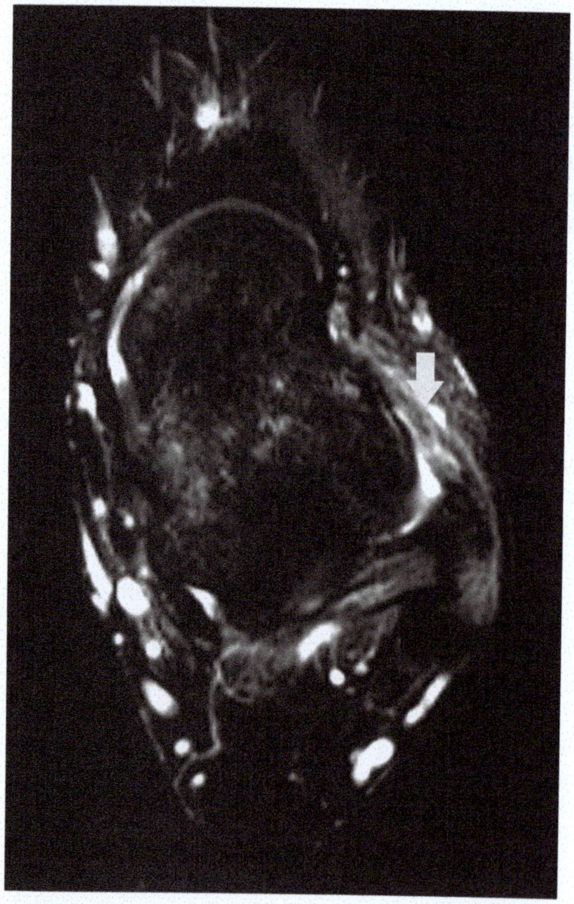

Fig. 5.51 Partial rupture of the anterior talofibular ligament (ATFL). Axial fat-suppressed intermediate-WI. There is focal thinning and increased signal along the course of the ATFL (*arrow*). Notice also associated soft-tissue edema

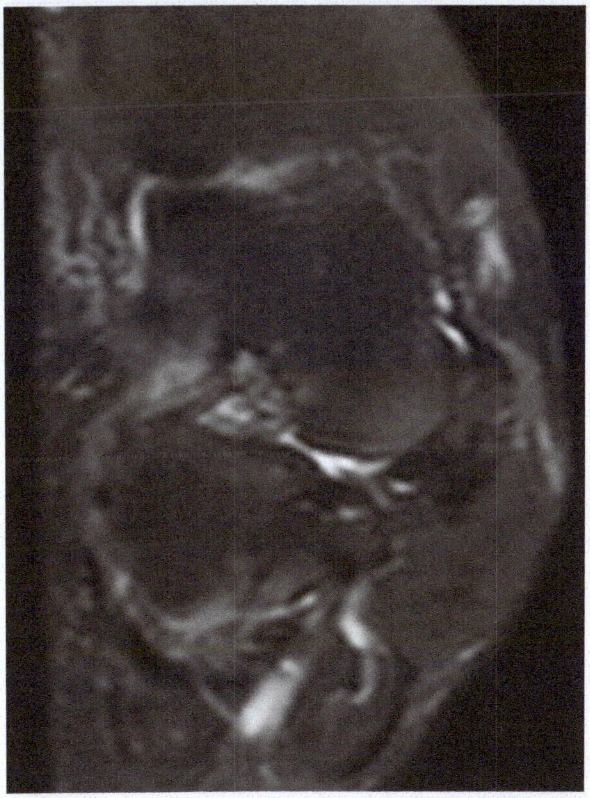

Fig. 5.52 Sinus tarsi syndrome. Coronal fat-suppressed intermediate-WI. There are high signal intensity changes within the sinus tarsi

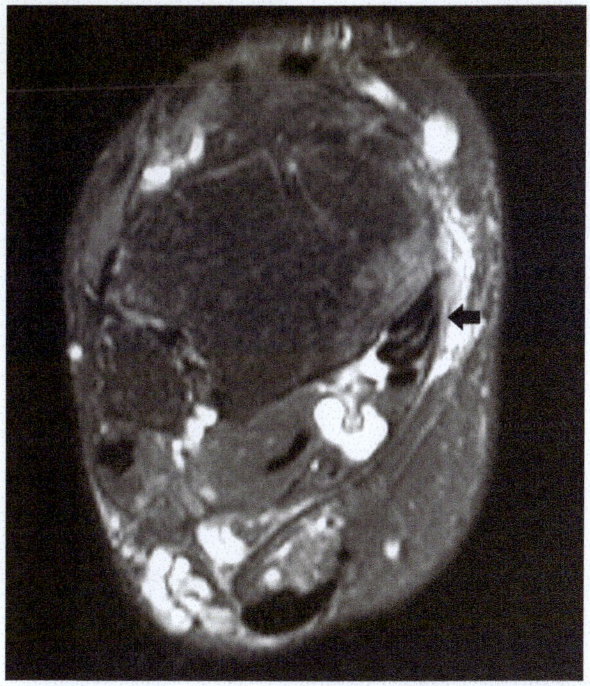

Fig. 5.53 Chronic tendon disease. Axial fat-suppressed intermediate-WI. Splitting (partial tear) of the posterior tibialis tendon (*arrow*) with associated bone and soft-tissue edema

On MRI, the fat in the sinus tarsi is replaced by low T1 and high T2 signal due to chronic synovitis and nonspecific inflammation (Fig. 5.52). The tarsal ligaments are usually not visualized by rupture or adjacent inflammation.

Late in the disease, fibrosis may result in low signal intensity on both MR pulse sequences.

5.3.3.2 Tendon Disorders

Ultrasound is the primary imaging modality to diagnose tendinosis due to tendon overuse, but MRI has the advantage to demonstrate predisposing factors, such as a prominent peroneal tubercle, shallow or convex osseous grooves responsible for chronic friction, and early tendon degeneration. Also, associated soft tissue and BME are easily demonstrated.

General MR features of tendon disease consist of caliber changes, signal intensity (SI) changes, associated soft tissue edema, and BME. Rosenberg described three grades of caliber changes according to the severity of the disease. Grade 1 consists of fusiform tendon thickening. In grade 2, the tendon is thinned, whereas tendon discontinuity is seen in grade 3. Areas of increased signal intensity within the tendon correspond to mucoid interstitial degeneration or partial longitudinal rupture. Edema-like signal around a tendon that is not invested by a tendon sheath, such as the Achilles tendon, is referred to as paratenonitis. Other tendons (e.g., peroneal tendons or posterior tibial tendon) are surrounded by a tendon sheath. Tenosynovitis is defined as an increased amount of fluid in the tendon sheath. Chronic tendon disease can be associated with reactive BME or periostitis, due to chronic friction of the diseased tendon against the adjacent bone (Fig. 5.53).

Achilles Tendon Injuries

Overuse and traumatic injuries of the Achilles tendon are among the most common tendinous disorders. Two groups are distinguished, noninsertional and insertional tendon injuries. Noninsertional injury is located between 2 and 6 cm above the tendon insertion on the

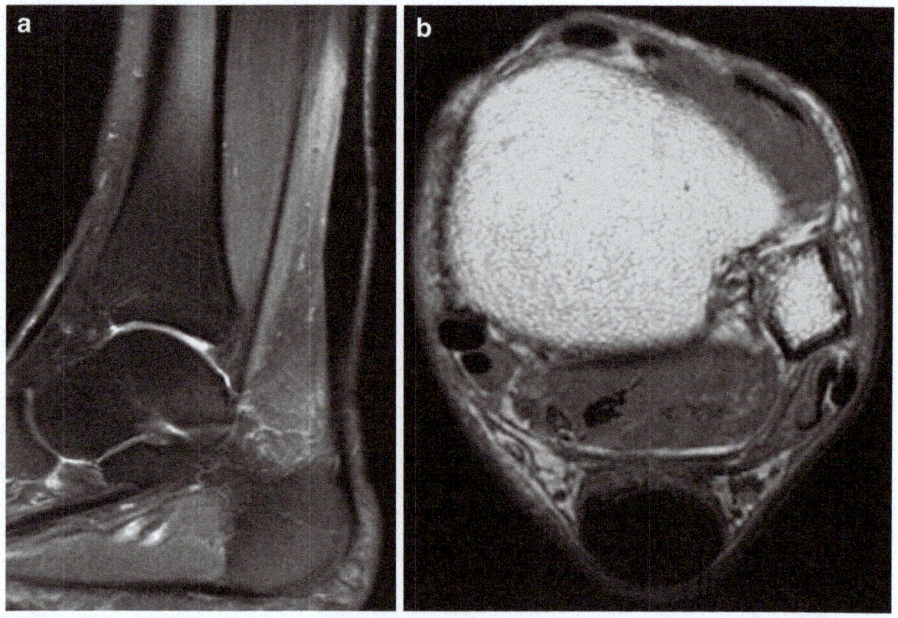

Fig. 5.54 Noninsertional Achilles tendinosis. Sagittal fat-suppressed intermediate-WI (**a**) Fusiform thickening of the Achilles tendon 3 cm proximally to its calcaneal insertion. Axial proton density image (**b**) showing thickening and convexity (instead of concavity) of the anterior contour of the Achilles tendon

calcaneus. Achilles tendinosis represents a degenerative process of the tendon with focal areas of intrasubstance microtearing and hemorrhage. On axial images, the normal anterior concave or flat surface of the tendon is lost, whereas sagittal images will demonstrate fusiform thickening. Rupture of the Achilles tendon occurs most often about 3–6 cm proximally to its calcaneal insertion, corresponding to the location of chronic tendinosis (Fig. 5.54). Paratenonitis manifests as a discrete zone of increased signal intensity limited to the posterior paratenon.

Insertional tendinosis occurs at the distal insertion of the tendon on the calcaneus and may be calcified or ossified or may be associated with a prominent posterosuperior calcaneal tuberosity, impinging on the Achilles tendon and retrocalcaneal bursa (Fig. 5.55). Retrocalcaneal bursitis is encountered in the majority of patients with insertional tendinosis, although it can occur as an isolated entity.

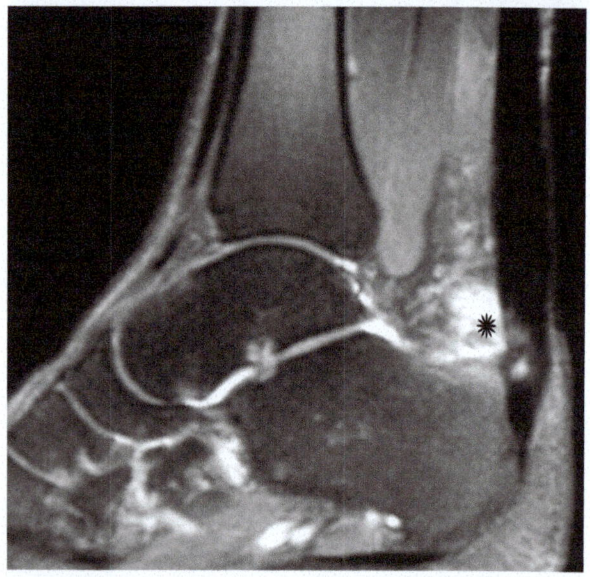

Fig. 5.55 Insertional Achilles tendinosis. Sagittal fat-suppressed intermediate-WI. Fusiform thickening of the distal Achilles tendon. Note also the presence of a focal area of high signal intensity within the tendon and associated fluid effusion within the retrocalcaneal bursa

Posterior Tibial Tendon Disease

The posterior tibialis tendon (PTT) is the second most commonly injured tendon in the foot and ankle (Fig. 5.56) and presents clinically as a progressive flatfoot deformity and weakness of inversion and inability to extend the toes (PTT dysfunction). A shallow retromalleolar groove may be a contributing factor. The tendon may dislocate medially if the flexor retinaculum is torn. Another anatomic variant that may predispose to PTT disorders is large accessory navicular bone connected to the navicular by a synchondrosis (type 2 accessory navicular bone) or a hypertrophied medial navicular tubercle (type 3 accessory navicular bone or cornuate

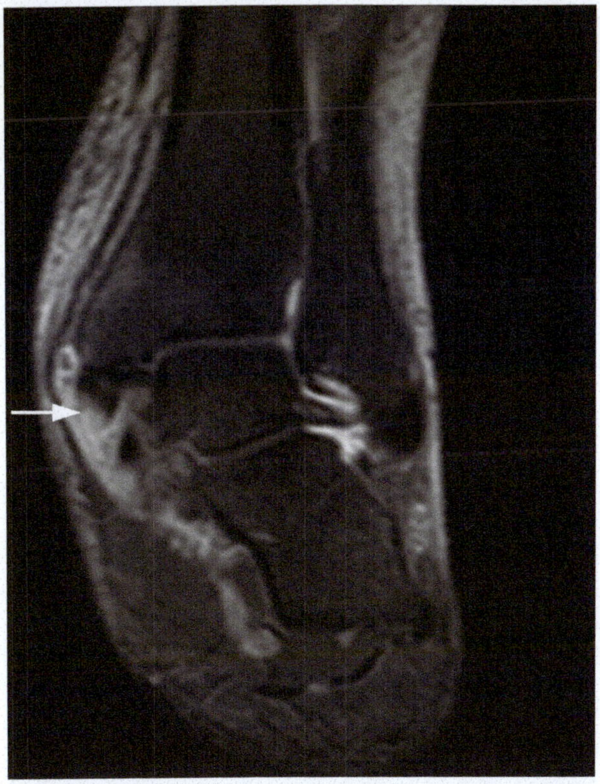

Fig. 5.56 Partial rupture of the posterior tibialis tendon. Coronal fat-suppressed intermediate-WI. Splitting (partial tear) of the posterior tibialis tendon (*arrow*) with associated BME at the medial malleolus

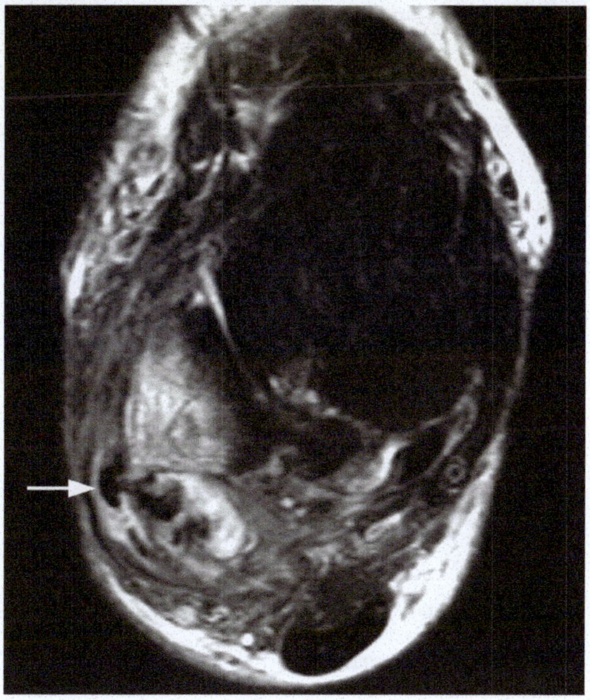

Fig. 5.57 Longitudinal split of the peroneus brevis (PB) tendon. Axial fat-suppressed intermediate-WI. There is spur formation at the distal fibula. High-signal intensity changes within the peroneus brevis tendon, indicating longitudinal splitting. There also is anterior subluxation of the PB with associated BME at the lateral malleolus. The peroneus longus tendon is also ill delineated

navicular). MRI may show PTT abnormalities and BME with the navicular and accessory bones. In case of a PTT disease, evaluation of the spring ligament is important for preoperative planning because this ligament offers additional stability to the arch.

Peroneal Tendon Disease and Other Tendon Disease

The peroneus brevis tendon is more frequently affected than the peroneus longus. Because of the shared tendon sheath, MRI will show fluid surrounding both tendons. A flat or convex peroneal groove may predispose to tendon (sub-)luxation. Repetitive ankle sprain or calcaneal fractures may cause (sub)luxation. This is best evaluated on axial FS T2-WIs. Furthermore, associated BME at the lateral distal fibula may be seen, secondary to friction or avulsion of the peroneal retinaculum. Longitudinal splitting of the peroneal brevis tendon may complicate repetitive peroneal subluxation (Fig. 5.57).

Anterior tibialis tendon tendinosis and rupture is rare and is usually located between the superior and inferior extensor retinaculum (Fig. 5.58). Flexor hallucis tendon disease may be seen in ballet dancers and athletes.

5.3.3.3 Osseous Disorders

Osteochondrosis Dissecans and Osteochondral Fractures

OCD and osteochondral fractures of the ankle are usually located at the talar dome.

Osteochondral fracture is secondary to acute trauma, whereas repeated trauma may be the cause of OCD. OCD most commonly involves the medial talar dome, less commonly involves the lateral talar dome, and rarely the central articular surface. MRI features of OCD of the talus are similar to OCD of the knee (Fig. 5.59).

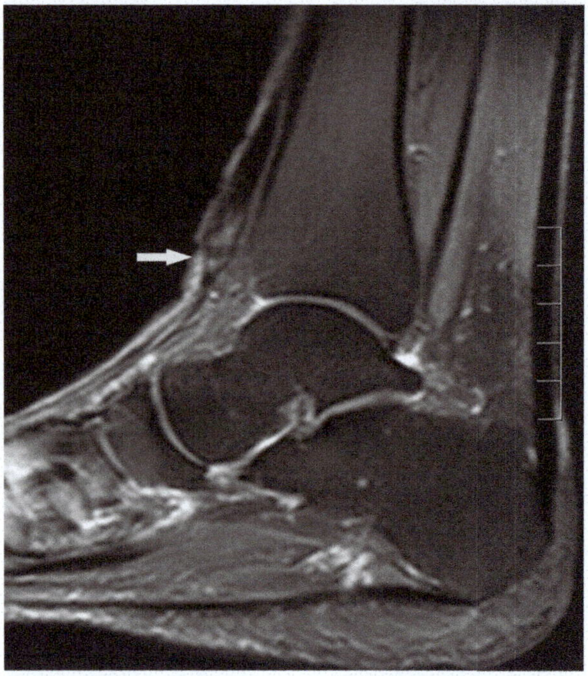

Fig. 5.58 Complete rupture of the anterior tibialis tendon. Sagittal fat-suppressed intermediate-WI. There is discontinuity and proximal tendon retraction with a typical location between the level of the superior and inferior extensor retinaculum

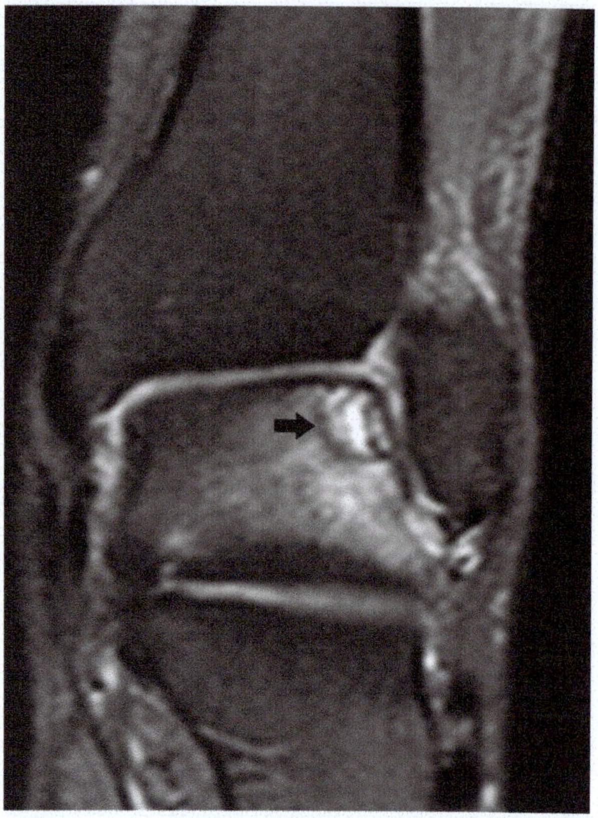

Fig. 5.59 OCD of the talus. Coronal fat-suppressed intermediate-WI. BME at the talar dome with irregular delineation of the articular cartilage (*arrow*). The presence of large cyst within the talus indicates lesion instability

Stress/Insufficiency Fractures and Occult Fractures

Stress or insufficiency fracture may involve the different bones of the foot, including the calcaneus, navicular bone, the metatarsal bones, and more rarely other tarsal bones.

The calcaneus is the most frequent location of a stress fracture, which is usually located at its posterior process, perpendicular to the stress lines of the spongious bone (Fig. 5.60). More rarely, it is anteriorly located.

Metatarsal stress fractures may be located at the base, the diaphysis, neck, and subchondral area of the metatarsal head (Fig. 5.61).

MRI is more sensitive in identifying stress fractures not detected on conventional radiographs. Before a stress fracture takes place, a stress response occurs. This corresponds to an ill-defined area of BME, without any visible fracture line. As the stress persists, a fracture develops, which is seen as an irregular line of low signal intensity on both pulse sequences surrounded by an area of BME.

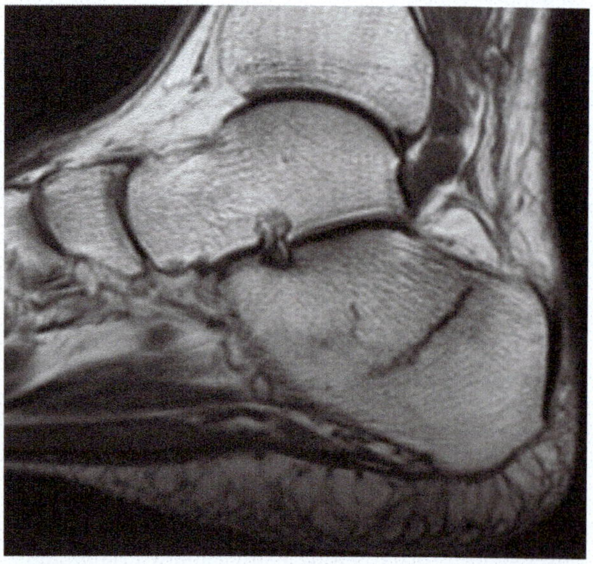

Fig. 5.60 Stress fracture of the calcaneus. Sagittal SE T1-WI showing a low signal intensity line, with typical course perpendicular to the stress lines of the calcaneus

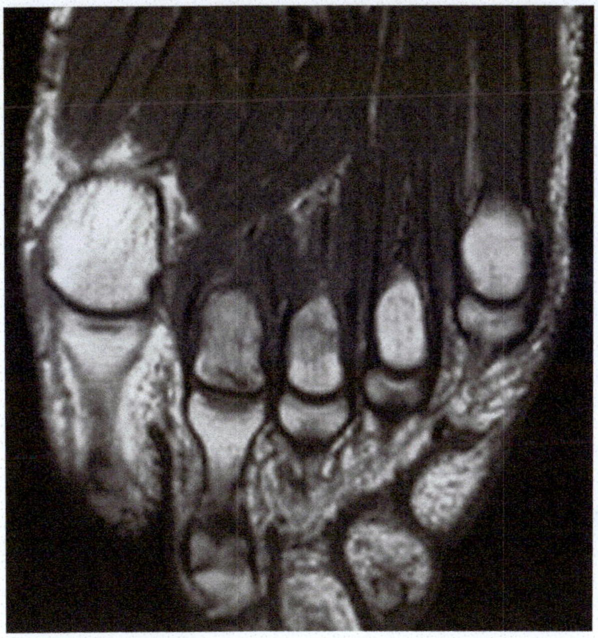

Fig. 5.61 Subchondral stress fracture of the metatarsal. Coronal SE T1-WI showing a linear subchondral low signal intensity line in the head of metatarsal 2

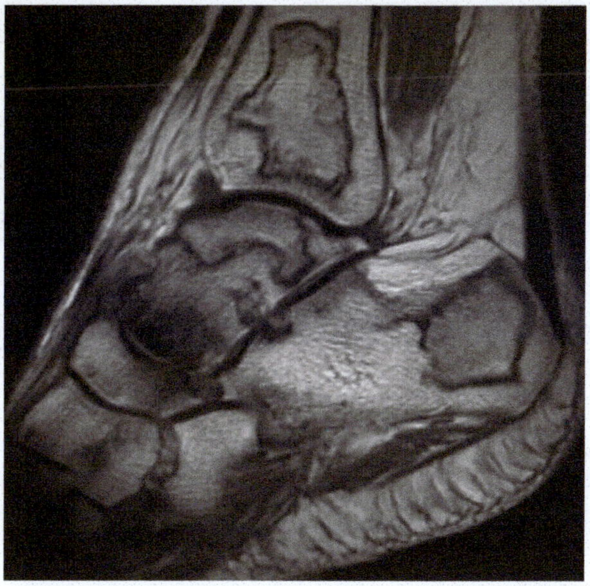

Fig. 5.62 Osteonecrosis in a patient with lupus. Sagittal SE T1-WI show multiple well-demarcated areas of osteonecrosis within the tarsal bones

In the metatarsal bones, there is often associated focal cortical thickening and periostitis and soft-tissue edema, which may mimic a tumoral appearance.

Osteonecrosis

Osteonecrosis (ON) of the talus may be idiopathic or secondary to trauma, steroid therapy, or any of the systemic causes of ON in other skeletal sites (hypercortisonism, ethylabusus, hyperlipidemia, underlying hemoglobinopathies, other coagulopathies, inflammatory bowel disease, lupus, etc.). The talus is particularly susceptible to ON, because the blood supply to the talar dome is mainly dependent on arteries of the tarsal sinus and the tarsal canal, which enter the bone on its plantar surface. This particular intraosseous blood supply is subject to interruption by fractures of the talar neck. The risk of posttraumatic ON of the talus increases with the degree of fracture displacement or subluxation of adjacent joints.

ON, due to a nontraumatic etiology is relatively rare in the foot (Fig. 5.62).

In the foot, ON is usually a secondary process to (repeated micro-) trauma.

Mueller–Weiss Syndrome

This entity represents ON of the navicular bone, occurring in adults, resulting from chronic compression of the adjacent bones.

Radiographs show a mediodorsal protrusion of part of the navicular bone, sclerosis, and later on superimposed talonavicular arthrosis.

MRI may have an interest in the diagnosis of early stages of the disease (Fig. 5.63).

Freiberg Infraction

Freiberg infraction affects the second or third metatarsal head and is characterized by subchondral collapse. The joint may appear normal or widened. It is most commonly seen in females in the second decade. The formerly used term infarction is considered as a misnomer, because the ON is secondarily to repetitive microtrauma.

In the early stage of the disease, MRI is most sensitive to detect the disease. Later in the course of the disease, subchondral collapse, irregularity of the epiphysis, sclerosis, and secondary osteoarthrosis may be seen on standard radiography.

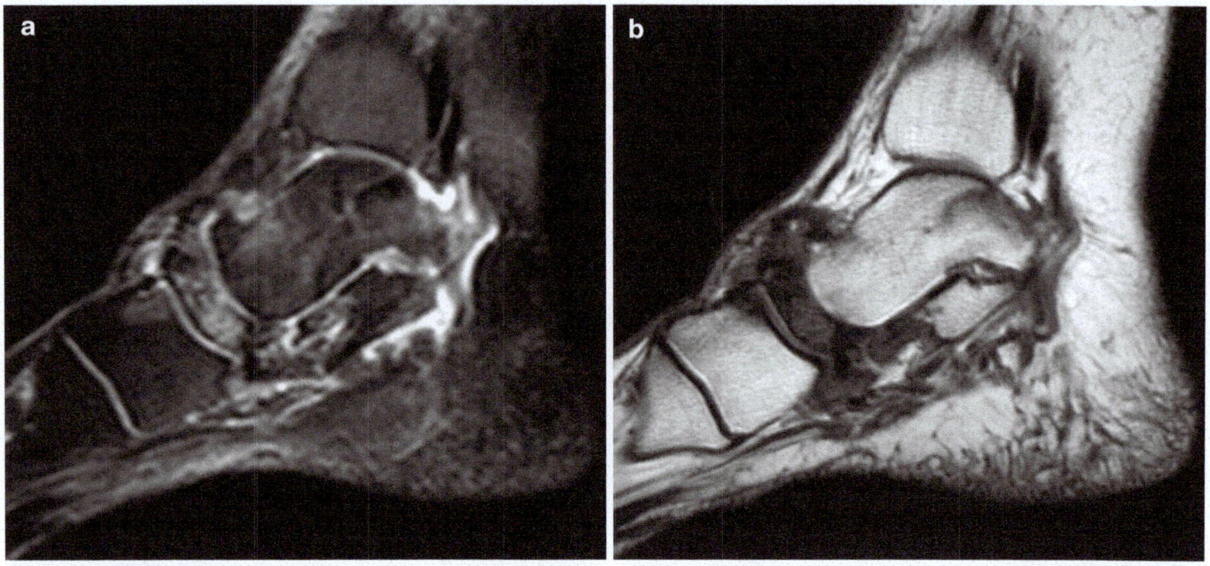

Fig. 5.63 Mueller–Weiss syndrome. Sagittal fat-suppressed intermediate-WI (**a**) shows collapse and and high SI BME in the navicular bone. Sagittal SE T1-WI (**b**) reveals a collapse of the navicular bone

Sesamoiditis

Sesamoiditis is a chronic condition, characterized by pain in the sesamoid region of the first metatarsal bone.

Its pathogenesis is still debated. Previously, it was believed that the condition starts by an interruption of the blood supply to the sesamoid bone, ultimately resulting in microfracture and collapse. According to others, repetitive trauma is the leading cause, secondarily resulting in an ischemic process of the bone. Therefore, this condition is referred in the literature with different terminology, such as osteochondritis or osteochondrosis, stress fracture, and ON of the sesamoid.

In reality, these conditions seem to be all part of the same disease spectrum, with chronic repetitive stress acting as the primum movens. Indeed, the sesamoids are subjects to forces exceeding three times the body weight during each cycle of normal gait. The tibial sesamoid receives most of this force because of its position directly under the first metatarsal head, and therefore it most frequently affected.

This microtraumatic hypothesis, regarding its etiology is further supported by the frequent occurrence of sesamoiditis in (young) women wearing high-heeled shoes. Other predisposing factors aggravating stress on the sesamoids are dancing or sports, and a cavus foot. To avoid any further nosological confusion, we advocate the use of the more neutral term "sesamoiditis," which is not a true inflammatory disorder but refers to a clinical syndrome of a painful sesamoid.

MRI findings include decreased signal intensity on T1-WIs and increased signal intensity on (fat suppressed) T2-WIs or STIR (Fig. 5.64). Associated soft tissue abnormalities include tendonitis, synovitis, and bursitis.

Initially, radiographs are negative, but late findings consist of microfracture, cortical irregularity, cyst formation, collapse of bone, and increased density. These late changes may be demonstrated on CT as well.

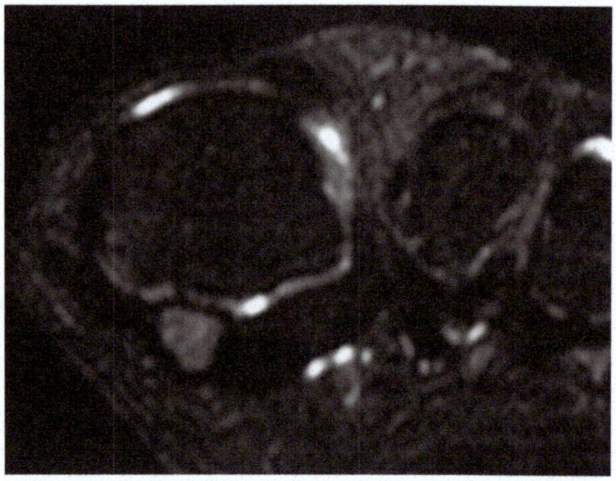

Fig. 5.64 Sesamoiditis. Coronal fat-suppressed intermediate-WI shows high SI BME in the medial sesamoid bone

As the process heals, residual sclerosis may persist and may cause low signal intensity on T2-WIs.

Tarsal Coalition

Tarsal coalition occurs in 1–2% of the population, and is bilateral in 25–50%. This condition is believed to represent a failure of segmentation of the cartilaginous primordium in utero. The ossific nuclei of two separate bones develop in one piece of cartilage, and the initially cartilaginous bridge between the two bones allows some movement of the hindfoot. The bridge may ossify totally or partially at a later age, causing motion deficit, flattening of the longitudinal arch, with stretching of the peroneus longus tendon and painful spasm.

The age of ossification differs for the different types of coalitions. Talonavicular coalitions ossify at 3–5 years of age, calcaneonavicular at 8–12 years, and talocalcaneal coalition at 12–16 years.

Calcaneonavicular and talocalcaneal coalitions are most frequent, whereas other types are rare.

On imaging, direct signs of coalition may be seen as total bony union (Fig. 5.65) or fibrous/cartilaginous union (Fig. 5.66). In the last type, a "pseudarthrosis" pattern is seen. Special views may be required to detect a coalition on standard radiographs, whereas CT scan is the best technique for confirmation. Although MRI may be as effective in the demonstration of complete fusion by marrow continuity across the joint, this is far more

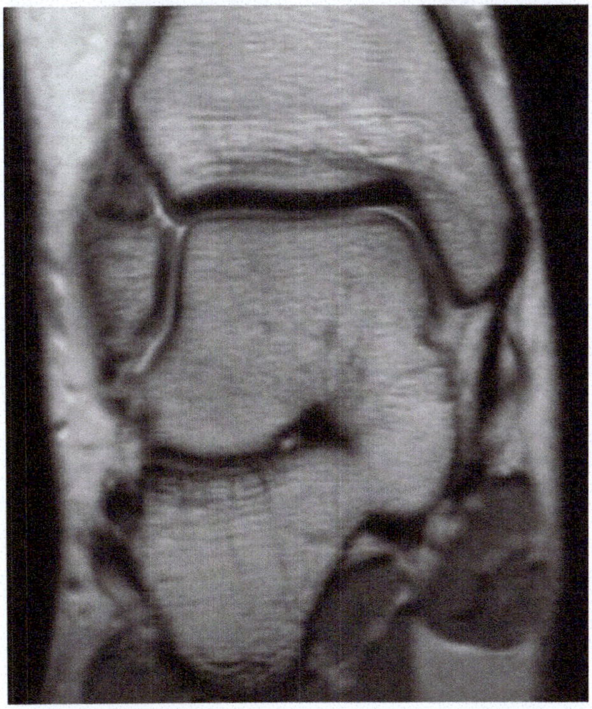

Fig. 5.65 Bony talocalcanael coalition. Coronal FSE PD-WI reveals continuity of the medullary bone of the medial aspect of calcaneus and talus

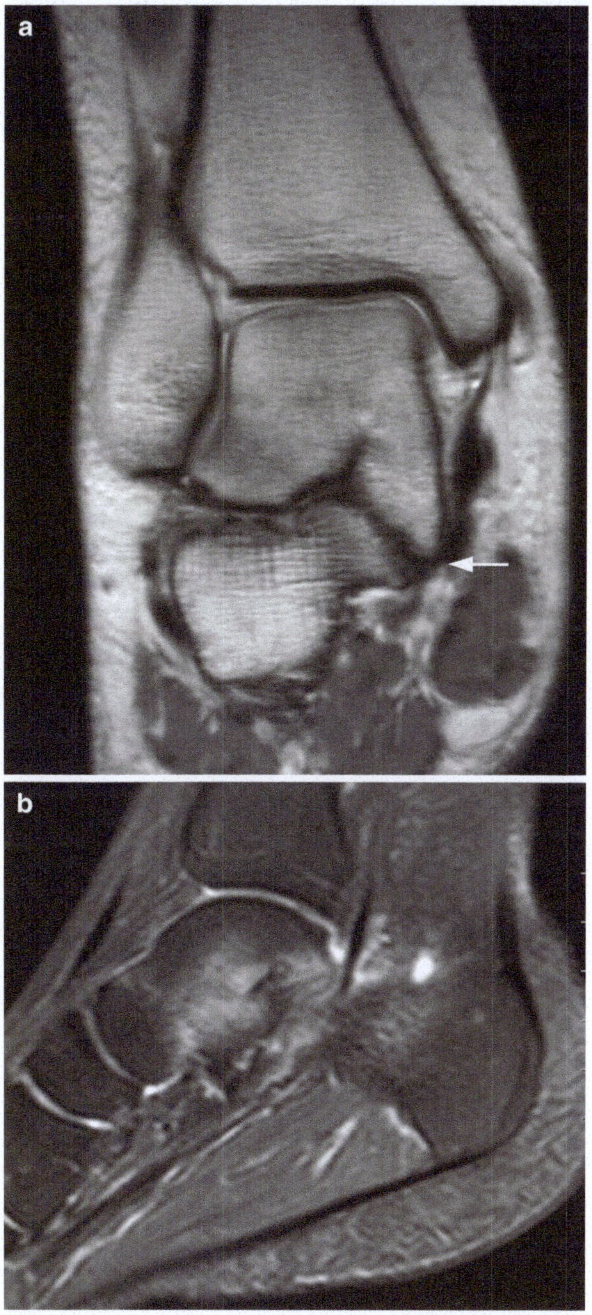

Fig. 5.66 Fibro-osseous talocalcanael coalition. Coronal SE PD-WI (**a**) demonstrates fibro-osseous coalition between talus and calcaneus. Notice associated BME in talus and calcaneus on sagittal fat-suppressed intermediate-WI (**b**)

difficult in fibro-osseous forms. On the other hand, MRI is superior to demonstrate the presence of stress changes (resulting in BME) in the adjacent joints as areas of high-signal intensity on fatsuppressed T2-WIs.

Other secondary signs are due to flattening of the longitudinal arch (with flatfoot deformity and C-sign in talocalcaneal coalition) or due to increased mobility of adjacent nonfused joints (resulting in ball-and-socket deformation of the tibiotalar joint and short talar neck and talar beaking).

5.3.3.4 Impingement Syndromes of the Ankle

Soft-Tissue Impingement

The most common type of soft-tissue impingement syndrome is anterolateral (AL) ankle impingement. Repetitive ligamentous trauma may lead to synovial hypertrophy and fibrosis in the lateral gutter of the ankle joint, between the lateral malleolus and talus. On axial T2-W images, a focal meniscoid lesion may be seen along the course of the thickened anterior talofibular ligament (Fig. 5.67).

Tarsal tunnel syndrome is a clinical entity consisting of numbness or paresthesias in foot as a result of compression of the posterior tibial nerve in the tarsal tunnel. It is most likely due to an overuse injury, but mass lesions (e.g., ganglion cysts or large varices) may also cause nerve compression.

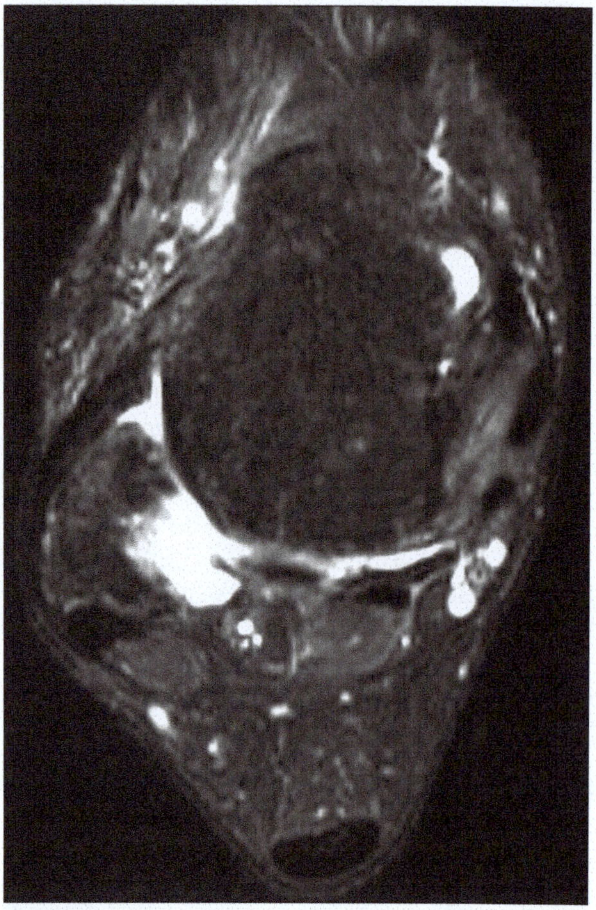

Fig. 5.67 Anterolateral impingement syndrome. Axial fat-suppressed intermediate-WI demonstrates a meniscoid lesion along the course of the anterior talofibular ligament;

Osseous Impingement

Osseous impingement may occur anteriorly or posteriorly.

Anterior impingement is due to osteophytes arising from the tibia or talus, blocking dorsiflexion of the ankle.

Posterior impingement is usually due to an enlarged os trigonum, irritating the flexor hallucis longus tendon, causing tenosynovitis, especially during activities that require repetitive plantar flexion. BME between the os trigonum and the posterior aspect of the talus may be seen on fat-suppressed T2-WIs (Fig. 5.68).

5.3.3.5 Other Disorders

Plantar Fasciitis

The normal plantar fascia is no more than 4 mm thick at its insertion. Plantar fasciitis is an overuse injury of the origin of the plantar fascia usually affecting the medial bundle of the fascia.

MRI may demonstrate inflammation within the adjacent perifascial soft tissues and BME in the calcaneus on fluid-sensitive sequences (Fig. 5.69).

Morton's Neuroma (Fibroma)

The term Morton's neuroma is a misnomer, because it is not a true tumor but represents perineural fibrosis around the interdigital nerve associated with pain and paresthesia on standing or compression of the metatarsal heads. Therefore, Morton's fibroma is the preferred terminology.

It is typically located in between the metatarsal heads on the plantar side of the transverse intermetatarsal ligament.

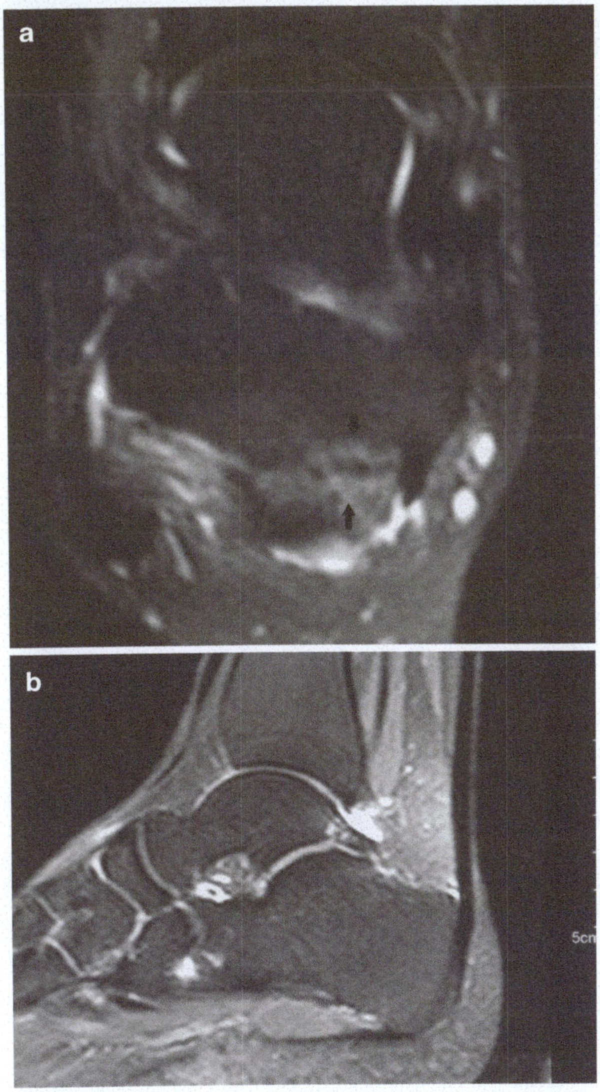

Fig. 5.68 Os trigonum syndrome. Axial fat-suppressed intermediate-WI (**a**). Sagittal fat-suppressed intermediate-WI (**b**). BME between the os trigonum and the dorsal aspect of the talus (*arrows in* **a**), due to chronic friction

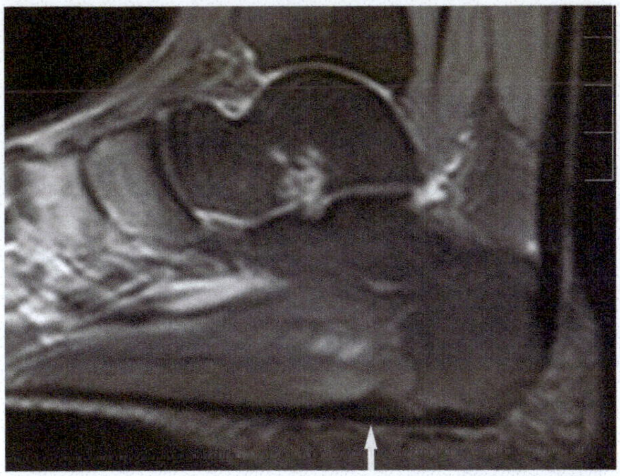

Fig. 5.69 Plantar fasciitis. Sagittal fat-suppressed intermediate-WI. Thickening and internal high signal (*arrow*) of the proximal part of the plantar fascia. Notice also minor adjacent soft-tissue edema and BME at the attachment of the plantar fascia at the calcaneus

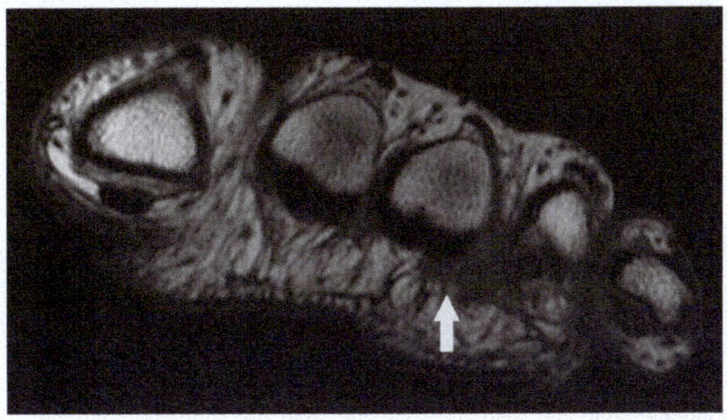

Fig. 5.70 Morton's fibroma. Coronal SE T1-WI showing a nodular hypointense mass lesion extending between the plantar aspect of head of metatarsal 3 and 4 (*arrow*)

On MRI, a typical Morton's neuroma is isointense to muscle on T1-WIs (Fig. 5.70), and homogeneously or heterogeneously hypointense to fat on T2-WIs.

Lesions less than 5 mm in diameter are usually asymptomatic.

Bursitis About the Forefoot

The differential diagnosis of Morton's neuroma includes a distended intercapitometatarsal and subcapitometatarsal bursitis. Distention results from (micro-) trauma or friction, inflammatory arthritis or infection.

Differential diagnosis can easily be obtained by analysis of their specific topography.

Intercapitometatarsal bursitis is best visualized on T2-W MR images as a fluid-filled structure between the metatarsal heads, on the dorsal side of the transverse intermetatarsal ligament. It can compress the interdigital nerve when the bursa exceeds a diameter of 3 mm.

Subcapitometatarsal bursitis is an adventitial bursitis located underneath the metatarsal heads (Fig. 5.71). It may be irregularly delineated, which supports its pathogenesis due to chronic friction. Both bursae may show peripheral enhancement after intravenous contrast administration.

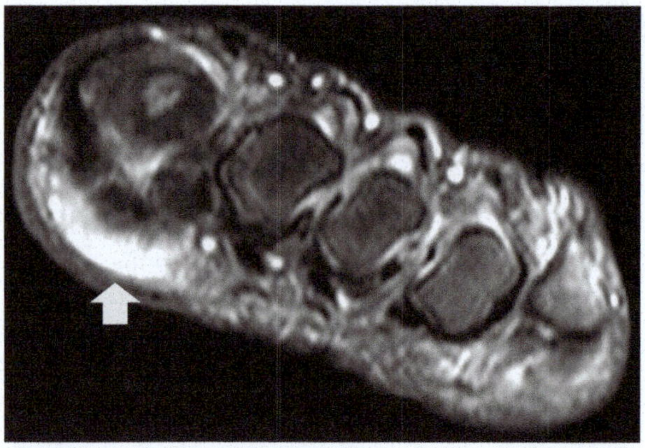

Fig. 5.71 Subcapitometatarsal bursitis. Coronal fat-suppressed intermediate-WI shows a hyperintense lesion at the plantar aspect of the first metatarsal (*arrow*)

Infectious Disorders

Infection of the foot includes skin ulceration, sinus tract formation, soft-tissue infection and necrosis, osteomyelitis, and septic arthritis.

Although standard radiography is usually the initial examination, radiographic findings of osteomyelitis do not appear for 10–14 days and until 35–50% of bone has been destroyed. Moreover, documentation of soft-tissue infection is poor on plain films.

MRI has largely replaced plain films in the evaluation of infection, because of its better sensitivity and anatomical depiction of soft tissue extent. The accuracy of MRI has even been improved due to the use of fat-suppressed T1-WIs before and after gadolinium and subtraction.

MRI is also a valuable tool for assessment of the diabetic foot and potential differential diagnosis between diabetic neuroarthropathy (Charcot) and osteomyelitis. The latter condition should be suspected in case of skin ulcerations, fistula, and abscess formation.

Inflammatory Disorders

MRI is usually not regarded as the first choice in the evaluation of rheumatologic and inflammatory disorder, although it may be helpful for early diagnosis and evaluation of disease activity by demonstration of BME (e.g., enthesis in seronegative spondyloarthopathy) and soft tissue changes such as an inflammatory etiology of retrocalcaneal bursitis. Administration of intravenous gadolinium contrast is necessary for differentiation between synovial pannus and joint fluid.

5.4 Shoulder Joint

5.4.1 Anatomy

5.4.1.1 *Biceps Tendon*

The biceps tendon originates from the superior tubercle of the superior portion of the labrum and passes through the joint, parallel to the superior glenohumeral ligament.

The tendon exits the joint anterosuperiorly at the anatomic neck of the humerus to enter the intertubercular sulcus. It is enveloped by a synovial sleeve over a variable length during its course in the intertubercular sulcus.

Near its exit point, the tendon is reinforced by the coracohumeral ligament (CHL) and by slips from the subscapularis and supraspinatus tendons, whereas the transverse ligament reinforces the tendon in the intertubercular sulcus below this point of exit.

A small amount of fluid in the biceps tendon sheath is normal.

On axial gradient-echo sequences, an increased signal in the lateral bicipital groove represents flow-related enhancement in the anterolateral (AL) branches of the anterior circumflex humeral artery and vein.

A magic angle phenomenon-with increased signal intensity in the substance of the biceps tendon on T1- and PD WIs, has been described.

5.4.1.2 Labral-Ligamentous Complex

The major benefit of MRA over conventional MRI of the shoulder is the visualization of the labral-ligamentous structures, consisting of three glenohumeral ligaments in combination with the labrum. This complex acts as the main stabilizer of the mobile glenohumeral joint.

The Glenohumeral Ligaments

These are best seen on axial and coronal oblique planes, although they can be identified in the three imaging planes.

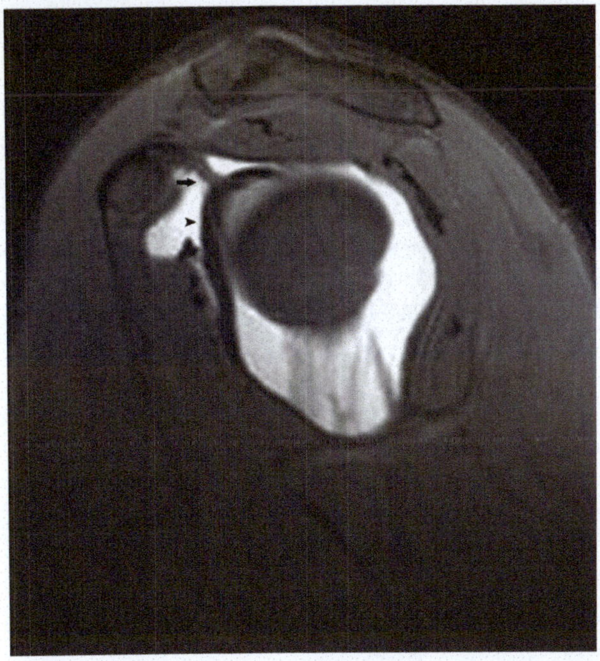

Fig. 5.72 Superior glenohumeral ligament. Sagittal fat-suppressed MR arthrogram. The superior glenohumeral ligament (*arrow*) has a conjoined origin with the middle glenohumeral ligament (*arrowhead*)

The Superior Glenohumeral Ligament (SGL)

This ligament has a conjoined origin with the middle glenohumeral ligament from the superior labrum immediately anterior to the labral-bicipital junction (Fig. 5.72). It courses anteriorly and parallel with the coracoid process and merges with the CHL in the rotator interval.

The Middle Glenohumeral Ligament (MGL)

This ligament is the most variable of the three ligaments. It can be absent or poorly defined. It shows normal variation in size from thread-like to cord-like, and there exists an inverse relationship between the size of the middle glenohumeral ligament and the adjacent anterior labrum: the larger the ligament, the smaller the labrum. A cord-like ligament in combination with an absent anterior labrum is known as the Buford complex (Fig. 5.73).

Its location depends on the shoulder positioning. The ligament lies medial to the anterior glenoid rim in internal rotation of the shoulder, and moves laterally to the glenoid rim in external rotation of the shoulder.

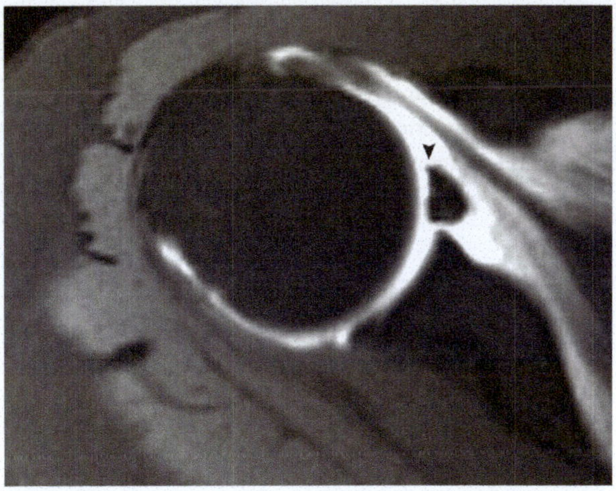

Fig. 5.73 Buford complex. Axial fat-suppressed MR arthrogram. Absence of the anterosuperior labrum and presence of a thick glenohumeral ligament (*arrowhead*)

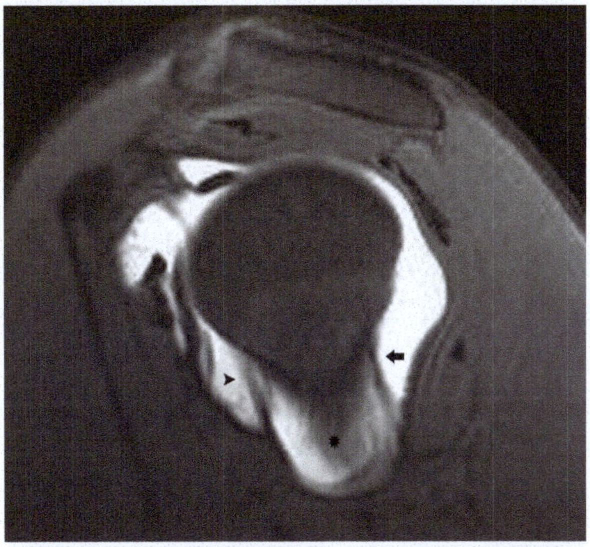

Fig. 5.74 Inferior glenohumeral ligament. Sagittal fat-suppressed MR arthrogram showing the different components of the glenohumeral ligaments, including the anterior band (*arrowhead*), the posterior band (*arrow*), and the axillary pouch (*asterisk*)

The ligament runs inferiorly and anteriorly to merge with the subscapularis tendon before insertion on the lesser tuberosity.

The Inferior Glenohumeral Ligament (IGL)

It consists of three components, the anterior, posterior, and intervening axillary pouch (Fig. 5.74). The anterior portion is the most important structure in maintaining passive anterior stability of the shoulder. This anterior band is thicker than the superior and middle glenohumeral ligaments. It runs inferiorly from a 2 cm segment of the anteroinferior glenoid labrum at the 4–6 o'clock position to its insertion on the anatomic neck of the humerus.

Glenoid Labrum

The glenoid labrum consists of a ring of fibrous tissue with interposed elastic fibers encircling the articular face of the osseous glenoid. It is hypointense on the different pulse sequences.

The Anterior Labrum

It shows normal variations in size and morphology. It can be triangular, rounded, flattened, notched (Fig. 5.75), or cleaved in appearance.

The Posterior Labrum

It is usually small and rounded.

Other anatomical variations in labral morphology that can cause diagnostic errors are:

- Articular cartilage undercutting the labral fibrocartilage.
- Normal insertion of glenohumeral ligaments vs. torn labrum.
- Sublabral sulci (Fig. 5.76).
- Sublabral holes (Fig. 5.77).

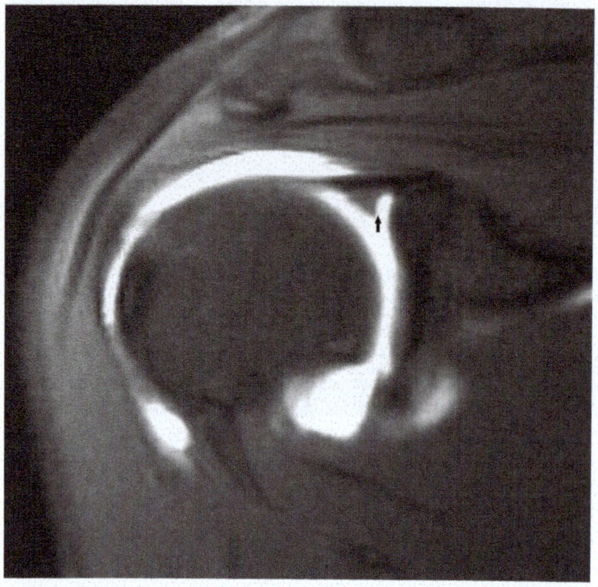

Fig. 5.76 Sublabral sulcus (recess). Oblique coronal fat-suppressed MR arthrogram. Well-delineated linear area of contrast extension between the superior labrum and the superior rim of the bony glenoid (*arrow*). The regular delineation and medial extension of contrast argue in favor of a normal variant

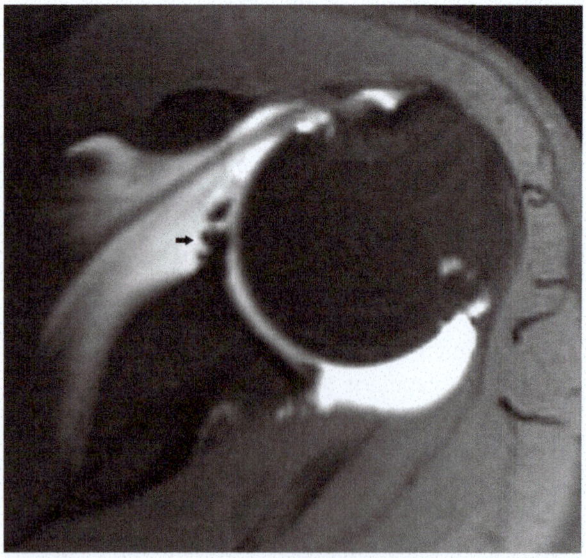

Fig. 5.75 Notched anterior labrum. Axial fat-suppressed MR arthrogram shows a notched morphology of the anterior labrum (*arrow*), which should be regarded as a normal variant

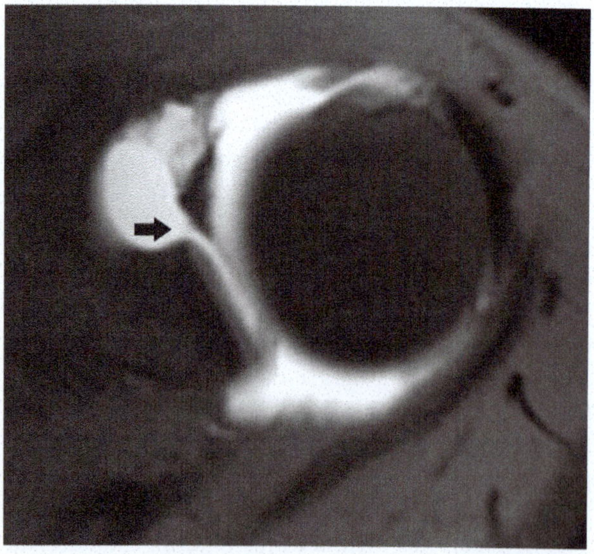

Fig. 5.77 Sublabral foramen. Axial fat-suppressed MR arthrogram demonstrates focal extension of contrast between the anterosuperior labrum and the bony glenoid (*arrow*)

Correct interpretation of these variations is much easier on MR arthrography (MRA) than on conventional MRI.

Articular Capsule

Anterior Capsule

The insertion of the anterior capsule is variable. Three types of capsular insertion have been described, but relationship of this variant with shoulder instability is questionable.

Posterior capsule

The insertion of the posterior capsule is constantly located on the base of the labrum at its junction with the glenoid rim.

5.4.2 Technique

Conventional MRI of the rotator cuff is useful for some types of shoulder pathology, but for imaging of the rotator cuff, it has some important limitations for the following indications:

- *Full-thickness tear:*

Conventional MRI does not provide sufficient information on the size of the tear and the amount of retraction, which is required for surgical therapy (arthroscopic subacromial decompression for massive tears, open surgery for large- or medium-sized tears, and arthroscopic repair for small tears).

- *Partial-thickness tear:*

Differentiation between tendinosis and partial-thickness tear may be difficult on conventional MRI due to: magic angle effect, muscle fibers, focal fat, subclinical degeneration, and anomalies of vascularization.

Direct MRA has proven to be the ideal solution for the limitations of conventional MRI of the shoulder. However, if a (large) full-thickness tear is present, an additional oblique sagittal T1-W sequence (without fat suppression!) is added in order to grade muscle atrophy and fatty degeneration on a semiquantitative basis. The ABER position is valuable in demonstrating lesions of posterior-superior impingement and (small) underface tears of the rotator cuff. Indirect MRA (after intravenous injection of gadolinium contrast) has been described as an alternative technique for diagnosis of rotator cuff disease, particularly in combination with ABER position to enhance the conspicuity for small rotator cuff tears. However, image interpretation is much more difficult (especially for differentiation of tendinosis vs. small tears, bursitis vs. small bursal tears …). Therefore, we do not rely on this technique. Additional advantages of direct MRA are better assessment of subscapularis lesions, lesions of the long head of the biceps tendon, and evaluation of the rotator cuff interval. Table 5.7. summarizes the pulse recommendations for routine imaging of the shoulder.

Table 5.7 Pulse recommendations for shoulder arthrography (1.5 T)

Pulse sequence	WI	Plane
FSE	PD	Oblique coronal
FSE	T2	Oblique coronal
FS SE	T1	Oblique axial
FS SE	T1	Oblique coronal
FS SE	T1	Oblique sagittal
SE contrast*	T1	Oblique sagittal through muscle belly

*Optional in case of large rotator cuff tear for evaluation of muscle atrophy and fatty infiltration

5.4.3 Pathology

5.4.3.1 Rotator Cuff (RC)

Radiological Semiology of Rotator Cuff Lesions on MRA

- Delineation of the superior recess with gadolinium contrast: articular partial-thickness tears (Fig. 5.78)
- Abnormal contrast opacification of the subacromial bursa: full-thickness tear (Fig. 5.79)
- Integrity of subacromial bursal fat stripe/fluid in bursa on PD/T2-WIs: partial-thickness bursal tears/subacromial bursitis (Fig. 5.80)
- Isolated signal changes within the rotator cuff on PD/T2-WIs for diagnosis of tendinosis (high SI on PD/less than fluid on T2) or intratendinous tears (higher on T2 than on PD) (Fig. 5.81)
- Calcifications: are often difficult to see on MRI (Fig. 5.82). Correlation with plain radiography (or ultrasound) is often required

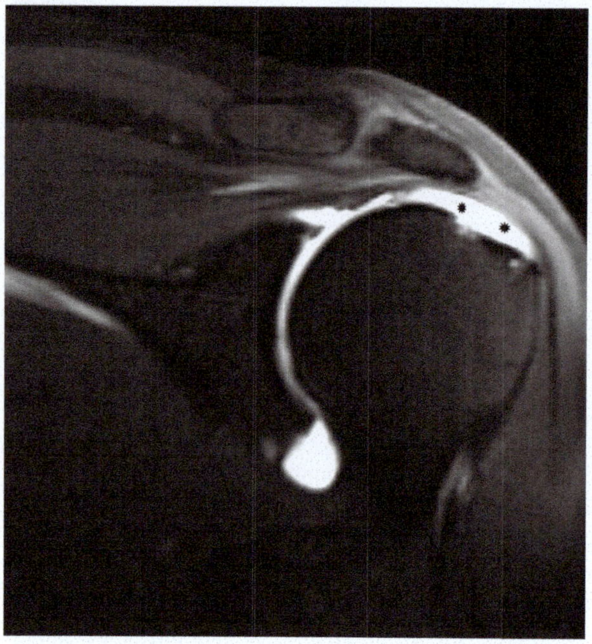

Fig. 5.78 Partial-thickness tear at the articular side of the supraspinatus tendon. Oblique coronal fat-suppressed MR arthrogram. Note contrast extension at the articular (undersurface) of the supraspinatus tendon (*asterisk*). There is absence of pathological filling of the subacromial-subdeltoid bursa

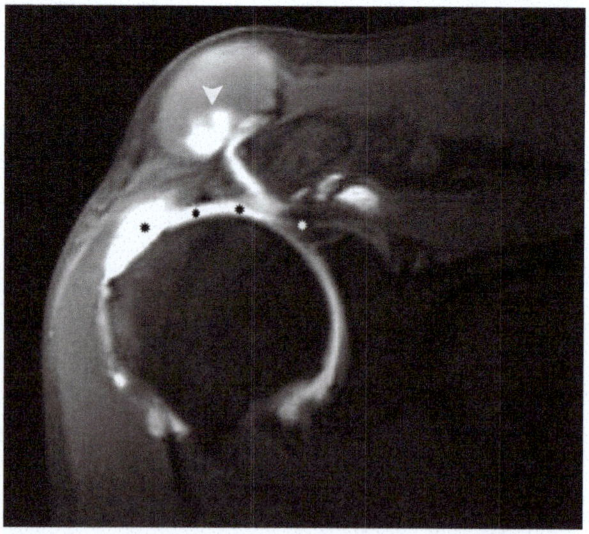

Fig. 5.79 Large full-thickness tear of the supraspinatus tendon with geyser phenomenon. Oblique coronal fat-suppressed MR arthrogram. There is a large contrast-filled gap in the supraspinatus (*black asterisk*) with extensive tendon retraction (grade 3; *white asterisk*) and ill delineation of the retracted tendon. Notice spilling of contrast into the subacromial-subdeltoid bursa, AC joint and a "cyst" on top of the AC joint (*arrowhead*)

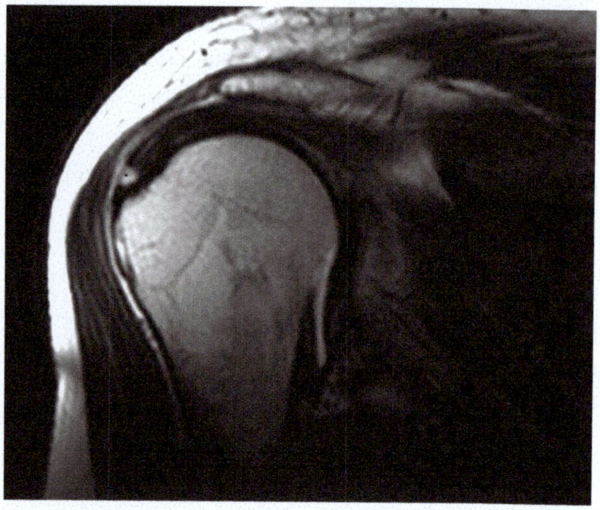

Fig. 5.80 Partial-thickness tear at the bursal side of the distal supraspinatus tendon. Oblique coronal T2-WI. Small area of high signal intensity within the distal supraspinatus (*asterisk*) and small amount of fluid within the subacromial-subdeltoid bursa. There was no spilling of contrast within the bursa on the MR arthrogram (not shown)

- Thickening (contour bulging) or thinning of the RC tendons
- Position of the myotendinous junction of the supraspinatus tendon: the normal myotendinous junction should lie within a 15° arc of the 12 o'clock position of the humeral head on coronal oblique imaging. If the myotendinous junction is more than 15° medial to the 12 o'clock position, there may be a full-thickness cuff tear
- Other important signs are the shape of the acromion and the presence of an os acromiale (Figs. 5.83 and 5.84) or degenerative changes on the acromioclavicular joint, causing RC impingement
- If a full-thickness cuff tear is present, the following parameters, important for the surgeon, should be assessed
  - Involved tendon(s)
  - Size: extent of the tear (small if less than 1 cm; intermediate: 1– 3 cm; large: 3–5 cm; massive if more than 5 cm)
  - Degree of tendon retraction (three grades according to position of free edge of the tendon compared to the AC joint (Fig. 5.79). Grade 3 retraction is surgically very difficult to repair
  - Quality of the free tendon edge (Fig. 5.79)
  - Muscle atrophy ("tangent" sign on sagittal T1-WIs; normal muscle should reach the level of

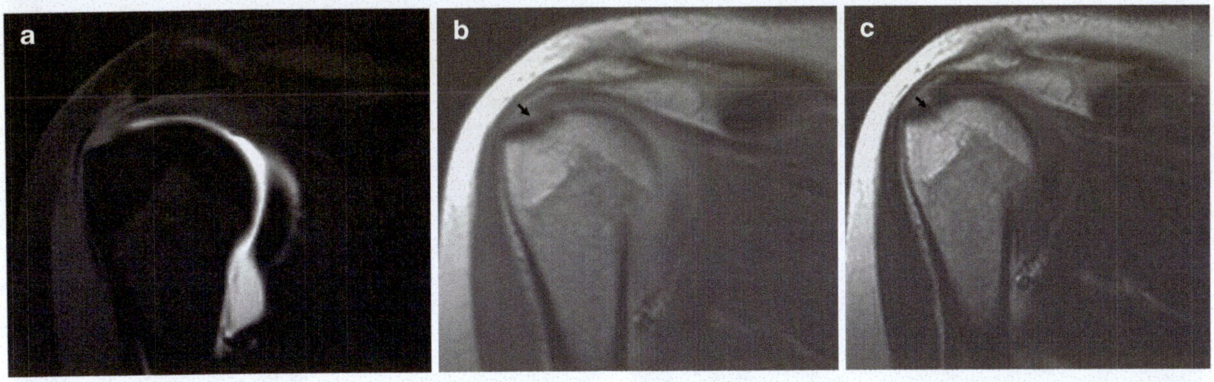

Fig. 5.81 Intratendinous tear of the supraspinatus tendon. Oblique coronal fat-suppressed SE T1-W MR arthrogram (**a**). Oblique coronal PD MR image (**b**). Oblique coronal FSE T2-W MR image (**c**). Normal delineation of the articular surface of the supraspinatus tendon (**a**). There is small focus of fluid-like signal (*arrows*) within the distal supraspinatus on the PD/T2 images (**b–c**). There is absence of communication with the subacromial bursa

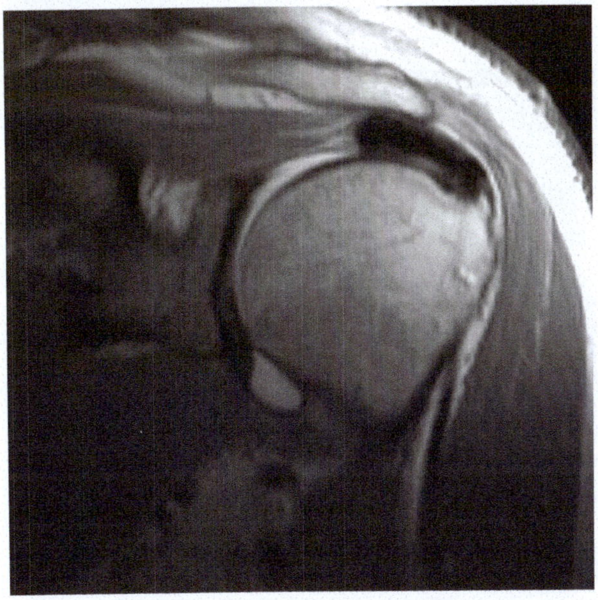

Fig. 5.82 Calcifications of the distal supraspinatus tendon. Oblique coronal T2-WI. Hypointense calcifications within the distal supraspinatus tendon

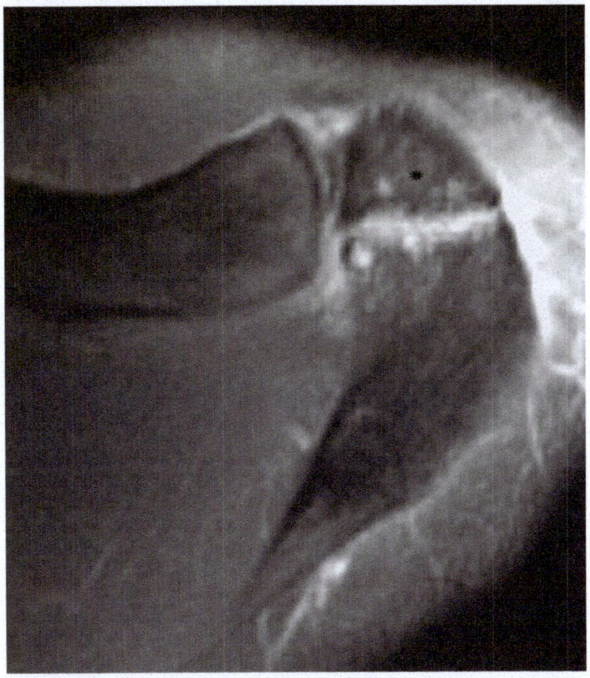

Fig. 5.83 Os acromiale. Axial fat-suppressed MR arthrogram shows absence of fusion of the mesoacomion, resulting in an os acromiale (*asterisk*). This morphological variant may predispose for rotator cuff disease

the superior border of "scapular Y") and fatty degeneration (grade 0: no fat; grade 1: streaks of fat; grade 2: less fat than muscle; grade 3: equal amounts of fat and muscle; and grade 4: more fat than muscle) (Fig. 5.85)

- Abnormal contrast spilling of the AC joint ("Geyser" phenomenon) and formation of AC cysts, which are negative prognostic factors for surgical repair (Fig. 5.79)
- Integrity and position of the long head of the biceps tendon. Biceps tendon (sub-) luxation or tears are particularly associated with Rotator cuff (RC) tears involving the subscapularis tendon (Fig. 5.86)
- Elevation of the humeral head, remodeling of the undersurface of the acromion and secondary glenohumeral osteoarthritis in longstanding RC tears (Fig. 5.87)

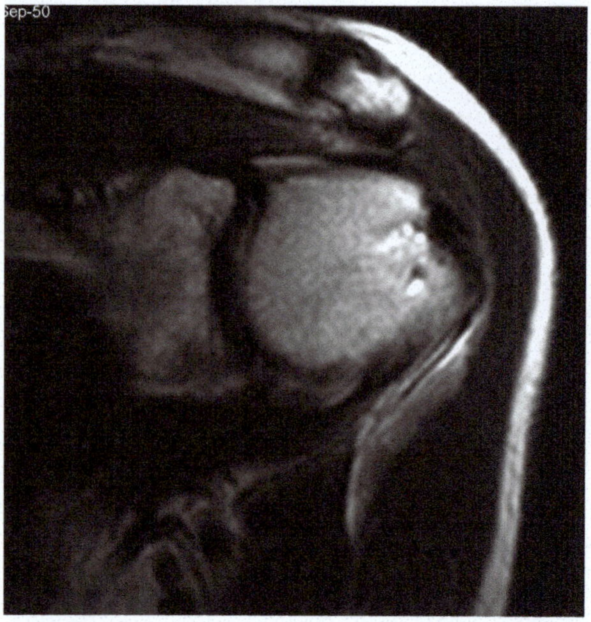

Fig. 5.84 Subacromial spur with impingement on the musculotendinous junction of the supraspinatus tendon. Oblique coronal FSE T2-W MR image. Note irregular delineation of the bursal surface of the supraspinatus tendon, indicating subtle partial-thickness tear on the bursal surface. There is also thickening of the coracoacromial ligament

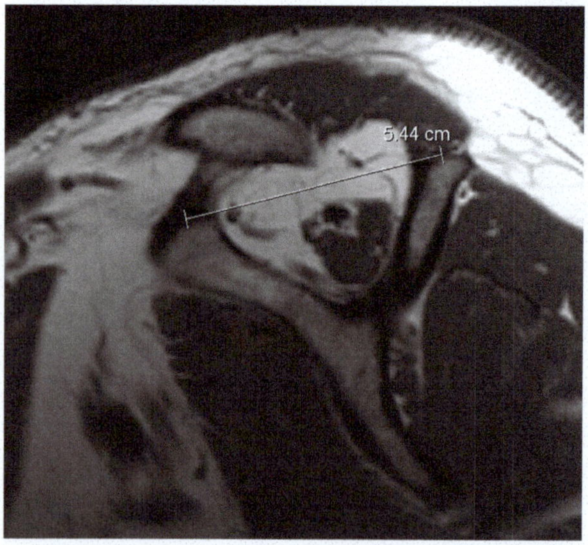

Fig. 5.85 Severe fat infiltration and muscle atrophy of the belly of the supraspinatus in a patient with a full-thickness tear of the rotator cuff (see also Fig. 5.79). Oblique sagittal SE T1-WI through the muscle belly. Notice that the tangent line is lying above the superior border of the supraspinatus muscle

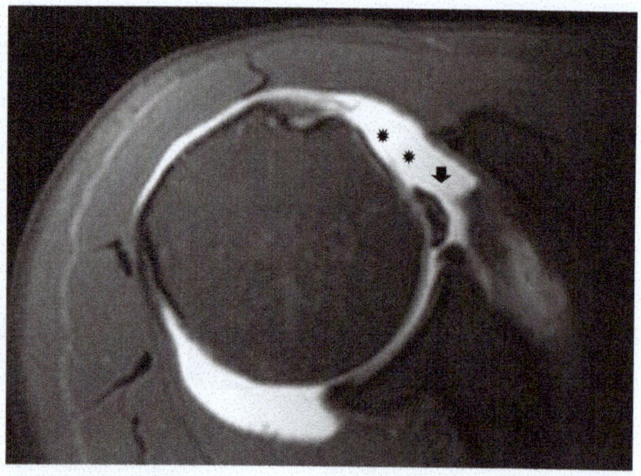

Fig. 5.86 Medial dislocation of the long head of the biceps tendon (*arrow*) and associated full-thickness subscapularis tendon tear (*asterisk*). Axial fat-suppressed SE T1-W MR arthrogram

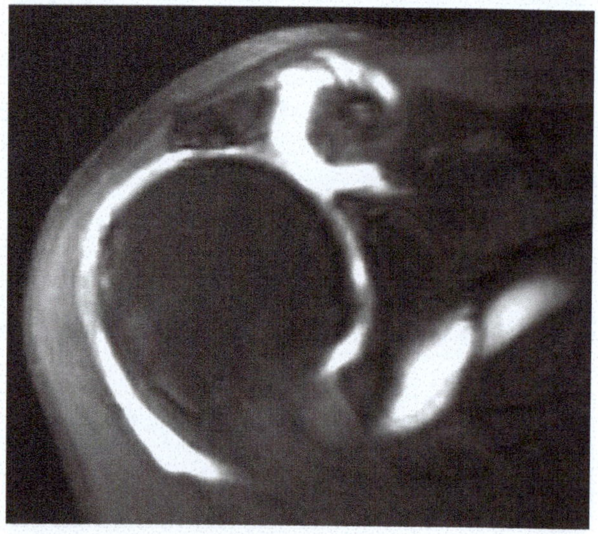

Fig. 5.87 Large longstanding full-thickness rotator cuff tear. Oblique coronal fat-suppressed MR arthrogram. Note elevation of the humeral head, secondary glenohumeral arthrosis and contrast within the AC joint (*geyser sign*)

MRI Findings of Rotator Cuff Tears

- Full-thickness tear: focal or diffuse contrast-filled gap in the entire thickness of the tendon, with contrast in the subacromial bursa. Tl-W fat-suppressed images avoid confusion among preexisting fluid (dark), with fluid extravasating from the joint (bright). Gadolinium is not confused with subacromial fat (dark). Easy assessment of the size of the tear can be made, which is helpful for deciding operative approach (see above).

The degree of tendon retraction and the amount of fraying of the ends of the tendon are findings that will assist the surgeon in the decision whether or not the tear is amenable to reparation.

- Partial tears: contrast imbibition in the supraspinatus tendon or irregularity of the articular surface of the tendon. Most partial tears can be found in the so-called critical zone (one centimeter medial to the greater tuberosity). Bursal tears are not so well seen on the Tl-WIs because gadolinium does not pass into the bursa. However, bursal tears are well seen on T2 or fat-suppressed T2 images.

Similarly, intrasubstance tears are characterized by intratendinous T2 fluid signal without extension to either bursal or articular surface. These lesions will not fill with gadolinium on MRA because of lack of communication between the tear and the articular surface of the tendon.

- Tendinosis: subjective thickening of the tendon on Tl-WIs. Other sequences can support this impression by showing brightening of the tendon most clearly seen on T2-WIs (with fat suppression) or STIR images. Further support comes from increased fluid in the subacromial bursa. The etiology may be evident on MR images, such as acromial spur formation, anterior hook of the acromion, acromioclavicular joint hypertrophic degenerative change, or thickening of the coracoacromial ligament (CAL).
- Subscapularis tears: subscapularis tears are best identified on axial and oblique sagittal images. Isolated full-thickness subscapularis tears are uncommon and typically occur in the setting of acute trauma. More frequently, subscapularis tears are found in association with supraspinatus tendon tears. Involvement of the cranial fibers is most frequent. MR arthrographic findings include tendon discontinuity, gadolinium filling a gap over the lesser tuberosity, atrophy of the subscapularis, or malposition of the tendon of the long head of the biceps tendon. Preoperative identification of subscapularis tears is important, as this may affect surgical planning.

Rotator Interval and Biceps Tendon Injuries

The rotator interval is the anatomic space along the anterosuperior aspect of the shoulder between the supraspinatus and subscapularis prior to their fusion. Oblique sagittal MR images are the most important in analyzing the interval. The interval is bridged by the rotator interval capsule and also, the coracohumeral ligament (CHL) contributes to the interval as it extends from the coracoid posteriorly and laterally and merges with the capsule. The fused capsule and CHL further merge with the anterior margin and superficial and deep fascial fibers of the supraspinatus. The capsule and ligament together serve as roof over the intraarticular course of the biceps tendon. As such, the CHL together with the superior glenohumeral ligament, which is a focal thickening of the glenohumeral capsule, contribute to the stability of the long biceps tendon within the sulcus.

The many structures that are involved with and course through the rotator interval can be injured together. The interval and biceps tendon are stressed in the athlete who uses repetitive and/or forceful overhead motions. Also, a fall on the outstretched hand may sprain or tear the rotator interval. The normal CHL should show thin and smooth with low SI on oblique sagittal images. As a result of acute injuries such as traumatic tearing, the rotator interval and CHL may show thickening and irregularity with heterogeneous higher SI. With more chronic derangement, such as in repetitive overuse situations, irregular scarring of the rotator interval capsule and CHL may be seen.

Prominent scarring of the CHL has also been thought to play a role in the clinical picture of an adhesive capsulitis. Besides thickening on the oblique sagittal images, one should be aware of synovitis within the rotator interval. Frequently, however, no specific MR abnormalities are noticed in patients with clinical symptoms of adhesive capsulitis.

The long tendon of the biceps extends from the superior glenoid tubercle or superior labrum, through the glenohumeral joint and rotator interval and exits the joint anteriorly. Extraarticularly, the tendon is located within the intertubercular sulcus. The biceps tendon together with the superior labrum attribute to prevention of superior dislocation of the humeral head.

The extraarticular appearance of the biceps tendon is best evaluated on axial MR images. Tears of the long head of the biceps tendon are usually a complication of a supraspinatus injury. In partial-thickness biceps tendon tears, fluid signal is appreciated within the tendon substance. Presence of two rather than one tendon slips, which is a normal variant, should not be misinterpreted as partial tearing. In complete tears, the tendon is absent or there is complete discontinuity.

Tearing most frequently occurs in the lateral intraarticular portion. In complete tears, the tendon is no longer visualized within the bicipital groove due to distal retraction of the muscle. A small proximal remnant at the biceps-labral anchor is frequently seen. Severe degeneration with thinning of the long biceps tendon may give rise to an apparently empty interval. An empty sulcus on the other hand can also exist without complete tear of the tendon, in case of medial dislocation. Intraarticular biceps tendon dislocation is usually associated with a full-thickness tear of the subscapularis tendon or rotator cuff interval injury, whereas extraarticular dislocation is associated with a partial-thickness tear of the subscapularis or tear of the transverse ligament.

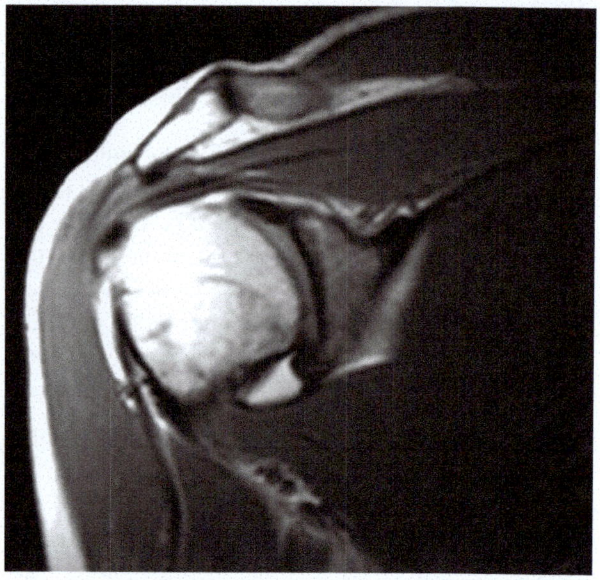

Fig. 5.88 Downsloping acromion, impinging on the supraspinatus tendon. Oblique coronal FSE PD WI

Shoulder Impingement Syndrome

Impingement reflects a clinical condition in which the subacromial soft tissues (supraspinatus tendon, biceps tendon, and bursa) are compressed between the humeral head and (components of) the coracoacromial arch. Mechanical impingement may lead to a compromise of tensile integrity and eventually rotator cuff tears. Several types of impingement can be distinguished: primary extrinsic impingement, secondary extrinsic impingement from instability, and internal impingement, particularly in throwing athletes.

1. *Primary extrinsic impingement*

Primary extrinsic impingement includes subacromial and subcoracoid impingement.

(a) *Subacromial impingement*

The arch that surrounds the rotator cuff is composed of the acromion, the acromioclavicular joint, the coracoid process, and the coracoacromial ligament (CAL). Anatomical variants and reactive degenerative irregularities of this osseous outlet may result in primary extrinsic impingement of the underlying cuff tendons and adjacent bursa with subsequent clinical impingement. Although rotator cuff degeneration and tearing may be due to intrinsic factors, such as diminished vascularity and overuse, it has been proposed that the vast majority of cuff tears are secondary to chronic impingement between the humeral head and coracoacromial arch. In this respect, the shape and aspect of the anterior acromion, assessed on the oblique sagittal and coronal MR images have been found to be of critical importance. The shape of the undersurface of the anterolateral (AL) acromion can be classified as flat (I), curved (II), anteriorly hooked (III), or convex (IV), however, variability among observers can be significant. Types II and III in particular are associated with higher incidence of impingement and rotator cuff abnormalities. Downsloping of the acromion (Fig. 5.88), either anteriorly (determined on sagittal images, immediately lateral to the AC joint) or laterally (on coronal images) may result in narrowing of the outlet and impingement of the distal part of the supraspinatus tendon. Another causing factor of impingement may be the presence of bony spurs on the inferior surface of the acromion (Fig. 5.84). Incidentally, a nonfused os acromiale may lead to osteophytic lipping at the acromial gap and as such, impingement of the rotator cuff, tendinopathy, and tearing of the supraspinatus. The nonfused ossification center of the acromion is best appreciated on axial MR images, the subsequent effects on the rotator cuff are best visible on the oblique coronal and sagittal images (Fig. 5.83).

Osteoarthritic changes of the A–C joint are frequently encountered after the age of 40. This may result in spur formation and synovial and capsular hypertrophy with scarring. Although these factors may influence the rotator cuff, it is usually less critical compared with changes of the anterior acromion.

The CAL is another component of the osseous outlet. This ligament is best appreciated on the oblique sagittal MR images, as it extends from the coracoid process to the acromion. The thickness of the normal ligament measures about 2–3 mm. The CAL can be congenitally thickened, or thickening can be reactive due to chronic pressure exerted by subacromial structures during arm abduction.

(b) *Subcoracoid impingement*

In subcoracoid impingement, the coracohumeral distance is narrowed (less than the normal 11 mm) on axial images, for instance due to developmental enlargement of the coracoid process or posttraumatic changes of the coracoid process or lesser tuberosity. This may result in entrapment of the subscapularis tendon between the humeral head and coracoid process.

2. *Secondary extrinsic impingement*

Secondary extrinsic impingement refers to instability of the glenohumeral joint resulting in dynamic narrowing of the coracoacromial outlet. The outlet itself can be morphologically normal. Repetitive microtraumata and weakening of the anterior capsule is quite commonly seen in overhead-throwing athletes. The instability itself is usually minor and by itself asymptomatic and may result from a lax capsule or stretched glenohumeral ligaments that develop over time. Due to superior translation of the humeral head in these throwers, there is dynamic impingement of the rotator cuff in the coracoacromial outlet, resulting in tendinosis and tearing.

Accurate assessment of the cause of impingement has critical consequences for further treatment: in the primary form of extrinsic impingement, open or arthroscopic surgery is warranted to remove osseous irregularities, whereas secondary impingement may be best treated by physical therapy aiming at strengthening of the cuff and avoidance of activities causing instability. Various surgical procedures are available to decrease the many factors that contribute to mechanical impingement of the rotator cuff, particularly the supraspinatus tendon: these include resection of a thickened coracoacromial ligament (CAL), anterior acromioplasty, resection of the distal clavicle, and resection of inferior osteophytes. Partial-thickness tears will be treated by arthroscopic debridement, whereas full-thickness tears should be repaired.

3. *Internal impingement*

Internal impingement may be classified as posterosuperior impingement or anterosuperior impingement.

(a) *Posterosuperior impingement*

Posterosuperior impingement is a condition which is encountered in throwing athletes. Impingement occurs of the undersurface of the posterior rotator cuff between the humeral head and the posterosuperior labrum and osseous glenoid. This position occurs during the late cocking phase of throwing with the arm in extreme abduction and exorotation. This may result in degeneration and partial cuff tears, particularly infraspinatus and posterior supraspinatus, fraying of the posterosuperior labrum and quite large subcortical cystic changes of the humeral head in the posterior greater tuberosity, due to repetitive impaction. Moreover, posterior capsular thickening and ossification (Bennett lesion) may occur under these circumstances.

(b) *Anterosuperior impingement*

Anterosuperior impingement is caused by the friction of the articular surface fibers of the subscapularis tendon along the anterosuperior glenoid rim. There is no relation with instability. MRA may demonstrate partial articular surface tears of the subscapularis tendon.

Miscellaneous Conditions that May Mimic Rotator Cuff Pathology

1. *Parsonage-Turner syndrome*

Parsonage-Turner syndrome (acute brachial neuritis) is a self-limiting disorder, which presents with sudden onset of shoulder pain and accompanying weakness. MRI usually shows characteristic edema of rotator cuff muscles and deltoid muscle.

2. *Quadrilateral space syndrome*

These patients present with pain that may simulate cuff pathology, presumably due to (posttraumatic) scar tissue and fibrous band in the quadrilateral space that may cause impingement on the axillary nerve.

MRI is rather typical, demonstrating fatty atrophy of the teres minor muscle.

3. *Spinoglenoid cyst*

A spinoglenoid notch is usually associated with tearing of the posterior labrum (Fig. 5.89).

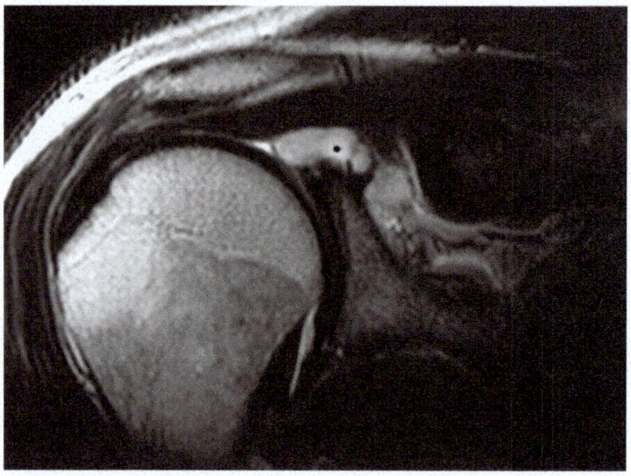

Fig. 5.89 Spinoglenoid cyst. Oblique coronal SE T1-W MR arthrogram demonstrating a well-delineated contrast-filled lesion (*asterisk*) and associated tear within the superior glenoid labrum

4. Other osseous lesions that may mimic rotator cuff (RC) tears are *greater tuberosity fractures and distal clavicular osteolysis* (Fig. 5.90).

5.4.3.2 Shoulder Instability

Because of its remarkable degree of mobility, the glenohumeral joint is inherently prone to instability.

The leading cause of instability about the glenohumeral joint relates to previous dislocations resulting from trauma. Direction of dislocation can be anterior, which is by far most commonly encountered (95%), posterior, superior, or inferior. These anteroinferior dislocations are usually associated with lesions of the anteroinferior bony glenoid margin (bony Bankart lesion), compression fracture of the superolateral humeral head (Hill–Sachs lesion), the anteroinferior labrum (Bankart lesion) with injury of the inferior glenohumeral ligament and/or stripping of the capsule and scapular periosteum. Nontraumatic shoulder instability may be caused by a congenital capsular hyperlaxity or hypoplasia of the glenoid. This may lead to multidirectional instability, which is often bilaterally encountered.

The impact of accurate imaging in the work-up of patients with glenohumeral instability is high. Results of (MR) imaging may directly influence the surgeon's strategy to perform an arthroscopic or open treatment for (recurrent) instability. Factors that are in favor of open treatment include a large bony Hill–Sachs defect, substantial bone erosion of the anterior glenoid rim, humeral avulsion of the glenohumeral ligament (HAGL), and hyperlaxity of the capsule. MRA is the optimal technique to detect, localize, and characterize injuries of the capsular-labrum complex.

There is extensive discussion in the literature regarding labral tears. The labrum is usually torn in its anterior-inferior portion. Tears of the superior labrum usually begin posteriorly and extend in an anterior direction (superior labral anterior to posterior (SLAP) lesion). Posterior tears are less common. The anterior–superior

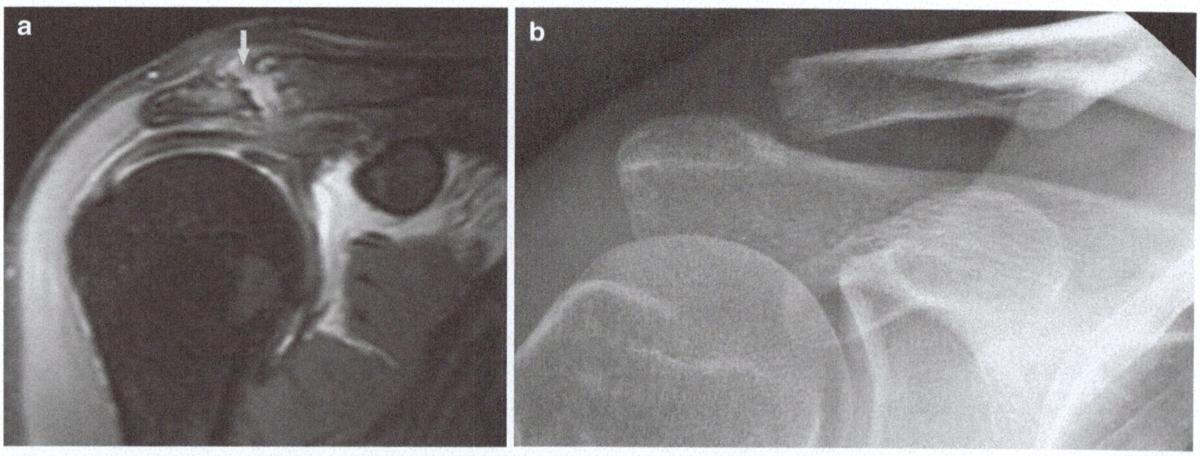

Fig. 5.90 Posttraumatic osteolysis 3 month following a blunt acromioclavicular (AC) joint trauma. Coronal fat-suppressed intermediate-WI (**a**) shows widening of the right AC joint (*arrow*), irregular delineation of the lateral clavicle and BME at the lateral clavicule and to a minor degree at the acromion. The corresponding radiograph (**b**) shows joint widening an irregular delineation of the lateral clavicle

portion of the labrum is almost never torn in isolation, and this should not be confused with the sublabral foramen (Fig. 5.77). The following paragraph will focus on the most frequently encountered labrum lesions.

Bankart Lesion

This is a tear involving the anterior-inferior portion of the labrum, with or without an associated fracture secondary to an anterior dislocation of the shoulder. A Hill–Sachs deformity is usually present and there may be a fracture of the inferior portion of the glenoid. Findings on MRA include the extension of contrast material between the labrum and glenoid, which is usually best visualized on the axial images (Figs. 5.91 and 5.92). The labrum may be totally avulsed and appear as a separate structure of low signal intensity along the anterior-inferior margin of the joint capsule. In the ABER position, the pull of the Inferior Glenohumeral Ligament (IGL) on the inferior portion of the labrum will allow easier detection of the Bankart lesion.

ALPSA Lesion

The anterior labroligamentous periosteal sleeve avulsion (ALPSA) lesion is a variant of the Bankart lesion, in which the labrum is torn but the periosteum remains intact. The mechanism of injury is the same as the Bankart lesion. The radiologist is required to discriminate between the ALPSA and Bankart lesions, because the surgical repair is not the same for both conditions. MR findings include the presence of contrast material between the labrum and the glenoid. The periosteum remains attached to the labrum, which may rotate medially along the glenoid (Figs. 5.93 and 5.94). Synovial tissue proliferates between the rotated glenoid and the displaced periosteum, and this has to be debrided prior

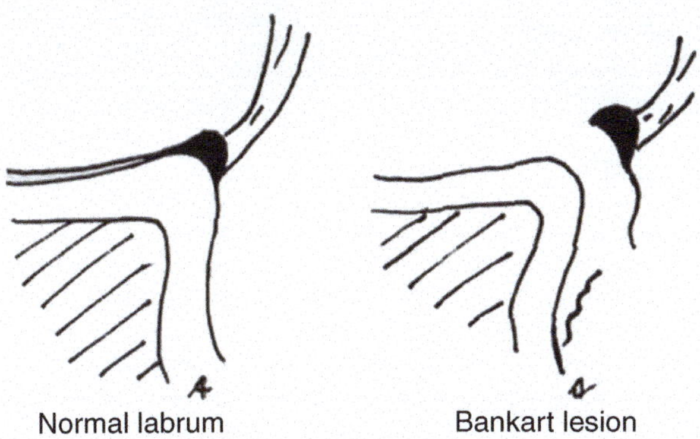

Fig. 5.91 Normal anterior labroligamentous complex vs. a Bankart lesion

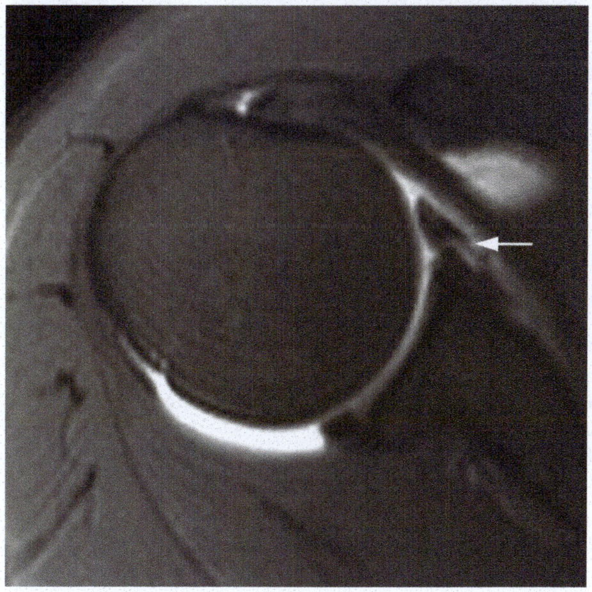

Fig. 5.92 Bankart lesion. Axial MR arthrogram. Extension of contrast between the antero-inferior labrum and the bony glenoid with disruption of the periosteal sleeve (*arrow*)

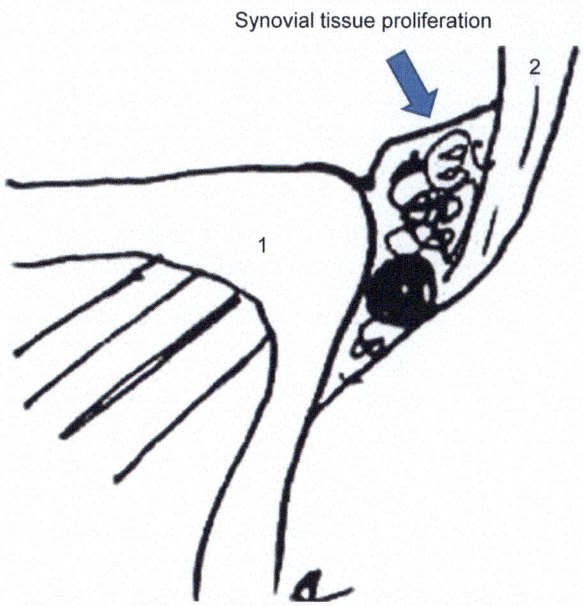

Fig. 5.93 Schematic drawing of an ALPSA lesion. Note the presence of synovial tissue proliferation (*arrow*) between the glenoid (1) and the anterior capsulolabral complex (2)

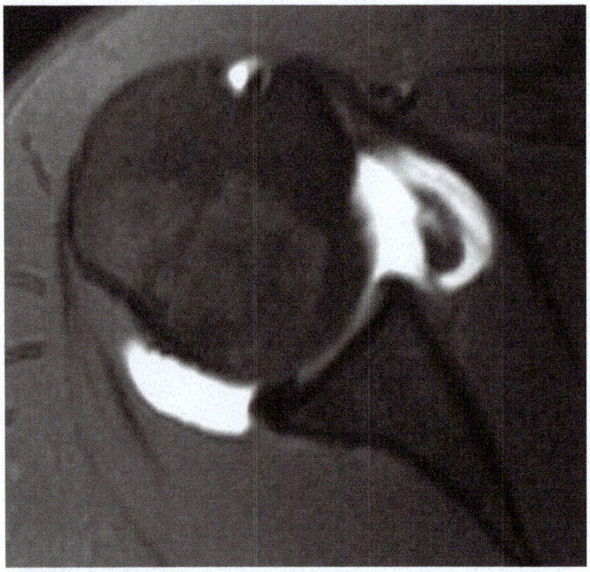

Fig. 5.94 Acute ALPSA lesion. Axial MR arthrogram. Note absence of disruption of the periost, in contradistinction to a Bankart lesion

to reattachment of the medialized labrum. A posterior variant of this lesion has been described (see posterior labro periosteal sleeve avulsion (POLPSA) lesion).

Perthes Lesion

This is a variant form of the Bankart lesion in which the torn labrum is not separated from the underlying bone and may be difficult to visualize without adequate joint distension or using the ABER technique. Some consider two forms of Perthes lesions: one as described above and a second type, the "detached" Perthes lesion, which can be considered as an anterior labroligamentous periosteal sleeve avulsion (ALPSA) lesion without medialization of the labrum.

SLAP Lesion

SLAP tear involves the superior portion of the labrum. It usually begins in the posterior-superior portion of the labrum and extends a variable distance anteriorly to the biceps-labral complex. Today, 12 grades of SLAP tears have been described (Table 5.8), only the first four are present in any significant abundance. Type 1(10%) represents fraying and can usually only be diagnosed if there is significant imbibed contrast within the labrum.

Table 5.8 Current classification of SLAP lesions

Type I: tear of the superior part of the labrum with intact Long Head of Biceps Tendon (LHBT)
Type II: avulsion of the LHBT with tear of the anterior and posterior labrum
Type III: bucket-handle tear of the labrum
Type IV: bucket-handle tear of the labrum with longitudinal tear of the LHBT
Type V: same as type II, but extension into the anterior-inferior labrum
Type VI: flap tear of the superior labrum
Type VII: same as type II, but extension into the Middle Glenohumeral Ligament (MGL)
Type VIII: same as type II, but more posterior extension
Type IX: circumferential involvement of the entire labrum
Type X: same as type VII, but associated with Rotator cuff (RC) interval tear
Type XI: same as type II, but extension into the Superior Glenohumeral Ligament (SGL)
Type XII: SLAC lesion

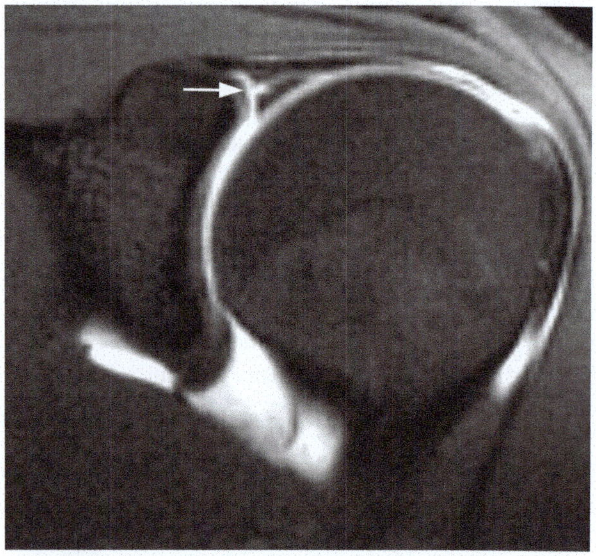

Fig. 5.95 SLAP lesion type 4. Coronal oblique MR arthrogram. There is an irregular delineated area of contrast extension at the superior labrum, with lateral extension toward the biceps tendon (*arrow*). The irregular delineation and lateral extension are in favor of a true SLAP lesion compared to a normal sublabral recess

Type 2 (40%) is a separation of the superior portion of the labrum and biceps anchor (Fig. 5.95).

Type 3 is a bucket-handle tear without involvement of the biceps. Type 4 is bucket-handle tear that extends into the biceps tendon.

Accurate identification of the specific type of SLAP lesion is extremely difficult, even with MRA. An accurate description of the lesion and adequate communication with the referring clinician seems more important than the exact designation of a specific type. It is –however – important to differentiate lesions with avulsion of the biceps anchor from other lesions.

The MR findings of an SLAP tear include the extension of contrast material between the labrum and the glenoid. Care should be taken when evaluating the superior portion of the labrum, because it has a deep cuff that may simulate a tear. If contrast material under the cuff extends toward the ipsilateral shoulder, it should be called a tear. Contrast material undercutting the labrum obliquely toward the patient's head is a normal finding in the labral cuff, unless the contrast then extends medial to the perpendicular superior surface of the glenoid. If the labrum is absent or small involving the anterior-superior location only, look for a large MGL and the Buford complex; if the labrum appears only to be separated at the anterior-superior portion of the glenoid, the diagnosis should be a sublabral foramen.

A specific combination of anterior-superior labral tear (SLAP lesion) and partial tear of the undersurface of the supraspinatus tendon has been described as a superior labrum anterior cuff lesion (SLAC). Other lesions found in this group include the anterior part of the biceps anchor and the superior glenohumeral ligament.

A posterior labral tear may result in formation of a ganglioncyst, similar to the mechanism found in a meniscal cyst associated with a meniscal tear (Fig. 5.96).

GLOM

The glenoid labral ovoid mass (GLOM) represents a torn labrum that has become separated from the glenoid. On MR, it appears as a structure of low signal intensity that is usually seen along the anterior joint space and often appears "floating" in the intraarticular contrast material. Care should be taken not to mistake the GLOM for a dislocated long head of the biceps tendon. MRA is also ideal for the evaluation of any possible loose body within the shoulder and can often demonstrate the site of an associated cartilage or bony defect.

HAGL

HAGL lesion is a disruption of the Inferior Glenohumeral Ligament (IGL) at its attachment to the anatomical neck of the humerus. It usually involves the anterior band. The MR appearance includes the extension of contrast material down the humeral shaft in a triangular manner. The torn IGL can usually be identified and is best seen on the oblique coronal (Fig. 5.97) and sagittal images.

The glenohumeral ligament may be torn at the labral side, midsubstance, or from the humeral side. Only the humeral side tear is called a HAGL. An associated bony avulsion of the humeral neck accompanying a HAGL has been designated a bony humeral avulsion of the Inferior Glenohumeral Ligament (IGL) lesion.

A floating anterior-inferior glenohumeral ligament (Floating AIGL) can be regarded as combined Bankart and HAGL lesion.

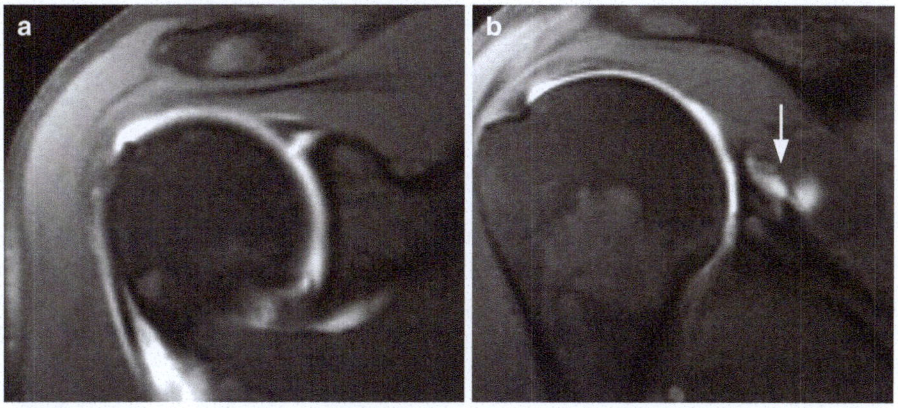

Fig. 5.96 SLAP lesion with associated paralabral cyst. Oblique coronal MR arthrogram. Posterosuperior labrum lesion (**a**) with extension in a small paralabral cyst (*arrow*, **b**)

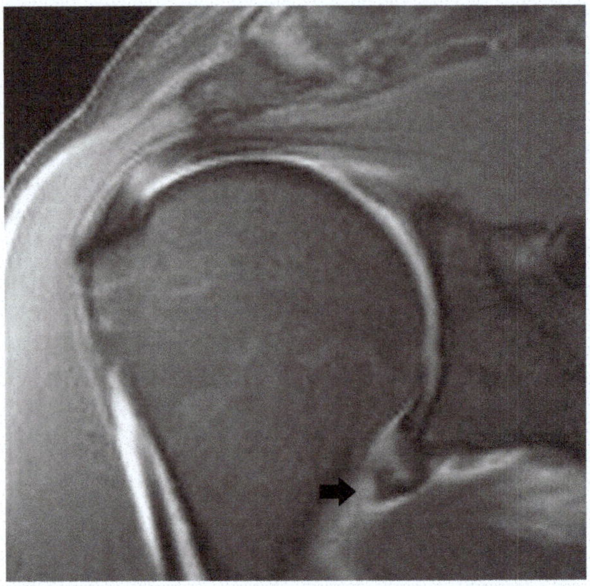

Fig. 5.97 HAGL lesion. Oblique coronal MR arthrogram showing the avulsion of the anterior band of the inferior glenohumeral complex (*arrow*)

Glenolabral Articular Disruption (GLAD) Lesion

Another variant consists of a labral tear with an associated articular cartilage divot that follows acute forced adduction. The lesion typically involves the anterior margin of the labrum and does not result in instability. It is called the GLAD lesion.

Posterior Labral Periosteal Sleeve Avulsion (POLPSA) Lesion

A POLPSA lesion is the posterior counterpart (located at the posterior labrum) of the anterior labroligamentous periosteal sleeve avulsion (ALPSA) lesion.

Bennett Lesion

Seen most frequently in baseball pitchers, the Bennett lesion leads to a peculiar excrescence developing on the posterior aspect of the glenoid cavity. It probably relates to an enthesophyte developing where the posterior band of the inferior glenohumeral ligament attaches to the scapula. Associated lesions include injuries to the posterior portion of the labrum and a partial tear of the rotator cuff.

Hypoplasia of the Glenoid Neck

Morphologically, this entity is characterized by a denticulate bony glenoid, which may result in multidirectional instability of the glenohumeral joint.

5.5 Hip Joint

5.5.1 Anatomy

The bony anatomy of the pelvis is complex, consisting of the sacrum, ilium, and ischium and pubis, all three contributing to the hip joint. The anatomy of the sacroiliac joints and its ligamentous attachments is discussed in Sect. 5.8.1.1.

The hip joint is a diarthrodial joint with a ball-and-cup configuration. The acetabulum is deepened by a fibrocartilaginous labrum that nearly surrounds the bony acetabulum. The capsule of the hip joint contributes to the stability of the joint, and has an area of thickening, the zona orbicularis. Numerous muscles take origin from the bony pelvis. Thorough understanding of their origins is important in understanding certain injuries.

Three main bursae are noted about the greater trochanter. The trochanteric bursa, also referred to as the subgluteus maximus bursa, is the largest of the three and covers the posterior facet and portions of the lateral facet of the grater trochanter. The second bursa is the subgluteus medius bursa, which is found deep to the lateral part of the gluteus medius tendon. It covers the superior part of the lateral facet. The third bursa is the subgluteus minimus bursa, lying beneath the gluteus minimus tendon, medial and superior to its insertion. When collapsed, these periarticular bursae cannot be identified in absence of pathology.

5.5.2 Technique

The pelvis should be imaged using a pelvic or torso phased-array coil, with a FoV covering the skin surfaces overlying both hips. Axial images are obtained from the top of the iliac crest to below the lesser trochanters.

If there is a specific complaint regarding one hip, surface coil can be used to examine the symptomatic side. Table 5.9 summarizes the proposed routine MR protocol of the pelvis and hip protocol.

Table 5.9 Pulse recommendations for routine imaging of the pelvis

Pulse sequence	WI	Plane
SE	T1	Coronal
FS FSE	T2	Coronal
FS FSE	T2	Axial
SE*	T1	Sagittal

*Optional in case of suspected osteonecrosis

Table 5.10 Pulse recommendations for direct hip arthrography

Pulse sequence	WI	Plane
FSE	PD	Oblique coronal
FSE	T2	Oblique coronal
FS SE	T1	Oblique axial
FS SE	T1	Oblique coronal
FS SE	T1	Sagittal
GRE	T2	Oblique Sagittal

If there is suspicion of labral pathology or femoro-acetabular impingement, an MR arthrogram is useful in evaluating intraarticular details. At our institution, we prefer the direct MR arthrographic technique. Prior to the MR examination, a fluoroscopic guide arthrogram of the symptomatic hip is performed. The MR examination consists of a coronal T2-W sequence of the entire pelvis, to evaluate extraarticular fluid collection of mass lesions and to identify bone marrow lesion. The MR arthrogram consists of a combination of T1-W sequences in three imaging planes, using a surface coil (Table 5.10).

5.5.3 Pathology

5.5.3.1 Trauma

Occult Acute Posttraumatic Fractures

Multidetector CT is the gold standard for evaluation of overt pelvic and acetabular fractures, but discussion of this topic is beyond the scope of this chapter.

Occult posttraumatic fractures in the elderly can occur in the femoral neck, greater trochanter, acetabulum or parasymphyseal, or ischial bone. These patients are usually osteoporotic and plain films may fail to demonstrate the fracture line. MRI is highly sensitive for detecting the fractures and the surrounding edema immediately after the traumatic event. The signal intensity changes are best documented by STIR or fat-suppressed T2-WI pulse sequences because of their high sensitivity for even small amounts of free water in the tissues.

Stress or Insufficiency Fractures

Stress or insufficiency fractures about the hip occur usually at the level of the internal aspect of the femoral neck, where the primary compression trabeculae are confluent toward the calcar. These fractures are most often incomplete and are seen on MRI as an area of BME at the inner aspect of the femoral neck with or without a fracture line (Fig. 5.98). Similar insufficiency fractures can be seen in the supra-acetabular area, pubic bones, and sacrum.

A special subtype of insufficiency fracture is the so-called subchondral (insufficiency) fracture (SIF) of the femoral head (Fig. 5.99). SIF is mostly occult on plain radiographs and is mostly seen in the elderly population or in patients with other causes of osteoporosis. Rarely, subchondral fractures may be related to stress in the population. This entity may be misdiagnosed as ON or transient osteoporosis of the hip (TOH) because of the extensive BME that is seen during the first few months. On the other hand, TOH and subchondral fracture may represent two manifestations of the same disease. Indeed, small subchondral linear low signal intensity lesions are often associated with TOH. The small size of these subchondral lesions is indicative for the transient pattern of the disease. Lesions thinner than 4 mm and shorter than 12.5 mm favor a good prognosis and spontaneous resolution of the symptoms within 4–9 months. Another disease that may be linked to subchondral fracture of the femoral head is rapidly destructive osteoarthritis of the hip or Postel's disease (Fig. 5.100). In these cases, subchondral fractures may lead to subsequent bone resorption and eventual collapse of the femoral head.

Osteochondrosis Dissecans and Osteochondral Fractures

OCD and osteochondral fractures are relatively rare in the femoral head and are mostly caused by shearing forces. MRI features are similar to OCD of the knee and ankle joint.

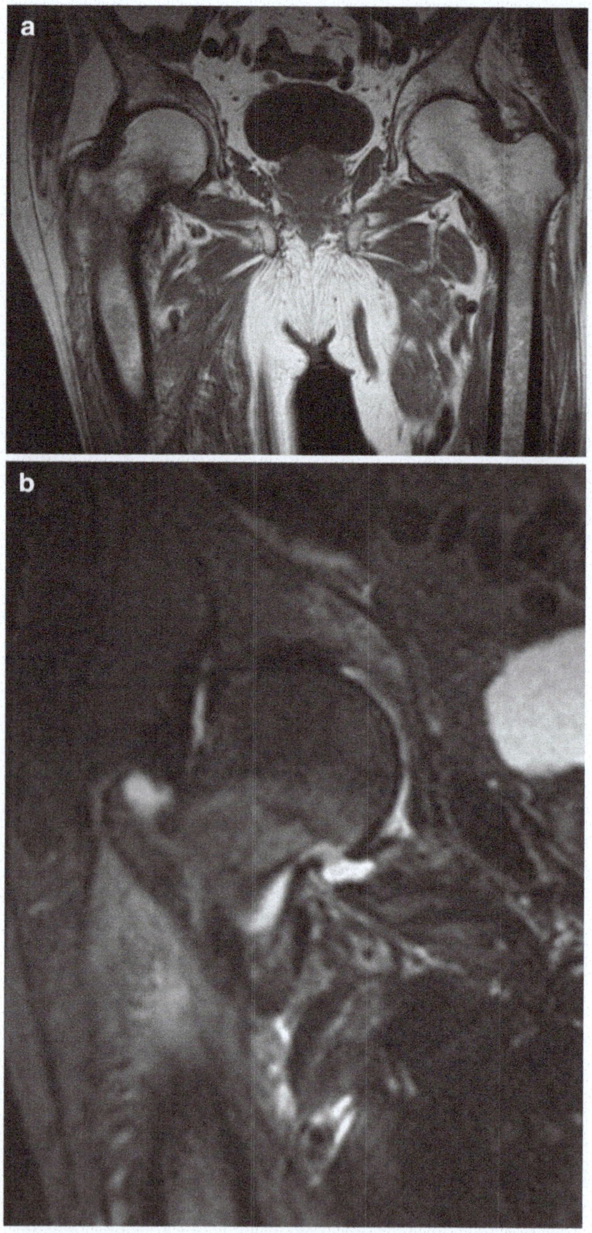

Fig. 5.98 Insufficiency fracture of the femoral neck. Coronal SE T1-WI (**a**) of the pelvis showing a hypointense fracture line at the inner aspect of the right femoral neck. Coronal fat-suppressed intermediate-WI (**b**) of the right hip confirms the fracture line, surrounded by hyperintense BME

Proximal Adductor-Gracilis Syndrome or Osteitis Pubis

Chronic traction on the pubic ramus by the adductor muscle, gracilis muscle may lead directly to disruption of the fibrocartilaginous symphyseal disc. This lesion is

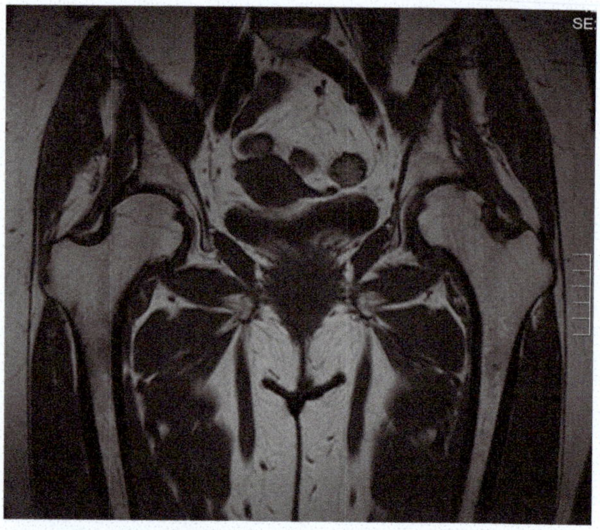

Fig. 5.99 Subchondral insufficiency fracture of the left femoral head. Coronal SE T1-WI of the pelvis showing a small hypointense fracture line at the subchondral area of the left femoral head

frequently seen in sporters (fencers, soccer, rugby, etc.) presenting with a history of increasing groin, pubic, or lower abdominal pain. Because of the radiographic similarity, the disorder was previously designated by the term "osteitis pubis," although not associated with infection.

On radiographs, there is variable diastasis of the symphysis pubis, periarticular cortical irregularity and erosion, sclerosis, and subchondral cyst formation with the subchondral bone.

MRI shows subperiosteal resorption and BME at the medial and inferior aspect of the pubic bone at the insertion of the adductor tendons. There is often increased fluid intensity within the joint and faint edema within the periarticular soft tissues. A secondary cleft sign (analogous to an annular tear of the intervertebral disc) consisting of hyperintense linear area of high-signal contiguous with the fluid-filled primary (central) cleft may be depicted at the symptomatic side on FS-T2 WI or STIR sequences. According to some authors, contrast enhancement correlates with the side of symptoms. Proximal adductor-gracilis syndrome may be associated with other causes of groin pain, such as sportsman's hernia. Abnormal motion of the symphysis pubis may also cause altered biomechanics at the other sites of the pelvic ring, i.e., the SI joints, resulting in simultaneous sacral stress fractures or degenerative changes at the SI joints (Fig. 5.101).

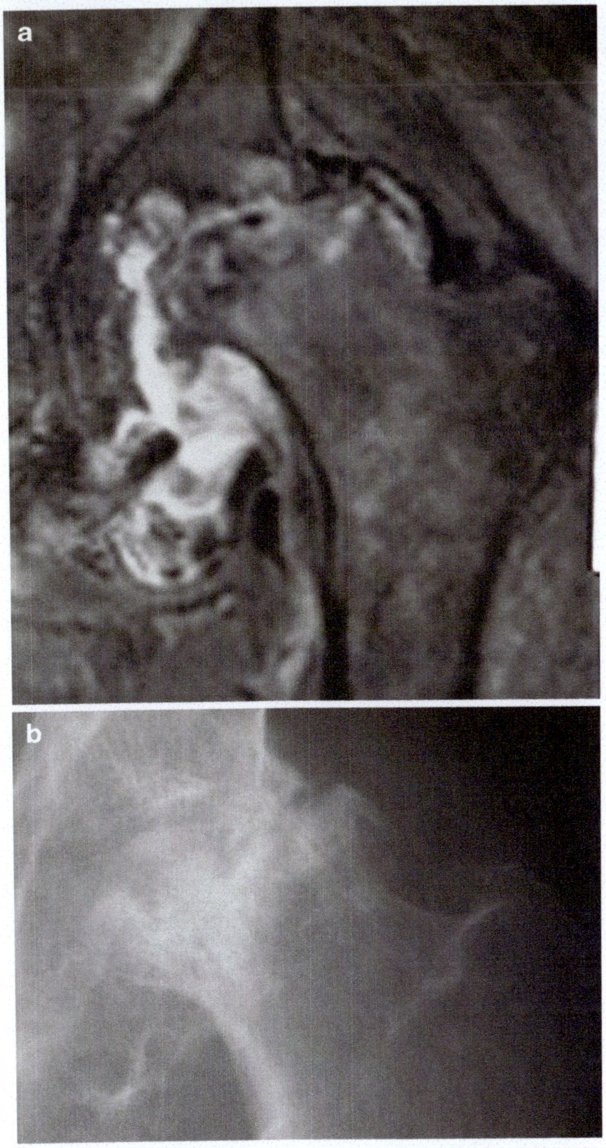

Fig. 5.100 Rapid destructive hip disease (RDHD) of the left femur. Coronal fat-suppressed intermediate-WI (**a**) of the left hip shows extensive destruction of the left hip. There is associated joint effusion. Corresponding radiograph (**b**) showing collapse of the femoral head. Previous radiographs (3 month earlier) were normal (not shown)

5.5.3.2 Nontraumatic Bone Marrow Lesions

Osteonecrosis or Avascular Necrosis of the Hip

ON of the femoral head is a very frequent indication forMRI of the hip. Due to its blood supply, the femoral head is particularly vulnerable to ON. ON is a progressive clinical entity, which may lead to destructive arthropathy. The risk factors and predisposing condition (i.e., steroid therapy, collagen vascular disease,..) are well known. Early diagnosis is mandatory for joint-preserving treatment. Currently, MRI is used in major classification systems solely for early detection when plain radiographs are normal.

MRI findings of ON include the following: bilateral involvement (seen in up to 72%) of patients), the presence of subchondral low signal intensity (with a thickness of at least 4 mm and length of more than 12.5 mm), the presence of a "double-line" sign on T2-WIs without fat suppression (seen in 80% of patients), and the "bandlike" low signal intensity demarcation line on T1-WIs (Fig. 5.102). This low signal intensity line demarcates the peripheral aspect of the necrotic segment. The "double-line" sign represents a chemical-shift artifact and is not seen when spectral fat suppression is applied with T2-W imaging. BME and joint effusion are additional but nonspecific findings of ON. The association of BME and ON has been a subject of controversy in the literature. In early ON, BME is never found before the appearance of the band-like pattern, suggesting that the latter are actually the initial changes of ON. BME appears to occur in a more advanced stage of the disease and seems to correlate highly with pain.

Other indications for evaluation of ON by MRI are accurate assessment of severity and prognosis, bilateral involvement and treatment evaluation.

Size and location of the lesions are important prognostic imaging signs. Large areas of ON do not respond to core decompression, and the femoral head eventually collapses, leading to osteoarthritis and subsequent need for joint replacement. Small lesions (less than 25% of the weight-bearing portion) have a better prognosis and may remain stable after core decompression. The location of focal ON involving less than 50% of the weight-bearing portion of the femoral head is also an important predictor of the disease outcome. Medially or centrally located lesions have a better prognosis than laterally located lesions.

Legg–Calvé–Perthes (LCP) Disease

LCP disease is the idiopathic counterpart of ON of the immature proximal femoral head. This entity will be discussed in detail in Chap. 15.

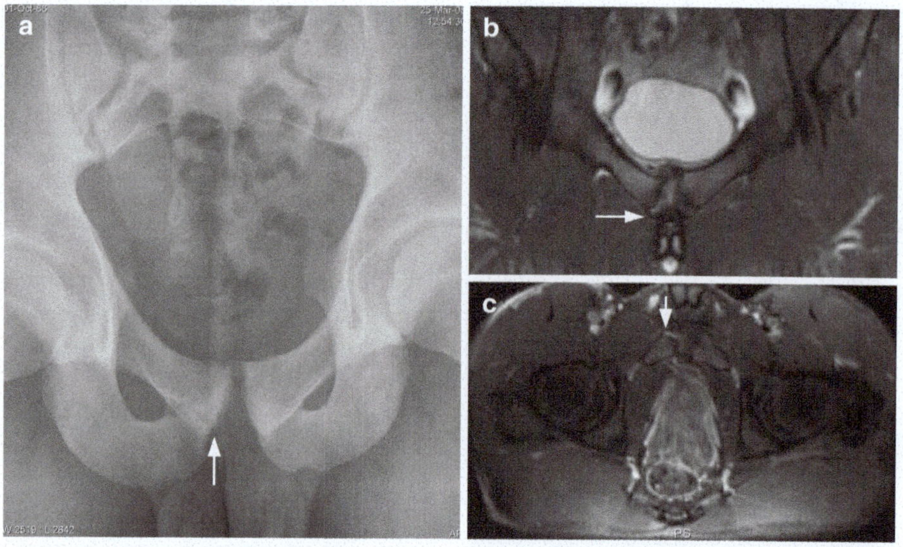

Fig. 5.101 Proximal gracilis-adductor syndrome. Anteroposterior radiograph (**a**) of the pelvis (spot view) shows articular surface irregularity, widening and subchondral sclerosis at the medial and inferior aspect of the right pubic bone (*arrow*). Coronal fat-suppressed T2-WI (FS T2-WI) (**b**) demonstrates fluid within the disc and the secondary cleft sign at the right side (*arrow*). There is also bilateral bone marrow edema at the pubic bones. Axial fat-suppressed T1-WI (FS T1-WI) (**c**) shows faint enhancement at the right right side (*arrow*), which correlates with the symptoms of the patient

Transient Osteoporosis of the Hip (TOH)

TOH is another frequent disorder of the hip, which is described in detail in subsection on bone marrow disorders (Sect. 5.9.6).

Rapidly Destructive Hip Disease (RDHD)

RDHD or Postel's disease is a relatively rare form of osteoarthritis that is more often seen in elderly women. It is characterized by radiographic findings of typical osteoarthritis progressing to bone resorption and joint collapse with destruction in a short period (Fig. 5.100). This entity may be linked to subchondral fracture or secondary ON.

Other Diseases Causing Nontraumatic Bone Marrow Edema

Inflammatory or infectious disorders of the hip joint can present with BME as well. Joint effusion and associated soft tissue changes (e.g., in osteomyelitis or spondylarthropathies) are other imaging clues to the diagnosis.

Some bone tumors and tumor-like conditions have a predilection for the proximal femur and may be accompanied by BME. Special mention is made of osteoid osteoma (OO), which may be the underlying cause for extensive bone and soft-tissue edema around the hip. MRI may be misleading, because the nidus of the tumor may be obscured by the extensive edema. If an OO is suspected, CT is mandatory to demonstrate the small nidus before surgical removal or percutaneous ablation.

Another tumoral lesion provoking extensive BME is chondroblastoma.

5.5.3.3 Labral Lesions

The labrum is a fibrocartilaginous structure that rims the horseshoe-shaped acetabulum. The labrum is widest anteriorly and superiorly. It is thickest superiorly and posteriorly. At the margins of the acetabular notch, the labrum blends imperceptibly with the transverse ligament. Clefts may be normally found at the junction of these structures and should not be confused with tears. The joint capsule inserts at the labral base anteriorly and posteriorly, creating small perilabral or labrocapsular sulci. Superiorly, the joint

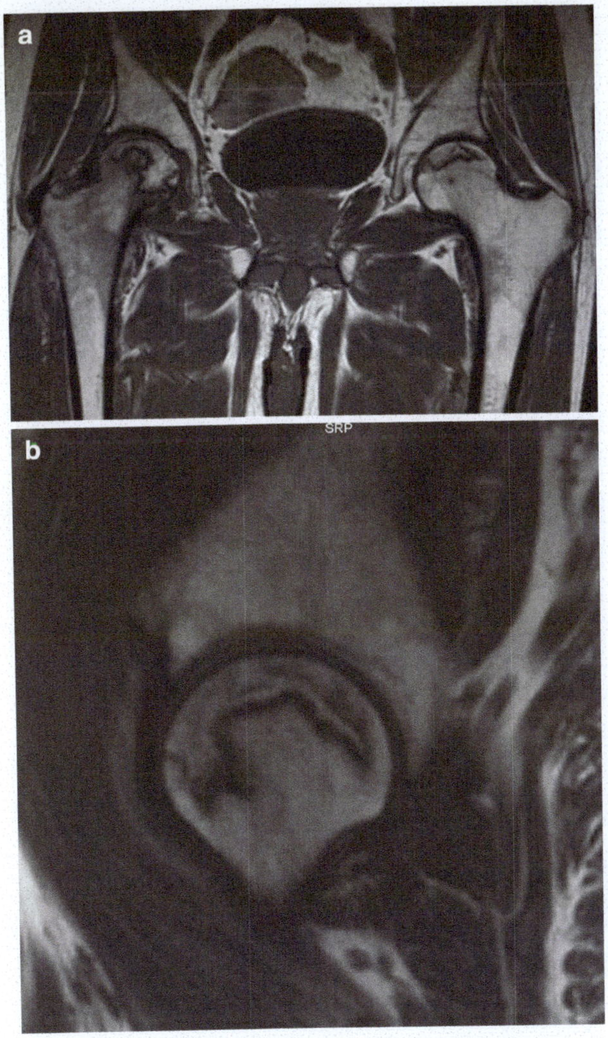

Fig. 5.102 Osteonecrosis. Coronal SE T1-WI (**a**) demonstrates bilateral well-demarcated areas of necrosis in both hips. There is hypointense BME within the femoral neck on the right side. Sagittal SE T1-WI (**b**) of the right hip. The extent of the lesion is better appreciated on sagittal images

capsule inserts several millimeters above the labrum, which creates a much larger perilabral sulcus or recess. At the junction of the articular cartilage and the labrum at the anterosuperior quadrant of the hip, another small cleft may be seen, the so-called labro-cartilaginous cleft.

The normal labrum has low signal intensity on all imaging sequences and has a triangular morphology in 66–94%. Variations in signal intensity and shape have been recognized and are most common in the superior labrum. Intermediate signal at the labral base may correlate with both intrasubstance fibrovascular bundles as well as degeneration. These signal variations may be globular, linear and may extend to the labral margin as well. These signal variations contribute to the relatively low sensitivity and specificity of conventional MRI for the assessment of labral pathology. Variations in labral morphology include flattening, rounding, blunting, and irregularity of the labral margins. Absent labra have been described as well in up to 14% of cases.

These normal variants should be considered when interpreting MR arthrograms.

As with the shoulder, MRA of the hip with its joint distention is the preferred imaging technique for evaluating the labrum. Labral lesions are most commonly located in the anterosuperior aspect. Two types of labral lesions have been described. Type I lesions or detachments occur between the articular cartilage and the labrum, resulting in interposition of contrast material at the acetabular cartilage-labral interface (Fig. 5.103). Type II lesions are true labral tears and occur within the substance of the labrum (Fig. 5.104). Tears are less frequent than detachments and are identified by intrasubstance collection of contrast material. Within the literature – however – the terms tear and detachment are often intermingled. Cartilaginous defects are frequently associated with labral pathology. MRA has only a moderate sensitivity for detection of cartilage lesions, because of the thin articular cartilage of the hip. Cartilaginous abnormalities are much more frequent on the acetabulum than on the femoral head. Other associated lesions are perilabral cysts and morphological factors predisposing to femoroacetabular impingement (see Sect. 5.5.3.4).

5.5.3.4 Femoroacetabular Impingement (FAI)

FAI is a distinct pathologic condition that occurs as a result of abnormal abutment between the proximal femur and acetabulum, arising from morphologic abnormalities affecting the proximal femur, acetabulum, or both. Repetitive mechanical conflict occurring in flexion and internal rotation will lead to lesions of the acetabular cartilage and acetabular labrum.

Two types of FAI can be distinguished, *Cam* and *Pincer* impingement.

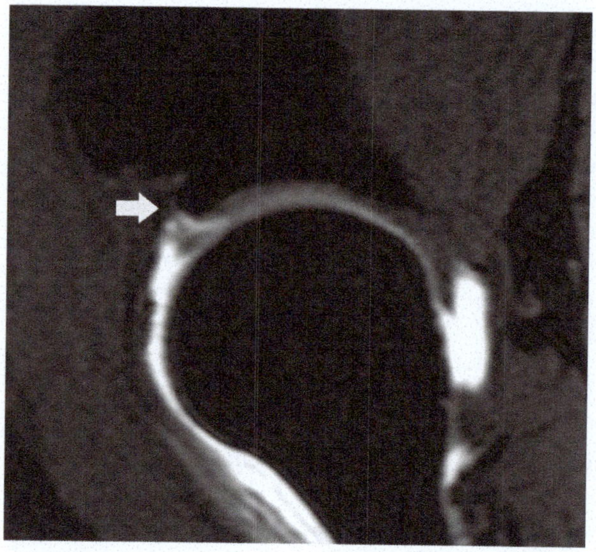

Fig. 5.103 Labral detachment. Sagittal MR arthrogram. Interposition of contrast material at the acetabular cartilage-labral interface (*arrow*)

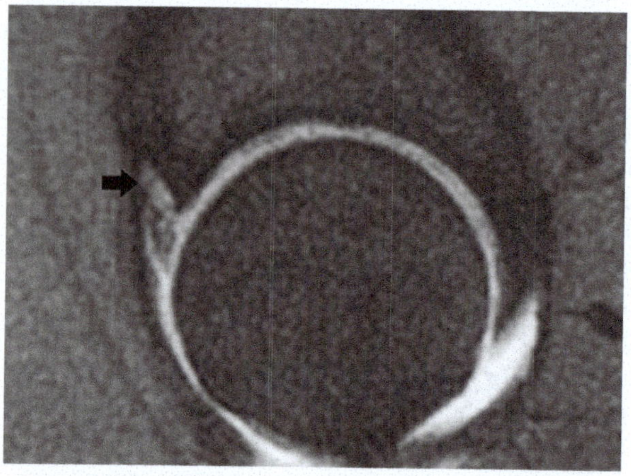

Fig. 5.104 Labral tear. Sagittal MR arthrogram. There is intrasubstance collection of contrast material as well as complete separation of the anterosuperior labrum from the acetabulum (*arrow*)

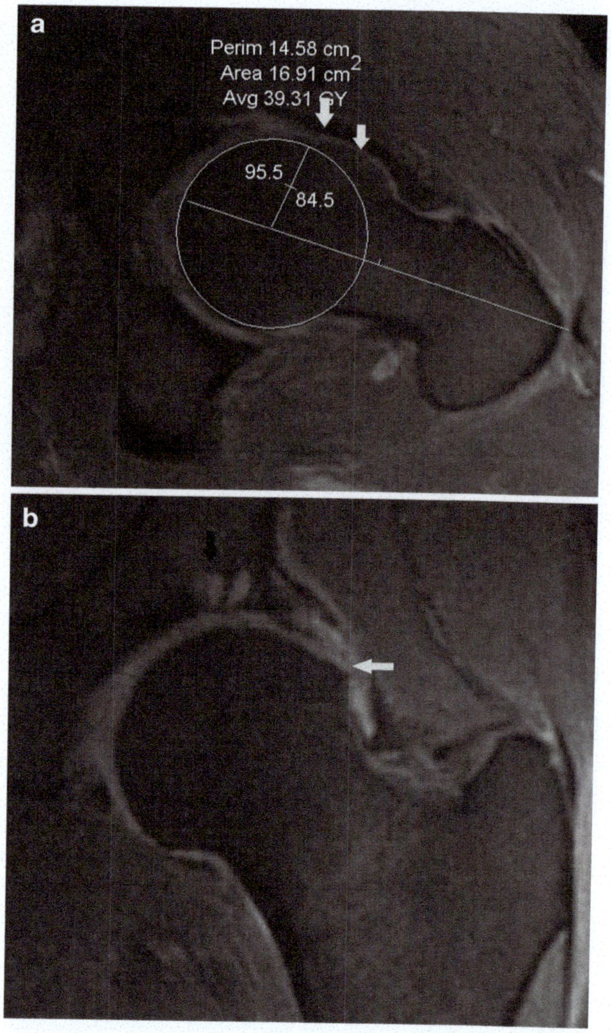

Fig. 5.105 FAI, type CAM. Axial oblique MR arthrogram (**a**) showing an increased alpha angle and reduced femoral head-neck offset with bump formation (*arrow*). The alpha angle is formed between the axis of the femoral neck and a line connecting the center of the head and neck at its narrowest point. An angle of more than 55° is considered to be abnormal. The coronal oblique MR arthrogram (**b**) shows thinning of the articular cartilage anterosuperiorly, an anterosuperior labral tear, an acetabular roof cyst (*black arrow*) and bump formation at the femur neck (*white arrow*)

Cam FAI

Cam impingement is caused by abutment of an abnormal femoral head (usually a deficiency of the femoral waist at the anterolateral (AL) portion of the femoral neck) against the acetabulum during forceful motion. This may result in abnormal forces on the acetabular cartilage and subchondral bone in the anterosuperior rim area, which leads to chondrolabral damage (cartilage abrasion and/or avulsion of acetabular cartilage from the labrum and subchondral bone). Chondral avulsion may evolve to tear or detachment of the fibrocartilaginous labrum. Cam impingement is more frequently seen in young athletic males.

Plain radiographs often show a bony prominence (*bump*) at the AL head and neck junction. Other findings include a reduced waist of the femoral neck and head junction, and changes at the acetabular rim such as os acetabuli or an acetabular rim ossification.

MRA is the imaging technique of choice to evaluate cam FAI. Oblique axial images are useful for the evaluation of the femoral waist contour. Notzli et al. described a method to quantify the concavity of the femoral head-neck junction (Fig. 5.105). Subchondral edema and subchondral acetabular roof cysts and femoral hernation pits may be seen and are best evaluated on fat-suppressed T2-WIs. The acetabular cartilage is hyperintense in areas of chondral softening. This softening progresses from articular cartilage fissures to frank chondral fragmentation, resulting in a full-thickness chondral defect in the superior portion on the acetabular roof. Anterosuperior labral tears or detachments may be easily evaluated by MRA. In a later stage of FAI, focal joint space narrowing and osteoarthritis may occur.

Pincer FAI

Pincer impingement results from a morphologic abnormality in the acetabulum, often a general (coxa profunda or protrusion acetabuli) or local anterior overcoverage (acetebular retroversion). Deepening of the acetabulum may lead to abutment of the femoral head against the acetabulum, resulting in labrum degeneration with ganglion cyst formation or ossification of the acetabular rim, leading to further increase in the relative depth of the acetabulum and worsening of overcoverage. Persistent abutment can result in chondral injury in the "contre-coup" region of the postero-inferior acetabulum. Pincer impingement is seen more frequently in middle-aged women.

Plain radiographs may show abnormal retroversion of the acetabulum (crossing sign between the lateral outlines of the anterior and posterior acetabular wall) or coxa profunda or protrusio acetabuli.

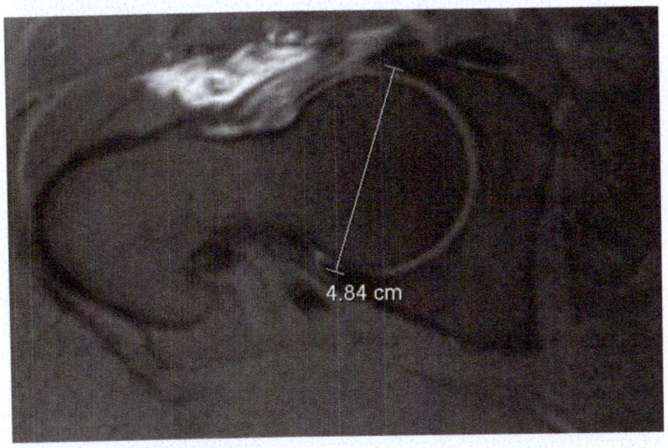

Fig. 5.106 FAI, type pincer. Oblique axial MR image showing an increased retroversion of the acetabulum. The depth of the acetubulum can be measured by drawing a line that connects the anterior and posterior acetabular rim. If this line runs laterally to the center of the femur head, there is increased acetabular coverage

Table 5.11 Differential diagnosis between cam and pincer FAI

	CAM	Pincer
Morphological abnormality	Femoral head	Acetabular overcoverage (focal or general)
Age/gender	Young male athletes	Middle-aged women
Early lesions	Articular cartilage	Labrum
Late lesions	Labrum	Articular cartilage

Characteristic MR features include labral tears, deepening of the acetabulum and posteroinferior cartilage lesions. Measurement of the acetabular depth may be performed on oblique axial MR images (Fig. 5.106).

Table 5.11 summarizes the basic pathogenetic morphological abnormalities, clinical findings, and major pathologic findings in cam vs. pincer FAI.

5.5.3.5 Periarticular Hip Pathology

Periarticular disease of the hip consists of variety of disorders, including trauma and degenerative disorders of the hamstrings, iliopsoas and rectus femoris musculotendinous junctions, and pathologic conditions about the greater trochanter. General principles on tendon and muscle pathology are discussed in Sect. 5.10. Detailed discussion of these disorders is beyond the scope of this chapter.

In clinical practice, lateral hip pain, also referred to as the greater trochanteric pain syndrome, is a commonly encountered problem with a broad spectrum of differential considerations. This entity was often attributed to trochanteric bursal inflammation. However, the cause of this pain syndrome may be due to a broad spectrum of articular, periarticular, and distant processes as sources of pain. Degenerative tendinosis of the abductor tendons, also designated as the rotator cuff of the hip, and bursal pathology are among the most frequent causes of periarticular pathology. Both conditions are often associated and rarely isolated. Damage to gluteal tendons at their insertion onto the greater trochanter may result in secondary involvement of the contiguous bursae. MRI demonstates high-signal intensity changes within the tendons and adjacent bursae on fluid-sensitive sequences. Sometimes, internal septations or irregular wall thickening can be identified within the distended bursae due to chronic inflammation (Fig. 5.107). Other less common causes of trochanteric bursal inflammation are tuberculosis and rheumatoid arthritis.

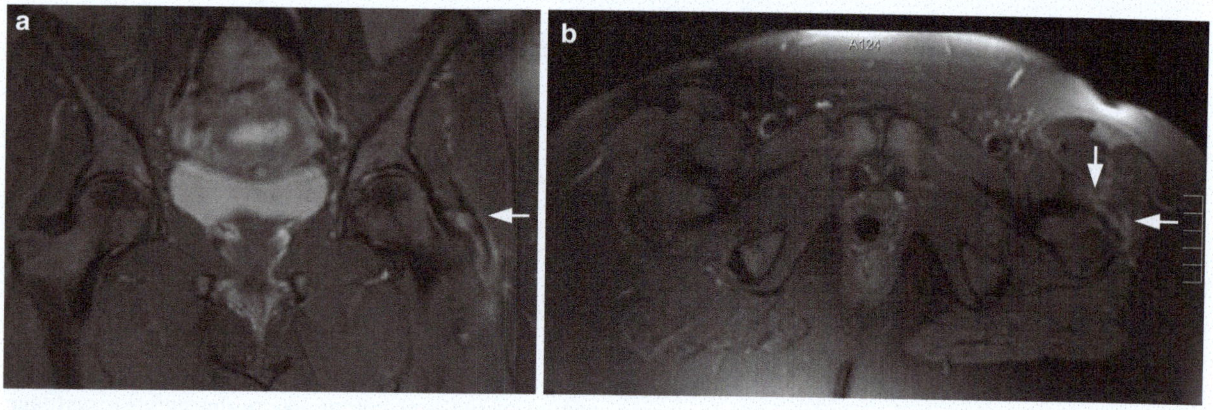

Fig. 5.107 Gluteus minimus (*black arrow*) and medius tendinosis (*white arrow*) and associated gluteus medius and minimus bursitis. Coronal (**a**) and axial (**b**) TSE FS intermediate-WI

5.6 Wrist Joint

5.6.1 Anatomy

The wrist comprises a series of separate joint compartments, including: radiocarpal compartment, distal radioulnar joint (DRUJ), midcarpal compartment, pisotriquetral joint, common carpometacarpal joint, first carpometacarpal compartment, and intermetacarpal compartments.

The extrinsic (radiocarpal) and intrinsic (interosseous) ligaments maintain carpal stability. Interosseous ligaments extend among the carpal bones of the proximal carpal row and prevent communication between the radiocarpal and midcarpal compartment (scapholunate, SL and lunotriquetral, and LT ligament). Both the SL and LT ligaments have three zones (dorsal, proximal, and volar). The most important soft-tissue structure of the wrist is the triangular fibrocartilage complex (TFCC), including the triangular fibrocartilage (preventing communication between the radiocarpal compartment and DRUJ, TFC), dorsal and volar radioulnar ligaments, meniscal homologue, ulnocarpal ligaments, ulnar collateral ligament (UCL), and extensor carpi ulnaris tendon/sheath.

5.6.2 Imaging Technique

For MRI of the wrist, a dedicated wrist coil is used. The wrist must be evaluated in the coronal, axial, and sagittal planes. Patients are positioned prone and semi-oblique, with the arm above the head in relaxed position, hand fixed with sand-bags, and fingers straightened.

For the detection of BME (occult fracture), FS TSE intermediate-WI are used. Direct (intraarticular administration of contrast medium) or indirect (intravenous administration of contrast medium) MRA should be used for the evaluation of articular cartilage, ligamentous injury, and TFC lesions. Furthermore, intravenous application of contrast media is indicated when there is clinical suspicion of AVN. Table 5.12. summarizes the pulse recommendations for routine imaging of the wrist.

Table 5.12 Pulse sequence recommendations for the wrist

Pulse sequence	WI	Plane
Intermediate TSE FS		Cor/ax/sag
SE	T1	Cor
Indirect MRA SE FS	T1	Ax/cor

5.6.3 Pathology

5.6.3.1 Ligamentous Injury and Carpal Instability

The extrinsic ligaments are best evaluated on sagittal images, and the intrinsic ligaments on coronal images. Classic dogma holds that, for carpal stability, the palmar extrinsic ligaments are more important than the dorsal extrinsic ligaments, and the SL and LT ligaments are the most important intrinsic ligaments. The most common causes of *carpal instability* are unstable fracture of the scaphoid, SL dissociation, and LT dissociation. MR signs of proximal intrinsic ligament injury include a discontinuity in the normal signal intensity of the intact ligament with fluid traversing the ligament entering the midcarpal compartment. While lesions of the dorsal and volar portions of the SL and LT ligaments are usually significant from a clinical and biomechanical point of view, small membranous perforations are degenerative and not thought to be biomechanically significant. Therefore, the radiological diagnosis of nonsymptomatic central ligamentous perforations remains questionable.

5.6.3.2 Triangular Fibrocartilage

Lesions of the TFCC may be confined to the TFC proper, or involve one or more components of the TFCC. There may also be associated DRUJ instability. The Palmer classification divides TFCC tears into traumatic (classes 1 A–D) and degenerative (classes 2 A–E) types. Traumatic tears are usually linear and occur at the edges of the TFCC at either the soft tissue attachments or attachment to the distal radius. Degenerative tears generally occur in ulnar impaction syndrome, in older people, and in the midportion of the TFC disc.

The "ulnar impaction syndrome" or "ulnolunate abutment syndrome" arises mainly in the ulnar-plus-variant, due to chronic contusion of the lunate. MR findings include the typically located edema in the lunate and possibly the triquetrum and distal ulna, degenerative tears of the TFC, and LT rupture.

5.6.3.3 Bone

Kienböck's disease (AVN of the lunate) is associated with ulnar minus variant in most cases. A definite diagnosis of necrosis can only be made when contrast-enhanced MR examination shows lack of enhancement (Fig. 5.108), as normal signal intensity on T1- and T2-WI does not exclude necrosis, and low signal intensity on T1-WI and high signal intensity on T2-WI does not prove necrosis. Moreover, low signal intensity on T2-WI, correlating well with necrosis, is a late finding. Also, for the evaluation of AVN of the scaphoid, administration of intravenous contrast is necessary.

5.6.3.4 Soft Tissue

The most common masses are *ganglia* (thin-walled cysts with viscous, mucoid fluid) and synovial cysts (containing joint fluid). They are frequently located at the dorsoradial wrist.

5.7 Elbow Joint

5.7.1 Anatomy

The elbow joint consists of three articulations joined in a common synovial compartment known as the humero-ulnar (flexion-extension), the capitello-radial, and the (proximal) radioulnar (prosupination) joint. Stability of the elbow joint is maintained by a specific congruent design of the articular surfaces and fortifications of the joint capsule on the medial (UCL) and radial (radial collateral ligamentous complex, RCL) side. The UCL consists of three separate structures, the anterior, posterior, and transverse bundle. The anterior bundle of the UCL is the primary stabilizer against valgus stress. The RLC is composed of the radial collateral ligament proper, anteriorly, and the ulnar band of the RCL (lateral ulnar collateral ligament, LUCL), more posteriorly, attaching to the ulna (Fig. 5.109b). The RLC protects the elbow against varus stress and posterolateral instability. The most important musculotendinous structures arising from the lateral and medial epicondyle are the common extensor and flexor/pronator tendon, respectively. Furthermore,the attachment of the distal biceps brachii tendon onto the tuberositas radii is a possible site of pathology. The ulnar nerve runs in a fibroosseous groove at the medial humeral epicondyle.

5.7.2 Imaging Technique

For MRI of the elbow, a wrap-around flexible coil is used. The elbow joint must be evaluated in the coronal, axial, and sagittal planes (Table 5.13). Patients are positioned supine, with the arm in supination and straightened, parallel to the body.

For the detection of both BME and cartilage lesions, FS TSE intermediate-WI are used. Some authors prefer the use of MRA – either direct or indirect – to

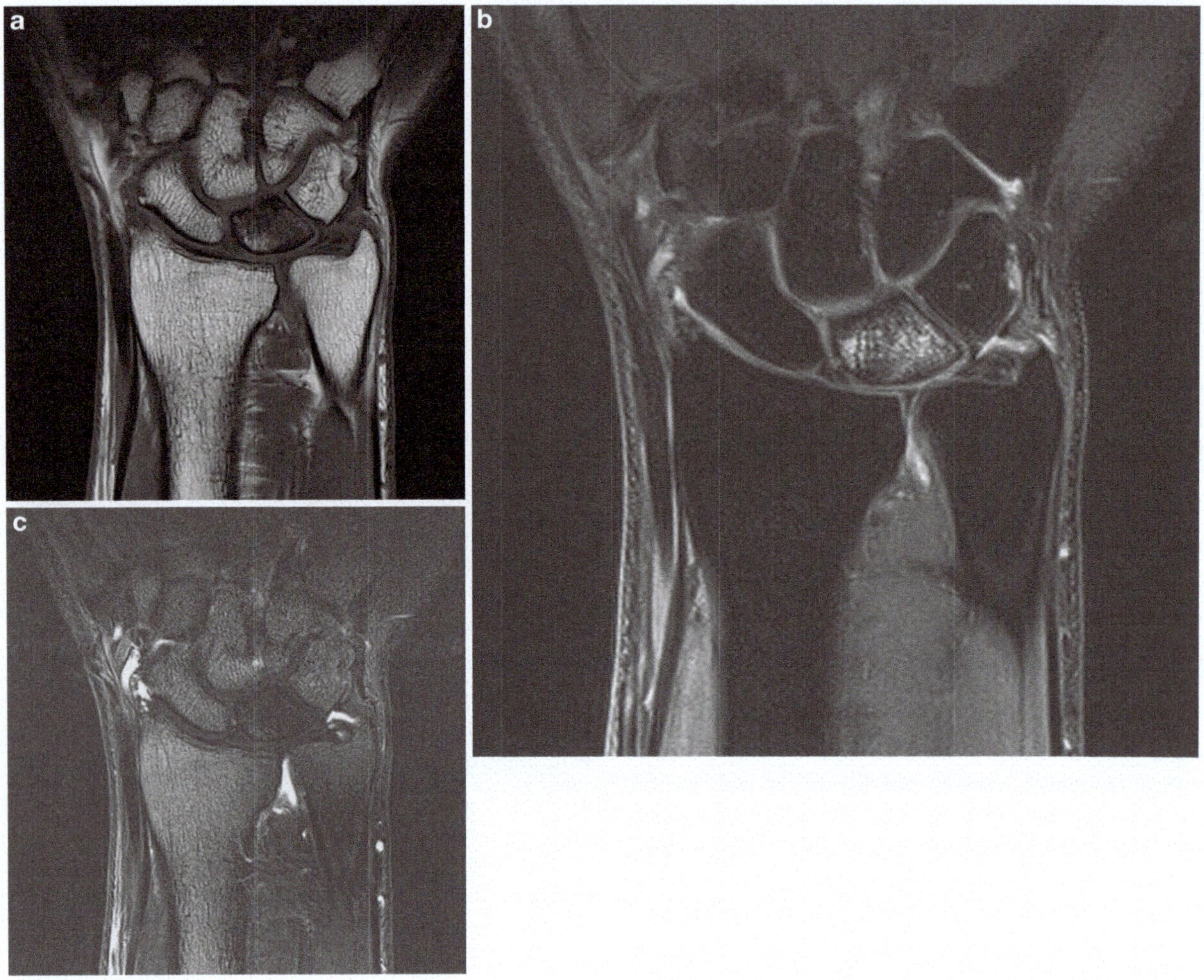

Fig. 5.108 Kienböck's disease (stage I). (**a**) Coronal SE T1-WI, (**b**) coronal TSE FS intermediate-WI, and (**c**) subtraction image, demonstrating low signal intensity replacement of lunate fatty marrow on T1-WI, hyperintense signal on intermediate-WI (reactive edema) and complete lack of contrast enhancement on the subtraction image due to necrosis

determine the stability of an osteochondral lesion or may be useful to differentiate partial from complete collateral ligamentous injury. Furthermore, intravenous application of contrast media is indicated in cases of (pseudo)tumoral pathology of the elbow.

5.7.3 Pathology

5.7.3.1 Ligaments

Injury to the UCL (anterior bundle) is most frequently encountered in throwing athletes (due to chronic repetitive valgus stress) or after joint dislocation. Chronic tensile overloading of the UCL causes inflammation and microscopic tears of the ligament, resulting in attenuation and eventually, partial or complete rupture. Tears are usually within the substance of the ligament. Distal ligament avulsions are rare and proximal avulsions even rarer. MR findings of a torn UCL (best demonstrated on coronal images) include redundancy, irregularity, poor definition of

Table 5.13 Pulse sequence recommendations for the elbow

Pulse sequence	WI	Plane
Intermediate TSE FS		Cor
SE	T1	Sag
TSE FS	T2	Ax

the ligament, and abnormal signal intensity within and adjacent to the ligament. Incomplete avulsive injuries of the distal attachment may be identified by the "T" sign. While conventional MRI has a high accuracy for detection of full-thickness UCL tears, its sensitivity for the detection of partial-thickness tears is rather low (57%). For better discrimination of complete from partial tears of the UCL, MRA is indicated.

Tears of the RCL lead to a condition referred to as "posterolateral rotatory instability of the elbow" (PLRI). PLRI is due to a tear of the LUCL, most commonly caused by a varus extension stress injury to the elbow. Also, tears of the LUCL may be seen after overaggressive release of the common extensor tendon origin for treatment of lateral epicondylitis (Fig. 5.109).

5.7.3.2 Tendons

Lateral epicondylitis or *tennis elbow* is associated with chronic excessive overuse of the hand and wrist extensor muscles. Usually, the origin of the extensor carpi radialis brevis tendon from the lateral epicondyle of the humerus is involved. In individuals who do not respond to conservative treatment, MRI may be helpful to determine the extent of tissue damage and to exclude other causes of lateral elbow pain. MR findings of lateral epicondylitis include common extensor increased tendon thickness and signal intensity in cases of tendinopathy. Partial-thickness tendon tear criteria on T2-WI include partial disruption of the tendon with high signal intensity. Complete tears are seen as a complete disruption of the tendon on both T1- and T2-WI. Furthermore, associated lesions of the LUCL may be found in patients who do not respond to conservative treatment.

Medial epicondylitis or *golfer's elbow* is an overuse injury of the common pronator/flexor origin from the medial epicondyle of the humerus. Medial epicondylitis is much less common than lateral epicondylitis. Unlike lateral epicondylitis (which is far more common in nonathletes), medial epicondylitis is mainly seen in athletes. Usually, the origins of the flexor carpi radialis and pronator teres muscles are involved. MR findings of medial epicondylitis are identical to those of lateral epicondylitis. Associated ulnar nerve neuropathy and injuries to the UCL may be seen in patients with medial epicondylitis.

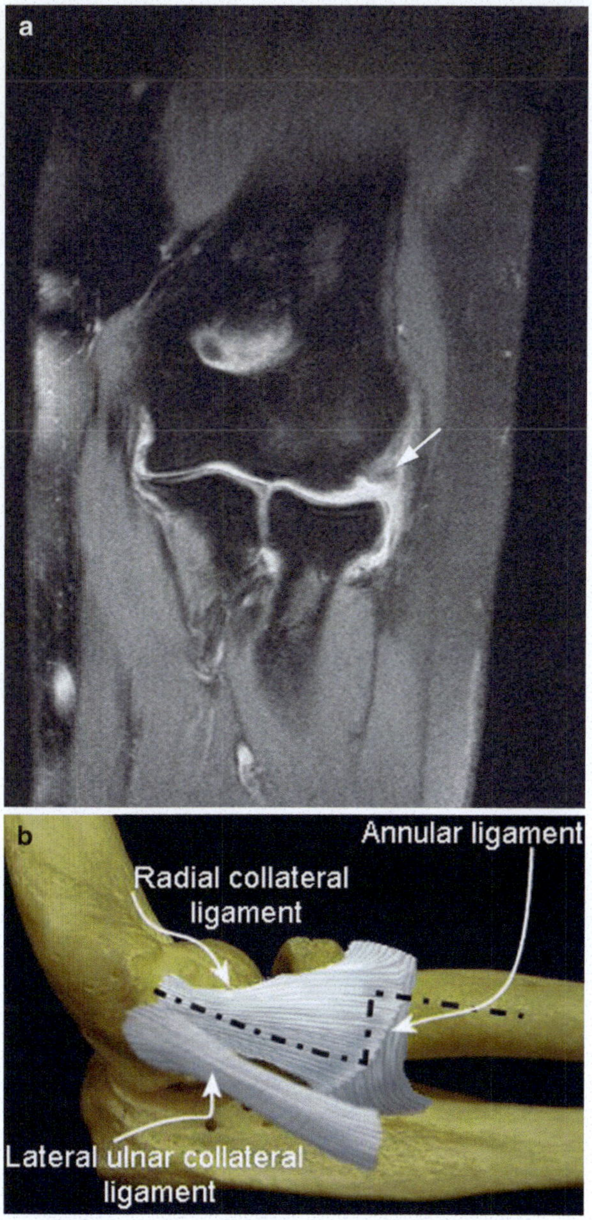

Fig. 5.109 (**a**) Torn lateral ulnar collateral ligament (LUCL) in a patient who developed posterolateral rotatory instability after extensor tendon release. Coronal TSE FS intermediate-WI demonstrates rupture of both the radial collateral ligament complex (RCL) and LUCL (*arrow*) adjacent to the lateral epicondyle of the humerus. (**b**) Schematic drawing of the radial collateral ligament of the elbow (reference: www.rcsed.ac.uk)

Rupture of the *distal biceps tendon* is relatively rare and accounts for less than 5% of all biceps tendon injuries. Complete rupture is almost always the result of a single traumatic event. Partial tears are rare. Most tears are degenerative, possibly due to repetitive mechanical

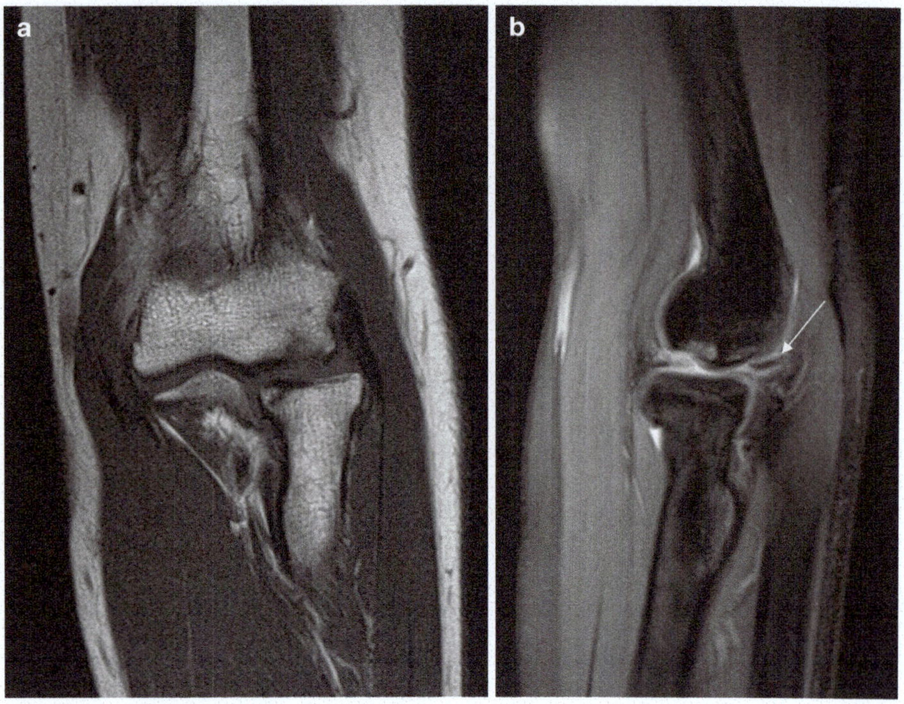

Fig. 5.110 Osteochondritis dissecans of the capitellum in a 15-year-old boy. (**a**) Coronal SE T1-WI. (**b**) Sagittal TSE FS intermediate-WI demonstrating a typical defect in the anteroinferior aspect of the capitellum with a loose body posteriorly (*arrow*)

impingement of the distal biceps tendon against the radial tuberosity during forearm rotation. MR findings of complete rupture include the absence of the low signal intensity biceps tendon at its insertion site, the presence of soft-tissue edema within the antecubital fossa with a variable amount of tendon retraction and, possibly, lesions of the lacertus fibrosus. Partial rupture is characterized by the presence of increased signal intensity within an abnormally thickened or thinned distal biceps tendon. Distinction between tendinopathy and partial rupture of the distal biceps tendon may be difficult on MRI. The presence of BME within the radial tuberosity and the presence of fluid within the bicipitoradial bursa are suggestive of a partially torn distal biceps tendon.

Rupture of the *triceps tendon* is very rare. They are caused by direct trauma or overuse (weight-lifter). Usually, there is an associated bony avulsion at the olecranon.

5.7.3.3 Bone and Cartilage

Osteochondritis dissecans of the elbow usually occurs in adolescents, due to repetitive valgus stress. The most common site is the capitellum, which normally is only involved in the anteroinferior or the inferior segment (Fig. 5.110). The posterior segment of the capitellum is the site of the pseudodefect. Panner's disease occurs between the age 5 and 10 and involves often the whole capitellum.

5.7.3.4 Neuropathy

MR may be helpful in evaluating patients with *nerve disorders* at the elbow (n. ulnaris, radialis and medianus). At the level of the elbow joint, compression of the ulnar nerve in the cubital tunnel is most common. MRI criteria for identification of neuritis include focal thickening, fascicular distortion, and increased signal of the ulnar nerve on T2-WI. Also, after a period of 1 month, denervation edema of muscles on the ulnar aspect of the forearm may be observed. Chronically denervated muscle may demonstrate significant atrophy and conspicuous fatty infiltration on T1-WI. Furthermore, MR may be useful for detection of possible causes of nerve compression in the cubital tunnel, e.g., osteophytes, synovitis, solid and cystic masses, posttraumatic deformities, and accessory muscles (m. anconeus epitrochlearis).

The median and radial nerves are much more difficult to visualize at the elbow and denervation edema may be the only abnormality detected at MRI.

5.7.3.5 Inflammation and (Pseudo) Tumoral Lesions

Contrast-enhanced MRI may be useful in inflammatory (e.g., rheumatoid arthritis), infectious (e.g., cellulitis, olecranon bursitis, osteomyelitis, and lymphadenopathy due to cat scratch disease) (Fig. 5.111) and (pseudo) tumoral (e.g., pigmented villonodular synovitis, synovial chondromatosis) pathology of the elbow.

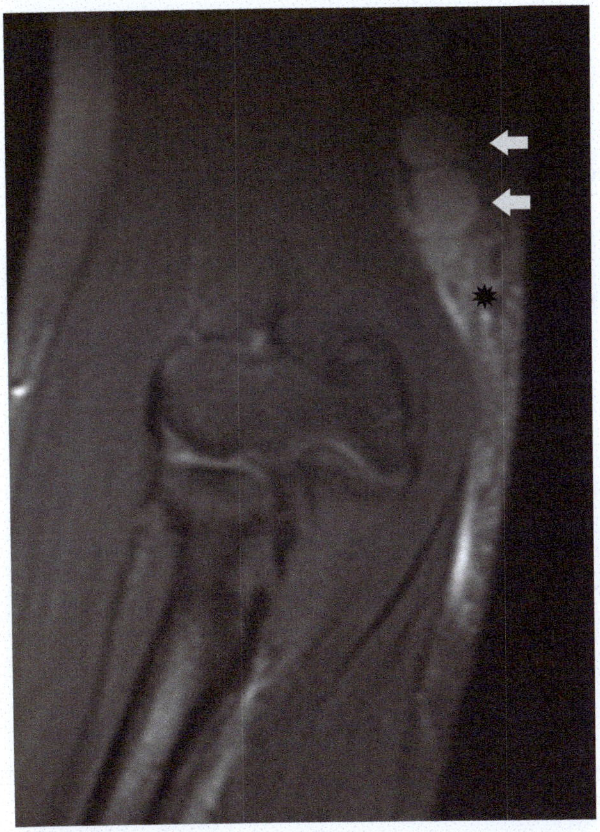

Fig. 5.111 Cat scratch disease. Coronal TSE FS intermediate-WI showing multiple high-signal intensity lymph nodes (*arrows*) and surrounding lymphadenitis (*asterisk*) within the subcutaneous fat at the medial aspect of the right elbow

5.8 Other Joints

5.8.1 Sacroiliac Joints

5.8.1.1 Anatomy

The sacroiliac joint is the largest joint of the axial skeleton. It is oriented mainly vertically, as well as anterolaterally in the transverse plane. The inferior two thirds of each joint is lined by articular cartilage, whereas the upper portion represents a syndesmosis. The lower portion is similar to a symphysis, covered by hyaline cartilage and held together by strong fibrous tissue. The cartilage is thinner on the iliac side than on the sacral side. Only a minor portion of this lower portion has a true synovial-lined joint capsule. In the syndesmotic upper third, the sacrum and ilium are held together by strong interosseous ligaments. The entire joint is further stabilized by strong superficial anterior and posterior sacroiliac ligaments.

5.8.1.2 Imaging Technique

Most authors perform a combination of oblique coronal (parallel to the upper sacrum), oblique axial (perpendicular to the upper sacrum) fast SE T1 sequences and oblique axial and coronal fluid-sensitive sequences (either STIR or fat-suppressed fast SE T2-WI). STIR is superior to detect BME than fat-suppressed fast SE T2-WI. In case of BME, active inflammation may be assessed by adding imaging after intravenous administration of gadolinium contrast. Table 5.14 summarizes the proposed MR protocol.

Table 5.14 Pulse recommendations for SI joints

Pulse sequence	WI	Plane
FSE FS	T2	Oblique coronal
FSE FS	T1	Oblique axial
FSE	T2	Oblique axial
SE after I.V. Gd contrast*	FS T1	Oblique coronal
SE after i.v. Gd contrast*	FS T1	Obique axial

*Optional (in case of bone marrow edema assessed on fluid-sensitive sequences)

5.8.1.3 Pathology

Trauma

The main physiological function of the joint is to resist vertical shearing forces and to allow supporting the weight of the entire torso. The SI joints are often involved in severe pelvic trauma. While multidetector CT is the imaging technique of choice to evaluate acute trauma, MRI is more useful to assess chronic trauma. Repetitive shear forces across the joint in athletes is often associated with asymmetric load on the pelvic ring, which can cause bone- and soft-tissue edema on MRI and subsequent joint widening due to subchondral bone resorption.

Sacral stress fractures are either associated with osteopenia or previous irradiation (insufficiency fracture) or result from excessive transmission of load from the spine to the lower extremities in sports (fatigue type) (see chronic overuse syndromes). Stress fractures typically run parallel to the sacroiliac joints, unilaterally (Fig. 5.112) or bilaterally, sometimes associated with transverse sacral fractures.

Inflammation

Seronegative spondylarthropathy consists of a spectrum of chronic inflammatory disorders that lack the presence of rheumatoid factor and that are clearly distinct from rheumatoid arthritis, ankylosing spondylitis (AS), and psoriatic arthritis (PA) being the most prevalent. Other less frequent spondylarthropaties consist of Reiter's syndrome, enteropathic arthropathies, and SAPHO (synovitis, acne, pustulosis palmoplantaris, hyperostosis, and osteitis).

Sacroiliitis is the hallmark of spondylartropathy and particularly of AS. Radiographically, inflammatory sacroiliitis appears as erosions, sclerosis, and eventually leading to ankylosis.

Symmetric or asymmetric distribution of the lesions allows further differential diagnosis of the different subtypes of spondylarthropathy. Sacroiliitis is usually bilateral but asymmetrical in Reiter's syndrome and PA. Furthermore, osseous ankylosis is less commonly seen in these subtypes of spondylarthropathy.

Although radiographs are the most cost-effective technique for imaging of sacroiliitis, they are not sensitive for depicting early inflammation.

MR has been reported as very sensitive for early detection of sacroiliitis, before bone changes are visible on radiographs or CT.

The presence of subchondral BME on fluid-sensitive sequences in the sacroiliac joints is very suggestive for early sacroiliitis (Fig. 5.113).

Recent studies have focused on the benefits of using dynamic enhanced MRI for early detection of sacroiliitis. Findings characteristic of AS include loss of the normal thin band of intermediate signal intensity representing cartilage on T1-WIs, with replacement by heterogeneous mixed signal intensity, which exhibits enhancement after gadolinium contrast administration.

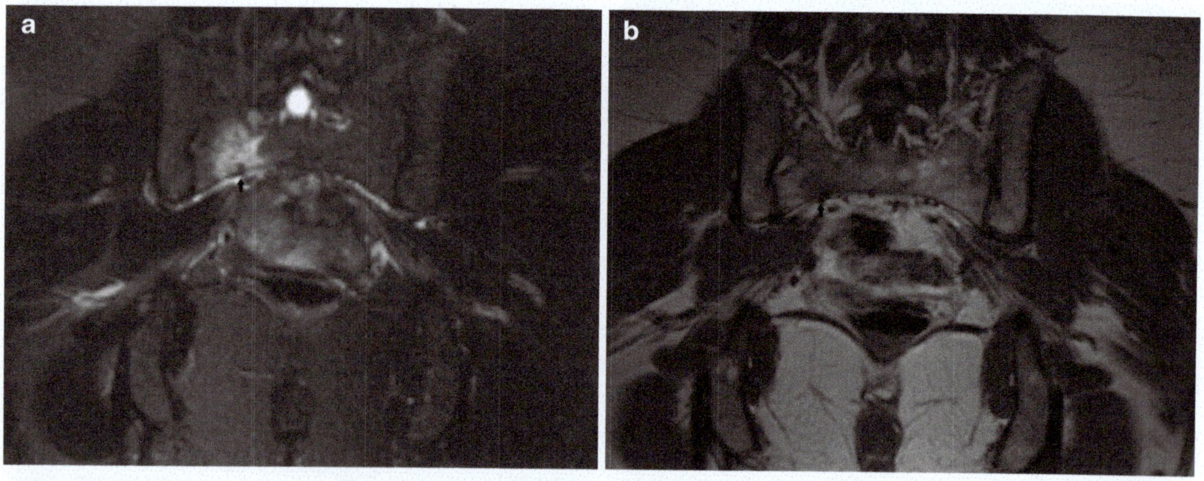

Fig. 5.112 Sacral stress fracture at the right side. Coronal TSE FS intermediate-WI (**a**) and coronal SE T1-WI (**b**) show a low signal intensity fracture line (*arrows*) parallel to the right SI joint with surrounding BME

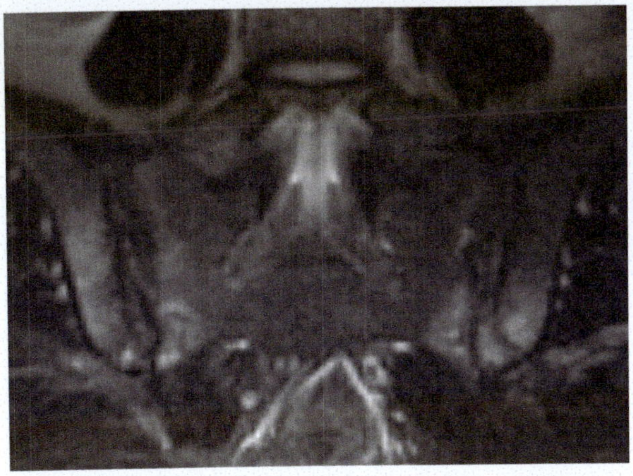

Fig. 5.113 Bilateral sacroiliitis in a patient with ankylosing spondylitis. Coronal TSE FS T2 WI shows BME at the ileal and sacral side of both sacroiliac joints

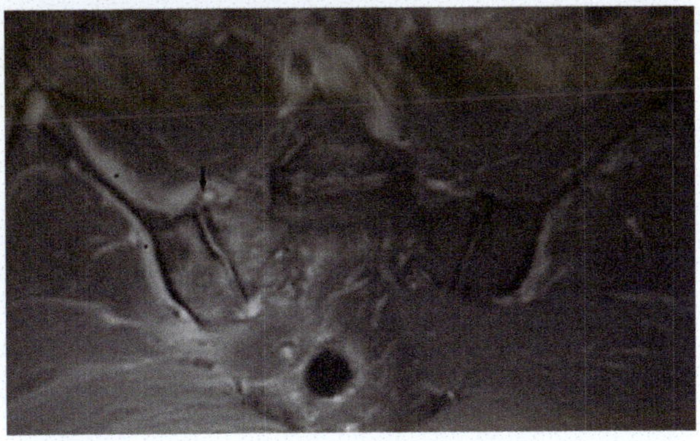

Fig. 5.114 Septic sacroiliitis on the right side. Coronal TSE FS T2 WI shows BME at both sides of right SI joint, as well as increased fluid within the joint (*arrow*) and adjacent soft-tissue edema (*asterisk*)

Dynamic enhanced MRI demonstrates distinct and rapid contrast enhancement of the joint space, both the degree and the rate of enhancement corresponding to the severity of the inflammation. However, the routine use of gadolinium is not required for diagnosis in all patients.

Initially, BME and enhancement are predominant on the iliac side, because of the thinner iliac-side hyaline cartilage compared to the sacral-side cartilage.

As the disease progresses, the marrow edema and enhancement becomes more extensive involving both sides of the joint. When the marrow edema resolves, a vertical band of high signal on T1-WIs may be seen adjacent to the joint representing conversion to fatty marrow.

Erosions on MRI are best seen on the oblique axial T1-WIs. Subchondral sclerosis appears as low signal intensity on all pulse sequences.

In advanced disease, ankylosis may be seen as continuity of the medullary bone across the obliterated joint space.

MRI is also helpful in identifying active disease and monitoring of therapy response.

Infection

Septic sacroiliitis is usually due to hematogenous spread of bacilli. Immunosuppression and intravenous drug abuse are risk factors. Children may also be affected, because the subchondral blood circulation in the adjacent ileum is sluggish, similar to that of the metaphysic of long bones.

Septic sacroiliitis differs from inflammatory arthritis, because it is usually unilateral and the erosions and subchondral resorption involves equally both the ileum and sacrum. Anterior and/or posterior subperiosteal infiltrations and transcapsular infiltrations of juxtaarticular muscle layers and periarticular BME are typical initial MR findings. In more advanced stages, additional abscess formation, sequestration, and large erosions may occur (Fig. 5.114).

5.8.2 Other Joints of the Axial Skeleton

Pathologic conditions of the joints of the spine are discussed in Chap. 3.

5.9 Bone Marrow

5.9.1 Normal Bone-Marrow Imaging

Yellow marrow contains aliphatic protons in fat cells (80%), whereas red marrow contains an overwhelming amount (60%) of water protons in hematopoietic cells. Because they have different physicochemical properties, MRI is able to demonstrate the proportion and distribution of yellow vs. red marrow under normal and pathological conditions. Otherwise, mineralized substances of bone (trabecular and cortical) lack mobile protons and yield little or no detectable signal; nevertheless, they may cause susceptibility artifacts on GE images.

In an adult, red marrow is located between the bony trabeculae and predominates in the axial skeleton, ribs, and proximal metaphyses of long bones (femur and humerus). Through aging and under normal conditions, red marrow will progressively be replaced by yellow marrow in the peripheral bones and, to a lesser degree, in the axial skeleton. This phenomenon is called marrow conversion. This process proceeds centripetally, i.e., from the peripheral to the axial skeleton; centrifugally, i.e., from the mid-diaphyses to the epimetaphyses; and symmetrically.

In SE T1-WI, conversion from red to yellow marrow results in an increasing signal intensity (SI) – from SI of muscle in the newborn to SI of fat in the adult. SI changes from high to intermediate on SE T2-WI and from high to low (the fat signal is nulled) on FS TSE T2-WI or intermediary (TE 30–40) WI or STIR images. Fatty marrow has a low SI on fat-presaturated SE T2-WI and GE out-of-phase images. Gd enhancement of normal bone marrow is subtle and only visible on subtracted images or FS SE T1-WI. With aging, increasing signal is found on SE T1-WI in the long bones and vertebrae, reflecting both the reduction of cellular components and the loss of cortical and trabecular bone (replaced by fat).

Hematopoietic marrow hyperplasia is a paranormal presentation in healthy individuals and is characterized by patchy, low-SI marrow in adults. It is more frequently seen in pregnant women, obese persons, and heavy smokers. Isolated islands of cellular marrow may be present in the fatty marrow and vice versa. This pattern is observed in the menstruating age group and under physical stress, i.e., in marathon runners.

5.9.2 Imaging Technique

Conventional radiography, CT, and bone scintigraphy have a low sensitivity for the detection of bone-marrow disorders. In contrast, MRI provides information about bone and about soft tissues that either surround the bones or fill in their medullary cavity. As such, MRI is a highly sensitive method for imaging normal and abnormal bone and can thereby differentiate between fatty, cellular, fibrotic, and hemosiderotic marrow.

SE T1-WI, short tau inversion recovery images (STIR or turbo STIR), fat-presaturated turbo SE (TSE) T2-WI, and chemical-shift imaging (in phase, out of phase) are used routinely in the axial skeleton, whereas SE T2-WI and GE T2*-WI are less suitable for marrow examination. A standard protocol includes also a coronal T1-WI and a STIR (or fat-presaturated TSE T2-WI) of the pelvis.

5.9.3 MRI of Marrow Disorders

Vogler and Murphy discerned four patterns of bone-marrow alteration: (1) red-marrow reconversion is the reversal of red-marrow conversion and is due to an increased demand for hematopoiesis (in hemolysis), (2) marrow infiltration or replacement, in which normal marrow is replaced by tumoral or inflammatory cellular infiltrates, (3) myeloid depletion, which is characterized by a decrease in hematopoietic cells (aplastic anemia) and an increase in fat content; these conditions include metastatic cancer and leukemia, infection, damage by chemical agents and ionizing radiation, and (4) marrow edema, which is due to an increased amount of interstitial water.

Vande Berg proposed a more logical approach to the understanding of MRI of bone marrow changes that is based on SI changes on T1-WI.

1. Red marrow depletion (increased SI on T1-WI). An increase in fat content can be seen as a consequence of radiation therapy, in aplastic anemia, in vertebral hemangiomas, and adjacent to degenerative bone changes.
2. Marrow infiltration (subtle or moderate decrease in SI on T1-WI and inhomogeneity of SI). This condition may be seen in marrow edema, transient osteoporosis, avascular necrosis, and reflex sympathetic dystrophy, and also in response to anemia, cyanotic heart disease, chronic infection, neoplastic infiltration, and storage disorders.
3. Marrow replacement (marked decrease in SI on T1-WI). This condition is mostly seen in primary marrow changes, such as neoplasms and infections.
4. Marrow signal void (dramatic decrease in SI on T1-WI). This condition is seen in compact bone islands and marrow hemosiderosis.

On T2-WI, the SI depends on the type of tissue that replaces fat. Fibrosis and osteoblastic metastases have low SI, cellular infiltration produces intermediate or high SI, and hemorrhagic material generates high SI on both SE sequences. Although MRI is a very sensitive method for detecting marrow disorders, it has a rather low specificity because there is a substantial overlap between various conditions. Therefore, factors such as clinical history, location of the abnormality, lesion multiplicity, and morphological features must be considered when marrow abnormality is assessed.

MRI can provide additional information in fracture healing (e.g., scaphoid), it can confirm bony union in a high proportion of patients deemed clinically non-united. Injection of intravenous gadolinium contrast may be helpful to evaluate the viability of the proximal pole of the scaphoid.

5.9.4 Osteomyelitis

In osteomyelitis, inflammatory cells replace bone marrow, and cellular material and fluid produce decreased SI on T1-WI and increased SI on T2-WI and STIR images (Fig. 5.115). In cases of osteomyelitis, parosseal edema is best demonstrated on STIR images. Enhancement of a thick, ill-defined abscess rim is best appreciated on T1-WI, following injection of Gd contrast.

In the case of Brodie's abscess, chronic recurrent multifocal osteomyelitis, or SAPHO, a sterile form of osteitis associated with pustulosis plantopalmaris and enthesitis and posttraumatic or exogenous osteomyelitis, MRI will be of additional value in demonstrating the presence or absence of marrow and soft-tissue involvement. Especially with children, MRI makes a significant additional contribution in the evaluation of the extent of epiphyseal involvement. As a consequence, plain SE T1-WI, FS SE T2-WI, and STIR images are the most suitable pulse sequences, whereas Gd contrast application with subtraction of pre- and postcontrast SE T1-WI or in combination with fat-presaturated SE T1-WI is mandatory to differentiate abscesses from edema and to demonstrate intralesional necrosis.

5.9.5 Bone-Marrow Edema and Stress Fractures

BME is characterized by increased fluid in the extravascular, interstitial compartment of the bone marrow. Increased capillary permeability is seen under variable conditions, such as inflammation, overuse, trauma (Fig. 5.116), ischemia, and also around tumoral processes (Fig. 5.117). MRI may be misleading, because the nidus of the tumor may be obscured by the extensive edema. If an OO is suspected, CT is mandatory to demonstrate the small nidus before surgical removal or percutaneous ablation.

The pattern of bone contusion after acute trauma is like a footprint; by studying the distribution of BME on MR images, one can frequently determine the type

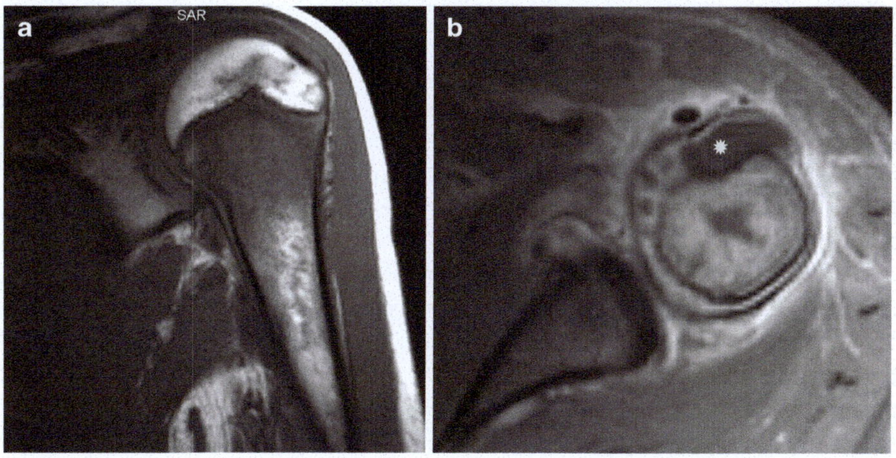

Fig. 5.115 Hematogeneous osteomyelitis of the left proximal humerus. Coronal SE T1-WI (**a**) shows marked bone marrow edema at the proximal metadiaphysis of the humerus. Axial fat-suppressed T1-WI after intravenous gadolinium contrast injection (**b**) reveals the presence of a subperiosteal abscess (*asterisk*) and surrounding soft-tissue edema

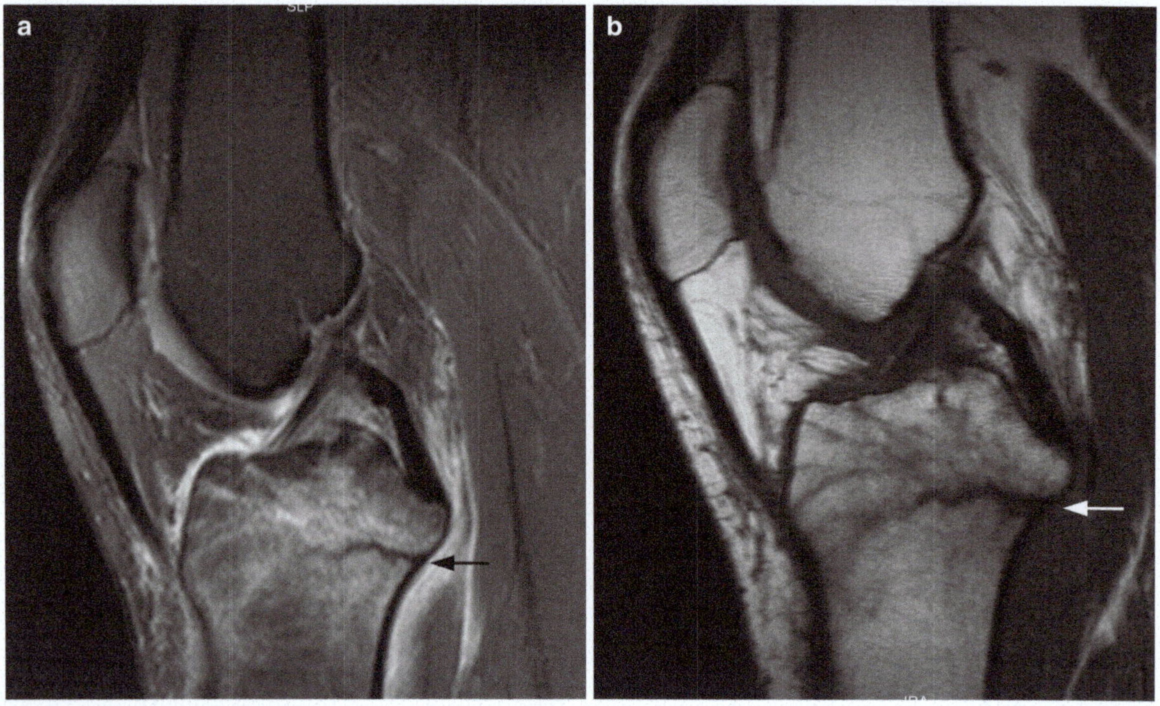

Fig. 5.116 Stress fracture of the proximal tibia. Sagittal TSE FS intermediate-WI (**a**) and sagittal SE T1-WI (**b**) show a low signal intensity fracture line (*arrows*) with surrounding BME at the proximal tibia. Note also the presence of soft-tissue edema

of injury that occurred (see also Sect. 5.2.3.3). Armed with the knowledge of the mechanism of injury, one can search more diligently for the commonly associated but sometimes less conspicuous MRI signs of soft-tissue injuries.

Chronic-overuse syndrome may cause stress fractures. These are called fatigue fractures if they occur in a normal mineralized bone (e.g., in professional sports activity) and are defined as an interruption of the cortical bone caused by repetitive and cyclic loads (Fig. 5.116). Insufficiency fractures are stress fractures in osteopenic bone (osteoporotic or osteomalatic). Previous irradiation is a well-known risk factor. Preferential locations are the metatarsals, the symphyseal and parasymphyseal area of the pubis, the lateral part of the sacral wings, the posteromedial part of the tibia, the tibial plateau, and the pars interarticularis (isthmus) of the vertebrae (see topographic discussion). Frequently, there is an associated involvement of the periosteum, the subperiosteal bone, and the fasciae. On MRI, the fracture line is seen as a low-SI line or zone in the medullary bone, surrounded by a zone of intermediate SI on T1-WI. On fat suppressed T2-WI (or STIR), a zone of high SI (BME) is seen, containing the fracture line. Conventional radiographs are normal in 72% of stress fractures in the initial phase.

Chronic avulsive lesion may also be associated with BME and periosteal edema. Typical examples include the Bufkin lesion of the knee (see Sect. 5.2.3.3), traction-induced stresses of the soleus muscle, rectus abdominis muscle, obturator muscle, proximal adductor and gracilis muscles (gracilis-adductor syndrome, see Sect. 5.5.3), the adductor brevis muscle at the medial femur (thigh splints), and the calf muscles along the posteromedial tibia (shin splints).

5.9.6 Transient Marrow Edema or Transient Osteoporosis

This disorder occurs mostly at the femoral neck, head, and intertrochanteric region (Transient Osteoporosis of the Hip-TOH), also known as BME syndrome, is another relatively frequent bone marrow condition seen on MRI. This entity was described in pregnant women during the third trimester of pregnancy but is now recognized to be more frequent in overweight

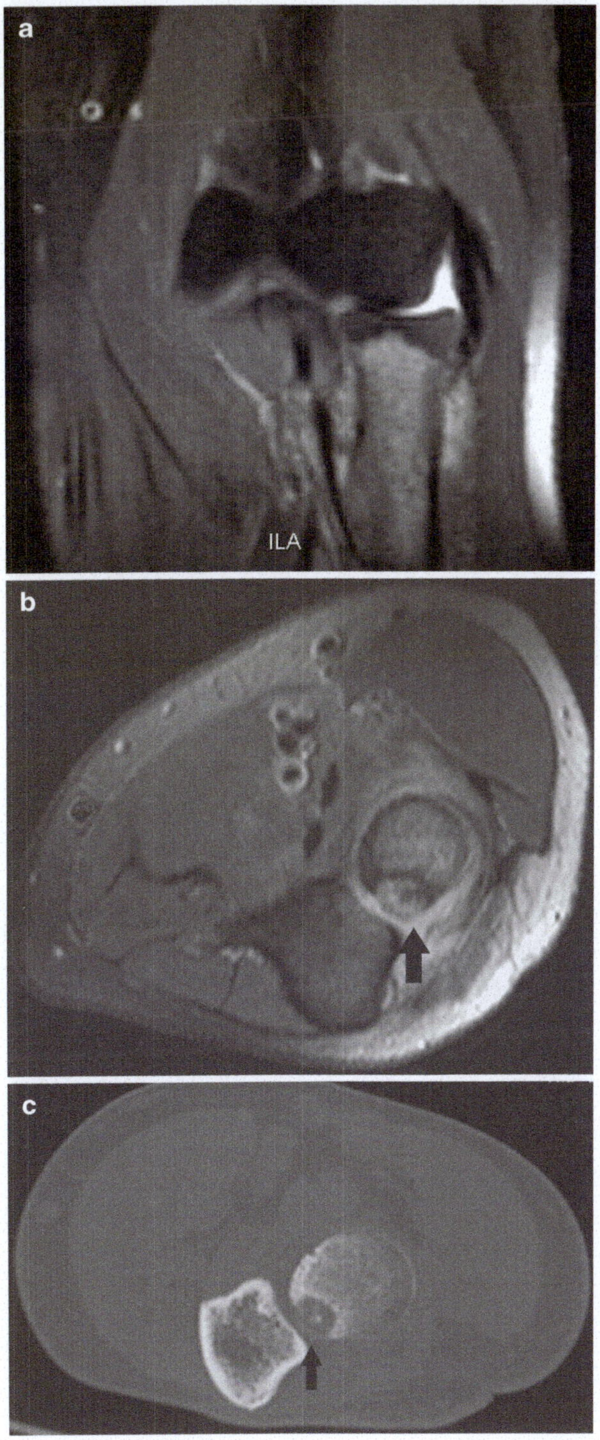

Fig. 5.117 Osteoid osteoma of the radial head. Coronal TSE FS intermediate-WI (**a**) shows marked BME at the proximal radius. Axial FS T1-WI (**b**) reveals contrast uptake within the radial head and the surrounding soft tissues. There is a lesion at the posterior aspect of the radial head (*arrow*), which proves to represent an osteoid osteoma (*arrow*) with central calcified nidus at CT (**c**)

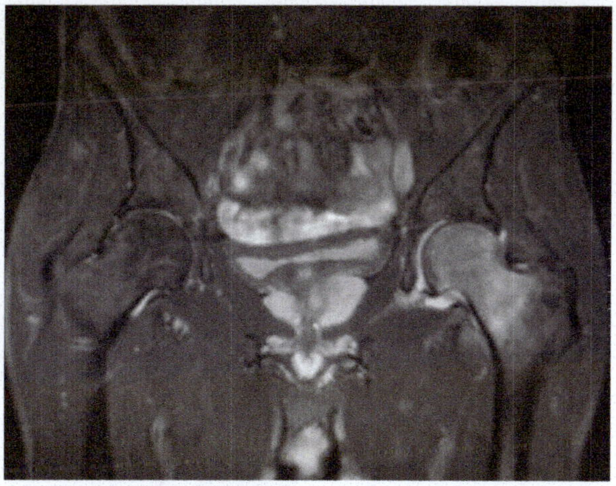

Fig. 5.118 Transient bone marrow edema (TOH) of the left hip. Coronal TSE FS intermediate-WI reveals marked BME within the left femoral head and neck. In contradistinction with osteonecrosis of the hip, there is absence of a demarcation line

middle-aged men (Fig. 5.118), and in the absence of risk factors for ON (steroid abuse, chronic alcohol abuse). Conventional radiography shows profound osteopenia 3–6 weeks after the onset of clinical symptoms. Laboratory findings are normal. On MRI, there are signs of diffuse BME with decreased SI on T1-WI and increased SI on (FS) T2-WI or STIR images. A subtle accompanying joint effusion may be seen. The disease is self-limiting, and clinical improvement occurs within 2–6 months. MRI will show complete resolution at that time. Possible causes of transient osteoporosis include trauma, synovitis, reflex sympathetic dystrophy, and transient ischemia or early reversible ON. Subchondral fractures as a consequence of the osteoporotic nature of Transient Osteoporosis of the Hip (TOH) were recently described. These findings suggest that TOH and stress or insufficiency subchondral fractures may be the same disease (see Sect. 5.5.3.1).

Other joints that may be involved are the knee, ankle, and foot. Another not well-defined behavior of BME in transient osteoporosis is the presence of a migratory pattern. Migration occurs in 5–41% of patients with hip BME. Migration may occur in the same joint, the contralateral hip or the knee and ankle, in an unpredictable time interval after the onset of the first symptoms. Usually, the joint nearest the diseased one is the next to be involved.

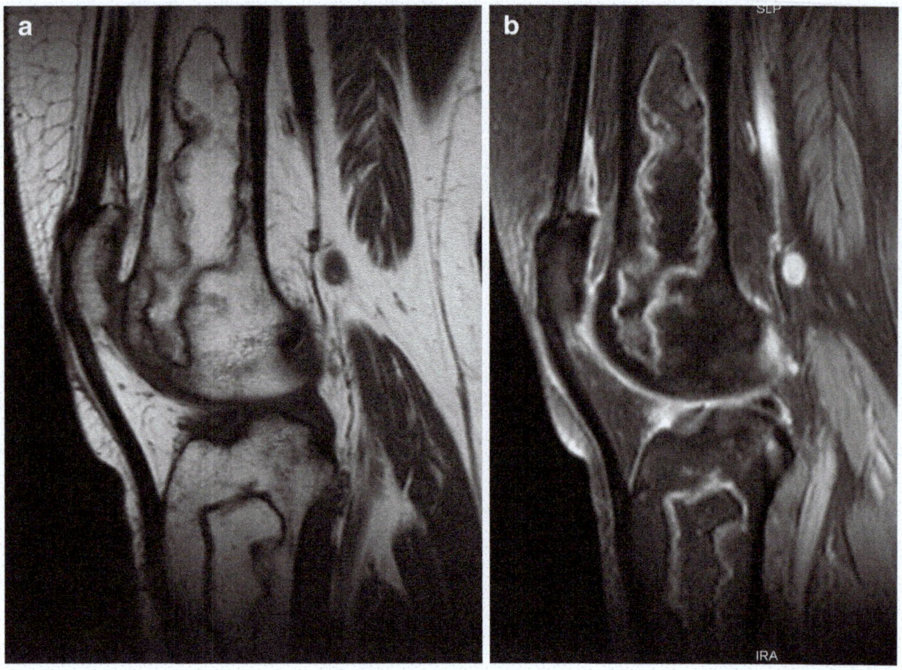

Fig. 5.119 Multiple bone infarctions in a patient receiving systemic steroid treatment. Sagittal SE T1-WI (**a**) and TSE FS intermediate-WI (**b**) show well-demarcated areas of necrosis within the distal femur and tibia

Table 5.15 Marrow pathology according to signal intensities on T1- and T2-weighted images

T1-WI	STIR/FS T2-WI	Bone marrow disorder
Very low SI	Low SI	Hemosiderosis (iron storage)
Low SI	High SI	Bone marrow edema (trauma, infection)
Low SI	Variable SI	Acute leukemia (homogeneous, diffuse, symmetric) Myeloma (diffuse or patchy) Metastases
Low SI	Intermediate	Marrow reconversion (patchy) Sickle cell anemia (+marrow infarction) Polycythemia vera
Low SI	Low SI	Gaucher's disease (patchy, coarse, diffuse) (+marrow infarction) Sclerotic metastasis (nodular)
		Myelofibrosis
Intermediate SI	High SI	Chronic leukemia Lymphoma (nodular or diffuse)
High SI	Intermediate SI	Irradiation (regional) Aplastic anemia (diffuse) Hemangioma (local) Degenerative bone changes (local)

5.9.7 Osteonecrosis

ON is an important cause of bone and joint pain. ON means "bone death," and different terms have been used to indicate ON depending on the etiology and location. Because loss of blood supply to the bone is considered to be the cause of ON, the terms avascular necrosis and ischemic necrosis are often used, particularly when it involves subchondral bone. The condition is referred to as bone infarction when it involves the diaphyses of the bones (Fig. 5.119). The disorder may be due to traumatic or atraumatic causes and may involve nearly any part of the skeleton, the hip joint being most frequently affected. Avascular necrosis of the hip is discussed in detail in Sect. 5.5.3.2. Further discussion on the specific topography, etiology, and pathogenesis is beyond the scope of this brief chapter.

In Table 5.15, marrow pathology is listed according to SI on T1-WI and T2-WI.

5.10 Tendon and Muscles

In this paragraph, general MR features of disorders involving tendon and muscles will be briefly reviewed. Further discussion of tendon disease on specific locations is previously done in the topographic section dealing with joint pathology.

5.10.1 Lesions of the Tendons and Tendo-Osseous Junctions

Ultrasound is the primary imaging modality to diagnose tendinosis due to tendon overuse, but MRI may demonstrate associated soft tissue and bone (marrow) abnormalities.

General MR features of tendon disease consist of caliber changes, signal intensity changes, associated soft-tissue edema and BME. Chronic tendon disease can be associated with reactive BME or periostitis, due to chronic friction of the diseased tendon against the adjacent bone. Subtendinous BME has a high association with pain. False-positive results consisting of intrasubstantial hyperintensity can be a consequence of the so-called "magic angle phenomenon" that results from changes in the direction of the collagen fibers and the orientation of the peroneal, tibial, and supraspinatus tendons. The "magic angle phenomenon" may cause a false-positive intratendinous SI increase on pulse sequences with short TE (T1-WI and PD-WI), which disappears on pulse sequences with long TE (T2-WI).

Because of their high collagen content, normal tendons demonstrate low SI on all MR pulse sequences. MRI of tendons and tendo-osseous junctions is performed in at least two orthogonal planes. Routinely used pulse sequences are SE T1-WI and FS T2-WI or STIR and GRE T2* images (low-grade flip-angle; see also imaging protocol for muscular diseases).

The following definitions apply to tendon disease:

- Tendinosis: degeneration of tendon due to loss of cross-linking between collagen fibers, edema, myxoid degeneration, angiofibroblastic hyperplasia, and reparative phenomena (collagenous type 3 matrix production). The term tendinitis should be avoided regarding tendon pathology, because the disease is rather (micro-) traumatic and reparative than inflammatory in nature. Neovascularization is easily seen on Doppler sonographic examination, which is an advantage of sonography over MRI.
- Insertion tendinosis: it is limited to the fibrocartilaginous insertion of the tendon to bone. Differentiation from tendinosis is very important because there is no indication for surgery for insertion tendinopathy. Most tendons may be affected by tendinosis at their tendo-osseous junction. More common sites of tendinosis are the gluteus medius and obturator tendon, adductor, rectus femoris, biceps femoris, sartorius and fascia lata, patellar (jumper's knee), Achilles, and peroneal and posterior tibial tendons, extensor tendons of the forearm (tennis elbow), and rotator cuff with the long head of the biceps muscle. In contradistinction to noninsertional tendinosis, insertion tendinosis is better detected with MRI than with sonography.
- Tenosynovitis: fluid in the tendon sheath in tendon invested with a tendon sheath. The tendon may be of normal thickness or slightly thickened. Typical examples are De Quervain stenosing tenovaginitis of the wrist, flexor hallucis longus tenovaginitis in posterior ankle impingement syndrome.
- Paratenonitis: in tendons without a synovial sheath, the epitendineum and surrounding paratenon can be involved, resulting in a paratenonitis. Edema and swelling is present in the paratenon surrounding the tendon. This is seen as a high signal on fat suppressed T2-WMRI (Fig. 5.120). The tendon itself is not always affected.

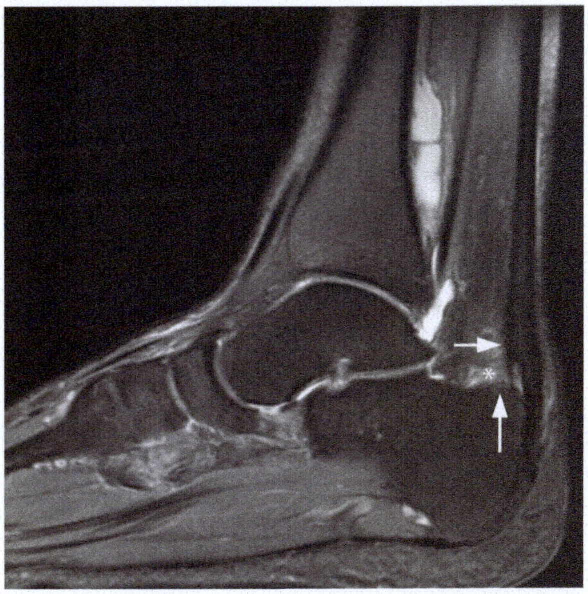

Fig. 5.120 Distal insertion tendinopathy of the Achilles tendon with associated retrocalcaneal bursitis (*asterisk*) and paratendonitis (*arrow*). Note also the presence of minor BME at the posterosuperior calcaneus (*white arrow*) on this sagittal TSE FS intermediate-WI

- Tendinobursitis: tendinosis may be accompanied by chronic bursitis (tendinobursitis), frequently seen in the trochanteric region (three largest bursae in the human body) and the Achilles tendon (Fig. 5.120).
- Tendon rupture: may be due to an acute injury or results from recurrent mechanical attrition or overuse syndrome. Tendon rupture is also frequently seen after repetitive injections of corticosteroids for tendinosis or bursitis. The tear may be partial or complete. Tendon discontinuity with fluid-filled gap will be seen in cases of complete rupture.
- Tendon (sub)luxation: luxation or subluxation of tendons is seen in acute injuries or as a result of chronic tendinosis. Common sites of luxation are the tendon of the long head of the biceps muscle and the peroneal tendons.
- Acute tendon avulsion: acute tendon avulsions are rare and are usually seen in the lower extremities. Acute lesions of the musculotendinous unit (MTU) are typical in muscles that span two joints. Typical locations include at the anterior-inferior iliac spine (rectus femoris muscle), the anterior-superior iliac spine (sartorius muscle and fascia lata), the ischial tuberosity (hamstrings), and the trochanter major (gluteus medius and obturator muscle).

Morphological changes and changes in SI in different tendinous diseases are listed in Table 5.16.

5.10.2 Diseases of the Muscle and Musculotendinous Junction

The region of lowest resistance at the MTU is age and activity dependent. In children, the most vulnerable area in acute trauma and chronic overuse is the apophyseal growth plate. In adults, the region of lowest resistance in acute trauma is the musculotendinous junction. In chronic overuse syndrome, the mid-tendinous region is particularly at risk, because of its poor vascularization.

Like tendon injuries, muscle injuries may be the result of a single acute traumatic event or of a more chronic, muscle-overuse syndrome. Increased intra- and extracellular water in muscle injuries correlates well with an increase in both T1 and T2 relaxation times.

Because muscles have a relatively short T2 relaxation time, even subtle changes in their composition will result in changes of SI on T2-WI. On (fast) STIR sequence or fat-suppressed T2-WI, muscle injuries appear hyperintense. GE sequences with a low flip angle generate a T2* effect and may be useful in demonstrating susceptibility effects.

Proposed protocols for MRI of the muscular system include: (1) axial STIR sequence or fat-suppressed T2 or intermediate-WI with 10-mm sections and a 2.5-mm interslice gap; this sectioning allows simultaneous visualization of the muscles; (2) coronal or sagittal STIR sequence (or fat-presaturated T2-WI); the

Table 5.16 Morphological and signal intensity changes in different tendinous diseases

Disease	Morphological changes	Changes in signal intensity
Early tendinosis	Increased diameter	Intermediate intrasubstance SI (T2-WI/STIR)
Early tendinosis with paratenonitis or tenovaginitis	Fluid accumulation	High SI (T2-WI/STIR) around the tendon or within the tendon sheath
Late tendinosis intermediate intrasubstance SI (T2-WI)	Fibrosis/mucoid degeneration	Intermediate intrasubstance SI (T1-WI),
	Fibrovascular repair	High SI (GE T2*)
	Decreased or increased diameter	Enhancing intrasubstance areas
Partial tear (incomplete rupture)	Increased or decreased diameter	Intermediate and heterogeneous intrasubstance SI (T1-WI)
	Ill-defined-feathery borders	Foci of high SI (T2-WI/STIR)
	Longitudinal splitting	
Acute complete rupture	Discontinuity	High SI (T2-WI/STIR) around the tendon or within the tendon sheath
	Retraction of ends	SI of hematoma within the tendon gap
Luxation/subluxation	Abnormal location	Normal

alignment of the image is parallel to the long axis of the involved muscles; and (3) axial or longitudinal SE T1-WI in case of acute or subacute hematoma. Surface coils are used for small sizes, providing excellent signal-to-noise ratio (SNR), whereas body coils afford a large field-of-view (FoV), allowing comparative examination of the contralateral side.

MRI will provide accurate information about muscle disease by demonstrating the integrity of strained muscles, the MTU, the tendon, and the tendo-osseous junction. As such, it allows for improved classification of the various types of muscle injuries.

5.10.3 Muscle Contusion

This disorder results in a combination of hemorrhage and edema and is due to a direct trauma. Hematoma pushing aside muscle fibers is frequently associated with muscle contusion and results in a volume increase of the muscle. MR image appearance is a direct reflection of superficial capillary rupture, interstitial hemorrhage, edema, and inflammatory reaction. SI of hematomas depends on the field strength used and on the age of the lesion itself. Variable signal intensities on different pulse sequences result from the variable influence of blood degradation products on relaxation times. Different SI of hematomas are listed in Table 5.17.

5.10.4 Muscle or Musculotendinous Junction Strain

Muscle strain is an indirect traumatic event caused by excessive stretching of the MTU. Certain muscles are more vulnerable to muscle strain, including those with the highest proportion of fast-twitch, type II muscle fibers and those that span more than one joint, i.e., the hamstrings, rectus femoris, gastrocnemius (tennis leg), adductor, and soleus muscles. The most frequent site of muscle strain is the musculotendinous junction of the lower extremity muscles. Multiple muscles may be involved at once. On MRI, muscle strain is characterized by a hyperintense signal on STIR or fat-presaturated T2-WI, with the degree of hyperintensity being related to the severity of the injury.

Muscles strains are graded as follows:

1. Grade I strain: low-grade inflammation without myofascial disruption. Mild T2-hyperintensity of the affected muscle is seen.
2. Grade II strain: muscle fiber tearing. This results in multiple foci of hyperintensity on a background of mildly elevated SI, with or without perifascial blood collection.
3. Grade III strain: complete disruption of the muscle or muscle-tendon unit. MRI reveals a fluid-filled gap surrounded by perimuscular hematoma. Muscle retraction and surrounding hematoma is best assessed on coronal or sagittal images. This pathological image is known as the bell-clapper sign.

Grade II and grade III strain may result in volume loss of the muscle.

5.10.5 Delayed-Onset Muscle Soreness

This condition is mostly the result of eccentric muscle lengthening. In this type of muscle injury, related symptoms develop following a delay of 24 h. Associated findings are increased intramuscular fluid pressure,

Table 5.17 Different SI of hematomas

	T1-WI	T2-WI (STIR)	Pathophysiology
Fresh hematoma(<24 h)	SI of muscle	Increased SI	Effect of oxyhemoglobin
Acute hematoma (1–7 days)	SI of muscle	Strongly decreased SI	Effect of desoxyhemoglobin
Subacute hematoma (1–4 weeks)	Increasing SI	Intermediate SI	Decreasing water content – increasing protein content – effect of intracellular methemoglobin
Chronic hematoma (>4 weeks)	High SI	High SI Peripheral rim of low SI (hemosiderin)	Lysis of erythrocytes-effect of hemosiderin

elevation of plasma enzymes, and myoglobinemia. Rhabdomyolysis is the extreme form of delayed-onset muscle soreness (DOMS). MRI of DOMS is very rarely required. DOMS follows a consistent pattern where signal intensity on T2-WIs increases gradually over few days after initial eccentric exercises, peaks after several days, and gradually returns to normal over as long as 80 days. Because DOMS is not associated with bleeding, it is assumed that the MRI changes are primarily due to edema. Muscle strain and DOMS frequently have similar appearance, and the two clinical conditions are difficult to differentiate on the basis of the imaging findings alone. Muscle strain often appears less extensive or uniform in its distribution within a muscle than DOMS by MRI.

5.10.6 Compartment Syndrome

In case of muscle injury, edema and hemorrhage may raise the intracompartmental pressure (40–60 mmHg) within intact fascial boundaries. Common locations affected by compartment syndrome are calf, arm, and thigh. Untreated compartment syndrome may result in myonecrosis and invalidating outcome. MRI is capable to visualize the early, prenecrotic stages of compartment syndrome, which sonography cannot. Postexercise MRI can show edema in the clinically affected muscles confirming the diagnosis.

5.10.7 Chronic Overuse Syndromes

These conditions consist of pain and stiffness as a result of repetitive movements used in certain occupational and recreational activities. Often, there is a combined pathology of tendons, muscles, bony structures, and adjacent soft tissues (e.g., lateral patellar-lateral femoral friction syndrome, see Sect. 5.2.3.4).

5.10.8 Muscle Fibrosis

Muscle fibrosis is a sequel of third-degree muscle strain or muscle contusion and is related to the severity of the muscle injury. Fibrotic areas present with hypointense signal on all MR sequences. Fibrosis occurs in close proximity to the musculo-tendinous junction. Distinguishing between hypointense tendon and fibrosis is sometimes difficult and requires comparative axial and coronal images. MRI is useful in differentiating chronic scar and recurrent acute muscle tear.

5.10.9 Myositis Ossificans

Myositis ossificans is generally a solitary, benign, self-limiting ossifying process occurring in the musculature of the extremities in young men and is related to direct trauma in about half of the cases. Infection and coagulopathy have been mentioned as other causative factors. Furthermore, the disease may also occur in association with burns, paraplegia, and quadriplegia or with other neuromuscular disorders such as tetanus.

Pain and tenderness are the first symptoms, followed by a diffuse swelling of the soft tissues. This swelling typically becomes more circumscribed and indurated after 2–3 weeks. Thereafter, it changes progressively into a firm, hard mass – approximately 3–6 cm in diameter – that is well outlined on palpation. Principal sites of involvement are the limbs, which are affected in more than 80% of cases. The quadriceps muscle and brachialis muscle are favored sites in the lower and upper extremity, respectively. Areas prone to trauma are more commonly afflicted.

Three different appearances of myositis ossificans are noted on MRI, corresponding to the stage of maturation. Early stages of myositis ossificans, the so-called acute form, present on MRI as a mass that is isointense or even slightly hyperintense to muscle on T1-WI, but hyperintense on T2-WI. The lesion is surrounded by variable amounts of edema, appearing hyperintense on T2-WI. Following administration of Gadolinium contrast, a well-defined rim of enhancement is observed. The MR appearance of the lesions during the intermediate or subacute stage is characterized by isointensity with muscle on T1-WI and by a mild increase in SI on T2-WI (Fig. 5.121). These findings correspond to a central fibrous transformation. Mature lesions (i.e., the "chronic stage") show more extensive signal voids on all sequences, corresponding to a considerable degree of peripheral calcification and ossification. In this stage, lesions demonstrate increased SI with an "onion-skin pattern" on T2-WI.

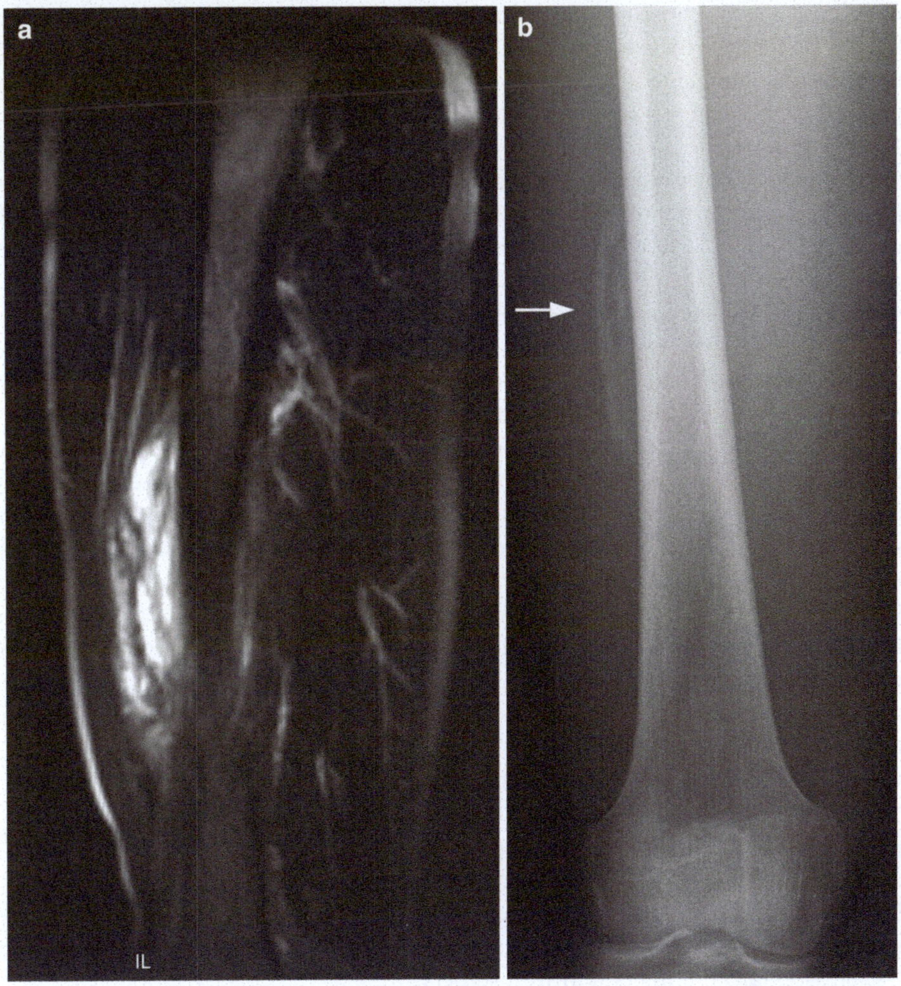

Fig. 5.121 Myositis ossificans. Sagittal TSE FS intermediate-WI (**a**) showing an ill-defined area of high signal intensity within the quadriceps muscle, with peripheral low signal intensity structures. The corresponding radiograph (**b**) confirms the presence of peripheral calcifications, indicating myositis ossificans

5.10.10 Muscle Denervation

The subacute stage of the denervation process reveals prolonged T1 and T2 values due to increased extracellular water with hyperintensity on T2-WI with or without fat suppression and STIR sequences (Fig. 5.122). In chronic denervation, muscles will atrophy with fatty infiltration.

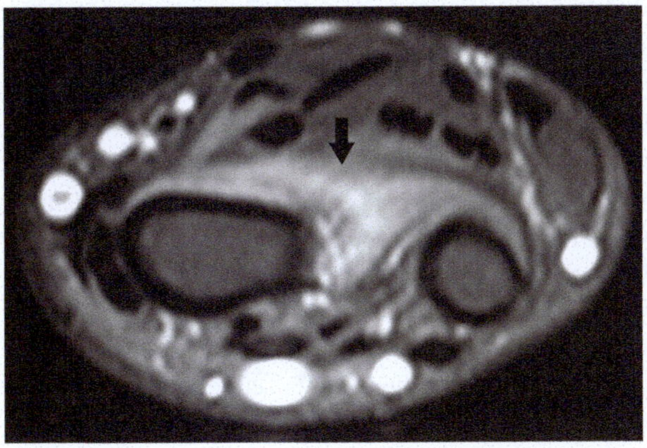

Fig. 5.122 Subacute muscle denervation. Axial TSE FS intermediate-WI. Notice a high signal intensity within the pronator quadratus muscle (*arrow*), due to denervation of the anterior interosseous nerve

5.11 Bone Tumors

5.11.1 Introduction

MRI has been recognized as a powerful diagnostic tool in the work-up of bone tumors. Plain films, however, remain of utmost importance in the analysis of bone tumors and tumor-like lesions, i.e., in detecting the lesion, differentiating between benign and malignant tumors, and predicting a correct histological diagnosis. When the lesion is not visible on radiography in a symptomatic patient, other imaging modalities should be applied, such as scintigraphy or MRI since they are more sensitive in detecting bone (marrow) abnormalities than radiography. MRI, however, became the cornerstone in locoregional staging of primary bone tumors. Because of its high spatial resolution, high soft-tissue contrast, and multiplanar imaging capabilities, MRI provides precise information about the intramedullary extent of the tumor and its relationship to adjacent extraosseous structures. Diffusion-weighted imaging (DWI) has been described as a useful technique for improved differentiation of acute benign and neoplastic vertebral compression fractures. Whole-body DWI (particularly on 3 T) seems to represent a highly sensitive technique for detection of metastasis monitoring treatment of multiple myeloma. DWI may also be useful in the differential diagnosis of bone neoplasms and soft-tissue tumors. As cellular changes are expected to precede morphologic changes in treated tumors, DWI can be used as a supplement to morphologic imaging for the evaluation of tumor response to anticancer therapy in patients with soft-tissue sarcomas. However, there is overlap between benign and malignant changes, and therefore, DWI remains controversial for the assessment of tumoral MSK disorders.

5.11.2 Imaging Technique

To avoid diagnostic errors and misinterpretations, plain films should be the first step in a diagnostic work-up of bone tumors. If possible, MRI should be performed with a dedicated surface coil to improve the SNR and spatial resolution. Imaging should be performed in at least two orthogonal planes. After scout views in three orthogonal planes, we perform mostly SE T1-WI in a sagittal or coronal plane, depending on the localization of the tumor in the bone. This sequence is necessary for accurate determination of any intraosseous extension. Afterward, axial SE or fast SE T2-WI is performed, covering the whole tumor volume. T2-WI is mandatory for adequate depiction of extension into the adjacent soft tissues.

The main drawback of fast SE T2-WI is the high SI of fat. Therefore, fat-presaturated T2-WI or STIR sequences should be performed. Thus, the inability of fast SE T2-WI sequences in detecting BME is resolved. On STIR images, lesion conspicuity is high, but delineation of the intra- and extraosseous extent is hampered since the tumor, peritumoral edema, and fracture all have high SI. Fat-saturated T2-WI may be reliable for determining the extension into the soft tissues, encasement of the neurovascular bundle, and visualizing intratumoral necrosis in osteosarcomas and Ewing's sarcomas. This sequence is a valuable alternative to T2-WI.

In most cases, SE T1-WI after i.v. injection of Gd-chelates is performed in the same imaging plane as that of the precontrast series and in the axial plane. Gd-enhanced T1-WI affords an excellent demonstration of intratumoral necrosis, differentiation of BME vs. tumor, depiction of extraosseous extension, and differentiation of recurrent tumor vs. postoperative fibrosis. Subtraction of post- from pre-Gd-enhanced images may be of use to demonstrate subtle enhancement and to delineate the tumor from fatty surrounding tissues.

5.11.3 Tissue Characterization

MRI has only a limited role in offering a tissue-related diagnosis. Plain films, indeed, are indispensable for characterization. They accurately depict calcification/ossification of the tumor matrix, cortical permeation or disruption, and faint periosteal reaction, less clearly visualized by MRI. Furthermore, most tumors have low SI on T1-WI and high SI on T2-WI.

In certain cases, however, a combination of distinctive findings (e.g., SI, enhancement patterns) allows for an accurate diagnosis or else narrows the differential diagnosis. Intratumoral fluid-fluid levels (Fig. 5.123) are often seen in aneurysmal bone cyst, but also in fibrous dysplasia, chondroblastoma, (telangiectatic) osteosarcoma, and giant-cell tumor. Ring-and-arc ("septal") enhancement is seen in immature enchondromas and low-grade chondrosarcoma, whereas high-grade chondrosarcomas show strong inhomogeneous contrast enhancement. Intraosseous lipomas are easily recognized by their high SI on T1-WI. Other fat-containing lesions are haemangioma and nontumoral lesions (Paget's disease and in focal bone marrow changes after radiation treatment). Giant-cell tumor and dense bone

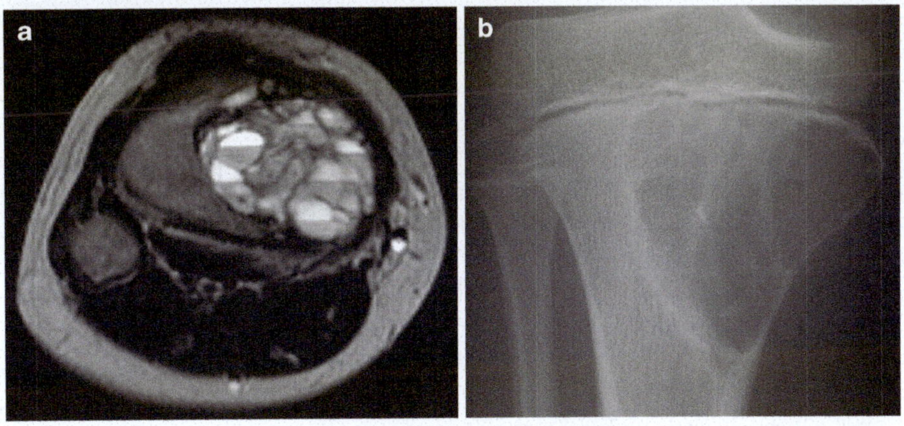

Fig. 5.123 Aneurysmal bone cyst of the proximal tibia. Axial FSE T2-WI (**a**). The lesions contain multiple fluid–fluid levels. The plain radiograph (**b**) shows an expansile lytic lesion at the medial aspect of the proximal tibia, causing thinning of the cortical bone. The epiphysis is spared

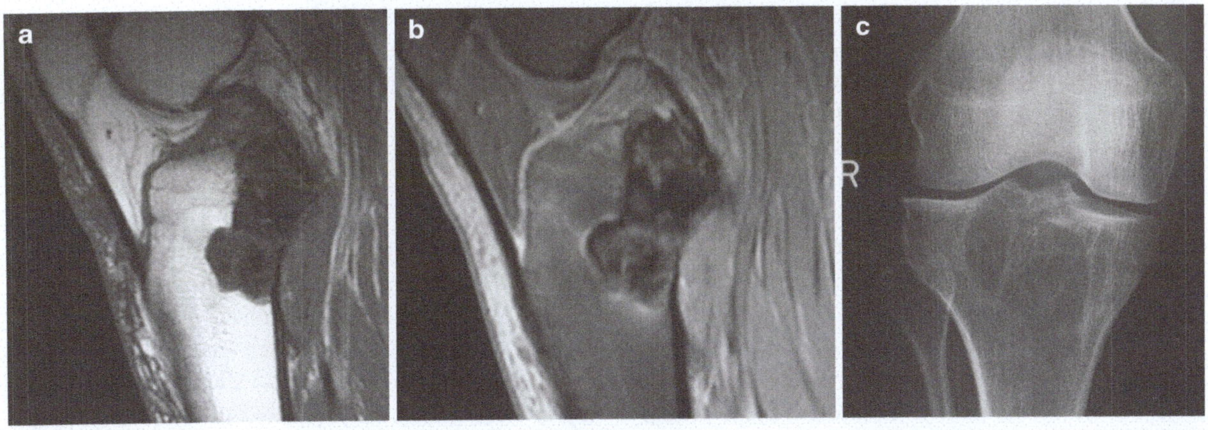

Fig. 5.124 Giant-cell tumor of the proximal tibia. Axial SE T1-WI (**a**). Sagittal TSE FS intermediate-WI (**b**). The lesion has a low signal on both pulse sequences. The corresponding standard radiograph (**c**) reveals a large lytic lesion within the proximal tibia with epiphyseal extension

islands are characterized by its low SI on T1-WI and T2-WI (Fig. 5.124). Flow voids resulting from signal loss due to rapidly flowing blood have been demonstrated in metastasis of renal cell carcinoma and hepatocellular carcinoma, but this sign is less specific for other types of hypervascular tumors. Eosinophilic granuloma manifests as an expansile, lytic lesion with rather high SI on T1-WI, abundant intramedullary and soft-tissue edema, and often firm periosteal reaction. Fibrous cortical defects are sharply circumscribed metaphyseal lesions with characteristic low SI on T1-WI, T2-WI, and STIR images. In general, MRI provides additional value in the diagnosis of bone tumors. In a study performed at our institution, lipoma, chondrosarcoma, and osteomyelitis were the three most common pathologies with the strongest gain concerning diagnosis. A diagnostic gain of MRI was seen in 50% of cases.

5.11.4 Grading

The role of MRI in grading bone tumors is limited, because plain films are highly accurate in differentiating benign from malignant tumors. In a study performed at our institution on 79 bone tumors in children, correct grading on plain films occurred in 89% of cases. One may never solely rely on MR images to distinguish benign from malignant tumors.

5.11.5 Locoregional Staging

Because of its unequaled soft-tissue contrast and spatial resolution, MRI is the cornerstone of locoregional staging. This means defining intra- and extraosseous extent and the relationship to adjacent soft tissues and neurovascular elements. Exact tumor extent can be determined most accurately by a combination of T1-WI, T2-WI, and Gd-enhanced T1-WI. On these Gd-enhanced images, intramedullary edema will enhance differently and can be differentiated from primary tumor. Some authors have reported the value of MR angiography in demonstrating tumor neovascularity. The promising initial results need to be confirmed in larger prospective series.

Correlative MRI histopathology contradicts the misconception of the ability of the growth plate to limit tumor spread. Indeed, transphyseal spread occurs in 50–88% of osteosarcomas in patients with an apparently normal growth plate. While plain radiography and even axial CT scan do not allow accurate visualization of the relationship between the tumor, physeal plate, and epiphysis, MRI is highly accurate in this regard. In contrast to transphyseal spread, involvement of an adjacent joint by a bone tumor is rarely seen, given that cartilage is an effective barrier against tumoral spread. When transarticular spread occurs, MRI can easily show it.

In the diagnostic work-up of malignant bone tumors, it is important to detect skip metastases (small intraosseous metastatic deposits beyond the reactive zone, but within the same compartment as the primary tumor). Therefore, a large FoV, T1-W sequence may be added to the imaging protocol to visualize the largest possible peritumoral area.

5.11.6 Dynamic MRI

Gd-chelates, currently used for musculoskeletal imaging, have a small molecular size and are distributed in the intravascular and interstitial space. This allows them to diffuse in necrotic tissue, leading to enhancement and, thus, underestimation of the presence and amount of intratumoral necrosis. Therefore, static Gd-enhanced MRI does not accurately show the amount of intratumoral necrosis.

Dynamic MRI after i.v. injection of Gd-chelates is a useful diagnostic tool that overcomes this problem. Different techniques have been developed, but the first pass and subtraction techniques are used most frequently. Fast or ultrafast sequences with a temporal resolution of 2–3 s per image or a set of parallel images are available and mandatory for the measurement of tissue enhancement during the first pass of the contrast agent. Various parameters, such as time of onset of enhancement, wash-out, maximal enhancement, and slope values can be measured. Because a large overlap exists in slope values of benign and malignant bone tumors, the role of dynamic imaging in grading and tissue characterization is limited.

5.11.7 Posttreatment and Detection of Recurrence

Dynamic Gd-enhanced MRI is well established in the detection of residual or recurrent tumors. In the postoperative follow-up of a patient with a malignant bone tumor, regular MR studies are mandatory when searching for evidence of residual or recurrent tumor. On plain films or CT, a large recurrent tumor can present as an osteolytic area that may be accompanied by a soft-tissue mass and periosteal reaction. When performing MRI, small recurrences can be detected, enabling early therapeutic actions.

First, MR examination after surgical intervention should be performed within 9–15 weeks. When imaging is done within the first 6 weeks after surgery, any residual mass cannot be differentiated from postoperative changes, such as edema, subacute hematoma, and inflammatory granulation tissue. The imaging protocol starts with a T2-W sequence. When no areas of high SI are seen, no tumor recurrence is present. When high SI areas are present, one must evaluate whether such areas are mass-like or not. An inhomogeneous high SI area without mass lesion may correspond to postoperative inflammatory changes. When a mass lesion is encountered, intravenous administration of Gd-contrast is necessary to differentiate between postoperative seroma/lymphocele and recurrence. Cystic space-occupying lesions, such as seroma or lymphocele, will show either no or only rim enhancement, whereas recurrences enhance more homogeneously.

A major problem arises when postoperative MRI must be performed in patients who have undergone reconstructive surgery with ferromagnetic osteosynthetic devices, such as nails, plates, and screws. Susceptibility artifacts will disturb the image quality. However, most recurrences will be detected by the meticulous comparison of pre- and postcontrast series.

Nowadays, most prosthetic devices consist of titanium, causing fewer artifacts. Further options available to minimize susceptibility artifacts are: (1) performing the examination with a magnet at low field strength and (2) accurately choosing and optimizing the sequence type and parameters (susceptibility artifacts are less pronounced on FSE sequences than on GE sequences, dedicated MR sequences such as tilted view angle, shortening the TE value, decreasing the voxel size, increasing band width, and avoiding spectral FS).

Soft-tissue edema poses another problem for the radiologist viewing MR follow-up studies of patients who have undergone radiation therapy for bone or soft-tissue sarcomas. Postirradiation edema of the soft tissues complicates the postoperative picture characterized by myositis, peritumoral edema, hemorrhage, fibrosis, and even toxic edema (due to chemotherapeutic agents). These changes will subside within 1 year posttreatment, whereas postirradiation edema persists for more than 2–4 years in 20–50% of the patients treated with photon or neutron radiation therapy. On T2-WI and STIR images, diffuse BME is seen very early and lasts for weeks to months, until fatty replacement occurs.

Different authors have reported on the role of dynamic Gd-enhanced MRI in the evaluation of preoperative chemotherapy of bone sarcomas. The ultimate goal is to reveal the presence and amount of intratumoral necrosis, in order to differentiate responders from nonresponders. This enables the prediction of definitive outcomes in individual cases. Accuracy levels of 86–100% in differentiating these two groups have been achieved using dynamic Gd-enhanced MR to depict tissue vascularization and nests of remaining viable tumor. By this means, the best biopsy site can be determined.

Further applications of this technique are being developed, for example, the use of dynamic MRI in distinguishing tumor and tumor-related edema, slope values for differentiating regions of microscopic intramedullary invasion from tumor-free bone marrow in patients with osteosarcoma after chemotherapy, and diffusion-weighted MR images to refine the assessment of intratumoral necrosis (differences in molecular diffusion and, thus, in membrane integrity between viable and necrotic tissue are easily detected). However, the clinical usefulness of these techniques in daily routine remains questionable.

5.12 Soft-Tissue Tumors

5.12.1 Introduction

The most recent World Health Organization (WHO) classification of tumors divides soft-tissue tumors (STT) into four categories according to the biological behavior of the lesion:

1. Benign STT: are characterized by absence of local recurrence or distant metastasis.
2. Intermediate-locally aggressive STT: locoregional infiltrative growth and recurrence may occur, but without metastatic potential. A typical example is a desmoid tumor.
3. Intermediate-rarely metastasizing: may show locoregional infiltrative growth, recurrence and occasionally distant metastases.
4. Malignant: typical features include locoregional infiltrative growth, recurrence, and high risk of distant metastases.

Although there is no definite correlation between these four categories and the findings on medical imaging, some STT present with more characteristic imaging features, allowing a more detailed tissue-specific diagnosis (Fig. 5.125). Another important task for the radiologist is to alert the referring physician when the imaging findings raise uncertainty regarding the exact diagnosis. Additional examination by genetic studies (if an underlying genetic disorder is suspected) or by biopsy is often mandatory in these cases. Last but not the least, imaging is of utmost importance for locoregional staging of STT.

5.12.2 Staging

Staging is defined as locoregional extent and distant metastasis. Important locaoregional staging parameters are grading, tumor size, and location (intra- vs. extra-compartmental extension; deep vs. superficial location; and relationship with adjacent structures such as fasciae, tendons, ligaments, joints, bone, and neurovascular bundle).

Local staging must be completed before a biopsy is performed. There is no doubt that MRI is by far the best imaging modality for local staging of soft-tissue tumors.

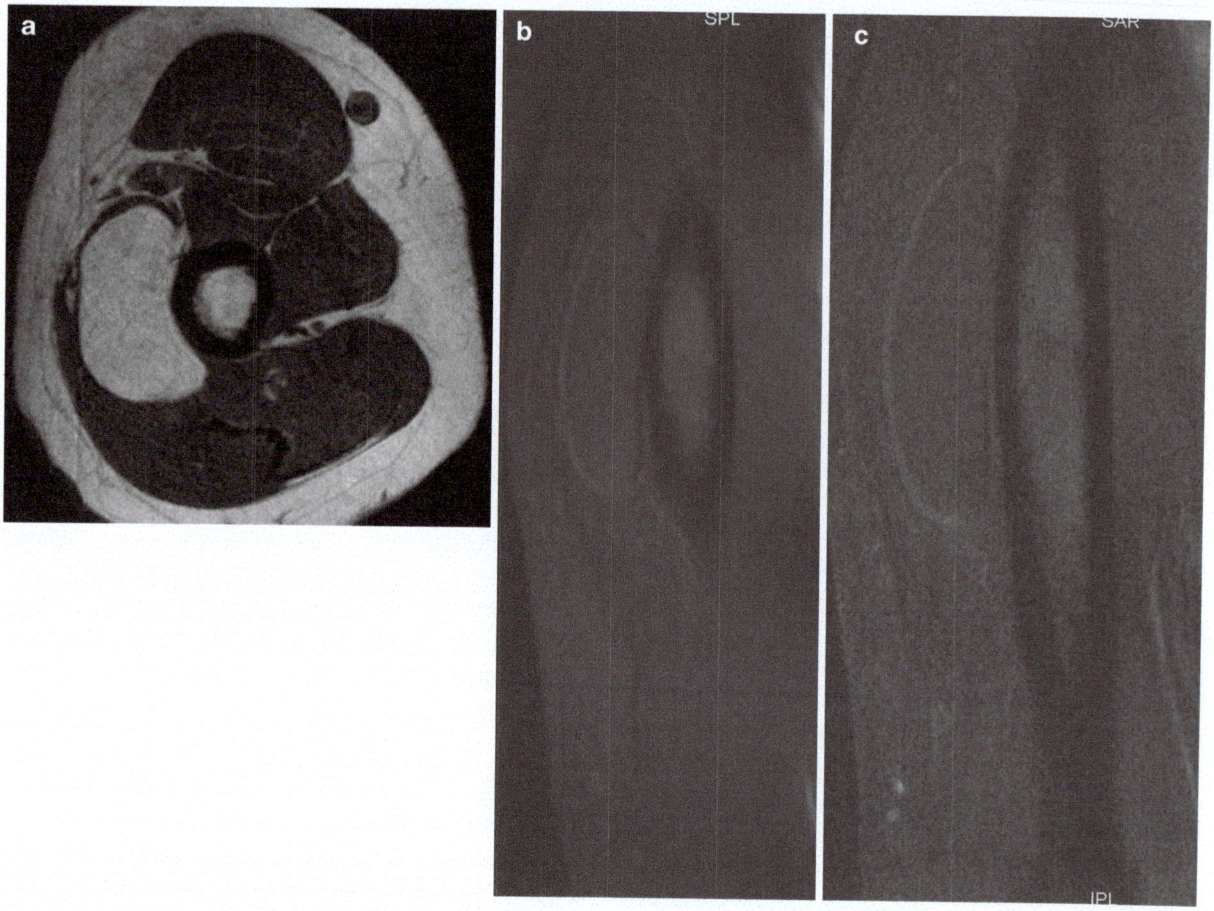

Fig. 5.125 Intramuscular lipoma within the medial head of the left triceps muscle. Axial SE T1-WI (**a**). Coronal FS T1-WI (**b**) before and after injection of gadolinium contrast (**c**). The lesion is well delineated and is similar to fat on all pulse sequences. There is only faint peripheral enhancement

5.12.3 Grading

Well-known histologic grading parameters, such as cellularity, mitotic rate, matrix, degree of pleiomorphism, vascular invasion, presence of necrosis, may influence SI, degree and pattern of contrast enhancement on MRI. Nevertheless, there is still much controversy regarding the value of MRI in the differentiation between the above-mentioned WHO categories of STT.

Table 5.18 summarizes the previously reported imaging parameters that suggest malignancy. The value of these signs, both alone and in combination, has been discussed by several authors. With a few exceptions, the grading of soft-tissue tumors on the basis of individual parameters is not useful. Combinations of different parameters guarantee higher sensitivity and specificity. Gielen et al. reported

Table 5.18 Grading parameters suggesting malignancy on imaging

Large size
Ill-defined margins
Extracompartmental extension
Broad contact with underlying fascia
Invasion of bone and/or neurovascular bundle
Heterogeneous signal intensity (SI) on all pulse sequences
High SI on T2-WI
Intralesional hemorrhage or necrosis
Contrast enhancement
Static studies (marked, merely peripheral)
Dynamic studies (fast enhancement with steep slope and long-standing plateau phase)

a sensitivity of 93%, a specificity of 82%, a negative predictive value of 98%, and a positive predictive value of 60% in differentiating between benign and malignant STT (Fig. 5.126). Van Rijswijk et al. reported even better accuracy, using a combination of nonenhanced, static and dynamic contrast-enhanced MR parameters. The most useful parameters in predicting malignancy consist of liquefaction, start of dynamic enhancement (time interval between start of arterial and tumor enhancement), and large lesion size.

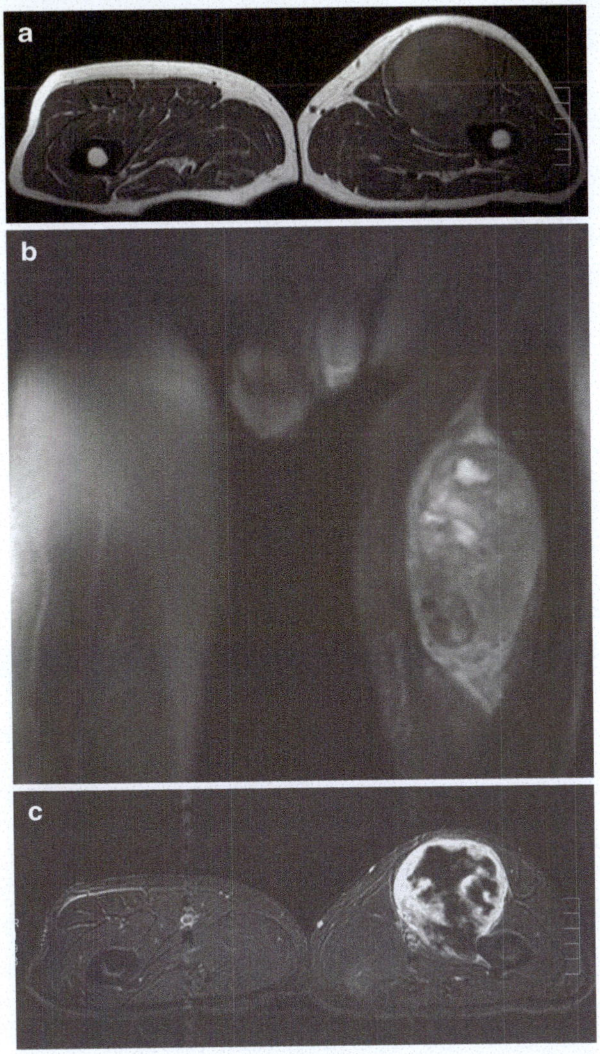

Fig. 5.126 Pleiomorphic leiomyosarcoma of the left thigh in an 82-year-old male. Axial SE T1-WI (**a**). Coronal FS T2-WI (**b**) and axial subtraction image after intravenous administration of gadolinium contrast (**c**). Huge lesion within the left adductor muscles, with heterogeneous signal intensity on T1- and T2-WI and irregular peripheral enhancement. The age of the patient, the location with the thigh, heterogeneous signal, large size, and the enhancement pattern are suspicious for malignancy

5.12.4 Tissue-Specific Diagnosis

Because of its high intrinsic contrast resolution, it was expected that MRI had great potential for the histological classification of soft-tissue tumors. Unfortunately, the basis for the initial enthusiasm has not been confirmed.

There are two reasons for this. First, by showing SI related to some physicochemical properties of tumor components (e.g., fat, blood, water, and collagen) and, consequently, reflecting gross morphology of the lesion rather than underlying histology, MR images provide only indirect information about tumor histology. Soft-tissue tumors belonging to the same histologic group may have a different composition or different proportions of tumor components, resulting in different MR signals. This feature is well exemplified by the group of liposarcomas that may be well differentiated (lipomatous), myxoid, round cell, or pleiomorphic, or contain different proportions of these components. Only well-differentiated liposarcomas are predominantly fatty, whereas the other histologic subtypes have less than 25% fat or no fat at all. As a consequence, there are no specific MR characteristics for liposarcomas as a group.

The second reason for the poor performance of MRI in characterizing tumors histologically involves time-dependent changes during natural evolution or as a consequence of therapy. Young desmoid tumors are highly cellular with high water content; this results in high SI on T2-WI. With aging, they become more collagenous and less cellular, which results in a decreasing SI. The same transformation has been described for many tumors of fibrous tissue and also for malignant fibrous histiocytomas. Furthermore, the SI of large malignant tumors undergoes changes as a consequence of intratumoral necrosis and/or bleeding.

These limitations have prompted Kransdorf to state “a correct histological diagnosis reached on the basis of imaging studies is possible in only approximately one quarter of cases.” More recently, Gielen et al. reported better results in a series of 548 histologically proven STT in which a correct tissue-specific diagnosis on MRI was made in 294 of 425 benign tumors and in 47 of 123 malignant tumors. As for grading, the best results are obtained by using a combination of different parameters. As a guideline for the reader, we have summarized the value of different parameters, such as preferential location (Table 5.19), shape (Table 5.20), presence of signal voids (Table 5.21), fluid-fluid levels (Table 5.22), signal intensities on different pulse sequences (Table 5.23), multiplicity (Table 5.24), and concomitant diseases (Table 5.25) in concise tables.

Other imaging modalities, such as plain films for detection of calcifications (Fig. 5.127) and ultrasound for superficially located cystic lesions may be helpful in the differential diagnosis.

The highest confidence in characterization is reached when the majority of the cases are benign lesions, such as lipomas (Fig. 5.125), hemangiomas (Fig. 5.127) and arteriovenous malformations, benign neural tumors, periarticular cysts, hematomas, pigmented villonodular synovitis, giant-cell tumors of tendon sheath, and abscesses. The use of intravenously injected paramagnetic contrast agents is valuable in the detection and staging of soft-tissue tumors, but neither the intensity nor the pattern of enhancement contributes to further histological characterization of these lesions. Dynamic contrast studies are useful for assessing the response of soft-tissue tumors to chemotherapy and for differentiating postoperative edema from recurrent tumor. "First-pass" imaging may aid in differentiating hemangioma from arteriovenous malformation.

Table 5.19 Preferential location of soft-tissue tumors

Location		Tumor
Neck	Infants	Cystic hygroma – lymphangioma capillary hemangioma
	Dorsal neck	Nuchal fibroma
	Sternocleidomastoid muscle (children)	Fibromatosis colli
	Carotid bifurcation	Glomus tumor
Trunk	Axilla	Cystic hygroma – lymphangioma
	Subscapular	Elastofibroma
	Paraspinal gutter	Neurogenic tumor
Abdomen	Rectus abdominis muscle (postpuerperal women)	Abdominal desmoid
	Paraspinal gutter	Neurogenic tumor
	Psoas muscle, parapsoatic	Plexiform neurofibroma
Pelvis	Presacral	Plexiform neurofibroma
	Buttock, lateral aspect	Desmoid
		Injection granuloma
	Coccyx	Extraspinal ependymoma
Upper limb	Deltoid, subcutaneous	Desmoid
		Injection granuloma
	Wrist	Ganglion cyst
	Wrist, volar aspect	Fibrolipohamartoma of median nerve
	Hand	(Gouty tophi)
	Hand, volar aspect	Palmar fibromatosis
		Fibrolipohamartoma of median nerve
	Finger, volar aspect	Giant-cell tumor of tendon sheath
	Finger, dorsal aspect (children)	Digital fibroma
	Finger, tip	Epidermoid cyst
		Glomus tumor
Lower limb	Flexor aspect, along major nerves	Schwannoma
	Thigh (older men)	Sarcoma (liposarcoma)
	Thigh (adults)	Alveolar soft part sarcoma

(*continued*)

Table 5.19 (continued)

Location		Tumor
	Thigh (infants)	Fibrohamartoma of infancy
	Knee	Synovial hemangioma
	Knee (young, middle-aged men)	Pigmented villonodular synovitis
	Knee (older men)	Lipoma arborescens
	Knee, popliteal fosa	Pigmented villonodular synovitis Baker's cyst Synovial cyst Ganglion cyst Meniscal cyst Nerve sheath tumors (Aneurysm of popliteal artery)
	Knee, tibio-fibular joint	Ganglion cyst
	Ankle	Ganglion cyst
	Foot, extensor aspect	Ganglion cyst
	Sole (young adults)	Synoviosarcoma Plantar fibromatosis
	Heel	Clear cell sarcoma
	Metatarsals (women)	Morton's neuroma
	Toes	Giant-cell tumor of tendon sheath
Upper and lower limbs	Extensor aspect (young adults)	Fibrous histiocytoma Myxofibrosarcoma (Myositis ossificans) Leiomyoma
Tendons	Achilles tendon, bilateral	Xanthoma Giant-cell tumor of tendon sheath Clear cell sarcoma
Joints, periarticular		Synovial hemangioma Pigmented villonodular synovitis Synoviosarcoma
Cutis, subcutis		Desmoid Neurofibroma Nodular fasciitis Dermatofibrosarcoma protuberans

Table 5.20 Distinguishing shapes of soft-tissue tumors

Fusiform (ovoid)	Neurofibroma Lipoma
Dumbbell	Neurofibroma
	Desmoid
Moniliform	Neurofibroma
Round	Cyst Schwannoma
Serpiginous	Hemangioma
Soap bubbles	Lipoma arborescens
Nodular	Fibromatosis (plantaris, palmaris)
Branching (bilateral) finger-like, bag of worms	Plexiform neurofibroma

Table 5.21 Intratumoral signal void

Flow	Hemangioma (capillary) Arteriovenous malformation
Calcification	Hemangioma (phlebolith) Lipoma (well-differentiated and dedifferentiated) Desmoid Cartilaginous tumors Osteosarcoma of soft tissue Synoviosarcoma (poorly defined, amorphous) Chordoma Alveolar soft part sarcoma Myosilis ossificans (marginal)

Table 5.22 Fluid-fluid levels

Hemangioma
Hematoma
Cystic lymphangioma
Synoviosarcoma
Myxoma
Myositis
Metastasis

Table 5.23 Signal intensities on spin echo sequences

High SI on T1-WI + intermediate SI on T2-WI	Lipoma
	Liposarcoma Lipoblastoma Hibernoma Elastofibroma Fibrolipohamartoma Metastasis of melanoma (melanin) Clear cell sarcoma (melanin)
High SI on T1-WI + high SI on T2-WI	Hemangioma
	Lymphangioma Subacute hematoma Myxoma Small arteriovenous malformation
Low SI on T1-WI + high SI on T2-WI	Cyst
	Myxoma Myxoid liposarcoma Sarcoma
Low to intermediate SI on T1-WI + low SI on T2-WI	Desmoid and other fibromatoses Pigmented villonodular synovitis Morton's neuroma Fibrolipohamartoma Giant-cell tumor of tendon sheath Acute hematoma (few days) Old hematoma Xanthoma High flow arteriovenous malformation Mineralized mass Scar tissue Amyloidosis
Intermediate SI on T1-WI + high SI on T2-WI	Neurogenic tumor Desmoid

Table 5.24 Multiplicity

Venous malformation
Lipoma (5–8%)
Lipoma of tendon sheath (50%)
Desmoid
Neurofibroma
Myxoma
Metastasis
Dermatofibrosarcoma protuberans
Kaposi's sarcoma

Table 5.25 Concomitant diseases

Concomitant osseous involvement	Pigmented villonodular Synovitis
	Lymphoma Desmoid Angiomatosis Parosteal lipoma
Concomitant osseous involvement + nodular soft-tissue tumors	Infantile myofibromatosis Infantile fibromatosis Fibrosarcoma multiforme
Concomitant osseous involvement + nodular soft-tissue	Juvenile hyalin fibromatosis tumors + hypertrophic gingiva + flexion contractures + acroosteolysis
Maffucci's disease	Cavernous hemangioma(s)
Fibrous dysplasia (Mazabraud) Neurofibromatosis	Myxoma(s) Schwannoma(s) Neurofibroma(s)
Gardner's syndrome	Fibromatosis
Dupuytren's disease (flexion contractures)	Palmar fibromatosis
Macrodystrophia lipomatosa of the digits	Fibrolipohamartoma of the median nerve
Familial hypercholesterolemia	Xanthoma
Normolipidemia + lymphoma or granuloma	Cutaneous xanthoma
Turner's syndrome	Lymphangioma
Noonan's syndrome	
Fetal alcohol syndrome	
Down's syndrome	
Familial pterygium colli	
Diabetes + degenerative joint disease + trauma	Lipoma arborescens
Multiple myeloma	Amyloidosis

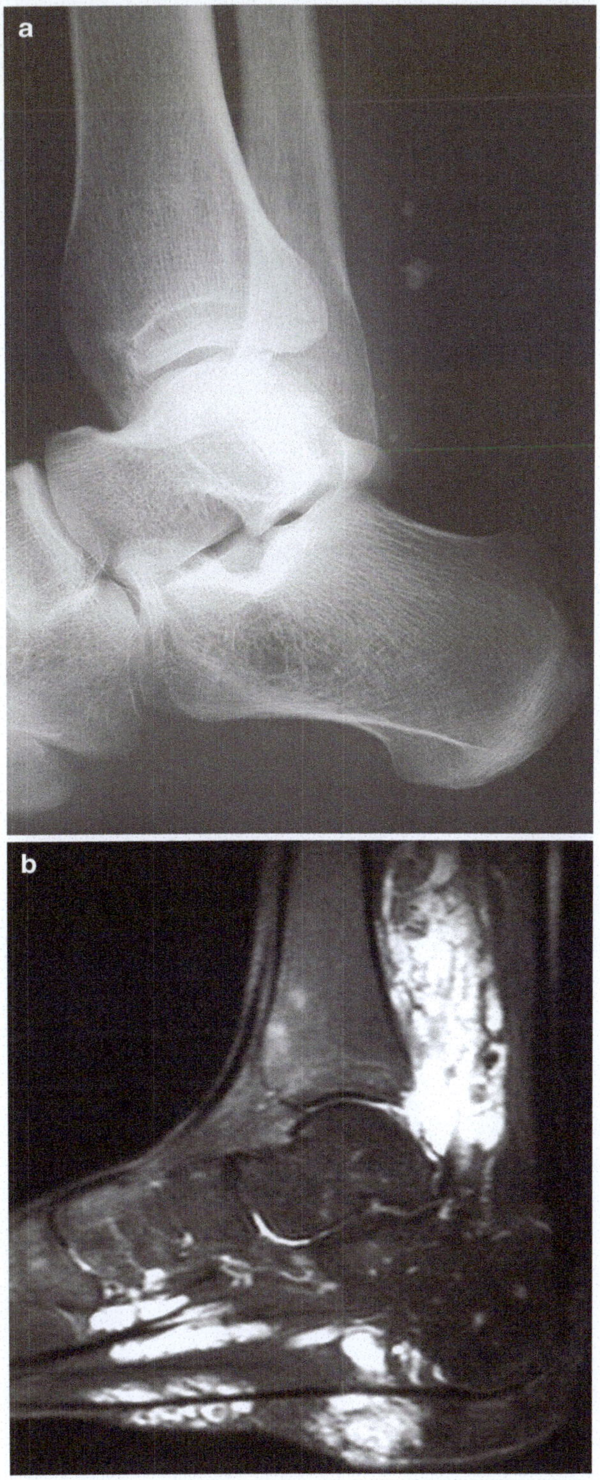

Fig. 5.127 Soft-tissue hemangioma. Sagittal TSE FS intermediate-WI (**a**). The lesion involves multiple compartments (posterior and plantar aspect of the ankle) with a lobular morphology and predominantly high T2-signal. Note the presence of characteristic phleboliths on the plain film (**b**)

Further Reading

Alyas F, James SL, Davies AM, Saifuddin A (2007) The role of MR imaging in the diagnostic characterization of appendicular bone tumors and tumor-like conditions. Eur Radiol 17:2675–2686

Cerezal L, Abascal F, Canga A et al (2000) Usefulness of gadolinium-enhanced MRI in the evaluation of the vascularity of scaphoid nonunions. AJR 174:141–149

De Schepper AM, Bloem JL (2007) Soft-tissue tumors: grading, staging, and tissue-specific diagnosis. Top Magn Reson Imaging 18:431–444

De Schepper AM, Vanhoenacker F, Gielen J, Parizel PM (2006) Imaging of soft tissue tumors, 3rd edn. Springer, Berlin

Gielen JL, De Schepper AM, Vanhoenacker F et al (2004) Accuracy of MRI in characterization of soft-tissue tumors and tumor-like lesions. A prospective study in 548 patients. Eur Radiol 14:2320–2330

Herold T, Bachthaler M, Hamer OW et al (2006) Indirect MR arthrography of the shoulder: use of abduction and external rotation to detect full-and partial-thickness tears of the supraspinatus tendon. Radiology 240:152–160

Karantanas AH (2007) Acute bone marrow edema of the hip: role of MR imaging. Eur Radiol 17:2225–2236

Kassarjian A, Bencardino JT, Palmer WE (2006) MR Imaging of the Rotator Cuff. Radiol Clin N Am 44:503–523

Kijowski R, Tuite M and Sanford M (2005) Magnetic resonance imaging of the elbow. Part II: abnormalities of the ligaments, tendons, and nerves. Skeletal Radiol 34:1–18

Kransdorf MJ, Murphey MD (2006) Imaging of soft tissue tumors, 2nd edn. Lippincott Williams & Wilkins, Philadelphia

Manelfe C, Vanhoenacker FM (2007) Seronegative spondylarthropathy. In: Van Goethem J, Parizel PM, Van den Hauwe L (eds) Spinal imaging: diagnostic imaging of the spine and spinal cord. Springer, Berlin, pp 541–563

McNally E (2007) Knee: ligaments. In: Vanhoenacker FM, Maas M, Gielen JL (eds) Imaging of orthopedic sports injuries. Springer, Berlin, pp 283–305

Miller TT, Schweitzer ME (2005) Diagnostic musculoskeletal imaging. McGraw-Hill, New York

Morag Y, Jacobson JA, Miller B, De Maeseneer M, Gandikota G, Jamadar D (2006) MR imaging of rotator cuff injury: what the clinician needs to know. Radiographics 26:1045–1065

Ouellette H, Bredella M, Labis J et al (2008) MR imaging of the elbow in baseball pitchers. Skeletal Radiol 37:115–121

Peterson JJ (2007) The knee. Magn Reson Imaging Clin N Am 15:1

Resnick, Kang, Pretterklieber (2007) Internal derangements of joints, 2nd edn. Saunders Elsevier, Philadelphia

Rosenberg ZS (2001) Update on the ankle and foot. Magn Reson Imaging Clin N Am 9:3

Rosenberg ZS (2005) MR Imaging of the hip. Magn Reson Imaging Clin N Am 13:4

Stoller DW (2007) Magnetic resonance imaging in orthopaedics and sports medicine, 3rd edn. Lippincott Williams & Wilkins, Philadelphia

Timins ME, Jahnke JP, Krah SF et al (1995) MR imaging of the major carpal stabilizing ligaments: normal anatomy and clinical examples. Radiographics 15:575–587

Tuite MJ (2008) Sacroiliac joint imaging. Semin Musculoskelet Radiol 12:72–82

Van der Woude H-J, Franssen-Franken DG (2007) Rotator cuff and impingement. In: Vanhoenacker FM, Maas M, Gielen JL (eds) Imaging of orthopedic sports injuries. Springer, Berlin, pp 149–168

Van Rijswijk CS, Geinaerdt MJ, Hogendoorn PC et al (2004) Soft-tissue tumors: value of static and dynamic gadopentate dimeglumine-enhanced MR imaging in prediction of malignancy. Radiology 233:493–502

Vanhoenacker FM, Maas M, Gielen JL (2007) Imaging of orthopedic sports injuries. Springer-Verlag, Berlin

Vanhoenacker FM, Van der Woude HJ, Vanhoenacker PK, De Praeter G (2007) MR arthrography of the rotator cuff. JBR-BTR 90:338–344

Waldt S, Bruegel M, Mueller D et al (2007) Rotator cuff tears: assessment with MR arthrography in 275 patients with arthroscopic correlation. Eur Radiol 17:491–498

Abdomen: Liver, Spleen, Biliary System, Pancreas, and GI Tract

6

Peter Reimer, Wolfgang Schima, Thomas Lauenstein, and Sanjay Saini

Contents

P. Reimer (✉)
Department of Radiology, Klinikum Karlsruhe,
Moltkestrasse 90, 76133 Karlsruhe, Germany
e-mail: p.reimer@web.de

P. Reimer et al. (eds.), *Clinical MR Imaging*,
DOI: 10.1007/978-3-540-74504-4_6,

6.1 General Introduction

Peter Reimer and Wolfgang Schima

6.1.1 General Clinical Indications

Magnetic resonance imaging (MRI) is a widely used modality for the evaluation of diffuse liver disease and detection, as well as further characterization of focal liver disease. The same principles apply to the spleen. Furthermore, MRI represents a comprehensive approach for the biliary system, the pancreas, and the GI tract. The different technical options make MRI a useful but also challenging technique. MRI competes with ultrasound (US) and MDCT, which have also improved considerably.

6.1.2 Coils

Patients are scanned in supine position (feet or head first) with a variety of phased-array coil options depending on the vendor's philosophy. Phased-array coils combine a number of small coils, typically positioned anterior and posterior to the patient and wrapped together (wrap-around coil) providing a higher signal-to-noise ratio and a better image quality (see also Chap. 1). Since the anterior–posterior diameter of patients varies considerably, scanning technicians need to adjust the signal amplification of the middle third of the body specifically to patients' anterior-posterior diameter to avoid a layering effect with a higher signal toward the coil and a lower signal toward the middle of the body (noise break through). The inhomogeneous signal within phased-array coils makes signal measurements for signal quantification complex. Newer coils allow for the acquisition of parallel imaging techniques (e.g., SENSE, GRAPPA, etc.) with different terms and technical approaches by the different vendors to speed up acquisition times as described in Chap. 1.

6.1.3 Pulse Sequences

The minimum protocol for the parenchymal organs of the upper abdomen consists of 2D or 3D-T1-weighted (T1-W) and 2D or 3D-T2-weighted (T2-W) sequences obtained in the axial plane. If a tumor is suspected, contrast-enhanced pulse sequences are mandatory, even if no abnormality is detected on the unenhanced sequences. The section thickness varies from 2–6 mm for the liver and spleen, 2–4 mm for the pancreas, and 1–3 mm for vessels and cholangiopancreatography. Breathing-related movements are the major source of artifacts of the upper abdomen. A variety of compensatory techniques have been developed, such as respiratory compensation, cranial, caudal, and anterior saturation pulses, multiple averaging, fat suppression, and navigator echoes. An effective and at the same time robust technique is to use breath-held sequences with acquisition times of 20 s or less, combined with cranial and caudal saturation pulses further minimizing pulsation artifacts. Typically, an expiratory breath hold is performed to ensure reproducible slice positioning. If patients cannot suspend respiration for around 20 s, a nonbreath-held sequence with multiple averaging or respiratory-triggering and saturation pulses is preferable. Fat suppression may be applied with both T1-W and T2-W pulse sequences, using the available technology for fat suppression on each scanner, providing more advantages for the pancreas and biliary system than for the liver and spleen. General pulse sequence recommendations are summarized in Table 6.1.

Breath-held spoiled-gradient echo (GRE) sequences, such as fast low-angle shot imaging (FLASH [Siemens], FFE [Philips], and SPGR [GE Healthcare]), are preferable for T1-W imaging (T1-WI) and are referred to within the text. The echo time (TE) of spoiled-GRE sequences should be chosen close to in-phase (1.0 T: 6.9 ms, 1.5 T: 4.6 ms, and 3.0 T 2.3 ms) and out-of-phase (1.0 T: 3.45 ms, 1.5 T: 2.3 ms, and 3.0 T: 1.1 ms) to characterize fatty tissue. TEs close to optimal in-phase echo times may be used, depending on specific pulse sequence optimization strategies. Traditional sequences allow for coverage of the entire liver during a single breath hold at the cost of some artifacts, because the increase in the number of sections is typically achieved by applying the spoiler pulses just before acquisition of the data set and not before each phase-encoding step. More advanced 3D-T1-W spoiled GRE sequences with fat saturation allow the acquisition of thin sections in the order of 2–4 mm. T1-W sequences are combined with extracellular gadolinium chelates, paramagnetic hepatobiliary agents, and also with superparamagnetic iron oxides.

Table 6.1 Overview of some commonly used MRI sequences for the abdomen (see also Chap. 1)

SSFP	Use breathhold to plan further breath-held sequences Good localizer Usually applied in axial and/or coronal imaging planes Provide signal in fluid and vessels
T1	Typically 2D or 3D GRE sequence Breathhold recommended Fat saturation improves image contrast
T2	TSE/FSE/HASTE with breathhold or free breathing Fat saturation may increase image contrast Long echo for detection of long T2 lesions Used for MRCP as 2D or 3D sequence Respiratory triggered 3D recommended for high spatial resolution MRCP
DWI/ADC	Is indicated in the evaluation of cystic lesions (e.g., to differentiate solid from cystic tumor or solid from necrotic tumor) Provides good detection of lymph nodes (inverting images giving PET like appearance) At 1.5 T use *b* values of 50 s/mm^2 and 600–800 s/mm^2 Future motto may be: "diffusion imaging for all patients"
T2*	Gradient echo sequence provides information about hemoglobin breakdown products and calcifications Sensitivity to susceptibility effects is proportional to TE and field strength Mandatory for RES-specific contrast agents (SPIO/USPIO)
T1 ± Gd	Part of many imaging protocols Usually applied in axial or coronal imaging planes, depending on indication Same imaging plane should be used before and after gadolinium-chelate injection For dynamic studies, 3D GRE with fat saturation most suited
Contrast-enhanced MRA	Indicated for specific vascular cases Allows for time-resolved angiography

A variety of sequences are available for T2-WI. Turbo spin echo (TSE) imaging are now standard, with different options for breath held and nonbreath-held sequences. Breath-held TSE sequences use increasing numbers of echoes per TR (echo train length, "ETL") to decrease the acquisition time at the same anatomical resolution or increase the anatomical resolution at the same temporal resolution. However, the use of sequences with increasing ETL with numerous 180° refocussing pulses, also decreases the susceptibility weighting, which is an important contributor to lesion contrast within parenchymal organs. Therefore, TSE sequences with a very long ETL (i.e., single-shot TSE) may provide lower lesion contrast for solid lesions than TSE sequences with a short ETL (i.e., respiratory-triggered TSE). Thus, nonbreath-held sequences with a limited number of echoes are still relevant for clinical MRI and provide stable image quality. Breath-held multishot rapid acquisition relation enhancement (RARE) imaging sequences have been recently improved by using fast read-outs, half Fourier acquisitions, and Half Fourier acquired single-shot turbo spin-echo sequence (HASTE) techniques and are becoming clinically useful because of their good display of liver anatomy. T2-W sequences with susceptibility weighting (T2*-W GRE) are combined with superparamagnetic iron oxides.

Diffusion-based sequences have gained considerable attention for the detection and characterization of focal lesions. Diffusion-weighted imaging (DWI) with b values of 50 and 600–800 s/mm^2 has matured into a substantial part of abdominal protocols, both for lesion detection and characterization. Additional calculation of ADC values may offer new applications for the assessment of treatment response or lesions characterization.

MR angiography (MRA) of the portal venous system, supplying visceral arteries and visceral veins, may be performed by means of contrast-enhanced MRA (ceMRA) techniques that utilize a combination of gadolinium chelates and breath-held coronal 3D-nonspoiled GRE sequences (see also Chap. 11). Individual angiographic sections should always be viewed together with postprocessed maximum intensity projection (MIP) angiograms. More recently, balanced nonspoiled GRE sequences have gained particular importance. Typically acquired as 2D sequences, this technique provides bright vessels almost irrespective of the flow direction and velocity as well as bright fluid-filled structures. Therefore, these sequences are useful in demonstrating the patency of a vessel without the use of contrast agents. Clinically, gadolinium-enhanced T1-W 3D GRE sequences with thin section obviate the acquisition of additional MRA sequences in most patients.

MR cholangiopancreatography (MRCP) has been improved with the refinement of TSE/FSE/HASTE pulse sequences. Current approaches differ from scanner technology and use predominantly either breath-held

2D sequences or nonbreath-held and often respiratory-triggered 3D sequences. Intraductal fluid is visualized, based on long TE compared with background tissues, which have already lost their signal. Individual sections should always be viewed together with postprocessed MIP cholangiograms and pancreaticograms.

More specific information is provided in Chap. 1.

6.2 Liver

Peter Reimer and Sanjay Saini

6.2.1 Liver Anatomy

The liver demonstrates higher signal intensity on T1-W sequences and lower signal intensity on T2-W sequences than the spleen on nonfat-suppressed images. Signal intensity from normal parenchyma is homogeneous on both sequences (Fig. 6.1).

6.2.2 Contrast Agents for Liver MR

Nonspecific low-molecular extracellular gadolinium chelates are still most frequently used for contrast-enhanced liver MRI and are useful for the detection and characterization of liver disease. A standard dose of 0.1 mmol Gd/kg bodyweight is sufficient (see Chap. 1). These compounds behave pharmacologically similar to iodinated X-ray contrast agents and can be bolus injected to perform dynamic studies using multisection spoiled GRE techniques covering the entire upper abdomen in a single breath hold. Gadolinium-enhanced images can be interpreted in a manner very similar to contrast-enhanced CT images, because gadolinium shortens T1-relaxation time, resulting in tissue signal enhancement on T1-WI. Contrast timing requires the acquisition of arterial phase (20–30 s following injection) images to detect and characterize hypervascular lesions [focal nodular hyperplasia (FNH), adenoma, hepatocellular carcinoma (HCC), hypervascular metastases: renal cell cancer, neuroendocrine tumors (NET), pheochromocytoma, etc.]. In the arterial phase, contrast

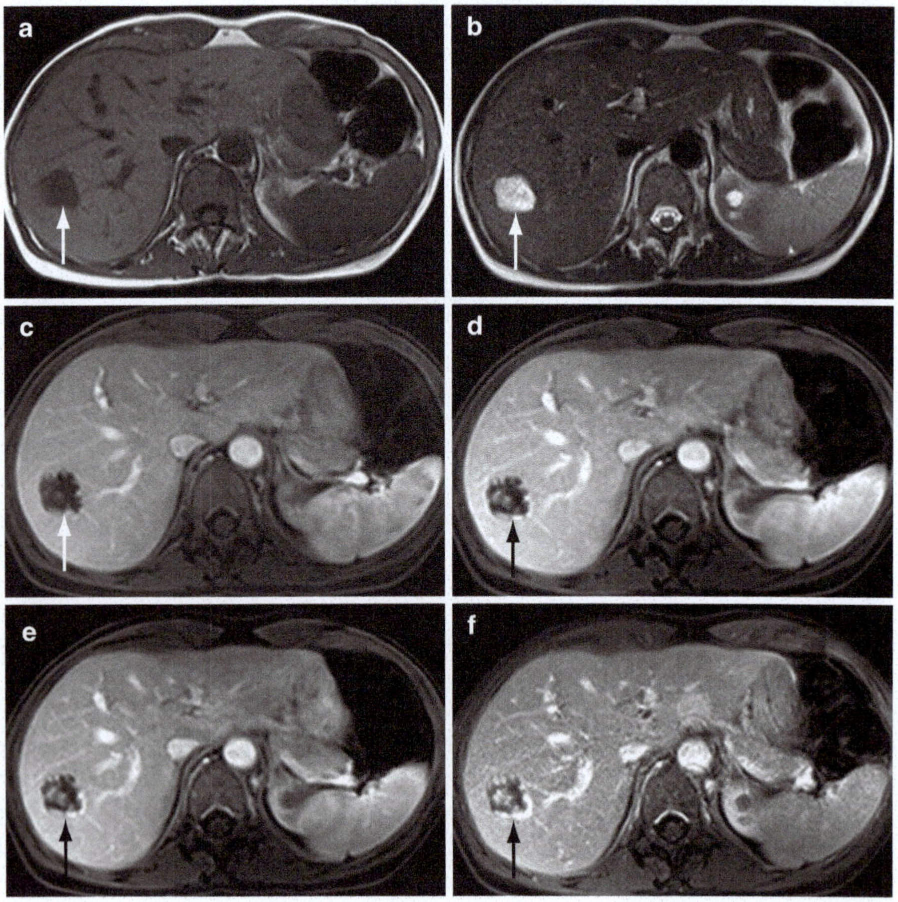

Fig. 6.1 Typical hemangioma (*arrows*). Plain T1-W spoiled 2D GRE (**a**), T2-W Haste (**b**), arterial phase gadobutrol-enhanced FS T1-W spoiled 3D GRE (**c**), portal venous phase-enhanced FS T1-W spoiled 3D GRE (**d**), venous-enhanced FS T1-W spoiled 3D GRE (**e**), and late phase FS T1-W spoiled 2D GRE (**f**) show a typical hemangioma centrally in the right liver. The tumor is hypointense on T1-W and hyperintense on T2-W. Dynamic imaging demonstrates a type-3 enhancement pattern with peripheral nodular gadolinium enhancement, followed by a centripetal progression on late gadolinium-enhanced T1-W images without complete uniform signal enhancement

material is present in the visceral arteries, with strong enhancement of the pancreas and renal cortex without opacification of the hepatic veins. The normal spleen should show an arciform or serpiginous enhancement pattern. Portal-phase images (60–90 s following injection) demonstrate strong parenchymal enhancement to detect hypovascular lesions with best conspicuity during this phase. Equilibrium phase images acquired more than 2 min following injection up to 10 min result in a diffuse enhancement that can be useful to allow hemangiomas to fill-in and cholangiocarcinoma (CCC) and inflammatory changes to enhance.

Liver-specific intracellular contrast agents have been developed to further improve liver imaging. Since clinical approval may vary among different countries, it is recommended to check approval and labels carefully.

Teslascan® (mangafodipir trisodium, formerly known as Mn-DPDP) was the first approved paramagnetic hepatocyte-specific MR contrast agent. It is partially excreted into the bile following uptake into hepatocytes and causes an increase of signal intensity on T1-WI. In Europe, the label allows a drip infusion; therefore, dynamic scanning cannot be performed. The compound enhances liver parenchyma and was advocated to detect nonhepatocellular lesions and differentiate tumors of hepatocellular origin from nonhepatocellular origin. Due to the lack of enhancement of nonhepatocellular tumors, metastases are better seen on postcontrast images. A perilesional rim (i.e., enhanced adjacent tissue due to compression by the tumor) may be visible. Enhancement patterns of different well-differentiated hepatocellular tumors appear not to be specific enough to further differentiate these tumors (see Chap. 1).

A second compound with comparable enhancement characteristics on T1-WI, MultiHance® (gadobenate dimeglumine, formerly known as Gd-BOPTA) is clinically available for liver imaging due to a 4% biliary excretion, but has gained more attention for vascular imaging as an off-label-use. The compound can be bolus injected and imaging studies may be designed as described for nonspecific gadolinium compounds combined with delayed scans 1–2 h later for tumor detection because of uptake into the liver parenchyma to increase conspicuity of metastases. (see Chap. 1).

A third compound, Primovist® (gadoxetic acid, formerly known as Gd-EOB-DTPA) is approved in Europe, Asia and the US for liver imaging. This compound provides a strong biliary excretion and can be bolus injected at a dose of 0.025 mmol/kg, with imaging studies as described for nonspecific gadolinium compounds combined with delayed scans as early as 20 min postinjection (see Chap. 1).

Superparamagnetic iron oxide particles (SPIO) accumulate efficiently within minutes of administration within phagocytic cells in the liver with approximately 80% and in the spleen with 5–10% of the injected dose. Malignant tumors are typically devoid of a substantial number of phagocytic cells, so they appear as hyperintense/bright lesions in a hypointense/black liver on T2-W sequences. Tumors with a substantial number of phagocytic cells, such as FNH, hepatocellular adenoma, well-differentiated HCC, may show sufficient uptake of SPIO and, thus, decrease in signal intensity on T2-W sequences. Likewise, hemangiomas may tend to show uptake of SPIO due to the blood pool effect with signal intensity drop on T2-WI. The signal decrease is related to the Kupffer cell activity and tumor vascularity. Clinically approved Endorem®/Feridex® is currently administered by drip infusion in glucose or saline at a dose of 10–15 μmol Fe/kg bodyweight over 30 min, with a flow rate of approximately 3 mL/min, since side effects (facial flash, dyspnea, rash, and lumbar pain) occur at higher injection rates. The patient is then brought back into the magnet, typically on the same day, with a large time window of several hours to acquire postcontrast images.

Resovist® is the second clinically available SPIO with approval in Europe and Japan. Resovist is bolus-inject able and patients may either be scanned within one session or up to 1–4 days postcontrast (see also Chap. 1).

6.3 Liver Pathology Diffuse Liver Disease

6.3.1 *Diffuse Liver Disease: Fatty Liver*

Fatty infiltration is a metabolic complication of a variety of toxic, ischemic, and infectious insults to the liver. In fatty infiltration, the hepatocytes accumulate triglycerides within cytoplasmic fat vacuoles. Fatty infiltration can be diffuse or focal and can have a lobar, segmental, or nodular distribution. Focal fatty infiltration, however, has no mass effect on the adjacent hepatic parenchyma, and vascular structures course normally through the

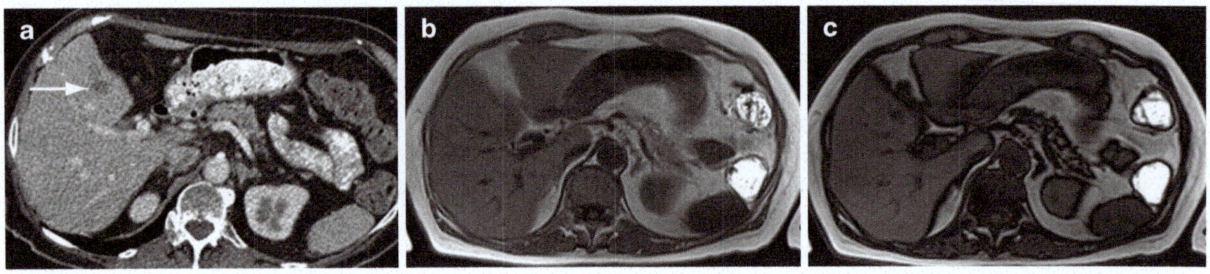

Fig. 6.2 Focal fatty infiltration (*arrow*) mimicking a metastasis on CT. Contrast-enhanced CT (**a**) in a patient with gastric cancer shows a focal lesion adjacent to the gall bladder in segment 5. In-phase (**b**) and out-of-phase 2D GRE (**c**) prove focal fatty infiltration by showing high signal on in-phase (**b**) and a complete signal decrease on out-of-phase (**c**)

fatty areas. Fatty liver may cause severe problems on US and CT by obscuring focal lesions; however, MR is very effective in fatty liver since fat contributes to the signal intensity, and a signal from fat can be eliminated selectively (fat suppression). Follow-up of patients for metastases with chemotherapy-induced fatty liver are therefore best evaluated by MR. High signal on T1-WI and decreasing signal with fat-suppression techniques proves the presence of fat. Opposed-phase GRE techniques are clinically useful to differentiate focal fatty infiltration and focal sparing in diffuse fatty infiltration from mass lesions (Fig. 6.2). Some lesions have to be considered for differential diagnoses. Well-differentiated HCC is typically better delineated and often encapsulated with spotted areas of fat. Hepatic adenoma can be differentiated by strong early enhancement following gadolinium injection, by late enhancement following hepatobiliary agents, or by contrast agent uptake on delayed images following SPIO. Hemorrhage, melanin, protein, and copper may also cause increased signal on T1-WI. Hepatic injury with nonmass like areas of signal changes may also occur in toxin- or drug-induced liver disease or following radiation therapy.

6.3.2 Diffuse Liver Disease: Hepatitis

Hepatitis can be divided into acute and chronic forms. In acute hepatitis, histological changes are present primarily in the intralobular portion of the liver with swelling of hepatocytes. Chronic hepatitis is characterized by a portal inflammatory infiltrate with additional fibrous and inflammatory changes. Acute viral hepatitis is a systemic infection that affects the liver and is usually caused by one of the following five viral agents: hepatitis A virus, hepatitis B virus (HBV), hepatitis C virus, the HBV-associated delta agent or hepatitis D virus, and hepatitis E virus. A vast array of other viruses may also produce hepatitis, including herpes viruses, yellow fever virus, rubella virus, adenovirus, or coxsackie virus.

The imaging features of acute hepatitis are nonspecific, and the diagnosis is usually based on serologic, virologic, and clinical findings. Probably, the most important role of imaging patients with suspected hepatitis is to help rule out other diseases that produce similar clinical and biochemical abnormalities, such as extrahepatic cholestasis, diffuse metastatic disease, and cirrhosis.

At MRI, periportal edema appears as hyperintense areas on T2-WI. Involved areas may be normal or demonstrate decreased signal intensity on T1-WI and increased signal intensity on T2-WI. Extrahepatic findings in patients with severe acute hepatitis include gallbladder wall thickening due to edema and, infrequently, ascites. In patients with chronic hepatitis, the MRI features resemble those of early stage liver cirrhosis. Periportal lymphadenopathy may be the sole detectable abnormality in both acute and chronic hepatitis.

6.3.3 Diffuse Liver Disease: Cirrhosis

A wide range of disease processes results in hepatic injury and may result in cirrhotic changes in the liver. The most common pathologic conditions worldwide are alcohol-related injury and viral hepatitis. Liver cirrhosis is characterized by irreversible fibrosis with destruction of the hepatic architecture. Atrophy of the right liver lobe and the medial segment of the left liver lobe with consecutive hypertrophy of the lateral segment of the left lobe and caudate lobe is frequently present. An irregular parenchymal pattern is often also present and the liver contour frequently has a nodular appearance (Fig. 6.3). Hepatic enhancement is characteristically inhomogeneous with abrupt tapering of intrahepatic portal and hepatic venous branches. Regenerative nodules develop from heterogeneous regeneration and dysplasia. MRI is superior to CT and US in depicting regenerative nodules presenting with lower signal intensity than the cirrhotic liver on T2-WI. SPIO-enhanced MRI and gadolinium-enhanced MRI can be used to differentiate regenerative nodules with higher signal intensity on T2-WI compared with HCC. Regenerative nodules appear hypointense on early gadolinium-enhanced T1-WI and reveal a substantial uptake of SPIO resulting in a signal decrease, which is rarely observed in well-differentiated HCC. The major benefit of MRI in these patients is identifying specific causes or complications of cirrhosis, including fat deposition, portal vein thrombosis (with or without splenic vein thrombosis), iron deposition, and HCC.

MRI is performed after rapid infusion of extracellular gadolinium chelates, hepatobiliary agents, or SPIO. Arterial phase imaging with gadolinium chelates typically demonstrates small HCCs as brightly enhancing lesions that may have signal intensity similar to that of adjacent liver on portal- or equilibrium-phase images. More recently, SPIO has been used as a contrast agent without or with additional gadolinium chelates at MRI, which may increase accuracy in the detection of small HCCs in cirrhotic livers. Liver cirrhosis is the most common cause of portal hypertension due to a sinusoidal obstruction with subsequent complications, such as variceal bleed, ascites, and splenomegaly (Fig. 6.3). The normal hepatopetal flow may reverse in severe cirrhosis and become hepatofugal, which can be easily demonstrated by MR phase-contrast flow measurements. Portal

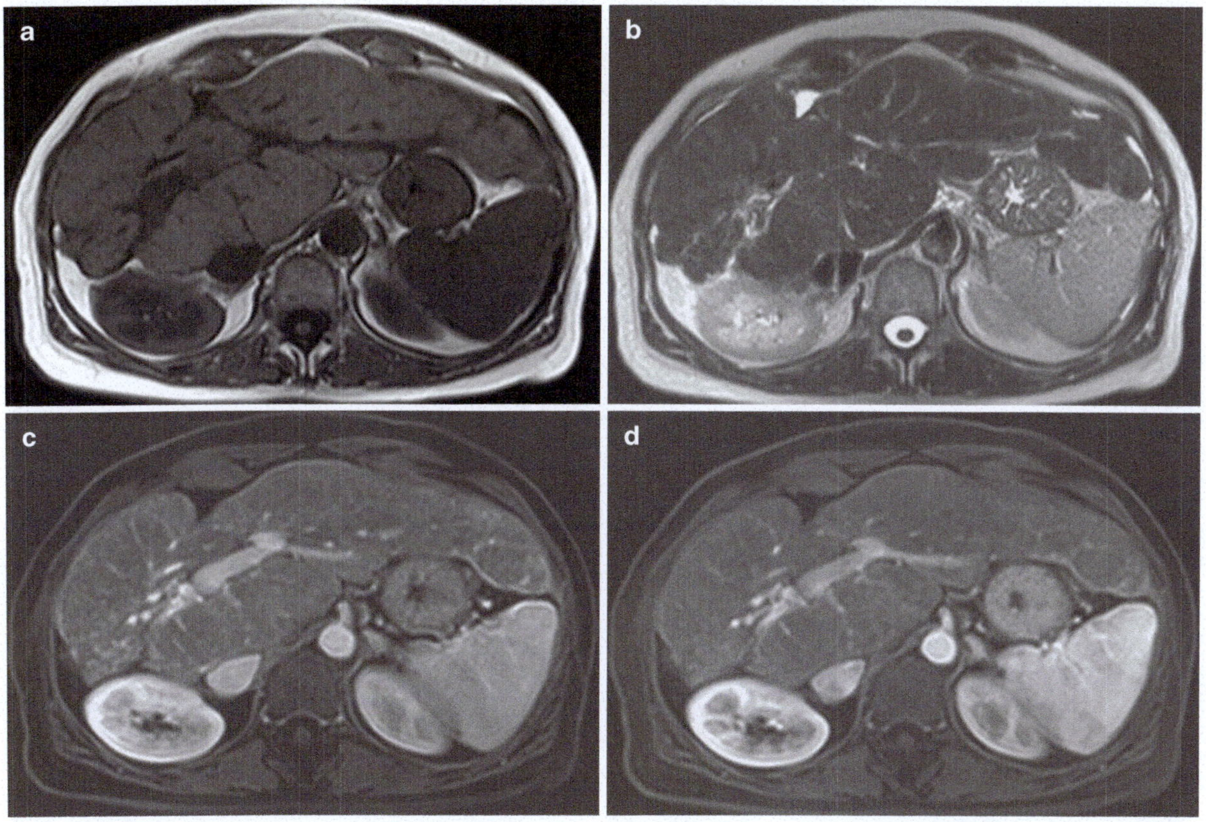

Fig. 6.3 Liver cirrhosis following chronic hepatitis C. Plain 2D T1-W spoiled GRE (**a**), T2-W HASTE (**b**), arterial phase gadolinium-enhanced FS 3D T1-W spoiled GRE (**c**), and portal venous phase gadolinium-enhanced FS 3D T1-W spoiled GRE, and (**d**) of a patient with chronic hepatitis C with liver cirrhosis. The liver demonstrates higher signal intensity than the spleen on T1-W sequences and lower signal intensity than the spleen on T2-W sequences. Liver cirrhosis with hypertrophy of the left lobe, splenomegaly, and ascites is present

varices and shunts (splenorenal, splenocaval, etc.) are demonstrated by True-FISP, PC-MR-, TOF-MR-, and gadolinium-enhanced MR angiography.

Differential diagnoses for liver cirrhosis include Wilson disease and Gaucher disease. Wilson disease is characterized by excessive copper retention. The hepatic manifestations predominate in children, whereas neuropsychiatric manifestations predominate in adolescents and adults. Even though copper is paramagnetic, signal intensity at T1-WI is usually within normal range. In later stages, patients develop liver cirrhosis, which is indistinguishable from cirrhosis due to other causes.

Gaucher disease is caused by a deficiency of glucosylceramidase that results in the accumulation of glucosylceramide in the reticuloendothelial cells such as in the liver and spleen. Imaging findings are nonspecific and characterized by fatty and cirrhotic changes in the hepatic parenchyma.

6.3.4 Diffuse Liver Disease: Iron Overload

The signal appearance of iron overload is quite similar to postcontrast SPIO-enhanced images with low signal intensity on T2/T2*-WI. Severe iron overload may also lead to low signal intensity on T1-WI (Fig. 6.4). MRI is the most sensitive imaging technique to demonstrate iron overload, with muscle and fat serving as inherent reference tissues. Hepatic iron overload is caused by idiopathic (primary) hemochromatosis, transfusional iron overload, hemolytic anemia, or associated with liver cirrhosis.

Idiopathic hemochromatosis (Fig. 6.5) results from increased absorption and accumulation of dietary iron affecting primarily the liver, pancreas, and heart. Iron accumulation can be fatal due to the development of liver cirrhosis, HCC, diabetes mellitus, and cardiomyopathy. Iron accumulation starts in the liver; it should be diagnosed early, since therapy before accumulation in the pancreas and heart may result in a normal life expectancy. The spleen is typically spared, and involvement of the pancreas typically presents when liver cirrhosis has already developed. Patients with liver cirrhosis are at risk of HCC, and nonsiderotic dominant nodules in patients with hemochromatosis should be considered as malignant until proven otherwise. Regenerative nodules contain iron and decrease in signal compared with HCC, which also serves as a test by means of SPIO-enhanced MRI to differentiate regenerative nodules from HCC in patients with liver cirrhosis but without iron overload. However, hepatocellular iron may also be mildly increased in patients with liver cirrhosis. Dysplastic nodules may show variable iron uptake and, thus, may also appear as relatively bright lesions within the hypointense liver as a differential diagnosis to HCC.

Transfusional iron overload (Fig. 6.4) results in iron deposition in the reticuloendothelial system (RES) of the liver, spleen, and bone marrow (so-called hemosiderosis), sparing hepatocytes, pancreas, heart, and other parenchyma. Involvement of the spleen (transfusional iron overload) vs. the pancreas (idiopathic hemochromatosis) helps to differentiate RES iron from hepatocellular iron overload.

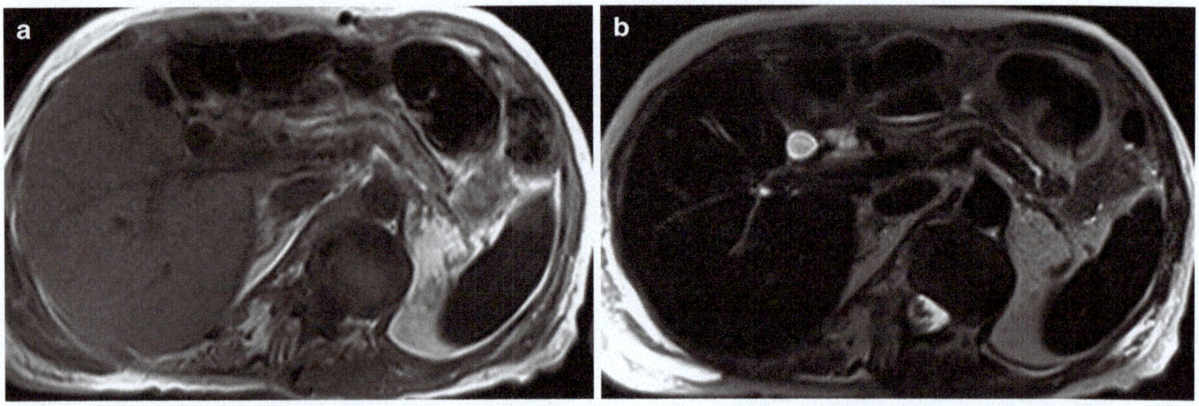

Fig. 6.4 Transfusion iron overload. Plain T1-W spoiled GRE (TE 5 ms) (**a**) and T2-W HASTE (**b**) in a patient with chronic kidney disease and kidney transplantation. The liver, spleen, and to some degree the bone marrow (**b**) demonstrate low signal intensity on T1- and T2-W sequences without a signal decrease within the pancreas or heart. There is no cirrhosis of the liver visible

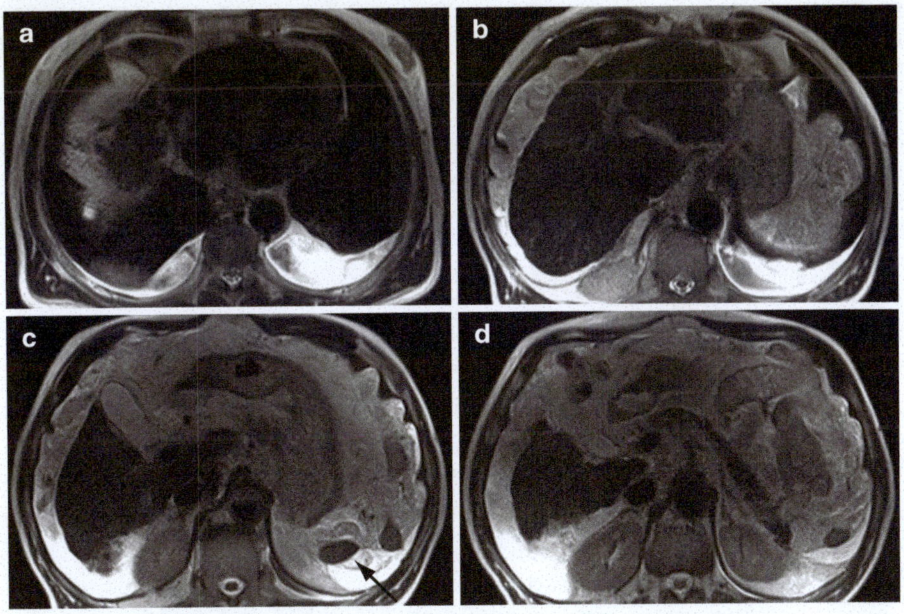

Fig. 6.5 Idiopathic hemochromatosis. T2-W HASTE (**a–d**) in a patient with idiopathic hemochromatosis who has developed severe liver cirrhosis, cardiomyopathy (**a**), and diabetes mellitus (**d**-*arrow*) based on iron accumulation. The spleen has been removed and an accessory spleen (*arrow*) is demonstrated (**c**)

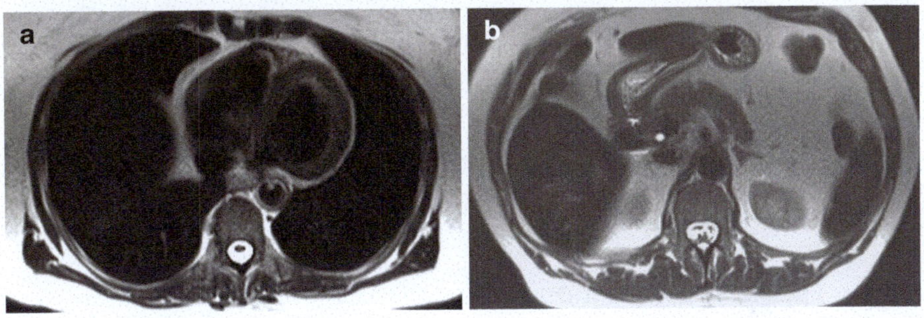

Fig. 6.6 Iron overload by thalassemia vera. T2-W HASTE (**a–b**) in a patient with thalassemia vera show a signal decrease in the liver and the spleen sparing the pancreas and the heart

Hemolytic anemia frequently require blood transfusions and, therefore, a coexisting transfusional iron overload is developed. Patients with thalassemia vera (Fig. 6.6) without transfusions with increased absorption of dietary iron may develop erythrogenic hemochromatosis, primarily affecting the liver. Filtration and tubular absorption of free hemoglobin in sickle cell anemia explain decreased signal of the renal cortex. Paroxysmal nocturnal hemoglobinuria often develops iron overload in the liver and renal cortex.

6.3.5 Diffuse Liver Disease: Vascular Liver Disease

Portal thrombosis may occur in malignant liver tumors (HCC), coagulopathies (cirrhosis), inflammation (pancreatitis), or extrinsic compression (CCC, metastases, lymphomas, etc.) of portal veins and may lead to a cavernous transformation of the portal vein (Fig. 6.7). Higher signal on T2-WI and enhancement on T1-W gadolinium images typically characterize tumor thrombus. Bland thrombus (see Chap.3) shows a lower signal on T2-WI and no gadolinium enhancement. Areas with decreased portal perfusion are usually wedge shaped and may demonstrate an earlier and stronger enhancement during the capillary phase due to a relative increase in arterial supply compared with liver regions with normal portal perfusion. The difference in parenchymal enhancement fades away on delayed contrast-enhanced images. Liver infarcts may occur following surgery, chemoembolisation, trauma, and portal thrombosis, resulting in hypoperfused wedge-shaped defects. Extrahepatic and intrahepatic liver vessels are well demonstrated on dynamic gadolinium-enhanced 3D-T1-WI or gadolinium-enhanced 3D-MRA. Intrahepatic vessels

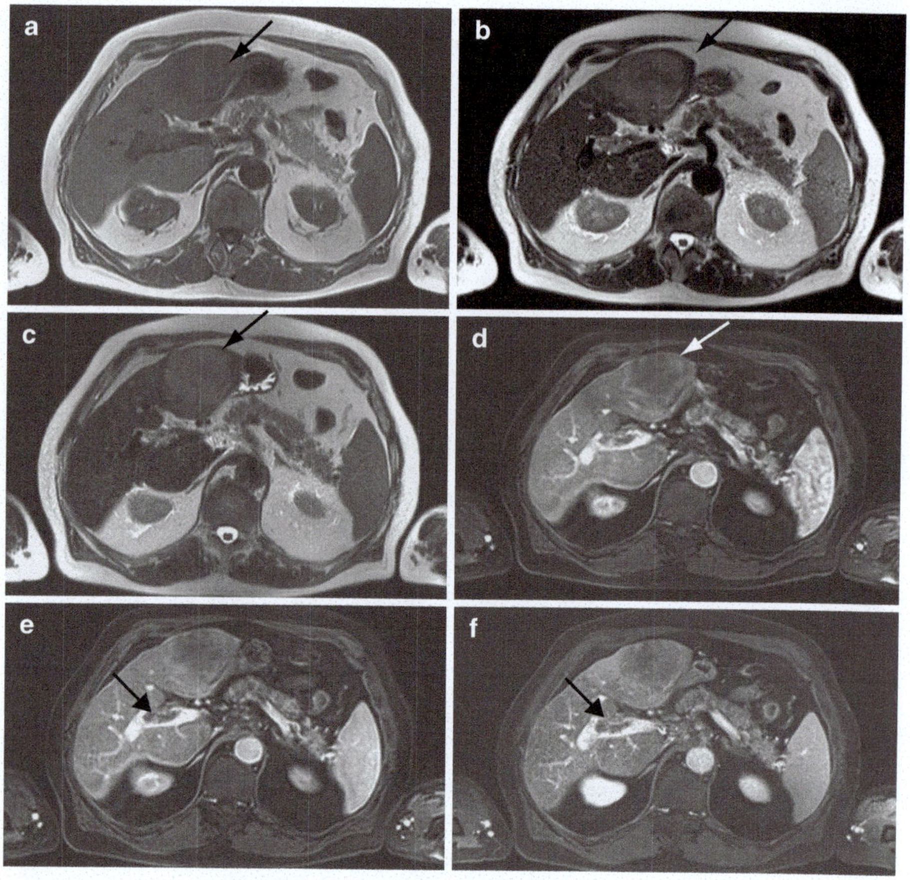

Fig. 6.7 Portal vein tumor thrombus and hepatocellular carcinoma. Plain T1-W spoiled 2D GRE (**a**), T2-W HASTE before ferucarbotran (**b**), T2-W HASTE 10 min following ferucarbotran (**c**), arterial phase gadolinium-enhanced FS T1-W spoiled 3D GRE (**d**), portal venous phase gadolinium-enhanced FS T1-W spoiled 3D GRE (**e**), and venous phase gadolinium-enhanced FS T1-W spoiled 3D GRE (**f**) in a patient with clinical history of alcoholic cirrhosis. A large HCC (*arrows*) is present in segments 2 and 3. The right main portal vein contains a tumor thrombus (*arrows*) with similar enhancement as the HCC

are also visualized on iron oxide-enhanced 2D-TOF images, contrasting the portal venous system against the dark liver parenchyma.

6.3.6 Diffuse Liver Disease: Budd–Chiari Syndrome

Venous outflow in Budd–Chiari's syndrome is often not completely eliminated due to accessory hepatic veins, segmental obstruction, or small veins. Shunting into the portal vein may cause reversed portal flow in patients with portal hypertension. Typically, the caudate lobe and central parts are spared and the right lobe is atrophic. Portosystemic shunts, intrahepatic collaterals, and capsular collaterals are often present. Gadolinium enhancement varies from acute disease with more decreased enhancement to chronic disease with increased enhancement relative to normal or hypertrophied segments. Central parts may, therefore, appear as low signal intensity mass-like lesions. Nodular regenerative hyperplasia may develop in chronic disease, demonstrating a similar signal pattern to adenomatous hyperplastic nodules with high signal intensity on T1-WI, intermediate to low signal intensity on T2-WI, and early enhancement on gadolinium-enhanced images. The differential diagnoses of HCC in individual patients may become quite difficult.

6.3.7 Diffuse Liver Disease: Granulomatous Disease

Granulomatous hepatitis is defined as an inflammatory liver disease associated with granuloma formation in the liver. Granulomatous hepatitis is most commonly associated with sarcoidosis, tuberculosis, and histoplasmosis. Diagnosis of granulomatous hepatitis is based solely on a finding of granulomas in the liver tissue. Hepatic granulomas usually appear as discrete, sharply defined nodular infiltrates consisting of aggregates of epitheloid cells or macrophages surrounded by a rim of mononuclear cells, predominantly lymphocytes.

In tuberculosis, the granulomas may undergo central liquefaction necrosis, and reticulin forms around the granuloma, which eventually undergoes fibrosis. This at MRI, the lesions are hypointense on T1-WI and hypo- to isointense on T2-WI. Percutaneous liver biopsy is necessary in almost all patients with liver lesions that are suspicious for tuberculosis. Sarcoidosis typically presents as multifocal small lesions in size (≤1 cm) in the liver and spleen. Granulomas are hypointense on T1- and T2-WI and show delayed gadolinium enhancement.

6.4 Liver Pathology–Focal Liver Disease

6.4.1 Focal Liver Disease: Cysts

Liver cysts appear as well-defined and frequently multiple focal lesions with a typical signal pattern demonstrating low signal–signal intensity on T1-WI, homogeneous high signal intensity on T2-WI, and no contrast enhancement with either extracellular or liver-specific contrast agents (Fig. 6.8). MRI is superior to CT and US in depicting and characterizing small cysts. Rarely, cysts may appear with higher signal on T1-WI due to a hemorrhagic or proteinaceous content.

6.4.2 Focal Liver Disease: Hemangioma

Hemangioma is the most common solid benign focal liver lesion and is typically detected incidentally. The prevalence in the general population ranges from 1 to 20% with a female-to-male ratio varying from 2:1 to 5:1. Cavernous liver hemangiomas are by far more common than capillary hemangiomas. Because hepatic hemangiomas are most often asymptomatic and have a very low rate of complications, these lesions do not require surgical resection. Therefore, the role of imaging is to characterize the lesion. MR is the best modality to detect and characterize liver hemangioma and should be recommended widely for this clinical question.

MRI is highly reliable for the diagnosis of typical hemangioma with a sensitivity and specificity of greater than 90%. Conversely, the presence of atypical features in cases of hepatic hemangioma may lead to misdiagnosis and confusion with other lesions. At MRI, typical hemangiomas appear as well-defined and lobulated focal lesions. The signal pattern on unenhanced MRI is very similar to cysts with low signal intensity on T1-WI and high signal intensity on T2-WI due to long T1- and T2 relaxation times (>120 ms), which is however less bright than

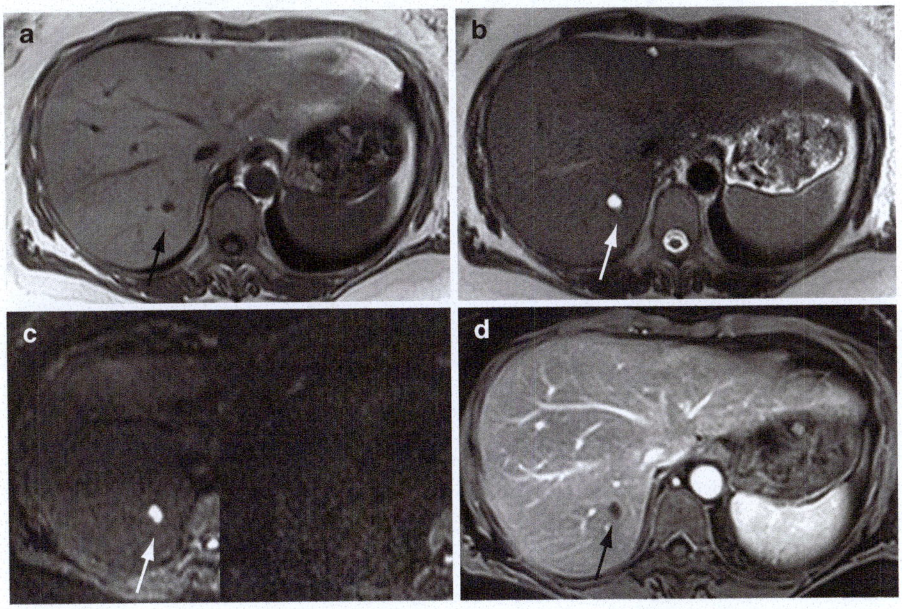

Fig. 6.8 Liver cyst. Plain T1-W spoiled 2D GRE (**a**), T2-W HASTE (**b**), diffusion-weighted imaging at b-values of 50 (*left*) and 800 (*right*) (**c**), and portal venous phase gadolinium-enhanced FS T1-W spoiled 3D GRE (**d**) show a typical cyst in the posterior section of the right liver lobe. The cyst is hypointense on T1-W, hyperintense on T2-W, shows high signal on the small *b*-value, no signal on the high *b*-value, and no contrast enhancement (*arrows*)

cysts. Dynamic and serial gadolinium-enhanced T1-WI is effective in distinguishing hemangiomas from malignant lesions, because hemangiomas typically enhance in a peripheral nodular fashion with subsequent complete or almost complete fill-in of the entire lesion over 5–10 min (Figs. 6.1 and 6.9). Three types of enhancement patterns for dynamic T1-WI have been described:

Type 1. Uniform high signal enhancement during the early phase, without washout

Type 2. Peripheral nodular signal enhancement during the early phase, followed by a centripetal progression to uniform high signal enhancement

Type 3. Peripheral nodular signal enhancement during the early phase, followed by a centripetal progression with a persistent central scar

Type 1. Enhancement is present in small hemangiomas (≤15 mm), type-3 enhancement typically in large hemangiomas (>5 cm) or giant hemangiomas (Fig. 6.10), and type-2 enhancement in hemangiomas of each size. The dynamic pattern of enhancement provides additional criteria to establish the diagnosis of a hemangioma. Nodular enhancement is demonstrated immediately following gadolinium enhancement, which is also frequently eccentric. Enhancement fades away over time without a peripheral or heterogeneous washout (see metastases). Some hemangiomas may also enhance fairly rapidly, within less than 2 min. Hypervascular malignant liver lesions (HCC, leiomyosarcoma, angiosarcoma, and islet cell tumors) may be indistinguishable from small hemangiomas on the

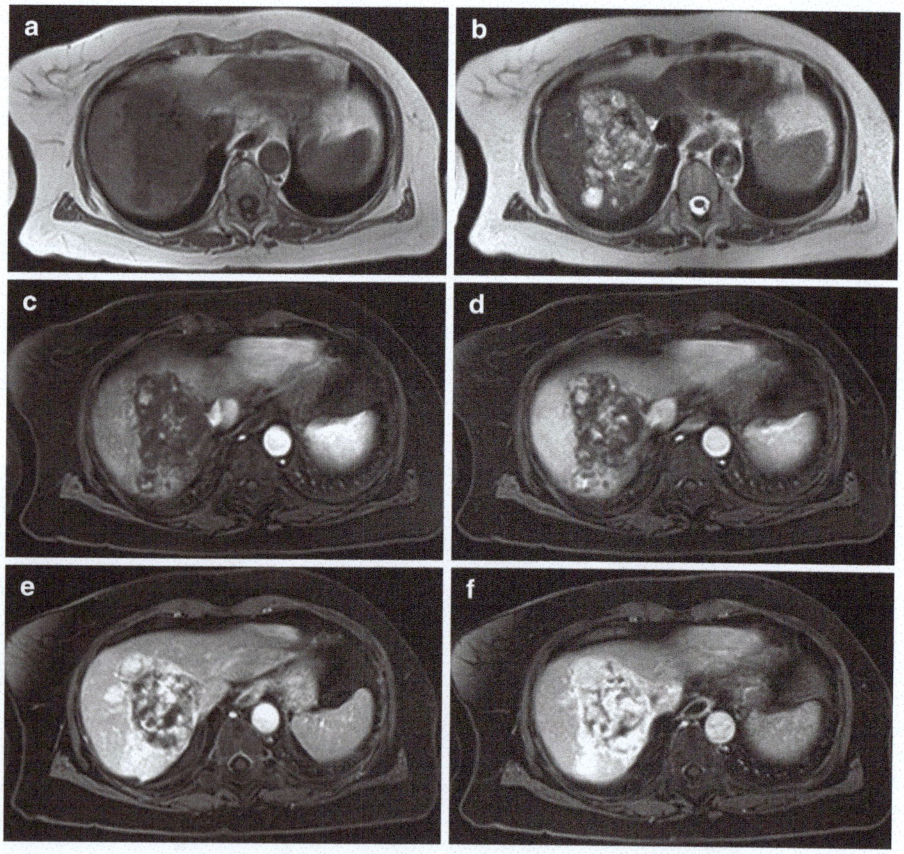

Fig. 6.9 Large hemangioma. Plain T1-W spoiled 2D GRE (**a**), T2-W HASTE (**b**), arterial phase gadobutrol-enhanced FS T1-W spoiled 3D GRE (**c**), portal venous phase-enhanced FS T1-W spoiled 3D GRE (**d**), venous-enhanced FS T1-W spoiled 3D GRE (**e**), and late phase FS T1-W spoiled 2D GRE (**f**) images demonstrate a large hemangioma within the right liver lobe with surrounding smaller hemangioma nodules. The smaller hemangiomas show a typical signal pattern on unenhanced images. The larger hemangioma demonstrates a type-3 enhancement pattern with peripheral nodular gadolinium enhancement, followed by a centripetal progression on delayed gadolinium-enhanced T1-W images without complete uniform signal enhancement. The smaller hemangiomas reveal a type-1 enhancement pattern with early uniform high signal enhancement and homogeneous signal intensity on delayed T1-W images

early arterial phase. However, these malignant tumors will display rapid washout on venous and equilibrium phase scans in contrast to the pooling of gadolinium in hemangiomas. The gadolinium-based hepatobiliary contrast agents demonstrate similar patterns of signal enhancement following bolus injection, such as feasible with MultiHance® or Primovist®. SPIO shows a decrease in signal intensity on heavily T2-WI, and dynamic imaging with Resovist® again may show similar signal patterns as described for T1-W gadolinium-enhanced images (signal increase) and a reversed pattern (signal decrease) on T2 or T2*-WI during the perfusion phase. Delayed T2 or T2*-WI will demonstrate hemangiomas hyopintense.

There are several subtypes of hemangiomas with atypical signal characteristics or morphology.

Large hemangiomas or giant hemangiomas (>7–10 cm) are often heterogeneous and may cause abdominal discomfort (Figs. 6.9 and 6.10). The MRI findings of giant hemangiomas are closely correlated with the macroscopic appearance, which demonstrates changes such as hemorrhage, thrombosis, extensive hyalinization, liquefaction, and fibrosis. Central cleft-like areas may be due to cystic degeneration or liquefaction. The internal septa may correspond to poorly cellular fibrous tissue. T2-WI shows hyperintense cleft-like areas and some hypointense internal septa within an otherwise hyperintense mass.

Following compression of the adjacent portal vein enhancement on immediate postgadolinium images may increase secondary to auto regulatory increased hepatic arterial blood supply. The absence of a central scar in an otherwise mass lesion appearing like a giant hemangioma should raise concern and a biopsy may be required (Fig. 6.10).

Hepatic hemangiomas rarely calcify and small calcifications are typically found incidentally on CT or US. Phleboliths may cause multiple spotty calcifications. Large and more organized calcifications have also been observed. The finding of a solid hepatic

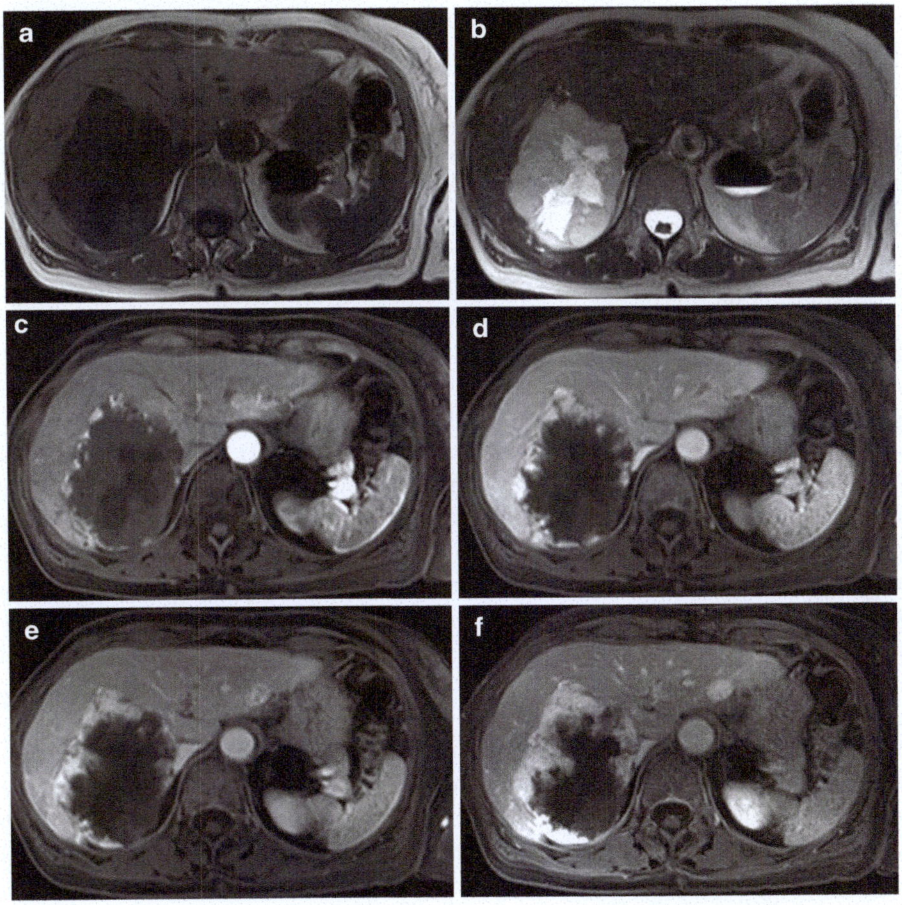

Fig. 6.10 Giant hemangioma. Plain T1-W spoiled 2D GRE (**a**), T2-W Haste (**b**), arterial phase gadobutrol-enhanced FS T1-W spoiled 3D GRE (**c**), portal venous phase-enhanced FS T1-W spoiled 3D GRE (**d**), venous-enhanced FS T1-W spoiled 3D GRE (**e**), and late phase FS T1-W spoiled 2D GRE (**f**) images demonstrate a giant hemangioma with a central scar showing high signal intensity on T2-W images and absent gadolinium enhancement. Dynamic imaging demonstrates a type-3 enhancement pattern with peripheral nodular gadolinium enhancement, followed by a centripetal progression on late gadolinium-enhanced T1-W images

tumor with minor or missing enhancement should not preclude the diagnosis of hemangioma. High signal intensity in noncalcified areas of the lesion on T2-WI can still help in characterizing the lesion.

Hyalinized hepatic hemangiomas are also rare. Pathologic examination reveals extensive fibrous tissue and obliteration of vascular channels. There is speculation that hyalinized hemangiomas represent an end stage of hemangioma involution, typically without clinical symptoms. Hyalinized hemangiomas show only slight hyperintensity on T2-WI and a lack of early enhancement on dynamic T1-WI with reduced peripheral enhancement in the late phase. MRI does not allow differentiation of hyalinized hemangiomas from malignant hepatic tumors. Percutaneous biopsy is indicated in these cases.

Hemangiomas may appear with atypical features such as cystic or multilocular fluid-filled cavities, fluid-fluid levels, or pedunculation. Potential adjacent abnormalities, mainly seen in malignant tumors, range from usually asymptomatic arterial-portal venous shunts, capsular retraction, hemangiomas developing in diffuse fatty liver, regenerative nodular hyperplasia, multiple hemangiomas in up to 10% of patients, or ill-defined borders in giant hemangiomas, particularly in children. There is no clear evidence for the malignant transformation of hemangiomas. Hemangiomas typically remain stable in size or may demonstrate minimal increase in diameter overtime. A relevant or significant enlargement of a hemangioma is rare and these hemangiomas may become symptomatic with a possible role of estrogens such as during pregnancy.

Complications are mostly observed in large hemangiomas and can be divided into alterations of internal architecture such as inflammation; coagulation, which could lead to systemic disorders; hemorrhage, which can cause hemoperitoneum; volvulus; and compression of adjacent structures. Inflammatory reactions may include low-grade fever, weight loss, abdominal pain, accelerated erythrocyte sedimentation rate, anemia, thrombocytosis, and increased fibrinogen level. Clinical and laboratory abnormalities may disappear after surgical excision of the hemangioma.

Kasabach–Merritt syndrome is a rare complication of hepatic hemangiomas in adults consisting of intravascular coagulation, clotting, and fibrinolysis within the hemangioma. The initially localized coagulopathy may progress to secondary increased systemic fibrinolysis and thrombocytopenia with a potentially fatal outcome in up to a quarter of patients.

Intratumoral hemorrhage is rarely encountered in hepatic hemangiomas with symptoms consisting of acute abdominal pain. Acute hemorrhage is suggested by hyperintensity on T1-WI (see Chap. 1). Similar imaging characteristics apply to spontaneous rupture of a hemangioma with hemoperitoneum, which is unusual.

In doubtful cases, percutaneous biopsy, including fine-needle aspiration biopsy, may be performed. Due to the hypervascularity of the lesion, care should be taken when performing the procedure and the needle should pass into the lesion via the hepatic parenchyma. The differential diagnosis of hypervascular hemangiomas includes all hepatic tumors that enhance during the arterial phase of contrast-enhanced MRI, including FNH, hepatocellular adenoma, HCC, or hypervascular metastases.

The coexistence of hepatic hemangioma and FNH (Fig. 6.11) is quite frequent occurring in up to 20% of patients. FNH is considered to be a hyperplastic response due to focal increased arterial flow in the hepatic parenchyma and, like hemangioma, is thought to have a vascular origin. The association between hemangioma and FNH has only been noted in women who had previously used oral contraceptives.

6.4.3 Focal Nodular Hyperplasia

FNH is the second most common benign liver tumor after hemangioma and has a reported prevalence in the order of 1%. FNH is more frequently diagnosed in female (80–90%) than male (10–20%) patients. Approximately 20–25% of the patients have multiple FNH lesions. The combination of multiple FNH lesions and hemangiomas is recognized as multiple FNH syndrome. FNH is often an incidental finding at imaging. Multiple FNH lesions may also be associated with other benign lesions, such as cysts and adenomas.

Distinction between FNH and other hypervascular liver lesions such as hepatocellular adenoma, HCC, and hypervascular metastases is critical to ensure proper treatment. FNH is asymptomatic in most patients, and in such cases, no treatment is necessary. FNH does not have a capsule. The thin (<5 mm) pseudocapsule of FNH results from compression of the surrounding liver parenchyma, perilesion vessels, and inflammatory reaction. The pseudocapsule typically shows high signal intensity on T2-WI and may enhance. A tumor capsule is a characteristic sign of HCC and is

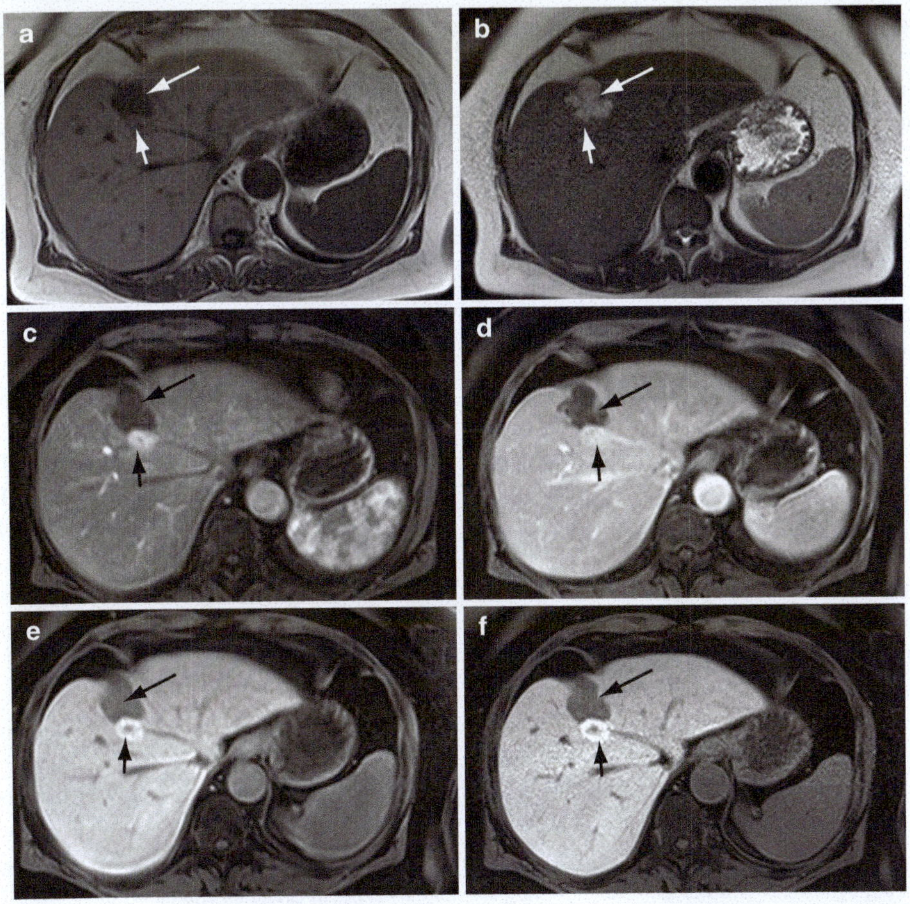

Fig. 6.11 Focal nodular hyperplasia (*long arrows*) with associated hemangioma (*short arrows*). Plain T1-W spoiled 2D GRE (**a**), T2-W HASTE (**b**), arterial phase gadoxetic acid-enhanced FS-T1-W spoiled 3D GRE (**c**), portal venous phase gadoxetic acid-enhanced FS T1-W spoiled 3D GRE (**d**), hepatocellular phase FS-T1-W spoiled 3D GRE (**e**) and high spatial resolution FS-T1-W spoiled GRE 2D (**f**) gadoxetic acid-enhanced FS T1-W spoiled 3D GRE 20 min following contrast injection. The liver demonstrates a lobulated hemangioma (*white arrows*), which is hypointense compared with liver on T1-W (**a**) and hyperintense compared on T2-W imaging (**b**). A solid lesion (FNH - *black arrows*) adjacent to the hemangioma is appreciated on dynamic images (**c, d**) and signal intensity stays high on late phase images due to hepatocellular uptake (**e, f**)

present in 60–80% of cases. This capsule mainly consists of fibrosis and has low signal intensity on bothT1- and T2-WI; it shows persistent enhancement on delayed contrast-enhanced images.

Currently, FNH is divided into two types, classic (80%) and nonclassic (20%). Classic FNH contains all of the components, including an abnormal nodular architecture, malformed vessels, and cholangiolar proliferation. The nonclassic type contains two of the three components but always shows bile ductular proliferation. Both types exhibit Kupffer cells. Typically, FNH contains one or more thick-walled, large arteries that run within the fibrous septa and divide into numerous capillaries that are connected to the sinusoids. Relatively large veins drain blood from the sinusoids toward the hepatic vein. FNH does not contain portal veins. The typical tumor contains hepatocytes, bile duct elements, Kupffer cells, fibrous stroma, and frequently possesses a central scar containing malformed vascular structures. Among classic FNH lesions, one or more macroscopic central scars may be present.

The arterial blood in FNH, as opposed to that in adenomas, flows centrifugally from the central arteries. Hemorrhage is very rare and there is no malignant potential of the lesion.

The typical signal pattern on plain MRI is either isointensity or minimal hyointensity on T1-WI and an isointensity or slightly higher signal intensity on T2-WI than normal liver parenchyma in the vast majority of patients (Fig. 6.11). The central scar is a relatively characteristic feature with high signal intensity on T2-WI, but may be missing in <20% of patients. Gadolinium-enhanced MRI is useful for the detection and characterization of FNH with multisection 2D or 3D GRE sequences featuring a strong uniform blush on arterial phase, and also with rapid fading of enhancement within less than 60 s (Fig. 6.11). A low signal intensity central scar may enhance over time. The delayed enhancement of the central scar relates to increased interstitial space and fluid content with slow diffusion of contrast material into this space. High signal intensity of the central scar may be caused by the inflammatory reaction around the ductular proliferation as well as the vessels within the septa and central scar. The central scar is not a specific finding of FNH and can be seen in a variety of other focal liver lesions such as giant hemangiomas an HCCs. The central scar in giant hemangiomas is typically larger and brighter on T2-WIs. Some HCCs may contain a central scar. Owing to the presence of scar tissue, calcifications, or necrosis, the central scar in HCC shows low signal intensity on T2- and T1-WI and does not enhance much on contrast-enhanced images. Although HCCs occur in noncirrhotic livers, the lesions show quite a different type of enhancement than FNH. In general, one should be very cautious to diagnose a FNH in a patient with cirrhosis, even if a central scar is present. Any hypervascular lesion in cirrhosis has to be suspected for HCC. Hepatocellular adenomas show less intense enhancement and lack a central scar.

The higher sensitivity and specificity of MRI for FNH than US or CT also may be due to the fact that MRI provides a number of unique possibilities concerning the technique of data acquisition and contrast medium administration.

Gadolinium-enhanced MRI is useful for the detection and characterization of FNH with a strong uniform blush on arterial phase gadolinium-enhanced T1-W spoiled GRE images, and also with rapid fading of enhancement within less than 60 s. A low signal intensity central scar enhances over time.

Rarely, FNH may show more than one atypical feature at MRI and cause difficulty in diagnosis. Such lesions may have exceptionally high signal intensity on T2-WI with a suggestion of lamellae, a central scar with low signal intensity on T2-WI, a prominent pseudocapsule, and incomplete intense enhancement of the lesion. In such cases, application of a specific type of contrast medium, such as hepatobiliary agents such as gadoxetic acid or SPIO such as ferucarbotran, may demonstrate the hepatocellular origin of the lesion. When there is homogeneous uptake of such an agent in combination with a normal α-fetoprotein level and normal results at viral serologic analysis, the patient may be safely followed up with imaging. If any doubt remains, one or more biopsies should be performed within the lesion as well as the surrounding liver to exclude malignancies, such as fibrolamellar carcinoma and HCC in a noncirrhotic liver. Hepatobiliary agents enhance FNH, similar to adenomas, reflecting the presence of well-differentiated hepatocytes with well-differentiated HCC or early dedifferentiation as a differential diagnosis (Fig. 6.11). The central scar may enhance to a lesser degree. It has been proposed using MultiHance® for differentiating FNH and adenoma since FNH enhances on delayed images, which is not regularly observed with adenoma.

All SPIO are effective for the characterization of FNH on T2-W accumulation phase images because of phagocytic cells within the tumor, resulting in a signal decrease. Therefore, lesions are less visible on SPIO-enhanced accumulation phase images than on plain images.

Diagnoses of typical FNH may be confirmed with at least one follow-up MRI examination at 6–12 months. Atypical cases may undergo additional imaging with specific contrast media to rule out malignancy. MRI is an ideal imaging modality for work-up of lesions in relatively young women suspected of having FNH because radiation and iodine-based contrast media are not used.

6.4.4 Focal Liver Disease: Adenoma

Liver adenomas have a strong association with oral contraception and more than 90% are found in young females. Further reported associations are familial diabetes mellitus, galactosemia, glycogen storage disease type 1, and anabolic steroids. Liver cell adenomas are composed of sheets of cells that may resemble normal hepatocytes and lack a central scar and radiating septa as described in detail for FNH. Necrosis and hemorrhage, which may be life threatening, are common causes of pain. In addition, according to the currently used terminology, Hepatocellular adenomas are more recently classified as premalignant nodules and preferably treated surgically.

Adenomas may contain fat, intracellular glycogen, may present with a thin pseudocapsule, and show a loose architecture. The hepatocyte origin explains why adenomas vary in signal from hypointense to hyperintense (fat content) on T1-WI and are typically slightly hyperintense on T2-WI. Some adenomas are almost isointense to normal liver. Fat-containing adenomas demonstrate a signal decrease on opposed-phase images, and hemorrhage causes mixed signal patterns.

Gadolinium-enhanced MRI (Fig. 6.12) shows a strong transient blush on arterial phase gadolinium-enhanced T1-W spoiled GRE images, also with rapid vanishing of enhancement within less than 60s. Hepatobiliary agents enhance adenomas, although usually to a lesser degree than FNH, reflecting the presence of well-differentiated hepatocytes within tumors, again with well-differentiated HCC or early dedifferentiation as a differential diagnosis.

SPIO again shows a similar pattern as described for FNH and observed for regenerating nodules with a signal decrease on T2-W accumulation phase images. Additional information for lesion characterization may be obtained by dynamic imaging.

6.4.5 Focal Liver Disease: Metastases

Metastases are the most common liver tumors in western countries. Contrast-enhanced MRI exceeds the diagnostic ability of contrast-enhanced MDCT to detect and subsequently characterize malignant focal liver lesions. Lesion characterization is of particular importance in patients with primary malignancies, because even in this selected population, up to 50% of small lesions (<10–15 mm) may be benign. Imaging protocols include transverse plain and contrast-enhanced T1- and/or T2-W pulse sequences, depending on the contrast agents administered. The acquisition of an additional T1- or T2-W sagittal or coronal plane may be useful to depict lesions at the diaphragmal surface of the liver.

Contrast enhancement with extracellular low-molecular gadolinium chelates requires rapid T1-W spoiled GRE imaging before, during the arterial phase (hypervascular lesions), during the portal venous phase (hypovascular lesions), and plain T2-W images with moderate (detection) and long (characterization) TEs. Fat saturation of T2-W TSE sequences may be advantageous to facilitate detection of superficial lesions. Delayed T1-W imaging is recommended to observe slow fill-in patterns.

Contrast enhancement with hepatobiliary agents is best performed with T1-WI before and at different time points following rapid contrast injection (MultiHance®

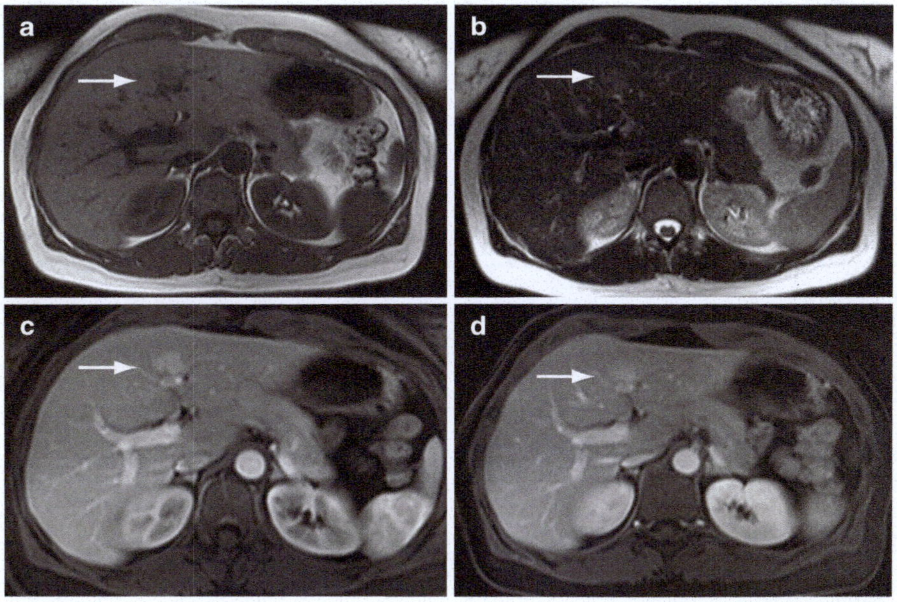

Fig. 6.12 Adenoma. Plain T1-W spoiled 2D GRE (**a**), T2-W HASTE (**b**), arterial phase gadolinium-enhanced FS-T1-W spoiled 3D GRE (**c**), and portal venous phase gadolinium-enhanced FS-T1-W spoiled 3D GRE (**d**). The liver demonstrates a single lesion in the left liver lobe (*arrow*), which is slightly hypointense compared with liver on T1-W spoiled 2D GRE and hyperintense on T2-W HASTE. Contrast-enhanced FS-T1 3D GRE shows strong enhancement during the arterial phase and decreasing enhancement during the portal venous phase (*arrows*)

and Primovist®) or infusion (Teslascan®). T2-WI with moderate (detection) and long (characterization) TEs is typically performed before contrast administration. With the gadolinium-based hepatobiliary agents (Primovist®, MultiHance®), dynamic T1-WI is helpful to study the perfusion phase of lesions comparable to extracellular low-molecular gadolinium chelates, and delayed imaging (>1 h for MultiHance® and ≥20 min for Teslascan® and Primovist®) has to be performed because of nonspecific enhancement of lesions during the perfusion phase. Malignant nonhepatocellular lesions exhibit constant signal on T1-W delayed images. However, the presence of hepatocytes within early stages of HCC may cause enhancement comparable to liver tissue (see adenoma and FNH).

It is recommended to acquire T1-WI in a second plane as part of the protocol for delayed scanning to look for small lesions close to the liver capsule beneath the diaphragm.

Metastases are typically hypointense on T1-WI and moderately hyperintense on T2-WI (Fig. 6.13). Lesion border may be either irregular or sharp, and lesion shape can be irregular, oval, or round. Hemorrhage may result in hyperintense lesions on T1- and hypointense lesions on T2-WI. Coagulative necrosis (colorectal metastases) results in a hypointense lesion center and hyperintense periphery (viable tumor) on T2-WI. Mucin-producing tumors demonstrate high signal intensity on T2. Cystic or extensive necrotic metastasis can appear strongly hyperintense on T2-WI and, thus, resemble hemangiomas or liver cysts. Most metastases of colorectal origin or other carcinomas appear hypointense on T1-WI. Metastases could show a signal intensity decrease when they are strongly fibrotic or contain calcifications. Hyperintense pseudolesions caused by fatty degeneration are found adjacent to the gallbladder, the falciforme ligament and in segment IV. In- and opposed-phase sequences or chemical shift imaging help to reach an accurate diagnosis noninvasively avoiding biopsy.

Hypovascular metastases (Fig. 6.13) represent the vast majority (colorectal) of metastases and the perfusion pattern is based on a diminished blood supply. Thus, similar to CT, lesions are typically best detected on the portal venous gadolinium-enhanced T1-WI. Plain images typically show low signal intensity on T1-WI and slightly higher signal intensity or almost isointensity on T2-WI. Metastases with large amounts of liquefactive necrosis may appear as cystic lesions with a signal void on immediate gadolinium-enhanced T1-WI. A peripheral enhancement is common on portal venous phase and delayed T1-WI. Typically, peripheral ring enhancement begins on immediate arterial phase contrast-enhanced images with potential enhancement toward the center of the lesion and peripheral washout on delayed T1-WI. It has been demonstrated that perilesional

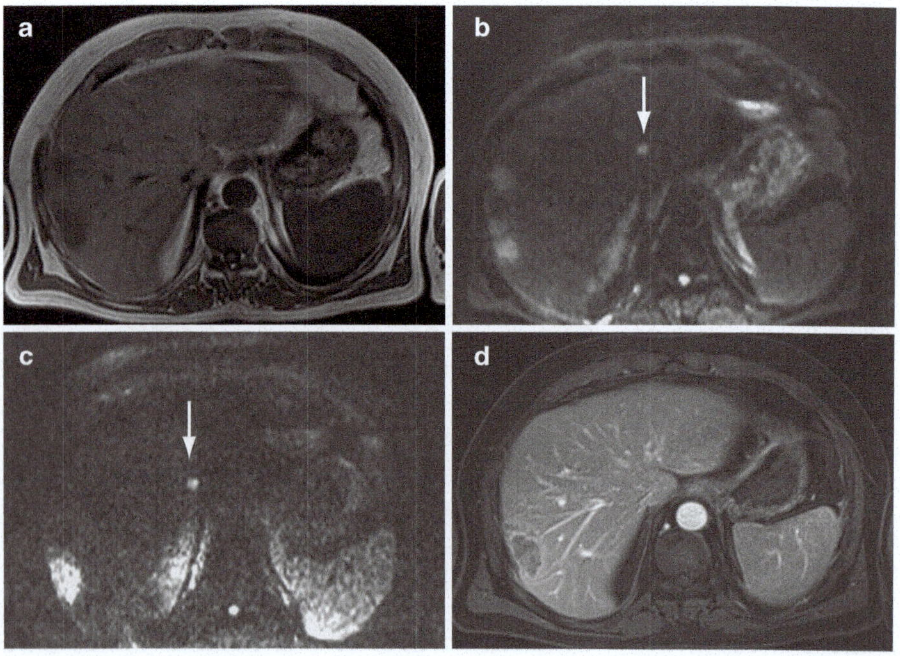

Fig. 6.13 Hypovascular metastases (colon cancer). Plain T1-W spoiled 2D GRE (**a**), DWI b 50 (**b**), DWI b 800 (**c**), and portal venous phase gadolinium-enhanced FS T1-W spoiled 3D GRE (**d**) in a patient with multiple liver metastases. The small metastasis on the DWI sequences adjacent to segment 1 (*arrows*) shows typical signal pattern of a solid lesion and is barely seen on the contrast-enhanced T1-W image demonstrating the added value of DWI

enhancement of metastases on early gadolinium-enhanced MR images correlates with histopathologic hepatic parenchymal changes, which include peritumoral desmoplastic reaction, inflammatory cell infiltration, and vascular proliferation. Approximately 10 min after application of contrast media, metastases often show a peripheral hypointense rim (peripheral washout sign) that is a specific sign for malignancy. In the case of metastases from adenocarcinoma, a multiplicity of lesions is characteristic. Some metastases show a complete uptake of nonspecific gadolinium contrast media and, thus, appear isointense compared with the normal surrounding liver parenchyma, which must not be confused with the enhancing properties of hemangiomas. These small metastases must be differentiated from hemangiomas on the basis of their appearance on T2-W and dynamic sequences.

Large colorectal metastases may show an additional inhomogeneous "cauliflower-enhancement." These enhancement features are also observed with dynamically scanned liver-specific contrast agents.

A variety of primary malignancies frequently cause hypervascular metastases (pheochromocytoma, renal cell, neuroendocrine, leiomyosarcoma, thyroid, or melanoma). Hypervascular metastases (Fig. 6.14) may appear with high signal on T2-WI, comparable with hemangiomas, and show an intense peripheral ring enhancement with a potential progressing centripetal enhancement. Small hypervascular metastases vary in contrast enhancement with immediate and often complete lesion enhancement.

The different melanin content of melanoma metastases causes different hyperintense/hypointense patterns on T1- and T2-WI, because the paramagnetic property of melanin presents hyperintense on T1-WI. Dynamic gadolinium-enhanced MRI is particularly useful for the detection and characterization of hypervascular liver lesions with immediate ring-type, uniform, or irregular enhancement and subsequent washout effects. The absence of nodular enhancement within the enhancing ring-type periphery, the uniform thickness of the enhancing ring, and the peripheral

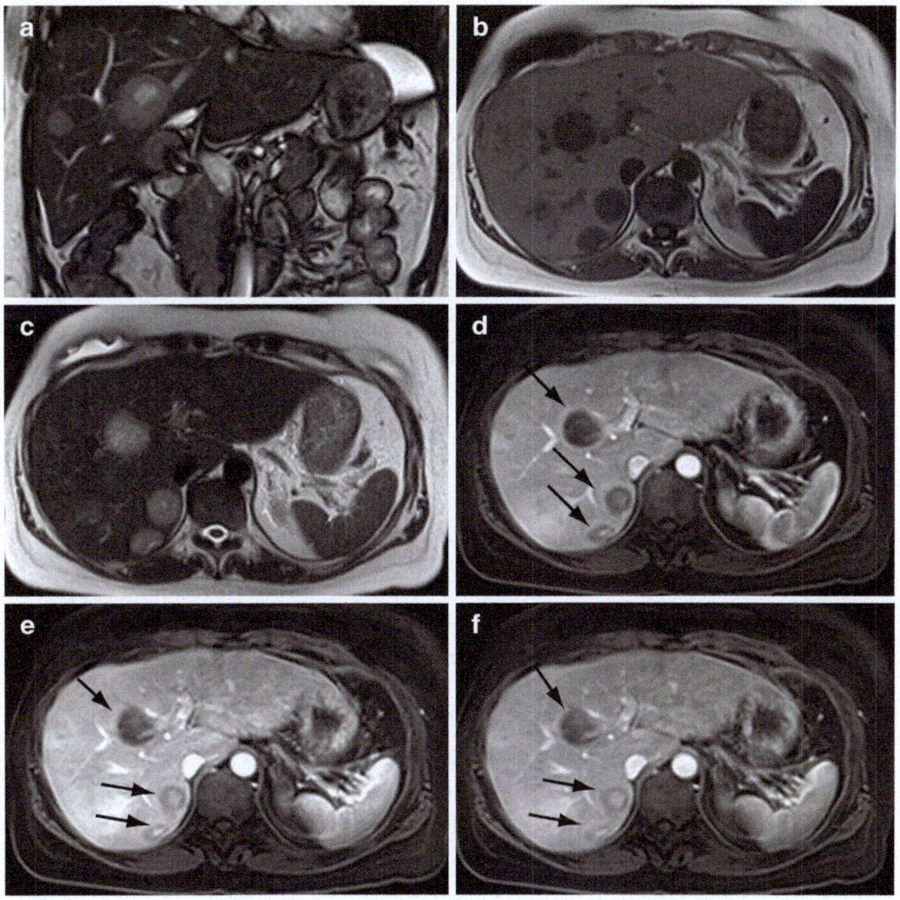

Fig. 6.14 Breast cancer metastases. Coronal True-FISP localizer (**a**), plain T1-W spoiled 2D GRE (**b**), T2-W HASTE (**c**), and multiple phase gadolinium-enhanced FS T1-W spoiled 3D GRE (**d–f**) in a patient with breast cancer liver metastases. Dynamic contrast-enhanced imaging shows a hypervascular ring-like enhancement in most lesions (*arrow*) with initial washout on the next phase and subsequent enhancement of metastases (*arrows*)

washout help to differentiate malignant lesions from hemangiomas, which also show enhancement of a longer period of time.

One of the major advantages of liver-specific contrast agents is the improved detection of hypovascular liver metastases as compared to gadolinium-enhanced MRI or contrast-enhanced CT techniques. The administration of SPIO or hepatobiliary contrast media improves the detection rate of metastases. In preoperative patients, hepatobiliary contrast-enhanced MRI is extremely helpful in the detection and delineation of small liver metastases, especially small metastases that are immediately adjacent to the venous system. The combined use of very thin slices, using T1-W 3D GRE sequences, and delayed contrast-enhanced hepatocyte-specific MR images improves the detection rate of liver metastases considerably, both, at 1.5 and 3.0 T. Furthermore, small liver metastases, which could imitate vessels, can be reliably identified by means of multiplanar reconstructions with near-isotropic imaging.

In principle, contrast-enhanced MRI is superior to CT with regard to the detection and characterization of small focal liver lesions. Small focal liver lesions <10 mm in patients with a history of cancer are of benign character in 80% of cases. MRI with liver-specific contrast media such as gadoxetic acid is the best modality for the detection and characterization of focal liver lesions and should be used for the characterization of equivocal lesions and for patients who are considered candidates for liver resection or oncologic liver intervention. Furthermore, fatty degeneration of the liver parenchyma, as a possible result of chemotherapy, reduces the CT detection rate of liver metastases considerably. Contrast-enhanced MRI of the liver can compensate for these limitations of MDCT.

6.4.6 *Focal Liver Disease: Hepatocellular Carcinoma*

Worldwide, HCC is the most common primary malignancy, because of the high prevalence in Asia and Africa. HCC in Europe and North America predominantly arises on the basis of chronic liver disease, such as chronic active forms of hepatitis, alcoholic cirrhosis, and hemochromatosis. A stepwise carcinogenesis for HCC has been proposed on the basis of gradually increasing size and cellular density among regenerative nodules, dysplastic nodule, early HCC, and early advanced HCC. The stepwise sequence of events includes the following steps: regenerative nodule, low-grade dysplastic nodule, high-grade dysplastic nodule, small HCC, and large HCC. Alternatively, a de novo pathway for HCC in cirrhotic as well as noncirrhotic livers with a single cell or a group of hepatocytes as a focus of small HCC that will grow into a large HCC is described. At some point during the whole process, formation of new tumor vessels (tumor angiogenesis, neovascularity) takes place.

Hepatic nodules are categorized into two groups: regenerative lesions and dysplastic or neoplastic lesions.

Regenerative nodules result from localized proliferation of hepatocytes and their supporting stroma, including monoacinar regenerative nodules, multiacinar regenerative nodules, cirrhotic nodules, segmental or lobar hyperplasia, and FNH. The diameter of monoacinar nodules is usually 0.1–10 mm, and that of multiacinar nodules should be at least 2 mm. Large multiacinar nodules are usually 5–15 mm in diameter. Cirrhotic nodules are regenerative nodules that are largely or completely surrounded by fibrous septa. Cirrhotic nodules can be monoacinar or multiacinar. Macronodular cirrhosis contains nodules larger than 3 mm in diameter. Dysplastic or neoplastic lesions are composed of hepatocytes that show histologic characteristics of abnormal growth caused by a presumed or proved genetic alteration.

Dysplastic or neoplastic nodules include hepatocellular adenoma, dysplastic foci, dysplastic nodules, and HCC. Dysplastic foci are common in cirrhosis and uncommon in noncirrhotic livers. Dysplastic nodules (>1 mm) with low-grade dysplasia may show an altered liver parenchymal structure as well as an increased number of cells with an increased nuclei-to-cytoplasm ratio. Nodules with high-grade dysplasia show increased thickness of the layers of hepatocytes, which contain nuclei that are variable in size and shape. HCC is a malignant neoplasm composed of cells with hepatocellular differentiation. A small HCC is defined as less than or equal to 2 cm in diameter. The criteria used to distinguish HCC from high-grade dysplastic nodules are not clearly defined. Therefore, the histologic differentiation between small HCCs and dysplastic nodules may become critical.

The signal intensity and enhancement characteristics of dysplastic nodules are not yet well established. Owing to a gradual stepwise transition from a regenerative nodule to a low-grade dysplastic nodule, a high-grade dysplastic nodule, and eventually to a small HCC and a large HCC, the hepatocytes within hepatic nodules undergo numerous changes that might not be reflected in their signal intensity or vascularity. Thus, current MRI sequences might not allow differentiation of regenerative nodules from dysplastic nodules. The majority of high-grade dysplastic lesions (formerly known as adenomatous hyperplasia) and well-differentiated small HCCs (Edmondson grade I or II) have high signal intensity on T1-WI.

Histologic grading differentiates among hepatocellular nodules depending on tumor differentiation from I to IV.

Grade I – cells are similar in size to normal hepatocytes, arranged in relatively thin trabeculae, some bile containing acini.

Grade II – cells that are larger than normal hepatocytes, more hyperchromatic nuclei, thicker trabeculae are, acini with bile are common.

Grade III – hepatocytes with larger nuclei (>50% of cytoplasm), trabeculae still dominant, present solid areas and isolated cells, giant and bizarre cells common, bile rarely present.

Grade IV – cells with nuclei occupying most of the cytoplasm, mostly solid, bile rarely found, intravascular and intrasinusoidal growth.

Grade I cell populations may be difficult to distinguish from hepatocellular adenomas, and grade IV cell populations may be difficult to distinguish from tumors of nonhepatocellular origin.

Small HCC is a solitary lesion ≤2 cm in diameter. High-grade dysplastic nodules and small HCC may have a nodule-within-a-nodule appearance on MR images, especially if a focus of HCC originates within a siderotic regenerative nodule. On T1-WI, such lesions typically show markedly low signal intensity of a large nodule, with internal foci that are isointense to the liver. On T2-WI, this appearance may consist of low signal intensity of a large nodule, with one or more internal foci of higher signal intensity. The recognition of HCC while still small is important because the tumor is aggressive and has a fast doubling time. Small HCC may also appear as small areas of slightly higher signal intensity than the surrounding liver on T2-WI. On T1-WI, such areas may be isointense, hypointense, or hyperintense to the liver. On arterial phase dynamic Gd-enhanced images, most small HCCs are well perfused, enhancing lesions during arterial phase images.

Large HCCs may have a number of characteristic features, such as a mosaic pattern, a tumor capsule (60–80%), extracapsular extension or intravascular invasion. HCC grows predominantly as a solitary tumor in 50% of patients or multifocal in 40% of patients, but is rarely diffuse (in less than 10% of patients).

The tumor capsule becomes thicker with increasing tumor size and is composed of two layers, an inner fibrous layer and an outer layer containing compressed vessels and bile ducts. The tumor capsule is hypointense on both T1- and T2-WI in most cases, although capsules with a thickness of more than 4 mm can have an outer hyperintense layer on T2-WI. The pseudocapsule appears hypointense on early Gd-enhanced T1-WI and with some enhancement on delayed T1-WI.

Extracapsular extension of the tumor, with partial projections or formation of satellite nodules in the immediate vicinity, is present in 40–80% of HCCs.

Vascular invasion occurs frequently and typically affects both the portal vein (20–30%) as well as the hepatic veins (50–60%) (Fig. 6.7). Vascular invasion may be seen as lack of a signal void unenhanced T1- or T2-WI with flow compensation. In postcontrast Gd-enhanced images, the tumor thrombus typically shows enhancement on images acquired during the arterial phase comparable to the intrahepatic component and a filling defect on images acquired during later phases.

In patients without cirrhosis or other underlying liver disease, HCC is usually diagnosed at a very late stage with larger lesion size, more often solitary, and more frequently containing a central scar.

HCCs show a variable signal pattern on plain MR images. As a rule of thumb, one-third appear hypointense, one-third isointense, and one-third hyperintense (fat, copper, or proteins) compared to liver SI on T1-WI. Signal intensity on T2-WI varies from almost isointensity to slight hyperintensity relative to liver parenchyma (Fig. 6.15).

Dynamic gadolinium-enhanced MRI with thin section 3D sequences demonstrates the hypervascular nature of tumors with often diffuse and intense enhancement, which typically involves the entire tumor stroma, while metastases predominantly reveal peripheral enhancement. The intensity of enhancement appears to correlate with tumor grading, and well-differentiated lesions may be completely hypovascular (Fig. 6.15).

Patients with preexisting cirrhosis require careful image analysis, and any mass lesion with either hyperintensity on T2-WI or diffuse enhancement on gadolinium-enhanced images should be considered as potential HCC

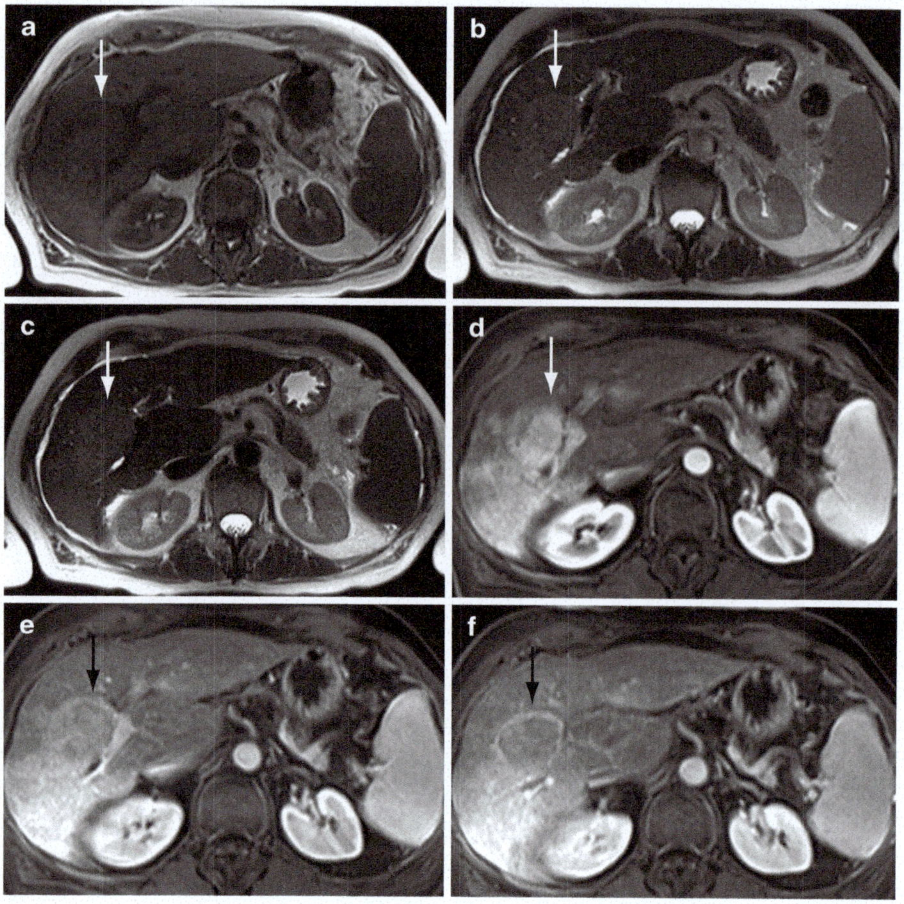

Fig. 6.15 Hepatocellular carcinoma (*arrows*) with dual contrast enhancement. Plain T1-W spoiled 2D GRE (**a**), T2-W Haste before ferucarbotran (**b**), T2-W HASTE 10 min following ferucarbotran (**c**), arterial phase gadolinium-enhanced FS T1-W spoiled 3D GRE (**d**), portal venous phase gadolinium-enhanced FS T1-W spoiled 3D GRE (**e**), and venous phase gadolinium-enhanced FS T1-W spoiled 3D GRE (**f**) in a patient with clinical history hepatitis C. Liver cirrhosis with hypertrophy of the left lobe, splenomegaly, and ascites is present. A well-demarcated mass with a pseudocapsule on T1-W (**a**) is present in the right liver lobe before and following ferucarbotran-enhanced T2-W images. Gadolinium-enhanced images following ferucarbotran (**d–f**) show a wedge-shaped portal perfusion defect based on compression of the inferior right portal vein and a satellite node adjacent to the main mass (**d**,**e**). The liver parenchyma within the perfusion defect enhances stronger during the capillary phase due to a relative increase in arterial supply compared with liver parenchyma that has normal portal perfusion. The difference in parenchymal enhancement fades away on portal venous phase images (**d**)

(Fig. 6.15). In general, dynamic gadolinium-enhanced pulse sequences are the best sequences to detect HCC.

SPIO are suited to improve the detection of HCC in cirrhosis because both, regenerating nodules and dysplastic nodules, contain RES cells and, therefore, show uptake of particles. Phagocytic cells may be present within early stages of HCC, which may then also show some enhancement. The combined application of SPIO followed by dynamic Gd-enhanced dynamic T1-WI during the intracellular phase of the SPIO with a hyopintense liver has become increasingly popular as an off-label application. Hepatobiliary contrast agents may not consistently add information to a dynamic gadolinium-enhanced study, because there is no clear-cut decrease or increase of hepatobiliary agent uptake with the gradual development from high-grade dysplasia into early HCC. Some HCCIS show uptake of gadoxeticaced (Primovist®, Eovist®) an late images (also called green HCC).

Fibrolamellar HCC represents a slow growing subtype with good prognosis that occurs predominantly in young females without underlying liver disease as a large and solitary lesion. At histologic analysis, the lesions consist of large eosinophilic, polygonal neoplastic cells arranged in sheets, cords, or trabeculae separated by parallel sheets of fibrous tissue (i.e., lamellae).

Therefore, fibrolamellar carcinoma should be considered a separate entity. Vascular invasion occurs in less than 5% of cases. Regional adenopathy may be present in up to 50–70% of patients, and distant metastases are uncommon (<20%). A central scar with radiating appearance is common. Lesions demonstrate heterogeneous hypointensity on T1-WI and heterogeneous hyperintensity on T2-WI. Gadolinium enhancement is diffuse without enhancement of the scar, which appears also hypointense on T2-WI (see also Sect. 6.4.3).

6.4.7 Focal Liver Disease: Cholangiocarcinoma

Intrahepatic CCC is the second most common form of primary hepatic malignancy and is derived from the biliary epithelium. However, CCC is by far not as common as HCC. Extrahepatic CCC deriving from the extrahepatic bile ducts is more common (90%) than intrahepatic CCC (10%).

Intrahepatic CCC typically presents as a large mass lesion in elderly patients with low signal intensity on T1-WI and moderate signal intensity on T2-WI. Signal intensity on T2-WI varies with fibrous content (lower SI) and mucin content (higher SI). Gadolinium-enhanced T1-WI typically demonstrates a hypovascular tumor with minimal to diffuse heterogeneous enhancement, which then persists on delayed images with some variation going along with fibrous issue components (Fig. 6.16). Enhancement patterns with gadobenate dimeglumine and gadoxetic acid during dynamic imaging are similar to imaging with extracellular gadolinium chelates. Since CCC is devoid of Kupffer cells, uptake of SPIO is not significant and

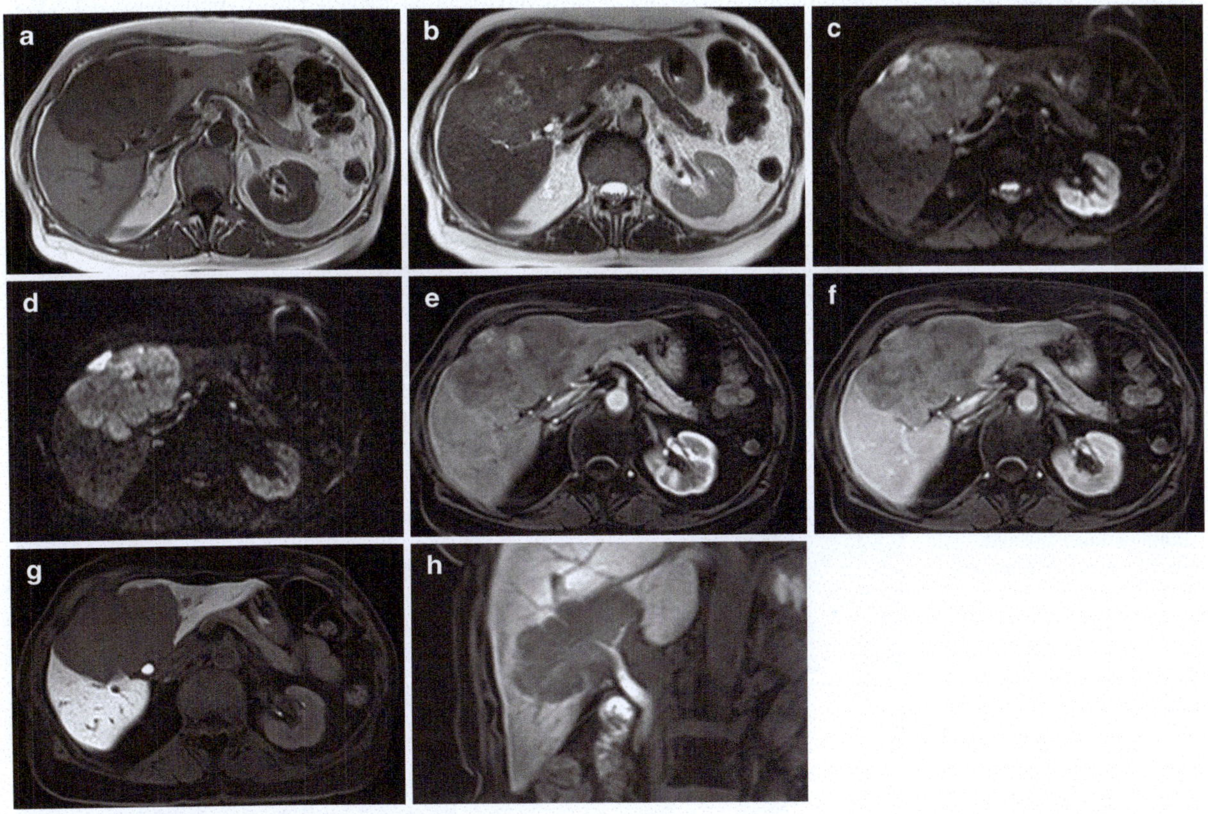

Fig. 6.16 Cholangiocellular carcinoma. Plain T1-W spoiled 2D GRE (**a**), T2-W HASTE (**b**), DWI with *b*-values of 400 (**c**) and 800 (**d**), arterial phase gadoxetic acid-enhanced FS T1-W spoiled 3D GRE (**e**), portal venous phase-enhanced FS T1-W spoiled 3D GRE (**f**), and late phase gadoxetic acid-enhanced axial (**g**) and coronal (**h**) FS T1-W spoiled images 3D GRE 20–30 min postcontrast show a large tumor centrally in the liver. The tumor is hypointense on T1, slightly hyperintense on T2, and shows persistent high signal with increasing *b*-values. Dynamic T1-weighted images (T1-WIs) demonstrate a hypovascular lesions and late phase T1-WIs absent uptake proving the nonhepatocellular nature of the lesion. Coronal images show encasement of the biliary hilum and proximal common bile duct, which are enhanced by biliary excreted contrast material (see Chap. 1)

CCC appears more conspicuous on T2-WI after injection of SPIO. CCC causes compression of portal veins and the biliary system.

6.4.8 Focal Liver Disease: Infectious Diseases

Pyogenic abscesses may exhibit variable signal intensity on T1-WI and T2-WI, however, typically show low signal intensity on T1-WI, moderate to high signal intensity on T2-WI (hyperintense necrotic center), and a thick rim of perilesional enhancement on gadolinium-enhanced T1-WI with an indistinct or irregular outer margin (Fig. 6.17). There may be an overlap of imaging features with hematoma, however, applying signal analysis as presented in Chap. 1 should lead to the correct diagnosis (Fig. 6.18).

Amebic abscesses have homogeneous low signal intensity on T1-WI and high signal intensity on T2-WI. Perilesional edema is seen on T2-WI in up to 50% of cases. Amebic abscesses are typically encapsulated with enhancement of the capsule.

Echinococcal disease presents as echinococus granulosus or echinococus multilocularis. MRI demonstrates features of echinococus granulosus like the pericyst, the matrix or hydatid debris, and the daughter cysts. The pericyst is seen as a hypointense rim on both T1-WI and T2-WI because of its fibrous composition and the potential presence of calcifications. MRI cannot reliably distinguish the fibrous tissue of the capsule from calcifications. The fibrous capsule and the internal septations are well shown on gadolinium-enhanced MRI. The hydatid matrix appears hypointense on T1-WI and markedly hyperintense on T2-WI; daughter cysts are hypointense relative to the matrix on both T1- and T2-WI.

Echinococus multilocularis presents with multiple irregular, ill-defined lesions scattered throughout the involved liver that are generally hyperintense at T2-WI. This signal pattern may mimic either metastases or

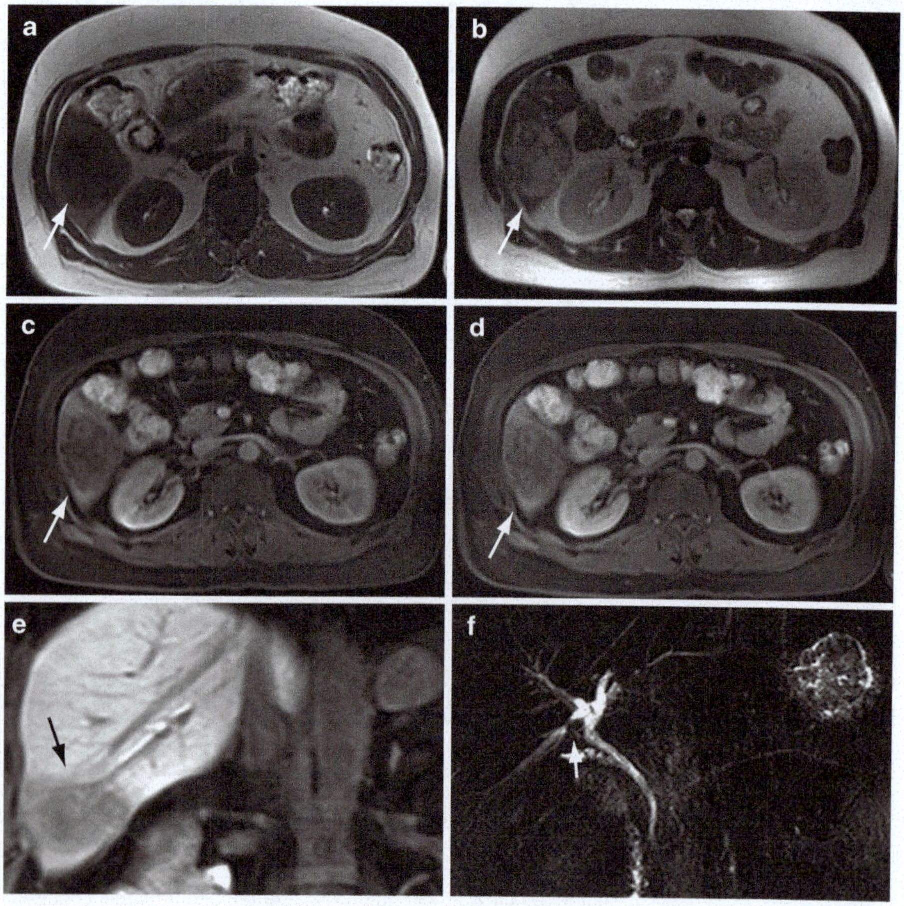

Fig. 6.17 Liver abscess. (*long arrows*). Plain T1-W spoiled 2D GRE (**a**), T2-W HASTE (**b**), portal venous phase gadoxetic acid-enhanced FS T1-W spoiled 3D GRE (**c**), venous phase gadoxetic acid-enhanced FS T1-W spoiled 3D GRE (**d**), coronal late phase gadoxetic acid-enhanced FS T1-W spoiled 3D GRE (**e**), and MRCP projection (**f**) in a patient with clinical history of cholangitis. Plain and dynamic contrast-enhanced images show a mass in segments 5 and 6 of the right liver lobe with hypointense appearance on T1-W, some hyperintensity on T2-W with peripheral and ring-like contrast enhancement. The potential cause of the subsequently drained abscess is visible on the late gadoxetic acid-enhanced image (**e**) and the MRCP (**f**) showing a central stenosis of the right inferior bile duct (*small arrow*)

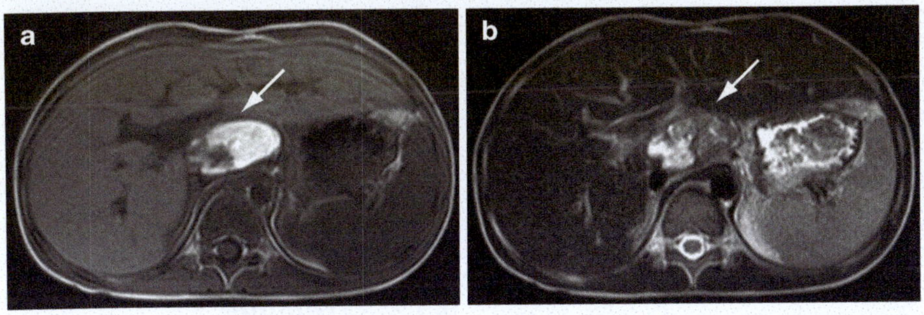

Fig. 6.18 Hematoma (*arrows*). Plain T1-W spoiled 2D GRE (**a**) and T2-W HASTE (**b**) in a child following blunt abdominal trauma with right upper quadrant pain. A mass is visible within the caudate lobe characterized by mostly hyperintense components in T1-W and hypointense components in T2-W. The different signal intensities reflect different stages of hematoma evolvement (see Chap. 1 for further details)

CCC. However, there is little or no enhancement after gadolinium administration. Advanced disease may cause hilar infiltration, dilatation of the intrahepatic bile ducts and invasion of the portal and hepatic veins, with subsequent atrophy of the affected liver segments due to hypoperfusion.

Hepatosplenic fungal infection is a clinical manifestation of disseminated fungal disease in patients with hematologic malignancies or compromise of the immunologic system. The reported prevalence of fungal dissemination in affected patients ranges from 20 to 40%. Microabscesses often also involve the spleen and, occasionally, the kidney. Most hepatic fungal microabscesses occur in leukemia patients and are caused by candida albicans; other fungus-related diseases include cryptococcus infection, histoplasmosis, and mucormycosis. Sporadic cases of liver infection by aspergillus species have also been reported. The imaging features of most types of fungal disease are similar.

Candida albicans typically begins at the untreated stage with small lesions <1 cm that are hypointense on T1-WI plain and Gd-enhanced images and markedly hyperintense on T2-WI. FS T2-WI and gadolinium-enhanced dynamic T1-WI is most useful in depicting lesions. Following initiation of treatment, lesions appear mildly to moderately hyperintense on T1-WI and T2-WI and demonstrate Gd enhancement with a hypointense ring around these lesions with all sequences. Completely treated lesions are minimally hypointense on T1-WI, isointense to mildly hyperintense on T2-WI, moderately hypointense on early Gd-enhanced images, and minimally hypointense on delayed Gd-enhanced images. Chronic lesions with scarring show low signal intensity on T1-W images and are typically invisible on T2-W images. Irregular lesions without gadolinium enhancement are best visualized on early gadolinium-enhanced T1-WI. Liver-specific agents do not provide additional clinically relevant information.

Acute schistosomiasis remains a significant health risk for travelers to endemic regions. Schistosoma japonicum, hematobium, and mansoni are the three most important species that infect humans. The schistosomes live in the bowel lumen and lay eggs in the mesenteric veins. The eggs may then embolize to the portal vein, where they cause an inflammatory reaction with areas of central necrosis in 60% of infected, granulomatous response, eventual fibrosis, and presinusoidal hypertension. At MRI, the periportal bands are isointense relative to normal liver parenchyma on T1-WI and hyperintense on T2-WI, with marked enhancement following gadolinium administration.

Bacillary angiomatosis is a manifestation of infection by *Bartonella henselae* in immunocompromised patients. The same organism causes cat-scratch disease in noncompromised patients. It is characterized by localized areas of vascular proliferation that may affect the skin, airway, mucous membranes, visceral organs, bone, and brain. Peliosis hepatis is the term used for liver infection by *B henselae*. This condition occurs almost exclusively in patients with acquired immunodeficiency syndrome. In the abdomen, multiple granulomas ranging from 3 to 30 mm may form in the liver and spleen, with or without hepatosplenomegaly. Peliosis hepatis is a condition in which irregular blood-filled spaces are seen in the liver. At histologic analysis, the lesions are seen to consist of irregular cystic spaces, either dilated sinusoids lined by endothelium or dilated spaces of Disse. The lesions appear as hypointense nodules on T1-WI and as hyperintense nodules on T2-WI. Peripheral enhancement may be seen on Gd-enhanced T1-WI.

The liver and biliary tracts are frequent sites of involvement during the course of HIV infection. A variety of viral, bacterial, fungal, and other opportunistic infections can manifest with hepatobiliary involvement as either the primary site of infection or secondary to a disseminated process. Co-infection with hepatitis B and C viruses is particularly common due to the shared means of transmission of these viruses with HIV.

6.4.9 Focal Liver Disease: Lymphomatous Disease

Focal lymphomatous disease demonstrates low signal on T1-WI and a slightly high signal on T2-WI. Gadolinium-enhanced T1-WI shows no significant increase in lesion signal intensity, but occasionally perilesional enhancement. Liver-specific agents offer a better delineation of lesions on accumulation phase images.

6.5 Spleen

Peter Reimer and Sanjay Saini

6.5.1 Spleen Anatomy

The spleen as the largest single lymphatic organ in the body is divided into two compartments, namely, the red and white pulps, separated by the marginal zone. The white pulp is made up of T and B-lymphocytes and located centrally, while the red pulp is composed of rich plexuses of tortuous venous sinuses. The spleen is an intraperitoneal organ with a smooth serosal surface, which are termed the diaphragmatic (phrenic) and visceral surfaces. The visceral surface is divided into an anterior or gastric ridge and a posterior or renal portion. The splenic hilum is directed anteromedially. The spleen is attached to the retroperitoneum by fatty ligaments that also contain its vascular supply. The splenic artery and vein emerge from the splenic hilum with six or more branches, with the splenic artery located slightly superior to the vein.

The spleen is hypointense on T1-WI and hyperintense on T2-WI (Fig. 6.1) based on a large fractional heme content characterized by long T1 and T2 relaxation. This signal behavior is unfortunately similar to the signal of many splenic lesions, limiting the value of plain MR for detecting focal or diffuse splenic disease.

6.5.2 Technique

Two different contrast techniques are available to further differentiate many splenic lesions, various gadolinium chelates, and alternatively SPIO.

Pulse sequences used for MRI of the spleen are similar to those used for standard upper abdominal MRI as described previously. Basically, T1-WI (GRE) and T2-WI (TSE, HASTE, RARE, and GRE) images are acquired in the axial plane preferably as breath-hold sequences. Additional coronal images may be acquired with T2-WI (RARE and HASTE). For T1-WI, a 2D GRE sequence in-phase and opposed-phase and axial 3D GRE with fat suppression such as volumetric interpolated breath-hold examination (VIBE) with precontrast and dynamic gadolinium-enhanced imaging is a robust strategy (see Table 6.1).

Gadolinium-enhanced images obtained during the arterial or early phase usually demonstrate different circulations as regions of alternating high and low signal intensity, resulting in a serpentine or arciform pattern. This pattern becomes homogeneous approximately 60–90 s after contrast material administration (Fig. 6.13).

Alternatively, delayed SPIO-enhanced T2-WI demonstrates a signal decrease in normal spleen based on the RES content without a signal change within lesions such as metastases or lymphoma. A similar contrast pattern may be present in hemosiderosis due to hemosiderin deposition. We also recommend postcontrast scanning in the coronal plane additionally to pre- and regular postcontrast images in the axial plane to better visualize the spleen.

6.5.3 Spleen Pathology

A wide range of pathologic conditions can affect the spleen. Further developments in MRI techniques have increased the role of MRI in detection and characterization of splenic diseases. MRI is an excellent tool for diagnosis and evaluation of focal lesions and pathologic conditions of the spleen whenever US or CT are not conclusive.

Specific topics discussed are normal variants and congenital diseases, trauma, inflammation, vascular disorders, hematologic disorders, benign neoplasms or cysts, malignant neoplasms, and diffuse enlargement.

6.5.4 Congenital Diseases and Variants

Congenital diseases cover the occurrence of accessory spleen, polysplenia, and asplenia. Accessory spleen may occur in up to 10% of patients typically located in the splenic hilum and has to be differentiated from other mass lesions. Accessory spleens may be solitary or multiple and are usually of limited size, <3–4 cm in diameter. Polysplenia is seen in association with other congenital diseases, typically abdominal situs and cardiovascular anomalies. Small masses may be seen in the right or left hypochondrium with masses resembling spleen like signal characteristics.

6.5.5 Trauma

The spleen is the most commonly involved organ in trauma and most commonly ruptured intraabdominal organ after blunt abdominal trauma. Trauma may lead to formation of hematoma, contusion, laceration, and infarcts, which may also develop based on thromboembolic disease (Fig. 6.19). Immediate US or CT typically detect or rule out splenic trauma in the acute trauma phase. However, subtle splenic injury or delayed hematoma may be detected at follow-up MRI. Therefore, the knowledge of MRI characteristics of splenic hematoma is clinically valuable. Acute hematoma demonstrates prolonged T2. The evolvement of blood products over time into methemoglobin, deoxyhemoglobin, and other paramagnetic degradation products with concomitant signal intensity changes is described in detail in Chap. 1.

6.5.6 Infection

Viral and bacterial infections may cause splenomegaly. The prevalence of abscesses has increased due to the increased number of immunosuppressed patients. Abscesses can be solitary, multiple, or multilocular. Splenic abscesses may also develop following infected thromboembolism, such as in patients with endocarditis. Larger bacterial abscesses show fluid-like signal behavior with hypointensity on T1-WI and hyperintensity on T2-WI. Postcontrast gadolinium-enhanced T1-WI typically shows enhancement of the abscess wall.

Fungal infection with candida albicans is the most common infection in immunocompromised patients

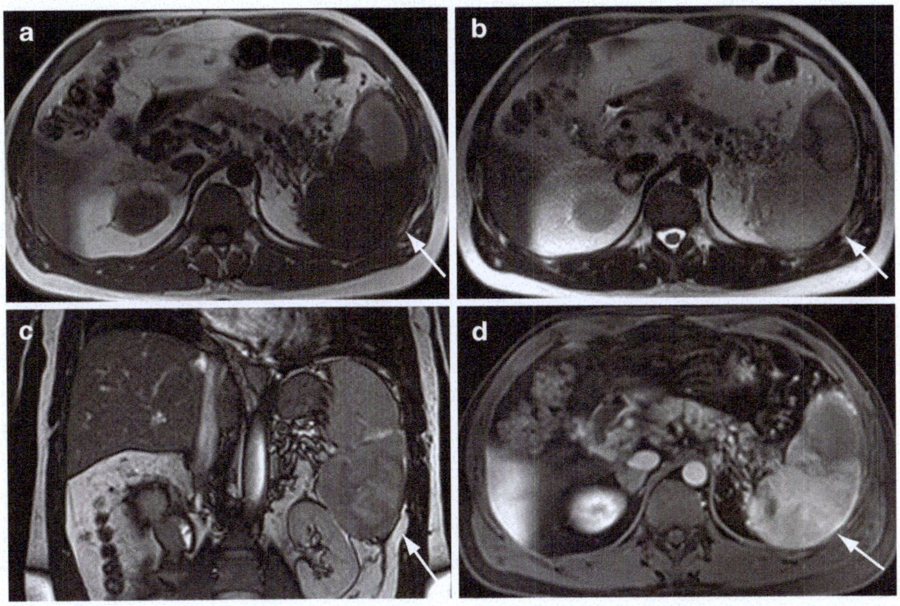

Fig. 6.19 Splenic hematoma (*arrows*). Plain 2D T1-W spoiled GRE (**a**), axial T2-W HASTE (**b**), and coronal T2-W HASTE GRE (**c**), portal-phase gadolinium-enhanced 2D T1-W spoiled GRE (**d**). A mass is visible within the lower part of an enlarged spleen. The mass is characterized by mostly hyperintense components on T1-W and mild hyperintense components on T2-W (see Chap. 1 for further details). The portal venous phase-enhanced GD FS-3D T1-WI (**d**) shows a cavernous transformation within the splenic hilum following an occlusion of the splenic vein

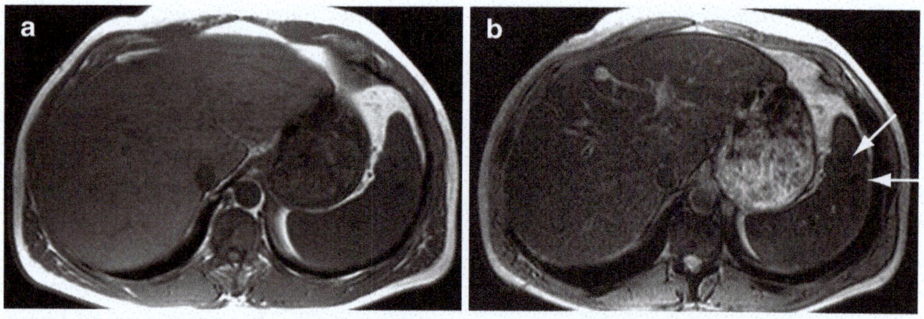

Fig. 6.20 Gamna–Gandy bodies/liver cirrhosis/HCC. Plain 2D T1-W spoiled GRE (**a**) and T2*-GRE (**b**) in a patient with severe liver cirrhosis following hepatitis B and C. The spleen contains foci of decreased signal intensity (*arrows*) corresponding to Gamna–Gandy bodies. Liver signal is decreased and an incidental liver lesion (*arrowhead*) is visible, which turned out to be a hepatocellular carcinoma

involving the liver and spleen. Fungal microabscesses are typically scattered throughout the liver and spleen, appear hypointense on T1-WI, hyperintense on T2-WI, and hypointense on gadolinium-enhanced T1-WI with subtle ring-like enhancement of typically small lesions <1–2 cm. Signal intensity of splenic abscesses is often altered due to underlying splenic hemosiderosis from transfusion overload in hematological patients (Fig. 6.4). Fat suppression may improve lesion conspicuity, and MR is superior to CT for the detection and follow-up of fungal microabscesses.

Histoplasmosis may occur in patients with competent immune systems, however, the prevalence of histoplasmosis is greater in immunocompromised patients. MRI demonstrates the acute and subacute phases of histoplasmosis with scattered hypointense lesions on both T1- and T2-WI. Calcifications within old granulomas may cause susceptibility effects with blooming artifacts. This appearance is best visualized on GRE T2*-WI.

6.5.7 Diffuse Diseases

Disease processes that affect the spleen diffusely are portal hypertension, sarcoid, malaria, lymphoma, leukemia, and metabolic diseases (e.g., Gaucher disease).

Portal hypertension represents the most common cause of splenomegaly in many countries. MRI may reveal associated signs of hepatic cirrhosis with or without change in liver size depending on the stage of hypertension. Dilated collateral veins are demonstrated at the splenic hilum or in the upper abdomen, particularly when using 3D GRE T1-WI for dynamic postcontrast scanning (Fig. 6.19). Patients with cirrhosis or portal hypertension may develop small (<1 cm) foci of iron deposition, appearing particularly hypointense on T2-W and T1-W GRE in about 10% of patients and are called Gamna–Gandy bodies (Fig. 6.20). T2-W TSE are much less susceptible to iron and, thus, often do not demonstrate the lesions readily displayed on GRE images.

Granulomatous lesions, such as sarcoid, infrequently involve the spleen. Sarcoid lesions are typically small (<1 cm) and hypovascular. They appear with low signal intensity on both T1-WI and T2-WI and almost no enhancement on arterial phase or portal venous phase gadolinium-enhanced T1-WI. Sarcoidosis lesions may enhance in a subtle and delayed pattern. Fat suppression may improve visibility on T2-WI.

6.5.8 Vascular Disorders

Some vascular disorders that affect the spleen are infarction, diseases affecting the splenic vasculature, and arteriovenous malformation.

Splenic infarcts are typically caused by arterial emboli such as in sickle cell anemia, Gaucher disease, hematologic malignancies, cardiac emboli, collagen vascular disease, and portal hypertension. Infarcts are identified as peripheral wedge-shaped defects that appear hypointense on both T1- and T2-WI and do not enhance after gadolinium administration (Fig. 6.21).

Splenic artery aneurysms are secondary to multiple causes such as medial degeneration with superimposed atherosclerosis, mycotic causes, fibromuscular dysplasia, and pseudoaneurysms from trauma and pancreatitis.

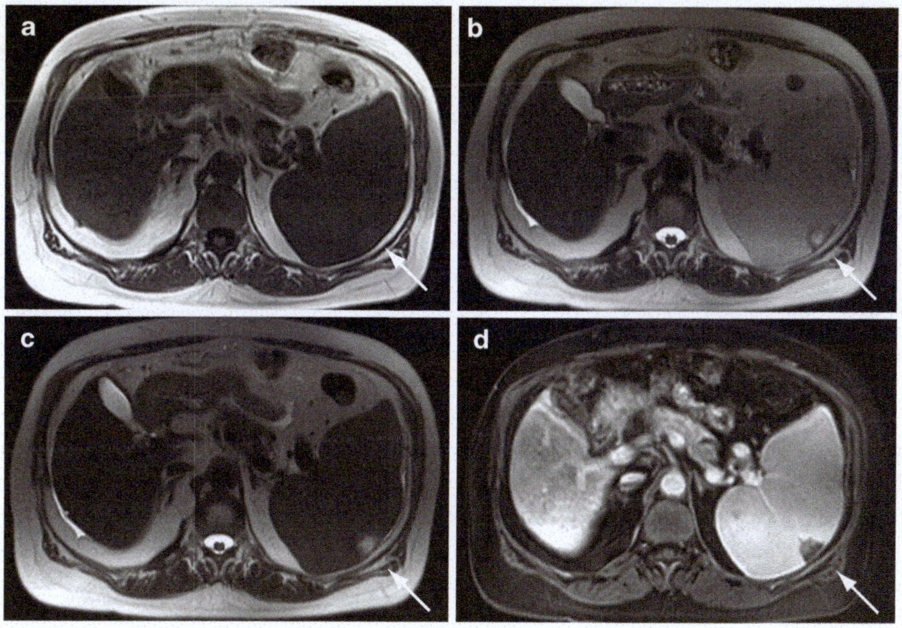

Fig. 6.21 Splenic infarct (*arrows*). Plain T1-W spoiled GRE (**a**), T2-W HASTE before Resovist (**b**), T2-W HASTE following Resovist® (**c**), and portal venous phase gadolinium-enhanced T1-W spoiled GRE (**d**) in a patient with a hematologic disease and left upper quadrant pain since a few days. A wedge-shaped defect is seen within the spleen with absent contrast perfusion. Signal intensity of the spleen on T2-W is decreased following Resovist®

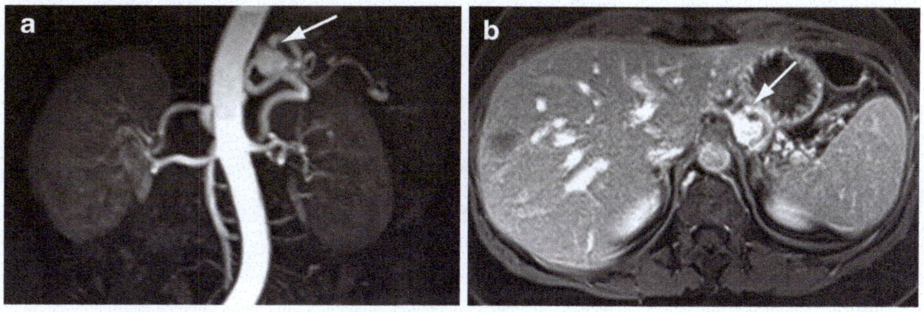

Fig. 6.22 Splenic artery aneurysm. Maximum intensity projection (**a**) and gadolinium-enhanced FS T1-W spoiled 3D GRE (**b**) show a splenic artery aneurysm with some wall thrombus (*arrows*)

Current 3D GRE T1-WI such as VIBE have obviated the acquisition of dedicated 3D MRA sequences since they exhibit aneurysms in great detail due to the improved spatial resolution (Fig. 6.22).

Splenic vein thrombosis is most commonly secondary to pancreatitis in up to 20% of patients with chronic pancreatitis due to compression and fibrosis. Splenic vein thrombosis may result in subsequent gastric, esophageal, or colonic varices. The intraluminal-filling defect is more easily detected on postcontrast dynamic 3D GRE T1-WI than on precontrast images. Arteriovenous malformations rarely occur in the spleen. MRI shows multiple signal voids with no enhanced pulse sequences and serpentine enhancement after gadolinium injection.

6.5.9 Hematologic Disorders

Hematologic disorders that affect the spleen are mainly sickle cell disease extramedullary hematopoiesis.

The spleen is the organ most commonly involved by sickle cell disease. Patients with sickle cell anemia may present with a hypointense spleen, mainly due to iron deposition following multiple blood transfusions. In this case, hyperintense lesions on T1-WI represent most likely secondary infarcts. Autosplenectomy is often found in patients with homozygous sickle cell disease.

Extramedullary hematopoiesis is a compensatory response to deficient bone marrow cells. It predominantly affects the spleen and diffuse infiltration, however, there may be focal mass-like involvement of both organs. The signal characteristics of these mass lesions mimic the signal of hematopoietic marrow. Active lesions demonstrate intermediate signal intensity on T1-WI, hyperintesity on T2-WI, and some enhancement after gadolinium injection. Older lesions may show low signal intensity on T1- and T2-WI and may not show any enhancement. Due to the presence of iron, any sequence susceptible to iron may show a signal decrease.

6.5.10 Benign Lesions

The spectrum of the most common benign tumors of the spleen consists of cysts, hemangioma, diffuse hemangiomatosis of the spleen, and hamartoma.

Cystic lesions are the most common benign focal splenic lesions, and three benign types exist: pseudocysts, epidermoid cysts, and hydatid cysts. Most cystic lesions in industrialized countries are posttraumatic pseudocysts without epithelial cell lining. Epidermoid cysts are true cysts with epithelial cell lining and are usually discovered incidentally in young patients. Hydatid cysts or echinococal cysts may show extensive wall calcification, which is better seen by CT. All cysts are well demarcated, hypointense on T1-WI, hyperintense on T2-WI, and show no contrast enhancement (Fig. 6.23).

Hemangioma is the most common benign solid focal splenic tumor and is composed of endothelium-lined vascular channels filled with blood. Splenic hemangiomas are typically cavernous hemangiomas and are smaller in size than liver hemangiomas. Hemangiomas are generally hypointense on T1-WI, hyperintense on T2-WI, and show contrast enhancement (Fig. 6.24). Gadolinium enhancement on T1-WI may be early and homogeneous or nodular with a filling-in pattern; however, these features are not as pronounced as those known for liver

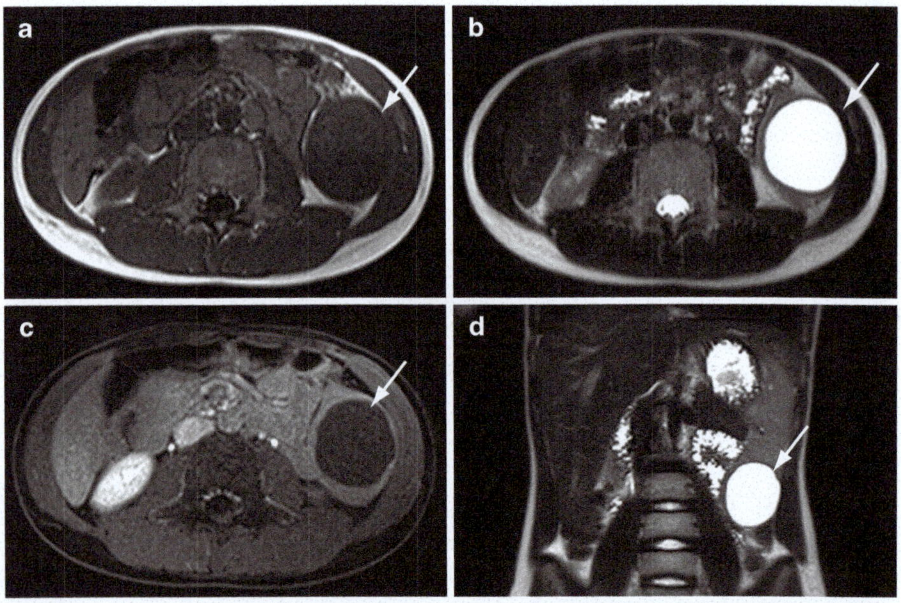

Fig. 6.23 Splenic cyst (*arrows*). Plain 2D T1-W spoiled GRE (**a**), axial T2-W HASTE (**b**), venous phase gadolinium-enhanced 2D T1-W spoiled GRE (**c**), and coronal T2-W HASTE. Plain and contrast-enhanced images reveal a large splenic cyst with homogeneous high signal intensity on T2-W images (**b, d**) and without contrast enhancement (**a, c**)

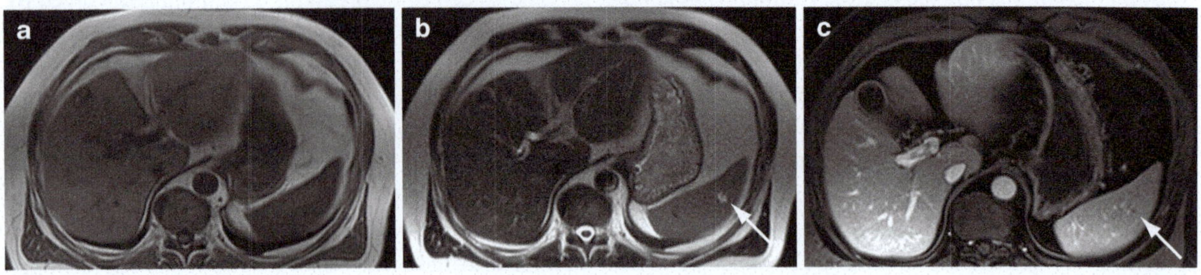

Fig. 6.24 Splenic hemangioma. Plain T1-W spoiled 2D GRE (**a**), and T2-W HASTE (**b**), and late gadolinium-enhanced FS T1-W spoiled 3D GRE (**c**) show a single lesion in the spleen. The hemangioma appears hypointense on T1-W (**a**), hyperintense on T2-W (**b**), and shows almost complete filling with contrast (**c**) (*arrows*)

hemangiomas. MRI is useful when US and CT results are equivocal. Iron oxides show a decrease in T2-WI due to pooling of particles within hemangiomas. Diffuse hemangiomatosis of the spleen is a rare benign vascular condition occurring as a manifestation of systemic angiomatosis and may present with severe coagulopathy. A location confined to the spleen is less common.

Cystic lymphangiomas and hamartoma are rare benign focal lesions. Cystic lymphangiomas appear as well-defined multiloculated masses hypointense on T1-WI and hyperintense on T2-WI. Hamartomas are composed of a mixture of normal splenic structures such as white and red pulp. Hamartomas are predominantly solid and commonly associated with tuberous sclerosis. Most splenic hamartomas show intermediate signal intensity on T1-WI, are heterogeneously hyperintense relative to the spleen on T2-WI, and demonstrate strong diffuse enhancement on early postcontrast images and more uniform enhancement on delayed images.

6.5.11 *Malignant Lesions*

Malignant lesions that affect the spleen are mainly sarcoma, lymphoma, and metastases.

Primary splenic angiosarcomas are extremely rare tumors with a very poor prognosis. These tumors are highly aggressive and manifest with widespread metastatic disease or splenic rupture. At MRI, the spleen is hypointense on T1-WI and heterogeneous hyperintense on T2-WI. Postcontrast gadolinium T1-WI demonstrate heterogeneous enhancement with multiple hyperintense nodular foci and hypointense regions.

Lymphoma is the commonest malignant tumor of the spleen. Lymphomatous disease (Hodgkin's and non-Hodgkin's lymphoma) often involves the spleen and, again, plain MR often fails to detect focal or diffuse splenic involvement because of similar contrast behavior of normal spleen and lesions. Visible lymphomas are typically isointense to hypointense on both T1-WI and T2-WI and enhance on early (≤30 s) gadolinium-enhanced T1-WI. Diffuse involvement may demonstrate a disturbance of the regular arciform perfusion pattern and diffusely scattered focal lesions appear as multiple hypointense lesions on early gadolinium-enhanced T1-WI. Iron oxides improve the conspicuity of splenic lymphoma presenting as hyperintense lesions compared with the hypointense spleen due to the uptake of particles in the RES present in the normal spleen. The dose of SPIO required to effectively decrease signal intensity of normal splenic tissue is somewhat higher than currently approved for the liver, however, a mild signal decrease is observed at approved doses.

Splenic metastases are relatively uncommon, however, may occur in advanced stages of cancer disease, typically originating from breast carcinoma, lung carcinoma, or malignant melanoma (Fig. 6.25). Isolated splenic metastases are rare. Plain MR often fails to detect lesions because of similar contrast behavior of

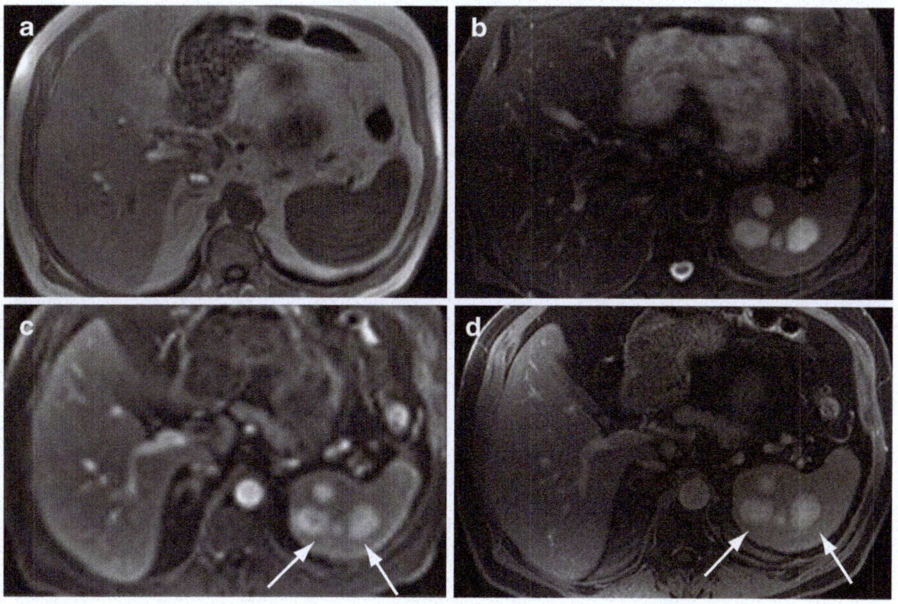

Fig. 6.25 Spleen metastases (melanoma). Plain T1-W spoiled 2D GRE (**a**), FS-T2-W TSE (**b**), portal venous phase gadolinium-enhanced FS T1-W spoiled 2D GRE (**c**), and delayed phase-enhanced FS T1-W spoiled 2D GRE (**d**) show multiple metastases in the spleen. Metastases are isointense on T1-W and hyperintense on T2-W with strong and persistent gadolinium enhancement (*arrows*)

normal spleen and lesions. Somewhat visible lesions may present isointense to mildly hyopintense lesions on T1-WI and mildly hyperintense on T2-WI. Contrast-enhanced techniques help to improve lesion conspicuity by means of hypointense lesions on early (≤30 s) gadolinium-enhanced T1-WI or hyperintense lesions on iron oxide-enhanced T2-WI with a time window of up to 3 days. Enhancement characteristics depend on the underlying primary neoplasm. Melanoma metastasis represents an exception since the melanin content may cause high signal intensity on T1-WI.

6.6 Biliary System

Wolfgang Schima

6.6.1 Biliary Anatomy and Variants

MRI of the intrahepatic and extrahepatic biliary system is tailored to visualize the biliary fluid, the duct walls, and adjacent soft-tissue structures. In contrast to ERCP, which demonstrates all ductal structuresthat can be cannulated and filled with contrast material, MRCP demonstrates all biliary ducts and the gallbladder, which are in vivo filled with fluid. MRCP uses heavily T2-W sequences with TEs longer than T2-relaxation times of soft tissue, which then do not contribute to the signal on images. This technique allows visualization of static fluid and may be considered as a fluid-W technique. T2-WI without or with fat suppression with moderate TE and gadolinium-enhanced T1-W GRE demonstrate duct wall and adjacent soft-tissue structures. Hepatobiliary agents (e.g., Teslascan®, GE Healthcare; MultiHance®, Bracco; Primovist®, Bayer Schering) are excreted into the bile and show a bright ductal system on delayed phase T1-WI GRE images. However, in addition to the disadvantage of increased examination time and cost, the use of hepatobiliary agents does not add information in patients with serum bilirubin level >5 mg/dL because of the lack of biliary excretion in these patients. T1-W MR cholangiography has been shown to be effective in patients with nondilated bile duct system (e.g., living related liver transplant donors), where conventional T2-W MRCP fails to visualize the small ducts.

Normally, the right anterior (for segments 6 and 7) and right posterior segmental ducts (for segments 5 and 8) merge to form the right hepatic duct, which together with the left hepatic duct forms the main hepatic duct. There are a variety of biliary anatomic variants, some of which are clinically relevant (Fig. 6.26). The right posterior segmental ducts may insert into the left hepatic duct. In this case, obstruction of the left hepatic duct will result in bile duct dilatation not only in the left lobe, but also in segments 6 and 7 of the right lobe. Deep insertion of the right anterior of posterior segmental duct into the main hepatic duct puts the patient at risk of inadvertent clipping of this duct during laparoscopic cholecystectomy.

6.6.2 Technique

A variety of MRCP techniques with different approaches depending on scanner hardware and software are available, including 2D, 3D T2-W pulse sequences with

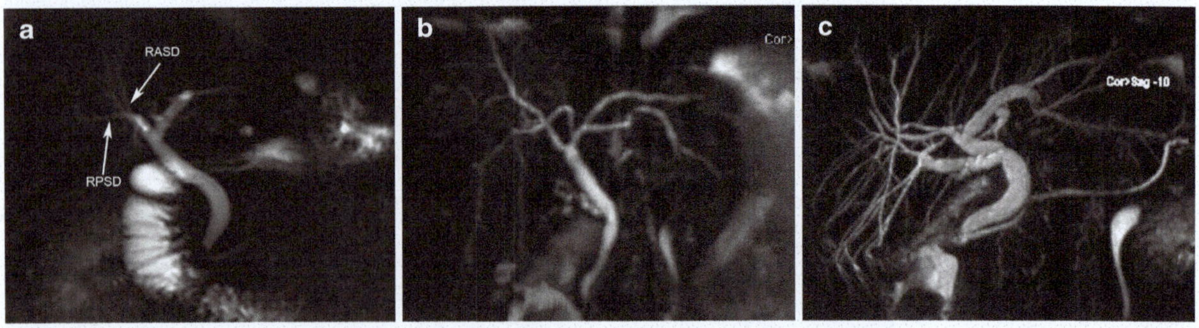

Fig. 6.26 Normal biliary anatomy and variants. (**a**) Coronal RARE of normal biliary anatomy: the right anterior segmental duct (RASD) and the right posterior segmental duct (RPSD) merge to form the right hepatic duct. (**b**) Variant anatomy: the RPSD merges with the left hepatic duct. In this case, there is no"normal" right hepatic duct. (**c**) Variant anatomy: there is deep insertion of the RPSD into the main hepatic duct. Patients are at risk of inadvertent clipping of this duct during laparoscopic cholecystectomy. Note prior cheolcystectomy in this patient, cystic duct stump comes off this aberrant duct

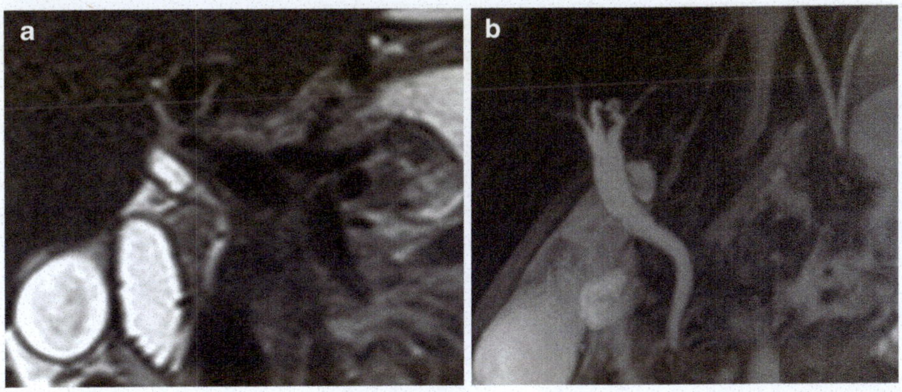

Fig. 6.27 Value of MRCP source images for evaluation of bile ducts. (**a**) The coronal thin source image shows a small stone in the dilated CBD, which (**b**) is not seen on the thick MIP reconstruction

breath holding, respiratory triggering with an abdominal belt or navigator. For a quick overview, a simple breath-hold thick-slab T2-W RARE sequence in radial orientation requires no further postprocessing. Still commonly used is multisection T2-W HASTE with thin sections and postprocessing to generate MIPs. New 3D techniques are typically based upon TSE sequences acquired with respiratory triggering using navigator techniques and thin near-isotropic voxels. However, consideration of thin source images together with postprocessed images is mandatory for clinical analysis (Fig. 6.27). The performance of these different approaches is somewhat vendor specific and depends on the equipment available. When administered for other indications, hepatobiliary contrast agents also exhibit high signal intensity within the bile and, thus, directly visualize the duct lumen. Gadolinium-enhanced T1-WI shows ducts with intraluminal low signal intensity and can be used as a "dark-fluid" technique. Gadolinium-enhanced FS T1-WI, preferably with breath-held techniques, is ideal to image the ducts and adjacent soft tissues. Secretin is a polypeptide hormone, which stimulates pancreatic secretions. Synthetic secretin can be used to enhance MRCP. By inducing pancreatic secretion, it causes temporary dilatation of pancreatic ducts and allows better visualization of strictures and ductal anomalies on dynamic MRCP.

6.6.3 Benign Biliary Disease

Acute and chronic cholecystitis is imaged with axial fat-suppressed T1-, T2-, and gadolinium-enhanced T1-W images. T1-WI show marked thickening of the gallbladder wall together with pericholecystic edema. Enhanced T1-WI demonstrates a strong enhancement of the gallbladder wall and pericholecystic tissues in acute cholecystitis. Chronic cholecystitis presents as a crumpled, irregularly shaped gallbladder with a thickened but only mildly enhancing wall. The degree of mural enhancement and enhancement of pericholecystic tissues reflects the activity and the degree of the inflammatory process. As differential diagnosis, gallbladder wall thickening may be seen secondary to a variety of liver diseases, such as acute hepatitis, acute liver failure, cirrhosis with ascites, etc.

Cholangitis occurs as infectious or sclerosing cholangitis. Infectious cholangitis, by biliary obstruction and ascending infection, presents with ductal wall thickening, which enhances on gadolinium-enhanced T1-WI. Ductal obstruction site and dilatation is best appreciated with MRCP techniques. A potential complication is the development of biliary abscesses, which are visualized best on FS T2-WI and FS gadolinium-enhanced T1-WI. Sclerosing cholangitis, either primary (primary sclerosing cholangitis, an autoimmune disorder) or secondary due to long-standing cholangiolithiasis or after prolonged treatment in intensive care units is characterized by a segmental dilatation of the biliary tree with interleaved narrowed segments resulting in a beaded and stenotic appearance that is best appreciated with MRCP techniques (Fig. 6.28). A second feature is mild ductal wall thickening, which is demonstrated best on FS gadolinium-enhanced T1-WI obtained during the portal venous phase. Enhancement correlates with the degree of inflammation. MRI follow-up helps to define dominant biliary strictures, which need ERCP intervention, and CCC, which is the most feared complication of PSC. Its differential diagnosis should be considered when ductal wall thickening exceeds 5 mm.

Calculous disease within the gallbladder and biliary ducts is best depicted with heavily T2-WI (e.g., MRCP), rendering the bile bright and stones dark. The bile is typically dark on T1-WI and bright on T2-WI

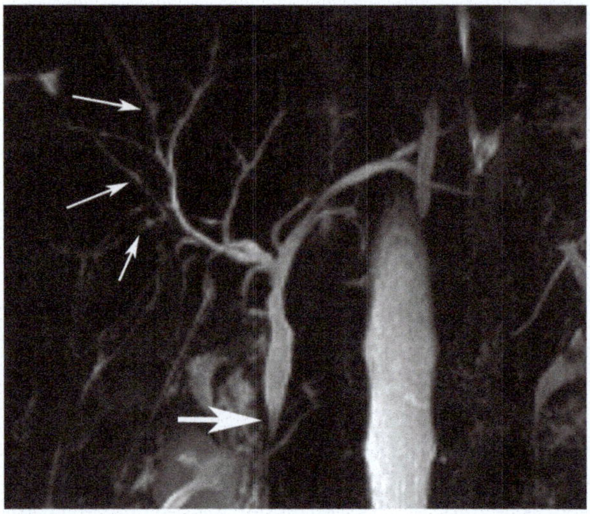

Fig. 6.28 Primary sclerosing cholangitis: the coronal MRCP (MIP reconstruction) shows multiple slight conout irregularities of the intrahepatic ducts (*arrows*) with a stricture of the distal CBD (*arrowhead*).

(Fig. 6.29). Signal intensity of the gallbladder content on T1-WI may vary from dark (water) to bright (fat and proteins) with fluid-fluid levels if sludge is present. Biliary obstruction is also best demonstrated using MRCP techniques, which are also helpful for planning of endoscopic or percutaneous interventions. The specificity, sensitivity, and accuracy for the detection of choledocholithiasis have been reported to be 90% or even higher. ERCP is still the gold standard, combining diagnosis and treatment. However, MRCP is valuable in patients prior to laparoscopic cholecystectomy to rule out choledocholithiasis, with surgical bypass procedures such as hepatojejunostomy or gastrectomy, and in patients with acute pancreatitis. Pitfalls in diagnosing calculous disease are biliary prostheses, clips, aerobilia, hematobilia, and incrustations.

MRCP studies should be performed prior to placement of biliary endoprostheses, because aerobilia renders MRCP assessment of bile ducts difficult. Plastic prostheses are diamagnetic and provide no signal on MR images isointense to stones or sludge. Metal stents show susceptibility artifacts depending on their structure and composition. The assessment of the duct over the length of the stent is subsequently at least significantly reduced, and in most stents, impossible (see Chap. 11). Patients with surgical complications following laparoscopic cholecystectomy may be scanned without any harm since surgical clips are MR compatible and the area of interest may be assessed without any restrictions. In patients with metallic stents or significant aerobilia, patency of bile ducts can be assessed with T1-W cholangiography after IV administration of hepatobiliary contrast agents, which are excreted into the bile and flow into the duodenum.

Cystic diseases, such as pancreatic cysts, choledochal cyst, choledochocele, or Caroli's syndrome (Fig. 6.30), are best visualized on coronal and axial MRCP images.

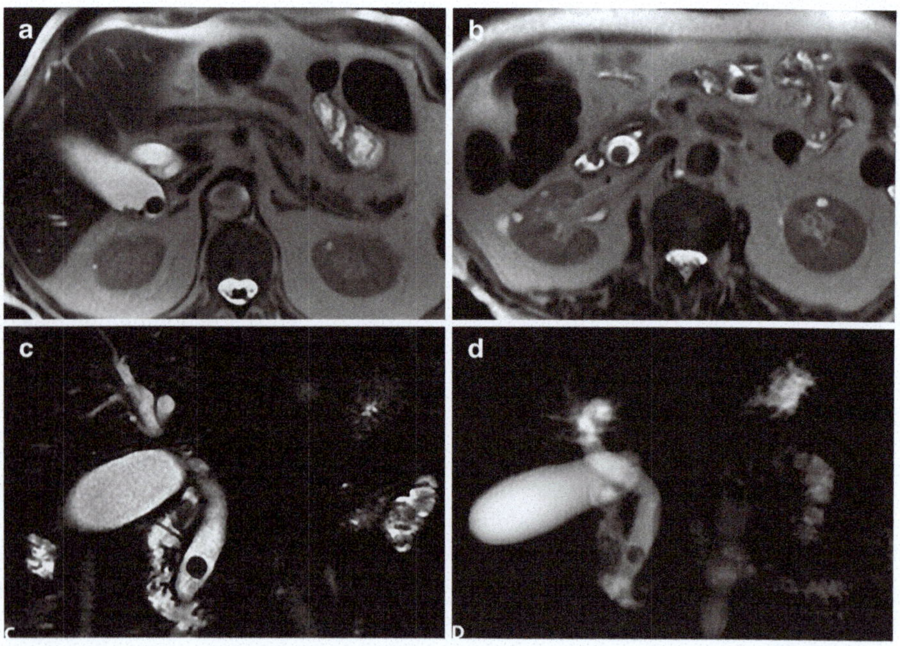

Fig. 6.29 Gallbladder and common bile duct stones. Axial T2-HASTE (TE90 ms) (**a**, **b**), thin coronal MRCP section (**c**), and MIP of MRCP images (**d**) demonstrate multiple stones in the gallbladder and a distal common bile duct stone. The hypointense stones are well demarcated in the otherwise hyperintense bile (**a**–**c**). The common bile duct stone is better visualized with the thin section technique (**b**, **c**) and the gallbladder stones are completely missed on the MIP (**d**)

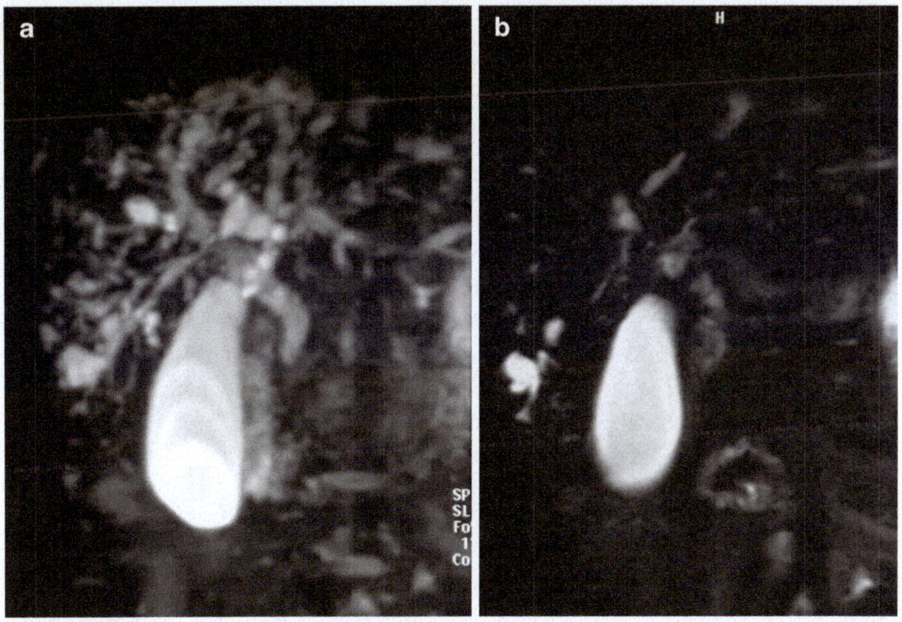

Fig. 6.30 Caroli's syndrome. (**a**) Coronal MRCP MIP reconstruction shows multiple cystically dilated bile ducts. (**b**) The thin source images better show the club-shaped bile ducts, which helps to rule out liver cysts adjacent to the bile ducts

6.6.4 Malignant Biliary Disease

Gallbladder cancer has a strong association with calculous disease, typically presenting as a defect within the gallbladder or a mass replacing the gallbladder. Focal or diffuse thickening (≥10 mm) of the gallbladder wall is suspicious. Invasion into adjacent liver, duodenum, and the pancreas occurs frequently. T2-WI and gadolinium-enhanced T1-WI are useful in depicting liver invasion (T4 stage). Advanced gallbladder cancer may also cause biliary obstruction at the hilum similar to a CCC, but the origin of the mass in the gallbladder helps in the characterization.

Extrahepatic CCC typically occurs in older patients presenting with jaundice and weight loss. The tumor represents a primary malignancy of the bile ducts and is classified as central or peripheral. Central tumors refer to lesions arising from main hepatic duct or bifurcation and peripheral tumors arise from intrahepatic branches. The most frequent location is the junction of the right and left hepatic ducts, the so-called Klatskin tumors. The role of imaging is to determine the proximal and distal extent of Klatskin tumors for planning of resectability (Fig. 6.31). Any mass leading to biliary duct obstruction at the hilum is suspicious for CCC, until proven otherwise. A combination of MRCP and gadolinium-enhanced FS T1-WI is useful to depict lesions that enhance moderately. For detection of CCC, SPIO-enhanced T2-W TSE with fat suppression has been found useful because of high contrast between

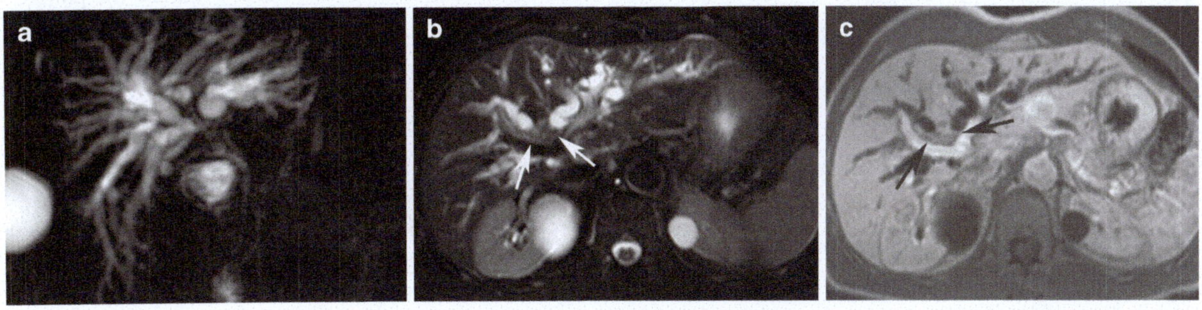

Fig. 6.31 Klatskin tumor. (**a**) The coronal MRCP shows a stricture of the main hepatic duct extending into the bifurcation of right and left hepatic ducts. (**b**) The axial T2-W TSE shows a mass (*arrows*) obstructing the central bile ducts. (**c**) The gadolinium-enhanced T1-W images shows the hypovascular tumor adjacent to the portal vein bifurcation, which was resected (right hemihepatectomy with portal vein bifurcation resection)

normal parenchyma, periductal tumor, and bile fluid. MRCP is particularly helpful in guiding palliative treatment and visualizes a 3D view of the intrahepatic and extrahepatic biliary tree, which is more difficult to obtain by ERCP. It is mandatory to obtain axial and coronal/oblique contrast-enhanced images in order to assess the presence or absence of infiltration of the Klatskin tumor into the hepatic parenchyma, which is important for tumor staging. A Bismuth type-1 tumor is defined as a tumor involving only the main hepatic duct, a type 2 affects the bifurcation of right and left hepatic ducts with separation of the two (Fig. 6.31). A type 3 tumor involves peripheral, secondary branch ducts in one lobe, and in type 4 tumors in both liver lobes. Inflammatory changes and susceptibility artifacts following stenting may complicate this diagnosis. The complete evaluation of Klatskin tumors includes imaging of the liver, the biliary ducts, adjacent soft tissues, lymph nodes, and vessels with focus on the portal vein. A comprehensive MRI and MRA protocol with conventional imaging, MRCP, and MRA is mandatory.

Distal tumors of the (intrapancreatic) common bile duct are difficult to differentiate from pancreatic adenocarcinoma. Tumors within the pancreatic head present as hypointense lesions within the otherwise hyperintense pancreatic head. Periampullary disease includes carcinomas, adenomas, and inflammatory changes. Tumors are best depicted using a combination of MRCP and gadolinium-enhanced T1-WI. Tumors typically present as hypointense lesions contrasted against the hyperintense pancreas on FS T1-WI and show mild contrast enhancement. Inflammatory changes, such as those observed following ERCP, demonstrate stronger contrast enhancement, which is also demonstrated best on FS T1-WI. The role of dedicated oral contrast agents as compared to water or studies without any additional oral contrast has not been clearly evaluated.

6.7 Pancreas

Wolfgang Schima

6.7.1 Pancreas Anatomy

The pancreas is best depicted on fat-suppressed T1-W sequences with thin sections (<6 mm), which provide good contrast of pancreatic tissue with high signal intensity against the low signal intensity of surrounding adipose tissue. Pancreatic signal intensity may be decreased by atrophy, pancreatitis, neoplasm, and iron overload. Signal intensity on T2-W sequences varies even more than on T1-W sequences; however, T2-WI is useful to demonstrate fluid-filled structures. Fat-suppressed T2-WI is useful to demonstrate peripancreatic edema in pancreatitis. MRA scans are preferably obtained as breath-held 3D CE-MRA sequences. MRCP visualizes ductal structures by means of intraluminal fluid and is performed with heavily T2-W 2D- or 3D-sequences (see Table 6.1).

6.7.2 Technique

Two different intravenous contrast techniques are available to improve pancreatic MR, especially for the depiction of small focal lesions and vascular invasion. Gadolinium-enhanced T1-W GRE show a stronger and earlier enhancement of the well-vascularized pancreas compared with the liver. Detection of adenocarcinoma, a hypovascular tumor, relies on the visualization of a T1-W low signal intensity lesion against the well-enhanced pancreas in the pancreatic parenchymal phase. Contrast is also helpful to depict nonperfused areas in necrotizing pancreatitis.

Alternatively, mangafodipir (Teslascan®) may be used to enhance the normal pancreatic parenchyma on T1-WIs over a longer period of time. Originally developed as a hepatobiliary agent with intracellular uptake into hepatocytes, Teslascan has subsequently been tested for CE-MRI of the pancreas and is clinically approved for this indication in Europe (see Chap. 1). The compound has been noted to enhance the pancreatic parenchyma, but does not show significant uptake into neoplasms and necrosis, which improves their delineation of postcontrast images. The exact clinical role of Teslascan-enhanced pancreatic MRI compared to gadolinium-enhanced pancreatic MRI has still to be defined by controlled clinical studies.

Delineation of pancreas from bowel can be improved by the administration of oral contrast media. The least expensive, well tolerated, and safest contrast agent is water with low signal intensity on T1-WI and high signal intensity on T2-WI. Some commercially available fruit juices, due to their high manganese content, can be used as oral T1-W contrast agents with high signal intensity. The effects of commercially available paramagnetic or superparamagnetic oral contrast agents on intraluminal signal intensity depend on the pulse sequences used. Paramagnetic oral contrast media show predominantly high intraluminal signal intensity on T1-W, and superparamagnetic oral contrast media show predominantly low intraluminal signal intensity on T2-WI (see Chap. 1).

6.7.3 Congenital Anomalies and Diseases

6.7.3.1 Pancreas Divisum

Pancreas divisum is the most clinically important anatomic variant with a lack of fusion of dorsal and ventral main pancreatic ducts (Fig. 6.32). The dorsal part of the main pancreatic duct (Santorini) drains into the minor papilla, separately from the common bile duct drains at the major papilla. The higher incidence of acute pancreatitis in patients with pancreas divisum is believed to be due to congestion in the duct from partial obstruction at the orifice of the minor papilla. MRCP is a tool to detect this anomaly in patients with acute pancreatitis obviating diagnostic ERCP.

6.7.3.2 Hemochromatosis

Primary or idiopathic hemochromatosis may show low signal intensity on T2/T2*-WI due to iron deposition within exocrine and islet cells causing diabetes mellitus. The liver is involved earlier and more substantially with formation of liver cirrhosis. Deposition of iron in the pancreas and heart tends to occur during late stages of disease. Secondary hemosiderosis due to blood transfusion or hemolysis involves the RES of the spleen and liver, but not the pancreas.

6.7.3.3 Cystic Fibrosis

Cystic fibrosis is the autosomal recessive congenital disorder that causes variable degrees of fatty replacement and atrophy. The fat content can be reliably demonstrated by T1-W sequences with and without fat suppression.

6.7.3.4 Lipomatosis and Lipoma

Severe lipomatous depositions within the pancreas may be observed in adult patients with overweight, senile atrophy, or cystic fibrosis. The parenchyma appears lobulated with preserved margins and a reduced volume. T1-W techniques without and with fat saturation are mostly used to demonstrate and prove these lipomatous depositions. Circumscribed lipomas of the pancreas are not that rare as previously thought and of no clinical significance. With thin-section MRI, you can see the intraparenchymal location of adipose tissue with the typical appearance on T1-W GRE images without and with fat suppression and no enhancement after gadolinium.

6.7.4 Pancreatitis

Acute and chronic forms of pancreatitis may be grouped according to their clinical course and severity (edematous or necrotizing).

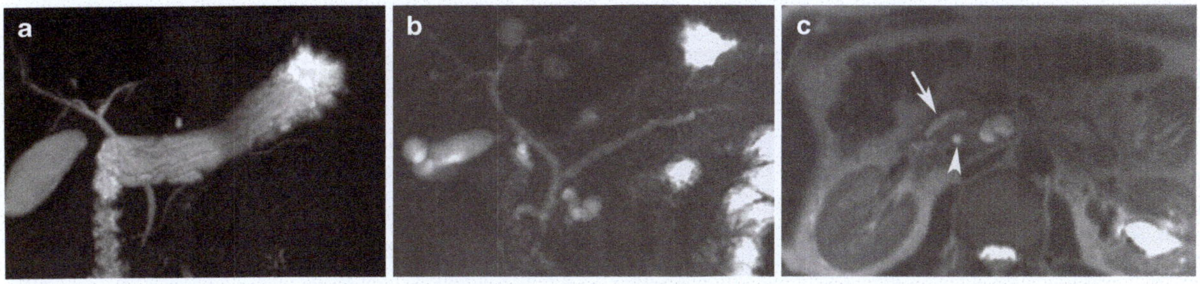

Fig. 6.32 Pancreas divisum. (**a**) MRCP in an asymptomatic patient demonstrates that the dorsal main pancreatic duct (Santorini) drains into the minor papilla, separately from the common bile duct, which course to the major papilla. (**b**) Chronic pancreatitis in pancreas divisum: the dilated duct shows contour irregularities and dilated side branches. (**c**) The axial T2-W HASTE image shows the typical course of the main pancreatic duct in pancreas divisum, anteriorly and superiorly (*arrow*) to the CBD (*arrowhead*)

6.7.4.1 Acute Pancreatitis

Patients with suspected or known acute pancreatitis are usually imaged by US or CT complementary to clinical and laboratory findings. These imaging modalities can be performed in intensive care units and therefore more accessible in clinical practice.

Edematous acute pancreatitis resembles features of normal pancreas with intermediate to slightly high signal intensity on T1-WI and homogenous gadolinium-enhancement. Diagnostic features are stranding of peripancreatic fat tissue, which is low in signal intensity on T1-WI without fat suppression and high in signal intensity on (fat-suppressed!) T2-WI (Fig. 6.33). In necrotizing pancreatitis, contrast-enhanced images, similar to the CT protocol for pancreatitis, are mandatory to define necrotic areas. Patients with necrotizing pancreatitis may develop complications, such as abscess, bleeding, and vascular complications such as thrombosis or aneurysm. The assessment of pancreatitis requires a comprehensive MR protocol with MRI and MRCP, and is more difficult to perform than CT in severely ill patients. Therefore, the most important indication for MRI in acute pancreatitis is suspected choledocholithiasis ("biliary pancreatitis") (Fig. 6.34). These patients should undergo emergency MRCP to confirm or rule out bile duct stones. It has been shown that patients with biliary pancreatitis will benefit, if endoscopic stone removal can be accomplished within the first 24 h after onset of pancreatitis. The patient should be able to sustain breath-hold acquisitions of up to 20 s. RARE or HASTE type sequences are very more robust to breathing artifacts due to their contiguous acquisition scheme. Alternatively, navigator-or respiratory-triggered T2-W pulse sequences will do the job.

6.7.4.2 Chronic Pancreatitis

Chronic pancreatitis is characterized by an irreversible damage of the endocrine and exocrine pancreatic function. Dilatation of the main pancreatic duct, parenchymal atrophy, parenchymal calcification, duct stones, pseudocysts, focal gland enlargement (Inflammatory pseudotumor), and eventually biliary ductal dilatation (Figs. 6.35 and 6.36) characterize chronic pancreatitis. MRCP with thin source images shows strictures and pancreatic duct stones not amenable to ERCP.

The most difficult diagnosis is the differentiation of adenocarcinoma from focal pancreatitis, which

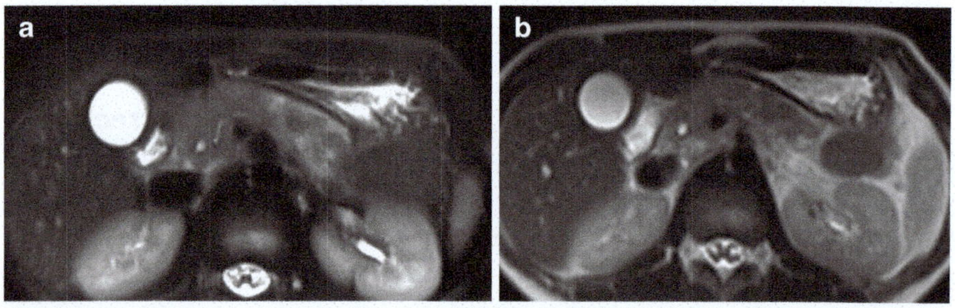

Fig. 6.33 Acute edematous pancreatitis. The axial T2-W TSE images with fat suppression (**a**) and without (**b**) both demonstrate swelling of the gland. However, the peripancreatic edema is better seen on the fat-supressed sequence (**a**)

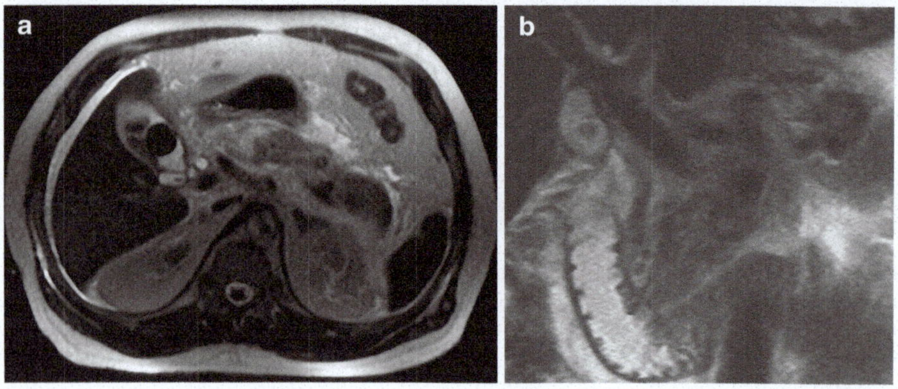

Fig. 6.34 Common bile duct stones with acute biliary pancreatitis. (**a**) The axial T2-HASTE (TE90 ms) demonstrates multiple stones in the gallbladder, and an enlarged pancreas with surrounding fluid. (**b**) The thin True-FISP section shows distal common bile duct stones, causing obstruction of the main pancreatic duct. Stones were subsequently removed

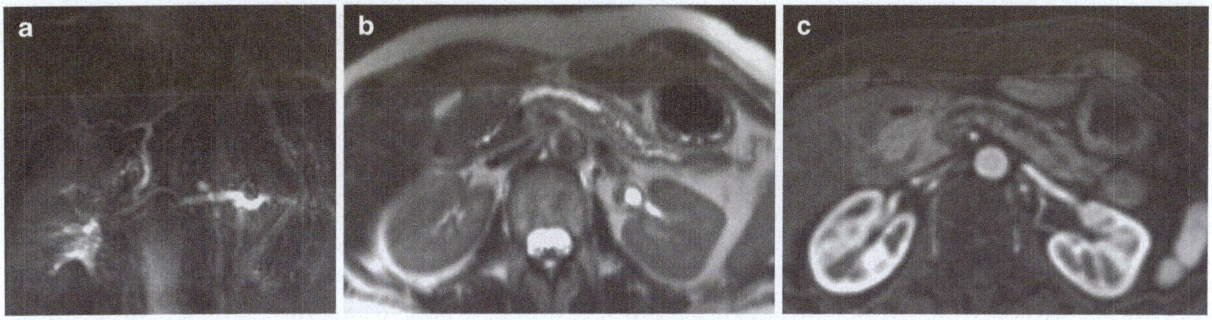

Fig. 6.35 Chronic pancreatitis with stricture. (**a**) Coronal MRCP shows a stricture in the body with pancreatic duct dilatation of the body and tail. (**b**) Axial T2-W TSE shows the stricture, there is no underlying mass causing the stricture. (**c**) The gadolinium-enhanced T1-W FS GRE image in the parenchymal phase shows less enhancement of the affected parenchyma of body and tail. A tumor obstruction of the duct can be ruled out.

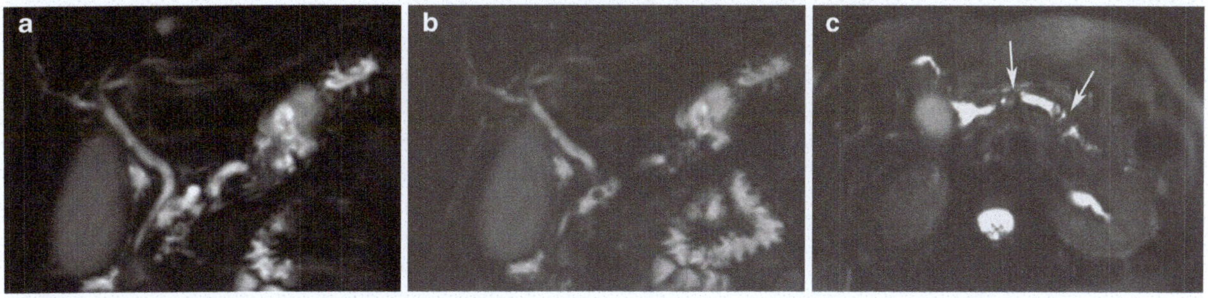

Fig. 6.36 Chronic pancreatitis with pancreatolithiasis and pseudocyst. (**a**) Coronal MRCP (MIP) shows severe strictures of the main duct with pseudocyst formation in the tail. Intraluminal content is not well seen. (**b**) Coronal subvolume-MIP and (**c**) axial thin source MRCP images depict the intraductal stones better than the thick MIP

presents with similar features (hypovascular mass with hypointense appearance on T1-WI). MR shows decreased signal intensity on T1-WI with decreased and more inhomogeneous gadolinium enhancement. Ductal dilatations and strictures can be well visualized with MRCP. Parenchymal calcifications cannot be directly demonstrated. CE-MRI with gadolinium chelates and Teslascan exhibit similar contrast effects with a lower enhancement within chronic pancreatitis than in normal pancreas and a sometimes even lower enhancement within areas of focal tumor. The best diagnostic feature to differentiate cancer and inflammatory pseudotumor is the "duct penetrating sign": the main pancreatic duct or side branches are likely to traverse an inflammatory pseudotumor (as seen on MRCP), whereas a densely fibrotic adenocarcinoma will show complete obstruction of the duct. The duct penetrating sign has an accuracy >90% for differentiation between inflammatory pseudotumor and adenocarcinoma. Still, characterization of focal masses in pancreatitis remains a diagnostic challenge, which often requires multimodality imaging, including MRI, CE-CT, endosonography, and biopsy.

Groove pancreatitis is a special form of chronic pancreatitis affecting the groove between the pancreatic head and the duodenum. The pancreatic head is usually spared or only minimally affected. The pathogenesis is most likely ectopic pancreatic tissue located in the duodenal wall, which undergoes inflammation with scar formation and cystic degeneration, hence the synonym "cystic dystrophy of the duodenum." At MRI, there is a mass located between the pancreas and the duodenum, which is T1-W hypointense, T2-W isointense to hypointense, and hypovascular to the pancreas on gadolinium-enhanced T1-W images. Typical features to differentiate it from cancer are the location not in the pancreas but between the head and the duodenum, and the appearance of small T2-W hyperintense cysts in the mass (Fig. 6.37).

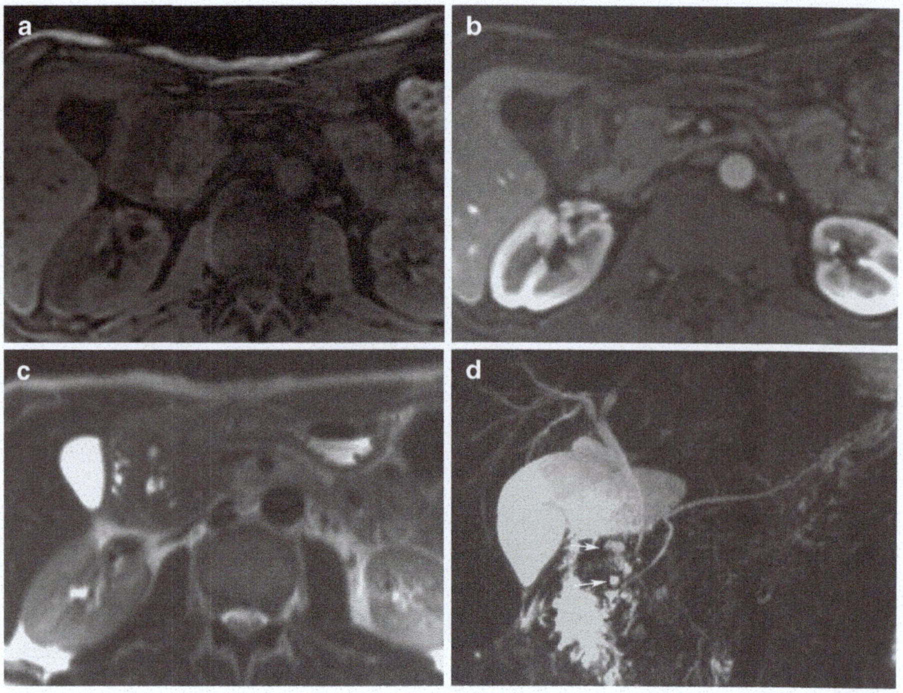

Fig. 6.37 Groove pancreatitis (synonym: cystic dystrophy of the duodenum). (**a**) Axial unenhanced and (**b**) gadolinium-enhanced T1-W GRE show a T1-W hypointense, hypovascular mass between the pancreatic head and the duodenum (in the"groove"). Rest of the pancreas seems unaffected. (**c**) T2-W TSE shows the solid mass with several small cysts, due to cystic degeneration of ectopic pancreatic tissue in the duodenal wall. (**d**) Small cysts between pancreatic head and duodenal lumen are best appreciated on coronal MRCP (*arrows*)

6.7.5 Tumors

6.7.5.1 Cystic Masses

Pseudocysts

Pseudocysts are still the most common cystic mass of the pancreas (>50%). Its reported prevalence has decreased with the development of thin-section CT and MRI to enhance recognition of cystic pancreatic masses as cystic neoplasms. Pseudocysts may develop during the course of acute or chronic pancreatitis within areas of necrosis or exudation with a surrounding wall of granulation tissue and without an epithelial cell lining (hence the name pseudocyst). The content consists of pancreatic debris, pancreatic secretion, or old blood. A spontaneous and typically early (<6–8 weeks) regression is possible. Imaging of acute pancreatitis and pancreatic pseudocysts is a domain of CT and pseudocysts are most often incidentally detected. Pseudocysts are typically unilocular, often thick-walled cysts. The signal intensity varies considerably going along with the potentially different components. They show typically low signal intensity on T1-WI and high signal intensity on T2-WI (Fig. 6.36). Hemorrhagic components cause a signal intensity increase on T1-WI and a decrease on T2-WI. The hypointense cystic wall may reach several millimeters and may demonstrate gadolinium enhancement due to the well-perfused granulation tissue. Although being quite prevalent in the parenchyma in chronic pancreatitis, calcifications of the cyst wall are not frequent and should raise the suspicion of the presence of a mucinous cystic neoplasm. In general, calcifications are best depicted at CT.

Serous Cystadenoma and Mucinous Cystadenoma/Cystadenocarcinoma

MR can be useful to differentiate benign serous adenoma (often referred to as microcystic cystadenoma) and potentially malignant mucinous cystic neoplasms (macrocystic cystadenoma or cystadenocarcinoma) besides clinical parameters such as age, location, and size. MR better evaluates cystic components of these tumors than CT or US.

Serous adenoma is a benign tumor characterized by multiple small cysts occurring in older patients (Fig. 6.38). The tumor may contain a central, calcified scar (approximately 50%), has an average diameter of approximately 5 cm without invasion of surrounding structures, and is well defined on MR with hypointense cystic components on T1-WI and multiple tiny hyperintense cystic components on T2-WI. Cystic wall may show contrast enhancement.

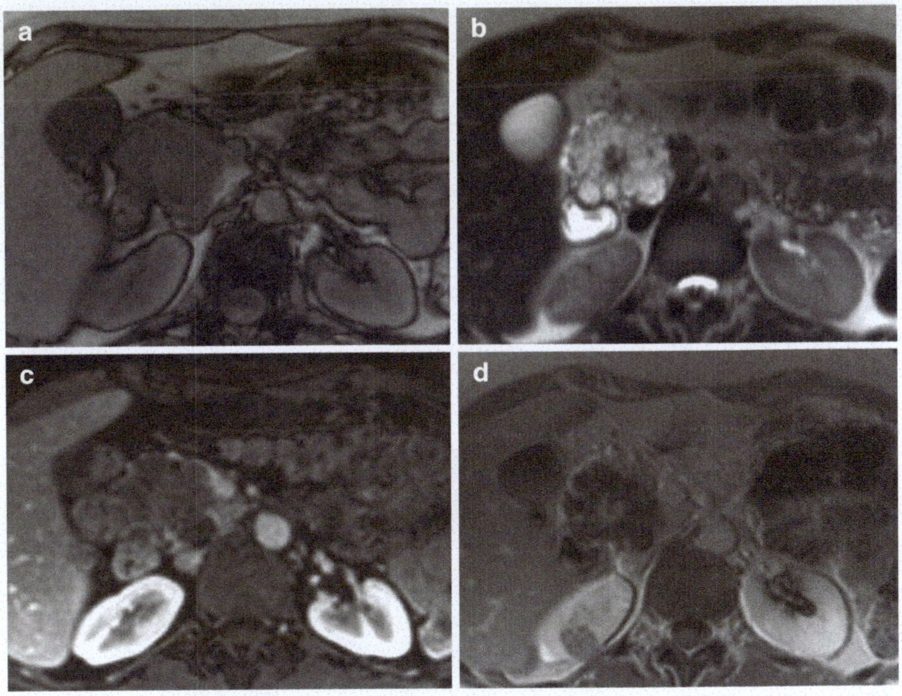

Fig. 6.38 Serous cystadenoma. (**a**) T1-W GRE shows a large hypointense mass in the pancreatic head with a pseudosolid appearance. (**b**) T2-W TSE shows the internal structure with innumerable tiny cysts and a central scar. (**c**) On the dynamic gadolinium-enhanced T1-W FS GRE image, only the septa enhance. (**d**) On the delayed enhanced image, contrast uptake into the central scar is seen

Mucinous adenoma or adenocarcinoma is a macrocystic potentially malignant mucin-containing tumor. Mucinous cystadenoma are unilocular or multilocular, usually located in the pancreatic body and tail, and occur more frequently in females. Single cysts are typically larger than 20 mm in diameter. The cystic structure is more readily visible with MRI than with CT. The cysts are hypointense on T1-WI and hyperintense on T2-WI. T1-W FS gadolinium-enhanced images show thick septa. Depending on the size and age of the patient, follow-up or resection of mucinous cystadenoma will be sought. At MRI, the appearance of thick irregular septations and nodular contrast-enhanced structures is suspicious for malignant transformations and should prompt histologic diagnosis. A differential diagnosis of macrocystic mucinous neoplasms is the rare entity of a solid and papillary epithelial neoplasm. This rather rare low-grade tumor with a low risk to metastasize is typically observed in young female patients during their second or third decade of life.

Intraductal Papillary Mucinous Tumor (IPMT)

Once considered a rare tumor, IPMT is now recognized with MRI and CT at increasing frequency. IPMT is a mucin-producing tumor, arising from the epithelium of the main pancreatic duct or side branches. Histologically, IPMT represents a spectrum of diseases, ranging from benign over borderline to frankly malignant tumors. According to their location, they are classified as main duct, branch duct, and combined type. Main duct type IPMT may show diffuse or segmental dilatation of the main duct due to mucin, typically hyperintense on T2-WI (Fig. 6.39). A branch duct type is a multilocular cystic lesion, most often in the uncinate process, with communication to the (nondilated) main duct, a feature to distinguish branch duct type IPMT from mucinous cystadenoma (Fig. 6.40). A combined type will involve the main duct as well as side branches and show massive duct dilatation. Main duct type IPMT have a higher risk for malignancy than branch duct type, which can be followed, if they are small (<3 cm) and asymptomatic. MRI features suggestive of malignant transformation are the presence of solid, contrast-enhanced nodules, main duct dilatation >10 mm, and diffuse involvement.

Simple Pancreatic Cysts

Simple pancreatic cysts with an epithelial cell lining are very rare and incidentally detected. They are more frequently associated with polycystic kidney disease

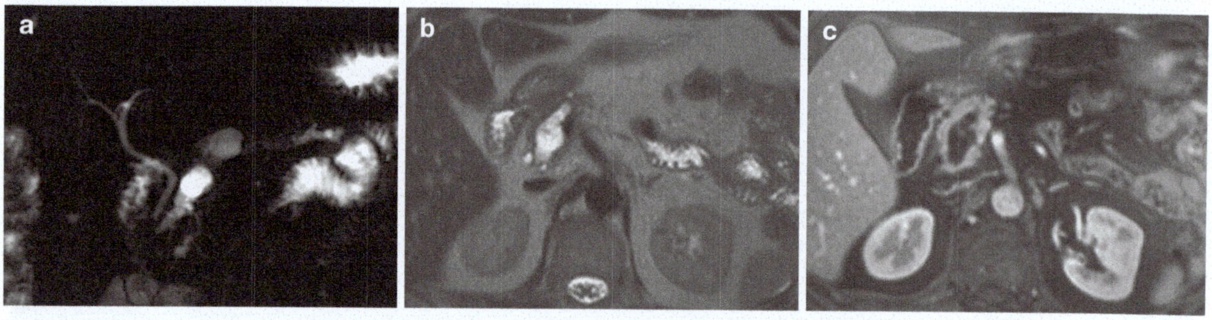

Fig. 6.39 IPMT (Intraductal Papillary Mucinous Tumor) of main duct type (malignant). (**a**) The coronal MRCP and (**b**) axial T2-W TSE show massive dilatation of the main duct with contour irregularities. (**c**) Axial gadolinium-enhanced T1-W GRE shows enhancing nodules in the duct, suspicious for malignant transformation

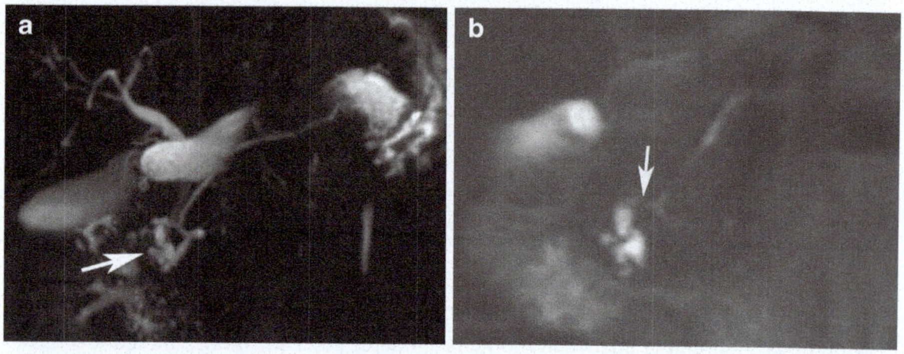

Fig. 6.40 IPMT of branch duct type. (**a**) Coronal MRCP shows a single dilated side branch in the head (*arrow*). (**b**) The thin section MRCP images show the communication of the side branch with the main duct (*arrow*), typical for IPMT

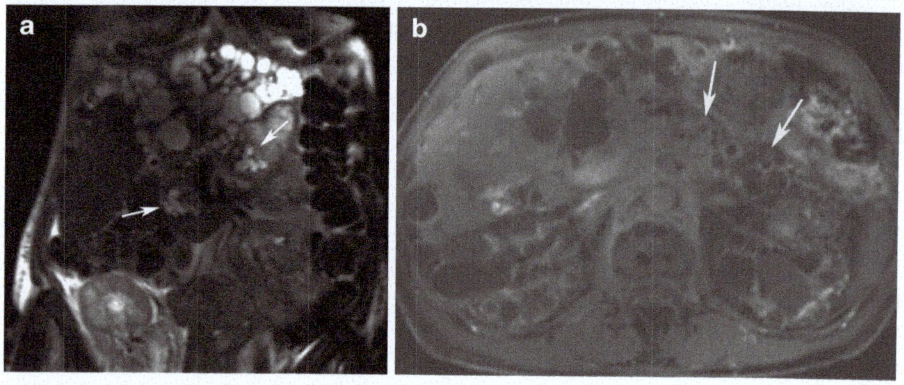

Fig. 6.41 Multiple simple cysts in polycystic kidney disease. (**a**) Coronal T2-W TSE and (**b**) axial gadolinium-enhanced T1-WI show multiple T2 hyperintense cysts without contrast enhancement (*arrows*). Note the innumerable cysts in kidneys and liver. Note renal transplant in right iliac fossa

and von Hippel-Lindau disease. MR features of these well-circumscribed, round, or oval cysts include low signal intensity on T1-WI, high signal intensity on T2-WI, and no contrast enhancement (Fig. 6.41).

6.7.5.2 Solid Tumors

Pancreatic Adenocarcinoma

The most common pancreatic tumor is ductal adenocarcinoma, accounting for more than 90% of primary malignant tumors of the pancreas and known for its dismal prognosis. Overall, only approximately 20% of pancreatic cancers are resectable at the time of diagnosis. Staging of disease is still the main role of imaging modalities to differentiate between resectable disease and locally advanced tumors and/or tumors with distant metastases. The incidental detection of a ductal adenocarcinoma is quite rare. Focal disease is present in 80% and diffuse involvement in 20%. Location of focal disease is predominantly confined to the pancreatic head in 60–70%. Since pancreatic carcinomas of the pancreatic head tend to obstruct the CBD and produce jaundice, these tumors are typically smaller than tumors of the body and tail at the time of diagnosis.

The standard imaging technique for staging of pancreatic cancer is MDCT with 3D reconstructions in many institutions. However, if CT is not possible or CT results are equivocal, MRI offers a comprehensive evaluation of the tumor, parenchymal organs, surrounding soft tissue, vessels, and ductal structures. Pancreatic adenocarcinoma is hypointense on T1-WI, and fat suppression improves conspicuity. Rapid scanning following gadolinium injection during the parenchymal phase (<30–50 s postinjection) should demonstrate tumors as hypointense (hypovascular) lesions (Fig. 6.42), and some enhancement of viable tumor may be visible on later scans in the venous and equilibrium phases. Consecutive pancreatic atrophy, causing low signal intensity of normal pancreas, may reduce contrast relative to focal tumors and, as a rule of thumb, the pancreas should only be considered normal if the signal intensity on T1-W GRE in-phase images (without or with fat suppression) is higher than that of the liver. Ductal obstruction is best visualized with MRCP techniques (Fig. 6.42). However, the depiction and differentiation of a pancreatic adenocarcinoma close to the ampulla of Vater, ampullary tumors, periampullary tumors, and distal bile duct calculi may still be difficult and require ERCP also for histopathologic proof and palliative intervention. T2-WI may help to rule out stones that appear with low signal intensity, while tumors appear with intermediate signal intensity; however, the detection of a stone does not rule out cancer.

Imaging analysis has to include all relevant structures. A dilatation of the pancreatic duct may already be suggestive for a tumor. Irregular ductal dilatations following the course of chronic pancreatitis and stone-related dilatations have to be considered. A pronounced tumor necrosis may mimic an abscess or pancreas necrosis in pancreatitis. Some tumors are associated with an inflammatory reaction and thus the tumor may appear larger. Regional peripancreatic lymph node metastases are observed in up to two third of patients. The presence of peripancreatic lymph node metastases does not preclude surgery. Irresectable disease is characterized by peritoneal carcinomatosis with ascites, tumor infiltration into the peripancreatic vasculature (i.e., celiac trunk, hepatic artery, and superior mesenteric artery) or surrounding organs (i.e., stomach) or liver metastases. The most difficult indication is to rule out or depict carcinoma within chronic pancreatitis (see Sect. 6.7.4.2).

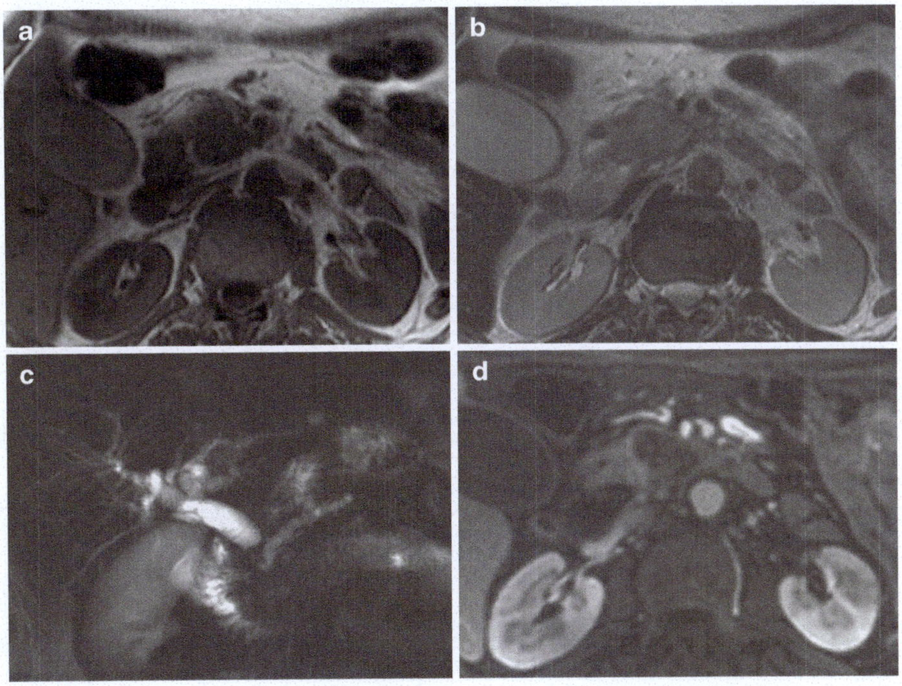

Fig. 6.42 Adenocarcinoma of the pancreatic head. (**a**) Axial T1-W GRE shows hypointense tumor in the head, which (**b**) is slightly hyperintense on T2-WI. (**c**) Typical double duct sign due to tumor obstruction of the CBD and main pancreatic duct. (**d**) On the gadolinium-enhanced T1-W GRE image in the parenchymal phase, the tumor is markedly hypointense to the parenchyma

Signs of inoperability (vascular involvement, involvement of adjacent organs, and distant metastases) are best identified by a comprehensive protocol, including plain FS T1-WI, T2-WI, gadolinium-enhanced MRI, MRCP, and ce-MRA. A capsule does not surround the pancreas and, thus, pancreatic carcinoma tends to invade along perivascular, lymphatic, and perineural structures. Therefore, the celiac axis, SMA, SMV, portal vein, and hepatoduodenal ligament are often encased or infiltrated at an early stage. Obliteration of perivascular fat planes and circumferential tumor growth around vessels or even vessel deformation by tumor are reliable signs of inoperability. Limited invasion into SMV or portal vein may be considered only a relative contraindication to surgery. The detection of lymph nodes is comparable to CT; however, nodes along the celiac axis and porta hepatis may be more readily visible with MR. Liver metastases are hypointense on T1-WI, slightly hyperintense on T2-WI, show rim enhancement on immediate gadolinium-enhanced T1-WI, and demonstrate no enhancement on delayed SPIO- or Teslascan-enhanced images (Fig. 6.43). MR offers the potential of a comprehensive test for the detection and staging of pancreatic adenocarcinoma; however, this requires that the study be specifically tailored to individual patients.

Neuroendocrine Tumors

The majority of NET, formerly known as islet cell tumors, arise from the pancreas. NET are classified as well differentiated, either functioning (i.e., histologically as insulinoma, gastrinoma, glucagonoma, VIPoma, and somatostatinoma) or nonfunctioning, well-differentiated endocrine carcinoma (functioning insulinoma, gastrinoma, glucagonoma, VIPoma, somatostatinoma, or nonfunctioning tumor), or poorly differentiated endocrine carcinoma. Most NET are well-differentiated, small tumors (<2 cm). Ninety percent of insulinoma are benign, but more than 50% of gastrinoma are malignant, and somatostatinoma, glucagonoma, VIPoma, and nonfunctioning tumors are almost always malignant. Functional tumors may be part of multiple endocrine neoplasm I syndrome. T1-W GRE FS, T2-W FS sequences, and dynamic gadolinium-enhanced T1-W GRE sequences are mandatory. Tumors are well defined, hypointense on T1-WI, demonstrate strong ring (larger tumors) or complete (smaller tumors) early gadolinium enhancement, and are mostly hyperintense on T2-WI (Fig. 6.44). This also differentiates NET from pancreatic adenocarcinoma. Liver metastases of NET tend to be tiny and multiple, and show hypervascularity on gadolinium-enhanced sequences. Vessels are typically not encased, no ductal dilatation is present, and central

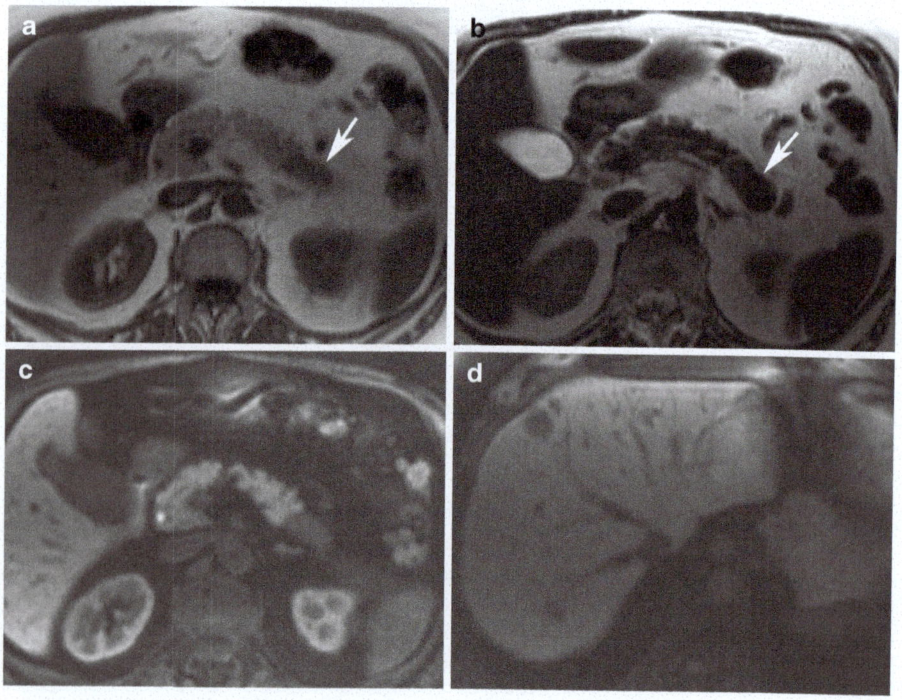

Fig. 6.43 Adenocarcinoma of the tail with liver metastases (*arrows*). The tumor in the tail is (**a**) hypointense on unenhanced T1-W and (**b**) isointense on T2-WI. (**c**, **d**) On the Teslascan-enhanced images, delineation of the tumor against the enhanced parenchyma is improved. There are several liver metastases present, which render the tumor irresectable

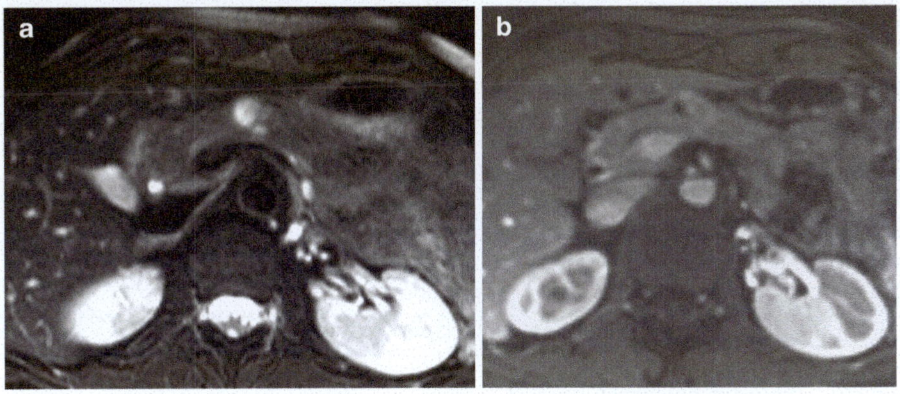

Fig. 6.44 Neuroendocrine tumor: insulinoma. (**a**) T2-W TSE FS images show a small hyperintense tumor in the body, which (**b**) is moderately hypervascular on the gadolinium-enhanced sequence

necrosis is rare compared with pancreatic adenocarcinoma. Insulinomas are usually more hypervascular than the other NET.

Lymphoma

Primary pancreatic lymphoma is very rare, but non-Hodgkin's lymphoma may directly involve the pancreas or peripancreatic lymph nodes during later stages of the disease, appearing with lower signal intensity than the pancreas on T1-WI and only mild contrast enhancement. Pancreatic lymphomas are typically large and present often with anterior displacement of the pancreas. Being a soft tumor, pancreatic lymphoma does not obstruct the common bile duct or the pancreatic duct early.

Metastases

Primary malignancies metastasizing to the pancreas or peripancreatic lymph nodes include melanoma, kidney, breast, lung, and gastrointestinal cancer. Melanoma metastases may display high signal intensity on T1-WI (due to melanin content) and RCC metastases tend to be multiple and very hypervascular (similar to the imaging features of a NET) (Fig. 6.45). In general, the patient history will lead to the diagnosis.

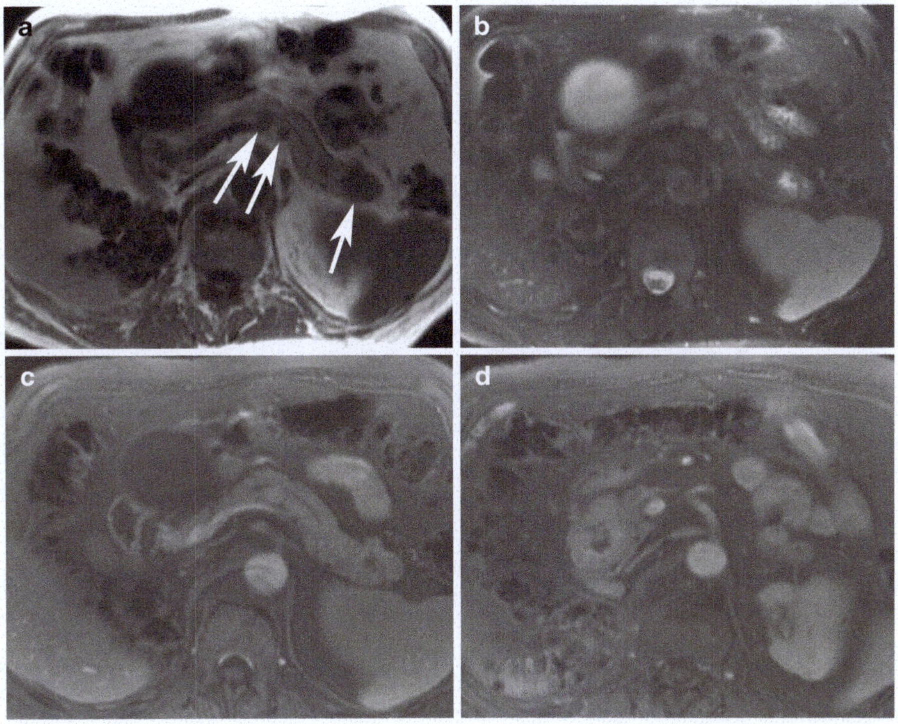

Fig. 6.45 Metastases from renal cell cancer. There are multiple masses in the pancreas (*arrows*), which (**a**) are hypointense on T1-WI and (**b**) hyperintense on T2-WI. (**c**, **d**) On the gadolinium-enhanced T1-W GRE FS in the arterial phase, the tumors are mostly hypervasular. Imaging features are similar to NET. Note right nephrectomy with typical position of right colon flexure

6.7.6 *Trauma and Surgical Complications*

6.7.6.1 Trauma

Since MRI with MRCP and ce-MRA is a comprehensive tool to assess all pancreatic components, it is also a valid means in acute trauma (Fig. 6.46). Lacerations show a broad range from contusion to complete transection of the parenchyma and duct, typically within the pancreatic body with development of peripancreatic fluid collections. Early pancreatitis is possible. Ductal injuries, typically evaluated by ERCP, may also be demonstrated by MRCP. Further complications are pseudocysts, strictures, aneurysms, or fistulas.

6.7.6.2 Pancreatic Surgery

Detailed information on surgical procedures performed in individual patients is helpful to interpret MR studies following pancreatic surgery. Surgical materials like vascular clips or clips from stapled intestinal anastomoses are no contraindication but may cause a signal void or susceptibility artifact. US and CT are the imaging methods of choice for imaging of most surgical complications. MR is useful to rule out or detect recurrent pancreatic tumor. However, surgical creation of a pancreatojejunostomy may pose a problem to the diagnostic radiologist, as the collapsed jejunal loop may mimic tumor recurrence at the anastomosis. In this case, secretin-enhanced MRCP will stimulate exocrine secretion to fill the jejunal loop with fluid for better differentiation. Problems located in the biliary ducts or pancreatic duct are a good indication since some surgical techniques do not always allow a postoperative ERCP.

6.7.6.3 Transplantation

MRI is typically performed to evaluate severe surgical complications such as transplant rejection or necrosis. The most common surgical technique connects afferent and efferent pancreatic vessels with iliac vessel and implants the pancreatic duct into the urinary bladder. Acute rejections are characterized by an edematous swelling of the organ and fluid collections. Dynamic perfusion studies with gadolinium chelates are useful to evaluate organ vascularization in chronic rejection and ce-MRA for the assessment of vascular complications.

6.8 GI Tract and Bowel

Thomas Lauenstein

6.8.1 *Anatomy: Stomach, Small Bowel, and Colon*

The stomach is typically J-shaped and is located in the left upper abdominal quadrant. It can show variable anatomical formations depending on the degree of gastric filling. Five main parts can be distinguished: (1) cardia, (2) fundus, (3) body, (4) antrum, and (5) pylorus. The latter connects the stomach to the duodenum. Due to its curved structure, a greater and lesser curvature of the stomach can be distinguished. Four different histological layers compromise the gastric wall, including (1) mucosa, (2) submucosa, (3) muscularis, and (4) serosa.

The small bowel encompasses the duodenum, jejunum, and ileum. Its length in adults can vary between 4 and 7 m. Although the small bowel is longer than

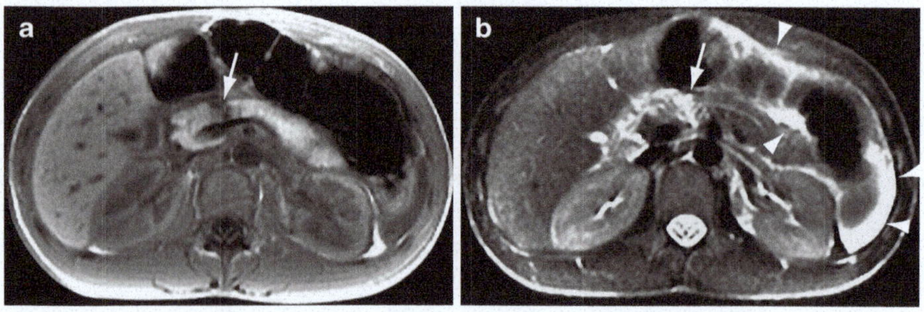

Fig. 6.46 Pancreatic trauma with transsection. Unenhanced T1-W GRE (**a**) and FS T2-W HASTE (TE 64ms) (**b**) in a child with abdominal pain following a bicycle accident. The pancreas shows a complete transsection (*arrows*) (T1-hypointense (**a**) – T2-hyperintense (**b**) anterior to the spinal column in the region of the pancreatic neck (between head and body). Free intraabdominal fluid (hemorrhage) is present (*arrowheads*) (**b**). Imaging findings were confirmed at surgery

the large bowel, the terminology "small" refers to its diameter. The proximal part of the small bowel, the duodenum, is divided into four parts: (1) the superior part, which passes from the pylorus to the superior duodenal flexure; (2) the descending part from the superior to the inferior duodenal flexure, which harbors the entrance of the hepatico-pancreatico duct at the duodenal papilla; (3) the inferior/horizontal part crossing the IVC, aorta, and vertebral column; and (4) ascending part terminating at the duodenojejunal flexure/ligament of Treitz where it joins the jejunum in the left upper quadrant. The first three parts describe a C shape around the pancreatic head. Except for the superior part, the duodenum is located in the retroperitoneum. The mesenteric small bowel encompasses the jejunum in the superior/left abdomen and ileum in the inferior abdomen. The ileum has fewer mucosal folds than the jejunum. The terminal ileum is separated from the cecum by the ileocecal valve.

The large bowel is divided into appendix, cecum, ascending colon, transverse colon, descending colon, sigmoid colon, and rectum. Its length amounts to approximately 150 cm in adults. Ascending, descending colon, and rectum are retroperitoneal, while cecum, transverse, and sigmoid colon are intraperitoneal.

6.8.2 MRI Technique

6.8.2.1 Patient Preparation

Residual stool or foodstuff may obviate the evaluation of gastrointestinal wall structures. Therefore, MRI should be performed following a 4–6 h fasting period to ensure a consistent assessment of the stomach and the small bowel. As transit times of the colon may widely vary, bowel cleansing needs to be performed in an identical way to that required for conventional colonoscopy if the colonic wall is to be visualized.

6.8.2.2 Bowel Distension

As stomach and bowel loops are collapsed in their physiological state, a reliable distension must be achieved to allow for a reliable evaluation of the gastric or bowel wall. Otherwise, insufficient distension may result in false-positive or false-negative findings: collapsed segments may mimic bowel wall thickening being misinterpreted as inflammation or tumor disease. On the flipside, smaller lesions may be missed.

Good distension of the stomach can be easily accomplished by oral administration of water or water-based contrast agents. The mere ingestion of 500 cc contrast leads to a good distension and a reliable assessment of the gastric wall. Due to the fast passage of liquids to the small bowel, image data should be collected without any time delay after contrast administration.

As for the small bowel, there are two different techniques available to achieve bowel distension. (1) Oral contrast agents can be administered via a nasoduodenal tube in a similar manner as for conventional enteroclysis. This technique leads to homogenously high bowel distension. However, the procedure may be perceived as traumatizing by patients. (2) The mere oral administration of contrast agents without intubation is noninvasive. As water is rapidly reabsorbed in the small bowel, water-based formulas with a high osmolarity have been used. These agents provide similar signal properties as water. However, in contrary to pure water, they are absorpted to a smaller fraction in the gastrointestinal tract. Mannitol and sorbitol are widely used carbohydrates and mix well with water. Solutions of mannitol or sorbitol have been shown to provide good bowel distension when used in concentrations between 1.5 and 2.5%. Another substance represents polyethylene glycol 4000 (PEG 4000), a strong hydrophilic molecule, which has no intestinal absorption. PEG 4000 has been shown to provide high luminal distension of small bowel loops. The oral administration of these solutions results in a consistently high small bowel distension. Ingestion should start approximately 45 min prior to the examination. A total volume of 1,200–1,500 cc is to be given at a steady, evenly distributed rate. Furthermore, gastric emptying enhancing substances (e.g., metoclopramide) should be used to allow for a fast transit through the stomach.

The administration of distending media including water solutions or gasiform media (room air, CO_2) via a rectal catheter results in a good distension of all colonic segments. Usually 1,500–2,000 cc of contrast should be applied when the colon is examined.

6.8.2.3 Imaging Protocol

Patients should be examined in prone position. This position has advantages for the depiction of bowel loops because a thinner slab in coronal plane can be used. A torso phased-array surface coil should be utilized for signal reception. The administration of spasmolytic agents (e.g., scopolamine or glucagon) has a proven

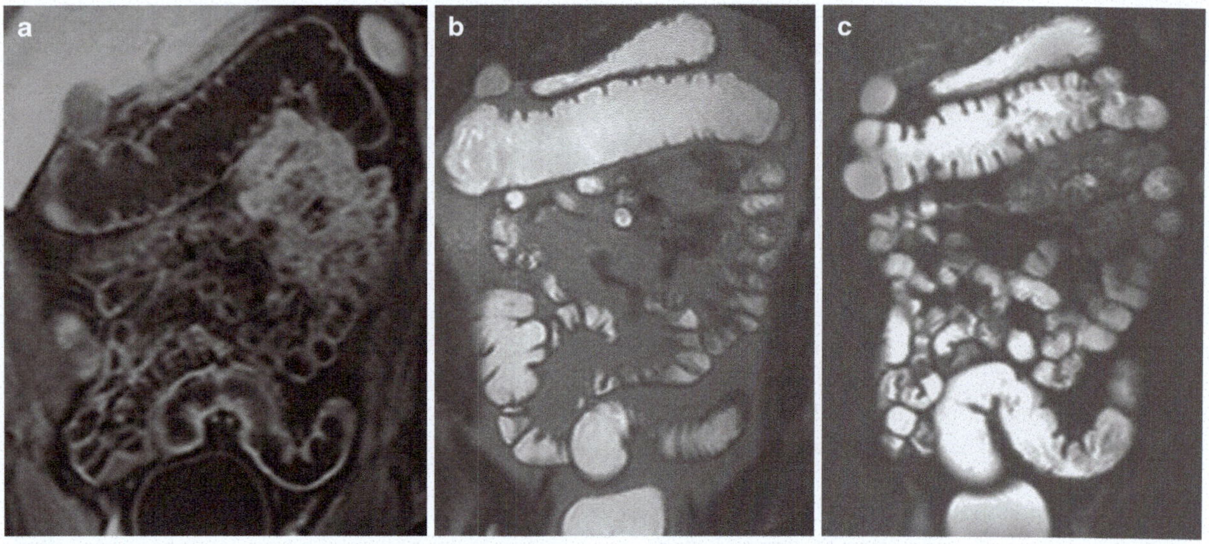

Fig. 6.47 Three main sequences types for MRI of the GIT. Contrast-enhanced T1-W GRE showing a hyperintense bowel wall and a hypointense bowel lumen (**a**); FISP imaging without fat saturation (**b**) and T2-W SSFSE imaging with fat saturation exhibiting a hypointense bowel wall and a hyperintense bowel lumen (**c**)

benefit for MRI of the GI tract: motion artifacts are significantly reduced. Besides, optimal bowel distension will be ensured. As spasmolytic agents have a short half-life, they only should be administered shortly before data collection.

MR data acquisition is performed under breath-hold conditions and can be limited to three sequence types. (1) Fast imaging with steady-state precession (FISP): this sequence provides a good anatomical overview and is motion insensitive, which can be particularly important in patients unable to hold their breath. Different vendor-specific names have been introduced: TrueFISP (Siemens Medical Solution), Balanced Fast Field Echo (Philips Medical Systems), and FIESTA (General Electric Medical Systems). FISP data should be collected without fat suppression, because it does not only ensure a good visualization of the GI tract itself, but also of adjacent mesenteric and retroperitoneal structures. (2) Single-shot T2-W imaging with fat saturation: this sequence type is helpful to depict edema in keeping with inflammatory processes. (3) 3D GRE T1-W MRI: this data should be acquired in conjunction with the intravenous administration of paramagnetic contrast. After a first precontrast T1-W 3D GE data set, paramagnetic contrast is administered i.v. (0.1–0.2 mmol/kg gadolinium) and the acquisition is repeated after a delay of 20 s (arterial phase), 70 s (portal venous phase), 120 s (venous phase), and 180 s (equilibrium phase). Imaging examples for all sequence types are shown in Fig. 6.47.

6.8.3 Stomach Pathology

6.8.3.1 Stomach–Inflammatory and Infectious disease

The main etiological factor for gastritis is the infection with *Helicobacter pylori*. However, causes may be related to drug therapy (especially NSAIDs), alcohol intake, radiation therapy, and severe stress. Ulcerations following chronic gastritis can particularly be found at the lesser gastric curvature. Inflammatory disease goes along with an increased contrast enhancement of the gastric wall on T1-W images. Furthermore, T2-W imaging with fat saturation exhibits an increased signal of the gastric wall in acute inflammatory disease.

Zollinger–Ellison syndrome is a severe peptic ulcer disease in conjunction with thickened gastric and duodenal folds (Fig. 6.48). Underlying reason is an increased gastric acid production due to a gastrin-producing pancreatic tumor. Similarly to features of gastritis, an elevated T2 signal of the gastric wall as well as increased enhancement after intravenous contrast administration can be seen. An important differential diagnosis includes Menetrier disease, presenting thickened

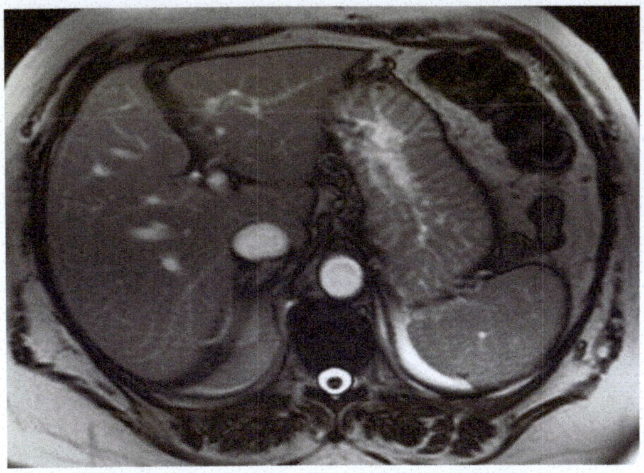

Fig. 6.48 Zollinger–Ellison syndrome. Axial FISP image exhibits a diffuse thickening of all gastric folds

Table 6.2 TNM classification of gastric adenocarcinoma

Primary tumor (T)
T1: tumor limited to mucosa/submucosa
T2: tumor reaching the serosa
T3: tumor surpassing the serosa. Adjacent organs are not involved
T4: tumor infiltrating neighbouring organs
Lymph node involvement (N)
N0: no lymph node metastases
N1: regional lymph nodes affected within 3 cm of the primary tumor
N2: regional lymph node metastases more than 3 cm from the primary tumor
N3: distant lymph node metastases (retroperitoneal, intraabdominal)
Distant metastases (M)
M0: no distant metastases
M1: distant metastases

tortuous gastric folds. The extension of disease is usually limited to the gastric fundus and body, while the antrum is mostly spared. The etiology of Menetrier disease is unknown.

6.8.3.2 Stomach–Benign Neoplasm

Most gastric polyps (80–90%) are hyperplastic and benign. Adenomatous polyps must be considered real neoplasm similar to adenomas in the colon. The malignant potential of adenomatous polyps is size-dependent and almost half of these lesions >2 cm contain a focus of adenocarcinoma. Polyps are mainly found in patients with chronic gastritis or polyposis syndromes. A sufficiently high gastric distension is mandatory for a good visualization of gastric polyps. Benign polyps show similar signal characteristics and enhancement patterns like the normal gastric wall. In presence of adenocarcinoma, a more heterogeneous contrast enhancement can be revealed. Retained food particles may simulate gastric polyps on unenhanced MRI. However, gastric polyps always show some form of contrast enhancement while food particles do not.

6.8.3.3 Stomach–Malignant Neoplasm

Adenocarcinoma

Adenocarcinoma is the most common malignant neoplasm of the stomach. Predisposing factors include chronic gastritis, adenomatous polyps, pernicious anemia, dietary nitrates, and Menetrier disease. Native Japanese have been found to have a higher risk of disease. The tumor may exhibit different growth patterns such as exophytic, ulcerative, or diffusely infiltrative. Metastases will spread mainly to liver, lungs, peritoneum, and regional lymph nodes. The TNM classification for gastric adenocarcinoma is shown in Table 6.2. The T1 signal of gastric adenocarcinoma is isointense to the normal gastric wall, while the T2 signal can be slightly increased. Gadolinium enhancement can be very variable in the tumor, depending on the size and presence of necrotic tissue (Fig. 6.49). However, most forms of gastric adenocarcinoma exhibit an increased gadolinium enhancement.

Gastrointestinal Stromal Tumors (GIST)

GIST is an entity of smooth-muscle tumors of the gastric and bowel wall. It is a well-circumscribed submucosal mass (Fig. 6.50). Although being rare and constituting only 2% of all gastric malignancies, it can mainly be found in the stomach (70%). Other locations include small bowel (20%) and esophagus (10%). Both benign and malignant forms of GIST can be found. Imaging characteristics are not leading to determine the malignant potential. An exophytic component with necrotic/hemorrhagic central area can often be found. High-grade GIST have an increased vascularity resulting in an elevated T2 signal and increased gadolinium enhancement. Low-grade tumors only show little

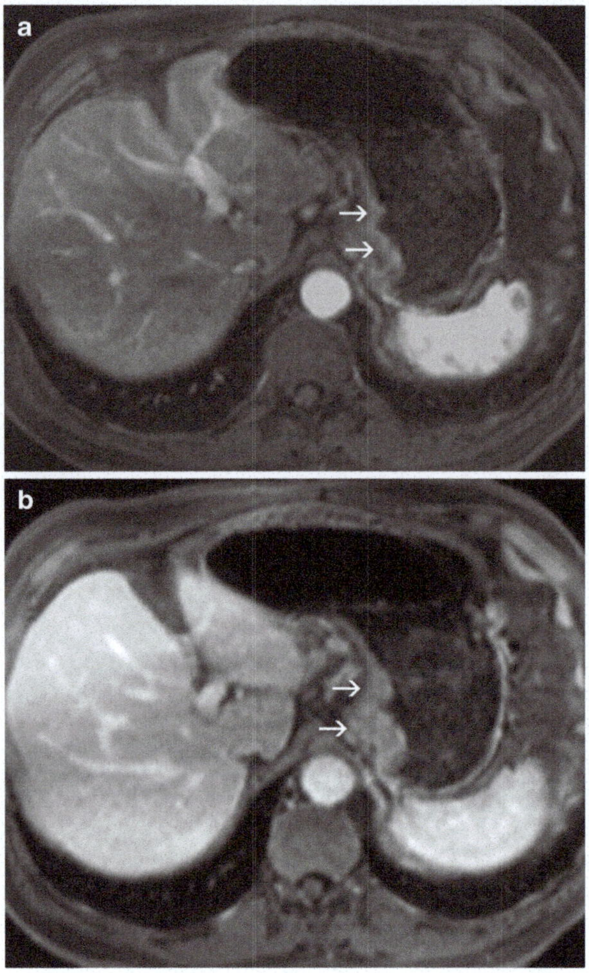

Fig. 6.49 Gastric adenomcarcinoma. Axial T1-W GRE images of a gastric adenocarcinoma: increased mucosal/submucosal enhancement during the arterial phase (**a**) and considerable gastric wall thickening shown on portalvenous contrast phase (**b**)

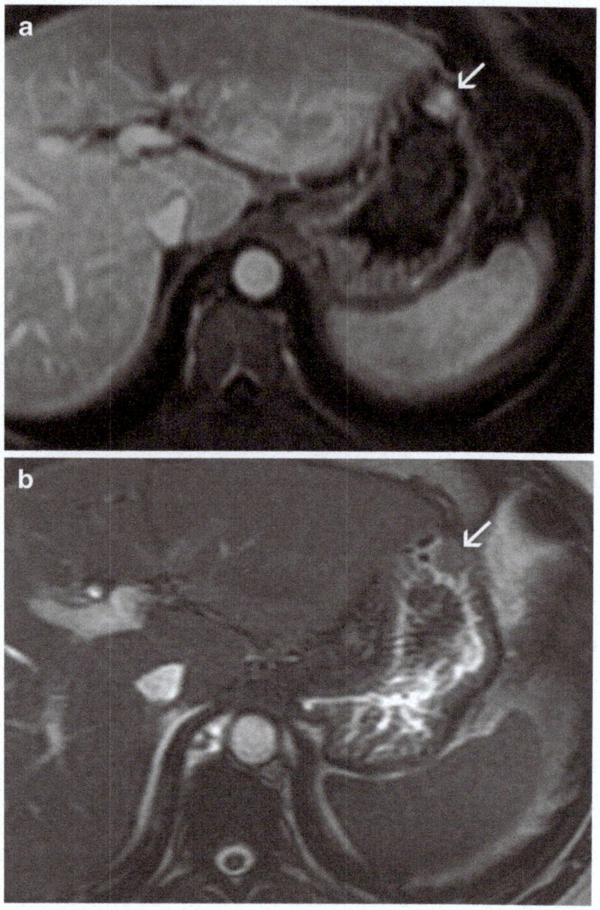

Fig. 6.50 Gastrointestinal stromal tumor. GIST in the ventral part of the gastric body: axial T1-W images after gadolinium administration exhibit a strong enhancement accounting for a high-grade neoplasm (**a**). T2-W images show an intermediate homogenous signal of a well-circumscribed lesion (**b**)

enhancement. It can be difficult to differentiate GIST from lymphoma or exophytic adenocarcinoma. The latter tumor is in general less vascular and often leads to focal thickening of adjacent gastric wall.

Lymphoma

As primary lymphomas are extremely rare, mostly spread of non-Hodgkin lymphoma (NHL) can be seen. Approximately 50% of gastrointestinal NHL can be found in the stomach, 40% in the small bowel and 10% in the large bowel. This form of lymphoma mainly arises from mucosa-associated lymphoid tissue (MALT). A diffuse thickening of the gastric wall with preservation of rugal folds can often be found, which is well displayed on T2-W and contrast-enhanced T1-W images (Fig. 6.51). Hodgkin lymphomas, however, may lead to a rigid, nondistensible stomach. A gastric lymphoma should be considered, especially in presence of regional and/or widespread adenopathy.

Metastases and Carcinoid Tumor

Gastric metastases are uncommon. Metastatic disease of the stomach can be mainly found by hematogenous spread of melanoma, bronchial carcinoma, and breast carcinoma. They are typically located in the submucosa. Imaging features are mostly comparable to the

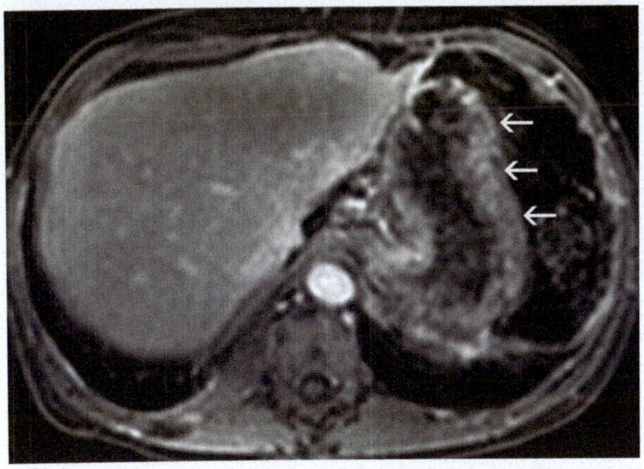

Fig. 6.51 Gastric lymphoma. A diffuse thickening of the gastric wall can be seen on axial contrast-enhanced T1-W images

primary malignancy. A direct invasion can be found in pancreatic cancer and cancer of the transverse colon as well as in HCC.

Carcinoids are well-differentiated NET. They are mainly found in the small bowel and in the appendix, but can rarely occur in the stomach. Hypergastrinemia may stimulate the growth of neuroendocrine cells and thus may lead to the development of carcinoid tumors. Imaging features are discussed in the small bowel section.

6.8.4 Small Bowel Pathology

6.8.4.1 Inflammatory and Infectious Disease

Inflammatory and infectious changes are the most common pathologies affecting the small bowel. A good distension is crucial to depict even tiny lesions of the small bowel wall. Numerous different imaging features can be found and it can be difficult if not impossible to differentiate between inflammatory and infectious disease (Table 6.3). Hereby, clinical features of the patient play a key role.

Table 6.3 MRI features of inflammatory and infectious small bowel disease

Transmural bowel wall thickening
Increased contrast enhancement of the bowel wall
Luminal narrowing
Increased number of periintestinal lymph nodes
Mesenteric stranding
Elevated T2 signal of bowel wall and adjacent tissue in active disease

FISP imaging may be particularly important to evaluate bowel wall thickening, depiction of mesenteric lymph nodes and periintestinal stranding. Besides, fistulae can be easily detected on these images. Gadolinium-enhanced T1-W data is helpful to detect inflammatory or infectious disease independent of its activity state with a high sensitivity of nearly 90%. However, specificity of T1-W imaging is limited. Thus, it is often difficult to differentiate between active and chronic inflammation/infection (Figs. 6.52 and 6.53). While active disease shows increased contrast enhancement due to increased perfusion and vascularity, chronic disease may also strongly enhance due to fibrotic changes. The latter observation is comparable to findings of late enhancement in infracted myocardial tissue. Therefore, the evaluation of disease activity remains one challenging task. This is often a key factor because therapeutic options are different, especially for active and chronic IBD. While active inflammation is treated with immunomodulator drugs such as corticosteroids, interventional or surgical therapeutic

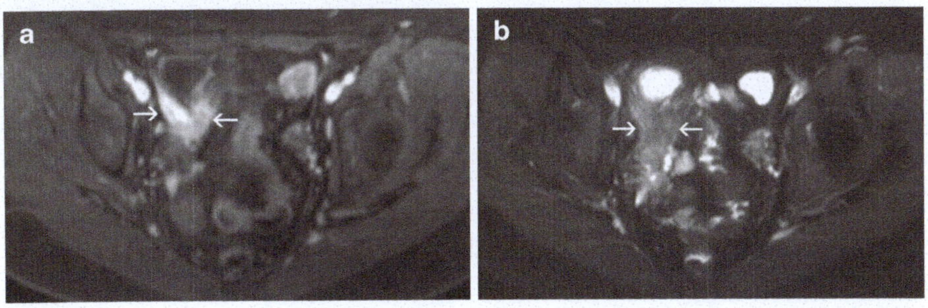

Fig. 6.52 Active Crohn's disease. A disease differentiation between active and chronic inflammation is difficult based on contrast-enhanced T1-W imaging due to the increased contrast uptake of the bowel wall (**a**). T2-W imaging in conjunction with fat saturation proves the diagnosis of active inflammation. High signal of the bowel wall and adjacent tissue due to edema can be found (**b**)

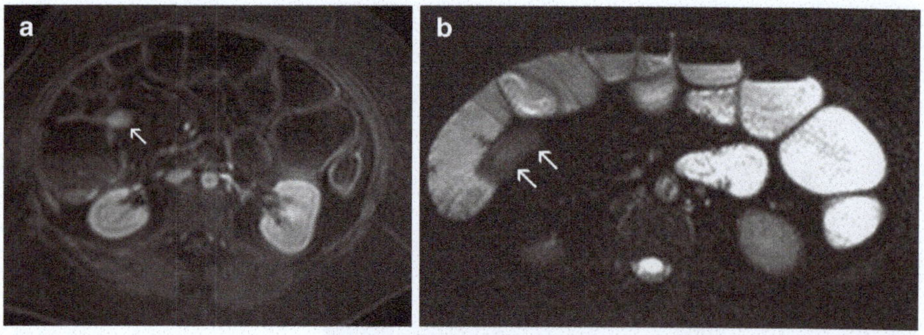

Fig. 6.53 Crohn's disease with chronic/fibrotic changes. Similar to active inflammatory disease, an elevated contrast enhancement of the bowel wall is present (**a**). However, there is only low to moderate signal on fat-saturated T2 images (**b**)

options are chosen for chronic disease. T2-W imaging with fat suppression can be used as a good marker for the detection of active inflammatory bowel disease, because edema in or adjacent to the bowel wall can be easily visualized (Fig. 6.52). Chronically inflamed/fibrotic bowel segments, however, do not show an increased T2 signal (Fig. 6.53).

Crohn's Disease

Crohn's disease (CD) is the most common chronic inflammatory pathology affecting the small bowel. There is a peak of incidence in the second and third decade of life and a smaller peak in the sixth and seventh decade of life. MRI should be preferred over CT for the diagnosis and follow-up of CD due to the high number of young patients and repetitive imaging for therapeutic monitoring. The exact etiology of CD is unknown. Several (co-) factors are considered to be relevant, including genetic, immunologic, environmental, and psychogenic mechanisms. All parts of the GI tract can be potentially affected. However, most common sites include the terminal ileum and proximal colon. The inflammation itself is mostly granulomatous and transmural. In early stages of CD, aphtoid ulcerations of the mucosa can be found. Other typical appearances of CD include skip lesions (areas of inflammation separated by unaffected areas), cobblestone mucosa, bowel wall fissures and fistulae (Fig. 6.54). As mentioned earlier, CD may be indistinguishable from infectious disease such as yersiniosis or tuberculosis. Clinical presentation and follow-up after treatment may help to distinguish between these entities. Another differential diagnosis is backwash ileitis in ulcerative colitis (UC). Backwash ileitis does not show strictures, it is continuous with affected adjacent colonic segments and the inflammation type is not transmural, but limited to the mucosa.

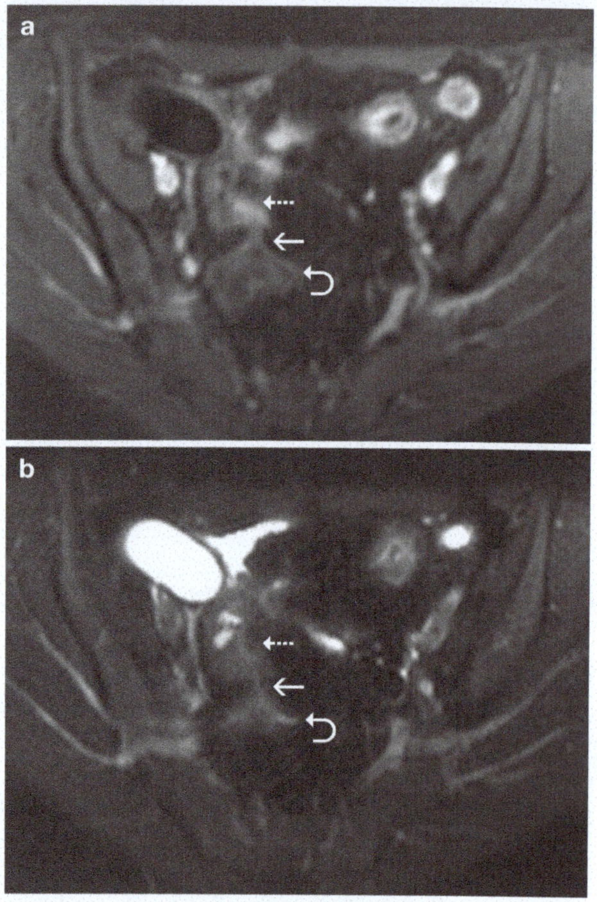

Fig. 6.54 Interintestinal fistula. Fistula (*arrow*) between distal ileum (*dashed arrow*) and sigmoid colon (*curved arrow*) shown on contrast-enhanced T1-W MRI (**a**). The fluid-containing fistula tract can also easily be depicted on T2-W MRI (**b**)

Infectious Enteritis

Different bacterial, viral, protozoal, and fungal pathogens can cause active infection of the small bowel. MRI features are nonspecific and often similar to those of CD. Most common infections are caused by *Campylobacter jejuni* or *Yersinia enterocolica*. Yersiniosis often manifests as ileitis terminalis, thereby mimicking CD or appendicitis. Due to the increasing number of immunecompromised patients, the spectrum of pathogens has become broader and also includes cytomegalovirus, mycobacterium avium-intracellulare, and cryptosporidium species.

Radiation Enteritis

The small intestine is very sensitive to radiation exposure. The radiation tolerance of the ileum is the lowest within the small bowel. Direct cytotoxic effects coupled with ischemic changes lead to radiation-based enteritis. Permanent radiological features may occur between 1 month and 2 years after radiation therapy. Typical changes include diffuse symmetric mural thickening and luminal narrowing with small bowel obstruction and prestenotic dilatation (Fig. 6.55). Furthermore, presence of adhesions may lead to an angulation between adjacent bowel loops. On T2-W images, a typical submucosal edema can be appreciated in early stage radiation enteritis. Differential diagnoses include lymphoma showing in general a widened bowel lumen and fewer strictures. In addition, primary bowel tumors can mimic radiation enteritis. However, they have a more irregular appearance and show more mass effects.

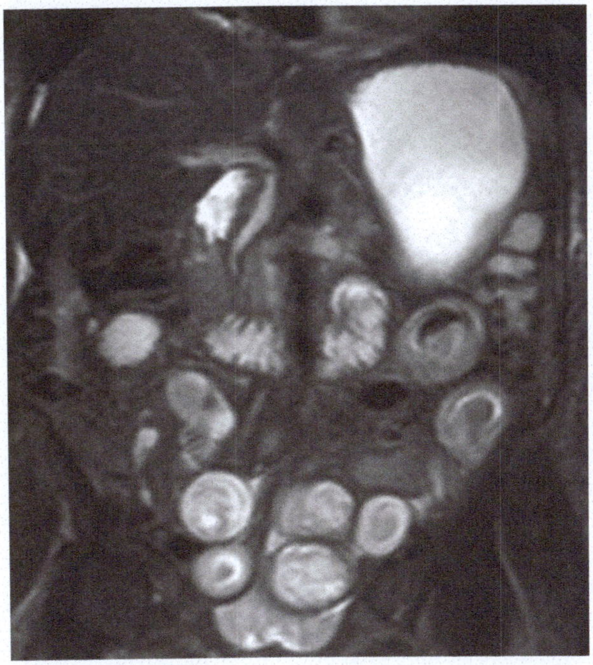

Fig. 6.55 Radiation enteritis. T2-W MRI exhibits diffuse symmetric mural thickening and with small bowel dilatation

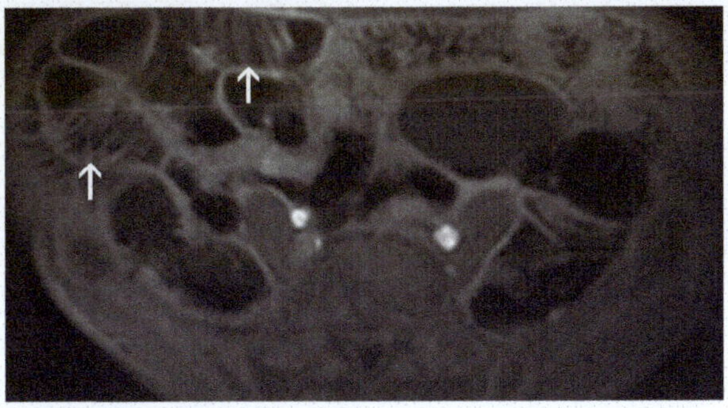

Fig. 6.56 Celiac disease. A typical jejunalization of the distal ileum with an increasing number of ileal folds is shown on T1-W contrast-enhanced images

Celiac Disease

Celiac disease is a malabsorption syndrome of the small bowel caused by an immunologically mediated inflammation as a response to dietary glutens. Most significant clinical symptoms are diarrhea and weight. It goes along with an atrophy of jejuna villi resulting in a numerical decrease of jejuna folds (ilealization). On the flipside, the number of ileal folds increase (jejunalization; Fig. 6.56). Thus, celiac disease leads to a jejunoileal fold pattern reversal.

6.8.4.2 Benign Neoplasm

Benign tumors of the small bowel are rare. Polyps are still the most frequent type of benign neoplasm. Adenomatous polyps can be seen in the setting of Gardner syndrome, familial polyposis syndrome, while hamartomatous polyps are found in patients with Peutz–Jeghers syndrome. They increase in frequency from duodenum to ileum. Although mostly asymptomatic, polyps can be a common localization for intussusceptions. Similarly to gastric and colonic polyps, they usually show a strong enhancement after gadolinium administration. This makes them distinguishable from residual foodstuff. Leiomyomas form another groups of benign small bowel tumors. They are proliferations of the smooth-muscle in the submucosa or muscularis externa and can either protrude into the bowel lumen or produce a mass effect on adjacent bowel loops.

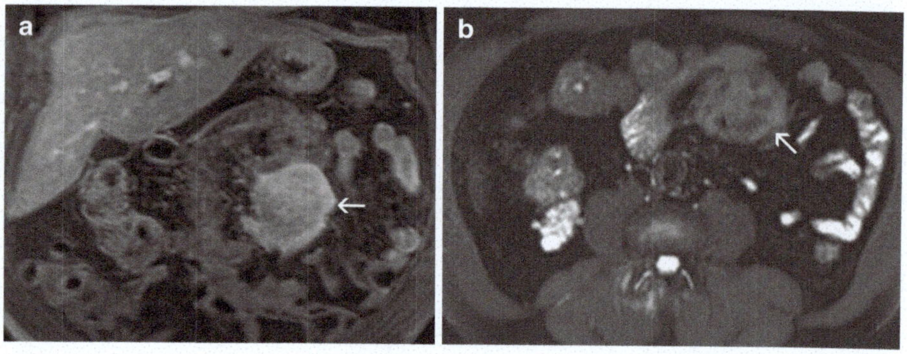

Fig. 6.57 Jejunal carcinoid tumor. A well-circumscribed lesion with increased contrast uptake (**a**) and moderate to increased signal on T2-W images (**b**) is seen

6.8.4.3 Malignant Neoplasm

Malignant neoplasm of the small bowel can be categorized in a similar way to malignant tumors of the stomach. Thus, adenocarcinoma, carcinoid tumor, and lymphoma need to be considered. GIST and metastases of the small bowel are very rare. As clinical information is presented in the gastric section, only mayor features and differences will be described below.

Adenocarcinoma

The most common site of adenocarcinoma of the small bowel is the duodenum. As the tumor often arises in close proximity to the papilla, jaundice may be one of the leading clinical symptoms. Furthermore, it can be found in the proximal jejunum. Similar to gastric and colonic adenocarcinoma, tumors may present with a variety of imaging patterns depending on the tumor's size and degree of necrosis. However, a moderate (albeit heterogeneous) enhancement can be seen after gadolinium administration.

Carcinoid Tumor

Carcinoid tumors represent the most common primary neoplasm of the small bowel. About 80% of carcinoid tumors arise in the distal and terminal ileum. Different features of carcinoid tumors can be found including submucosal involvement, bowel wall thickening or mesenteric extension. Large tumor can lead to bowel obstruction and intussusceptions. Small tumors can be easily missed on MRI, and concomitant lymphadenopathy/desmoplastic reaction of the mesenteries may be the only detectable manifestation. The tumor itself is hyperintense/isointense to musculature on T2-W images and shows a moderate to strong contrast enhancement (Fig. 6.57). Carcinoid tumors are in most cases asymptomatic, but a carcinoid syndrome can occur with cutaneous flushing, wheezing, and diarrhea. Hypervascular liver metastases can be almost always found in presence of the carcinoid syndrome.

Lymphoma

Lymphomas of the small bowel are usually non-Hodgkin-lymphoma of the B cell type, which arise from the MALT. They often are diffusely infiltrating several bowel loops causing bowel wall thickening (Fig. 6.58). However, they can rarely imitate polypoid or exophytic lesions. Despite the infiltrate character, bowel obstruction is only rarely seen. Rather dilated bowel segments are found assumingly due to the interference with the innervations of the enteric smooth muscles.

6.8.4.4 Miscellaneous

Diverticula

A diverticulum is defined as a mucosal outpouching, which communicates with gastrointestinal lumen. The duodenum is the most common site of small bowel diverticula. Especially large diverticula can cause a mass effect and therefore lead to a stenosis of the biliary and pancreatic tree. They can be depicted as air or air fluid-filled structures (Fig. 6.59). Depending on their filling state, they can considerably change in size between two examinations.

Meckel diverticulum is an ileal outpouching due to persistence of the congenital omphalomesenteric duct. Its prevalence is about 2% in the general population. It is located about 50 cm proximal of the ileocecal valve

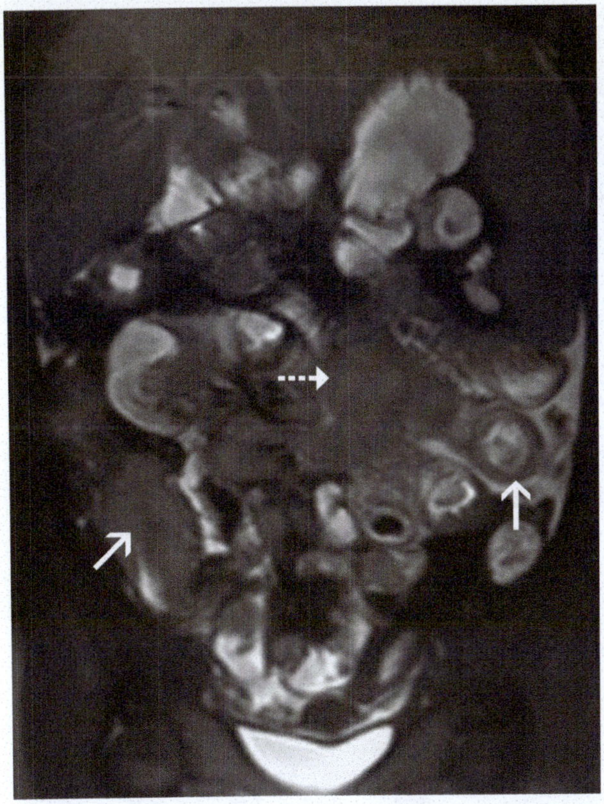

Fig. 6.58 Small bowel lymphoma. T2-W coronal MRI: a large mesenteric lymphoma manifestation (*dashed arrow*) is found with affection/thickening of several bowel wall loops (*arrows*)

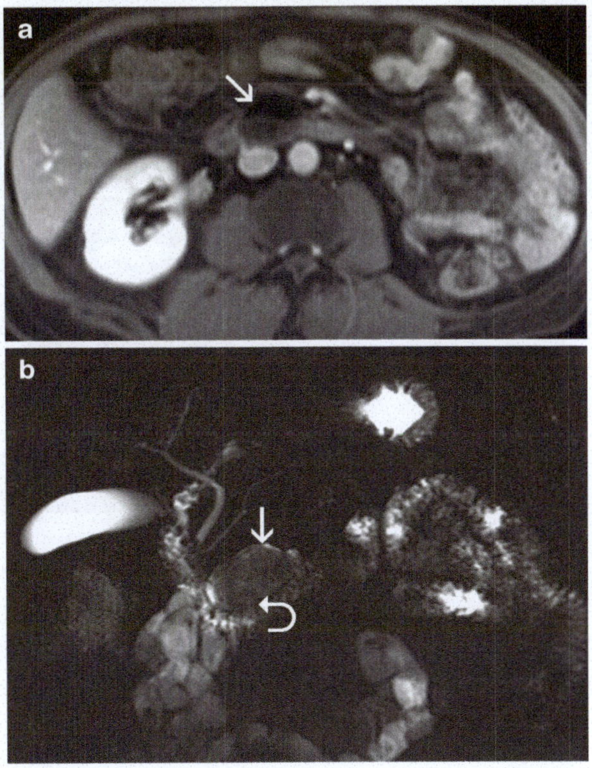

Fig. 6.59 Duodenal diverticulum. An outpouching with fluid/gas layer is seen in the horizontal part of the duodenum on the contrast-enhanced T1-W axial image (**a**, *arrow*). A communication between duodenum and diverticulum can be clearly seen on the MRCP image (**b**, *curved arrow*)

and arises from the antimesenteric border of the ileum. About 50% of Meckel diverticula contain ectopic gastric mucosa, and GI bleeding is one of the main complications. Diverticulitis and bowel obstruction represent other complications.

Ischemia

Mesenteric ischemia is caused by lack of oxygen supply to the small bowel due to vascular occlusion or hypoperfusion. This leads to capillary leakage and mural edema in an acute stage. Early imaging pattern include diffuse bowel wall thickening. The late phase of ischemia can result in mural hemorrhage, necrosis, pneumatosis intestinalis, and postmesenteric venous gas, particularly portal venous gas. Bowel wall hemorrhage from ischemia can be easily assessed due to the high signal on both T1-W and T2-W images.

6.8.5 Colon

6.8.5.1 Inflammatory and Infectious Disease

Main features of inflammatory changes including CD and radiation enteritis are described in the Sect. 6.8.4. CD can exclusively affect the large bowel in approximately 25% of all patients. CD is often difficult to be distinguished from UC. However, haustral markings are maintained in CD and often skip lesions are found. As for radiation enteritis, the rectosigmoid is most prone to be affected. While acute radiation induces edema, late changes include fibrosis and development of strictures.

Ulcerative Colitis

UC is a chronic diffuse inflammation involving colorectal mucosa. There is a peak of incidence in the second and third decade of life. Similar to the CD,

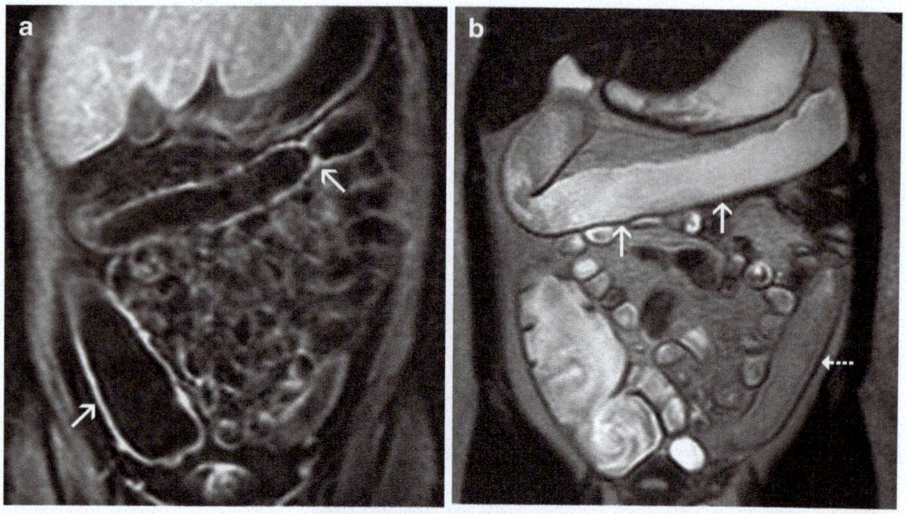

Fig. 6.60 Ulcerative colitis. A thickened bowel wall with increased contrast uptake is seen on T1-W MRI (**a**, *arrows*). Furthermore, a loss of haustral folds (lead pipe sign) is shown on T2-W images (**b**) in the transverse colon (*arrows*) and descending colon (*dashed arrow*)

the etiology of UC is not fully understood. Genetic, infectious, nutritional, and immunological factors are claimed to play a role. Associated abnormalities are primary sclerosing cholangitis, uveitis, and ankylosing spondylitis. Patients with UC have a highly increased risk of colorectal cancer and the development of a toxic megacolon. The disease originates in the rectum. It extends contiguously to more proximal colonic segments and may eventually affect the entire colon. Typical early imaging findings include edematous changes resulting in bowel wall thickening, and ulcerations leading to mucosal islands and pseudopolyps. As disease progresses, a luminal narrowing and loss of haustral folds (lead pipe sign) occurs (Fig. 6.60). In about one fourth of all patients, the terminal ileum is involved (backwash ileitis). As mentioned earlier, a differentiation between UC and CD may be difficult. It should be noted that there is lack of serosal/peri-colonic inflammatory involvement and lack of fistula in UC. Furthermore, UC does not result in a transmural inflammation and shows a continuous retrograde affection of the large bowel. Gadolinium-enhanced T1-W images are most helpful to depict UC. Increased contrast uptake is present both at acute and chronic stages of disease. However, fat-suppressed T2-W imaging helps to differentiate between active and chronic/fibrotic changes (Figs. 6.61 and 6.62).

Appendicitis

Although CT and US are main imaging tools for the diagnosis of appendicitis, there are certain features of MRI (lack of ionizing radiation, excellent soft-tissue contrast) making it an attractive alternative. A dilated appendix >7 mm is always suspicious for appendicitis. Focal bowel wall thickening at the cecal tip and increased gadolinium enhancement can be found. Furthermore, pericecal stranding and increased T2 signal of the bowel wall and the adjacent tissue is typical (Fig. 6.63).

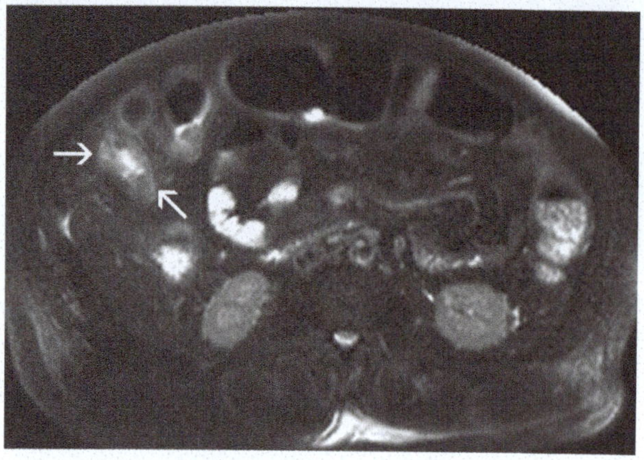

Fig. 6.61 Active colitis. An increased T2 signal is found in and adjacent to the affected bowel loop (*arrow*)

Diverticulitis

Colonic diverticula can be found throughout the colon. However, the descending and sigmoid colon are most frequently affected. The inflammation of colonic diverticula can lead to abscess formations, perforation, and peritonitis. Pericolonic stranding, thickening of

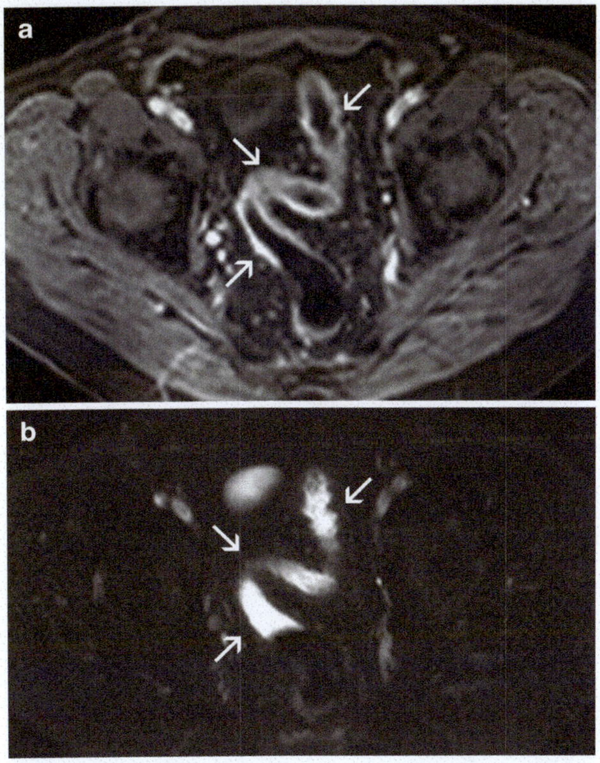

Fig. 6.62 Nonactive colitis with fibrotic changes. Contrast-enhanced T1-W MRI exhibits an increased signal of the bowel wall (**a**). However, T2 signal is not elevated (**b**), accounting for a lack of edema

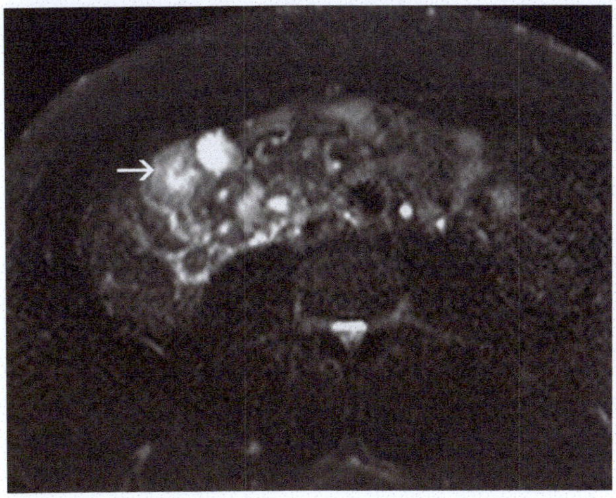

Fig. 6.63 Appendicitis. T2-W MRI shows a thickened appendix and increased T2 signal of the wall and surrounding tissues

the bowel wall, increased contrast enhancement, and elevated T2 signal in acute stages of inflammation are typical (Fig. 6.64). Segmental diverticulitis can

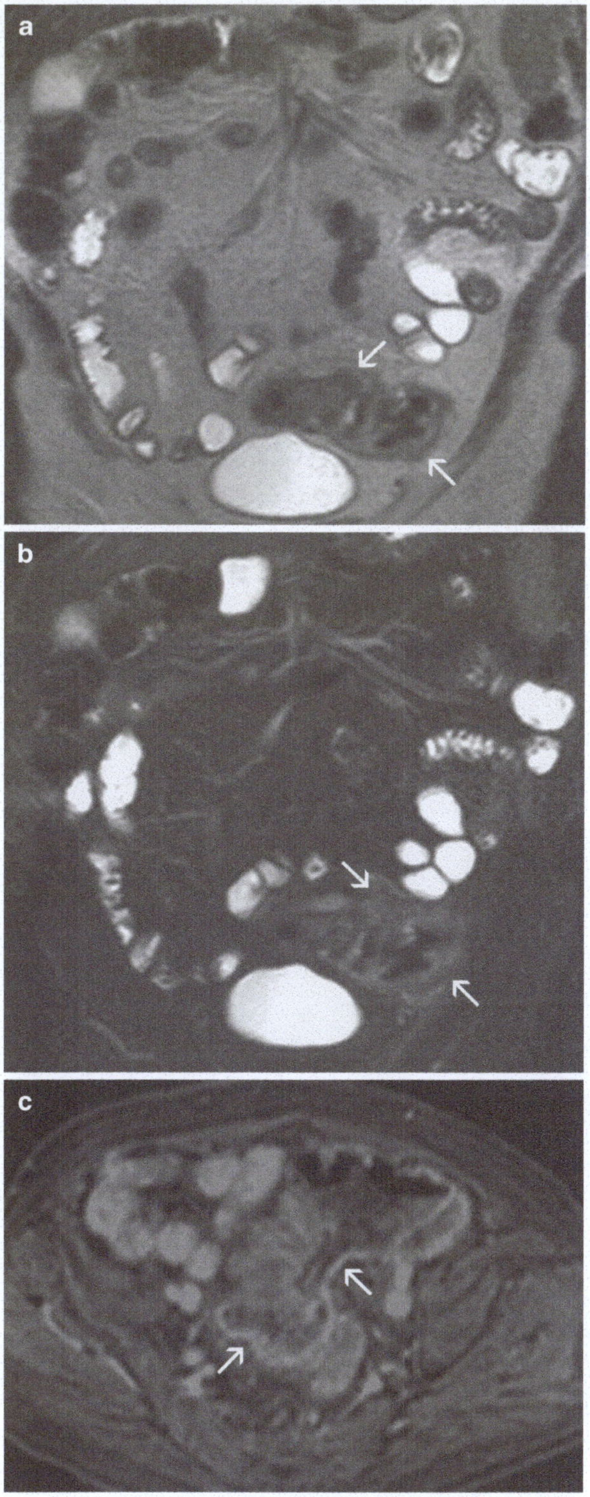

Fig. 6.64 Diverticulitis of the sigmoid colon. Typical features are presented, including bowel wall thickening (FISP, **a**), high T2 signal (T2 SSFSE, **b**), and increased contrast enhancement after gadolinium administration (T1-W GRE, **c**)

be difficult to be distinguished from colorectal carcinoma. However, carcinomas normally involve only a very short colonic segment and may present more as an asymmetric bowel wall thickening.

Infectious Colitis

Infectious colitis is caused by bacterial, viral, fungal, or parasitic pathogens, leading to a focal or diffuse thickening of the colonic wall and pericolonic stranding. Pseudomembranous colitis is found after antibiotic treatment mainly with Clindamycin. This results in an overgrowth of resistant enteric Clostridium difficile and the production of cytotoxins and enterotoxins. Imaging features include marked submucosal edema over a long colonic segment and the "accordeon sign," which is based on trapped contrast between thickened haustral folds.

6.8.5.2 Benign Neoplasm

Colonic polyps can be found throughout the large bowel. However, most common locations are sigmoid (40%), descending colon (20%), and rectum (20%). There are variable morphologies including flat polyps (Fig. 6.65), sessile polyps with a broad base, and pedunculated polyps with a stalk (Fig. 6.66). With regards to the potential

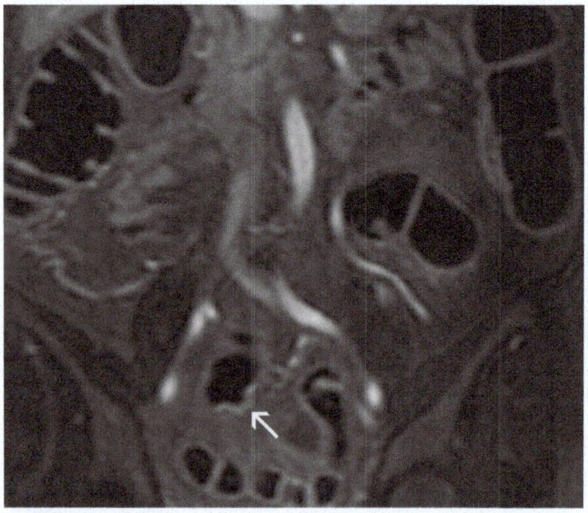

Fig. 6.65 Flat adenoma of the sigmoid colon. The lesion exhibits an increased gadolinium uptake on T1-W MRI compared to the remaining bowel wall

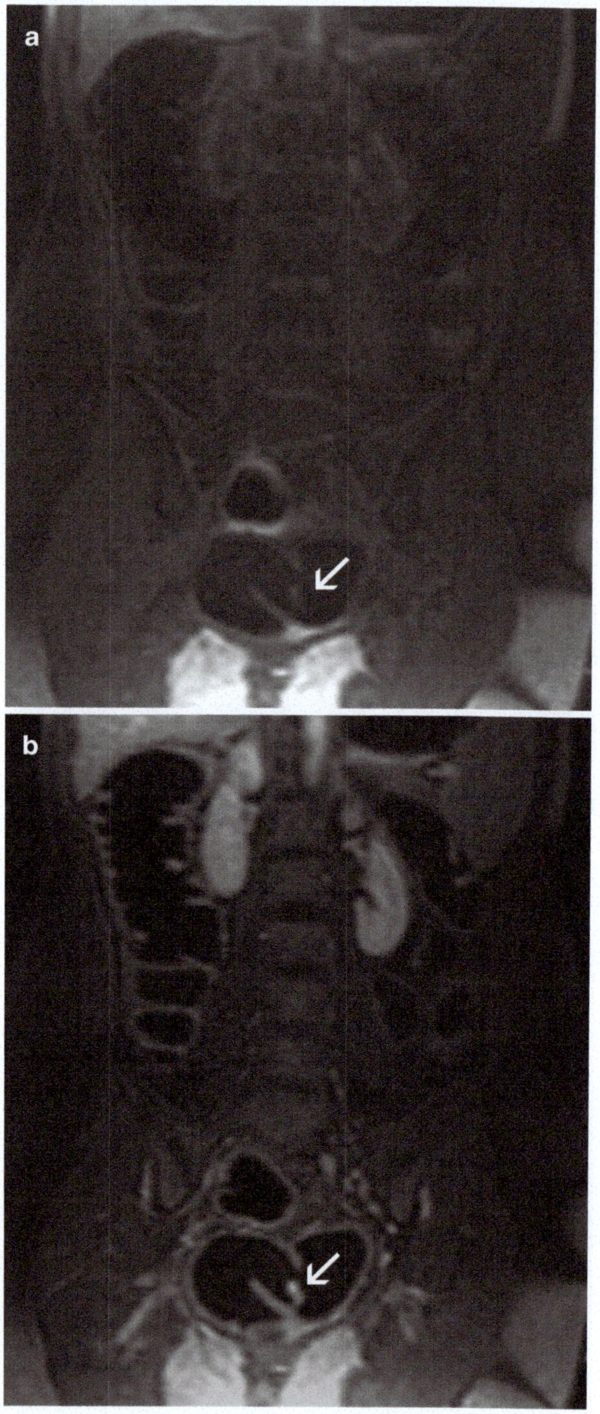

Fig. 6.66 Pedunculated polyp of the sigmoid colon. A high contrast uptake can be detected comparing precontrast T1-W MRI (**a**) and contrast-enhanced T1-W MRI (**b**). This feature ensures an easy differentiation between colonic masses and residual stool

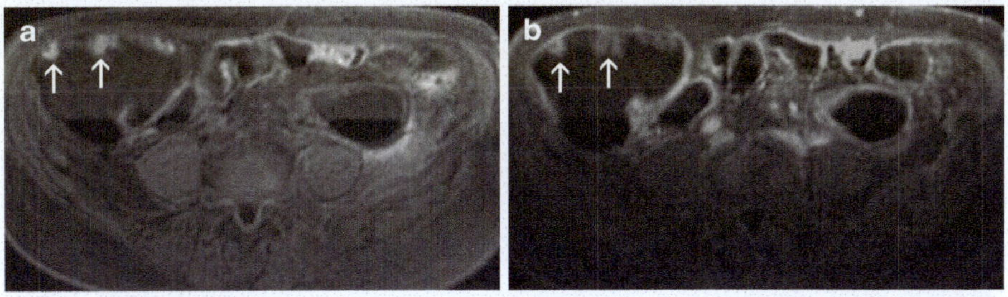

Fig. 6.67 Residual fecal material. Residual fecal material can mimic colorectal masses on contrast-enhanced T1-W MRI (**b**). However, no contrast enhancement is seen and fecal material exhibits a high signal on precontrast scans as well (**a**)

Table 6.4 Diagnostic value of MRI for the depiction of colorectal polyps

Author	Patients (*n*)	Sensitivity[a] (%)	Specificity[a] (%)	Polyps[a] 6–10 mm (%)	Polyps[b] >10 mm (%)
Hartmann et al. (2006)	100	89	96	84	100
Saar et al. (2006)	50	92	96	100	100
Kuehle et al. (2007)	315	36	90	85	81

[a]Results on a patient basis

[b]Sensitivity on a lesion basis for the depiction of adenomatous polyps

of malignant transformation, adenomatous (neoplastic) polyps must be differentiated from nonneoplastic lesions including hyperplastic, inflammatory, or hamartomatous polyps. Adenomas are precursors of colorectal adenocarcinoma. As the majority of colorectal cancers develop from benign lesions over a relatively long time range of up to 10 years, screening for colorectal polyps and subsequent polypectomy is a very effective approach for reducing the incidence of colorectal cancer.

Multiple colonic adenomas can be seen in patients with Gardner syndrome, familial adenomatous polyposis, and Trucot syndrome. One main imaging criterion of adenomatous polyps is the strong contrast enhancement after gadolinium administration. Thus, polyps >5 mm can be depicted both with a high sensitivity and specificity. Residual stool particles can mimic polyps on contrast-enhanced T1-W MRI. However, a high signal is already exhibited on precontrast T1-W images and no gadolinium enhancement is found (Fig. 6.67). An overview about diagnostic accuracy of MRI for the detection of colorectal polyps is shown in Table 6.4.

6.8.5.3 Malignant Neoplasm

Colorectal adenocarcinoma is the most common malignancy of the gastrointestinal tract and the cancer with the second highest mortality. They occur most often in the rectosigmoid colon. Most adenocarcinomas develop from benign adenomatous precursors (adenomacarcinoma sequence) over a long time range. Furthermore, patients with inflammatory bowel disease are at high risk for the development of colorectal adenocarcinoma. The TNM classification for colorectal adenocarcinoma is shown in Table 6.5. In 5% of all patients, there are metachronous colonic lesions. In presence of stenotic tumors, however, proximal colonic segments may not be accessible by optical endoscopy. Hereby, MRI provides considerable diagnostic advantages: the distending medium (water or gasiform contrast) can retrogradely pass even high-grade stenoses, enabling distension and visualization of prestenotic segments. Hence, a significantly higher completion rate than optical colonoscopy can be achieved.

Imaging features of colorectal adenocarcinoma include short segmental, asymmetric luminal wall thickening with an irregular surface (Fig. 6.68). A differentiation between adenocarcinoma, diverticulitis, and postinflammatory fibrotic changes can be difficult. The concomitant clinical history of the patient needs to be taken into account. As hepatic metastases are common, a simultaneous assessment of the liver should be performed. Lymph node metastases can often be smaller than 10 mm at the time of diagnosis. However, depiction of more than five lymph nodes in regional distribution is typical for metastatic spread.

Table 6.5 TNM classification for adenocarcinoma of the colon

Primary tumor (T) T1: tumor limited to mucosa/submucosa T2: tumor reaching the serosa T3: tumor surpassing the serosa. Adjacent organs are not involved T4: tumor with perforation and/or infiltration of neighboring organs
Lymph node involvement (N) N0: no lymph node metastases N1: 1–3 regional lymph nodes affected N2: 4 or more regional lymph metastases affected
Distant metastases (M) M0: no distant metastases M1: distant metastases

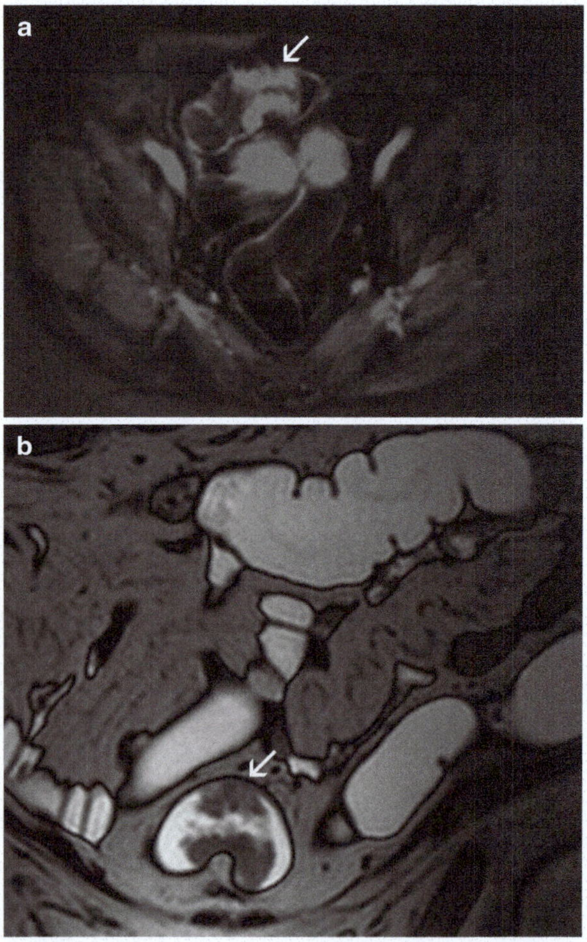

Fig. 6.68 Adenocarcinoma of the sigmoid colon. A typical apple core lesion is shown on contrast-enhanced T1-W MRI (**a**) and FISP imaging (**b**)

Acknowledgment We are indebted to Nadine Faucheron for collecting images.

Further Reading

Ba-Ssalamah A et al. (2007) Magnetic resonance imaging of liver malignancies. Top Magn Reson Imaging 18:445–455

Catalano OA, Sahani DV, Kalva SP, Cushing MS, Hahn PF, Brown JJ, Edelman RR (2008) MR imaging of the gallbladder: a pictorial essay. Radiographics 28:135–155

Chen F, Ward, J, Robinson PJ (1999) MR imaging of the liver and spleen: a comparison of the effects on signal intensity of two superparamagnetic iron oxide agents. Magn Reson Imaging 17:549–556

Edelman RR, Hesselink JR, Zlatkin MB, Crues JV III (2006) Clinical magnetic resonance imaging, 3rd edn. Elsevier, Amsteadam

Elsayes KM, Narra VR, Mukundan G, Lewis JS Jr, Menias CO., Heiken JP (2005) MR imaging of the spleen: spectrum of abnormalities. Radiographics 25:967–982

Fidler J (2007) MR imaging of the small bowel. Radiol Clin North Am 45(2):317–331

Glockner JF (2007) Hepatobiliary MRI: current concepts and controversies. J Magn Reson Imaging 25:681–695

Gourtsoyianni S, Papanikolaou N, Yarmenitis S, Maris T, Karantanas A, Gourtsoyiannis N (2008) Respiratory gated diffusion-weighted imaging of the liver: value of apparent diffusion coefficient measurements in the differentiation between most commonly encountered benign and malignant focal liver lesions. Eur Radiol 18(3):486–492

Gourtsoyiannis NC, Papanikolaou N (2005) Magnetic resonance enteroclysis. Semin Ultrasound CT MR 26(4):237–246

Gourtsoyiannis NC, Papanikolaou N, Karantanas A (2006) Magnetic resonance imaging evaluation of small intestinal Crohn's disease. Best Pract Res Clin Gastroenterol 20(1): 137–156

Horsthuis K, Lavini Mphil C, Stoker J (2005) MRI in Crohn's disease. J Magn Reson Imaging 22(1):1–12

Hussain SM et al. (2002) Benign versus malignant hepatic nodules: MR imaging findings with pathologic correlation. Radiographics 22:1023–1036; discussion 1037–1039

Hussain SM et al. (2004) Focal nodular hyperplasia: findings at state-of-the-art MR imaging, US, CT, and pathologic analysis. Radiographics 24:3–17; discussion 18–19

Kinner S, Lauenstein TC (2007) MR colonography. Radiol Clin North Am 45(2):377–387

Krinsky GA, Lee VS, Theise N. D et al (2001) Hepatocellular carcinoma and dysplastic nodules in patients with cirrhosis: prospective diagnosis with MR imaging and explantation correlation. Radiology 219:445–454

Laghi A, Paolantonio P, Iafrate F, Altomari F, Miglio C, Passariello R (2002) Oral contrast agents for magnetic resonance imaging of the bowel. Top Magn Reson Imaging 13(6):389–396

Lauenstein TC, Saar B, Martin DR (2007) MR colonography: 1.5T versus 3T. Magn Reson Imaging Clin N Am 15(3):395–402

Lavelle MT, Lee VS, Rofsky NM, Krinsky GA, Weinreb JC (2001) Dynamic contrast-enhanced three-dimensional MR imaging of liver parenchyma: source images and angiographic reconstructions to define hepatic arterial anatomy. Radiology 218:389–394

Lim JH et al (2001) Conspicuity of hepatocellular nodular lesions in cirrhotic livers at ferumoxides-enhanced MR imaging: importance of Kupffer cell number. Radiology 220:669–676

Maccioni F, Colaiacomo MC, Parlanti S (2005) Ulcerative colitis: value of MR imaging. Abdom Imaging 30(5):584–592

Martin DR, Danrad R, Herrmann K, Semelka RC, Hussain SM (2005) Magnetic resonance imaging of the gastrointestinal tract. Top Magn Reson Imaging 16(1):77–98

Morana G, Guarise A (2006) Cystic tumors of the pancreas. Cancer Imaging 13(6):60–71

Mortele KJ, Segatto E, Ros PR (2004) The infected liver: radiologic-pathologic correlation. Radiographics 24:937–955

Paolantonio P, Tomei E, Rengo M, Ferrari R, Lucchesi P, Laghi A (2007) Adult celiac disease: MRI findings. Abdom Imaging 32:433–440

Park MS, Yu JS, Kim KW et al (2001) Recurrent pyogenic cholangitis: comparison between MR cholangiography and direct cholangiography. Radiology 220:677–682

Pedrosa I, Saiz A, Arrazola J, Ferreiros J, Pedrosa CS (2000) Hydatid disease: radiologic and pathologic features and complications. Radiographics 20:795–817

Ramani M, Reinhold C, Semelka, RC et al (1997) Splenic hemangiomas and hamartomas: MR imaging characteristics of 28 lesions. Radiology 202:166–172

Robertson F, Leander P, Ekberg O (2001) Radiology of the spleen. Eur Radiol 11:80–95

Schima W (2006) MRI of the pancreas: tumors and tumor-simulating processes. Cancer Imaging 6:199–203

Schima W, Ba-Ssalamah A, Goetzinger P et al (2007) State-of-the-art magnetic resonance imaging of pancreatic cancer. Top Magn Reson Imaging 18:421–429

Schmidt G P, Kramer H, Reiser MF, Glaser C (2007) Whole-body magnetic resonance imaging and positron emission tomography-computed tomography in oncology. Top Magn Reson Imaging 18(3):193–202

Schreyer AG, Scheibl K, Heiss P, Feuerbach S, Seitz J, Herfarth H (2006) MR colonography in inflammatory bowel disease. Abdom Imaging 31:302–307

Semelka RC (2002) Abdominal-pelvic MRI. Wiley-Liss, New York

Semelka RC, Hussain SM, Marcos HB, Woosley JT (2000) Perilesional enhancement of hepatic metastases: correlation between MR imaging and histopathologic findings-initial observations. Radiology 215:89–94

Tanaka M, Chari S, Adsay V, Fernandez-del Castillo C, Falconi M, Shimizu M, Yamaguchi K, Yamao K, Matsuno S (2006) International consensus guidelines for management of intraductal papillary mucinous neoplasms and mucinous cystic neoplasms of the pancreas. Pancreatology 6:17–32

Ward J, Guthrie JA, Scott D J et al (2000) Hepatocellular carcinoma in the cirrhotic liver: double-contrast MR imaging for diagnosis. Radiology 216:154–162

Yu JS, Kim KW, Jeong MG, Lee JT, Yoo HS (2000) Nontumorous hepatic arterial-portal venous shunts: MR imaging findings. Radiology 217:750–756

Abdomen: Retroperitoneum, Adrenals, Kidneys, and Upper Urinary Tract

7

Gertraud Heinz-Peer

Contents

G. Heinz-Peer
Department of Radiology, Medical University of Vienna, Allgemeines Krankenhaus (AKH), Währinger Gürtel 18–20, 1090 Wien, Austria
e-mail: gertraud.heinz@meduniwien.ac.at

7.1 Retroperitoneum

7.1.1 Introduction

The retroperitoneum is the compartmentalized space located external to and predominantly posterior to the posterior parietal peritoneum.

Magnetic Resonance Imaging (MRI) has advantages of high spatial resolution, multiplanar tomographic or volumetric image display, relatively good soft tissue contrast between normal structures and disease processes, a short examination time (generally less than 20–30 min), and the capability for whole-body imaging (related to parallel imaging technologies).

CT is frequently used for initial cross-sectional imaging evaluation of the retroperitoneum, particularly when the underlying etiology of a patient's symptoms or signs is unclear. Although CT has higher spatial resolution than MRI, MRI has superior contrast resolution, does not utilize ionizing radiation, can be used when there are contraindications to obtaining an iodinated contrast-enhanced CT such as contrast allergy, and allows for acquisition of multiple image sequences that may each be useful to depict different inherent characteristics of disease processes affecting the retroperitoneum. As such, if the diagnosis of a retroperitoneal malignancy is suspected, particularly when the pelvis is the primary site of disease, MRI may be used as the initial imaging test to potentially better delineate the nature and extent of disease.

P. Reimer et al. (eds.), *Clinical MR Imaging*,
DOI: 10.1007/978-3-540-74504-4_7, © Springer-Verlag Berlin Heidelberg 2010

7.1.2 Normal Anatomy

7.1.2.1 Retroperitoneal Anatomy

The abdominal retroperitoneum is bounded anteriorly by the posterior parietal peritoneum and posteriorly by the transversalis fascia, and extends craniocaudally from the diaphragm to the pelvic brim. It is divided by fascial planes into three compartments: the anterior pararenal space, the perirenal (or perinephric) space, and the posterior pararenal space.

The anterior pararenal space contains the retroperitoneal portions of the colon, duodenum, and pancreas, is continuous with the transverse mesocolon and root of the small bowel mesentery, and is confined by the posterior parietal peritoneum anteriorly, the anterior renal fascia posteriorly, and the lateroconal fascia laterally. While the anterior pararenal space is potentially continuous across the midline, fluid collections are generally confined to their side of origin without crossing the midline, with exception of pancreatic fluid collections related to the presence of pancreatic enzymes.

The perirenal space contains the kidney, renal vessels, adrenal gland, renal pelvis, proximal ureter, perirenal lymphatics, and perirenal fat, is confined by the anterior and posterior renal fascia that comprise the renal fascia (also called Gerota's fascia), and has the shape of a cone superiorly and an inverted cone inferiorly. The anterior renal fascia also extends cranially to the diaphragm, but may be deficient superiorly on the right side posterior to the bare area of the liver. As a result, lacerations of the liver involving the hepatic capsule adjacent to its bare area may be associated with hemorrhage that extends posteriorly into the right perirenal space. Furthermore, perirenal fluid collections may extend from the right perirenal space anteriorly to the bare area of the liver. Similarly, the splenorenal ligament may serve as a conduit for hemorrhage from the bare area of the spleen to the left anterior pararenal space in the setting of splenic trauma.

The perirenal space is contiguous superiorly with the mediastinum through splanchnic foramina of the diaphragmatic crura and through small transdiaphragmatic perforations and lymphatic vessels, providing conduits of potential disease spread between the thorax and the abdomen. The perirenal space is further divided into multiple compartments by fibrous lamellae, the bridging septa, which are of three types: those that arise from the renal capsule and extend to the renal fascia, those that are attached only to the renal capsule and are arranged more or less parallel to the renal surface, and those that connect the anterior renal fascia to the posterior renal fascia. These septa can exert an important influence on pathologic processes by either limiting the spread of disease or by serving as bidirectional conduits for spread of disease between the renal fascia, the perirenal space, and the central prevertebral space.

The posterior pararenal space almost always contains only fat, is confined by the posterior renal fascia anteriorly, the transversalis fascia posteriorly, and by the psoas muscle medially, and continues laterally external to the lateroconal fascia as the properitoneal fat of the abdominal wall. Inferiorly, the posterior pararenal space is open to the pelvis, and superiorly, it continues as a thin subdiaphragmatic layer of extraperitoneal fat.

The retroperitoneal fascia are not composed of single membranes, but are laminated because of variable embryonic fusion of discrete layers of dorsal mesenteries. In addition, retroperitoneal fascial layers may not be intact in all patients due to congenital variation, traumatic or iatrogenic disruption, or dissolution due to infected fluid or enzymatic digestion, allowing for fluid collections and other pathologies to involve multiple retroperitoneal or peritoneal compartments.

The normal thickness of the retroperitoneal fascial planes is 1–3 mm. On MRI, retroperitoneal fascial planes are more frequently detected when there is an abundance of retroperitoneal fat. In general, the posterior renal fascia is more often seen than the anterior renal fascia, and the anterior renal fascia is more commonly seen on the left side than on the right side. Fascia that is focally thickened or greater than 3 mm in width is considered abnormal, and it can be caused by a large variety of pathologic conditions involving the retroperitoneal organs or nonparenchymal retroperitoneum.

7.1.2.2 Pelvic Extraperitoneal Anatomy

The pelvic extraperitoneal connective tissue is organized into groups of fascia that are fused together to demarcate the pelvic extraperitoneal spaces. The parietal pelvic fascia (PPF) is the variable dense fascial system that covers the structures limiting the pelvic cavity including the levator ani, obturator, coccygeus, and piriformis muscles, the anterior surfaces of the sacrum and coccyx, and structures contiguous to the pelvic walls such as internal iliac vessels and sacral roots.

The visceral pelvic fascia (VPF) is the fascial system derived from the visceral reflection of the PPF. It envelops the pelvic organs and attaches them to the pelvic walls. On CT and MRI, it is best seen posteriorly where it is the thickest - the appearance is that of thin continuous lines enveloping the perirectal fat. An additional group of fascia is oriented in the coronal plane that originates from the genital artery sheaths and the inferolateral extensions of the peritoneal layer of the cul-de-sac. The anterior layer separates the urinary bladder and genital tract, and the posterior layer separates the genital tract from the rectum. These fascial planes are not well seen on CT or MRI due to a paucity of surrounding fat.

The obliterated urachus is also often visible in the axial plane in the location of the median umbilical fold.

The perirectal space, which contains the rectum, hemorrhoidal vessels, and fat, is limited by the posterior portion of the VPF, continues superiorly into the abdominal extraperitoneal space, and is continuous with the sigmoid mesocolon. The Denonvillier's fascia is comprised of the anterior portion of the perirectal fascia and the posterior layer of the prostatic fascia.

7.1.3 MR Imaging Techniques

Pulse sequences used for MRI examination of the retroperitoneum are similar to those of standard abdominal MRI (Table 7.1). T1-weighted images (T1-WIs) are useful for demonstrating high signal intensity (SI) fat or hemorrhage, lymphadenopathy, and vascular invasion by tumors. Fat-suppressed T2-weighted images (T2-WIs) are useful for demonstrating lymphadenopathy, muscle invasion by a disease process, cystic change or necrosis, fluid collections, bone marrow edema, and dilation or obstruction of fluid containing hollow structures such as the biliary tree and gallbladder, bowel, or genitourinary system. Precontrast, arterial phase, and parenchymal/venous phase contrast-enhanced T1-WI may be obtained to provide information that is often useful to characterize retroperitoneal pathology. However, delayed contrast-enhanced T1-WI is the most useful imaging sequence for rapid screening of the extraparenchymal abdomen and pelvis as there is increased conspicuity of pathology. The solid or cystic/necrotic nature of lesions, the extent of disease, and the presence and nature of vascular thrombosis or tumor encasement of abdominal vessels are demonstrated well on this sequence.

7.1.4 Retroperitoneal Masses

7.1.4.1 Retroperitoneal Sarcoma

Soft tissue sarcomas are rare mesenchymal neoplasms accounting for less than 1% of adult malignancies. About 15% of sarcomas originate within the retroperitoneum.

Retroperitoneal sarcomas may develop at any age, but are most commonly present in the sixth and seventh decades of life, occurring slightly more commonly in men. They are often of high histologic grade and have a mean size of 17 cm at presentation. As these reports indicate, retroperitoneal sarcomas are often very large in size before producing any symptoms or signs, leading to a delay in diagnosis and subsequent poor prognosis. Symptoms are related to compression of adjacent organs and can include early satiety, nausea, vomiting, constipation, urinary frequency, neurologic symptoms in the lower extremities, and pain in the flank, back, or radicular pain.

Table 7.1 Some commonly used MRI sequences for imaging of the retroperitoneum

T1w	Typically 2D or 3D GRE sequence breathold and breathing independant sequences may be acquired. Fat saturation improves image contrast
T2w	TSE/FSE/HASTE with breathold or free breathing. Fat saturation may increase image contrast. Used for MRU as 2D or 3D sequence
DWI/ADC	May be helpful in the evaluation of cystic lesions, e.g. to differentiate solid from cystic lesion or solid from necrotic tumor. Provides good detection of lymphnodes
Post i.v. admin. of GBCA	
T1w	Usually GRE sequences applied in axial and/or coronal imaging planes, depending on indication. Same imaging plane should be used before and after gadolinium-chelate injection. MR angiographic techniques (usually breathold 3D GRE) have important role in imaging the aorta and its branches

MRI can define the extent of the primary tumor, evaluate for direct involvement of adjacent organs and vessels, and detect and delineate the extent of distant metastatic disease. Imaging features that suggest unresectability include extensive vascular involvement, peritoneal implantation, and distant metastatic disease.

There are approximately 50 histological subtypes of soft tissue sarcoma (Fig. 7.1–7.4). In the retroperitoneum, the histologic subtypes in descending order include liposarcoma (40%), leiomyosarcoma (30%), and malignant fibrous histiocytoma (MFH) (15%). In contrast to its occurrence in the extremities, MFH is uncommonly found in the retroperitoneum.

MRI may occasionally suggest a specific histologic diagnosis. For example, the presence of macroscopic fat within a large retroperitoneal mass favors the diagnosis of a well-differentiated liposarcoma, whereas caval involvement favors a leiomyosarcoma, particularly if cystic or necrotic intratumoral components and/or metastases are present. Similarly, a large retroperitoneal mass that contains calcifications, extensive hemorrhage without fatty components, or central necrosis favors a diagnosis of MFH. Although cross-sectional imaging cannot accurately predict the grade of a retroperitoneal sarcoma, the visualization of tumor necrosis suggests the presence of a high-grade tumor and a poorer prognosis.

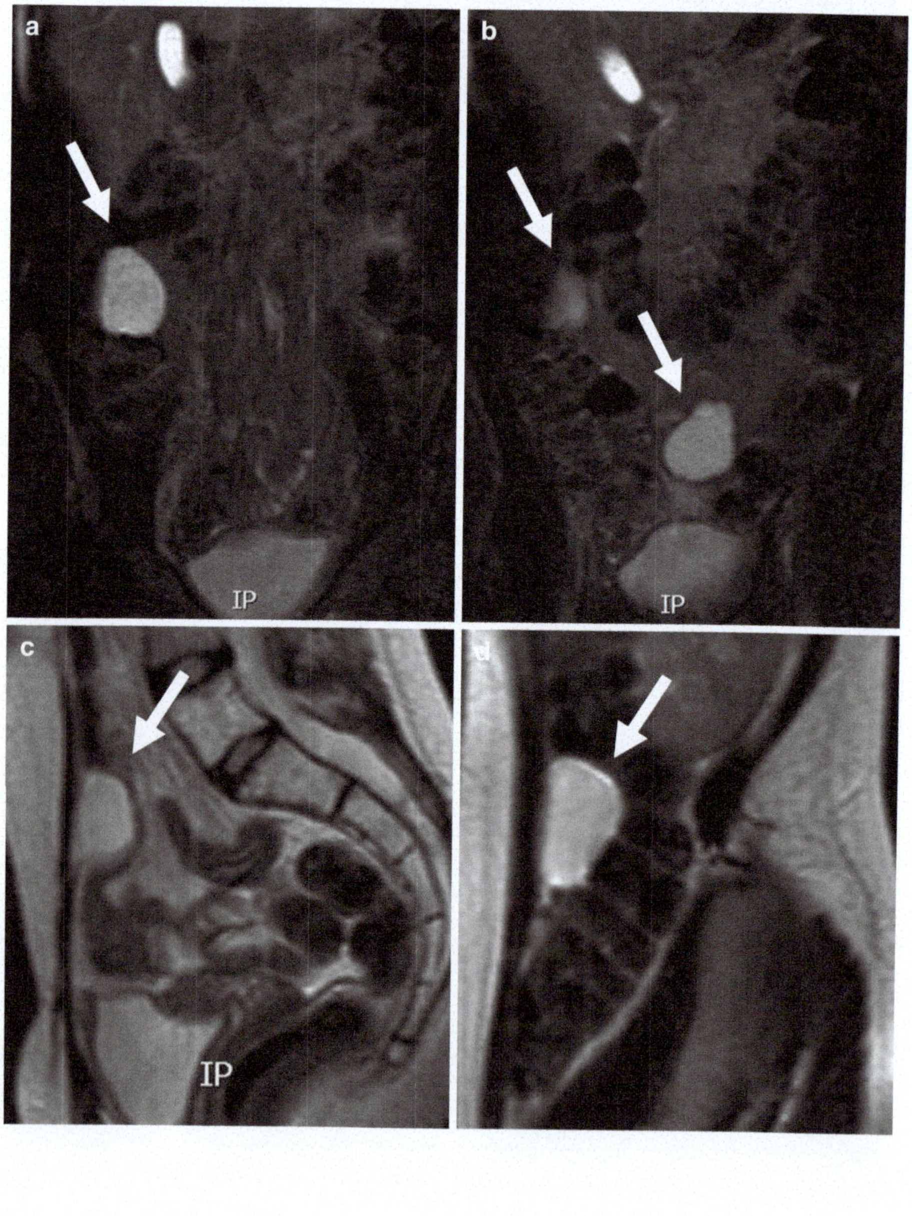

Fig. 7.1 Retroperitoneal liposarcoma. On coronal T2-W TSE with fat saturation images (**a**, **b**) and sagittal T2- W TSE (**c**, **d**) images, two separated cystic lesions were demonstrated in a 23-year-old female patient in the anterior pararenal space and superior to the urinary bladder, which proved to be a multicentric liposarcoma with myxoid components

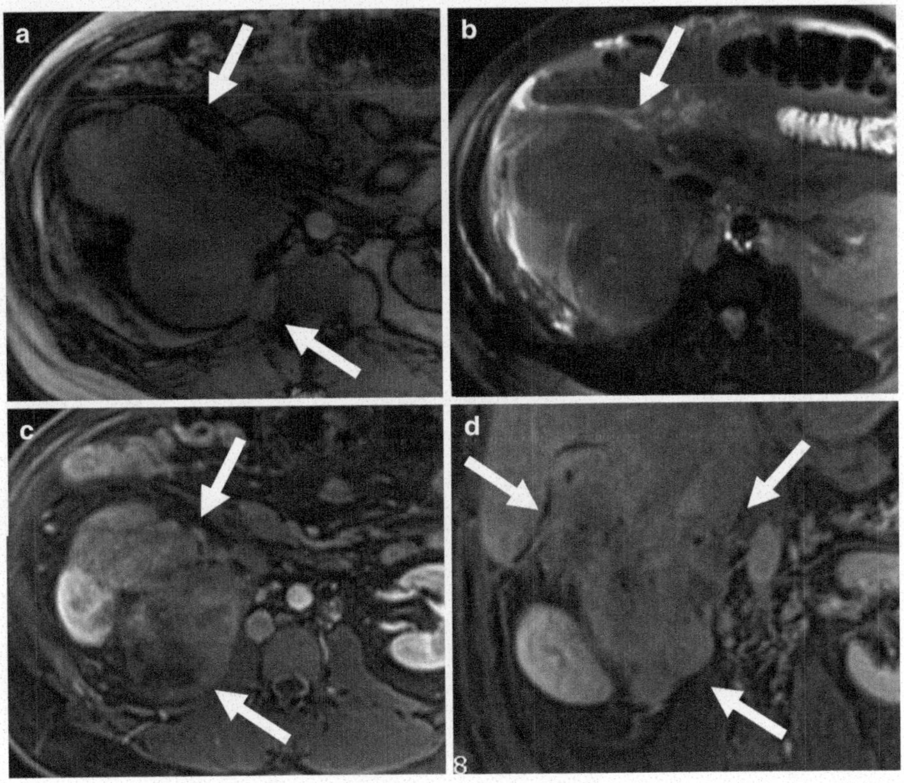

Fig. 7.2 Retroperitoneal leiomyosarcoma. Axial T1-W spoiled 2D GRE (**a**), axial T2-W TSE with fatsat (**b**), axial and coronal T1-W spoiled contrast-enhanced 2D GRE with fatsat (**c, d**) show a huge inhomogeneous mass in the right posterior pararenal space invading the perirenal space, expanding to the anterior pararenal space, crossing the midline and infiltrating renal vessels and the vena cava inferior in a 36-year-old male patient. On MR images, there was no evidence of fat-containing structures; histology showed a leiomyosarkoma

The attenuation and SI features of recurrent sarcoma may differ from those of the original primary sarcoma.

7.1.4.2 Primary Retroperitoneal Extragonadal Germ Cell Tumor (EGCT)

Primary EGCTs represent between 1–3% of all germ cell tumors, occurring most commonly within the mediastinum and slightly less commonly within the retroperitoneum. Primary EGCTs are more common in men than women with a peak occurrence in the fourth and fifth decades of life, which is a slightly older age group compared to patients who develop primary testicular germ cell neoplasms.

As the majority of retroperitoneal germ cell tumors are metastases from primary testicular tumors, careful clinical and imaging evaluation should be performed in affected men to exclude a coexistent primary testicular neoplasm.

Seminomatous EGCTs account for 15% of EGCTs and are not associated with elevated tumor markers. Nonseminomatous EGCTs are associated with elevated tumor markers in 70–94% of cases. Levels of serum alpha-fetoprotein may be elevated due to the presence of yolk sac tumor or embryonal carcinoma, or human chorionic gonadotropin levels may be elevated due to the presence of components of choriocarcinoma. Serial levels of tumor markers correlate with the clinical course and therapeutic response, and high levels are associated with a poor survival.

On gross examination, seminomas are usually homogeneous lobulated masses whereas mixed and nonseminomatous tumors are heterogeneous with solid and cystic areas, necrosis, and hemorrhage. On MRI, primary retroperitoneal EGCTs are typically large, with mean size of 7–8 cm, midline enhancing retroperitoneal masses of soft tissue attenuation that are of low-intermediate SI on T1-WI and intermediate or high SI on T2-WI relative to skeletal muscle. Areas of cystic change or necrosis are seen as very high SI foci on T2-WI. Seminomatous EGCTs tend to be homogeneous in attenuation and SI, whereas mixed and nonseminomatous EGCTs tend to be heterogeneous in attenuation and SI, with areas of cystic necrosis or hemorrhage. A midline location of a retroperitoneal mass is probably the most helpful finding to suggest this diagnosis, whereas metastatic retroperitoneal

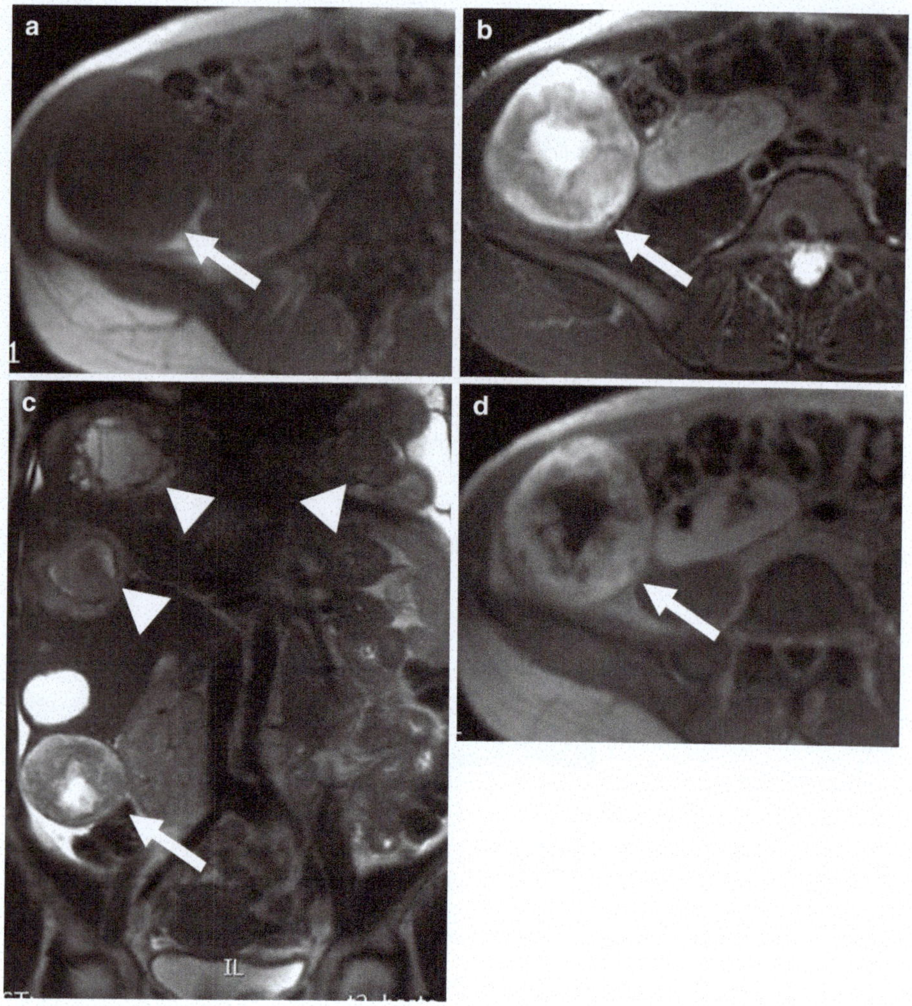

Fig. 7.3 Retroperitoneal fibrosarcoma (*arrow*). On axial T1-W TSE (**a**), axial T2-W TSE with fatsat (**b**), coronal T2-W TSE (**c**), and axial T1-W contrast-enhanced TSE (**d**) a well-defined mass with central necrosis is demarcated in the right posterior pararenal space in a 38-year-old female patient, and it proved to be a fibrosarcoma with myxoid components. On coronal T2-W TSE (**c**) large metastases to the liver and the lung are depicted (*arrowheads*)

lymphadenopathy from a primary testicular neoplasm tends not to be midline in location.

7.1.4.3 Retroperitoneal Neurogenic Tumors

Paraganglioma

Paragangliomas, sometimes called extraadrenal pheochromocytomas (Fig. 7.5), are rare neurogenic tumors that arise from highly vascularized specialized neural crest cells called paraganglia, which are symmetrically distributed along the aortic axis in close association with the sympathetic chain in the neck, chest, abdomen, and pelvis. The largest collection of paraganglia includes the paired organs of Zuckerkandl that overlie the aorta at the level of the inferior mesenteric artery, and have an uncertain physiologic role. They are prominent during early infancy and regress after 12–18 months. Ten to twenty percent of pheochromocytomas are extraadrenal in location, and most often arise in the retroperitoneum from the organs of Zuckerkandl. Only a few tumors develop at other locations along the aorta or its branch vessels.

On gross examination, paragangliomas are partially encapsulated solid and/or cystic brown masses that usually measure several centimeters in diameter, and are commonly hemorrhagic.

Patients with paragangliomas present in the fourth and fifth decades of life, although malignant paragangliomas may sometimes arise in younger patients. Men and women are affected equally. Paragangliomas may be multicentric, particularly if there is a family history of paraganglioma, or may be associated with other

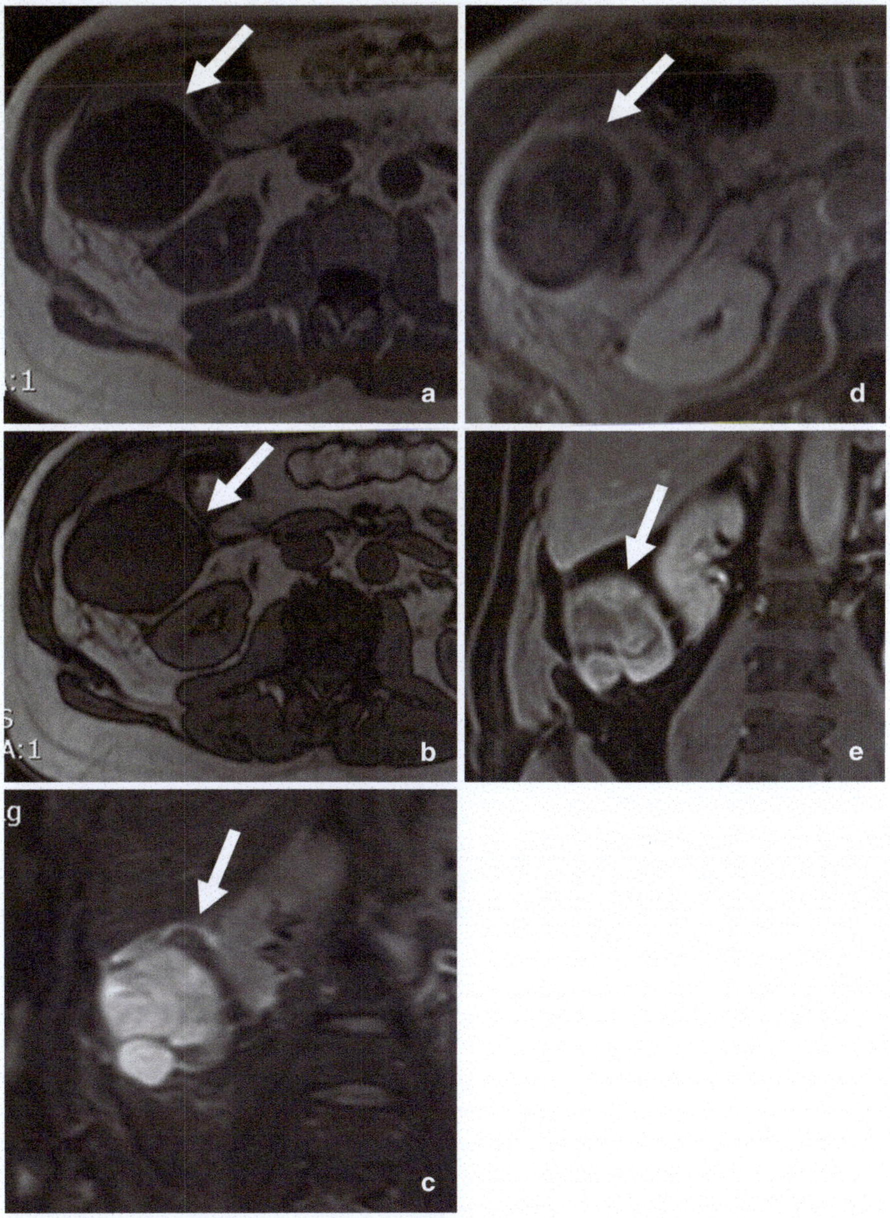

Fig. 7.4 Retroperitoneal chondrosarcoma. On axial T1-W spoiled GRE in-phase (**a**), and opposed phase (**b**), coronal T2-W TSE with fatsat (**c**), axial T1-W contrast-enhanced TSE (**d**), and coronal T1-W contrast-enhanced TSE with fatsat (**e**) a nonfatty inhomogeneous mass is delineated in the right anterior pararenal space in a 67-year-old male patient, and it proved to be a chondrosarcoma

tumors such as gastric malignant gastrointestinal stromal tumors and pulmonary chondromas as a component of Carney's triad. Ten percent of paragangliomas are familial, occurring in conditions such as multiple endocrine neoplasia (MEN) types IIA and IIB and neuroectodermal syndromes such as tuberous sclerosis (TS), neurofibromatosis type I (NF-1), and von Hippel-Lindau (VHL) syndrome.

Up to 40% of paragangliomas are malignant as compared to 10% of adrenal pheochromocytomas. Malignant nature is recognized by metastatic spread or locally aggressive behavior; approximately 10% of patients initially present with metastatic disease. The most common sites of metastatic disease are lymph nodes, bone, lung, and liver.

Paragangliomas may be considered to be functional or nonfunctional, depending on whether catecholamines are secreted or not. Nonfunctional abdominal paragangliomas present with nonspecific symptoms and signs and are rarely diagnosed as such prior to surgery. Paragangliomas may be functional in up to 60% of patients, and may cause chronic or intermittent

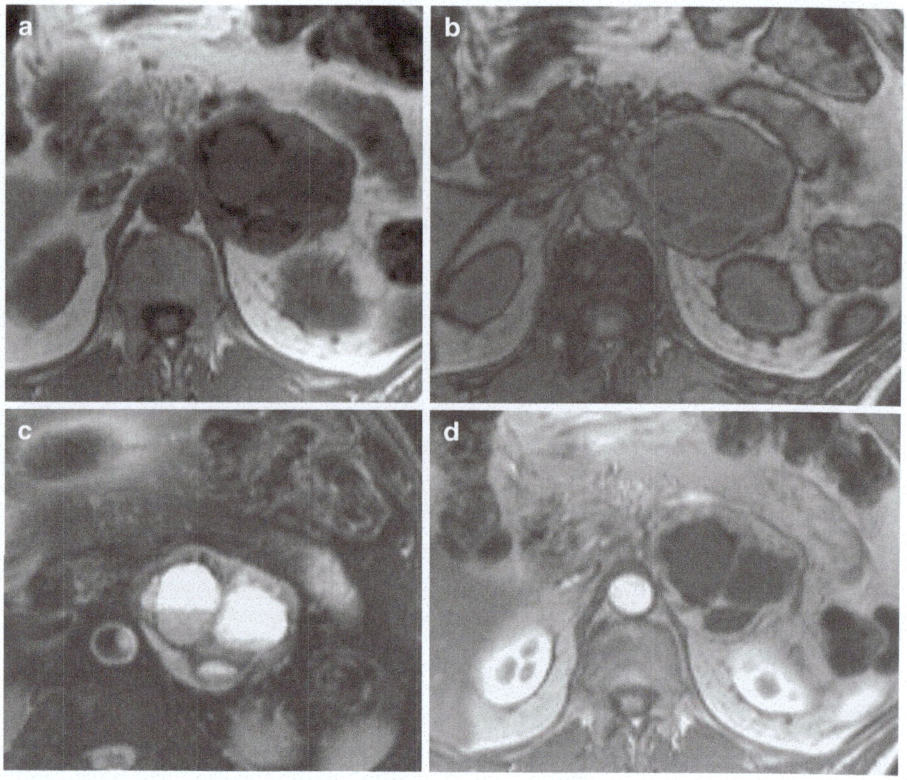

Fig. 7.5 Retroperitoneal collision tumor (pheochromocytoma and ganglioneuroma. On axial T1-W in-phase GRE (**a**), axial T1-W opposed-phase GRE (**b**), axial T2-W TSE (**c**), and axial T1-W contrast-enhanced TSE (**d**), a well-defined mass with central fluid levels (*arrow*) is demarcated in the left adrenal region in a 49-year-old female patient. Histology showed a benign neurogenic collision tumor consisting of a paraganglioma (pheochromocytoma) and ganglioneuroma. There is no evidence of intracellular lipid on chemical shift images (**a**, **b**)

hypertension, headaches, or palpitations. In affected patients, detection of elevated urinary catecholamines is the most efficacious way of characterizing an abdominal mass as a paraganglioma.

On MRI, SI and enhancement characteristics of paragangliomas are similar to those of adrenal pheochromocytoma. The masses generally have low-intermediate SI on T1-WI and moderately high SI on T2-WI relative to skeletal muscle, and are commonly heterogeneous secondary to foci of intratumoral necrosis or hemorrhage. Low SI intratumoral septa and a low SI peripheral capsule are also commonly seen on T2-WI. Progressive enhancement is present on parenchymal/venous and delayed phases of enhancement, but arterial phase enhancement is variable.

Ganglioneuroma

Ganglioneuromas (Fig. 7.5) are uncommon benign neurogenic tumors that arise from sympathetic ganglia and represent 1–2% of all primary retroperitoneal tumors, outnumbering neuroblastomas by about 3:1. They occur slightly more commonly in women than in men at a ratio of 1.5:1, most commonly in the first through fifth decades of life, with a mean age of 7 years at diagnosis. Although some ganglioneuromas result from maturation of neuroblastomas and ganglioneuroblastomas, the majority arise de novo.

Most patients with ganglioneuromas are asymptomatic and have normal levels of urinary catecholamines. When symptomatic, abdominal pain and a palpable abdominal mass are the most frequent symptoms and signs. Patients with hormonally active ganglioneuromas may clinically present with episodic hypertension, sweating, flushing, or diarrhea due to the excess catecholamine production. Secretion of androgenic hormones may lead to virilization with some tumors.

Retroperitoneal ganglioneuromas are typically well-defined longitudinally oriented masses that are lobulated or oval in shape. On MRI, ganglioneuromas have relatively homogeneous attenuation similar to or lower than that of skeletal muscle with low SI on T1-WI and heterogeneous intermediate-high SI on T2-WI. Intratumoral hemorrhage or fatty components may cause mixed intermediate-high SI on T1-WI. SI on T2-WI is influenced by the proportion of myxoid stroma to cellular components and collagen fibers.

Intermediate SI on T2-WI occurs when there is an abundance of cellular components and collagen fibers relative to myxoid stroma, whereas high SI on T2-WI occurs when there is a large amount of myxoid stroma with relatively few cellular components and collagen fibers. A whorled appearance may be present on T2-WI and sometimes on T1-WI, due to interlacing bundles of Schwann cells and collagen fibers. In contrast to schwannomas, cystic degeneration is not present. On T1-WI and T2-WI, a low SI peripheral rim may be visualized, but is more often identified on contrast-enhanced images. Calcifications are seen in 42–60% of tumors and appear as low SI foci on T1-WI and T2-WI. In contrast, the calcifications in neuroblastoma are amorphous and coarse in appearance.

After contrast administration, ganglioneuromas show gradual progressive enhancement, although linear septa may enhance early. The MRI characteristics of ganglioneuroma overlap with those of ganglioneuroblastoma and neuroblastoma, and distinguishing between these lesions is not possible unless metastatic disease is present. Approximately 57% of ganglioneuromas may be functional and produce increased amounts of catecholamines.

Ganglioneuroblastoma and Neuroblastoma

Ganglioneuroblastoma most often develops in children who are 2–4 years old. It is rare in adults and affects men and women equally. Neuroblastoma (Fig. 7.6) most commonly occurs in the first decade of life, with 80% occurring in children under 5 years of age and 42% under 1 year of age. It is slightly more common in boys than girls, and is rare in adults. Neuroblastoma is the third most common pediatric malignancy, after leukemia and central nervous system tumors, accounting for close to 15% of childhood cancer fatalities.

Two-thirds of neuroblastomas are located in the abdomen. Two-thirds of abdominal neuroblastomas are located in the adrenal gland, and the remainder in the extraadrenal retroperitoneum. Locally advanced tumors or distant metastases may be present at the time of diagnosis in 50% of patients with ganglioneuroblastoma and over 70% of patients with neuroblastoma with involvement of bone, bone marrow, liver, lymph nodes, and skin.

On gross examination, ganglioneuroblastomas may be partially or totally encapsulated, whereas neuroblastomas are unencapsulated with variable amounts of hemorrhage, calcification, and necrosis present. There is remarkable heterogeneity observed in neuroblastoma phenotype, ranging from spontaneous regression to relentless progression, and there are dozens of clinical and biologic markers that have been proposed as being predictive of disease outcome. Children who present with neuroblastoma at an age of less than 12 months have a better prognosis than those who present after the age of 12 months. Even with metastatic disease, infants younger than 12 months of age can have a favorable outcome with treatment. The majority of children older than 12 months of age with advanced neuroblastoma at presentation will die from progressive disease.

On MRI, ganglioneuroblastomas and neuroblastomas are less than 10 cm in size and have similar attenuation and SI characteristics to ganglioneuromas. They

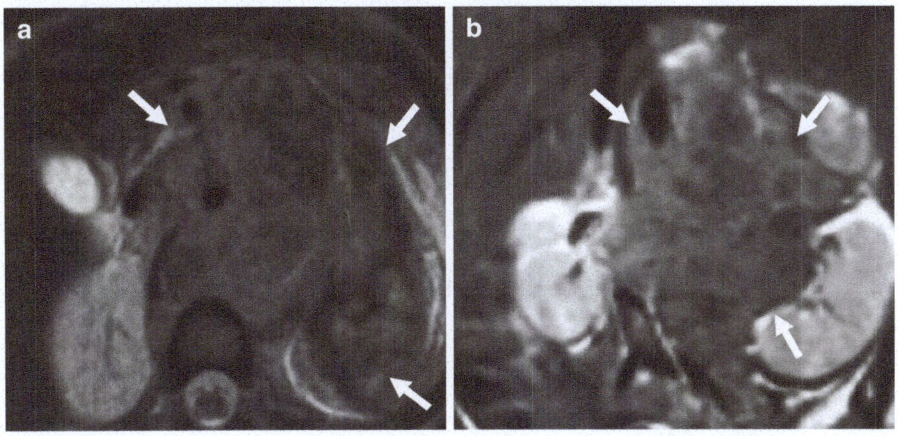

Fig. 7.6 Retroperitoneal neuroblastoma. Axial T2-W TSE (**a**) and coronal T1-W contrast-enhanced TSE (**b**) show a poorly defined, inhomogeneous, retroperitoneal mass with invasion of the left kidney and encasement of retroperitoneal and mesenteric vessels in a 3-year-old boy, and it proved to be a neuroblastoma

tend to have poorly defined margins with invasion of adjacent organs and encasement or occlusion of vessels. There may be cystic change or foci of hemorrhage.

Schwannoma

Schwannomas (Fig. 7.7) are benign tumors of nerve sheaths of peripheral nerves that account for up to 4% of all retroperitoneal tumors. They occur in the third through sixth decades of life, usually as solitary sporadic lesions that arise sporadically, and are twice as common in women as in men. Most patients are asymptomatic and present with a slowly growing painless soft tissue mass. Malignant transformation is rare. Schwannomas are usually less than 5 cm in diameter at presentation, but retroperitoneal schwannomas are typically larger than 8 cm at the time of presentation.

On MRI, schwannomas are sharply circumscribed fusiform, round, or oval masses, usually located in the paravertebral or presacral portions of the retroperitoneum. They are of low-intermediate SI on T1-WI, high SI on T2-WI, and have solid enhancing components. A low SI capsule may sometimes be seen on T1-WI and T2-WI. Heterogeneous attenuation and SI are much more common in schwannomas than in neurofibromas, and may be due to the mixture of Antoni A and B areas along with hemorrhage, cystic degeneration, or punctate, mottled, or curvilinear calcification that is often difficult to visualize on MRI prospectively. A "target sign" may be present in both schwannomas and neurofibromas on T2-WI, which consists of a central area of low-intermediate SI fibrous tissue surrounded by peripheral high SI myxoid tissue. A target-like enhancement pattern, with greater enhancement centrally than peripherally may be seen on contrast-enhanced T1-WI. If the parent nerve of a schwannoma can be identified, the schwannoma can be seen to have an eccentric position in relation to the nerve.

Neurofibroma

Neurofibromas are benign tumors of nerve sheaths of peripheral nerves that represent 5% of all benign soft tissue neoplasms. They occur sporadically in the third through fifth decades of life and are more common in men, and may develop in up to 10% of patients with NF-1 in a younger age range. Approximately one-third of patients with a solitary neurofibroma and almost every patient with multiple or plexiform neurofibromas have NF-1. Neurofibromas commonly occur in deep anatomic locations in patients with NF-1 (especially in retroperitoneal and paraspinal locations), and are commonly associated with neurologic symptoms. Other nonspecific symptoms and signs may also be seen with abdominal neurofibroma.

Sporadic neurofibromas are usually less than 5 cm in size, whereas neurofibromas in those with NF-1 tend to be multifocal and larger in size.

On MRI, they are of low SI on T1-WI and high SI on T2-WI. The SI on T2-WI may be homogeneous, or may be heterogeneous with either a "target sign" as described with schwannomas, or with a whorled appearance consisting of linear or curvilinear low SI Schwann cell bundles and collagen fibers in a background of high SI.

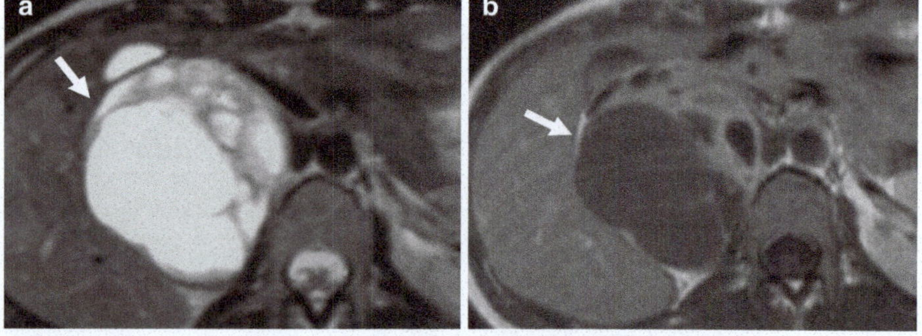

Fig. 7.7 Retroperitoneal schwannoma. On axial T2-W TSE (**a**) and axial T1-W contrast-enhanced TSE (**b**), a well-defined predominantly cystic lesion with left peripheral enhancing solid part is demarcated in the right adrenal region in a 27-year-old female patient. There was no drop of SI on opposed-phase images (not demonstrated), and there was no underlying malignant disease, thus indicating a benign neurogenic tumor. A schwannoma was proved on histological examination

After contrast administration, enhancement may be homogeneous or heterogeneous. Areas of fluid attenuation may be seen due to regions of myxoid degeneration, and this may cause confusion with necrotic lymphadenopathy or other cystic lesions in the retroperitoneum.

Malignant Peripheral Nerve Sheath Tumor (MPNST)

MPNSTs occur in 2–5% of patients with NF-1, and arise from preexisting neurofibromas, usually after a latent period of at least 10 years. Conversely, about 50% of patients with MPNST have NF-1. 10–20% of MPNSTs are related to prior radiation exposure, occurring after a latent period of more than 15 years. Most MPNSTs occur during the third through sixth decades of life, which is earlier than other retroperitoneal sarcomas. On MRI, benign and malignant neural tumors cannot be reliably differentiated, as SI and enhancement characteristics overlap.

7.1.4.4 Retroperitoneal Fibrotic Lesions

Retroperitoneal Fibrosis (RPF)

RPF is a rare fibrotic reactive process with a prevalence of about 1 per 200,000 of population. It is considered as a member of a family of disorders referred to as chronic periaortitis. Two-thirds of all cases of RPF are considered idiopathic (also called Ormond's disease), and approximately one-third of cases develop in response to various medications, malignancies, or other etiologies.

The exact etiology of idiopathic RPF is unclear although an underlying systemic autoimmune process is believed to be responsible instead.

Malignant RPF is an unusual subtype of RPF, and is clinically difficult to distinguish from RPF due to benign or idiopathic causes. Malignant RPF occurs when small metastatic foci to the retroperitoneum (usually from lymphoma) elicit a desmoplastic response. Malignant RPF is distinct from malignant retroperitoneal lymphadenopathy. Infections due to tuberculosis, syphilis, actinomycosis, or fungi, nonspecific gastrointestinal inflammation including appendicitis, Crohn's disease, or diverticulitis, retroperitoneal hemorrhage, urine extravasation, or prior irradiation or surgery may also lead to RPF.

On MRI, the T2-W SI of RPF is dependent on the activity of the disease. RPF has low-intermediate SI on T1-WI, and on T2-WI, mature fibrotic plaque in benign RPF has low SI whereas immature fibrotic plaque in benign RPF and malignant RPF has higher SI due to inflammatory edema or hypercellularity. Enhancement of RPF on MRI is variable, and depends upon the maturity of the fibrous process, with immature plaque enhancing to a greater degree due to greater vascularity. After corticosteroid therapy and with maturation, there is a decrease in inflammatory reaction with a subsequent decrease in T2-W SI as well as decreased enhancement on dynamic contrast-enhanced T1-WI.

Desmoid Tumor

Desmoid tumors are uncommon neoplastic lesions, comprising 0.1% of all tumors and 3.5% of fibrous tumors, occurring either sporadically or in association with familial adenomatous polyposis (FAP). The incidence of desmoid tumor in FAP ranges from 3.6–34%, and patients with FAP are at an approximately 1,000-fold increased risk compared to the general population. Sporadic desmoid tumor occurs more commonly in women by a ratio of 2–5:1 whereas FAP-associated desmoid tumor occurs with equal gender frequency. Both types of desmoid tumor have a peak incidence in the fourth decade of life.

Sporadic desmoid tumors are solitary in >90% of patients, are often present in the retroperitoneum, pelvis, and anterior abdominal wall, and tend to be large in size with a mean diameter of 13.8 cm. In contrast, FAP-associated desmoid tumors are multiple in 40% of patients, are more likely to involve the mesentery and the abdominal wall, and tend to be smaller, with a mean diameter of 4.8 cm.

Retroperitoneal desmoid tumors are rare and principally originate from the connective tissue of the muscles and their overlying fascia or aponeuroses. They tend to be infiltrative, may be asymptomatic or may have a variable clinical presentation due to ureteral obstruction or bowel invasion. Minor bone malformations such as exostoses, enostoses, and incomplete spinal segmentation maybe seen on imaging in 80% of sporadic desmoid tumor patients compared to 5% of the general population.

On MRI, desmoid tumors are typically infiltrative and cross fascial boundaries, have homogeneous low-intermediate attenuation and low-intermediate SI on T1-WI and T2-WI relative to skeletal muscle, are uncommonly calcified, and tend to appear aggressive although they are not malignant. However, as desmoid tumors may have a variable degree of cellularity, fibrosis, myxoid stroma, vascularity, and infiltration, they may be either well defined or poorly defined, and may have variable SI. Slightly high SI components on T1-WI relative to skeletal muscle are also not infrequently seen. The presence of high SI on T2-WI does not exclude a diagnosis of a desmoid tumor, as immature lesions with higher cellularity and less mature fibrosis can be of higher SI than skeletal muscle on T2-WI. Occasionally, a low SI fibrous capsule may be partially or completely visualized on T1-WI, and low SI bands of collagen may be present on T1-WI and T2-WI. Both mature and immature desmoid tumors tend to enhance and the enhancement can be variable. Associated encasement of the bowel or mesenteric vessels or hydronephrosis may also be seen.

7.1.4.5 Primary Retroperitoneal Fat-Containing Lesions

Lipoma

Lipomas (Fig. 7.8) are benign mesenchymal tumors composed of mature fat and represent the most common mesenchymal neoplasm. Even though retroperitoneal lipomas are rare, they are the most common benign tumor of the retroperitoneum. Variants of lipoma include angiolipoma, myolipoma, angiomyolipoma, myelolipoma, chondroid lipoma, spindle cell and pleomorphic lipoma, and benign lipoblastoma, and are found much less commonly in the abdomen. Lipomatous tumors account for half of all soft tissue tumors in surgical series.

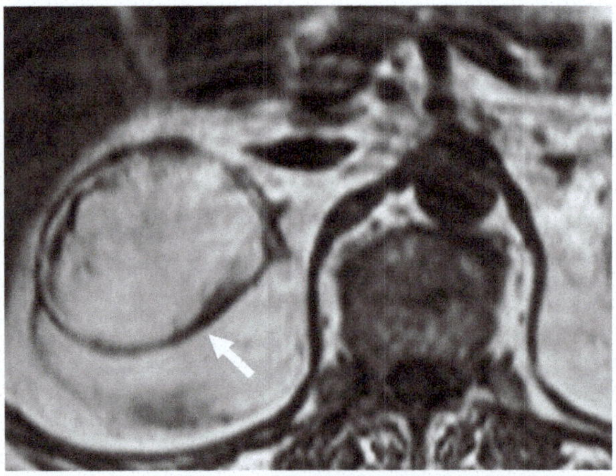

Fig. 7.8 Retroperitoneal lipoma. On axial T1-W TSE, a hyperintense well-defined lesion is demarcated in the right pararenal space most likely indicating a lipoma in a nontraumatic patient without underlying malignant disease (melanoma)

Solitary lipomas occur in the fifth through seventh decades of life, at a significantly younger peak age range compared to that of well-differentiated liposarcomas.

On MRI, lipomas typically have homogeneous attenuation and SI identical to that of macroscopic fat on all pulse sequences, without enhancing components, in contrast to well-differentiated liposarcomas. In up to 49% of cases, however, a few thin, <2 mm, septae that have minimal-moderate enhancement may be seen, and mild enhancement of a thin fibrous capsule may also be seen. Many lipomas also have prominent nonadipose areas that may demonstrate enhancement, and the imaging appearance then overlaps with that of well-differentiated liposarcomas. These nonadipose components may be seen in up to 31% of lipomas, and are secondary to fat necrosis and associated calcification, fibrosis, inflammation, and areas of myxoid change. Lipomas tend to be smaller in size than well-differentiated liposarcomas, and most remain stable in size.

Extrarenal Angiomyolipoma (AML)

AMLs are choristomas, which are lesions composed of ectopic rests of normal tissue in an abnormal arrangement, containing fat, abnormal blood vessels, and smooth muscle in varying relative proportions, and are most often found in the kidneys. They are rarely encountered in the extrarenal retroperitoneum. Approximately 90% of AMLs occur sporadically in the kidney, most frequently in middle-aged women, while 20% of renal AML cases have TS; 80% of TS patients have AMLs, which tend to be multiple and bilateral. Up to 57% of patients with lymphangioleiomyomatosis (LAM) have AMLs. Although benign, some AMLs exhibit aggressive features that may mimic malignancy. These include vascular invasion, lymph node involvement, nonrenal organ involvement, and local recurrence after resection. Multicentric or extrarenal retroperitoneal AMLs are thought to be caused by the congenital presence of cell precursors in multiple sites or by a form of benign metastases similar to that in benign metastasizing leiomyoma. Similar to renal AMLs, extrarenal AMLs have a propensity to undergo spontaneous hemorrhage, with a risk which correlates with the size of the lesion.

On MRI, extrarenal AMLs typically appear as masses that contain areas of macroscopic fat. Soft tissue components and vascular components are frequently present, and there is a variable amount of enhancement. The major differential diagnosis is retroperitoneal liposarcoma, but preoperative cross-sectional imaging combined with tissue sampling may permit a nonoperative diagnosis in lesions that pose a diagnostic problem.

Extraadrenal Myelolipoma

Myelolipomas are uncommon benign well-circumscribed tumors that are composed of mature adipose cells and hematopoietic tissue. They are of uncertain etiology, but usually arise in the adrenal gland. Extraadrenal retroperitoneal myelolipomas are rare, occurring most often in the presacral space. They are more common in women than in men by a ratio of 2:1, with a peak occurrence in the seventh decade of life.

Extraadrenal myelolipomas can range in size from 2 to 26 cm with a mean size of 8.2 cm. Smaller lesions are typically asymptomatic while larger lesions are frequently symptomatic due to mass effect or hemorrhage. Associated hemorrhage is more common with larger lesions than with smaller lesions. The natural history of extraadrenal myelolipoma is unknown, but adrenal myelolipomas can enlarge with time and become symptomatic.

On MRI, myelolipomas contain areas with attenuation and SI characteristics similar to macroscopic fat, often with enhancing soft tissue components due to mixed hematopoietic tissue, and, less commonly, may have foci of calcification. A thin peripheral rim of mild enhancement is often seen on contrast-enhanced T1-WI. Associated retroperitoneal hemorrhage may occasionally be seen as well. Extraadrenal myelolipomas tend to have smaller amounts of macroscopic fat compared to adrenal myelolipomas.

7.1.4.6 Primary Retroperitoneal Teratoma

Primary retroperitoneal teratomas are rare lesions that represent 6–11% of primary retroperitoneal tumors. The majority occur in children. They are 2–4 times more common in women than in men. Teratomas in adults have a greater chance of being malignant than in children (14–26 vs. 6–7%, respectively). Primary retroperitoneal teratomas tend to be asymptomatic, but may cause nonspecific symptoms as seen with other retroperitoneal masses when large in size. Alpha-fetoprotein levels are normal in patients with benign teratomas but may be elevated with malignant teratomas.

Primary retroperitoneal teratomas may be cystic and/or solid, and frequently contain mature tissues including skin and dermal appendages, cartilage, bone, teeth, or fat. Cystic teratomas are benign, well-defined lesions that contain multiple solid and cystic areas along with mature tissues, sebaceous material, and/or mucoid fluid. Solid teratomas are frequently malignant and contain immature embryonic tissue in addition to the mature components. Retroperitoneal teratomas tend to be located near the upper poles of the kidneys, with preponderance on the left side. Sixty to eighty percent of all primary retroperitoneal teratomas have calcifications; up to 74% of benign teratomas and up to 25% of malignant teratomas may contain calcifications. Therefore, the presence of calcifications does not predict benignity.

On MRI, teratomas are usually heterogeneous, well-defined solid and/or multiloculated cystic lesions that may contain fatty components, calcifications, ossifications, or teeth. Other tumoral components have less specific MRI features. Occasionally, a low SI fibrous pseudocapsule may be visualized on T1-WI and T2-WI, and a dermoid plug or Rokitansky nodule may also be seen along the inner surface of a cystic component with variable attenuation and SI depending on components present within it. An almost pathognomonic finding of a mature cystic teratoma is an internal fat-fluid level, with the nondependent fat layer following the attenuation and SI of fat on all pulse sequences. This finding is usually seen in ovarian teratomas, but may rarely be present in teratomas developing at other anatomic sites.

7.1.4.7 Pseudomyxoma Retroperitonei

The term pseudomyxoma peritonei or "false mucinous tumor of the peritoneum" has been used historically as a pathologic diagnostic term to describe any benign or malignant condition that results in intraperitoneal mucin accumulation. However, pseudomyxoma peritonei should be used strictly as a clinical descriptor for patients with mucinous ascites originating from a primary appendiceal mucinous adenoma with pathologic features of disseminated peritoneal adenomucinosis. Pseudomyxoma peritonei is a rare condition that occurs twice as often in men than in women, with a peak presentation in the sixth decade of life. Pseudomyxoma retroperitonei (or pseudomyxoma extraperitonei) occurs very rarely, and is caused by retroperitoneal rupture of a primary appendiceal mucinous adenoma in a retrocecal appendix, and fixation of the lesion to the posterior abdominal wall. It most often occurs in men in the fourth through ninth decades of life, with a peak occurrence in the sixth decade of life. Histologically, the lesions are lined with glandular epithelium and are filled with thick gelatinous mucinous material.

On MRI, multicystic lesions with low attenuation, low-intermediate SI on T1-WI, and high SI on T2-WI as well as thickened walls or septations that displace and distort adjacent structures are seen. Curvilinear or punctate mural calcifications may also be present. The primary appendiceal mucinous adenoma may be indistinguishable from adjacent mucinous fluid.

7.1.4.8 Lymphangioma

Lymphangiomas (Fig. 7.9) are uncommon cystic lesions that are very rare in the abdomen and pelvis. The most common location of an abdominal lymphangioma is in the mesentery, followed by the omentum, mesocolon, and retroperitoneum. Rare multisystemic involvement and extensive intra-abdominal cystic lymphangiomatosis may occur, and has a poor prognosis. Up to 40% of retroperitoneal and other abdominal lymphangiomas occur in older children or adults. Lymphangiomas tend to occur slightly more commonly in men than in women.

The etiology and pathogenesis of lymphangioma is not entirely clear. Some consider them to be acquired malformations resulting from obstruction of lymphatic vessels, whereas others consider them to be congenital malformations of lymphangiectasia related to failure of communication with the lymphatic system. Histologically, lymphangiomas are large, thin walled, usually multiloculated, cystic lesions that are lined by attenuated endothelium resembling that of

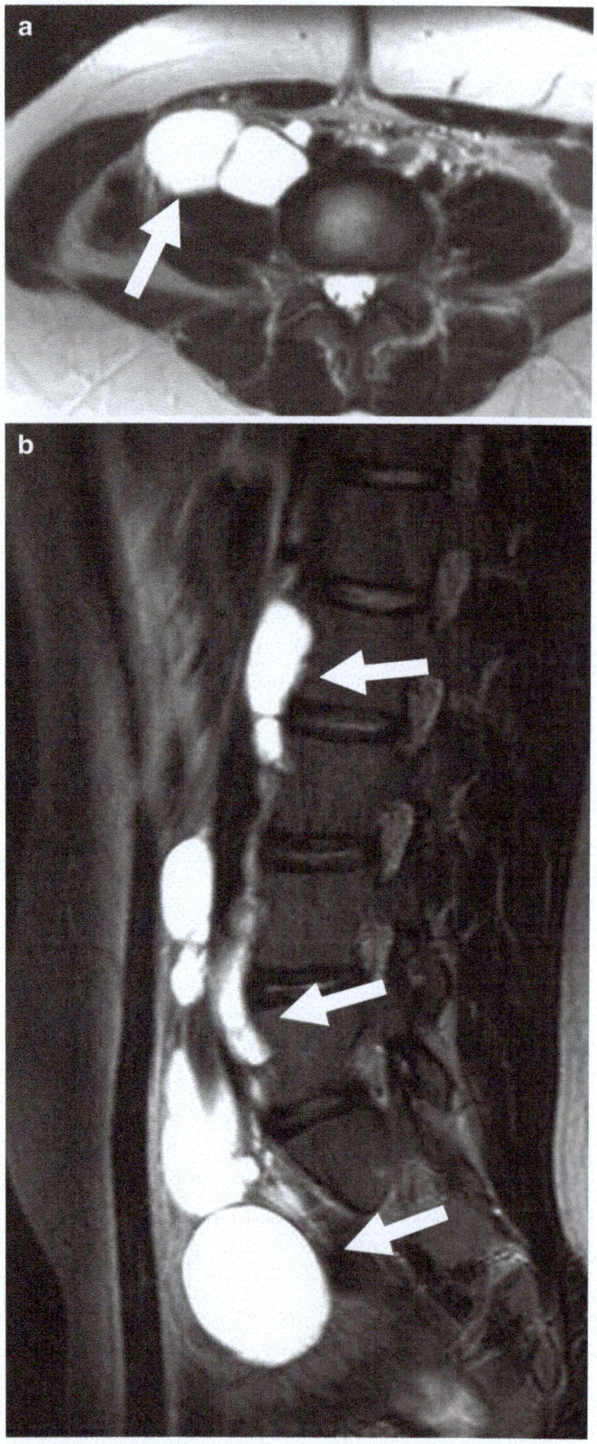

Fig. 7.9 Retroperitoneal lymphangioma. On axial T2-W TSE (**a**) and sagittal T2-W TSE (**b**) a multilocular cystic lesion is demarcated in the posterior pararenal space in a 16-year-old girl, and it proved to be a lymphangioma on histological specimen

normal lymphatics, with a stroma formed by a delicate meshwork of collagen punctuated by small lymphoid aggregates. Lymphangiomas are classified into capillary (simple), cavernous, and cystic (hygroma) types, depending on the size of the lymphatic spaces. Retroperitoneal lymphangiomas are usually asymptomatic and are discovered either incidentally on cross-sectional imaging, or during surgery for unrelated conditions. This is in contradistinction to lymphangiomas of the mesentery, omentum, or mesocolon, which tend to be symptomatic.

On MRI, lymphangiomas usually appear as large, cystic, unilocular, or multilocular thin-walled lesions, with multiple cystic components of various sizes that tend to invaginate between rather than displace structures, and may cause bowel dilation due to obstruction. Serous fluid contents have water attenuation and low SI on T1-WI and very high SI on T2-WI relative to skeletal muscle. Sometimes, the fluid contents may be chylous with water or fat attenuation, increased SI on T1-WI, and high SI on T2-WI, or proteinaceous/hemorrhagic with high attenuation, increased SI on T1-WI, and high SI on T2-WI. Loss of SI of the internal fluid contents from in-phase to out-of-phase T1-W gradient echo images may sometimes be seen in chylous lymphangiomas of the mesentery. Occasionally, a small amount of fat may be detected within the septations of a lymphangioma, with high SI noted on T1-WI and loss of SI with both fat suppressed and out-of-phase T1-WI. Rarely, calcifications may be present, which appear as foci of very high attenuation and very low SI on both T1-WI and T2-WI. Mild septal or wall enhancement may be present. With complications of infection or hemorrhage, the outer wall and internal septations tend to be thicker.

7.1.5 Retroperitoneal and Pelvic Lymphadenopathy

There are approximately 400–500 lymph nodes in the human body, with approximately half located in the abdomen and pelvis. Retroperitoneal and pelvic lymph nodes are generally present in a perivascular distribution about the aorta, inferior vena cava (IVC), and iliac vessels. Both normal and malignant lymph nodes appear as small oval or flat structures that have soft tissue attenuation, intermediate SI on T1-WI and intermediate-high SI on T2-WI relative to skeletal muscle, and enhance. Fatty hila with SI similar to that of subcutaneous fat may also be present. Conventional MRI has shown to be equally effective to or slightly superior to CT in the detection of abdominopelvic lymph nodes, and can more easily distinguish lymph nodes from vessels.

Attenuation and SI characteristics of lymph nodes on conventional imaging sequences are not accurate in differentiating between benign and malignant lymph nodes. Calcifications may sometimes be present, appearing as foci of very high attenuation and very low SI on T1-WI and T2-WI when visualized, and may be secondary to neoplastic or inflammatory conditions. Hemorrhagic lymphadenopathy or lymphadenopathy due to metastatic melanoma may demonstrate increased SI on T1-WI.

Fatty lymphadenopathy may be seen with lipoplastic lymphadenopathy, cavitary lymph node syndrome, and Whipple's disease. Lipoplastic lymphadenopathy has a benign course and typically occurs in obese middle-aged women. The lymph nodes are enlarged and replaced by fat, with attenuation and SI similar to macroscopic fat on all pulse sequences, sometimes with thin rim of nodal tissue remaining. In the pelvis, this can mimic the appearance of pelvic lipomatosis, but can be differentiated at lymphangiography. Cavitary lymph node syndrome is sometimes found in association with celiac disease along with splenic atrophy, and appears as low attenuation lymphadenopathy that sometimes contains fat-fluid levels. Necrosis of lymph nodes suggests malignant lymphadenopathy, such as from metastatic squamous cell carcinoma, or less commonly, lymphoma or testicular carcinoma, but may also occur in benign inflammatory diseases including mycobacterial infections, bacterial infection, Whipple's disease, histoplasmosis infection, and systemic lupus erythematosus. On MRI, necrotic lymph nodes have central low attenuation, central high SI on T2-WI, and lack of central enhancement.

Short axis size estimation is the imaging criterion used most often to differentiate benign from malignant lymph nodes. In patients with a primary cancer, lymph nodes <10 mm in short axis dimension are considered benign, whereas nodes ≥10 mm are suspicious for malignancy. However, overlap exists as malignant lymph nodes can sometimes be <10 mm, and benign reactive or hyperplastic lymph nodes can be ≥10 mm. Lymph node location may also affect the criteria used to assess nodal size. For example, normal retrocrural and porta hepatis nodes should not exceed 6 mm, and gastrohepatic ligament nodes should not exceed 8 mm, whereas normal pelvic lymph nodes (particularly inguinal lymph nodes) may normally be up to 10–15 mm in size. The presence of multiple, slightly smaller lymph nodes in the 8–10 mm range should be viewed with suspicion for underlying pathology, e.g., chronic lymphocytic leukemia. Most normal lymph nodes have an oval shape, whereas malignant lymph nodes are often round in shape.

Malignant neoplasms tend to spread initially to their regional nodal groups, although it is not unusual for lymphadenopathy to involve several contiguous or even widely separated nodal chains, as there are complex intercommunications between regional groups of lymph nodes. Virtually any abdominal or pelvic neoplasm may lead to retroperitoneal lymphadenopathy, but the most common are lymphoma, renal cell carcinoma, testicular carcinoma, cervical carcinoma, and prostatic carcinoma. Carcinomas of the bladder, prostate, cervix, and uterus initially spread to the pelvic nodes, as may anorectal carcinoma, after first involving nodes in the perirectal space. Testicular, ovarian, and fallopian tube malignancies spread first to the retroperitoneal nodes adjacent to or near the renal hila, but may involve the pelvic nodes via retrograde spread. Testicular carcinoma of the right testis tends to involve aortocaval and paracaval lymph nodes and can cross over to the left side of the aorta, whereas testicular carcinoma of the left testis tends to involve left paraaortic lymph nodes. Anterior displacement of the aorta or IVC or lateral ureteral displacement may be seen when malignant retroperitoneal lymphadenopathy is present.

Ultrasmall superparamagnetic iron oxide particles such as ferumoxtran-10 (not yet FDA approved) may be used as a nontargeted MRI negative lymph node contrast agent to differentiate between benign and malignant lymph nodes, as benign lymph nodal tissue accumulates iron particles within macrophages and has very low SI on T2*-WI, whereas foci of malignancy within lymph nodes remain intermediate-high SI on T2*-WI. Use of this approach increases the sensitivity and specificity for detecting nodal metastatic disease, compared to CT or conventional MRI, as micrometastases within normal sized lymph nodes can be indirectly detected. However, false-positive results can occur because of focal nodal lipomatosis or a prominent fatty hilum, as well as by reactive lymphoid follicular hyperplasia or nodal necrosis, and false-negative results can occur because of limitations in spatial resolution. Lymphoma and metastatic disease are by far the most common causes of abdominopelvic lymphadenopathy. Other less common causes of abdominopelvic lymphadenopathy include leukemia, Kaposi's sarcoma, tuberculosis, atypical mycobacterial infection, bacterial, viral, or fungal infection, AIDS, mesenteric lymphadenitis, idiopathic retroperitoneal fibrosis, sarcoidosis, cat-scratch disease, Whipple's disease, amyloidosis, Castleman's disease, mastocytosis, celiac sprue, and Crohn's disease, amongst numerous other infectious or inflammatory etiologies. Several of these etiologies will be discussed below.

7.1.5.1 Lymphoma

Lymphoma (Fig. 7.10) is the most common retroperitoneal malignancy, and it accounts for one-third of

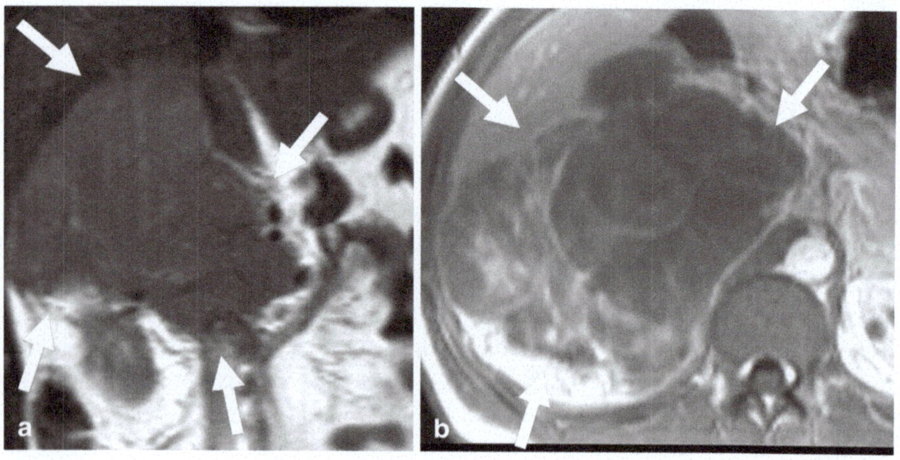

Fig. 7.10 Retroperitoneal Hodgkin lymphoma. Coronal T2-W TSE (**a**) and axial T1-W contrast-enhanced TSE (**b**) images show a poorly defined, huge mass in the right anterior pararenal space and right adrenal region with higher signal intensity on T2-W image (**a**) relative to muscle and very inhomogeneous contrast enhancement (**b**). Primary Hodgkin lymphoma was diagnosed by core needle biopsy

retroperitoneal malignant neoplasms. Patients of all ages may be affected, although the incidence of non-Hodgkin's lymphoma increases with age, whereas Hodgkin's lymphoma has a bimodal age distribution in young adults and the elderly. The clinical course may range from indolent to highly aggressive, depending partly on the histology of the tumor. Lymphoma typically begins as local lymph node enlargement, and then spreads via lymphatics to adjacent lymph nodes, commonly in the retroperitoneum, and sometimes becomes systemic. Conglomerate mesenteric and retroperitoneal masses may form, and they characteristically infiltrate the perinephric spaces of the retroperitoneum. Whereas abdominal Hodgkin's lymphoma tends to be confined to the spleen and retroperitoneum with spread of disease to contiguous lymph nodes, non-Hodgkin's lymphoma more commonly involves a variety of nodal groups and extranodal sites. Approximately 50% of patients with non-Hodgkin's lymphoma have mesenteric lymphadenopathy at presentation, which may become confluent with characteristic encasement of the mesenteric vessels. In contrast, enlarged lymph nodes due to other conditions tend to remain discrete, rarely forming a conglomerate mass.

The Ann Arbor staging system for lymphoma is used to help to predict the prognosis and survival of patients. This staging classification is less useful for non-Hodgkin's lymphoma than for Hodgkin's lymphoma, as non-Hodgkin's lymphoma more frequently disseminates hematogenously. The prognosis worsens as the stage increases, and the prognosis within each stage also worsens when B symptoms are present. The Revised European-American Classification of Lymphoid Neoplasms and the World Health Organization classification provide systems for classification of lymphomas. Studies have shown that these classification systems separate patients with clinically different types of lymphoma and stratify them into different prognostic groups.

On MRI, lymphoma is typically intermediate-slightly high in SI on T1-WI and high in SI on T2-WI relative to muscle. Associated involvement of the bone marrow, gastrointestinal tract, and other parenchymal organs such as the liver or spleen may be present.

Assessment of the SI of lymphomatous nodal masses after therapy on T2-WI may be useful, as low SI on T2-WI within treated lymph node masses represents nonviable tumor or fibrosis. However, most of the published literature on using T2-W SI to document response to treatment has focused on patients with mediastinal Hodgkin's lymphoma. In addition, one should be cautious in diagnosing residual tumor when there is high SI on T2-WI, as high SI may persist up to 12 months following therapy due to edema, granulation tissue, hemorrhage, or immature fibrosis. MRI and CT show equivalent accuracies for staging of abdominal lymphoma. However, MRI outperforms CT in the detection and characterization of bone marrow involvement by lymphoma.

7.1.5.2 Tuberculosis

Tuberculosis is endemic in most developing countries but is also globally increasing in incidence in both immunocompetent as well as immunocompromised patients, in part related to AIDS and multidrug-resistant tuberculosis. Although the thorax is the most frequently involved site, any of a number of organ systems may be involved. The abdomen is the most common site of extrapulmonary tuberculosis. Lymphadenopathy is the most common manifestation of abdominal tuberculosis, and is the only abdominal finding in up to 55% of patients. Mesenteric, omental, peripancreatic, periportal, pericaval, and upper paraaortic lymph nodes are commonly involved, due to lymphatic drainage from the small bowel and right colon, in addition to disease spread along the hepatoduodenal ligament. More extensive lymphadenopathy may be present in patients with AIDS.

Pathologically, active tuberculous lymphadenopathy passes through multiple stages: (1) lymphoid hyperplasia with formation of tubercles and granulomata without caseation necrosis, (2) caseation necrosis, (3) lymph node capsular destruction, adherence of multiple lymph nodes, and perilymphadenitis, (4) rupture into surrounding soft tissue forming a confluent abscess cavity, and (5) healing with subsequent fibrosis and calcification.

On MRI, the lymph nodes are usually multiple and large with mean size of 2–3 cm, and of low attenuation, low-intermediate SI on T1-WI, and central high SI on T2-WI relative to skeletal muscle in active disease, without associated urinary, biliary, or gastrointestinal tract obstruction. The degree of low attenuation and high SI on T2-WI within lymph nodes generally parallels the amount of central necrosis, and the degree of nodal necrosis correlates with clinical signs and symptoms. Low T2-W SI nodes may be present due to inactive or fibrotic tissue in later stages of disease or due to calcification. Homogeneous or mildly inhomogeneous enhancement of lymph nodes is seen if there is none or minimal central necrosis. However, peripheral intermediate SI on T1-WI and high SI on T2-WI with delayed peripheral enhancement are often present because of granulation tissue, inflammation, hypervascularity, and edema, along with central lack of enhancement due to caseation or liquefaction necrosis in up to 40% of cases. Nonenhancement of lymph nodes may be seen in AIDS, presumably due to a diminished inflammatory reaction association with this condition. Although the coexistence of findings of pulmonary tuberculosis may be seen, only 40% of patients with abdominal tuberculosis have findings of associated pleuropulmonary disease on chest radiography.

7.1.5.3 Castleman's Disease

Castleman's disease (Fig. 7.11), also known as angiofollicular lymph node hyperplasia or benign giant lymph node hyperplasia, is a hyperplastic-dysplastic-neoplastic lymphoproliferative process of uncertain etiology that is a rare cause of abdominopelvic lymph node enlargement. Individuals with Castleman's disease can present clinically with either unicentric or localized lymphadenopathy that remains relatively stable, or with multicentric or disseminated disease characterized by generalized lymphadenopathy, constitutional symptoms, organomegaly, and a more aggressive clinical course with 30% of patients developing malignant transformation. Patients with unicentric disease present at a significantly younger age with peak presentation in the third decade of life than those with multicentric disease who present in the sixth decade of life. Unicentric disease occurs equally in men and women, whereas multicentric disease occurs twice as commonly in men as in women. Patients with unicentric disease usually have intrathoracic disease most commonly involving mediastinal or hilar lymph nodes, whereas in patients with multicentric disease, the mesentery, retroperitoneum, and pelvis are involved in 7–12% of patients. Multicentric Castleman's disease is frequently associated with POEMS syndrome (polyneuropathy, organomegaly, endocrinopathy, M proteins, and skin changes), Kaposi's sarcoma, and AIDS, and less commonly with amyloidosis and monoclonal gammopathy.

Grossly, homogeneous, encapsulated, highly vascular masses are present, which are often adherent to surrounding structures.

On MRI, the lesions of Castleman's disease generally have soft tissue attenuation similar to muscle attenuation, low-intermediate SI on T1-WI and high SI on T2-WI relative to the skeletal muscle, and mild-marked enhancement, particularly in the arterial phase, with slow washout. Lesions smaller than 5 cm tend to have homogeneous attenuation and enhancement, whereas larger lesions tend to have more heterogeneous attenuation and enhancement. A peripheral rim of even greater enhancement may sometimes be visualized as well, related to a greater quantity of small or capillary vessels in the periphery, and dilated feeding

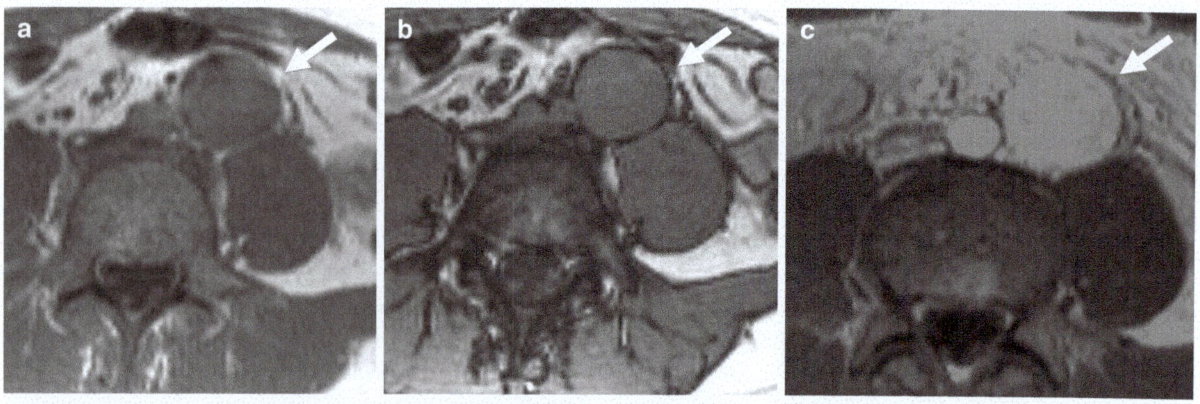

Fig. 7.11 Retroperitoneal Castleman disease. On axial T1-W inphase GRE (**a**), axial T1-W opposed-phase GRE (**b**), and axial T1-W contrast-enhanced TSE (**c**), a well-defined lesion is demarcated in the left paraaortic, infrarenal region in a 35-year-old male patient with mild hypertension. There is no evidence of intracellular lipids on chemical shift images (**a**, **b**) and a marked hypervascularity on contrast-enhanced image (**c**). A core needle biopsy was performed; however, final diagnosis of benign Castleman disease was gained by surgical excision

arteries may be seen due to lesional hypervascularity. Calcification may be present in one-third of cases of abdominal Castleman's disease.

7.1.6 Lymphangioleiomyomatosis

LAM, a forme fruste of TS, is a rare idiopathic disorder that occurs in women of childbearing age, and predominantly affects the lungs, and less often the mediastinum and retroperitoneum. The disease is characterized by a hamartomatous proliferation of smooth muscle cells that involves lymph nodes and lymphatics, resulting in dilation of lymphatic spaces with cyst formation.

On MRI, cystic lung disease, chylous pleural effusions, pneumothoraces, and renal angiomyolipomas are most frequently encountered. Retroperitoneal or pelvic lymphangioleiomyomas are less common, occurring in up to 20% of patients, which appear as high T2W SI cystic masses with enhancing walls, sometimes with delayed enhancement of the internal contents. Diurnal variation in size of lymphangioleiomyomas (with an increase in lesion size during the day) is frequently encountered on cross-sectional imaging, and is thought to be related in part to an increase in abdominopelvic lymph flow during the day related to an increase in chyle production after meals. Abdominopelvic lymphadenopathy may be seen in up to 40% of patients, some of which contains low attenuation high T2W SI areas due to chylous lymph collections, or hamartomatous hyperattenuating areas that enhance. Chylous ascites may also be seen infrequently.

7.2 Adrenal Glands

7.2.1 Normal Anatomy

The adrenal glands are paired retroperitoneal endocrine glands that are composed of an outer cortex and inner medulla. The adrenal cortex is derived from the mesoderm and is responsible for the secretion of aldosterone, cortisol, and androgens, while the adrenal medulla is derived from neural crest cells and secretes norepinephrine and epinephrine. The normal adrenal medulla and cortex cannot be distinguished with routine MR imaging. On high-resolution ex vivo T2-W MR images, the adrenal medulla can be seen as a band of higher SI compared to the adrenal cortex.

7.2.2 Adrenal Imaging Techniques

7.2.2.1 Plain MRI

Differentiation between benign and malignant adrenal masses is possible using T2-WIs. On such images, malignant primary and secondary adrenal neoplasms display high SIs. On the other hand, regardless of the hormonal activity, low to medium relative SIs may be found in adenomas irrespective of the repetition time, echo time (TE), and flip angles used. There is, however an important overlap between relative SI values of malignant and benign adrenal tumors, leading to equivocal findings in about one-third of cases.

7.2.2.2 Chemical Shift MR Imaging Techniques

The two most common neoplasms involving the adrenal gland are adrenal cortical adenomas and metastatic disease. The adrenal cortical cells that give rise to adenomas contain intracellular lipid. The ability to detect and characterize intracellular lipid makes chemical shift MR imaging (Fig. 7.12) an ideal imaging technique for evaluating adrenal masses and distinguishing between metastatic disease and benign cortical adenomas. A small number of adenomas may not contain substantial amounts of intracellular lipid and are referred to as "lipid-poor adenomas."

The term *chemical shift* refers to the difference in behavior of lipid and water protons when placed in a magnetic field. The chemical shift of lipid and water protons is approximately 3.5 ppm, with water protons precessing at a slightly higher frequency.

According to the Larmor equation, at 1.5 T, protons precess at approximately 63 × 106 times per second. The chemical shift difference between lipid and water protons at 1.5 T is approximately 220 Hz (63 × 3.5 ppm). At 1.5 T, lipid protons precess at a frequency of 63 million times per second, and water protons precess at 63,000,220 times per second. A 220-Hz frequency corresponds to a period of once every 4.4 ms. Imagine the precessing lipid and water protons within a voxel of

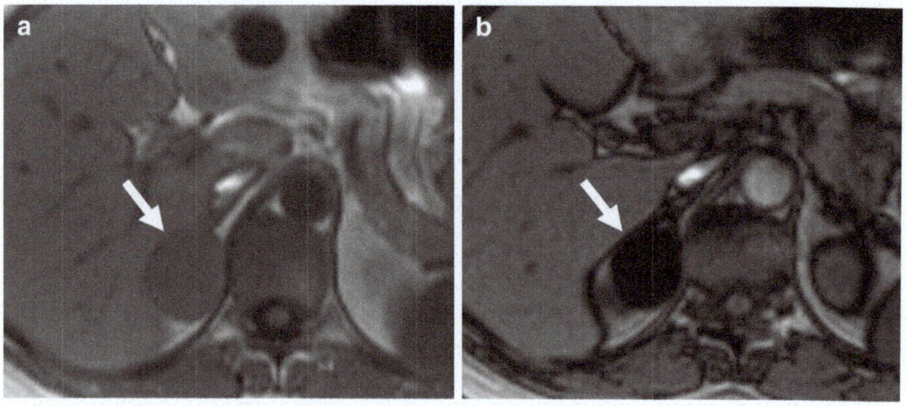

Fig. 7.12 Adrenal adenoma demonstrated by chemical shift imaging. On axial T1-W in-phase GRE (**a**) and axial T1-W opposed-phase GRE (**b**) images, a well-defined small right adrenal mass is delineated, which shows a marked drop of signal intensity on opposed-phase image (**b**)

tissue in a 1.5-T magnet as individuals running around a racetrack. Every 4.4 ms, both the lipid and water protons would cross the finish line at the same instant, even though they were running (precessing) at different speeds (frequencies). At 1.5 T, gradient echo sequences with an TE of 4.4 ms result in the addition of SI from lipid and water protons contained within the same voxel (termed *in-phase*). With a TE of 2.2 ms (and odd multiples of 2.2), the SI of lipid and water protons are at opposite sides of the racetrack; thus, their respective signals will be destructive, not additive. Such gradient echo sequences are termed *opposed phase*. At 3 T, protons precess at twice the frequency as they do at 1.5 T. Thus the chemical shift difference between water and lipid protons would then be approximately 440 Hz, and the shortest in-phase and opposed-phase TEs are 2.2 and 1.1 ms, respectively. Demonstration of loss of SI within an adrenal mass on an opposed-phase MR image when compared with a corresponding in-phase image establishes the presence of intracellular lipid and a presumptive diagnosis of an adrenal adenoma. If one wanted to use quantitative measurements to diagnose a cortical adenoma, a chemical shift index of more than 0.15 has been shown to be the most reliable method; chemical shift index is defined as SI of adrenal lesion on in-phase image - SI on opposed-phase image/SI on in-phase image, where SI is signal intensity. Many MR imagers are now capable of performing a dual-echo gradient echo sequence in which both the in-phase and opposed-phase images are obtained in a single breath-hold. The opposed-phase image can be subtracted from the corresponding in-phase image; the resulting chemical shift subtraction image is a map of those voxels that contain both lipid and water protons. This technique has been used to characterize the lipid within adrenal adenomas and does not require calculation of a chemical shift index. At 3 T, the shortest TEs for the first in-phase and opposed-phase images are 2.2 and 1.1 ms, respectively. It is unclear if a TE of 1.1 ms is obtainable in routine clinical practice secondary to issues of specific absorption rate. It is desirable to have the opposed-phase TE less than the in-phase TE because loss of SI on an opposed-phase image is specific for the presence of lipid and water in the same voxel. If the TE of the opposed-phase image is longer, then susceptibility effects (e.g., hemorrhage) can also result in SI loss and result in a potential false-positive diagnosis of adenoma.

There are several ways of assessing the degree of loss of SI. Quantitative analysis can be made using a variety of ratios, essentially comparing the loss of signal in the adrenal mass with that of the liver, paraspinal muscle, or spleen on in-phase and out-of-phase images. However, fatty infiltration of the liver and iron overload make the liver an unreliable internal standard. Fatty infiltration might also affect skeletal muscle, although to a lesser extent. The spleen has been shown to be the most reliable internal standard, although this might also be affected by iron overload.

To calculate the adrenal lesion to spleen ratio (ASR), regions of interest are used to acquire the SI within the adrenal mass and the spleen from in-phase and out-of-phase images. The ASR reflects the percentage signal drop-off within the adrenal lesion compared with the spleen and it can be calculated as follows:

$$\mathrm{ASR} = \frac{\text{SI lesion}\left(\text{out-of-phase}\right)/\text{SI spleen}\left(\text{out-of-phase}\right)}{\text{SI lesion}\left(\text{in-phase}\right)/\text{SI spleen}\left(\text{in-phase}\right)} \times 100$$

An ASR ratio of 70 or less has been shown to be 100% specific for adenomas, but only 78% sensitive. Simple visual assessment of relative SI loss is just as accurate, but quantitative methods might be useful in equivocal cases. A SI loss of greater than 20% within an adrenal mass on out-of-phase images is diagnostic of an adenoma.

7.2.2.3 Dynamic Contrast-Enhanced MRI

Dynamic Gadolinium-enhanced studies of the adrenal glands allow a further differentiation of even equivocal cases, as there is a distinct difference between the enhancement and wash-out pattern of adenomas on the one hand and of malignant lesions on the other. As with CT, adenomas display contrast enhancement after administration of gadolinium with quick wash-out (Fig. 7.13), whereas malignant tumors show a slower washout (Fig. 7.14). Uniform enhancement (capillary blush) on post gadolinium capillary phase has been reported in up to 70% of adenomas, but is rare in other adrenal masses. In addition, adenomas often show a rim of enhancement in the late phase of gadolinium-enhanced images. Metastases frequently have heterogeneous enhancement. Pheochromocytomas display nonuniform enhancement and washout characteristics. Also taking into account the variable SI on T2-WIs, the term of "imaging chameleon" has been introduced for pheochromocytoma.

The combination of spin-echo signal characteristics, gadolinium enhancement, and CSI is currently around 90% accurate in distinguishing adenomas from nonadenomas. In Table 7.2 imaging parameters for state-of-the-art imaging of adrenal lesions on a 1.5 T MR unit are outlined.

7.2.3 Neoplasms of the Adrenal Cortex

7.2.3.1 Adrenal Cortical Adenoma

Adrenal cortical adenomas are benign neoplasms of the adrenal cortex. Between 2 and 9% of autopsies demonstrate adrenal tumors, and 2–7% of patients have incidental adrenal masses discovered at cross-sectional imaging. Most of these adrenal lesions are nonhyperfunctioning benign adrenal cortical adenomas that require no treatment. There are clinical and imaging features independent of chemical shift MR imaging and attenuation values that are helpful in distinguishing adenomas from metastases. Adenomas tend to be smaller, demonstrate homogeneous MR SI and CT attenuation, and are well marginated. Adrenal metastases tend to be larger, heterogeneous, and poorly marginated, and they

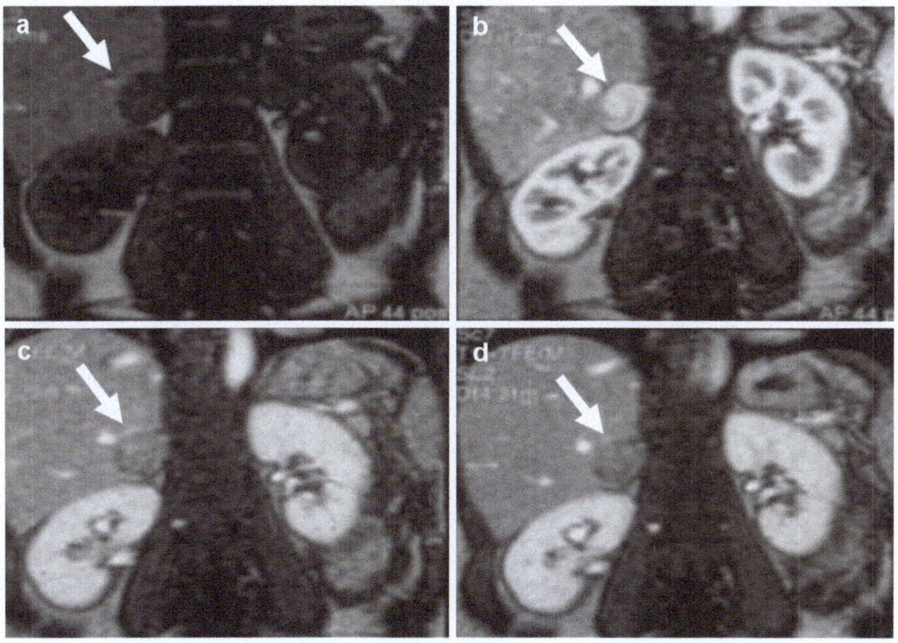

Fig. 7.13 Dynamic contrast-enhanced adrenal imaging. Dynamic contrast-enhanced adrenal imaging shows a small right adrenal mass (**a**–**d**) with marked contrast uptake in the corticomedullary phase (**b**) hyperintensity on the nephrographic phase (**c**) and a rapid washout in a 10 min delayed series (**d**) indicative of a benign adrenal lesion, most likely an adrenal adenoma

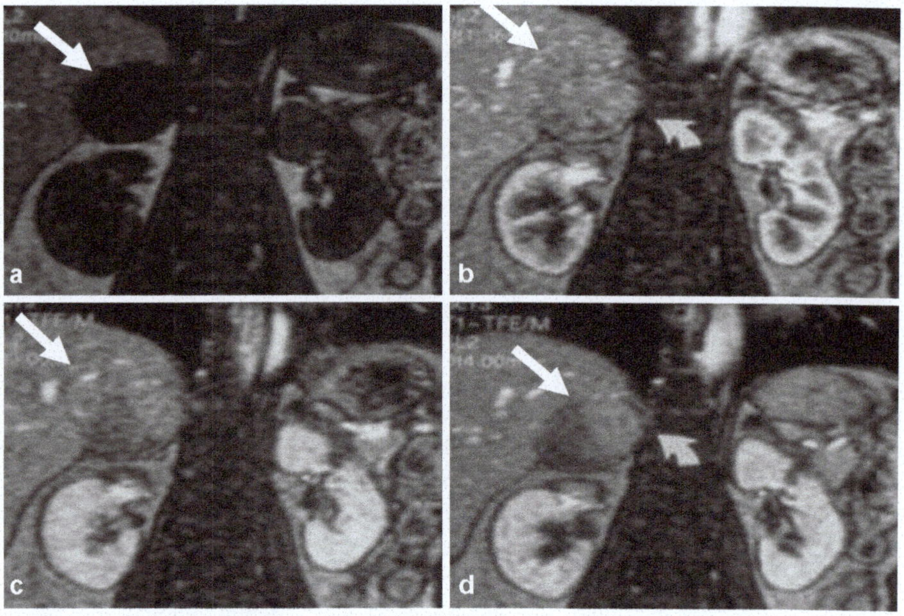

Fig. 7.14 Dynamic contrast-enhanced adrenal imaging. Dynamic contrast-enhanced adrenal imaging shows a medium size, well-defined right adrenal mass (**a–d**) with moderate contrast uptake in the arterial/corticomedullary phase (**b**), further enhancement on the nephrographic phase (**c**), and a slow washout in a 10 min delayed series (**d**) indicative of a malignant adrenal lesion. Histologically an adrenal cortical carcinoma was proven

Table 7.2 Commonly used sequences for imaging of the adrenals

T1w GRE inphase T1w GRE out-of-phase	Combined use with inphase gradient-echo technique (chemical shift imaging) to evaluate the presence of intracellular lipids and thus differentiate benign and malignant adrenal lesions
T2w	TSE/FSE sequences in axial and/or coronal plane. Fat saturation improves image contrast
T1w	Typically 2D or 3D GRE sequences in axial plane breathold recommended. Fat saturation may be used
Post i.v. admin. of GBCA	
T1w	Same sequence and imaging plane should be used before and after gadolinium-chelate injection Additionally a 15 min. delayed series should be included for evaluation of contrast enhancement washout

occur in patients with known primary malignancies. Adrenal metastases grow with time, while cortical adenomas tend to remain the same size or grow slowly.

Hypersecreting Adrenal Cortical Adenoma

When a clinician receives an imaging report that describes an adrenal cortical adenoma, he or she should obtain a history and perform a physical examination in an attempt to elicit signs or symptoms of hormonal hypersecretion. There is an increasing prevalence of cortisol- and aldosterone-secreting adenomas in patients who do not present with classic signs and symptoms of Cushing and Conn syndromes.

Cushing syndrome. The absence of obesity and hypertension excludes a diagnosis of Cushing syndrome with a high specificity, and thus additional testing is not necessary. However, in the presence of hypertension, obesity, or type 2 diabetes, it is recommended that a dexamethasone suppression test be performed to determine if there is autonomous cortisol production by the adrenal glands. A syndrome of subclinical Cushing syndrome has been described that is much more common than classic Cushing syndrome and may be present in as many as 20% of the patients who have adrenal cortical adenomas detected at imaging. Although such patients do not have overt signs and symptoms of classic Cushing syndrome, they may benefit from adrenalectomy. One investigator considers surgery for younger patients (<50 years) and for those with recent onset of weight gain, obesity, hypertension, diabetes, or osteopenia. Patients need to be treated with perioperative hormone therapy to prevent a postoperative addisonian crisis. A prospective study is yet to be performed to determine whether medical therapy or adrenalectomy is the optimal form of therapy for patients with subclinical Cushing syndrome. CT and MR imaging cannot be used to routinely distinguish between hypersecreting and nonhypersecreting adrenal cortical adenomas. One imaging clue, which is present only in some patients with Cushing syndrome secondary to a cortisol-producing adrenal adenoma, is relative atrophy of the contralateral adrenal gland secondary to feedback inhibition by a hyperfunctioning adrenal adenoma on the pituitary gland. In the absence of this imaging sign, one must again rely on the history and the findings at physical examination.

Conn syndrome. Primary aldosteronism is the most common cause of secondary renal hypertension. Two-thirds of the patients with aldosteronism have a single aldosterone-secreting adrenal cortical adenoma; these patients benefit from adrenalectomy. The remaining third of the patients have forms of adrenal hyperplasia that would not benefit from surgery, and these patients are treated medically. If an MR examination demonstrates a single adrenal adenoma in a patient who is clinically suspected of having Conn syndrome, then adrenalectomy can be performed with the expectation that most patients shall benefit. If a patient with primary aldosteronism has enlarged adrenal glands without a focal mass, then they are likely to have hyperplasia and not a single hypersecreting adenoma. In equivocal instances, renin sampling from the adrenal veins can be performed to detect a unilateral aldosterone-producing adenoma. Previously, it had been advocated that when an adrenal cortical adenoma was detected at imaging, only those hypertensive patients with hypokalemia should be further evaluated for Conn syndrome. However, more than half of the patients with Conn syndrome have normal potassium levels. It is now recommended that all hypertensive patients with an adrenal cortical adenoma should undergo laboratory evaluation of aldosterone and plasma renin activity, to identify a greater number of individuals who may benefit from adrenalectomy or targeted antihypertensive therapy.

Nonhypersecreting Adrenal Cortical Adenoma

Even with the recent insights into subclinical Cushing syndrome and normokalemic Conn syndrome, it is still the nonhypersecreting adrenal cortical adenoma that is the most commonly encountered adrenal mass at cross-sectional imaging. Although some investigators have emphasized the importance of excluding a pheochromocytoma, such an evaluation is unnecessary if MR imaging or CT is suggestive of the presence of lipid within an adrenal mass. Pheochromocytomas originate from the adrenal medulla and typically do not accumulate intracellular lipid or fat. The rare reported exceptions reinforce this rule. Certainly, if the patient has a known primary malignancy or if an MR imaging examination does not indicate the presence of intracellular lipid, then follow-up imaging or tissue sampling should be considered.

If the findings from a chemical shift MR examination establish a diagnosis of a cortical adenoma (Figs. 7.15 and 7.16) and if initial testing does not show signs, symptoms, or laboratory findings of cortical hyperfunction, then conservative observation can be performed. Some investigators recommend "ignoring" the lesion and not obtaining follow-up imaging. In one study in which 75 patients with adrenal "incidentaloma" were followed up, an initial size of more than 3 cm was associated with an increased probability that an adenoma would become hyperfunctioning.

7.2.3.2 Adrenal Cortical Carcinoma

Adrenal cortical carcinoma (Fig. 7.17) is a rare aggressive malignancy with an estimated annual incidence of one in one million. There is a bimodal age distribution of adrenal cortical carcinomas, with an initial peak in the pediatric population and a second peak in the fourth to fifth decades of life. Patients with hyperfunctioning cancers present with signs and symptoms of cortisol or androgen excess. Nonhypersecreting tumors either are discovered incidentally or are found secondary to localized mass effect or symptomatic metastatic disease. Three pathologic features that predict poor prognosis include large tumor size (>12 cm), intratumoral hemorrhage, and high mitotic rates. Patients who have undergone successful resection of a localized tumor have the best long-term prognosis. Individuals who undergo a complete resection have a median survival rate of 74 months, while those who undergo an incomplete primary resection have a median survival of only 12 months. MR imaging can often be used to detect adrenal cortical carcinomas, localize the masses to the adrenal gland, and evaluate for local extension and

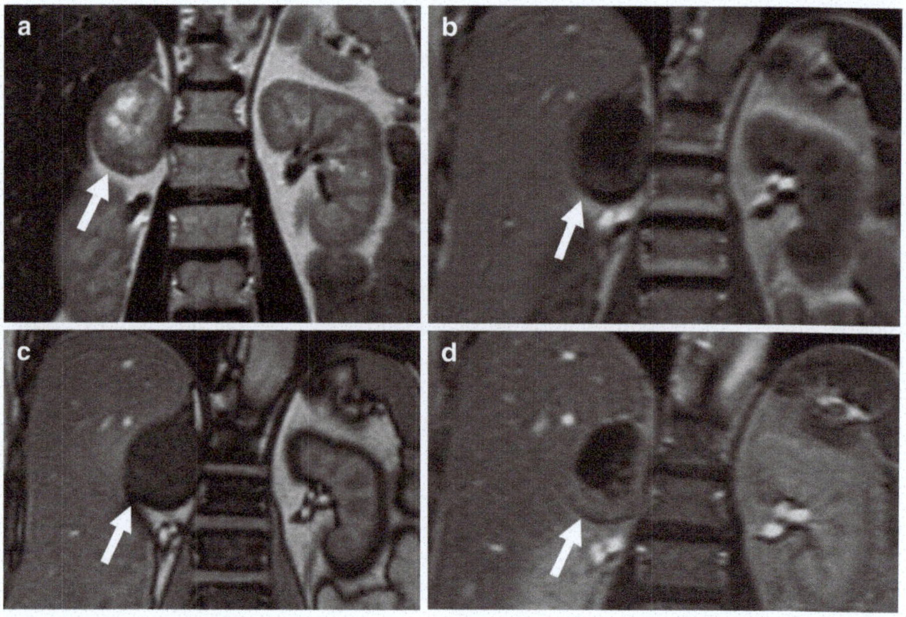

Fig. 7.15 Atypical adrenal adenoma. On coronal T2-W TSE (**a**), coronal T1-W in-phase GRE (**b**), coronal T1-W opposed-phase GRE (**c**), and coronal T1-W contrast-enhanced TSE (**d**), a 5 cm well-defined lesion with central hyperintense (cystic/necrotic) areas (**a**) is delineated in the right adrenal gland in a 52-year-old female patient with history of breast cancer. Chemical shift imaging shows a peripheral signal drop on the opposed-phase image (**c**) compared to the in-phase image (**b**) indicative of an adrenal adenoma

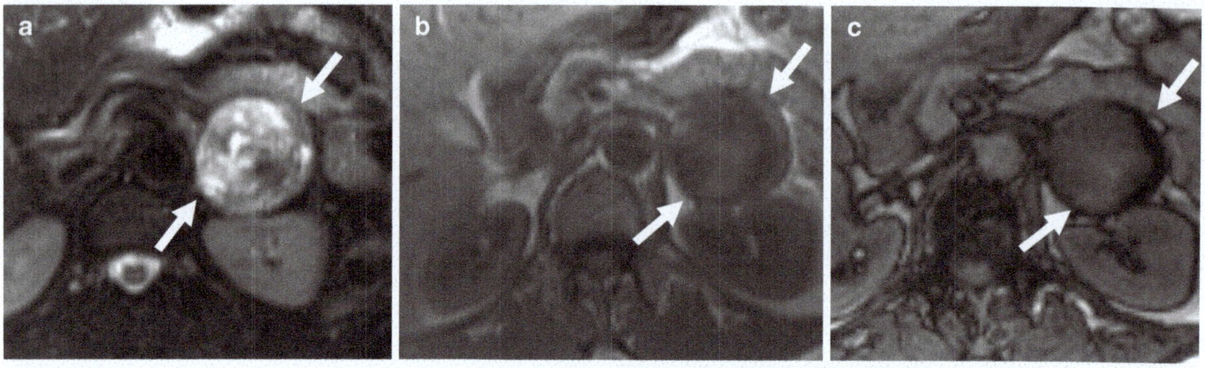

Fig. 7.16 Necrotic adrenal adenoma. On axial T2-W TSE (**a**), axial T1-W in-phase GRE (**b**), and axial T1-W opposed-phase GRE (**c**), a well-defined left adrenal lesion is demarcated in a 53-year-old female patient with history of cervical cancer. The lesions is very inhomogeneous on T2-W image (**a**); however, a significant drop of signal intensity is visible in the periphery of the lesion on the opposed-phase image (**c**) compared to the in-phase image (**b**) indicative of an adrenal adenoma. The central part of the lesion appears cystic/necrotic (**b, c**)

metastatic disease. At MR imaging, adrenal cortical carcinomas appear aggressive and infiltrative. On T1-WI, intratumoral hemorrhage is seen as foci of high SI that persist on fat-saturated T1-WI. Imaging can be used to detect growth of adrenocortical carcinoma into the left renal vein, IVC, or the right atrium. Chemical shift images of adrenal cortical carcinomas have demonstrated that some masses may focally lose SI. This finding reflects the origin of the tumor from the adrenal cortex. This should not create confusion with an adrenal adenoma because these masses are usually large (>5 cm) and heterogeneous and have only small foci of lipid. Unusual examples of degenerated large adrenal cortical adenomas have been described that are indistinguishable from adrenal cortical carcinoma at imaging. Fortunately, these benign adrenal cortical neoplasms with atypical imaging findings are uncommon. Surgical removal is still required, with the determination of benignancy or malignancy to be made by the pathologist.

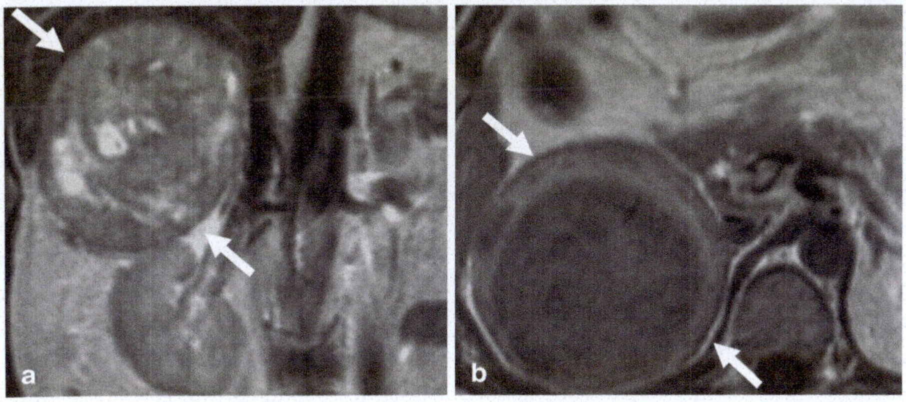

Fig. 7.17 Adrenal cortical carcinoma. Coronal T2-W TSE (**a**) and axial contrast-enhanced T1-W TSE (**b**) show a well-demarcated large right adrenal mass in a 63-year-old female patient without history of malignant disease. The lesion is very inhomogeneous on T2-W image (**a**) without drop of signal intensity on the opposed-phase images compared to the in-phase images (not demonstrated). On contrast-enhanced image (**b**), a predominantly homogenous enhancement of solid peripheral parts and an inhomogeneous central enhancement are visible. Histology showed an adrenal cortical carcinoma

7.2.4 Adrenal Pheochromocytoma

Pheochromocytomas (Fig. 7.18) are catecholamine-producing neoplasms that originate from the sympathetic nervous system. Patients can present with signs or symptoms of excess catecholamines. If a clinician suspects this diagnosis, the initial screening test of choice is measurement of the plasma-free metanephrines. Approximately 85–90% of pheochromocytomas are located within the adrenal medulla. Ten to fifteen percent of pheochromocytomas are located outside the adrenal gland; these tumors, which are termed *paragangliomas*, can occur anywhere from the brain to the bladder (see also MRI of the retroperitoneum). Often it is the radiologist, and not the pathologist, who determines whether the primary tumor is benign or malignant on the basis of the presence or absence of metastatic disease. Pheochromocytoma can occur sporadically or manifest as a part of a hereditary syndrome. Hereditary pheochromocytoma is associated with four syndromes: MEN types 2A and 2B, VHL syndrome, neurofibromatosis, and isolated familial pheochromocytoma. One should think of a hereditary syndrome in patients with bilateral pheochromocytomas because the lesions may be the first finding in VHL syndrome and MEN type 2A. Twenty-five percent (and not the widely quoted 10%) of the patients with sporadic pheochromocytomas are found to have one of four responsible genetic mutations. The treatment of choice for pheochromocytoma is laparoscopic adrenalectomy. Before surgery, patients are treated with α-adrenergic blocking agents to prevent a potential hypertensive

Fig. 7.18 Adrenal pheochromocytoma. On axial T2-W TSE (**a**) and axial contrast-enhanced T1-W TSE (**b**), a well-demarcated predominantly cystic, large, left adrenal mass is delineated in a 39-year-old female patient with attacks of severe hypertension and elevated catecholamines indicating a benign pheochromocytoma which was proved histologically

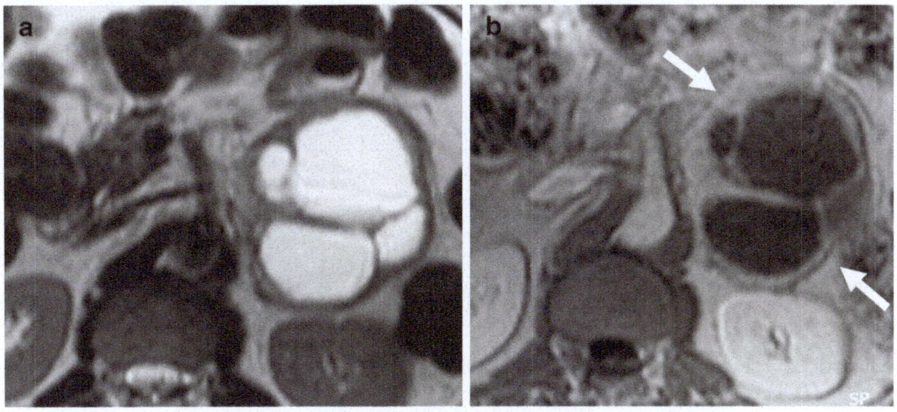

crisis. In a patient with hereditary pheochromocytoma and an identifiable unilateral adrenal mass, prophylactic contralateral adrenalectomy is not recommended because there is a long interval for those individuals who do develop a second pheochromocytoma. The initial MR appearance of pheochromocytoma was described as a "lightbulb" because lesions showed homogeneous high SI on T2-W MR images. However, the MR lightbulb sign is neither sensitive nor specific. With refinements in contemporary MR techniques, pheochromocytoma can show heterogeneous low, intermediate, and high SI on T2-W MR images. Tumor heterogeneity on T2-W MR images is, in part, secondary to intratumoral hemorrhage and cyst formation. Some pheochromocytomas are mostly cystic. Pheochromocytomas neither contain intracellular lipid nor show loss of SI on chemical shift MR images. In a patient with signs or symptoms of a pheochromocytoma, MR imaging is an ideal imaging modality for detection and localization of pheochromocytoma, with detection rates approaching 100%.

7.2.5 Metastases to the Adrenal Glands

The adrenal gland is a common site of metastatic disease (Fig. 7.19). Primary tumors that commonly metastasize to the adrenal gland include lung cancer, breast cancer, renal cell carcinoma, and melanoma. Benign adrenal masses are common not only in the general population but also in patients with cancer. For example, in patients with lung cancer, less than half of the adrenal masses are metastases. It is important to differentiate adrenal metastases from benign adrenal masses because it may determine whether patients can undergo curative resection of their primary tumor. As described previously, metastatic lesions do not lose SI at chemical shift MR imaging. In a patient with other findings of metastatic disease, the characterization of an adrenal mass usually does not alter therapy. However, in patients with bilateral adrenal metastases, signs or symptoms of Addison disease should be identified and treated with hormone replacement. How should one approach a patient with a known primary and no metastatic disease who has an adrenal mass that does not lose SI at chemical shift imaging? Documenting lesion stability by obtaining the results of previous cross-sectional imaging studies is the most cost-effective method. No growth of an adrenal lesion for more than 6 months excludes the diagnosis of an occult metastasis with high negative predictive value. Interval growth of a lesion is highly suggestive of metastatic disease. If prior imaging studies are not available, then one could consider performing contrast-enhanced CT with delayed imaging or PET scanning as described previously. Alternatively, one could consider performing an image-guided needle biopsy or laparoscopic adrenalectomy to prove a diagnosis of metastatic disease and thus guide appropriate therapy.

7.2.6 Adrenal Myelolipoma

Myelolipomas (Fig. 7.20) are uncommon benign encapsulated neoplasms that are composed of variable amounts of mature fat and bone marrow elements. Most myelolipomas originate within the adrenal gland. Uncommon extraadrenal myelolipomas have been reported in the retroperitoneum and liver. Most

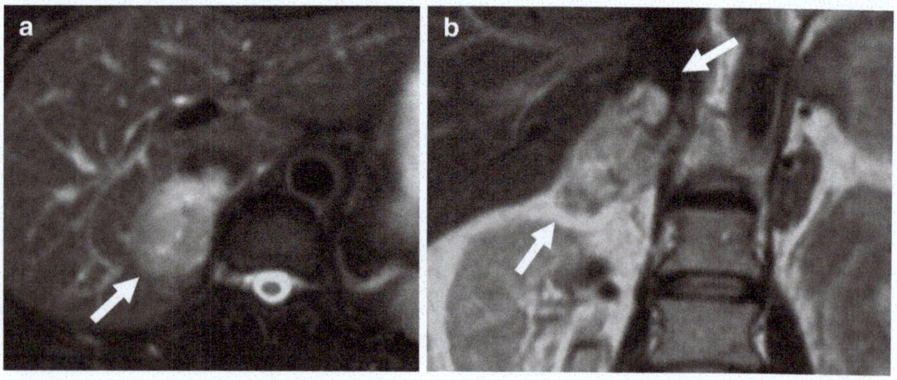

Fig. 7.19 Adrenal metastasis. On axial T2-W TSE with fat saturation (**a**) and coronal T2-W TSE (**b**), a right adrenal lesion is delineated in a 72-year-old male patient with history of left renal cell carcinoma. Infiltration of the vena cava inferior (*arrow* in **b**) is indicating a malignant lesion, most likely adrenal metastasis from renal cell carcinoma

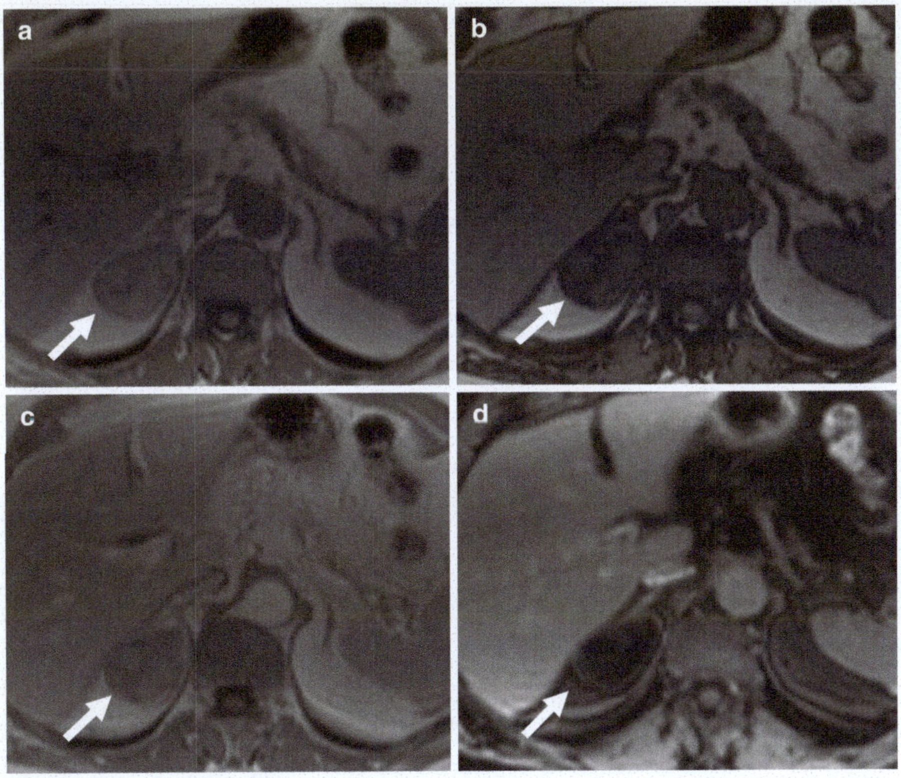

Fig. 7.20 Adrenal myelolipoma. Axial T1-W in-phase GRE (**a**), axial T1-W opposed-phase GRE (**b**), and axial contrast-enhanced T1-W TSE without (**c**) and with fat saturation technique (**d**) show a well-defined right adrenal lesion with areas of signal drop on the opposed-phase image (**b**) compared to the in-phase image (**a**) and a significant loss of signal intensity on the fat-suppressed image (**d**) indicating the presence of a myelolipoma

myelolipomas are asymptomatic and can be followed conservatively if a diagnosis can be established with imaging. Myelolipomas may become symptomatic due to localized mass effect or hemorrhage and are treated with surgical excision. Some investigators advocate elective surgical resection of larger myelolipomas because of the unknown risk of catastrophic hemorrhage. The detection and characterization of macroscopic fat within an adrenal mass establish a diagnosis of myelolipoma with high diagnostic certainty. Macroscopic fat can be demonstrated at MR imaging by the loss of SI with a fat-suppressed pulse sequence when compared with an identical sequence without fat suppression. It is not unusual to demonstrate adipocyte-rich and adipocyte-poor regions within the same myelolipoma. The adipocyte-rich regions show similar SI changes at chemical shift imaging when compared to the "pure fat" within the adjacent retroperitoneum. The adipocyte-poor regions of the neoplasm (where adipocytes and marrow elements are contained within the same voxel) can have identical chemical shift imaging findings of an adrenal adenoma. On T1-W MR images, the unusual complication of peritumoral hemorrhage will appear as high SI that persists with fat saturation secondary to the T1-shortening effects of methemoglobin.

7.2.7 Adrenal Hematoma

Adrenal hemorrhage (Fig. 7.21) and/or hematoma can result from either traumatic or nontraumatic causes. Traumatic causes include severe abdominal trauma, right-sided hepatic surgery, and child abuse. Nontraumatic causes include coagulation disorders, stress, and hemorrhage into an underlying adrenal neoplasm. When hematomas are bilateral, one should evaluate for signs and symptoms of adrenal failure (Addison disease), which is often not obvious clinically and can result in unnecessary morbidity and mortality. The specific MR imaging finding of subacute hematoma is the high-signal intensity rim sign, indicating the presence of methemoglobin within the periphery of the hematoma. In the absence of a known primary tumor, it is unusual to detect an adrenal hematoma as the initial finding of occult metastatic disease. In questionable cases, follow-up imaging should show a decrease in size of a benign hematoma.

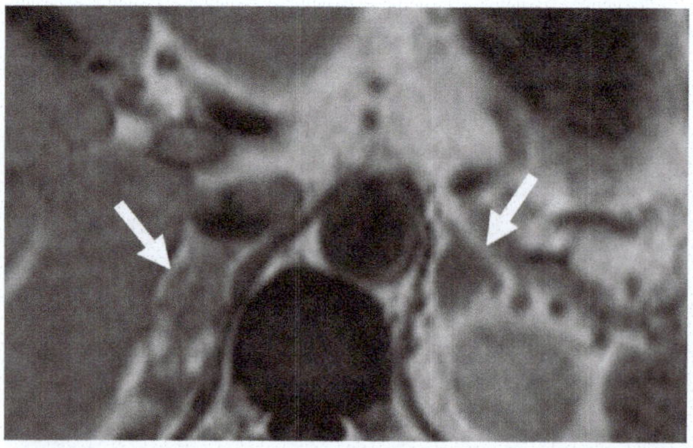

Fig. 7.21 Bilateral adrenal hemorrhage. On axial T1-W TSE image, ill-defined hyperintense bilateral adrenal lesions are demarcated in a patient with known coagulopathy indicating hemorrhage

7.2.8 Adrenal Cysts

Adrenal cysts are rare and have been categorized as endothelial, epithelial, parasitic, and pseudocysts. Most of these cysts are asymptomatic and can be managed with observation or aspiration. Symptomatic adrenal cysts or cysts larger than 5 cm can be removed laparoscopically. Adrenal pseudocysts are the result of prior hemorrhage (Fig. 7.22) into either a normal adrenal gland or a gland that contained a benign neoplasm. Adrenal cyst characterization with MR imaging is similar to cyst characterization in other organs. At MR imaging, one would expect high SI on T2-W and heavily T2-WIs. There should be no enhancement in the lesion after contrast administration at MR imaging.

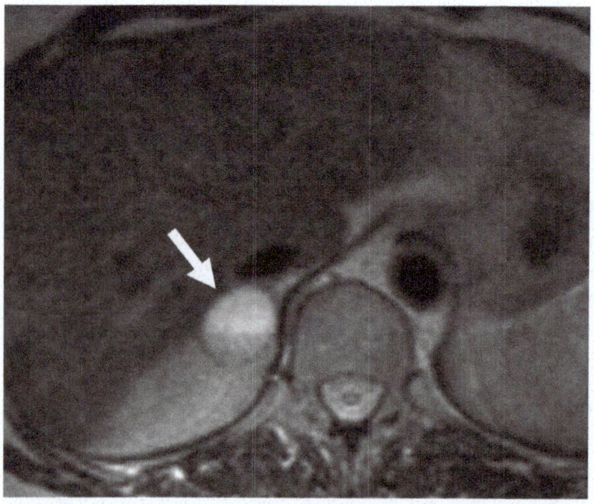

Fig. 7.22 Adrenal hemorrhagic cyst. Axial T2-W TSE image shows a small, round, right adrenal lesion with a fluid-fluid level. Signal intensity of the fluid components is suggestive of hemorrhagic cyst

7.2.9 Adrenal Granulomatous Disease

In very rare cases adrenal glands may be affected in granulomatous disease like tuberculosis (Fig. 7.23) or histoplasmosis.

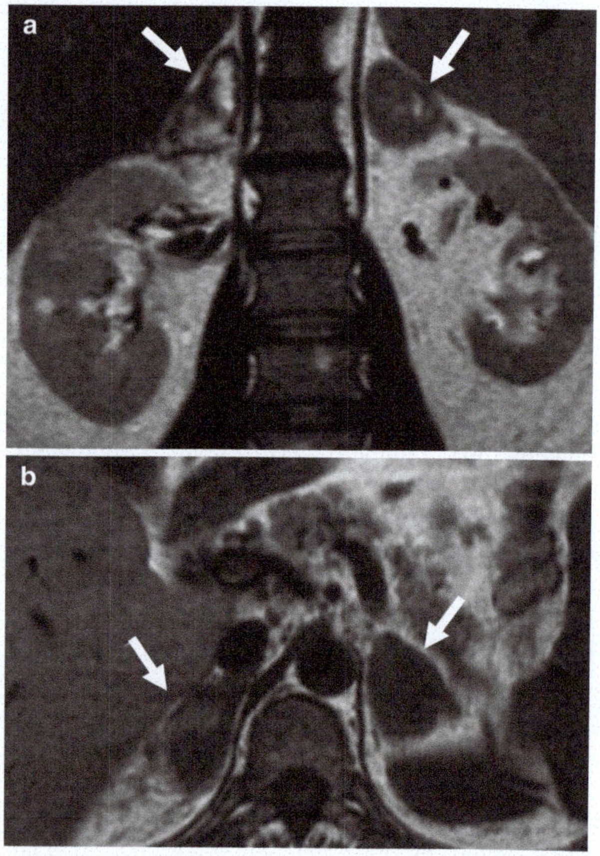

Fig. 7.23 Adrenal tuberculosis. On coronal T2-W TSE image (**a**) and axial T1-W TSE image (**b**) bilateral, not sharply demarcated adrenal lesions are delineated in a 28-year-old male patient with recent history of bicycle trauma. Hyperintense areas on both T2-W (**a**) and T1-W images (**b**) may indicate bilateral hematoma (hemorrhage). On follow-up examinations, no regression of the lesions was observed. Histology from core needle biopsy showed granulomatous disease, most likely tuberculosis. The lesions resolved with antimycobacterial therapy

7.3 Kidneys and Upper Urinary Tract

7.3.1 Introduction

The kidneys are the most important organs for maintaining homeostasis in the human body. Consequently, the diagnosis of renal diseases must cover not only possible morphological changes in the organs, but also, and in particular, any functional disturbances. The use of a contrast material permits the assessment of different states of perfusion and, consequently, a better delineation or differentiation of pathological processes. On the other hand, the visualization of the passage of a renally eliminated contrast agent also provides information about the excretory function of the kidneys. Conventional radiological procedures with iodinated, renal contrast agents allow only a qualitative functional evaluation. Conclusions are possible only with regard to mechanical obstruction and reduced perfusion, whereas the functional state may be evaluated only indirectly. Contrast-enhanced MRI of the kidneys therefore differs fundamentally from these imaging techniques, as CE-MRI permits simultaneous assessment of macroscopic changes and evaluation of functional derangements.

MRI examination of the kidneys is rendered difficult by artifacts due to respiratory motion and the nearby abdominal vessels. On the other hand, most of the pathological lesions of the kidneys display the same SI as the surrounding unaffected structures, leading to a decreased soft tissue contrast in plain examinations.

In order to provide morphological information that may compete with the results of CT and ultrasound (US), special techniques such as artifact compensation and fast imaging have to be employed. The additional use of renally eliminated paramagnetic contrast agents (Gd-based contrast agents) makes it possible to assess different states of perfusion and to visualize the passage of the contrast medium, providing information about hyper- or hypoperfusion of lesions and about the excretory function of the kidneys. Fat suppression techniques, fast spin-echo sequences, ultrafast imaging, chemical shift imaging techniques, diffusion-weighted (DW) imaging, blood oxygen level dependent (BOLD) imaging, and the use of specific contrast agents (e.g., ultrasmall paramagnetic particles of iron oxides) have further expanded the list of potential applications of MRI in the kidneys.

7.3.2 Anatomy

MR imaging can demonstrate detailed anatomy of the kidneys, urinary tract, and surrounding structures. T1-WI demonstrates distinct corticomedullary contrast of the kidney by higher intensity of the renal cortex and lower intensity of the medulla. On T2-WI, the signal intensities of both renal cortex and medulla are increased and they cannot be differentiated. The SI of sinus fat is high on both T1-WI and T2-WI. The SI of urine-containing renal pelvis is low on T1-WI and high on T2-WI. The signal intensities of the renal vessels are low on both T1-WI and T2-WI except for the high SI of slow venous flow on T2-WI.

7.3.3 Imaging Techniques

7.3.3.1 Plain MRI of the Kidneys

MRI, as well as other noninvasive modalities such as ultrasound and CT, can provide morphological information on kidneys. The size of the kidneys can be an indicator of the underlying disease. Small kidneys are generally the result of renal artery or glomerular disease, irregular-shaped kidneys are seen in interstitial kidney disease, and enlarged kidneys are due either to obstruction, diabetes mellitus, infection, amyloidosis, or renal vein thrombosis. The characterization of masses and cysts, such as polycystic kidney disease, is usually easy. Several renal diseases may cause spontaneous abnormal SI on MR images, the appearance of which being sufficiently characteristic to allow a specific radiologic diagnosis. Low signal MR images are seen in three main categories: hemolysis (paroxysmal nocturnal hemoglobinuria, cortical hemosiderin deposition from mechanical hemolysis, and sickle cell disease), infection (hemorrhagic fever with renal syndrome), and vascular disease (renal arterial infarction, acute renal vein thrombosis, renal cortical necrosis, transplanted kidney rejection, and acute nonmyoglobinuric renal failure). Frequently used MR-imaging protocols of kidneys are listed in Table 7.3.

Conventional contrast-enhanced MR imaging protocols of the kidneys may have limitations. A recent study showed that the loss of corticomedullary differentiation was independent of serum creatinine level on patients with acute renal failure. Therefore, there is need for other, more specific MR techniques.

Table 7.3 Commonly used sequences for renal imaging

T1w	Typically 2D or 3D GRE sequences in axial and/or coronal plane. Breathold recommended. Fat saturation may be used
T2w	TSE/FSE sequences in axial and/or coronal plane. Fat saturation improves image contrast
DWI/ADC	Provides information on diffusion and perfusion simultaneously. Hydration increases ADC values, RAS and obstruction decrease ADC values. May be helpful in differentiating solid from cystic tumor or solid from necrotic tumor
T2*	GRE sequence provides information about hemoglobin breakdown products and calcifications. Prerequisite for BOLD MRI. Sensitivity to susceptibility effects is proportional to TE and field strength. Mandatory for RES specific contrast agents (SPIO/USPIO)
Post i.v. admin. of GBCA	
T1w	GRE/TFE sequences in axial and/or coronal imaging planes. Same imaging plane should be used before and after gadolinium-chelate injection. MR angiographic techniques (usually breathold 3D GRE with fat saturation most suited) have important role in evaluation of RAS (renal artery stenosis)

7.3.3.2 Diffusion-Weighted MRI

The diagnosis of various renal diseases such as chronic renal failure, renal artery stenosis (RAS), and ureteral obstruction can benefit from measuring the diffusion characteristics of the kidneys. DW MR imaging of the kidneys is able to provide information on renal function and can be suggestive of the presence and degree of obstruction or inflammation (Fig. 7.32). The apparent diffusion coefficient (ADC), a quantitative parameter calculated from DW MR images, combines the effects of capillary perfusion and water diffusion in the extracellular extravascular space. Thus, DW MR imaging provides information on perfusion and diffusion simultaneously. Hydration is an important factor to increase global ADC values, whereas RAS or ureteral obstruction decreases those values. In case of acute or chronic renal failure, the cortical and medullary ADC values are significantly decreased when compared with normal kidneys and the cortical value seems to be well correlated with serum creatinine levels. In a rat study, the intravenous administration of the high-viscosity iodinated contrast agent iodixanol was found to significantly decrease the ADC, this effect occurring earlier in the cortex and lasting less than in the medulla.

7.3.3.3 BOLD (Blood Oxygen Level Dependent) MRI

This MR-technique is increasingly used to noninvasively evaluate intrarenal oxygenation levels.

The human kidneys, together weighing less than 1% of the total body mass, receive 25% of the cardiac output. Most of the blood passing through the kidneys is directed to the cortical regions to facilitate glomerular filtration. On the other hand the medulla operates in a hypoxic environment.

For renal BOLD MRI, the parameter R2* is commonly used to quantitatively assess oxygenation changes. R2* (= 1/T2*), the apparent spin-spin relaxation rate, is directly related to the tissue content of deoxyhemoglobin and can be estimated from the SI measurements made at several different TEs. The intensity vs. TE data is fit to a single exponential decay function to determine the rate constant R2*.

Decreases in R2* values imply an increase in the oxygenation of hemoglobin and thus, improved blood oxygenation. Assuming blood oxygenation to be in a dynamic equilibrium with the surrounding tissue oxygenation, estimated changes using BOLD MRI can be interpreted as changes in tissue pO_2.

Promising results have been reported recently using 3.0 T MR units and a newly implemented three-dimensional (3-D) version of the multiple gradient-recalled echo (mGRE) sequence for BOLD MRI of the kidney.

7.3.3.4 Conventional Gd-Enhanced MRI of the Kidneys

7.3.3.5 Patterns of Contrast Enhancement in Normally Functioning Kidneys

The paramagnetic GBCA is completely filtered in the glomerulus. The distinct concentration-dependent change in the tissue relaxation times brought about by GBCA allows an insight into the excretory kinetics.

According to the arterial perfusion, an increase in the SI in the renal cortex can be observed just 10–20 s after injection. A maximum value is reached about 20–50 s after the first signs of perfusion, followed by a slow, constant fall in the SI. This finding is due to the pronounced arterial perfusion of the renal cortex that leads to an early appearance of GBCA in this region. The T1-shortening effects of gadolinium chelates produce a visible increase in the SI; the onset of glomerular filtration and the dilution in the extravascular space manifest themselves as a subsequent slow decrease in the SI.

SI changes are different in the medulla: an increase can be observed about 10–20 s later than in the cortex. The maximum SI reaches the same, or slightly higher, values as in the cortex. 30–40 s after the first visible signs of perfusion, the SI decreases steeply to a minimum value which is comparable to the initial value of the precontrast image. Only when the contrast agent passes into the calyces and is diluted with noncontrasted glomerular filtrate does the SI increase again to values approximately equal to those in the cortex. Excretion into the calyces may usually be demonstrated at this point: it is characterized by a SI decrease in the region of the renal pelvis which is also followed by susceptibility artifacts.

These changes in the SI must be interpreted with reference to the effects of GBCA on the relaxation times of tissues. Since medulla accounts for only about 1–6.5% of the entire blood supply to the kidneys, it is understandable that contrast perfusion of the medullary structures is delayed in comparison with the cortex. The onset of glomerular filtration of the contrast agent and the reabsorption of water in the proximal convoluted tubule, in the loop of Henle, and, particularly, in the collecting duct results in a marked concentration of the GBCA (50–100-fold concentration). Depending on the sequence used, however, contrast reversal occurs because of the now predominant T2-shortening effects of gadolinium chelates. SI drop in the medullary pyramids is therefore an effect of the high concentration of the paramagnetic contrast agent.

The described alterations of SI in renal cortex, medulla, and calyces are characteristic of undisturbed renal function and can be evaluated using signal vs. time plots. On the other hand, an excellent delineation of the corticomedullary junction is possible in the early perfusion phase (10–20 s after injection) and in the early excretory phase (50–90 s after injection) allowing accurate detection of the internal structural derangements of the kidney.

7.3.3.6 Functional Assessment of the Kidneys by MRI

MRI is able to noninvasively provide a functional assessment of the kidney, such as glomerular filtration rate (GFR), tubular concentration and transit, blood volume and perfusion, diffusion, and oxygenation. These approaches can be achieved using endogenous contrast agents such as water protons or desoxyhemoglobin or require exogenous contrast agents such as gadolinium ($Gd3^{+}$) chelates or superparamagnetic iron oxide nanoparticles. Actually, $Gd3^{+}$ chelates are good markers of the renal function in that they are freely filtered by the glomerulus and are neither secreted nor reabsorbed by the nephron. In a pig model of RAS, MRI associated with the intravenous administration of a $Gd3^{+}$ chelate allowed the measurement of GFR as well as that of the extraction fraction.

Renal perfusion is one of the most common useful methods to detect renal impairment. It can be evaluated with contrast agents, based on tracer kinetic methods such as scintigraphy. By injecting a GBCA and following the change in image intensity over time, it is possible to obtain qualitative or semiquantitative information on the renal microcirculatory blood flow on a regional basis. Fast acquisition techniques such as T1-W gradient echo or echo plan sequences allow sufficient temporal resolution to monitor intrarenal signal changes during the first pass of the agent through the kidneys. $Gd3^{+}$ chelates diffuse into the interstitial space (about 10% during the first pass) and are freely filtered by the glomeruli (20% through the first pass). However, the quantitative assessment of renal perfusion is impaired by the rapid diffusion of the contrast agent in the extracellular space and thus, only iron oxide particles or blood pool $Gd3^{+}$ chelates can be considered as blood pool contrast agents and thus reliably applied to the measurement of renal perfusion. Recently, P792, a macromolecular $Gd3^{+}$-based blood pool agent, has been shown to improve renal functional MRI assessment in rats by inducing less T2* effect without compromising T1 enhancement.

Gadolinium-based dendrimers proved to be valuable for evaluation of proximal tubule dysfunction, since these Gd compounds accumulate in the proximal tubules after early glomerular filtration.

Ultrasmall superparamagnetic particles of iron oxide which have a specific uptake by macrophages may be used for the diagnosis of inflammatory and degenerative disorders associated with high macrophage phagocytic activity. At low concentrations they act as positive contrast agents (such as gadolinium), but at higher concentrations they result in a negative enhancement.

7.3.4 MR Appearance of Renal Disease

7.3.4.1 Renovascular Disease

Renovascular disease is a complex entity, encompassing atherosclerotic arterial lesions, renal disease, and hypertension leading to high renal and cardiovascular risk. The relationships among RASRAS, hypertension, and renal function vary from patient to patient and are difficult to assess. For evaluation of RAS (Fig. 7.24), in a recent meta-analysis (3-D), magnetic resonance angiography (MRA) performed significantly better than the other diagnostic tests and seemed to be preferred in patients referred for evaluation of renovascular hypertension.

MRA has now moved from flow-enhanced (time-of-flight or phase-contrast) sequences to T1-W contrast-enhanced acquisitions. Its performance is excellent, with a sensitivity and specificity for diagnosis of significant stenosis between 88 and 100% and between 71 and 99%, respectively. Other pathologies of renal arteries like aneurysms (Fig. 7.25), fibromuscular dysplasia, and most accessory arteries are also shown by this technique.

The clinical value of diffusion-weighted MRI and BOLD imaging in evaluation of RAS is still under debate.

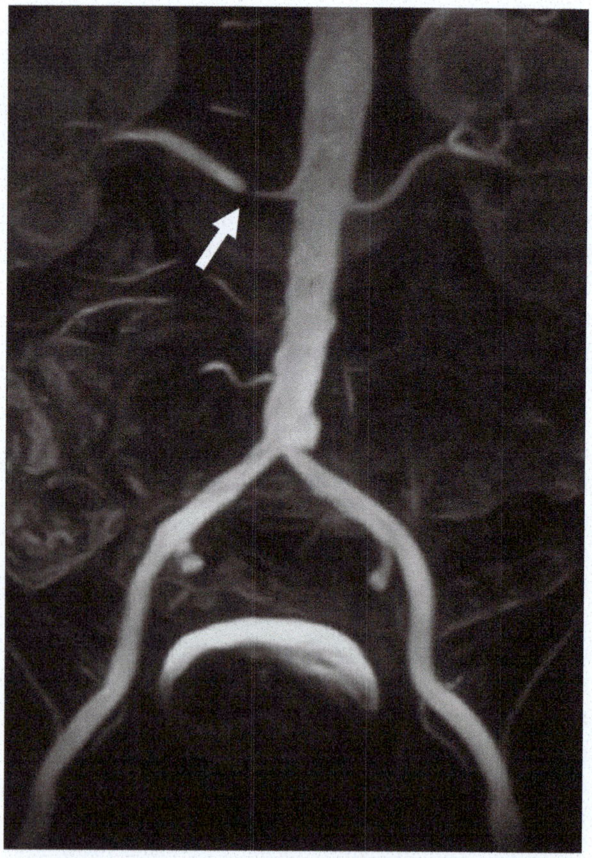

Fig. 7.24 Renal artery stenosis. On coronal contrast-enhanced T1-W GRE image, a high-grade stenosis of the proximal right renal artery is depicted

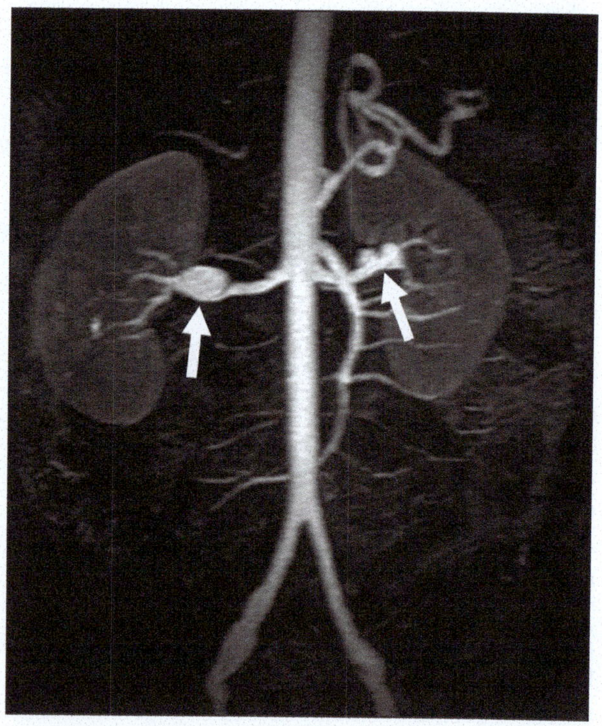

Fig. 7.25 Renal artery aneurysms. Coronal contrast-enhanced T1-W GRE image shows bilateral small to moderate aneurysms of both renal main arteries (*arrows*) in a patient with Ehlers-Danlos syndrome

7.3.4.2 Renal Masses

On plain MR images, solid as well as cystic renal and pararenal masses often present the same signal intensities as the adjacent renal tissue. Detection of such tumors is therefore based only on the visible displacement or alteration of organ contours. Delineation from the surrounding renal parenchyma is successful with the aid of contrast-enhanced examinations. Hyperperfused masses are easily distinguishable on early dynamic scans, while hypo- or nonperfused lesions may be detected better on late postcontrast images. State-of-the-art MRI with optimal technical skills allows delineation of even very small lesions, with a diameter of approximately 1 cm. Additional techniques like fat suppression provide a further improvement of lesion detection, allowing demonstration of small cysts or hypoperfused solid masses with diameters less than 1 cm.

7.3.4.3 Differentiation of Renal Tumors

Plain and, especially, contrast-enhanced MRI can help to differentiate renal and pararenal lesions. A nonenhancing mass with low signal intensities on the T1-WI and marked signal increase on T2-W scans represents a simple cyst in the majority of cases (Fig. 7.26). For this classification, however, MRI is needed only if the patient has a contraindication for

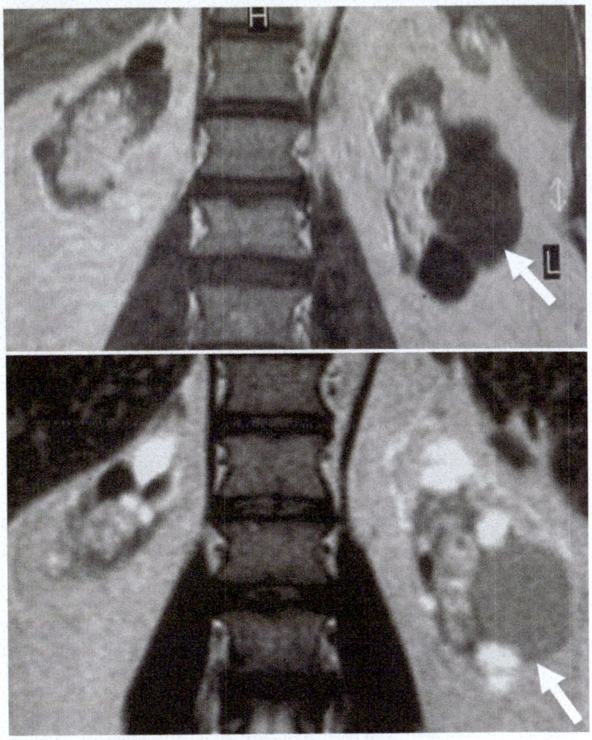

Fig. 7.27 Renal cysts. Coronal T1-W and coronal T2-W TSE images show multiple small cysts in a renal insufficient patient with acquired cystic renal disease indicating increased risk for development of renal cell carcinoma. A medium-sized lesion on the left shrunken kidney (*arrow*) shows higher signal intensity on T1-W and lower signal intensity on T2-W images compared to simple renal cysts as can typically be seen in high density cysts (Bosniak II)

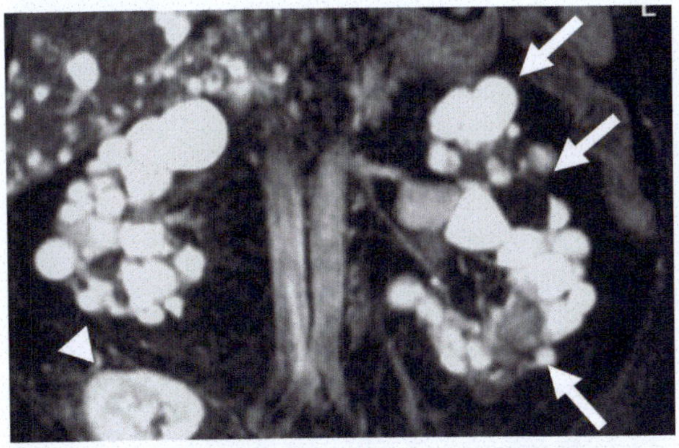

Fig. 7.26 Renal cysts. On coronal T2-W TSE image with fat saturation technique, multiple renal cysts are depicted in a patient with adult polycystic kidney disease. Note different signal intensities of various cysts in both kidneys indicating high density cysts and hemorrhagic cysts containing hemosiderin (Bosniak II). A renal transplant is delineated in the right fossa iliaca (*arrowhead*)

the use of iodinated contrast agents. Other cystic lesions may display similar signal intensities and, although MRI is highly sensitive in demonstrating hemorrhage (Figs. 7.26 and 7.27), one cannot differentiate between hemorrhagic cysts and cystic tumors with hemorrhage in rare cases.

Among solid tumors of the kidney, MRI allows accurate detection and characterization of fat-containing angiomyolipoma (Figs. 7.28 and 7.29). Other solid lesions such as oncocytoma, adenoma, or renal cell carcinoma (Fig. 7.30) show very similar signal intensities and enhancement patterns. However, chemical shift gradient echo MR imaging (CSI) can detect a small amount of fat as signal loss on opposed-phase images as compared to in-phase images. Cytoplasmatic fat in clear cell renal carcinoma (RCC) or interstitial histiocytic fat in papillary cell RCC can be successfully

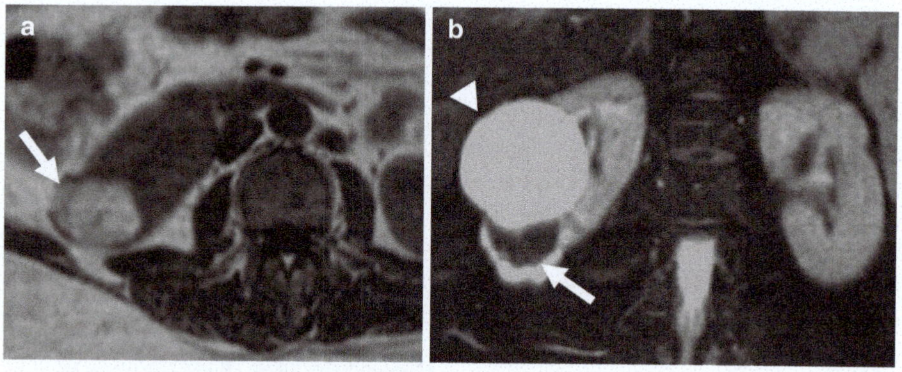

Fig. 7.28 Renal angiomyolipoma (AML) and renal cyst. On axial T1-W GRE and coronal T2-W TSE images a fatty lesion and a simple cyst (*arrowhead*) can be observed in the right kidney. The noncystic lesion (*arrows*) shows high signal intensity on T1-W image and presents with a significant drop of signal intensity on T2-W image with fat saturation technique indicating an AML

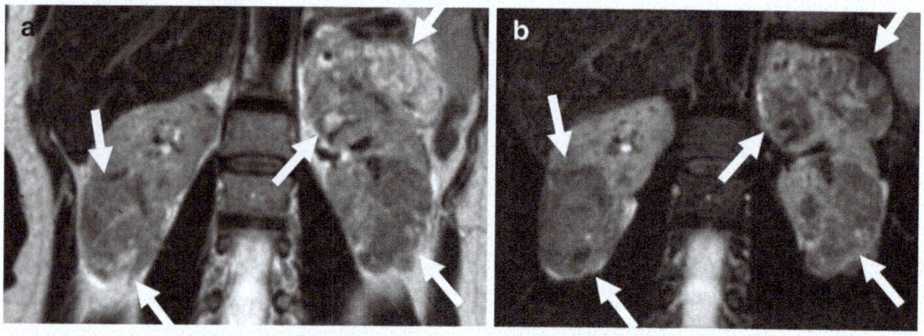

Fig. 7.29 Multiple renal AML in a patient with tuberous sclerosis. Coronal T2-W TSE (**a**) and coronal T2-W TSE with fat saturation technique (**b**) show multiple lesions in both kidneys of a patient with known tuberous sclerosis. Significant loss of signal intensity of the lesions (*arrows*) is delineated on the fat-saturated image (**b**) as typical finding in angiomyolipomas

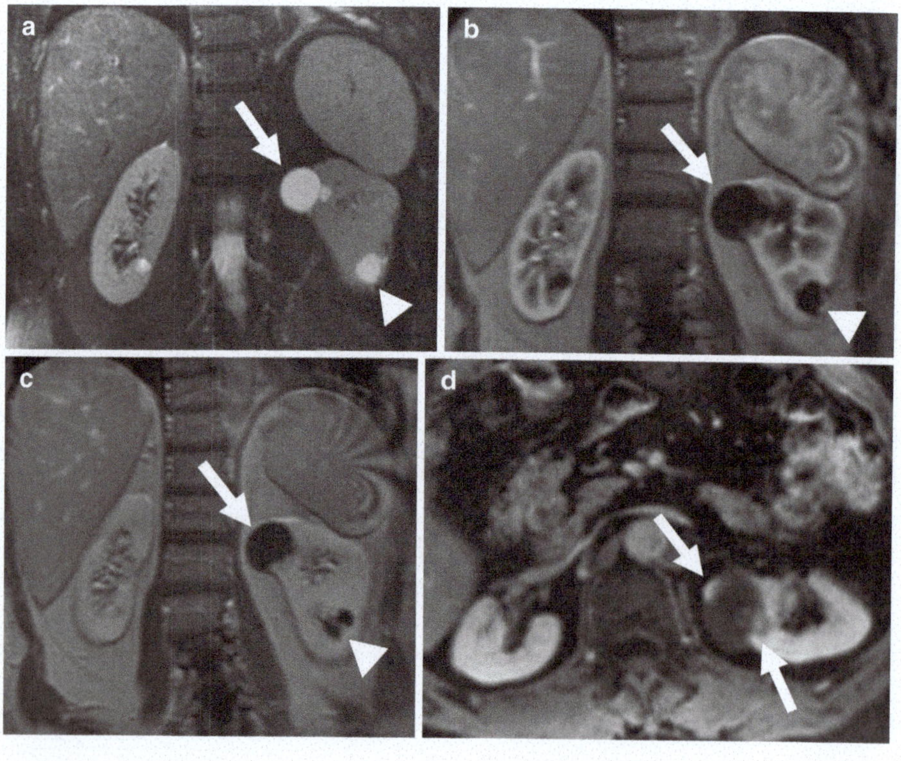

Fig. 7.30 Renal cell carcinoma. On coronal T2-W TSE image with fat saturation (**a**) and coronal dynamic contrast-enhanced T1-W GRE images (**b**, **c**), a small lobulated cystic lesion is depicted on the upper pole of the left kidney as well as a small simple cystic lesion on the lower pole of the left kidney in a 71-year-old male patient with previous history of colon and lung cancer. Dynamic contrast-enhanced images performed in the corticomedullary and nephrographic phase (**b**, **d**) show peripheral nodular enhancement in the upper pole lesion indicating a Bosniak type IV lesion. On histology, a renal cell carcinoma of Bellini duct type was confirmed. The lower pole lesion proved to be a simple cyst

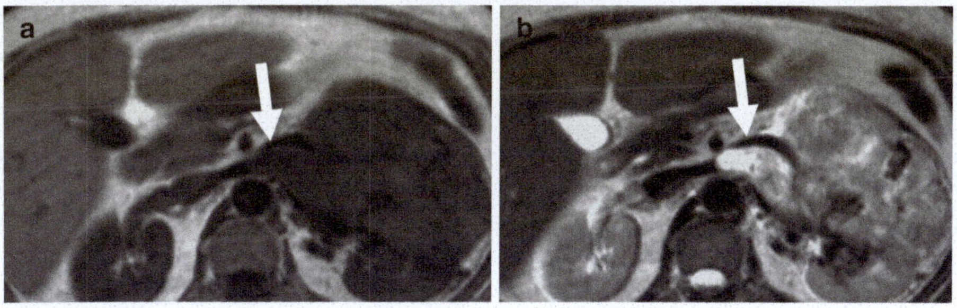

Fig. 7.31 Renal cell carcinoma. On axial T1-W TSE (**a**) and axial T2-W TSE (**b**), a huge mass is demarcated in the left kidney of a patient with allergy to both iodine and gadolinium-based contrast agents. On both unenhanced images, infiltration of the left renal vein is nicely depicted, indicating a renal cell carcinoma stage T3b, which was confirmed on the histological specimen after nephrectomy

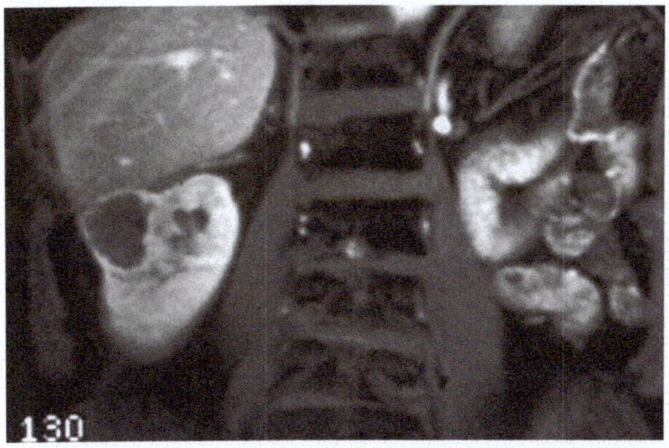

Fig. 7.32 Renal abscess. Coronal contrast-enhanced T1-W image shows a cystic right upper pole lesion with a thick rim enhancement in a female patient with urinary tract infection, right flank pain, and fever indicative for a renal abscess

demonstrated by this technique. T2*-W gradient echo or echo-planar MR imaging can detect local susceptibility, for example, due to cytoplasmic or interstitial histiocytic hemosiderin deposition in papillary cell RCC. Dynamic MRI following administration of Gd-DTPA, however, allows optimal delineation of the normally functioning renal parenchyma and good visualization of the corticomedullary junction. Delayed enhanced series allow us to differentiate between tumors arising from renal parenchyma and transitional cell cancer (Fig. 7.33). Using such sequences, renal and extrarenal masses can be differentiated accurately. Additional imaging planes may help to differentiate retroperitoneal masses which are only displacing and compressing the renal parenchyma.

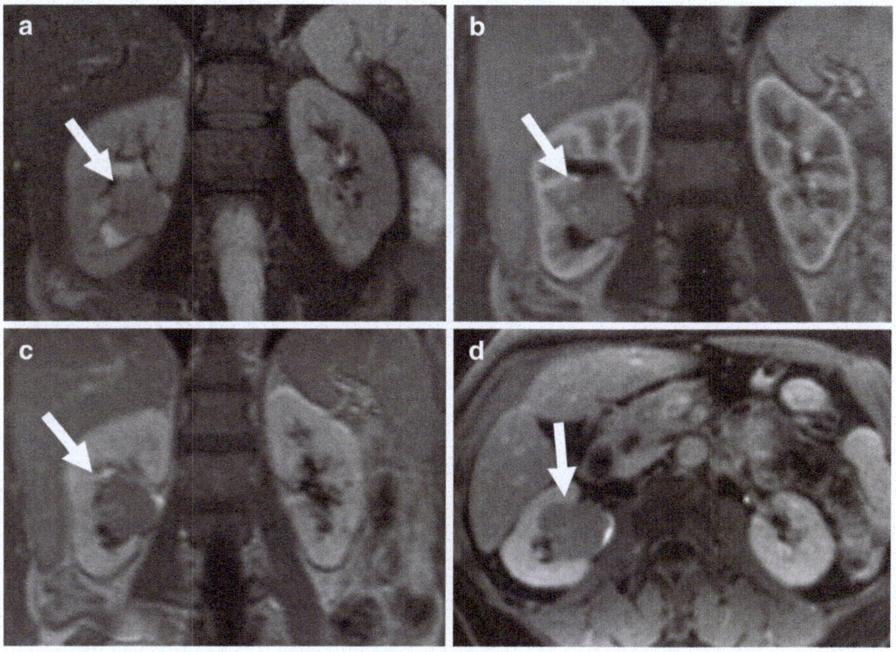

Fig. 7.33 Renal transitional carcinoma. On coronal T2-W TSE image with fat saturation (**a**) and coronal dynamic contrast-enhanced T1- W GRE images (**b**, **c**), a centrally located mass is depicted in the right kidney in a 68-year-old male patient with gross hematuria. Dynamic contrast-enhanced images performed in the corticomedullary, nephrographic, and urographic phase (**b–d**) show mild to moderate contrast uptake of the lesion and no washout in the nephrographic phase (**c**). Additionally, the mass is located in the renal pelvis as shown by the urographic phase (**d**), allowing to characterize the lesion as a transitional cell carcinoma

7.3.4.4 Staging of Renal Cell Carcinoma

The most important issues that are raised during preoperative staging of renal cell carcinoma are the evaluation of the intra- and extrarenal extent of tumor, involvement of perirenal fat, of renal veins and IVC, and of regional lymph nodes. Most of these problems can be already solved using CT, but MRI seems to be the method of choice in patients with renal impairment and patients with known allergic reaction to iodinated contrast agents.

Dynamic MRI studies are also useful for delineation of the intrarenal extent of primary renal malignancies. Although this does not help in terms of correct staging of the tumor, it may allow planning of a partial resection, if indicated. A differentiation between stage T2 and T3A is very important, since tumors that are not confined to the kidney lead to a more than 50% decrease in 5-year survival. Invasion of perinephric fat may be visualized clearly with gradient echo MRI using adequate TEs. When fat and water protons are out-of-phase, a signal loss marks the presence of tumor cells in perirenal fat. Similar alterations can however, be observed simply due to lymphatic or venous edema around the kidneys. In such cases, detection of perirenal invasion can be improved using fat-suppressed contrast-enhanced images. Enhancement of previously dark areas in perirenal tissue is indicative of extrarenal tumor invasion.

MRI allows evaluation of tumor thrombi in the renal veins or the IVC (Fig. 7.31). MRI is a noninvasive method that provides the same information as conventional venography. Gradient echo images even allow delineation of thrombi in nondilated veins due to a lack of high SI of flowing blood. Using gradient echo images, retroperitoneal lymphadenopathy may be detected as accurately as with CT or US. However, as with CT and US, the only criterion for diagnosis of malignant involvement remains the measurement of lymph node size. However, MR-lymphography with superparamagnetic particles of iron oxide may further increase the sensitivity of MRI in detection of lymphadenopathy.

7.3.4.5 Renal Functional Disorders

Due to the almost complete (>98%) elimination of GBCA by glomerular ultrafiltration, a correlation between enhancement patterns in the renal parenchyma and GFR can be expected. Dynamic examinations can be quantitatively evaluated by plotting the SI values in the renal cortex and medulla as a function of time. Time intervals between the first signs of cortical perfusion and maximal or minimal SI in the medullary pyramids can be calculated in this way.

In the majority of cases with acute obstruction of the urinary tract, no SI alterations are demonstrable at MRI. The SI plots display a pattern similar to that in patients without functional impairment. The preserved SI decrease in the renal medulla proves the preserved ability of the kidney to concentrate the contrast agent. Delayed excretion can be observed in the case of already affected renal function. In these patients, a normal perfusion of the renal cortex is followed by a delayed increase in the SI in the medulla. Maximal SI is reached here only after 40–70 s; the SI drop is less pronounced and the minimal value is seen after 60–100 s.

In chronic obstructed, nonfunctioning kidneys, SI alterations are even more evident. A normal enhancement in the renal cortex is followed by a delayed SI increase in the medulla that forms a plateau without demonstrable concentration of the contrast agent in the collecting ducts. Thus there is no SI decrease in the medulla and no time intervals can be measured on the SI plots.

In patients with bilateral functional damages, the bilaterally delayed concentration of GBCA in the collecting ducts or complete loss of the ability to concentrate the contrast agent in the renal medulla correlates well with the creatinine clearance. However, the temporal resolution of 10 s/ slice allows only an approximate splitting of the results. Using dynamic MRI, patients with a creatinine clearance between 50 and 80 mL/min display a 10–20 s delay in the SI drop in the medulla compared to patients with a normal excretory function. A delay of more than 20 s can be expected in patients with creatinine clearance values of about 30–50 mL/min, whereas time intervals are not measurable because of a complete loss of the GBCA concentration in patients with clearance values under 30 mL/min.

7.4 MR-Urography

7.4.1 Indications

MR-urography has become an established imaging tool for depicting the urinary tract, both in adults and in children. Its potential to assess anatomy and function make it ideally suited for evaluation of urinary tract malformations or anomalies, renal cysts or tumors, infections, and renal transplants. MR-urography does not utilize ionizing radiation and therefore is favored in patient populations such as pregnant women, children, and patients who need repeated examinations of the urinary tract. In addition, because the number of acquisitions is not limited by factors other than the examination time, repeated acquisitions can be used to generate time intensity curves as a means of assessing renal function or characterizing abnormalities after intravenous contrast material administration.

7.4.2 Techniques

7.4.2.1 Static-Fluid MR-Urography

Early practitioners of MR-urography used T2-W technique alone, such as rapid acquisition with relaxation enhancement (thick-slab, RARE) and half-Fourier acquisition single shot turbo spin echo, or respiratory-triggered 3-D echo-train spin-echo sequences to image the renal collecting systems, ureters, and bladder, essentially treating the urinary tract as a static collection of fluid. These are essentially the same techniques used routinely for MR-cholangiopancreatography. T2-W MR techniques rely on the intrinsically high SI of urine for image contrast, and therefore do not require the administration of intravenous contrast material. Static-fluid MR-urography sequences are typically used in the coronal plane, although other imaging planes can be used. In addition, multiple, sequential static-fluid acquisitions can be obtained to ensure visualization of the entire ureters and assess for a fixed narrowing or obstruction (Figs. 7.34 and 7.35). Oral hydration is discouraged, as the high T2 SI of fluid within the bowel can interfere with the visualization of the urinary tract during static-fluid MR-urography, particularly when maximum intensity projections are rendered.

The main appeal of these techniques is that they can be performed quickly and in any plane. Furthermore, because T2-W MR-urography can be performed without ionizing radiation or intravenous contrast material, they have their greatest utility in children, pregnant women, or other patients in whom intravenous contrast material is contraindicated. However, the clinical utility of MR-urography performed with T2-W imaging alone is limited in patients with nondistended urinary collecting systems. For

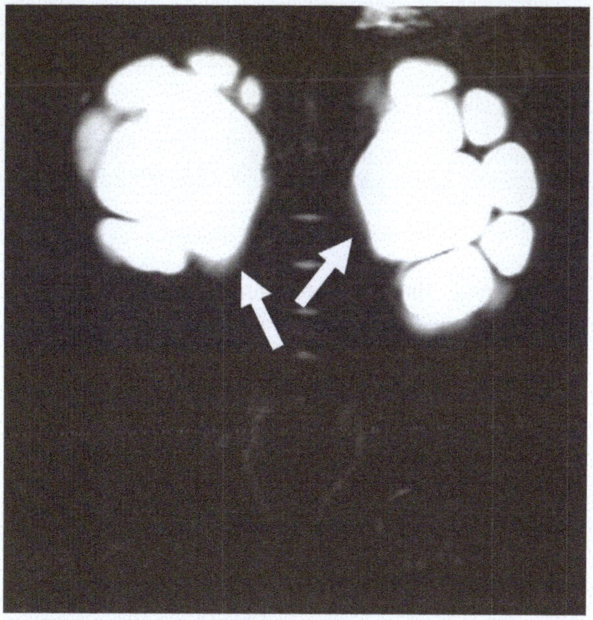

Fig. 7.34 Static-fluid MR-urography–bilateral congenital UPJ stenosis. Heavily coronal T2-W static-fluid MR-urography shows bilateral high-grade stenosis of the ureteropelvic junction with consecutive bilateral hydronephrosis grade IV in a newborn child

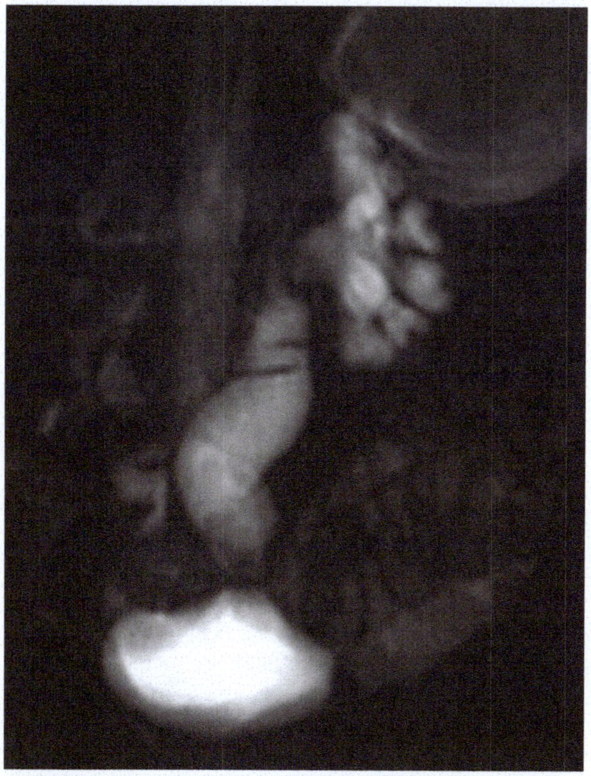

Fig. 7.35 Static-fluid MR-urography–congenital megaureter. On heavily coronal T2-W static-fluid MR-urography, a congenital megaureter is nicely depicted in this infant

Table 7.4 Imaging sequences used for MR-urography

T2w	TSE/FSE/HASTE usually applied in coronal plane
Post i.v. admin. of GBCA	
T1w	3D GRE/TFE sequences with fat saturation most suited. Usually applied in coronal plane. Breathhold recommended

urinary tracts that are not distended, imaging with a full urinary bladder can improve upper tract visualization, but additional techniques are often needed.

The introduction of nonpharmacologic interventions, such as intravenous hydration and ureteral compression, and of pharmacologic interventions, such as intravenous diuretics and gadolinium chelates administration, expanded the utility of MR-urography techniques to include the assessment of nondistended collecting systems. By combining sequences designed to evaluate the collecting systems, ureters, and bladder with sequences designed to evaluate the kidneys (especially for renal masses), a comprehensive assessment of the urinary tract became possible. However, the more complex techniques require a higher level of patient cooperation and radiologist supervision. A combined MR-urography imaging protocol is outlined in Table 7.4.

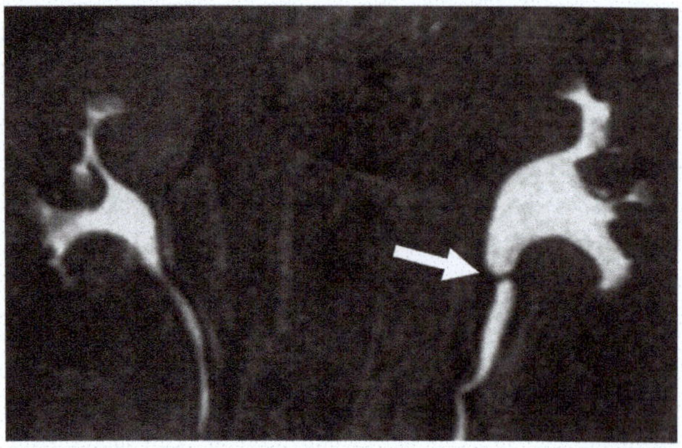

Fig. 7.36 Contrast-enhanced MR-urography - mild left UPJ stenosis. On contrast-enhanced MR-urography using a coronal T1-W GRE image, a signal void is delineated at the left UPJ indicating a crossing vessel, which causes mild obstruction in a 45-year-old male patient

7.4.2.2 Excretory MR-Urography

When intravenous gadolinium-based contrast material is administered to patients for excretory urography, some form of dynamic, multiphase T1-W sequence is typically performed of the kidneys. When information about vascular structures is critical, such as evaluation of congenital ureteropelvic junction obstruction in which a crossing vessel is suspected (Fig. 7.36), an additional MRA sequence is performed in the coronal plane. Alternatively, a dynamic axial, fat-suppressed sequence can be performed through the kidneys to capture the precontrast, corticomedullary, nephrographic, and excretory phases. Excretory phase images are then typically obtained approximately 5 min after intravenous gadolinium chelate is administered at a dose of 0.05–0.1 mmol/kg and are usually accomplished with some type of fat-suppressed 3-D gradient echo sequence. As with static-fluid MR-urography, any imaging plane can be chosen. Most authors prefer the coronal or axial plane and supplement with additional planes as needed. Having patients raise their arms over their heads during coronal acquisitions reduces wrap around artifact.

Excretory MR-urography performed after intravenous gadolinium chelate administration without pharmacologic intervention is often lacking due to suboptimal ureteral distention, uneven distribution of the contrast material in the collecting systems, and the hypointense T2* effect of concentrated gadolinium. Therefore, some combination of intravenous hydration and diuretic administration is typically used adjunctively. Furosemide is the diuretic usually used for excretory MR-urography and can be used successfully in adults at doses as low as 5 mg. In most centers, excretory MR-urography is performed in adults after 250 mL of intravenous normal saline and 5 mg of intravenous furosemide are administered.

For excretory MR-urography, the thinnest partitions that maintain acceptable signal-to-noise ratio (SNR) and anatomic coverage could be prescribed. Breath-holding is essential for excretory phase imaging, as acquisition times of 20–30 s are typical with most widely available 3-D gradient echo sequences. A through-plane resolution of 2–3 mm is usually achievable with currently available MR systems operating at 1.5–3.0 T. The use of parallel imaging techniques reduces acquisition times with a modest penalty in

SNR. For patients with limited breath-holding capacity, the urinary tract can be imaged in segments.

MR-urography is best performed with a phased-array surface coil; these coils increase SNR. Exceptions include some gravis patients in the latter stages of pregnancy and large patients whom the imager bore cannot accommodate with a surface coil in place. Depending on the MR imaging system, some surface coils limit the field of view to less than that required to encompass the kidneys and the bladder in a single acquisition. In such cases, the urinary tract is imaged in segments, repositioning the surface coil as necessary.

Further increases in SNR can be achieved by imaging patients with higher field strength, 3.0 T MR systems. The SNR gained when moving from 1.5 to 3.0 T can be used to improve spatial or temporal resolution. Improvements in spatial resolution could improve detection of small urothelial lesions; however, this has not been systematically studied to date. Additionally, there is evidence to suggest that the conspicuity of enhancement related to gadolinium chelates increases at 3.0 T relative to 1.5 T, although the impact of this difference is unknown for MR-urography. The potential benefits of 3.0 T MR imaging must be weighed against the limitations inherent to higher field strength imaging, such as increased specific absorption, prolonged T1 relaxation times, and worsening of some artifacts.

For many applications, MR-urography is accomplished by combining T2-W techniques (static-fluid MRU) with excretory images obtained after intravenous administration of gadolinium-based contrast agents (excretory MRU). When MR-urography is combined with assessment of the renal parenchyma and soft tissues of the abdomen and pelvis, precontrast axial T1- and T2-WI of the abdomen and pelvis (Fig. 7.37) are obtained. For T1-W imaging, most authors prefer a dual-echo gradient echo sequence with in- and opposed-phase TEs. The addition of fat-suppression techniques to T2-W sequences improves visualization of perinephric fluid due to obstruction and also helps to better delineate lymph nodes.

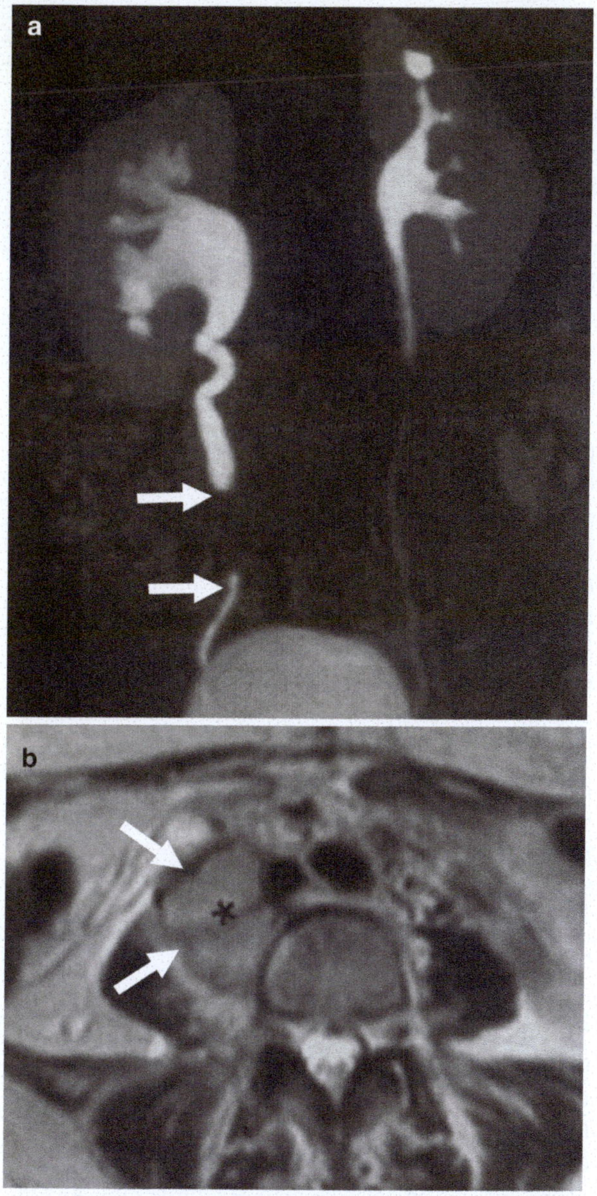

Fig. 7.37 Contrast-enhanced MR-urography–extrinsic ureteral stenosis. Contrast-enhanced MR-urography using a coronal T1-W GRE image shows a short distance stenosis of the distal part of the right ureter (*arrows*) with consecutive moderate hydroureteronephrosis grade II (**a**). On axial T2 W TSE image, multiple nodular retroperitoneal masses are demarcated (*arrows and asterix*), causing extrinsic stenosis of the right distal ureter (**b**). Histology revealed lymphnode metastases from gonadal cancer

7.4.3 Urinary Tract Disorders

7.4.3.1 Stone Disease

Because MR is relatively insensitive for the detection of calcification, the diagnosis of ureteral calculi often relies on detecting secondary signs of obstruction such as ureteral dilatation and perinephric fluid. Sometimes a persisting filling defect can be identified. Nonetheless, sensitivities in excess of 90% have been reported for the diagnosis of ureteral calculi with MR-urography techniques. The sensitivity of MR-urography is technique dependent, with higher sensitivities reported for excretory MR-urography than for static-fluid T2-W techniques. MR-urography is more sensitive for diagnosing the cause of urinary obstruction due to causes other than urolithiasis compared with unenhanced CT.

7.4.3.2 Pediatric Uropathies

MR-urography is the imaging modality of choice to depict a wide range of congenital urogenital tract abnormalities in pediatrics, including an abnormally positioned, rotated, duplicated, dysplastic, or absent kidney, as well as ectopic ureter, retrocaval ureter, primary megaureter, and ureteropelvic junction obstruction.

MR-urography additionally allows assessment of ectopically positioned or draining systems as well as associated pathology such as genital anomalies. Furthermore MR-urography may be used to evaluate urogenital tract infection, renal cysts, renal parenchymal pathology or tumors. MR-urography offers a "one stop shop" strategy for comprehensive assessment of all relevant aspects including assessment of non or poorly functioning moieties in the pediatrics obviating the need for intravenous urography and scintigraphy in most cases.

7.4.3.3 Urothelial Neoplasms

MR-urography yields a high sensitivity for diagnosing the cause of urinary obstruction due to causes other than urolithiasis; however, currently, no study comparing CT-urography and MR-urography for detection of urothelial neoplasms is available. Although urothelial neoplasms can be detected with MR-urography, its sensitivity remains to be determined. Presumably the sensitivities for detecting small urothelial carcinoma are lower for MR-urography compared to CT-urography largely due to the inferior spatial resolution relative to CT.

However, dynamic contrast-enhanced MR imaging yields higher accuracy than other imaging techniques in detection and staging of urothelial tumors of the urinary bladder (also see MR imaging of the urinary bladder).

7.4.3.4 Differentiation of Physiologic Dilatation and Obstructive Uropathy

In pregnant patients, MR-urography allows to differentiate between physiologic dilatation and obstructive uropathy caused by a calculus without administration of intravenous contrast agents. Because most static-fluid MR-urography techniques are quick and relatively easy to perform, the examination is well tolerated, even in the advanced stages of pregnancy.

Further Reading

Retroperitoneum

Bechtold RE, Dyer RB, Zagoria RJ et al (1996) The perirenal space: relationship of pathologic processes to normal retroperitoneal anatomy. Radiographics 16:841–854

Bellin MF, Lebleu L, Meric JB (2003) Evaluation of retroperitoneal and pelvic lymph node metastases with MRI and MR lymphangiography. Abdom Imaging 28:155–163

Bessell-Browne R, O'Malley ME (2007) CT of pheochromocytoma and paraganglioma: risk of adverse events with i.v. administration of nonionic contrast material. AJR Am J Roentgenol 188:970–974

Burrill J, Williams CJ, Bain G et al (2007) Tuberculosis: a radiologic review. Radiographics 27:1255–1273

Cormier JN, Pollock RE (2004) Soft tissue sarcomas. CA Cancer J Clin 54:94–109

Engin G, Acunas B, Acunas G et al (2000) Imaging of extrapulmonary tuberculosis. Radiographics 20:471–488; quiz 529–430, 532

Harisinghani MG, McLoud TC, Shepard JA et al (2000) Tuberculosis from head to toe. Radiographics 20:449–470; quiz 528–449, 532

Harisinghani MG, Saksena MA, Hahn PF et al (2006) Ferumoxtran-10-enhanced MR lymphangiography: does contrast-enhanced imaging alone suffice for accurate lymph node characterization? AJR Am J Roentgenol 186:144–148

Hrehorovich PA, Franke HR, Maximin S et al (2003) Malignant peripheral nerve sheath tumor. Radiographics 23:790–794

Kransdorf MJ, Bancroft LW, Peterson JJ et al (2002) Imaging of fatty tumors: distinction of lipoma and well-differentiated liposarcoma. Radiology 224:99–104

Lee JC, Thomas JM, Phillips S et al (2006) Aggressive fibromatosis: MRI features with pathologic correlation. AJR Am J Roentgenol 186:247–254

Lonergan GJ, Schwab CM, Suarez ES et al (2002)Neuroblastoma, ganglioneuroblastoma, and ganglioneuroma: radiologic-pathologic correlation. Radiographics 22:911–934

Nishimura H, Zhang Y, Ohkuma K et al (2001) MR imaging of soft-tissue masses of the extraperitoneal spaces. Radiographics 21:1141–1154

Pallisa E, Sanz P, Roman A et al (2002) Lymphangioleiomyomatosis: pulmonary and abdominal findings with pathologic correlation. Radiographics 22: S185–S198

Rha SE, Byun JY, Jung SE et al (2003) Neurogenic tumors in the abdomen: tumor types and imaging characteristics. Radiographics 23:29–43

Saksena MA, Saokar A, Harisinghani MG (2006) Lymphotropic nanoparticle enhanced MR imaging (LNMRI) technique for lymph node imaging. Eur J Radiol 58:367–374

Sherer DM, Abulafia O, Eliakim R (2001) Pseudomyxoma peritonei: a review of current literature. Gynecol Obstet Invest 51:73–80

Song T, Shen J, Liang BL et al (2007) Retroperitoneal liposarcoma: MR characteristics and pathological correlative analysis. Abdom Imaging 32(5):668–674

Teh HS, Lin MB, Tan AS et al (2000) Retroperitoneal Castleman's disease in the perinephric space-imaging appearance: a case report and a review of the literature. Ann Acad Med Singapore 29:773–776

Ueno T, Tanaka YO, Nagata M et al (2004) Spectrum of germ cell tumors: from head to toe. Radiographics 24:387–404

Vaglio A, Salvarani C, Buzio C (2006) Retroperitoneal fibrosis. Lancet 367:241–251

Vandevenne JE, De Schepper AM, De Beuckeleer L et al (1997) New concepts in understanding evolution of desmoid tumors: MR imaging of 30 lesions. Eur Radiol 7:1013–1019

Adrenals, Kidneys, and Upper Urinary Tract

Charagundla SR, Siegelman ES (2006)) Adrenal glands. In: Edelman RR, Hesselink JR, Zlatkin MB, Crues JV III (eds) Clinical magnetic resonance imaging, 3rd edn. Philadelphia, Saunders/Elsevier, 2863–2888

Choyke PL, Frank JA, Girton ME, Inscoe SW, Carvlin MJ, Black JL, Austin HL, Dwyer AJ (1989) Dynamic gadolinium-DTPA-enhanced MRI of the kidneys: a physiologic correlation. Radiology 170:713

Eilenberg SS, Lee JKT, Brown JJ, Mirowitz SA, Tartar VM (1990) Renal masses: evaluation with gradient-echo Gd-DTPA-enhanced dynamic MR imaging. Radiology 176:333

Fujiyoshi F, Nakajo M, Fukukura Y, Tsuchimochi S (2003) Characterization of adrenal tumors by chemical shift fast low-angle shot MR imaging: comparison of four methods of quantitative evaluation. AJR Am J Roentgenol 180: 1649–1657

Grenier N, Basseau F, Ries M, Tyndal B, Jones R, Moonen C (2003) Functional MRI of the kidney. Abdom Imaging 28: 164–175

Grenier N, Pedersen M, Hauger O (2006) Contrast agents for functional and cellular MRI of the kidney. Eur J Radiol 60:341–352

Haider MA, Ghai S, Jhaveri K, Lockwood G (2004) Chemical shift MR imaging of hyperattenuating (>10 HU) adrenal masses: does it still have a role? Radiology 231(3): 711–716.

Israel GM, Korobkin M, Wang C, Hecht EN, Krinsky GA (2004) Comparison of unenhanced CT and chemical shift MRI in evaluating lipid-rich adrenal adenomas. AJR Am J Roentgenol 183:215–219.

Kawashima A, Sandler CM, Ernst RD et al (1999) Imaging of nontraumatic hemorrhage of the adrenal gland. Radiographics 19(4):949–963.

Leyendecker JR, Childs DD (2007) Kidneys and MR urography. Magn Reson Imaging Clin N Am 15:373–382

Mayo-Smith WW, Boland GW, Noto RB, Lee MJ (2001) State-of-the art adrenal imaging. Radiographics 21(4): 995–1012

Merkle EM, Dale BM (2006) Abdominal MRI at 3.0 T: the basics revisited. AJR Am J Roentgenol 186:1524–1532

Mitchell DG, Crovello M, Matteucci T, Petersen RO, Miettinen MM (1992) Benign adrenocortical masses: diagnosis with chemical shift MR imaging. Radiology 185(2):345–351

Namimoto T, Yamashita Y, Mitsuzaki K, et al (2001) Adrenal masses: quantification of fat content with double-echo chemical shift in-phase and opposed-phase FLASH MR images for differentiation of adrenal adenomas. Radiology 218(3):642–646

Rescinito G, Zandrino F, Cittadini G Jr, Santacroce E, Giasotto V, Neumaier CE (2006) Characterization of adrenal adenomas and metastases: correlation between unenhanced computed tomography and chemical shift magnetic resonance imaging. Acta Radiol 47:71–76

Silverman S, Leyendecker JR, Amis ES (2009) What is the current role of CT urography and MR urography in the evaluation of the urinary tract? Radiology 250:309–323

MRI of the Pelvis

8

Dow-Mu Koh and David MacVicar

Contents

D. MacVicar (✉)
Department of Diagnostic Radiology, The Royal Marsden Hospital, Downs Road, Sutton, Surrey, SM2 5PT, UK
e-mail: david.macvicar@rmh.nhs.uk

8.1 Introduction

Magnetic resonance imaging (MRI) is now a widely validated technique for the evaluation of pelvic diseases in both men and women. Compared with other techniques such as ultrasound and computed tomography (CT), MRI offers superior image contrast between soft tissues, thus enabling better tissue and disease characterization in the pelvis.

The MRI hardware has continued to improve over the last decade with the introduction of surface and parallel imaging coil arrays. As a result, it is now possible to acquire detailed high spatial resolution images of pelvic structures such as the bladder, prostate, uterus, cervix, ovaries, and rectum on most commercial 1.5 T MR systems, which enhances image interpretation and radiological assessment. More recently, clinical pelvic imaging at higher field strength of 3.0 T has become viable on many MRI platforms, offering further improvements in image signal-to-noise, scanning spatial resolution, and the potential to reduce image acquisition times.

The most common clinical pathway to pelvic MRI examination is when an unsuspected or uncertain abnormality is detected at clinical examination, ultrasound or CT in patients presenting with pelvic symptoms. MRI has been shown to be useful for the detection and characterization of both benign and malignant pelvic diseases. However, MRI is also increasingly used for the primary evaluation of clinical symptoms, such as menorrhagia in females, to exclude sinister gynecological malignancies. In patients with pathological proven malignancies in the bladder, prostate, rectum, cervix, uterus, and rectum, MRI has an established role in staging of the primary tumor and in delineating the disease extent, thus providing critical information for

P. Reimer et al. (eds.), *Clinical MR Imaging*,
DOI: 10.1007/978-3-540-74504-4_8, © Springer-Verlag Berlin Heidelberg 2010

treatment planning. MRI is also employed to monitor the effects of treatment in the patient with cancer and to detect disease recurrence following primary treatment. Of course, MRI referrals for hip symptoms or traumatic injury to the pelvis from orthopedic practice are also common, but these are beyond the scope of this chapter.

In the following sections, we will review the techniques and instrumentation required to obtain high quality diagnostic images in the pelvis. The rationales for the imaging sequences to evaluate the pelvis are discussed. The relevant pelvic anatomy for image interpretation is emphasized. This is followed by discussions of the MR findings of pelvic diseases common to both males and females, and of those that are unique to each sex. Last but not least, emerging new MR techniques for pelvic imaging will be highlighted.

8.2 Techniques and Instrumentation

The patient is usually requested to empty the bladder 2–3 h prior to MRI examination of the pelvis, and then to drink normally afterwards. Assessment of the bladder is facilitated by bladder distension. However, overfilling of the bladder has to be avoided as this may become distressing over the course of the MR examination. In assessing gynecological conditions, emptying of the bladder prior to scanning is sometimes preferred. If there are no contraindications, intramuscular or intravenous injection of an antiperistaltic agent should be considered as this decreases motion artifacts and improves image quality. In our practice, 20 mg of intramuscular or intravenous hyoscine butylbromide (Buscopan, Boerhinger, Ingelheim) is routinely given for MR examination of the uterus, cervix, ovaries, bladder, or rectum. Hyoscine butylbromide is a smooth muscle relaxant, and once injected parenterally, it results in reduced peristalsis and smooth muscle contraction lasting about 30 min. Reflex hyperperistalsis may ensue as the effects of the drug wear off, and a repeat dose may be administered if the examination is prolonged. The drug should not be used if there is a history of glaucoma or acute urinary retention. An alternative smooth muscle relaxant that may be administered is glucagon. A dose of 1 mg, administered intramuscularly or intravenously, can inhibit peristalsis for up to about 1 h. However, glucagon appears to be less effective on the colon and is considerably more costly compared with hyoscine butylbromide.

Depending on the clinical indication, gastrointestinal luminal contrast agents may be prescribed. Both positive and negative T1 and T2-weighted contrast agents are available for use. In our practice, rectal enema (using water, barium, superparamagnetic iron oxide particles contrast) is usually not necessary for imaging of the rectum or the rest of the pelvic viscera. However, if inflammatory bowel disease is suspected, assessment of the small bowel loops in the pelvis may be enhanced by the administration of oral contrast. Nevertheless, the choice of luminal contrast is influenced by local clinical practice and experience.

MRI of the pelvis is usually performed with the patient in the supine position, with the feet toward the magnet. As short and wide bore magnets are progressively introduced into newer MR systems, the scan experience for the patient has become much less claustrophobic, compared with the older and narrower long bore MR systems. Nowadays, the head of the patient usually lies just outside the bore of the magnet, when the pelvis is optimally positioned in the centre of scanner, making the test a less stressful experience. Consequently, sedation is rarely required for pelvic imaging.

Increasingly, the use of external pelvic phased-array coils is standard, which allows parallel imaging to be utilized during image acquisition. The use of parallel imaging is advantageous, as it reduces k-space filling time and results in more rapid image acquisition. The use of these surface coils also maximizes the signal-to-noise ratio (SNR) and allows scanning to be performed at a high spatial resolution. Thus, high quality images of the pelvis using a combination of imaging sequences can be achieved in 30–40 min, improving scanner throughput and patient acceptability.

In the pursuit of even better imaging detail, some radiologists choose to use endocavitary coils. In imaging the prostate, using an endorectal coil places the receiver array just behind the prostate gland in the rectum, thus further improving SNR, and optimizes high resolution imaging of the prostate. Such detailed images can be helpful for assessing extracapsular spread in patients with prostate cancer. Endorectal coils also improve the quality of the magnetic resonance spectroscopy (MRS) data, a technique that is increasingly available on newer MR systems, which is used to detect prostate cancer based on metabolic alterations in the gland. It is also possible to combine the use of surface phased-array coils with endorectal coil simultaneously on some MR systems to maximize image quality.

Likewise, using an endovaginal coil in females can be advantageous for visualizing cervical pathologies such as early cervical cancer, and for assessing the presence of parametrial invasion. Some radiologists also apply endocavitary coils to study anorectal conditions, such as anorectal fistula, injury to the anal sphincter complex, and anorectal cancers. Again, the proximity of the receiver coil to the region of interest improves visualization of the anal sphincter complex and associated pathologies. The degree of tumor involvement of the rectal wall is also well delineated using this technique. However, the disadvantages of endocavitary probes include a limited field of view (FoV) and the inability to assess the pelvic sidewall; the technique may also not be suitable in patients with bulky or stenotic tumors of the anorectal region. In patients with rectal cancer, the presence of an endorectal probe also distort local anatomy and, combined with the limited FoV, may not allow accurate assessment of the relationship of tumor to the mesorectal fascia, which is critical to local tumor assessment and treatment planning.

The key advantages of applying MRI in the pelvis are its multiplanar capabilities, absence of ionizing radiation, and excellent soft tissue contrast. Even though multiplanar reformats are now possible using datasets from multichannel CT, MR still offers superior intrinsic soft tissue contrast. Using a combination of T1-weighted (T1-W), T2-weighted (T2-W), and sometimes fat-suppressed images may be sufficient for tissue characterization and disease assessment. High spatial resolution T2-W imaging is the key to pelvic MR assessment as normal anatomical details of pelvic viscera such as the uterus, cervix, ovaries, prostate, urinary bladder, rectum, and anus are clearly depicted. As such, many pelvic conditions can be accurately assessed without the administration of intravenous contrast medium. Although intravenous contrast medium usage is almost routine for CT assessment, the use of intravenous gadolinium-based contrast medium is more judicious for pelvic MRI. The specific indications for their use will be discussed later in the chapter.

8.3 Imaging Sequences

Each imaging department will derive its own MR study protocols for pelvic imaging. These, no doubt, will have evolved through everyday use and clinical experience but are also likely to be influenced by the MR scanner capabilities and the demands of service delivery. As such, it is difficult to be prescriptive about an exact imaging protocol as a reference standard to be widely adopted. Nevertheless, there are some guiding principles that help to ensure that high quality images of the pelvis are consistently attained, and that the combination of imaging sequences acquired is sufficient for clinical diagnosis.

Gradient-echo (GE) and turbo spin-echo (TSE) sequences are most frequently used in the pelvis. These sequences result in images of good SNR, and crucially, are relatively quick to perform. The most commonly applied MRI sequences for pelvic imaging and the rationale for their use are discussed below. These may be viewed as the "building blocks" to a complete pelvic MR examination. Some details relevant to optimization and interpretation of these sequences are discussed.

- *T2-W sagittal imaging*. A turbo spin-echo T2-W sequence is used, employing a large FoV (typically 380–420 mm), to include the lower lumbar spine above, down to at least the symphysis pubis below. Thin partitions of 3–5 mm are acquired from one to the other pelvic sidewall. An echo-time of about 120–130 ms results in good T2-W contrast. It is helpful to use the same echo-time for all T2-W scans in the imaging protocol to facilitate comparison. Sagittal scans are helpful to evaluate midline structures such as the bladder (particularly the bladder dome), uterus, rectum, and sacrum. The normal zonal anatomy of the uterus is best demonstrated on these images.
- *Large FoV T1 and T2-W axial imaging*. Axial imaging is performed from the level of iliac crest down to below the symphysis pubis. T1-W images are acquired using a GE sequence, whereas T2-W scans are acquired using TSE technique. Partition thickness of 5–8 mm is typical. These scans are useful to survey the entire pelvis and to detect suspicious areas that would benefit from more targeted high spatial resolution imaging. Although T2-W scans are sensitive

to pathological processes, T1-W imaging may be more helpful for the following:

1. The detection and evaluation of lymph nodes in the pelvic sidewall compartment. This is because lymph nodes can return very high signal intensity on T2-W imaging, making them difficult to be distinguished from the surrounding high signal intensity pelvic fat.
2. Bleeding or hemorrhage can be detected on T1-W imaging as by-products such as deoxyhemoglobin and methemoglobin return high signal.
3. The detection of marrow infiltration or metastatic deposits in the pelvic bones.

- *Small FoV, high spatial resolution oblique axial and coronal T2-W imaging.* Small FoV (140–180 cm) high spatial resolution (typically 3 mm partition thickness) T2-W imaging obliquely orientated either perpendicular or parallel to the long axis of the pelvic viscera (e.g., uterus, cervix, prostate, rectum, and anus) (Fig. 8.1) is essential for disease assessment. For the urinary bladder, these are usually acquired in the normal MR axial scan planes. As these images are prone to motion degradation and lower SNR, multiple signal averaging (typically 6–12) and administration of antiperistaltic agents help to reduce artifacts and improve image quality. Incorrect orientation of the imaging plane with respect to the targeted area or organ of interest (e.g., uterus, cervix, or rectum) can confound image interpretation because of partial volume effects, and therefore it should be avoided (Fig. 8.2).
- *Fat suppressed sequences.* Suppression of the high signal intensity returned from fat increases the sensitivity of the imaging to pathological processes that prolong T2-relaxation time. Fat suppression in the pelvis can be effected using a short-tau inversion recovery (STIR) technique or using spectral chemical fat suppression, e.g., chemical shift selective imaging sequence (CHESS). Over a larger FoV, it is usually easier to achieve a uniform fat suppression using the STIR technique. However, the disadvantages of STIR are poorer SNR, and because signal nulling is dependent on the inversion time, tissue signal suppression may not be chemically specific. This has to be borne in mind, particularly in the evaluation of ovarian masses, since hemorrhagic cysts, depending on the nature of the blood products, may show signal loss on STIR imaging, and be mistakenly thought to contain fat (Fig. 8.3). For this reason, spectral chemical fat-suppressed T2-W imaging is most useful in the pelvis for the evaluation of adnexal masses. Nevertheless, STIR imaging, acquired in oblique axial and coronal planes in relation to the anal canal, are very useful for the evaluation of perianal fistulae. One common disadvantage of STIR and spectral fat suppression techniques is that both lead to a loss of normal anatomical planes outlined by fat. For this reason, although fat suppressed imaging can be useful for identifying pathological processes, the relationship of an abnormality to adjacent structures may be better appreciated on the corresponding T1 or T2-W images.
- *Post contrast (Gadolinium-chelate) T1-W MRI.* There is likely to be significant variation in the extent to which gadolinium-chelate enhanced MRI

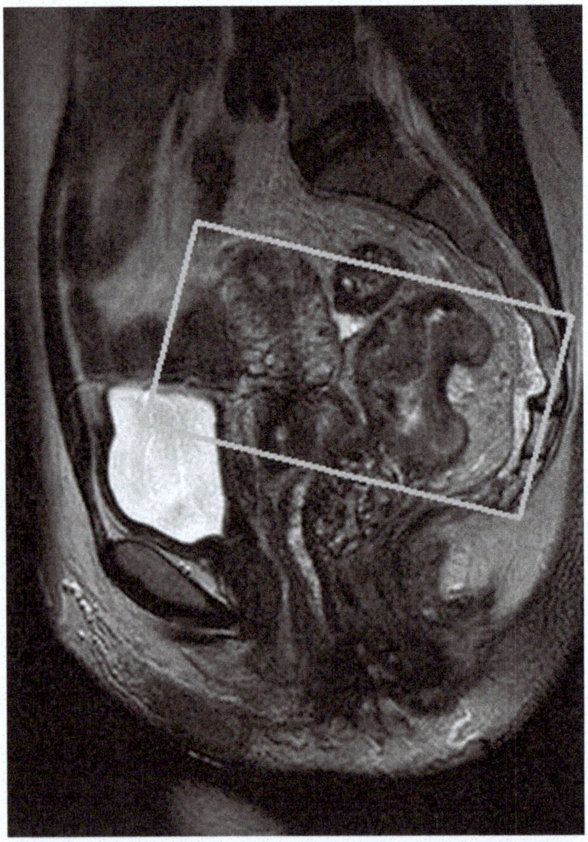

Fig. 8.1 Plane of orientation for the acquisition of small field of view paraxial images. In this example in a female with a mid-rectal cancer, note that the scans are acquired orthogonal at right angle to the rectum at the site of tumor

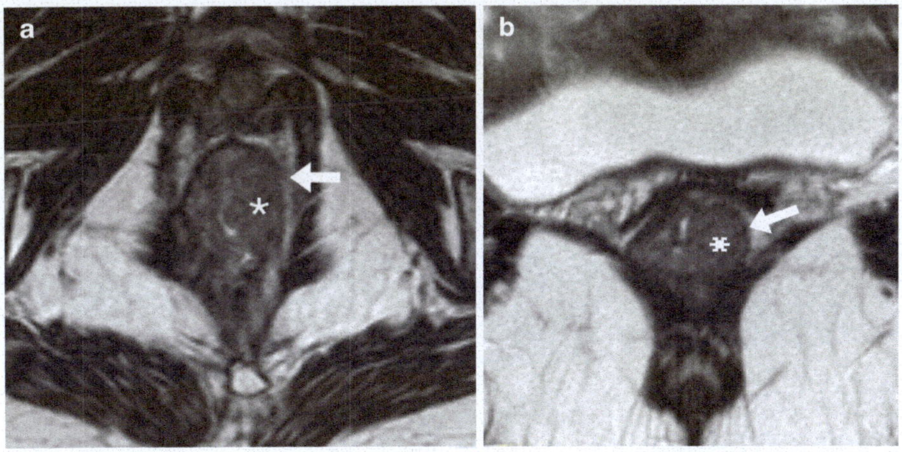

Fig. 8.2 Partial volume effect. (**a**) T2-weighted (T2-W) MR image acquired obliquely through the lower rectum shows intermediate signal intensity tumor (*asterisk*), which appears to extend through the wall of the rectum (*arrow*). However, the same area on the (**b**) T2-W image obtained orthogonal to the rectal wall shows that the tumor (*asterisk*) is entirely confined within the rectal wall (*arrow*). Partial volume effects can lead to spurious overstaging of pelvic tumors

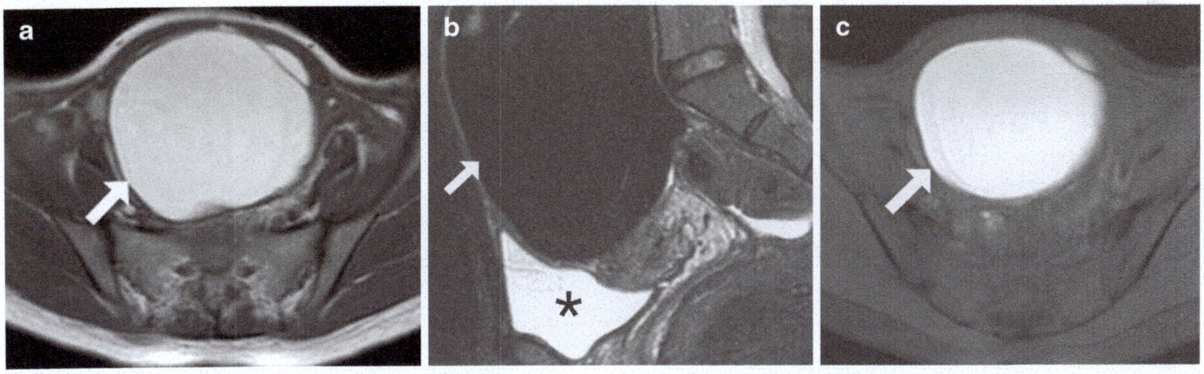

Fig. 8.3 The use of STIR vs. fat-suppression in the pelvis. (**a**) T1-W axial imaging shows a large cyst with a thin eccentric septum on the left returning high signal intensity (*arrow*). (**b**) The high signal intensity of the cyst content (*arrow*), as well as the signal from fat, is suppressed on the STIR sagittal image. Note that high signal intensity persists within the fluid in the bladder (*asterisk*). (**c**) However, using frequency selective fat suppression on T1-W imaging, the high signal intensity within the cyst is maintained (*arrow*), indicating that cyst does not contain fat. The high T1-signal in the cyst is due to hemorrhage, consistent with an endometrioma. The STIR inversion pulse is nonselective and results in signal nulling from blood, which can lead to misinterpretation. Hence, for lesion characterization of ovarian masses in the pelvis, chemical fat suppression is more useful than STIR imaging (Courtesy Dr. Paul Burn, Taunton, UK)

is performed in the pelvis. In our own practice, T2-W imaging remains the workhorse of pelvic imaging, and gadolinium-chelate enhanced T1-W imaging is reserved for specific indications. Contrast-enhanced scans are useful for the assessment of uterine, ovarian, cervical, and bladder tumors, although the presence and extent of disease may often be inferred on the T2-W imaging. In the post surgical pelvis, contrast-enhanced imaging can be helpful to detect tumor recurrence. In addition, contrast-enhanced imaging is also valuable for visualizing peritoneal pathologies, and for the assessment of inflammatory bowel disease.

A typical example of an imaging protocol that is used for evaluating pelvic diseases is shown in Table 8.1.

Table 8.1. Overview of some commonly used MRI sequences for the pelvis

Fast gradient echo T1 localiser	• Usually applied in axial, coronal and sagittal imaging planes • T1 weighted, dark fluid with bright signal in vessels
T2 Sagittal whole pelvis survey	• Plan from one pelvic sidewall to the other • Typically 250-300 mm FOV and 4mm slice thickness • 2D TSE / FSE sequence for female and male pelvic anatomy • High signal from fluid in urinary bladder and pelvic fat provides excellent contrast with soft tissues of bladder, prostate, rectum and uterus. Small FOV high resolution scans to be planned from sagittal images
T2 Axial whole pelvis Survey	• Plan Iliac crest to pelvic floor, large FOV, 5mm slice thickness • 2D TSE / FSE sequence • Excellent depiction of fluid filled bladder, ovarian follicles, cystic lesions • Zonal anatomy of prostate and uterus can be displayed • Black blood sequence
T1 Axial whole pelvis survey	• Plan iliac crest to pelvic floor, large FOV, 5mm slice thickness • 2D TSE / FSE sequence • Short T1 species (fat, blood, proteinacious fluids) display high signal • Good anatomical depiction of pelvic lymph nodes and sidewall, owing to natural contrast with fat • Black blood sequence
Axial / oblique high resolution	• 2D or 3D TSE / FSE sequence • Small FOV (140-180 mm) targeted to anatomy of choice • Thin slices / partitions 1-3mm for high resolution anatomy • Imaging plane selected according to anatomy and pathology to be investigated (e.g., rectal cancer prior to surgery, select plane perpendicular to long axis of rectum)
DWI / ADC	• Indicated in the evaluation of cystic lesions (e.g. to differentiate solid from cystic tumour or solid from necrotic tumour) or to evaluate tumour recurrence • Provides good detection of lymph nodes • Can be done as a whole pelvis survey b-values of 0-900s/mm^2 • Gaining wider acceptance in body imaging
T1 +/- Gd	• Usually applied in axial or sagittal imaging planes, depending on indication • Same imaging planes should be used before and after gadolinium-chelate injection • For dynamic studies 3D GRE with fat saturation most suited (VIBE, THRIVE, LAVA)

8.4 Pelvic Diseases Common to Males and Females

8.4.1 Urinary Bladder

8.4.1.1 Anatomy

The bladder lies within the pelvis and is roughly spherical in shape when distended. It is an extraperitoneal structure, but the dome of the bladder is covered by peritoneum. The ureters are inserted near the bladder base posteriorly, on either side of the trigone, and the bladder neck leads inferiorly into the urethra. In males, the peritoneum extends over the posterior surface of the bladder and is reflected over the anterior rectal wall to form the rectovesical pouch. In females, the peritoneum is reflected over the uterus to form the pouch of Douglas.

The bladder wall comprises four layers: an outer adventitia layer, a detrusor muscle (muscularis propria) layer comprising loosely packed outer and more densely organized inner smooth muscle fibers, the lamina propria (submucosa), and the innermost mucosal layer that is lined by transitional cell epithelium. The muscle layer can be recognized at T2-W MRI, appearing as low signal intensity, in contrast to the mucosa and submucosa, which usually returns high signal intensity. It is sometimes possible to discern a slight difference in the signal intensity within the muscle layers, with the more densely organized inner fibres appearing as lower signal intensity. However, it may be difficult to differentiate the normal mucosa and submucosa from the high signal intensity urine filling the bladder on T2-W imaging. On T1-W imaging, the bladder wall appears as intermediate signal intensity, and identification of the individual layers of the bladder wall is usually not possible.

After administration of gadolinium-chelate, there is differential enhancement of the normal bladder wall, and three layers can be observed on T1-W imaging: an inner thin layer of low signal intensity, a middle layer of marked enhancement, and a thick outer layer of lower intermediate intensity. These have been shown to correspond to the mucosa, submucosa, and muscularis propria, respectively.

The bladder wall is variable in thickness, depending on the degree of distension. As a guide, it should not measure more than 5 mm in thickness. For MR assessment, the bladder should be reasonably distended as an empty or poorly filled bladder can hide small polyps and tumors.

8.4.1.2 Practical Tips for MR Evaluation

In assessing the bladder, small FoV TSE T2-W imaging performed in the axial and coronal planes are particularly useful. The anterior, posterior, and lateral walls of the bladder are best assessed in the axial plane, whereas the coronal images are best for evaluating the dome and the base of the bladder. The sagittal images are also useful for visualizing the bladder outlet and proximal urethra.

Frequently, the nature and site of disease are already known when the patient is referred for MRI. Hence, it is easy to target imaging towards the region of interest. However, occasionally, a patient may be referred for urinary symptoms, such as dysuria or hematuria. If a suspicious tumor is diagnosed on MRI, it is important to also survey the sites of potential locoregional nodal spread. Bladder cancers disseminate most frequently to the obturator lymph nodes (40%), but also to nodes along the external iliac and internal iliac chain. These should be carefully scrutinized for possible involvement.

Benign and malignant conditions of the bladder can manifest as focal thickening or mass lesions, or as diffuse bladder thickening. While some of these have characteristic features on MRI, enabling confident diagnoses to be made, cystoscopy and biopsy are still frequently needed for a definitive diagnosis.

8.4.1.3 Benign Bladder Pathology

Although the majority of tumors arising from the bladder are malignant, benign conditions can result in bladder masses or wall thickening that mimics malignancy.

Inflammatory pseudotumor arises from nonneoplastic proliferation of myofibroblastic spindle cells. The etiology is uncertain, and the condition usually afflicts adults, although pediatric cases have been reported. The clinical presentation and cystoscopy findings may resemble bladder carcinoma. At MRI, inflammatory pseudotumor frequently appears as a solitary polypoidal or exophytic mass. Unusually, extravesical extension may be observed, making it difficult to differentiate from bladder carcinoma. On T2-W imaging, pseudotumors may show central high signal intensity, reflecting central necrosis, and low signal intensity peripherally. Following intravenous contrast administration, a rim enhancement pattern can be observed, due to poor enhancement of the necrotic centre. These features on MRI may help to suggest the diagnosis of inflammatory pseudotumors. However, as the imaging features overlap with bladder carcinoma, biopsy is often required for diagnosis.

Another benign condition that results in focal bladder masses in females is bladder endometriosis. Approximately 1–15% of women with endometriosis have bladder involvement. Bladder endometriosis is often deeply infiltrating, and occurs most frequently along the vesico-uterine pouch. As these infiltrate and grow within the bladder wall, they usually appear as submucosal masses. Rarely, an endometriotic deposit may grow through the submucosa as an intraluminal mass within the bladder. Fortunately, the MR findings are usually characteristic, enabling a confident diagnosis to be made. Endometriotic deposits show areas of high signal on T1-W (fat-suppressed or non fat-suppressed) images because of the presence of hemorrhage. The deposits typically also show regions of low T1- and T2-signal intensity because of fibrosis. Areas of high T2-signal intensity may also be present. Endometriotic deposits enhance following intravenous gadolinium contrast medium administration.

Some of the other focal lesions that occur in the bladder include leiomyomas, neurofibromas, harmatomas, nephrogenic adenomas, and papillary lesions of the bladder. Papillary lesions that are in the spectrum of "benign" include papilloma, inverted papilloma, and papillary urothelial neoplasm of low malignant potential (PUNLMP). PUNLMP is a low-grade, small and usually solitary neoplasm that does not invade or metastasize (Fig. 8.4). However, these have a propensity to recur or progress in grade, and hence surveillance is recommended.

Diffuse bladder wall thickening can result from many nonneoplastic processes such as infection with bacteria

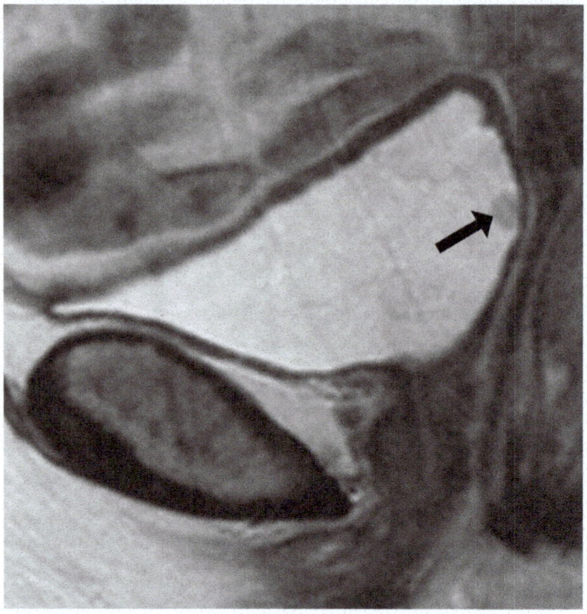

Fig. 8.4 Papillary urotherial neoplasm of low malignant potential (PUNLMP). T2-W sagittal MR image shows a small solitary polypoidal tumor arising from the posterior bladder wall (*arrow*), which was endoscopically removed

(cystitis), adenovirus, schistosomiasis, tuberculosis, and exposure to chemotherapy (e.g., cyclophosphamide) or irradiation. Unfortunately, MR findings in these conditions are often nonspecific. The bladder wall can also be thickened as a result of inflammatory processes adjacent to the bladder, such as inflammatory bowel disease. Crohn's disease may be complicated by ileovesical fistula, which can be visualized using T2-W, STIR or gadolinium-enhanced fat-suppressed T1-W MRI.

8.4.1.4 Bladder Carcinoma

Malignant epithelial neoplasms of the bladder are common, particularly in the elderly. These are classified according to the cell type, pattern of growth, and histological grade. Over 90% of all bladder cancers are transitional cell carcinomas. Squamous cell carcinoma, adenocarcinomas, and carcinosarcomas account for the remaining 10%. Although uncommon in the Western world, the incidence of squamous cell carcinoma of the bladder is higher where bladder schistosomiasis is endemic. The growth pattern of bladder carcinomas may be papillary, sessile or nodular, and can be invasive or noninvasive. Noninvasive tumors are confined to the mucosa or lamina propria. A tumor is considered invasive when it involves the muscularis propria. Histological grading ranges from I to III, with grade III (high-grade) tumors more likely to be sessile and invasive. Sessile lesions are also more likely to invade the muscle; however, the prognosis correlates more with tumor grade than with tumor morphology. Patients with tumors arising within bladder diverticula are also at higher risk of developing extravesical invasive disease due to the absence of the muscularis propria acting as a barrier to tumor growth.

The diagnosis of bladder carcinoma is usually made at cystoscopy and biopsy. At diagnosis, most transitional cell bladder carcinomas are found at the bladder base; the majority are single and measure more than 2 cm in size. However, multicentric disease occurs in up to 40% of cases, and careful scrutiny of imaging is therefore important to avoid missing a synchronous lesion. Once diagnosed, MRI is the best way of staging the disease prior to treatment. The tumor node metastasis (TNM) staging system is used to stage bladder tumors. In bladder cancer, the T-stage relates to the degree of tumor infiltration through the bladder wall and involvement of adjacent organs. The N-stage relates to the degree of nodal enlargement (nodal size) in locoregional lymph nodes.

On unenhanced T1-W imaging, bladder carcinoma returns intermediate signal intensity and is of higher signal intensity than the urine within the bladder lumen. Although the tumor is usually isointense compared with the normal bladder wall, unenhanced T1-W images can be helpful for the assessment of disease extension into the perivesical fat, bone metastases, and lymph nodes. However, the degree of bladder wall involvement is best assessed using T2-W imaging. On T2-W imaging, bladder carcinoma returns intermediate signal intensity, compared with the high signal intensity of urine in the bladder lumen and low signal intensity of the muscularis propria. By using the appropriate plane for the location of disease, the extent of disease within the bladder wall can be assessed. Disruption of the low signal intensity of the muscularis propria at the site of disease on T2-W imaging may be interpreted as muscle invasive disease (Fig. 8.5). The depth of invasion of the bladder wall is of considerable importance to the prognosis. If the deep layer of the muscle is involved, the incidence of nodal involvement is increased, and the 5-year survival is diminished. T2-W images are also useful to distinguish tumor from

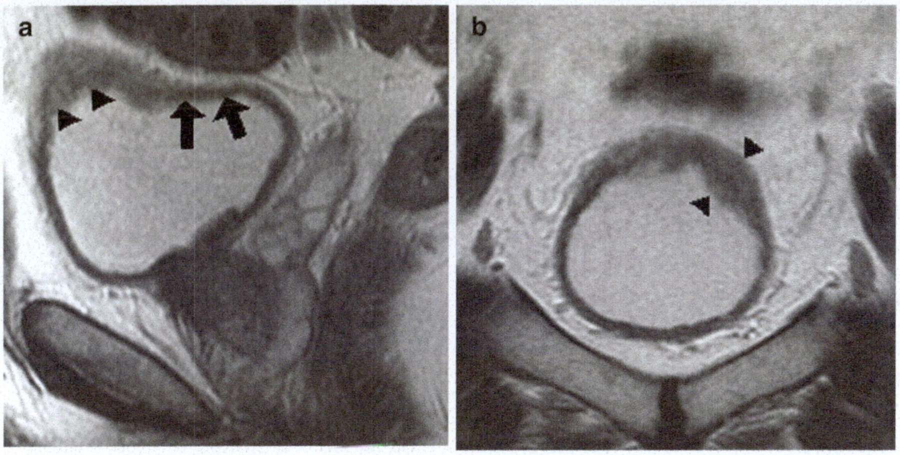

Fig. 8.5 Muscle invasive bladder carcinoma. T2-W (**a**) sagittal and (**b**) coronal images showing eccentric wall thickening at the left dome of the bladder. The *black line* of the muscularis propria (*black arrows*) can be traced into but is effaced at the site of tumor (*arrowheads*). The appearance indicates muscle invasive disease

fibrosis, and for the assessment of tumor invasion of adjacent organs.

Patients with tumor invasion of the deep layer of muscle can still be treated by radical cystectomy. It has been shown that the prognosis of patients whose disease shows microscopic extravesical spread following cystectomy is not significantly worse than patients with invasion of deep muscle without extravesical spread. By contrast, radical cystectomy is contraindicated in patients with evidence of macroscopic disease extending beyond the bladder wall because of the high likelihood of systemic dissemination (Fig. 8.6). Hence, one of the critical issues in MR staging is to determine the presence or absence of visible macroscopic extravesical disease. For this purpose, both the T1 and T2-W scans are helpful.

When the organ-confined disease is diffuse, or the degree of bladder wall involvement is uncertain on T2-W imaging, or when there has been recent instrumentation and biopsy, dynamic gadolinium contrast-enhanced T1-W imaging can be very helpful. Bladder cancer enhances early and allows the extent of tumor involvement of the bladder wall to be delineated (Fig. 8.7). After contrast administration, the muscularis propria appears lower in signal intensity compared with the tumor. Thus,

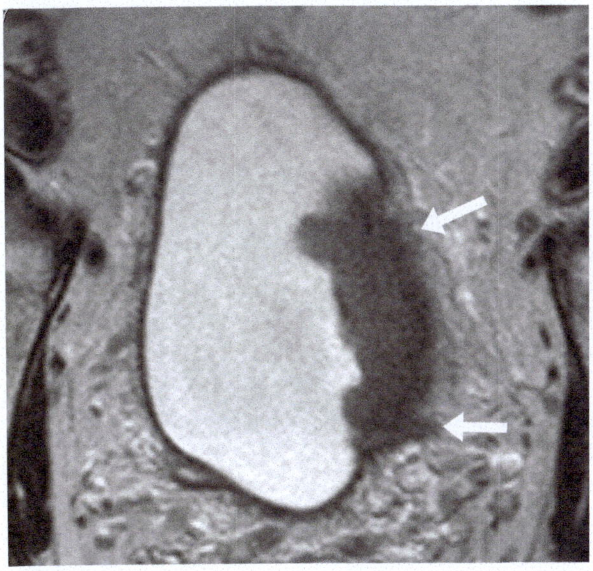

Fig. 8.6 Stage T3 disease. T2-W axial image showing tumor invasion (*arrows*) beyond the wall of the urinary bladder. Surgery is contraindicated in such patients

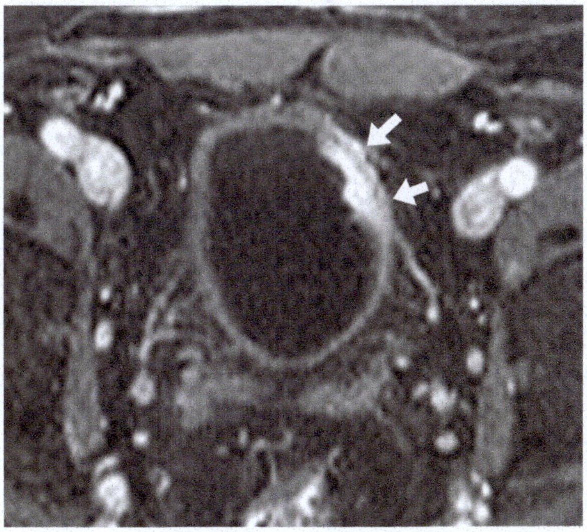

Fig. 8.7 Gadolinium contrast-enhanced T1-W imaging with fat-suppression showing a tumor arising eccentrically from the left bladder wall. The tumor enhances to a greater degree compared with the normal submucosa or muscularis propria (*arrows*), which may help to define tumor extent

preservation of this layer on contrast-enhanced imaging makes deep muscle invasion unlikely. The technique may also help to differentiate tumor from fibrosis/ edema, as the latter show little enhancement. However, contrast-enhanced imaging adds little value when there is clear evidence of extravesical disease or nodal dissemination.

8.4.2 The Rectum

8.4.2.1 Normal Anatomy

The rectum is continuous with the sigmoid colon above and the anal canal below. It is approximately 15 cm in length and is divided into three parts, which lie within the curve of the sacrum. The anterior surface and lateral sides of the upper third of the rectum are covered by peritoneum, which reflects laterally onto the pelvic sidewall. The middle third is covered by peritoneum anteriorly but the lower third is devoid of a peritoneal covering.

The connective tissues surrounding the rectum constitute the mesorectum, which is enclosed by the mesorectal fascia. The mesorectum contains fat, lymph nodes, blood vessels, and nerves supplying the rectum. The mesorectal fascia is also known as the fascia propria. The mesorectal fascia is a continuous fascia and surgical dissection is possible along this avascular plane to achieve a total en-bloc removal of the rectum and mesorectum. This technique of surgical dissection is known as total mesorectal excision (TME) surgery. The mesorectal fascia is clearly seen as a thin grey line on high spatial resolution T2-W MRI, and this fascial plane is important for assessing the potential resectability of rectal cancer (Fig. 8.8). At the pelvic inlet, the fascia lies deep to the hypogastric nerves and pelvic plexus. The mesorectal fascia fuses posteriorly with the presacral fascia at the level of S4 to form the rectosacral ligament. The Denonvillier's fascia contributes to the mesorectal fascia anteriorly, and is more distinct in males compared to females. The distal mesorectum has a bilobed appearance due to a posterior groove caused by the ano-coccygeal raphe. The mesorectal plane ends inferiorly at the intersphincteric plane between the internal and external sphincter of the rectum.

The predominant lymphatic drainage of the rectum is to lymph nodes embedded within the mesorectum. These in turn drain into nodes along the superior rectal vessels, which follow the inferior mesenteric artery to drain into retroperitoneal nodes. There is a lesser pathway of nodal drainage, accompanying the middle rectal veins, into the internal iliac group of pelvic sidewall nodes.

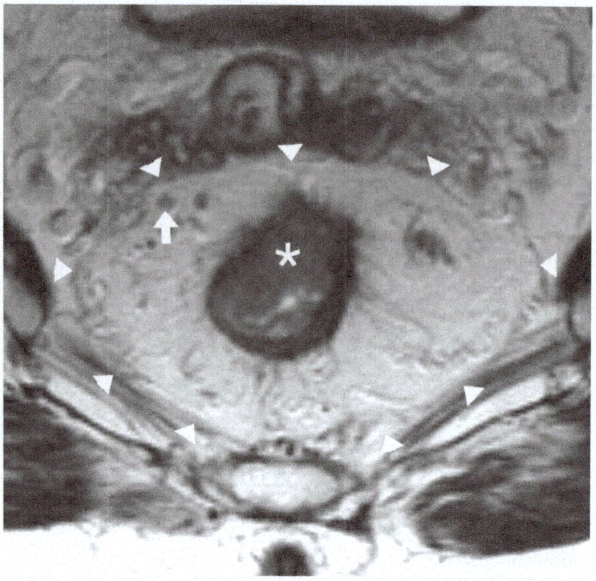

Fig. 8.8 The normal mesorectal fascia is seen as a *thin-grey line* (*arrowheads*) on the small field of view 3 mm section thickness T2-W imaging, which envelopes the rectum, the perirectal fat, as well as lymph nodes (*arrow*) and blood vessels embedded within the mesorectal fat. Note the intermediate signal intensity tumor in the wall of the rectum (*asterisk*). The mesorectal fascia represents the plane of surgical dissection at total mesorectal excision surgery for rectal cancers

On high spatial resolution T2-W imaging, a five-layer structure of the rectal wall may be recognized (Fig. 8.9). The mucosa, inner circular muscle, and outer longitudinal muscle layers of the bowel wall return low to intermediate signal intensity. By contrast, the submucosa and the fat, which is sometimes visible between the inner circular and outer longitudinal muscle layers, return higher signal intensity. However, the circular and longitudinal muscle layers cannot be separated in most instances, and the low signal intensity mucosa may be difficult to discern from air within the rectal lumen. Thus, the rectal wall often appears to comprise a higher signal intensity submucosal layer and a lower signal intensity outer muscularis layer. Hence, T2-W imaging is particularly helpful to assess the degree of invasion of the rectal wall by tumors. Unenhanced T1-W imaging is less helpful because the bowel wall appears as uniformly intermediate signal intensity, making it difficult to assess the degree of tumor involvement of the rectal wall.

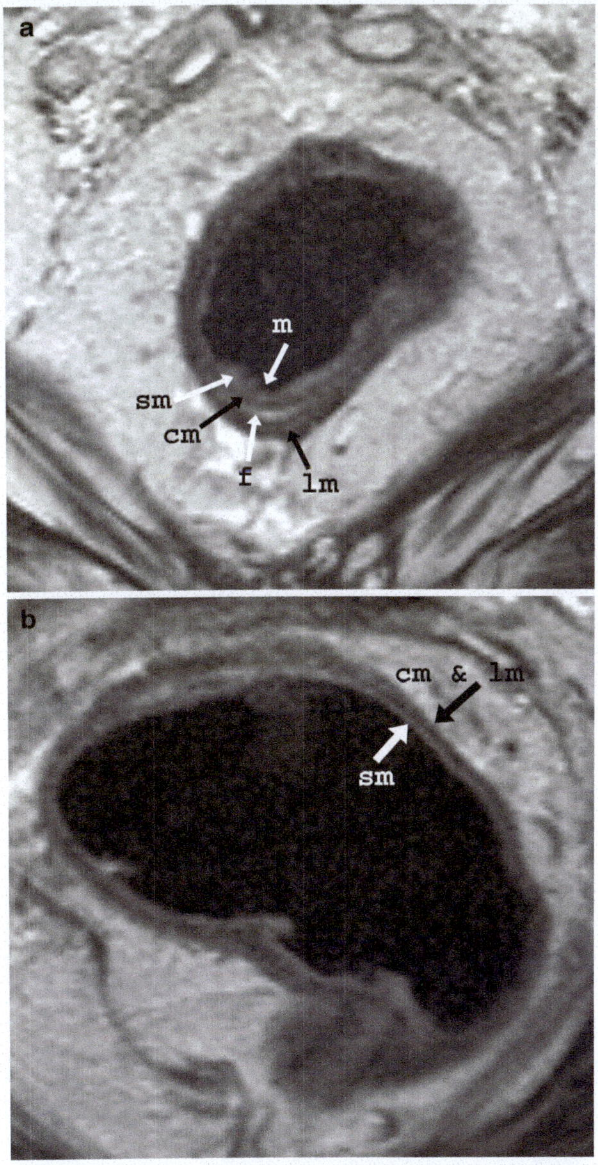

Fig. 8.9 Normal mural stratification of the rectal wall on T2-W imaging. (**a**) Up to five layers may be recognized in the rectal wall on high spatial resolution T2-W MRI. The mucosa (m), circular smooth muscle (cm) and longitudinal smooth muscle (lm) layers return lower signal intensity compared with the submuscosa (sm) and fat intervening between the smooth muscle layers (f). (**b**) However, frequently, only the higher signal intensity submucosa (sm) can be clearly distinguished from the muscularis layers (cm & lm)

8.4.2.2 Practical MRI Tips

Thin-section (3 mm) high spatial resolution T2-W MR images are most useful for assessing the rectum. Sagittal images are usually acquired first and are used to plan the acquisition of the axial and coronal images. The position of a rectal abnormality is best assessed on the sagittal images, which can be described in terms of measurement distance from the anal verge, thus providing a consistent method for disease localization. The distance from the anal verge is also used by surgeons and endoscopists to describe their clinical or endoscopic findings, and the MR localization can help to corroborate these findings. Sagittal images are also useful in revealing the relationship of a mass in the upper rectum to the bladder, prostate, uterus, and vagina.

Once an abnormality has been detected, thin section, small FoV (160–180 cm) oblique axial T2-W images are acquired perpendicular to the rectal wall over the length of the abnormality. Meticulous care should be taken to ensure that oblique axial scans are acquired orthogonal to the rectal wall, so as to minimize partial volume effects, which may result in misinterpretation. In patients with a low rectal abnormality, which can be defined on imaging as occurring below the level of the origins of the levator ani muscle from the pelvic sidewall, small FoV (160–185 mm) T2-W coronal imaging acquired parallel to the long axis of the anal canal enables accurate assessment of its relationship to the anal sphincter complex.

8.4.2.3 Benign Conditions

Ulcerative colitis and Crohn's disease can involve the rectum, and results in rectal wall thickening. However, it may be difficult to distinguish between the two entities based on imaging studies alone. In active disease, there is usually thickening and avid enhancement of the rectal wall following intravenous gadolinium contrast administration. On T2-W imaging, mural stratification may be observed, with increased signal intensity of the submucosa, attributed to submucosal edema (Fig. 8.10). Fistulae and perianal inflammation are frequently observed in patients with Crohn's disease, and there may be associated peri-enteric abscess or enlarged lymph nodes. Fibro-fatty proliferation is a feature of Crohn's disease and can result in widening of the presacral space. In patients with chronic or quiescent inflammatory bowel disease, high T1 signal intensity may be observed in the submucosa, which is believed to result from fat replacement of the bowel wall.

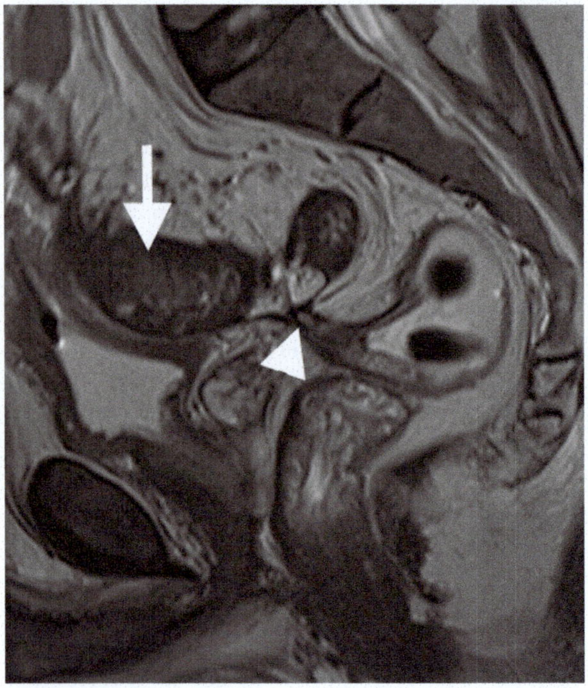

Fig. 8.10 Crohn's disease. T2-W sagittal image showing thickened segment of sigmoid colon due to Crohn's disease (*arrow*). Note the entero-enteric fistula between the sigmoid and the anterior wall of the rectum (*arrowhead*). There is also a pocket of air seen within the urinary bladder due to a sigmoid-vesical fistula (not shown on this image)

Radiation treatment to the pelvis can also result in rectal changes. Thickening of the rectal wall after radiation treatment is not uncommon if the rectum is included within the radiation field prescribed for the treatment of other pelvic tumors. This is characterized by increased T2 signal intensity in the submucosa, while the low to intermediate signal intensity of the outer muscular layer is usually preserved.

Infection of the rectum is relatively uncommon, although this may occur following instrumentation or trauma. The imaging changes are usually nonspecific, although focal abscess or collections may be associated.

Developmental cysts, including rectal duplication cysts, may be found in close proximity or contiguous with the rectum. These are usually asymptomatic, although the patient may present with symptoms resulting from its mass effect, or complications such as bleeding or infection. Uncomplicated cysts usually have a thin wall, may be unilocular or multilocular, demonstrate low T1 and high T2 signal intensity, and are nonenhancing.

8.4.2.4 Malignant Conditions

Rectal Carcinoma

Colorectal adenocarcinoma is common in the Western world, and is an important cause of cancer mortality and morbidity. The incidence of disease appears to be still rising. Surgery is potentially curative in patients with early stage good prognosis disease. MRI is increasingly used, not only to stage the tumor according to the TNM classification but also to stratify patients into prognostic groups, in order to identify patients with increased risk of local recurrence so that more intensified treatments may be prescribed to these patients.

High spatial resolution T2-W MRI technique is valuable in assessing the primary tumor. The technique is applied to evaluate the degree of tumor wall involvement (T-stage), predict the involvement of the circumferential resection margin, and identify pathological features (e.g., extramural venous invasion and depth of extramural disease infiltration), which predicts for an increased risk of local recurrence.

Rectal carcinomas usually appear as intermediate signal intensity on T2-W imaging, replacing the normal layers of the bowel wall (Fig. 8.11). However, mucinous carcinoma, a poor prognosis variant, returns high signal intensity on T2-W images. The morphology of the tumor may be polypoidal, semiannular, or annular. The tumor edge may be well-defined and

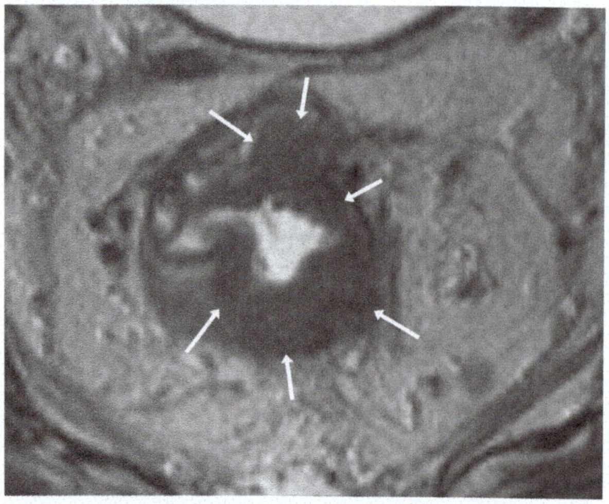

Fig. 8.11 Axial T2-W image showing a semiannular tumor of intermediate signal intensity (*arrows*) effacing the normal mural stratification of the rectal wall on the left. The tumor involves the submucosa and muscularis propria, indicating stage T2 disease

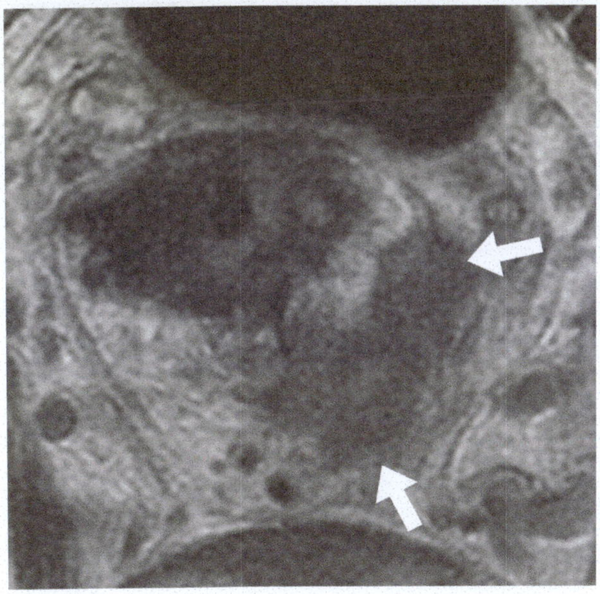

Fig. 8.12 Stage T3 tumor. T2-W paraxial image shows tumor arising in the rectum, which extends beyond the rectal wall into the mesorectum to come into contact with the mesorectal fascia (*arrows*). Primary surgery in such a patient would result in a tumor positive surgical resection margin. Thus, the patient was offered neoadjuvant chemoradiotherapy

pushing or diffusely infiltrating. The T-stage is assessed by evaluating the degree of involvement of the rectal wall. Stage T1 is confined to the submucosa. Stage T2 involves the muscularis propria. Stage T3 extends beyond the rectal wall into the mesorectum, and stage T4 involves adjacent structures or organs.

However, stage T3 represents a heterogeneous group as the degree of extramural tumor growth is not taken into account in the TNM classification. A stage T3 tumor with evidence of tumor extension out to the mesorectal fascia is likely to result in a tumor positive circumferential resection margin if primary surgical resection of the tumor is undertaken (Fig. 8.12). It has been shown that if tumor is visible within 1 mm of the mesorectal fascia on MRI, this predicts the involvement of the circumferential surgical margin. In addition, patients with tumors showing an extramural growth of more than 5 mm has also been shown to have worst long-term outcome and higher risk of local recurrence, compared with those with tumors showing extramural growth of 5 mm or less. Thus, it is possible to identify these groups of patients using MRI, with a view to administering preoperative chemoradiation to downsize and downstage tumors prior to surgery.

Invasion of the peritoneal surface (Fig. 8.13), pelvic sidewall, or adjacent organs represent T4 disease, and can be diagnosed on MRI. Another feature that has been shown to be associated with an increased risk of local failure is extramural venous invasion. This can be recognized on thin section T2-W imaging as intermediate signal intensity expansion of venules in the mesorectum adjacent to the tumor (Fig. 8.14).

Nodal disease is an independent poor prognostic factor in patients with rectal cancer. Patients with stage N2 disease (four or more involved nodes) have a significantly poorer long-term survival compared with patients with stage N0 or N1 disease. Nodal size is a poor discriminator between malignant and nonmalignant mesorectal nodes in rectal cancer because although malignant nodes are generally larger than nonmalignant nodes, there is substantial overlap. Approximately 30%

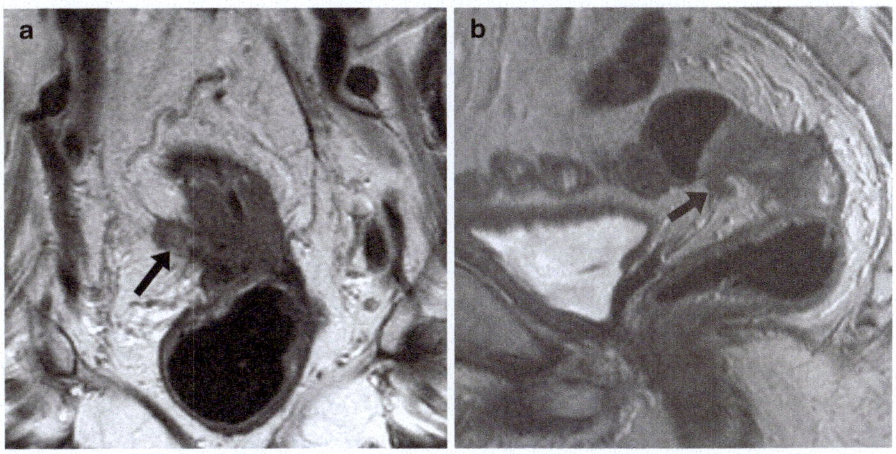

Fig. 8.13 T2-W (**a**) sagittal and (**b**) axial images showing tumor extension along the right peritoneal reflection (*arrows*), indicating stage T4 disease

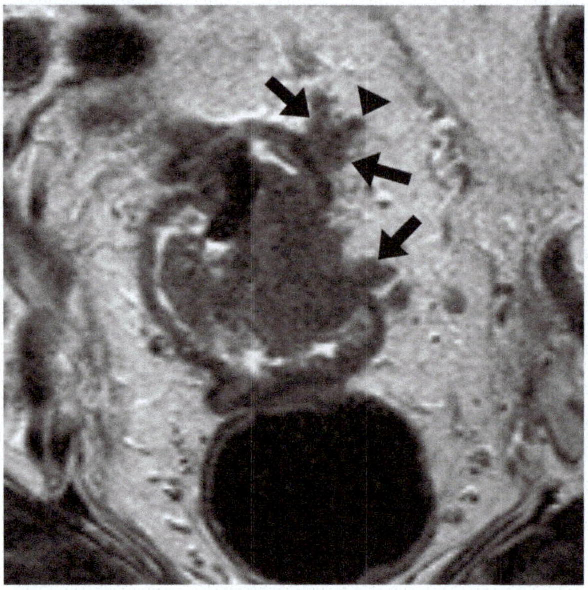

Fig. 8.14 Extramural venous invasion. T2-W axial image showing extramural tubular extensions adjacent to the left rectal wall (*arrows*), which are contiguous with and isointense to the primary rectal tumor. These represent extramural venous invasion and extension of disease. The ghost remnant of a perirectal vessel is just visible (*arrowhead*)

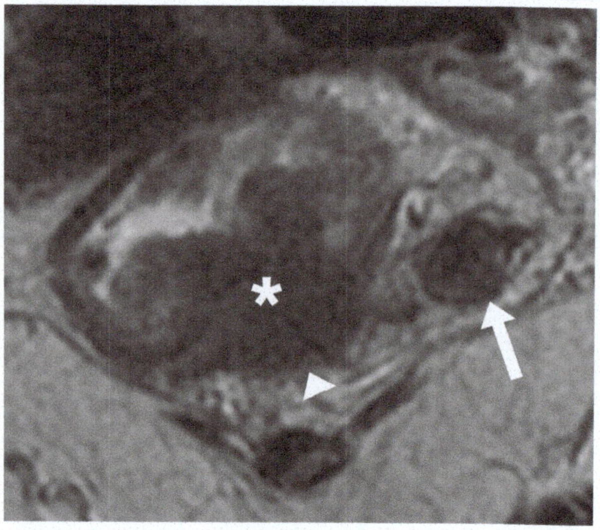

Fig. 8.15 Malignant mesorectal lymph node. T2-W axial image showing a tumor (*asterisk*) invading beyond the rectal wall (*arrowhead*). Note the malignant node (*arrow*) in the left mesorectum which demonstrates irregular outline and heterogeneous signal intensity

of malignant lymph nodes associated with rectal cancer measure less than 5 mm in diameter. Furthermore, benign reactive nodal hyperplasia is also common, which leads to nodal enlargement. Hence, applying the widely used criteria of 5 mm to discriminate between malignant and nonmalignant nodes would result in substantial misclassification.

More recently, it has been shown that assessing nodal morphology on T2-W imaging is more accurate than nodal size in distinguishing malignant from nonmalignant nodes. Malignant nodes were found to have irregular outlines or to exhibit heterogeneous signal intensity on T2-W MRI. Irregular nodal outline was related to extracapsular extension of disease, while signal heterogeneity reflected tumor foci within the involved node (Fig. 8.15). If either of these criteria was present, a sensitivity of 85% (95% CI: 74–92%) and a specificity of 97% (95% CI: 95–99%) was achieved for detecting nodal metastases in nodes ≥3 mm. Another technique that is being evaluated is ultrasmall superparamagnetic iron oxide (USPIO) particles enhanced MR lymphography, which appears to show substantial promise.

With the increasing application of neoadjuvant chemoradiation in rectal cancer, MRI is also used to evaluate the downsizing and downstaging of tumors after treatment. Apart from regression in tumor size, chemoradiation treatment also induces fibrosis, which can be observed as low signal intensity replacing previous intermediate signal intensity tumor on T2-W imaging. In some instances, chemoradiation may induce necrosis or mucinous change within the tumor, resulting in areas of high T2 signal intensity after treatment. However, it can still be difficult to predict the presence or absence of microscopic disease in areas showing apparent treatment response since these are beyond the resolution of MRI to detect confidently.

Other Malignancies

Other malignant tumors of the rectum include rectal stromal tumors, carcinoid tumors, melanoma, lymphoma, and squamous cell carcinoma. The rectum can also be involved by extension of malignant disease from adjacent pelvic organs, such as the prostate, bladder, uterus, cervix, and ovaries.

Rectal stromal tumors arise within the wall of the rectum and are usually well-circumscribed, although an exophytic component can be frequently identified. The centre of these tumors may appear necrotic or hemorrhagic. Lymphoma usually appears as diffuse thickening of the rectum. The disease is more frequent in patients who are infected with the human immunodeficiency virus, and is often bulky, but rarely causes obstruction.

8.4.3 The Anus

8.4.3.1 Anatomy

The anal canal is approximately 2.5–4 cm long. The upper anal canal is lined by columnar epithelium, and the lower anal canal by squamous epithelium. Two landmarks are of particular importance to the surgeon: (1) The palpable rather than visible intersphincteric groove, which defines the plane separating the involuntary internal sphincter from the voluntary external sphincter, and (2) the dentate line, which is defined by the columns of Morgagni. The positions of these may be estimated on MRI, but difficult to pinpoint exactly.

For practical application, the transition between the anal canal and the rectum may be taken to be at the level of anorectal ring, where a complete puborectalis sling is visible on axial MRI. The sphincter anatomy of the anal canal is best demonstrated on coronal MRI (Fig. 8.16). These include the levator ani muscle, the internal sphincter, the external sphincter, the intersphincteric plane, and the ischiorectal and ischioanal fossae. The internal sphincter is the continuation of the rectal circular smooth muscle, while the external sphincter is composed of striated muscles and blends in with the rectal longitudinal muscle. The two sphincters are separated by the intersphincteric plane, which contains fat. These structures are exquisitely shown using endoanal ultrasound and endoanal MRI, and normal variations of these have been described. A good understanding of the radiological anatomy of the anal canal is critical to the accurate assessment of fistula-in-ano and anal cancers.

8.4.3.2 Practical MRI Tips

For the assessment of the anal canal, small FoV (160–180 cm) imaging is essential. These are acquired perpendicular and parallel to the anal canal, and usually using T2-W and STIR sequences. However, for the assessment of perianal fistula, the use of gadolinium-enhanced fat-suppressed T1-W imaging can be useful to outline small focal collections and fistulous tracks.

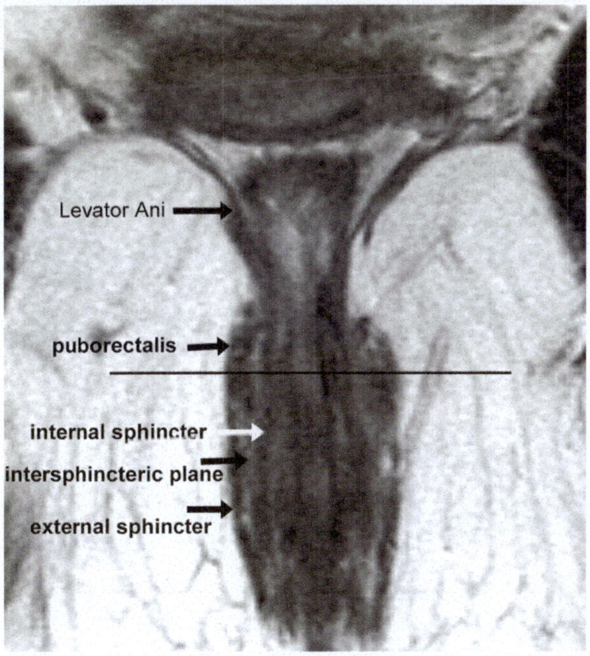

Fig. 8.16 Normal anatomy of the anal canal on T2-W coronal imaging obtained using a pelvic phased-array coil. Radiologically, the anal canal can be said to begin at approximately the level of the puborectalis (*black line*). Note the low signal intensity layers of the internal and external sphincter, with a higher signal intensity intersphincteric plane in between

8.4.3.3 Benign Conditions

Fistula-In-Ano

The "cryptoglandular theory" is widely accepted as the basis for the pathogenesis of perianal fistula. A focus of sepsis arising from cryptoglandular inflammation in the intersphincteric plane will attempt to drain, and the path (primary track) formed as a consequence determines the nature of the fistula. Perianal fistulae can be classified into four categories according to the system proposed by Park et al., which is based on the relationship of the track to the anal sphincter complex. These categories are: intersphincteric, transphincteric, suprasphincteric, and extrasphincteric.

In many institutions, perianal fistulae are assessed without using an endorectal coil due to their limited FoV, which can result in missed sepsis. Instead, pelvic phased-array coils are preferred. Intersphincteric fistulae are most common, and the primary tracks reach the perianal skin by extending along the intersphincteric plane (Fig. 8.17). Transphincteric fistulae by contrast, extend

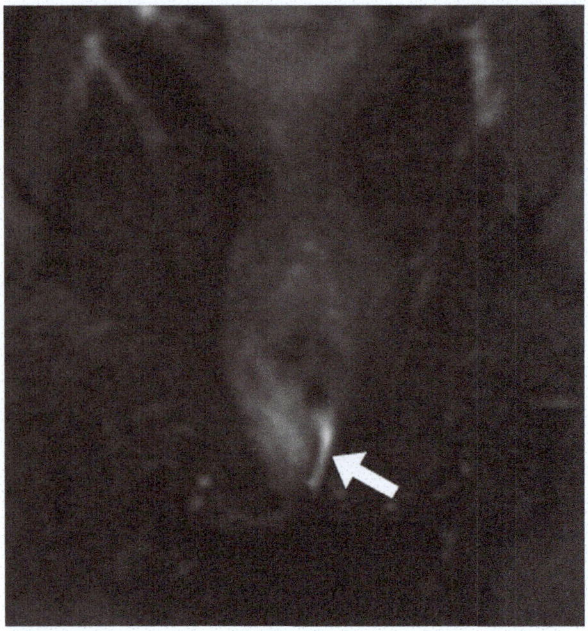

Fig. 8.17 Intersphincteric fistula. Coronal STIR image showing a high signal intensity intersphincteric fistula

across the external sphincter and track within the ischio-anal fossa to reach the perianal skin. Suprasphincteric fistulae ascend within the intersphincteric plane, but extend across the levator ani muscle to descend through the ischiorectal and ischioanal fossa to reach the perianal skin. Extrasphincteric fistulae are uncommon. These tracks bypass the anal sphincter complex, resulting in direct communications between the rectum and the perianal skin. Extrasphincteric fistulae are more frequently associated with Crohn's and inflammatory bowel disease. Although primary tracks can be identified and classified accurately using MRI, secondary tracks extending or communicating with the primary track can be complex, and may be described as infralevator or supralevator, depending on whether these extend below or above the levator ani muscle. However, these should also be clearly documented since they have a bearing on the nature of surgery or treatment prescribed.

MRI is increasingly used prior to surgery, as it enables careful surgical planning by demonstrating the pathways of the primary tracks, the presence of secondary tracks (if any), and associated complications. Axial imaging is best for establishing the nature and type of the primary tracks. Identification of the course of a track may be facilitated by heeding the positions of the internal and external openings. This is usually recorded using a clock face nomenclature, the 6 o'clock position being posterior with the patient lying supine. The position of the internal opening (e.g., in relation to the anal verge/ dentate line) should be noted, as this has a bearing on the extent of sphincter division that is undertaken during fistulotomy or fistulolectomy.

8.4.3.4 Malignant Conditions

Anal Carcinoma

Carcinoma of the anal canal is uncommon, accounting for less than 2% of large bowel malignancies and 1–6% of anorectal tumors. Anal carcinoma originates between the anorectal junction above and the anal verge below. Not surprisingly, the majority of anal canal cancers are squamous cell carcinoma. Treatment using combination chemotherapy and radiotherapy is curative in the majority of patients. However, radical surgery, such as abdomino-perineal resection, may still be necessary to treat local failure or recurrence after chemoradiation.

T2-W TSE and STIR MRI using external pelvic phased-array coil has been found useful for demonstrating the local extent of pelvic disease for both primary anal cancers as well as for recurrent diseases. Clear delineation of the anatomical boundaries of local disease enables optimal planning of radiation fields. The main advantages of using pelvic phased-array MRI over endoanal sonography include better visualization of mesorectal nodes beyond the depth of view of endoanal ultrasound and the ability to simultaneously assess the primary tumor, the pelvic sidewall, and the inguinal area. The internal iliac nodes and inguinal nodes are not infrequent sites of nodal dissemination.

Anal carcinomas are also staged using the TNM classification system, but unlike rectal carcinomas, the local tumor T-stage is dependent on tumor size rather than the degree of involvement of the anal canal and sphincter complex. T1 denotes a tumor less than 2 cm in maximum diameter, T2 tumors are 2–5 cm in size, T3 tumors are greater than 5 cm in diameter, and T4 denotes involvement of adjacent structures such as the vagina or prostate.

Prior to treatment, anal carcinomas appear mildly hyperintense on both T2-W and STIR imaging

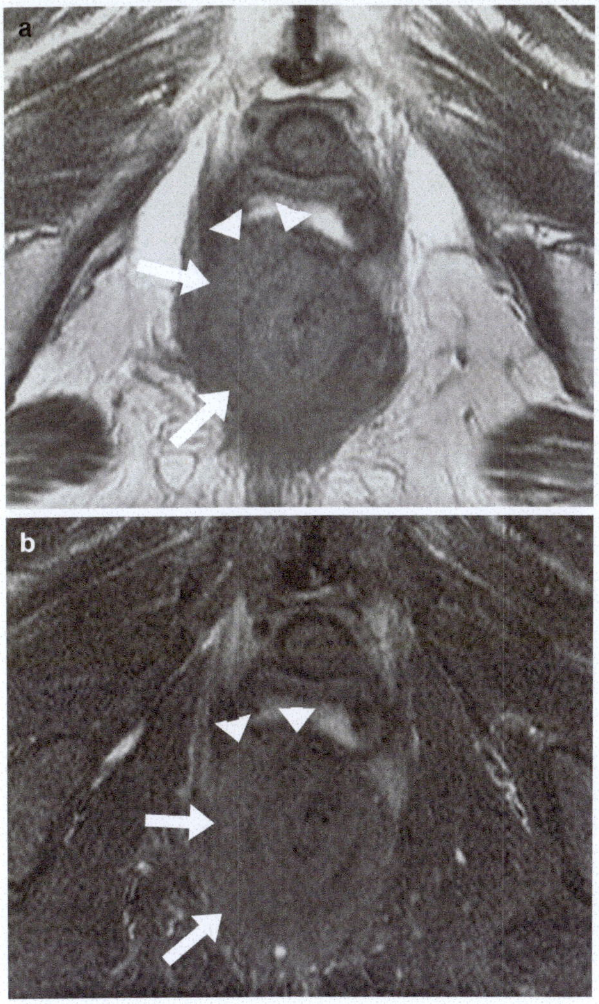

Fig. 8.18 (**a**) T2-W and (**b**) STIR axial imaging in a patient with anorectal cancer showing a tumor arising in right anal canal (*arrows*). The tumor is invading the posterior wall of the vagina (*arrowheads*). However, note that the normal anatomical planes are better seen on T2-W imaging compared with STIR imaging (Permission to reproduce from BJR)

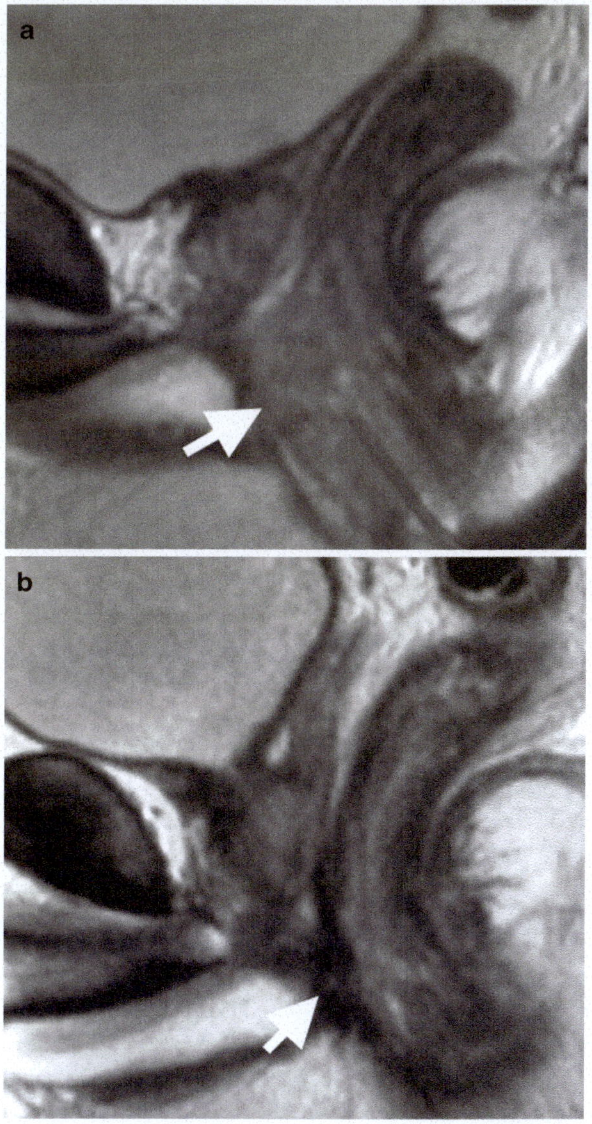

Fig. 8.19 T2-W sagittal images of anal cancer (**a**) before and (**b**) after chemoradiation. The intermediate to high signal intensity tumor in the anterior anal canal (*arrow*) showed a good response to chemoradiation treatment. Following treatment, low signal intensity fibrosis was observed at the site of previous disease (*arrow*)

(Fig. 8.18). However, T2-W imaging is better in demonstrating the relationship of the tumor to adjacent structures since there is greater homogenization of the soft tissue signal intensity on STIR imaging, making it more difficult to delineate tissue and anatomical boundaries. The most common direction of local tumor extension appears to be anterior into the urogenital triangle, as the levator ani muscle may act as a relative barrier to lateral tumor growth.

MRI can also be used to monitor treatment response to chemoradiation therapy. Chemoradiation results in tumor shrinkage, but tumor signal intensity may also decrease due to fibrosis (Fig. 8.19). However, these changes may be complex and slow to occur. However, it has been found that following chemoradiation, a reduction in tumor size accompanied by complete resolution or stabilization of the T2 signal intensity at the site of tumor more than 1 year after treatment was associated with a favorable outcome.

8.5 Pelvic Diseases in Males

8.5.1 Prostate

8.5.1.1 Anatomy

The lobar concept of prostatic anatomy, first described by Lowsley in 1929, has now been replaced by the zonal concept of prostatic anatomy, first described by McNeal in 1966. The zonal anatomy is well-demonstrated on T2-W SE/TSE sequences. The prostate is a cone-shaped glandular organ, with the apex of the cone lying caudally and the base lying cranially, abutting the bladder where the urethra starts. The prostatic urethra runs through the gland to the apex, where it becomes the membranous urethra. The muscular wall of the membranous urethra forms the external sphincter. At midgland level, the transition zone surrounds the urethra. The transition zone contains a relatively high proportion of stromal elements compared with glandular tissue and, therefore, has intermediate signal intensity on T2-W imaging. When the transition zone enlarges with age, benign prostatic hypertrophy develops, which is common enough to be considered virtually normal in patients over the age of 45 years. As prostatic hypertrophy increases, cystic spaces and discrete nodules may develop, but the zonal anatomy of the prostate should remain recognizable. Around the transition zone lies the peripheral zone. This area has a high glandular content, is relatively lacking in stromal elements and returns a high signal on T2-W imaging. At the apex of the gland, below the transition zone, it accounts for virtually the entire gland. However, if there is a significant degree of benign prostatic hypertrophy at midgland level, the peripheral zone is compressed into a horseshoe shape. The central zone is an area of gland lying in the midline, cranial to the transition zone. The ejaculatory ducts run through the central zone to the verumontanum, a small ovoid structure, which returns high signal. The central zone is frequently indistinguishable as a separate structure and accounts for only a small percentage of prostatic volume. The anterior border of the prostate is marked by a band of thickened fibromuscular tissue, which thins laterally to form the capsule of the prostate. This is frequently only a few cells thick, and, in places, is completely deficient, glandular tissue merging directly with periprostatic fat. The neurovascular bundles are located posterolaterally. The seminal vesicles lie immediately superior to the base of the gland.

8.5.1.2 Practical MRI Tips

T2-W sequences are crucial to the demonstration of zonal anatomy. TSE sequences function extremely well, although the degree of contrast between transition and peripheral zone is slightly reduced, compared with standard SE sequences. T2-W GRE sequences and STIR have been found less useful. T1-W sequences demonstrate good contrast between the prostate and surrounding periprostatic fat, but the zonal anatomy is obliterated by lack of contrast. T1-W images are helpful for identifying hemorrhage within the prostate gland following prostatic biopsy, since the accompanying low T2 signal intensity change could be misinterpreted as disease.

8.5.1.3 Benign Diseases

Severe congenital anomalies, such as agenesis and hypoplasia, are rare and are usually associated with other congenital abnormalities of the genital or urinary tract. However, developmental cysts, such as utricular and Müllerian-duct cysts may be seen. They return high signal on T2-W images and low signal on T1-W images. Benign prostatic hypertrophy results from enlargement of the transition zone (Fig. 8.20). Signal characteristics may be variable on T2-W imaging,

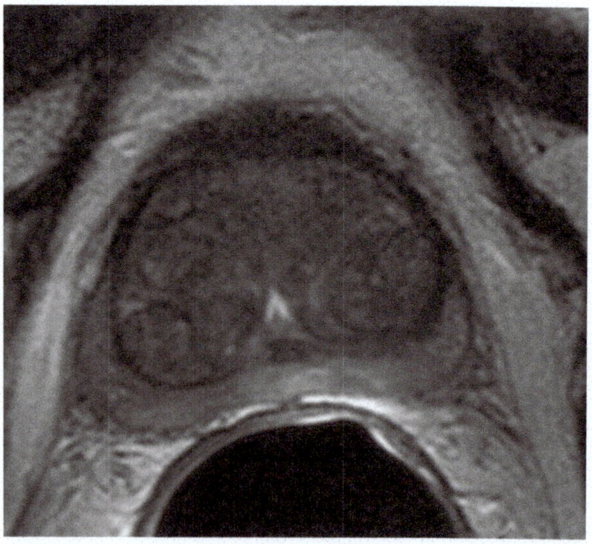

Fig. 8.20 Benign prostatic hypertrophy. T2-W imaging showing nodular enlargement of the transition zone of the prostate gland, typical of benign prostatic hypertrophy

depending on the relative preponderance of glandular hyperplasia, compared with interstitial or stromal hyperplasia. Cystic ectasia, resulting from dilatation of glandular elements, shows up as small areas of high signal intensity. Areas of infarction may cause low signal intensity. The appearance of benign prostatic hypertrophy is usually characteristic. Infiltration of the peripheral zone by benign prostatic hypertrophy has been described, but it is extremely rare, and for practical purposes, an abnormality visible on MRI in the peripheral zone is not benign prostatic hypertrophy.

8.5.1.4 Malignant Diseases

Adenocarcinoma of the prostate accounts for over 95% of malignant prostatic tumors. It is frequently latent, and its clinical behavior depends on histological grade, disease stage, and tumor bulk. Of all prostate carcinomas, 70% arise in the peripheral zone, 10% in the central zone, and 20% in the transition zone. Tumors are frequently small or diffusely infiltrative. Benign prostatic hypertrophy is common enough that the diseases may coexist, and therefore the typical appearance of benign prostatic hypertrophy does not exclude coexistent carcinoma.

Prostatic carcinoma is typically low signal, relative to the glandular tissue of the peripheral zone (Fig. 8.21). They are rarely isointense or hyperintense, and these tumors usually have mucinous elements. There is some overlap between the appearance of prostatic carcinoma and chronic inflammatory conditions of the prostate, e.g., chronic granulomatous prostatitis, and the diagnosis must always be confirmed by biopsy. Patients may be referred for MRI following biopsy. Ideally 6 weeks should be allowed for artifacts to resolve, but this is often impractical and biopsy artifacts may cause confusion (Fig. 8.22). Once the diagnosis is confirmed, MR is the most accurate method of staging prostate cancer. Staging accuracy reported in the literature exceeds that of transrectal ultrasound and CT, and nodal staging can be accomplished at the same investigation. The sensitivity and specificity of T2-W MRI for prostate cancer detection varies widely in the reported literature. Using pelvic phase-array coil, a sensitivity of 45% and specificity of 73% has been reported. However, even with the use of endorectal coil, there is still considerable variation with sensitivity of 27–61% and specificity of 77–91% being reported.

The TNM system is used for staging prostatic carcinoma. This is similar to the American Joint Committee on Cancer Staging system, but differs markedly from the American Urological Association system. Tumor spread initially penetrates the capsule, and the first route of spread is frequently to the neurovascular bundles or seminal vesicles. Locally advanced disease is common at

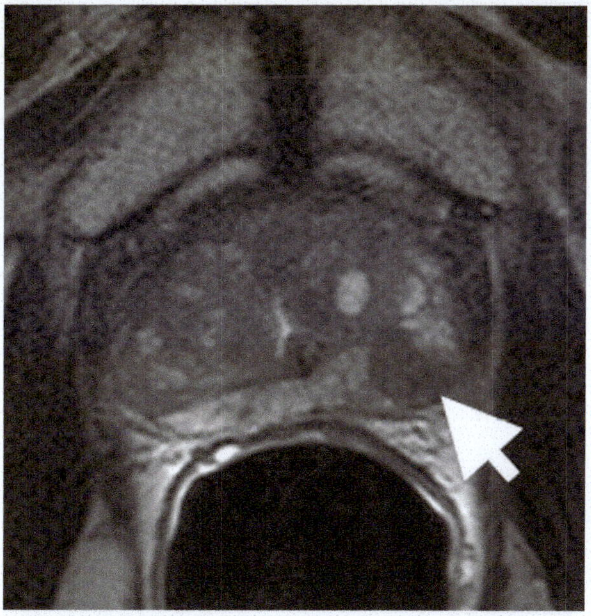

Fig. 8.21 Prostate carcinoma. T2-W axial image shows a discrete low signal intensity nodule in the left prostate gland (*arrow*), which was confirmed to be malignant at biopsy. There is no evidence of extracapsular extension of disease

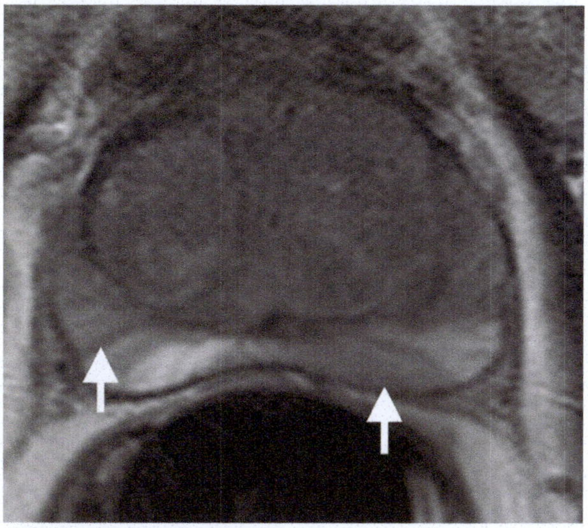

Fig. 8.22 Postbiopsy changes in the prostate gland. T2-W image showing geographical areas of low signal intensity (*arrows*) in the peripheral zone of the prostate gland related to previous biopsy. These should not be misinterpreted as disease infiltration

presentation, although if routine screening of asymptomatic men becomes prevalent, early-stage disease may be picked up. The tell-tale signs of extracapsular spread are the bulging of the prostatic outline (Fig. 8.23) and "beaks" pointing out toward the neurovascular bundle. These signs correlate well with the discovery of extracapsular spread in pathological specimens following radical prostatectomy. In general, the unequivocal detection of an extracapsular tumor mass is considered a contraindication to radical prostatectomy. Infiltration of the seminal vesicles and extracapsular spread near the apex of the gland can be difficult to diagnose, and for this reason, coronal images may be used to supplement the routine axial images. In some centers, sagittal images are recommended for evaluation of spread to the seminal vesicles.

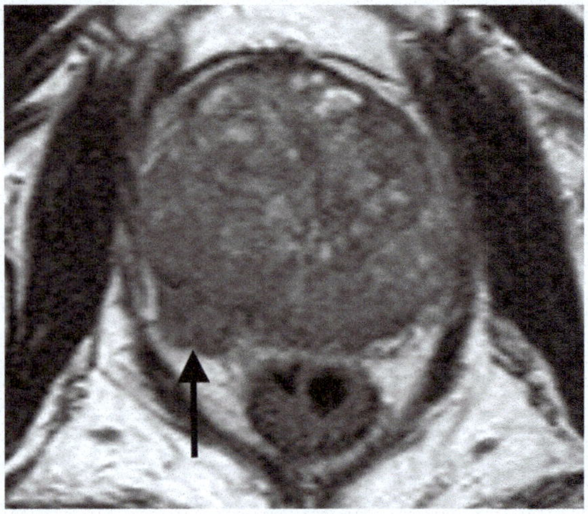

Fig. 8.23 Extracapsular extension of prostate cancer. T2-W axial image showing focal bulge due to extracapsular extension of tumor (*arrow*) from the right prostate gland

The key morphological MR criterion for identifying prostate cancer is low T2 signal intensity in an otherwise high T2 signal intensity peripheral zone of the gland. However, reliance on this MR feature has significant limitations since both benign (e.g., prostatitis, post-biopsy, postradiation, and hormone treatment) and malignant conditions can result in a similar appearance. Furthermore, prostate cancer arising in the transitional zone is often not distinguishable from benign prostatic hypertrophy on T2-W imaging. For these reasons, functional imaging techniques such as MRS and dynamic contrast-enhanced MR imaging (DCE-MRI) are used at some specialist centers to improve diagnostic accuracy.

To perform MRS on a 1.5 T system, endorectal coil imaging is mandatory, although at 3 T it may be possible to obtain satisfactory spectra using pelvic phased-array surface coils. The use of the endorectal coil is time-consuming; however, patient tolerance is surprisingly good, although this depends on age, attitude and educational background. MRS detects changes in the relative concentrations of metabolites in the prostate gland. The normal prostate gland contains a high concentration of citrate. In prostate cancer, the citrate level is decreased, but the level of choline is increased. The increase in choline concentration in prostate cancer reflects a high turnover of cell membranes in the tumor tissue. Hence, tumor tissues show an increase in the choline to citrate ratio compared with normal prostate gland (Fig. 8.24). A detailed description of MRS

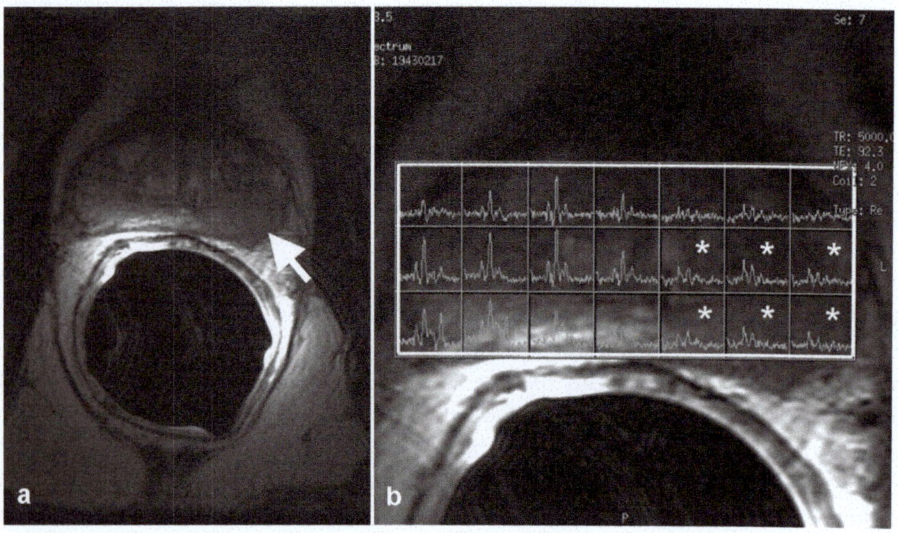

Fig. 8.24 Magnetic resonance proton spectroscopy (MRS) of prostate cancer. (**a**) T2-WI shows low signal intensity tumor in the left prostate gland (*arrow*). (**b**) 3D CSI MRS voxels overlaid on T2-WI show increased choline to citrate ratios in the voxels corresponding to the tumor regions (*asterisks*). Note normal spectra on the right side of gland (Courtesy Dr. Thng, Singapore)

techniques and interpretation is beyond the scope of this chapter, and the readers may want to refer elsewhere. MRS protocols and data analysis packages for prostate imaging are now available from most major commercial MR vendors, which should facilitate the adoption of the technique into clinical practice. However, the radiologist should attempt to enlist the help of an experienced physicist to quality assure the technique so as to have confidence in the data acquired. In experienced hands, the combined use of MRS and T2-W MRI has been shown to improve cancer detection and localization in the peripheral zone. Scheidler et al. demonstrated 91% sensitivity and 95% specificity for cancer detection for combined MRS and T2-W MRI, which was better than T2-W MRI (sensitivity 77–81%, specificity 46–61%) or MRS (sensitivity 63%, specificity 75%) alone.

Using DCE-MRI, prostate cancer is distinguished from normal prostate tissue by the differential rate of contrast uptake or tissue enhancement. Tumor tissue exhibits increased angiogenesis, which results in an increased number of blood vessels in the tumor, which are usually poorly formed and hyperpermeable. As a result, quantitative vascular parameters that are derived using DCE-MRI (e.g., blood volume, exchange constant *Ktrans,* and interstitial volume) are higher in tumor tissues (Fig. 8.25). Studies have also found that use of DCE-MRI can also improve cancer detection in the peripheral zone of the prostate. Although there is considerable research interest in the field of tumor vascularity and extracellular leakage of contrast in prostate cancer, the role of DCE-MRI is not firmly established in clinical practice.

MRI following hormonal or radiation therapy for prostate cancer usually demonstrates reduction in size and loss of contrast within the gland. Following radical prostatectomy, recurrence can be difficult to detect. The postsurgical prostatic bed returns low signal, and a local recurrence produces an enhancing mass (Fig. 8.26).

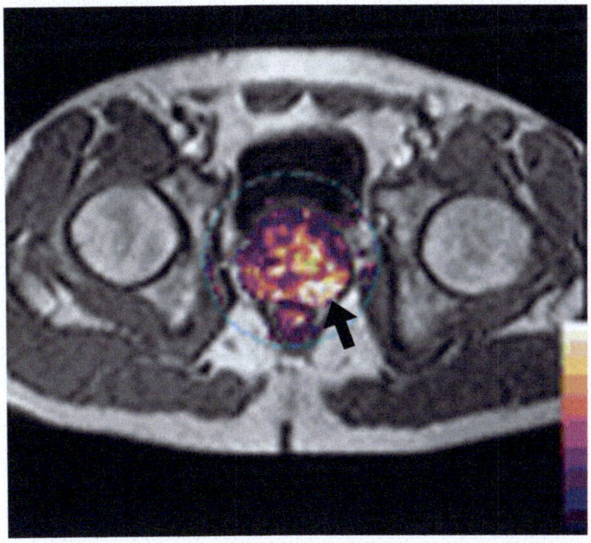

Fig. 8.25 Dynamic contrast-enhanced MRI of the prostate cancer. Parametric map of Ktrans showing increased vascular efflux of contrast in the left peripheral zone corresponding to the site of tumor (*arrow*)

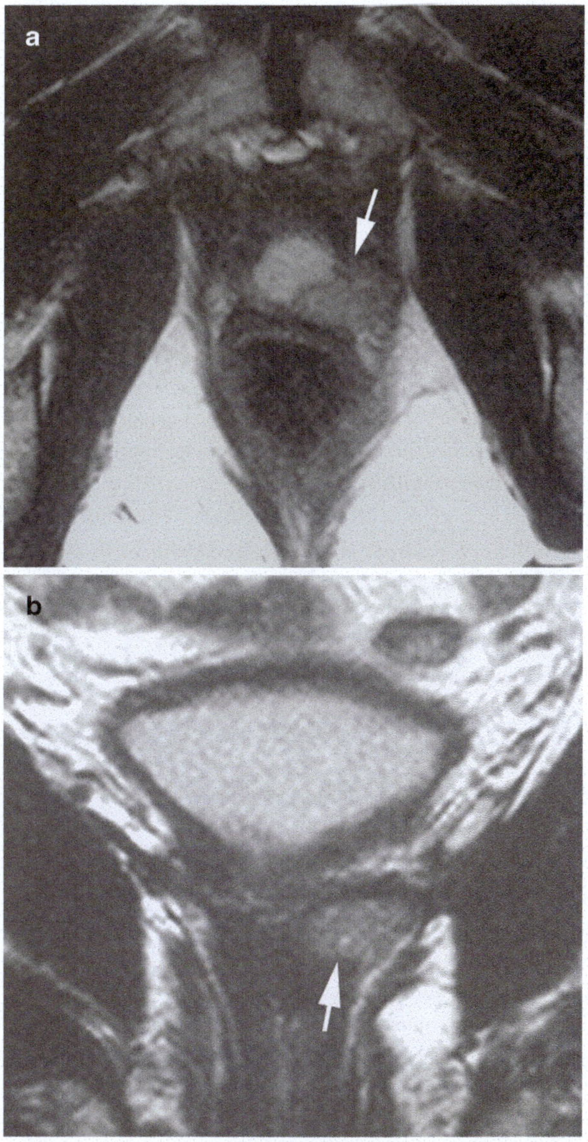

Fig. 8.26 Local disease relapse in the prostate bed. (**a**) T2-W axial and (**b**) coronal images showing soft tissue recurrence of intermediate to high signal intensity within the left prostatic bed (*arrow*)

Most local recurrences following surgery need TRUS guided biopsy confirmation.

8.6 Male External Genitalia

8.6.1 *Penis and Scrotum*

8.6.1.1 Anatomy

The anterior urethra runs through the corpus spongiosum, which is enveloped by a thin layer of tunica albuginea. These structures comprise the ventral compartment of the penis. The dorsal compartment contains the paired corpora cavernosa. The two compartments are separated by Buck's fascia, which also surrounds both compartments and their tunica albuginea. The posterior portion of the corpus spongiosum expands to form the bulb, and the anterior part expands to form the glans.

The testes lie within the scrotum, a sac comprised of internal cremasteric and external fascial layers, the dartos muscle, and skin. The testes are encased by tunica albuginea, which invaginates the testis posteriorly to form the mediastinum. The seminiferous tubules, coiled within each testis, converge to form the rete testis and the efferent ductules. These ductules form the epididymis, which lies posterior to the testis. The tail of the epididymis leads into the vas deferens. The supplying vessels pass into the mediastinum.

8.6.1.2 Practical MRI Tips

The anatomy of the male external genitalia is considered by some to be at its most beautiful when demonstrated by MRI using T2-W SE/TSE sequences. Following careful positioning to orientate the penis in a craniocaudal direction, thin sagittal slices (3 mm) should be obtained, supplemented by images perpendicular to the long axis of the penile shaft.

When imaging the testes, the scrotal contents should be supported by a towel placed between the thighs. Axial and coronal T2-W and T1-W SE/TSE sequences will demonstrate the anatomy. The normal testis returns homogeneous intermediate signal intensity on T1-W images and high signal intensity on T2-W images. The tunica albuginea appears as a thin low signal intensity band surrounding the testis on both T1 and T2 W sequences. On T2-W images, thin low signal intensity septa can be seen within the substance of the testis radiating back toward the mediastinum testis, which forms a band along the posterior edge of the testis. The epididymis is isointense or slightly hypointense compared with the testis on T1-W images and also hypointense on T2-W images. Following gadolinium enhancement, the epididymis will be enhanced to a greater extent than the normal testis.

8.6.1.3 Benign Conditions

Congenital abnormalities of the penis are usually clinically apparent. The characteristic signal returned by the testis makes MR a useful technique for hunting the testis in cases of cryptorchidism. Fat-suppression techniques such as STIR can be very helpful in this clinical setting. Most benign conditions of the penis can be evaluated clinically. MRI can be used to make the diagnoses of urethral diverticulum, fistulae, or the degree of damage following urethral injury. The rare but fascinating Peyronie's disease (induratio penis plastica) is caused by focal inflammation of the tunica albuginea and corpora cavernosa. The condition is painful and eventually leads to fibrosis, which, if unilateral, leads to deviated erections and, if bilateral, to shortening of the penis. On T2-W images, low signal intensity fibrotic plaques are visualized within the corpora cavernosa. These plaques will be enhanced following gadolinium, particularly where there is an element of active inflammation.

A number of prostheses are available for treatment of impotence. Some of these contain silicone and some are inflated with fluid. Care should be taken to ensure that no metallic prosthetic structures are present.

Hydrocele, varicocele, torsion, and epididymoorchitis may all be identified, but clinical examination and ultrasound are sufficient for diagnosis in the vast majority of cases. One unusual benign condition that can be recognized on MRI in the testis is an epidermoid cyst. Epidermoid cysts constitute approximately 1% of testicular tumors. Although they are cysts, they are usually filled with laminated material making them appear solid on imaging. An epidermoid cyst has a "target" appearance on MRI: A low signal intensity capsule surrounds the high-signal lipid-rich centre on both T1- and T2-W images.

8.6.1.4 Malignant Conditions

MRI is extremely useful in the evaluation of tumors of the penile urethra. The majority of penile urethral carcinomas are squamous (approximately 80%), with transitional cell carcinomas and adenocarcinomas accounting for the rest. Squamous cell carcinomas are, to some extent, radiosensitive, and the extent of disease can be well demonstrated by MRI (Fig. 8.27).

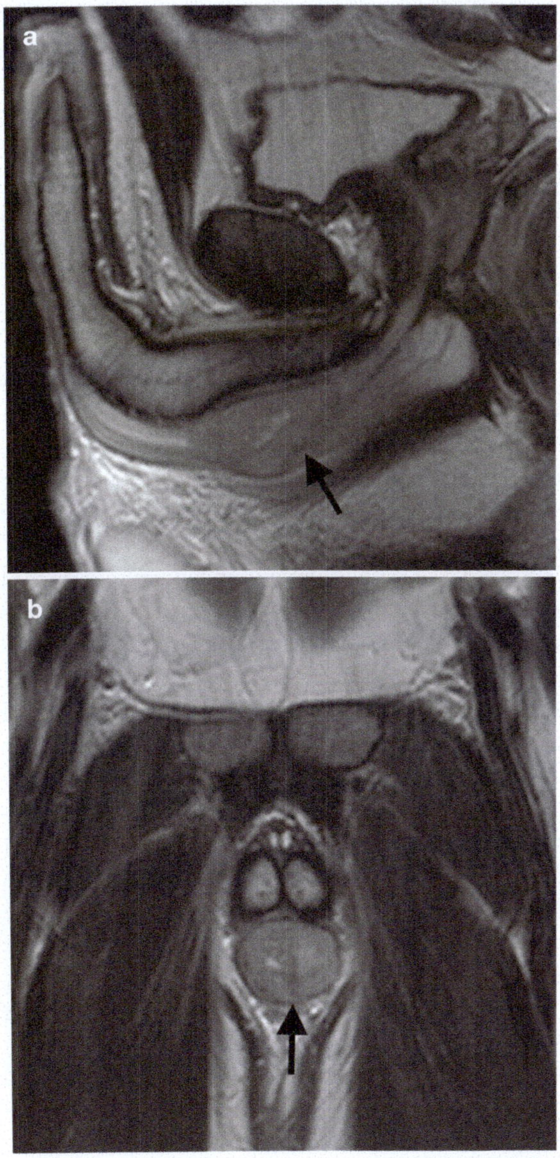

Fig. 8.27 Carcinoma of the urethra. T2-W (**a**) sagittal and (**b**) coronal images showing an irregular mass (*arrows*) arising from the penile urethra. Sagittal images are useful to demonstrate the extent of disease

Tumor masses are usually of a signal intensity slightly lower than the adjacent corpus spongiosum and corpora cavernosa on T2-W imaging. T1-W imaging following gadolinium is useful. Tumors show moderate enhancement, and there is often a flare of adjacent enhancement in the corpus spongiosum due to increased vascularity and extracellular diffusion locally. Extension of prostatic carcinoma down the urethra may also be demonstrated. Squamous cell carcinoma of the glans can usually be evaluated clinically, but depth of infiltration can be assessed using MR.

Malignant tumors of the testes are well-demonstrated by MRI. When small, they return slightly lower signal than normal testes on T2-W images. However, frequently, they are large, and teratoma may be hemorrhagic or cystic, resulting in heterogeneous signal intensity. Interestingly, one particular histological variant that appears to have a characteristic MRI appearance is the Leydig cell tumor. These tumors show striking enhancement on T1-W imaging following gadolinium contrast administration, a feature unusual amongst testicular neoplasms. It is also possible to visualize microlithiasis of the testes on MRI, which is associated with an increased risk of testicular malignancy (Fig. 8.28).

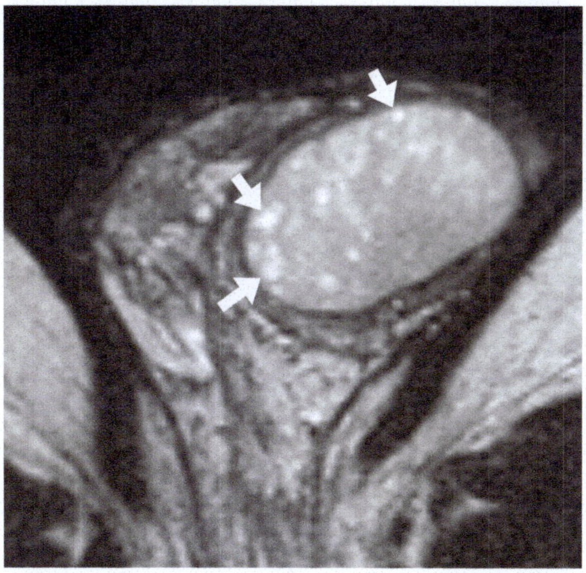

Fig. 8.28 MRI of the left testes. T2-W fat-suppressed images showing multiple hyperintense foci within the left testes due to microlithiasis (*arrows*)

8.7 Diseases of the Female Pelvis

8.7.1 Uterus and Cervix

8.7.1.1 Anatomy

The uterus is divided into three segments: the fundus lies above the cornua; the body or corpus uteri lies between the fundus and the most caudal part of the uterus, which is the cervix. Histologically, the uterine corpus has three tissue layers: the serosa, which is a covering of peritoneum draped over the uterus; the myometrium, which consists of smooth muscle; and the endometrium. The inner third of the myometrium is composed of smooth-muscle bundles, which are densely packed and orientated mostly along the long axis of the uterus. The outer myometrium contains more loosely packed and randomly orientated smooth-muscle fibres. The MRI anatomy of the uterine body and fundus is well-demonstrated by sagittal T2-W SE/TSE sequences (Fig. 8.29). A high signal intensity stripe represents normal endometrium and secretions within the cavity. The width of the endometrial stripe varies with the menstrual cycle, and the average thickness has been reported to be from 3 to 6 mm in the follicular phase and 5–13 mm during the secretory phase. Below the endometrial stripe, there is a band of low signal referred to as the junctional zone. Beyond this is an outer layer of myometrium, which returns intermediate signal intensity on T2-W images. There is some controversy about the histological basis for the low signal intensity of the junctional zone. The hypothesis that it represents the densely packed muscle bundles of the inner layer of the myometrium is attractive; however, some in vitro studies have demonstrated that the thickness of the inner layer of myometrium does not correspond exactly to the junctional zone on either MR or ultrasound. Some authors have attributed the low signal from the junctional zone to lower water content, while others have drawn attention to an increase in the percentage of nuclear area within the cells of the junctional zone compared with that of the outer myometrium.

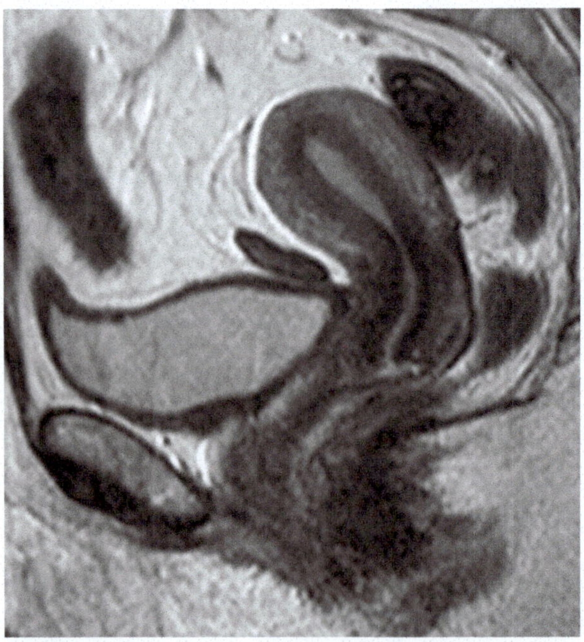

Fig. 8.29 Normal zonal anatomy of the uterus. T2-W MR sagittal image showing zonal anatomy of the uterus. Note the high signal intensity endometrium centrally, followed by the low signal intensity junctional zone, and the intermediate signal intensity outer myometrium

The cervix is separated from the uterine corpus by the internal os, which corresponds to a slight constriction, marked by the entrance of the uterine vessels. The cervical canal is lined by the columnar epithelium of the endocervix. Small folds can sometimes be seen (*plicae palmatae*). Surrounding the cervical endothelium is a dense fibrous stroma. The outermost layer of the cervix is composed of muscle, which becomes increasingly thin in the lower cervix toward the external os and is marked histologically by the squamocolumnar mucosal junction. On T2-W images, the secretions in the canal form a zone of very high signal. The cervical mucosa itself returns slightly lower signal, and the *plicae palmatae* may be seen. The fibrous stroma is of very low signal, and the muscular outer cervix is of intermediate signal. This muscular layer is continuous with the outer myometrium of the uterine corpus. The MR appearance of the cervix varies little with the menstrual cycle.

The parametrium and suspensory ligaments of the uterus may serve as pathways for local spread of disease. The parametrium lies between layers of the broad ligament, which is a folded double sheet of peritoneum that reflects from the ventral and dorsal surface of the uterus, and extends to the pelvic sidewall. The lower border of the broad ligament is thickened by a condensation of connective tissue and muscle, forming the cardinal ligaments. The paired uterosacral ligaments are fused anteriorly with the cardinal ligaments and extend posteriorly to the sacrum. The uterovesical ligaments extend from the cervix to the base of the urinary bladder. These are the main suspensory ligaments of the uterus. The round ligaments run from the posterolateral aspect of the uterine fundus, through the inguinal canal to the labia majora. The ligaments are of low signal intensity on T1-W imaging and of variable intensity on T2-W imaging. The parametrium contains multiple venous plexuses and some loosely packed connective tissue, which is of intermediate signal intensity on T1-W sequences and isointense with fat on T2-W sequences.

8.7.1.2 Practical MRI Tips

The pelvis is surveyed using T2-W sagittal scans, as well as T1 and T2-W axial imaging. However, small FoV (20–26 cm) T2-W imaging using a surface pelvic phased-array coil is essential for accurate assessment of the uterus and cervix. Oblique axial and coronal imaging are important as these allow the uterus and cervix to be assessed in their short and long axes. Gadolinium contrast-enhanced is not routine, and is usually reserved for evaluation of endometrial, cervical or ovarian cancers.

8.7.1.3 Congenital Anomalies

The fallopian tubes, uterus, and upper two-thirds of the vagina are derived from the paired Müllerian ducts. Agenesis or hypoplasia may affect any part of the female genital tract. A variety of partial and complete duplications may also result from embryological aberrations. MRI is very useful for demonstrating the presence and type of Müllerian duct abnormality. The more commonly encountered conditions include unicornuate uterus (complete or incomplete arrest of development of one Müllerian duct), uterus didelphy (complete non-fusion of the two Müllerian ducts leading to two separate uteri and cervix), bicornuate uterus (partial non fusion of the two Müllerian ducts leading to two uteri but one common cervix), and septate uterus (failure of resorption of central septum between the Müllerian ducts). The oblique coronal plane using T2-W sequences is frequently the most informative sequence.

8.7.1.4 Benign Pathology

Endometrial polyps and hyperplasia can usually be detected using transvaginal ultrasound, at which time endometrial sampling may be undertaken. MRI is usually not used in the initial investigation of endometrial pathology, although the MR findings may be corroborated with the ultrasound appearances. Thickening of the endometrial stripe is of pathological significance, particularly in postmenopausal women, but the abnormal ranges are not clearly defined. However, in a postmenopausal woman, a double-layer endometrial thickness of less than 5 mm without focal thickening excludes significant pathology and is compatible with atrophy. It has also been suggested that the postmenopausal endometrial thickness should not exceed 3 mm in women not receiving hormone-replacement therapy, and should not exceed 6 mm in women on hormone-replacement treatment.

On T2-W images, endometrial polyps appear as low signal intensity intracavitary masses surrounded by high signal intensity fluid and endometrium. When they are large, endometrial polyps may be markedly heterogeneous with areas of high and low signal. They show variable degrees of enhancement on T1-W sequences following administration of gadolinium. Typically, they enhance less than endometrium but more than adjacent myometrium.

Leiomyoma is the most common type of uterine tumor and is estimated to be present in 20–30% of premenopausal women over the age of 35 years. Following menopause, they may regress, as they are oestrogen dependent. Most leiomyomas exhibit some form of degeneration pathologically, particularly if they are large. Degeneration may be hyalin, myxomatous, cystic, fatty, or hemorrhagic. In addition, they may calcify and these diverse degenerative features account for the variable signal changes seen on MRI. T2-W sequences provide optimal contrast between leiomyomas and adjacent myometrium or endometrium. T1-W sequences may be useful in depicting hemorrhagic degeneration, and may be helpful in demonstrating clear fat planes between the uterus and adnexal structures in cases where difficulty is encountered in discriminating a uterine leiomyoma from an ovarian mass. Leiomyomas typically appear as well-marginated masses of low signal intensity relative to myometrium on T2-W sequences and may demonstrate a speckled internal architecture (Fig. 8.30). Very small lesions are

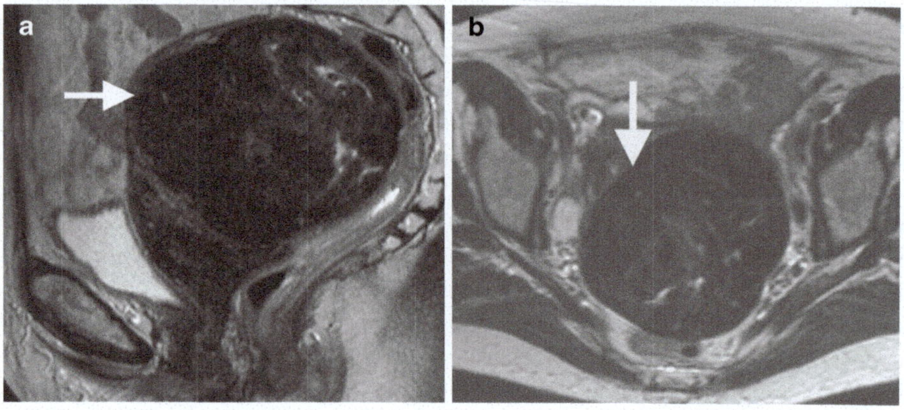

Fig. 8.30 Benign leiomyoma of the uterus. T2-W (**a**) sagittal and (**b**) axial image showing a well-circumscribed predominantly low signal intensity intramural mass typical of leiomyoma

frequently identified, and MR is more sensitive than transvaginal ultrasound. The details available on MRI may help demonstrate the myometrial origin of a submucosal leiomyoma protruding into the endometrial cavity, thus assisting in discrimination from an endometrial polyp.

The cellular subtype of leiomyoma and those with significant myxoid, cystic, or red degeneration are the most likely tumors to cause confusion, as they may return high signal on T2-W sequences. The appearance of leiomyomas following administration of gadolinium is variable. The majority enhance to a lesser degree than surrounding myometrium on both early and delayed contrast-enhanced images. However, early intense enhancement may be seen with the cellular subtype. Bizarre signal change in large leiomyomas should raise the possibility of sarcomatous degeneration, which is rare and cannot be reliably diagnosed by MR alone. The greatest utility of MRI in diagnosis of uterine leiomyoma is in demonstrating, unequivocally, the myometrial origin of a lesion, where other investigations such as transvaginal ultrasound are indeterminate.

Uterine adenomyosis is a common condition caused by heterotopic endometrial gland and stroma in the myometrium. This ectopic tissue appears to be independent of hormonal stimuli, and the clinical presentation usually involves irregular or excessive bleeding, pelvic pain, and sometimes uterine enlargement. Adenomyosis may be focal, diffuse or microscopic, and is frequently found incidentally following hysterectomy for other indications. Because the presenting symptoms are nonspecific, imaging is of value if the diagnosis is to be made preoperatively. In this clinical setting, MR has some advantages over transvaginal ultrasound, primarily the reproducibility and relative lack of operator dependency involved in MRI. T2-W sequences are ideal for diagnosing adenomyosis. The heterotopic endometrium generates adjacent myometrial hyperplasia and this is represented as diffuse or focal thickening of the junctional zone (Fig. 8.31) forming an ill-defined area of low signal intensity, occasionally with embedded bright foci on T2-W images. The low signal intensity results from smooth muscle hyperplasia, while the bright foci on T2-W images are related to islands of ectopic endometrial tissue and cystic dilatation of glands. On T1-W sequences, these bright T2-W foci may appear hyperintense when

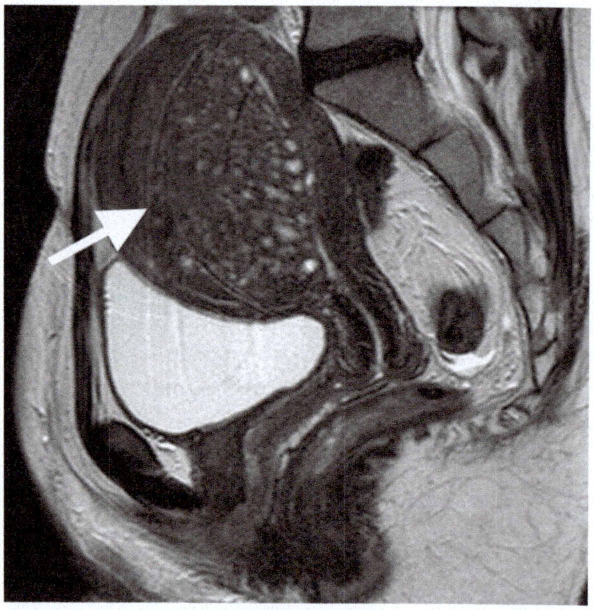

Fig. 8.31 Adenomyosis. T2-W sagittal image showing an ill-defined mass that is widening the junctional zone of the uterus (*arrow*). Note the foci of high T2 signal intensity in the mass, which is related to entrapped endometrial tissue and cystic dilatation of the glands

they contain hemorrhage. Gadolinium enhancement does not assist in diagnosis. Various values for the maximum thickness of the junctional zone have been proposed, but the consensus view is that it should be no thicker than 12 mm. A value in excess of this is highly predictive of the presence of adenomyosis. If the junctional zone is less than 8 mm, adenomyosis is very unlikely. Between 8 and 12 mm, diagnosis may rely on other features, such as the presence of localized hemorrhagic areas, poor definition of the junctional zone, and focal thickening of the junctional zone. The main differential diagnosis, clinically and radiologically, is with leiomyoma. MR, despite some overlap of features, is the most reliable method of preoperative diagnosis. This is an important point, since uterine leiomyoma may be treated conservatively, whereas the treatment for clinically debilitating adenomyosis is hysterectomy. Of note is that normal myometrial contractions can result in apparent thickening of the junctional zone, thereby mimicking adenomyosis. Another interesting fact is that in patients with adenomyosis treated and responding to GnRH agonist therapy, the lesion may become more demarcated resembling a leiomyoma.

Benign conditions of the cervix include Nabothian cysts, cervical stenosis, and cervical incompetence. Nabothian cysts result from distension of endocervical glands, and these very common lesions return high signal on T2-W images and are usually asymptomatic. Cervical stenosis may be congenital, inflammatory, iatrogenic, or neoplastic. MRI can identify the location of cervical stenosis and demonstrate neoplasms. It can also demonstrate the degree of distension of the proximal uterus by retained secretions.

8.7.1.5 Malignant Disease

Endometrial Carcinoma

Endometrial carcinoma is a common malignancy of the female genital tract in the developed world. Its peak incidence occurs between the ages of 55 and 65 years. Most patients present with postmenopausal bleeding or irregular bleeding, usually early in the course of disease. Patients are referred for dilatation and curettage if no obvious cause is found on clinical grounds. This allows for prompt diagnosis and treatment. Approximately 85% of endometrial carcinomas are adenocarcinomas, although papillary serous and clear-cell carcinomas, which carry a worse prognosis, may also be found. Endometrial carcinoma may spread locally. Lymphatic spread may be directly to para-aortic nodes. Most clinicians use the staging system of the Federation Internationale de Gynaecologie et d'Obstetrique (FIGO).

Tumor grade, stage of disease, and depth of myometrial invasion are the most important prognostic factors. Endometrial carcinoma usually manifests as a mass that, relative to normal endometrium, is hypo- to isointense on T1-W images and hyperintense or heterogeneous on T2-W images. Although MRI cannot reliably distinguish endometrial carcinoma from hyperplasia, it is helpful in cancer staging. Tumors are staged on the basis of depth of myometrial invasion. T2-W sequences in sagittal and transverse planes, as well as T1-W gadolinium-enhanced MRI are most helpful in demonstrating myometrial invasion. At contrast enhanced T1-W imaging, a carcinoma enhances less than the normal endometrium. The MR appearance of noninvasive endometrial carcinoma (stage IA) is nonspecific. Thickening of the endometrial stripe in postmenopausal women is a suspicious sign.

In patients with myometrial invasion (stage IB and IC), segmental or complete disruption of the junctional zone by a mass of intermediate signal intensity on T2-W sequence should be seen (Fig. 8.32). Using DCE

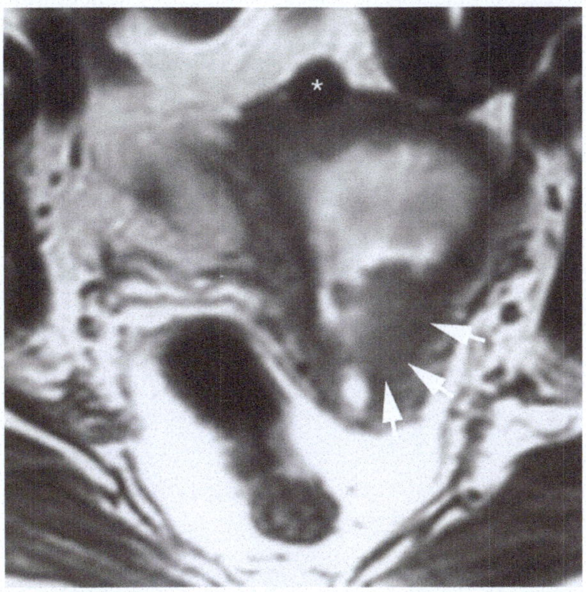

Fig. 8.32 Myometrial invasion of endometrial carcinoma. Axial T2-W image showing a mass arising from the left lower uterine segment (*arrows*). The intermediate signal intensity mass extends into the myometrium with loss of the normal junctional zone, indicating deep myometrial invasion. Incidental note is made of a fibroid (*asterisk*) at the fundus of the uterus

T1-W imaging, superficial invasion involves only the inner half of the myometrium, whereas deep invasion involves the outer half of the myometrium or beyond. If the normal low signal intensity junctional zone is intact, myometrial invasion is unlikely. If the junctional zone is thinned due to atrophy or distension from fluid/ tumor and poorly visualized, the presence of myometrial invasion may be inferred by an irregular endometrium-myometrium interface. For confidence in diagnosing myometrial invasion, disruption of the junctional zone should be seen on two imaging planes. There is overlap with the MR findings in adenomyosis, but once a histological diagnosis of carcinoma has been made, the MR signs can be interpreted with reasonable confidence. The percentage of myometrial invasion is estimated, separating patients into stage IB (less than 50% wall invasion) or stage IC (greater than 50% wall invasion). Superficial extension of endometrial carcinoma into the cervical mucosa (stage IIA) can be demonstrated on T2-W imaging by widening of the endocervical canal and internal os. If the low-signal intensity fibrous stroma of the cervix is invaded, stage IIB disease is diagnosed. MRI has been demonstrated to be an accurate technique for staging of early endometrial carcinoma. Fewer data are available in the literature regarding stage III and stage IV endometrial carcinoma, but MR is certainly capable of demonstrating bulky tumors with parametrial invasion, invasion of the vagina, and regional lymphadenopathy. It is less reliable in demonstrating peritoneal spread.

Endometrial sarcoma is a rare entity that often results in diffuse enlargement of the uterus. Although they can be difficult, if not impossible, to distinguish from myometrial invasive endometrial carcinoma, a feature that has been described in low-grade stromal sarcoma is bands of low signal intensity within the area of myometrial invasion on T2-W images. These bands represent strands of remnant myometrium in the tumor replaced mass.

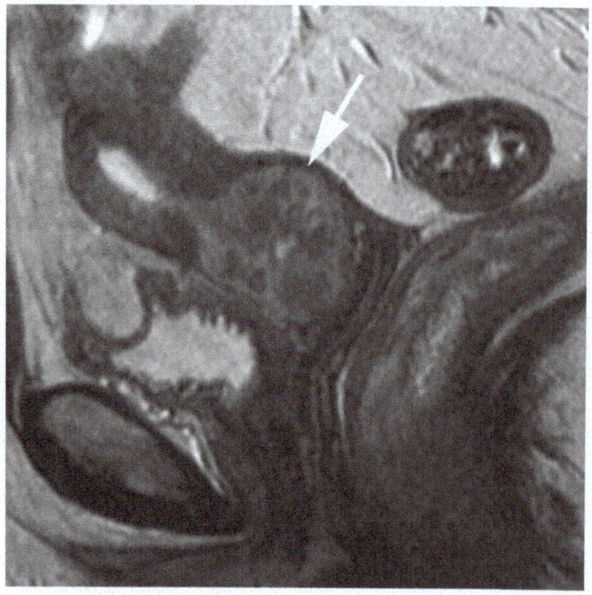

Fig. 8.33 Polypoidal growth of cervical cancer. T2-W sagittal image shows a polypoidal heterogeneous mass arising from the cervix which extends into the lower uterine segment (*arrow*). The appearance is typical for cervical cancer

Cervical Carcinoma

Cervical carcinoma is the third most common malignancy of the female genital tract in the developed world, but it is also extremely common in Africa. Screening by cytology picks up cervical intraepithelial neoplasia, which is considered to be a precursor of cervical carcinoma. The disease may, therefore, be picked up when asymptomatic. It is estimated that 80–90% of cervical carcinomas are squamous cell carcinomas, but adenocarcinoma is undoubtedly becoming more common and carries a worse prognosis. In women under 35 years of age, most cervical carcinomas arise from the squamocolumnar junction, which lies on the vaginal surface of the cervix. These tumors grow in a polypoid fashion (Fig. 8.33). In older women, most tumors occur within the endocervical canal, resulting in a barrel-shaped cervix. Tumors located within the cervical canal are more difficult to evaluate clinically and have a high incidence of parametrial invasion (Fig. 8.34). Cervical carcinoma is usually staged clinically, using the FIGO system, despite its well-known limitations.

T2-W sequences provide optimal contrast between tumors and the normal cervical structures. Cervical cancers appear as hyperintense masses on T2-W images regardless of histopathological type. Sagittal and oblique transverse imaging planes will normally evaluate local tumor extension accurately. Oblique coronal sections may be useful in providing additional information regarding the parametrium and the lateral vaginal fornices. It has been suggested that DCE T1-W studies may be helpful in diagnosing parametrial invasion and predicting radiosensitivity.

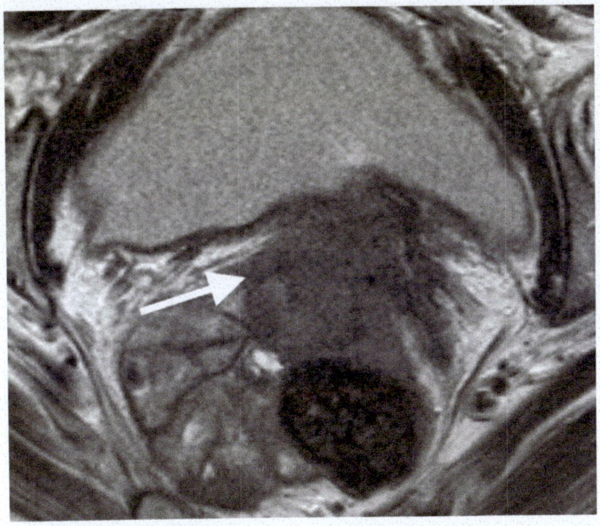

Fig. 8.34 Parametrial invasion by cervical cancer. T2-W axial image showing right parametrial invasion (*arrow*) by cervical cancer

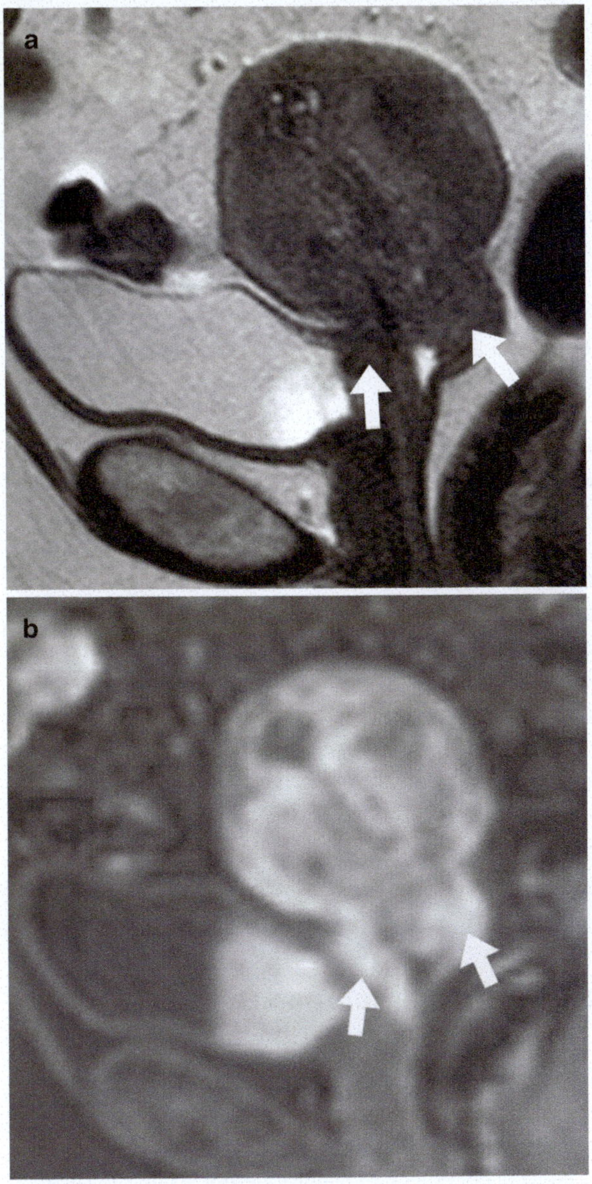

Fig. 8.35 Increased enhancement of cervical cancer. (**a**) T2-W image and (**b**) contrast enhanced T1-W fat-suppressed image showing increased contrast uptake of the cervical cancer (*arrows*)

Carcinoma in situ or microinvasive tumors (stage IA) are not normally identified by MRI. However, MR will identify tumors that invade the fibrous stroma, despite relatively normal-appearing epithelium. Macroinvasive cervical carcinoma (stage IB) is defined as an invasive component greater than 5 mm in depth and 7 mm in horizontal spread; these appear on T2-W imaging as masses of intermediate or high signal intensity that deform the canal or disrupt the very low signal intensity fibrous band. The lateral margins of the cervix, which are formed by muscle in continuity with the outer myometrium, should remain smooth in stage IB disease. On T1-W imaging, cervical tumors are usually isointense with normal cervix, and the zonal anatomy is difficult to appreciate. Small tumors are, therefore, not visible on T1-W sequences unless gadolinium is given. Cervical carcinoma will demonstrate increased enhancement relative to cervical stroma (Fig. 8.35), which is most marked on images acquired within 60s of administration, using a dynamic sequencing technique.

Cervical carcinoma is classified as stage IIA when it invades the upper two-thirds of the vagina. On T2-W imaging, disruption of the vaginal wall or diffuse thickening with high signal intensity is a sign of tumor invasion. One of the crucial clinical decisions is in the diagnosis of stage IIB disease, in which parametrial invasion is present. Under most circumstances, surgery is not considered for these patients and radiotherapy is the treatment of choice. It has been shown that a complete intact ring of cervical stroma accurately excludes parametrial extension. However, full thickness disruption of the fibrous stroma with abnormal signal intensity in the parametrium has a significant false-positive rate in stage I tumors, and it seems that overstaging results from peritumoral inflammatory change.

Locally advanced (stage III or stage IV) disease is usually diagnosed clinically and can easily be confirmed with MRI. There is relatively little histologically correlated data in the literature, as these tumors are rarely removed. Large masses frequently invade the pelvic sidewall, bladder, and rectum. When large, cervical carcinomas return mixed signal on T2-W and low signal on T1-W imaging. T2-W imaging is useful in demonstrating tumor invading muscles, such as levator ani, obturator internus, or pyriformis, as the muscles are usually of lower intensity than the invading tumor. T1-W sequences maximize contrast if there is sufficient fat in the pelvis. Fat-suppression techniques may also be helpful in clarifying anatomy.

Following radiotherapy for cervical carcinoma, diagnosis of suspected recurrent disease is a frequent and difficult clinical problem. Later than 12 months after completion of radiation treatment, the uterus and cervix should return low signal. However, during the initial 6–12 months after treatment, developing radiation changes may return high signal, due to inflammation and increased vascularity. Enhancement with gadolinium is not normally seen later than 12 months after radiation treatment. However, the rate of development of the typical hypointense signal from radiation fibrosis is extremely variable from patient to patient, and abnormal signal may persist for years. Recurrent tumor should, therefore, be diagnosed on the basis of a demonstrable mass, rather than on signal change alone.

8.7.2 Parametrium and Ovaries

MRI is capable of diagnosing adnexal masses as cystic or solid, and can characterize the components as fluid, fatty, or hemorrhagic. Up-to-date machinery using pelvic phased-array coils can usually demonstrate the ovaries and parametrial structures on T2-W SE sequences, axial and coronal planes being most useful. T1-W SE sequences following gadolinium may be helpful, as may fat-suppressed images. The fat suppressed T1-W sequences are helpful in distinguishing the presence of fat vs. hemorrhage. Transvaginal ultrasound remains the investigation most commonly performed first for investigation of the ovaries. However, in selected cases, MRI can yield additional information.

In women of reproductive age, the normal ovaries may demonstrate zonal anatomy on T2-W imaging. The medulla has slightly higher signal intensity than the cortex. Cysts are frequently seen, returning high signal on T2-W sequences. On T1-W sequences, follicular cysts have thin walls, which enhance variably (Fig. 8.36). Thick enhancing rims are typical of the corpus luteum, which is also prone to hemorrhage. Bizarre and complex cystic structures with irregular thickening and enhancement should raise a suspicion of malignant disease. Solid tumors are also frequently malignant (Fig. 8.37), although benign teratoma masses may demonstrate areas of signal intensity consistent with fat.

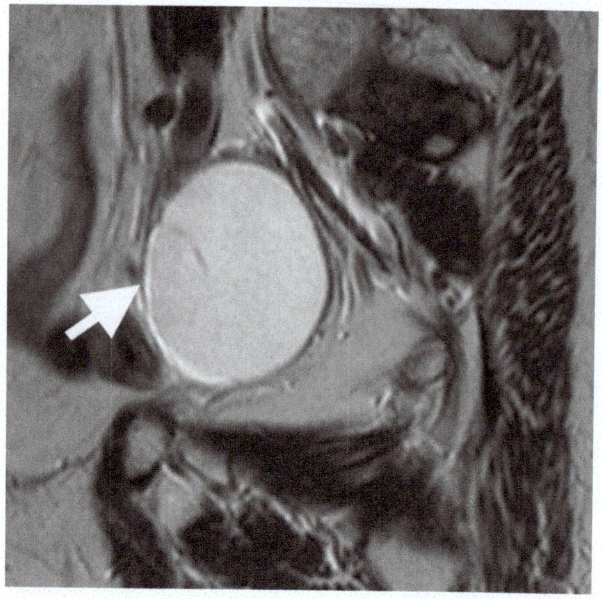

Fig. 8.36 Benign ovarian cyst. T2-W sagittal image reveals a large thin walled left adnexal cyst with a thin internal septum. No solid soft tissue component detected. The appearance is benign

Pelvic inflammatory disease is fundamentally a clinical diagnosis. Tubo-ovarian abscess, a well-recognized complication of pelvic inflammatory disease, can be demonstrated by MR, although transvaginal ultrasound remains the imaging investigation of first choice.

Endometriosis is defined as the presence of functional endometrial glands and stroma outside the uterine cavity. The condition afflicts women of childbearing age, with a mean age of diagnosis in the mid to late twenties. However, about 5% of endometriosis reportedly occurs in postmenopausal women and this is believed to be related to hormone replacement therapy. The most widely used staging system for endometriosis is that proposed by the American Fertility Society based on the 1985 Revised Classification of Endometriosis. Three components are assessed using

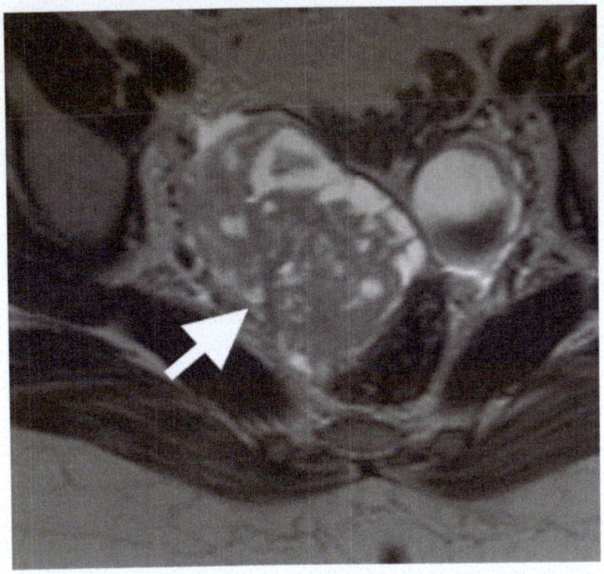

Fig. 8.37 Malignant ovarian tumor. T2-W axial image showing a predominantly solid right ovarian mass. Histopathology revealed small cell carcinoma of the right ovary. Incidental benign ovarian cyst also noted on the left

this system: evaluation of the endometrial implants (location, size, and depth of penetration), degree of cul-de-sac obliteration, and evaluation of adhesions (amount of surface area involvement and appearance).

In addition to standard T1-W and T2-W sequences, a T1-W fat-suppressed sequence should always be performed, which improves the sensitivity of lesion detection (Fig. 8.3). Administration of gadolinium-based contrast material is not always helpful as normal enhancing parametrium may be misinterpreted as disease. Endometriotic implants are usually multiple and often have a multilocular appearance. Endometriotic deposits contain blood products, thus often appearing as high signal intensity on T1- and T2-W images. However, endometriomas may also return high T1 signal but lowT2 signal. This is due to the chronic nature of many of these deposits, and this characteristic is used to differentiate them from other blood-containing lesions. Longstanding endometriomas become viscous and contain high concentrations of iron and protein, thus reducing their T2-relaxation time. Hemosiderin-laden macrophages along the fibrotic cyst wall can also result in a low signal intensity rim on both T1- and T2-W images. However, the diagnosis of small endometriotic implants remains challenging.

8.8 Future Developments

Diffusion-weighted imaging (DWI) is an MRI technique that is increasingly being applied in the body for disease assessment. Cellular tissues in the body restrict the mobility of water which is detected at DWI. The key advantages of this technique are that it is relatively quick to perform, does not require the administration of an exogenous contrast, and yields both qualitative and quantitative information.

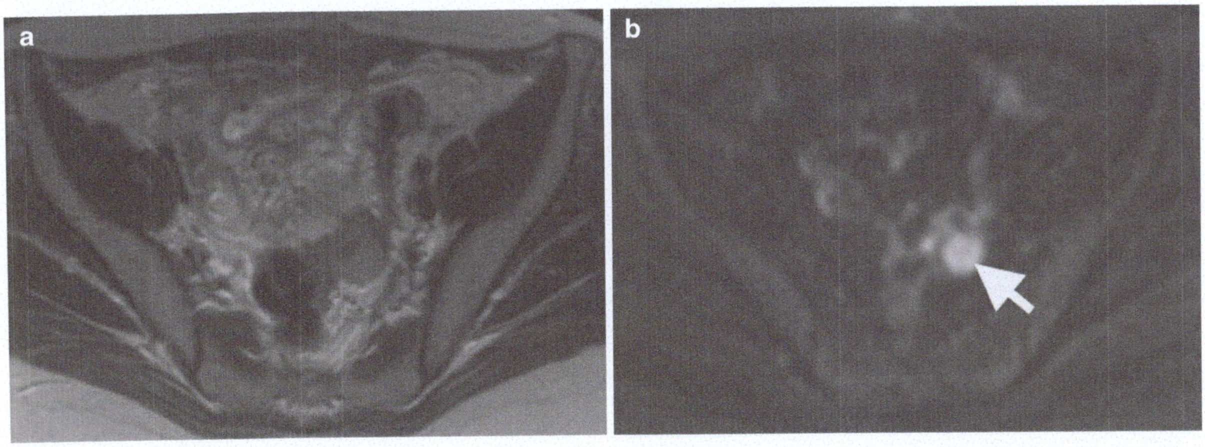

Fig. 8.38 Detection of peritoneal disease using diffusion-weighted MRI in a woman with history of ovarian cancer. (**a**) T2-W axial and (**b**) diffusion-weighted axial MR image acquired with a strong diffusion-weighting (b = 900 s/mm²). A high signal intensity focus of peritoneal/serosal disease is readily detected on the diffusion-weighted imaging (*arrow*), but is more difficult to discern on the T2-W image

Early experience with the technique has shown that DWI can be used to detect prostate, cervical, and endometrial carcinomas. In prostate cancer, it has also been shown that the addition of DWI to conventional T2-W imaging improves the detection of tumor compared with T2-W MRI alone. The technique has also been found to be helpful for the detection and characterization of uterine and cervical pathologies, as well as demonstrating sites of peritoneal disease in patients with gynecological malignancies (Fig. 8.38). Research is also being undertaken to evaluate the potential of this technique for the diagnosis of nodal metastases, and for the evaluation of treatment response. A recent study has also highlighted the potential of DWI for the detection of malignant lymph nodes in patients with uterine and cervical cancers.

Further Reading

Brown G (ed) (2008) Contemporary issues in cancer imaging: colorectal cancer. Cambridge University Press, Cambridge

Futterer JJ, Engelbrecht MR, Jager GJ et al (2007) Prostate cancer: comparison of local staging accuracy of pelvic phased-array coil alone versus integrated endorectal-pelvic phased-array coils. Local staging accuracy of prostate cancer using endorectal coil MR imaging. Eur Radiol 17:1055–1065

Hricak H, Scardino P (eds) (2008) Contemporary issues in cancer imaging: prostate cancer. Cambridge University Press, Cambridge

Imaoka I, Wada A, Kaji Y et al (2006) Developing an MR imaging strategy for diagnosis of ovarian masses. Radiographics 26:1431–1448

Koh DM, Dzik-Jurasz A, O'Neill B, Tait D, Husband JE, Brown G (2008) Pelvic phased-array MR imaging of anal carcinoma before and after chemoradiation. Br J Radiol 81:91–98

MacVicar D (ed) (2008) Contemporary issues in cancer imaging: bladder cancer. Cambridge University Press, Cambridge

MERCURY Study Group (2007) Extramural depth of tumor invasion at thin-section MR in patients with rectal cancer: results of the MERCURY study. Radiology 243:132–139

Reznek R (ed) (2007) Contemporary issues in cancer imaging: cancer of the ovary. Cambridge University Press, Cambridge

Seidenwurm D, Smathers RL, Lo RK, Carrol CL, Bassett J, Hoffman AR (1987) Testes and scrotum: MR imaging at 1.5 T. Radiology 164:393–398

Sohaib SA, Reznek RH (2007) MR imaging in ovarian cancer. Cancer Imaging 7(Spec No A):S119–S129

Vilanova JC, Barcelo J (2007) Prostate cancer detection: magnetic resonance (MR) spectroscopic imaging. Abdom Imaging 32:253–261

9 MRI of the Chest

Hans-Ulrich Kauczor and Edwin J. R Van Beek

Contents

H.-U. Kauczor (✉)
Department of Diagnostic and Interventional Radiology, University of Heidelberg, Im Neuenheimer Feld 110, 69120 Heidelberg, Germany
e-mail: Hans-Ulrich.Kauczor@med.uni-heidelberg.de

An excellent soft tissue contrast and the capacity to produce cross-sectional images or three-dimensional data sets in any orientation designate magnetic resonance imaging (MRI) as an ideal tool to evaluate chest wall masses or tumors of the mediastinum. However, traditionally, MRI of the lung was limited because of the combination of motion artifacts of both lungs and heart and the low number of protons. Furthermore, the susceptibility artifacts as a result of the interface of air and soft tissues were hampering efforts to perform MRI in the lungs. More recently, the development of fast (breath-hold) sequences, introduction of novel contrast agents and contrast mechanisms, has caused chest MRI to gain ground in the imaging of an increasing range of chest pathologies. As X-ray and computed tomography (CT) are increasingly criticized for the associated radiation exposure, particularly when applied for frequent follow-up examinations, during pregnancy, in children, and in clinical trials, a noninvasive method lacking ionizing radiation is desirable. In this chapter, we present the technical requirements, a comprehensive routine protocol, current clinical indications, and ongoing developments of chest MRI.

9.1 Technical Demands

9.1.1 Coils, Planes, and Positioning

Chest MRI relies on positioning of radiofrequency (RF) coils in close proximity to the body. This requires advanced array coil design, which has to take into account both the size and shape of the body, as well as the changing diameters due to respiration. This generally implies that coils are made of at least two parts or are made of flexible material. Thus, most RF coils used

P. Reimer et al. (eds.), *Clinical MR Imaging*,
DOI: 10.1007/978-3-540-74504-4_9, © Springer-Verlag Berlin Heidelberg 2010

consist of phased array design, albeit some modifications (such as wrap around coils) are also increasingly used. Additionally, high-resolution imaging of the chest wall sometimes requires dedicated surface coils, e.g., spine coil, or the selective use of individual arrays of the phased-array body coil.

The traditional CT imaging methods relied heavily on axial planes, albeit the introduction of multislice CT makes it possible to reconstruct in other planes. For MRI, axial images remain useful, especially when comparison with CT has to be made. However, the coronal plane has a major advantage because it covers the entire chest and can show delineation of structures such as the diaphragm more clearly. For possible chest wall involvement, one may have to rely on the sagittal plane, and this is also true for superior sulcus masses where vascular or brachial plexus involvement is suspected. Furthermore, MRI has the inherent advantage of lack of ionizing radiation, which is a current topic in view of legal requirements.

In general, the patient is positioned supine and will enter the MR system head first. In most situations, patients will be requested to keep the arms down along the body. However, for high-resolution imaging of the mediastinum or blood vessels, it is usually better to have the arms up as this reduces wraparound artifacts.

9.1.2 Factors Affecting Image Quality

The visualization of the normal lung parenchyma using MRI is extremely difficult. The spatial resolution, which can be obtained by MRI, is inherently lower than that obtained with CT. CT, performed as either spiral CT with high resolution CT or multislice CT, is generally accepted as the radiological gold standard for visualization of the morphology of the lung parenchyma. It yields excellent results of almost isotropic voxels at 0.4–1 mm. Several technical challenges need to be addressed in order to obtain diagnostic quality MR images of the chest. These are discussed in the following paragraphs.

9.1.2.1 Signal Loss Due to Physiological Motion

The major problem in imaging thoracic organs is the continuous physiological motion, which comes from several sources. The main contributors are (1) the lungs, (2) the heart and large blood vessels, and (3) blood motion. These adverse effects are most prominent in the lower and anterior sections of the chest. Technical difficulties to overcome these effects are one major reason why MRI of the chest was, for a long time, confined to the posterior chest wall and the thoracic outlet. Both locations are relatively static and can be examined with classical T1- and T2-weighted (T2-W) spin-echo and fast spin-echo techniques.

Respiratory Motion

Respiratory motion is the most important influence on image quality in chest MRI. It leads to blurring, loss of delineation, and decreased resolution. The simplest technique, which is very effective in reducing motion artifacts, is breath-hold imaging. This requires sequences with acquisition times well below 30 s. For this purpose, half-Fourier single-shot sequences (such as fast low-angle shot sequence, FLASH or half Fourier acquired single-shot turbo spin-echo sequence, HASTE) have been used successfully. As a result of its simplicity and good results, this approach has gained wide acceptance and application. Longer acquisitions can be split and acquired within several breath holds. However, splitting the acquisition introduces additional artifacts if the breath holds are not reproducible. The disadvantage of breath-holding is the usually lower spatial resolution and higher signal-to-noise ratio (SNR). For the chest wall and the mediastinum, clear T1- and T2-contrast can be mandatory, particularly for the characterization of mediastinal masses. Since conventional spin-echo- and fast spin-echo imaging requires acquisition times of several minutes, dedicated techniques are needed.

The most straightforward method to directly compensate for respiratory motion is a simple pneumatic belt or a compressible cushion placed at the upper abdomen or the chest of the patient. The ideal position of the device depends on the individual breathing pattern of the patient at rest. The changes of pressure during inspiration and expiration lead to compression and decompression of the device, which is fed back into the MR scanner. The trigger signal is usually set to expiration as this is the longest and most reproducible phase of the respiratory cycle. Imaging at end-expiration might be favorable for imaging lung parenchyma disease, since signal intensity increases with deflation. However, appropriate instructions of the patient remain the key to high image quality without respiratory motion artifacts.

More sophisticated techniques apply navigator sequences for monitoring the movements of the diaphragm with continuous real-time image acquisition from a small volume placed at the top of the diaphragm. The images are evaluated electronically, and trigger settings can be applied interactively. As a disadvantage, respiratory motion cannot be monitored during acquisition of the diagnostic images when the navigator has to be suppressed. It is therefore recommended to additionally apply a respiratory belt, if available, for uninterrupted control of the breathing maneuvers. Similarly, navigator techniques can be also used to adjust several slice blocks of a multibreath-hold acquisition in case of a variable depth of inspiration.

Higher number of acquisitions will also reduce the severity of breathing artifacts by averaging. A weakness of these methods is the fact that it prolongs the data acquisition time, thus resulting in extended overall imaging time. This can be especially problematic in dyspneic patients and when fast physiological effects (such as blood flow or respiratory motion) need to be assessed.

Cardiac and Large Blood Vessel Motion

Cardiac pulsation may be overcome with single-shot techniques such as T2-HASTE or ultra fast turbo-spin-echo (UTSE) using very short echo times (TE). ECG triggering has been widely advocated to reduce cardiac and vascular pulsation artifacts, such as ghosting artifacts in the phase-encoding direction and blurring. Triggering in diastole gives more time to obtain data, whereas triggering in systole has the advantage of a more constant time profile. Reordering of phase encoding is mainly employed to reduce blurring of lung parenchyma adjacent to the heart and great vessels. Similar to respiratory gating methods, ECG triggering will prolong the imaging time. Simultaneous double-triggering or gating for respiration and cardiac pulsation is usually not favorable. Fast sequences such as single-shot-turbo-spin-echo, fast low angle shot gradient echo, and T1-W 3D gradient echo such as volume interpolated breath hold examination (VIBE) are usually quite robust to cardiac motion. Their image quality largely depends more on the breath-hold capability than on compensation for cardiac motion.

Blood Motion

ECG triggering in systole can be used to obtain images during higher blood velocity, thus resulting in a greater flow void effect (black blood imaging). However, a disadvantage is the reduction in data acquisition time, thus leading to longer imaging intervals. Increasing the number of RF pulses can also be used to reduce blood motion effects, although this can interfere with the technique one wishes to employ.

9.1.2.2 Susceptibility Artifacts

Susceptibility artifacts are very closely related to specific morphology of ventilated lung. The unique combination of air and soft tissue that constitutes inflated lung is the cause for significant susceptibility artifacts since air-tissue interfaces induce local gradients. These gradients lead to inhomogeneities of the magnetic field, producing a complex spectrum of frequencies, which are spread across up to 9 ppm. They also lead to signal loss from intravoxel phase dispersion reflected by a short T2*. While imaging of the normal parenchyma is rather difficult due to susceptibility artifacts, it is much easier to image consolidations within the lung. The loss of air and the concomitant increase of tissue, cells, or fluid significantly reduce the number of air-tissue interfaces and subsequently the degree of susceptibility artifacts. T2* values increase from 7 ms in normal lungs to 35 ms in atelectatic lung and to more than 140 ms in lung tumors. This very short T2* in the normal parenchyma has an important impact on gradient-recalled echo (GRE) sequences, wherein they lead to blurring of pulmonary structures, which is much more obvious than when using spin-echo (SE) sequences. At the same time, the short T2 relaxation time of the pulmonary parenchyma influences GRE and SE sequences in the same way.

Different strategies have been proposed to reduce susceptibility artifacts. Use of short TE for T1-W SE or GRE sequences have been employed. Ultra-short TE (50–250 μs), as part of projection-reconstruction techniques, have been successfully applied to the lung parenchyma. They result in a significant improvement of the SNR. Alternatively, one can apply T2-W turbo-spin-echo (TSE) sequences or T2-W ultra-fast TSE sequences with high turbo factors. Finally, one can minimize susceptibility artifacts by using multiple 180° RF refocusing pulses.

9.1.2.3 Signal-to-Noise Ratio

Since about two thirds of the lung consists of air and only one third is tissue and blood, hence, the density of spins is markedly lower than in any other organ. The low spin density is the major drawback for MRI of the lung, especially for the visualization of lung diseases with loss of tissue, such as emphysema. In other lung diseases, however, pathological processes result in an increased amount of tissue, fluid, and/or cells. Thus, a higher number of protons (spins) become available, and significant improvements of the SNR can be achieved. To benefit from the higher number of spins, T1-W SE sequences with short TE (<7 ms), T1-W GRE sequences, like fast low angle single shot half Fourier (FLASH), with short TE (3 ms), or a higher number of acquisitions are recommended. The short TE are particularly important to avoid signal loss from T2 relaxation resulting in a significant increase of the SNR. For this purpose, GRE sequences are superior to SE sequences.

9.2 Pulse Sequences and Contrast Mechanisms

9.2.1 Pulse Sequences

When imaging the chest, the pulse sequences used are relatively limited due to constraints of motion and susceptibility artifacts. Generally, fast imaging sequences using short TR and short TE have been most successfully applied. Parallel imaging techniques are now capable to acquire 3D data sets of the whole chest with voxel sizes of down to 1.6 × 1.6 × 4 mm or isotropic voxels of 2 × 2 × 2 mm within one breath hold. The result of parallel imaging is a substantial (two- or threefold) improvement in image acquisition speed. The recommended protocols of Table 9.1 are based on parallel acquisition techniques, but, alternatively, multibreath-hold acquisitions can be applied if parallel imaging techniques are not available. Fat-suppressed imaging using inversion recovery (IR) techniques are

Table 9.1 Overview of some commonly used MRI sequences for the lung

T2	• FSE/HASTE with breathhold • Fat saturation may increase image contrast • Coronal orientation; TE = 550 ms; TR = 30 ms; FA = 180°; TA = 25 s • TSE multishot with motion correction (BLADE): TE = 4600 ms; TE = 100 ms; FA = 150° • TSE with respiratory triggering: TE = 1700 ms (approximately Resp/2); TE = 122 ms; FA = 150°
T1	• 3D GRE sequence (FLASH) • Breathhold recommended • TR = 3–7 ms; TE = 1.8–2.2 ms; FA = 15–30°
SSFP	• To be applied in breathhold and continuous breathing • TR = 318 ms; TE = 1.2 ms; FA = 80° • Provide signal in fluid and vessels
Inversion recovery	• Fat saturation (STIR, TIRM) • TR = 3500 ms; TE = 106; FA = 150°
T1 +/– Gd	• 3D GRE with breathhold; volume interpolation (VIBE) • Fat saturation • TR = 3.4–5.2 ms; TE = 1.4–1.9 ms; FA = 8–12° • Same imaging plane should be used before and after gadolinium-chelate injection
Contrast-enhanced MRA	• 3D GRE with high spatial resolution (FLASH) • Breathhold recommended • TR = 3.0–5.5 ms; TE = 1.1–1.8 ms; FA = 25–40°
Multiphasic MRA; perfusion	• 3D GRE with high temporal resolution (TREAT, TRICKS) • Allows for time-resolved angiography and perfusion MRI of the lung • TR = 1.64 ms; TE = 0.64 ms; FA = 40°

useful to assess mediastinal and chest wall masses. It will also yield relative signal enhancement from the lung. Furthermore, Gadolinium (Gd) chelates have been used for vascular and mass enhancement. Postcontrast images should include fat-suppression techniques in the assessment of masses. Dynamic contrast techniques may be used for vascular studies and in the assessment of pulmonary masses or nodules. Newer contrast agents are also undergoing clinical trials, which are described elsewhere.

Table 9.1 gives an overview of the sequences that are most commonly employed. Some variation may exist between the various MR systems, and they should be seen as a rough guide to successful MRI of the chest.

9.2.2 Contrast Mechanisms

9.2.2.1 Natural Contrast

In all lung diseases with an increase of the amount of tissue, fluid, and/or cells, the number of protons is increased, and a higher signal can be obtained. This is referred to as the disease-related contrast mechanism leading to a higher SNR. Unfortunately, T1-W contrast of fluid inside lung tissue is too low to be diagnostic, and T2-W sequences, such as single-shot techniques with partial-Fourier acquisition (e.g., HASTE) or ultra short TE (UTSE), have to be used. It may be favorable for particular purposes such as imaging of the mediastinum to apply such sequences with a dark blood preparation pulse, but this may reduce the sensitivity for lung infiltrates.

However, in many cases, such a disease-related increase of spin density is not sufficient for accurate delineation, characterization, and diagnosis of the disease process. For this purpose, different contrast agents and more advanced contrast mechanisms can be used.

9.2.2.2 Contrast Agents

The most common technique is the intravenous administration of contrast agents, like Gd-chelates, which lead to an iatrogenic increase of the relaxivity of existent spins. These contrast agents are used for the enhancement of nodules or opacifications, MR angiography (MRA), or perfusion imaging. Newer contrast agents, such as Gd-based blood pool agents and ultra-small super-paramagnetic iron oxide (USPIO) particles, are also under development. Gadolinium in the form of a diethylene triamine pentaacetate (DTPA) chelate has also been applied in aerosolized form to assess the airways. Hyperpolarized noble gases can be inhaled, giving rise to novel information of lung morphology and function. Finally, the application of inhaled oxygen has been investigated for ventilation imaging.

Gadolinium-Chelates Intravenous Administration

The basic principles of Gd-contrast are described in Chap. 1. Paramagnetic contrast agents enable better characterization and delineation of pathological processes, such as identification of benign vs. malignant nodules and in the definition of tumors from essential structures. Finally, it is possible to investigate disease activity, such as pulmonary fibrosis and alveolitis. The standard Gd-chelates have the disadvantage that they are rapidly excreted and leave the blood compartment. So-called blood pool agents remain in the blood compartment and offer advantages in terms of sequence design for MRA.

Aerosolized Gadolinium-Chelates

Commercially available Gd-DTPA can be diluted, aerosolized, and applied using a nebulizer. This method has only been applied in animal models, but did show a 70–120% increase in signal intensity of lung parenchyma. This technology offers good potential for the future use in assessment of small airway diseases.

Oxygen Enhancement

Higher oxygen concentrations administered via inhalation will induce different paramagnetic effects and lead to a dose-dependent increase of signal intensity. Scans acquired after breathing normal room air (20% oxygen) are subtracted from scans acquired after breathing 100% oxygen using an inhalation mask. Subtraction is indispensable because the increase in signal intensity is rather low. The increase of signal intensity is explained by enhancement of lung parenchyma due to the presence of dissolved molecular oxygen. The highest increase of signal is found in the pulmonary veins. This technique seems to be applicable in clinical routine if adequate postprocessing tools are available. It might be a complementary technique in the diagnosis of pulmonary embolism (PE) and in the assessment of oxygen uptake in obstructive and interstitial lung disease.

Iron Compounds

A number of agents, which are based on USPIO crystals or particles, are under development and undergoing preclinical and clinical trials. They are kept in solution by means of a coating. They can be applied for MR lymphography (as discussed below) or as blood pool agents for MRA.

9.2.2.3 Nonproton MRI

The use of hyperpolarized noble gases (He-3 and Xe-129) is a new approach to overcome the low spin density in the airspaces when administered as an "inhaled contrast agent." The spin density of the noble gases that represents the source of the MR signal is significantly increased by optical pumping (five magnitudes above thermal equilibrium), which compensates for the 2,500 times lower density of the gas as compared to proton concentrations in tissue. The decay of the hyperpolarization as given by the T1 relaxation time is dependent on the environment. For MRI of pulmonary ventilation, 300–1,500 mL of hyperpolarized He-3/Nitrogen mixture is inhaled. Normal ventilation corresponds to a homogeneous high signal intensity visualization of the airways and airspaces with rapid filling and distribution of He-3 gas within trachea and lungs. This technology is currently undergoing clinical trials with the use of hyperpolarized He-3 for ventilation imaging. The main disadvantages are the limited availability of He-3 gas, the complexity of producing hyperpolarization, and the need for multinuclear MR capabilities. However, there are great expectations for this technology, as shown below.

9.2.3 MR Angiography

In general, 3D techniques with minimum relaxation time (TE) of less than 5 ms and TE of less than 2 ms are used for contrast-enhanced MRA (CEMRA) of the pulmonary arteries. A short TR allows for short breath-hold acquisitions. A short TE minimizes background signal and susceptibility artifacts. Different flip angles were proposed ranging from 15 to 40°, and up to 70°. Adequate timing of the contrast agent (0.1–0.2 mmol/kg) administered by an automatic power injector is essential to achieve high contrast between pulmonary artery branches and surrounding structures. In general, arterial opacification should be predominant since the pulmonary veins are of minor diagnostic importance. Since the time gap between opacification of pulmonary arteries and veins is very short, selective visualization of vascular territories is difficult. To achieve a compact bolus, flow rates between 2 and 5 mL/s followed by a saline flush (20 mL) are recommended. The saline flush will ensure that the whole amount of contrast medium contributes to vessel opacification.

CEMRA is especially useful for imaging complex and slow flow with different spatial orientations, which is rather common in the pulmonary vascular system. In the clinical setting, shortening of acquisition time is of paramount importance for dyspneic patients suspected of PE. This holds particularly true since breath-holding in deep inspiration is strongly recommended for CEMRA. In adults, up to 18 s breath-hold periods are usually achieved; however, in concomitant pulmonary disease, this may be substantially less. If breath-holding is not possible, imaging during shallow breathing will still be diagnostic in most cases despite significant deterioration of image quality. The quality criteria for pulmonary CEMRA are (in decreasing importance) as follows: (1) complete visualization of the central (pulmonary trunk, main, and lobar arteries) and segmental pulmonary arteries with high signal, (2) high signal visualization of peripheral pulmonary arteries (subsegmental branches), (3) virtually selective visualization of the pulmonary arteries without significant superimposition by lung veins or the aorta and its side-branches. Several strategies have been advised to differentiate arteries and veins in case of superimposition: (1) cine or stack-mode viewing, (2) continuous rotation, (3) multiplanar reformation (MPR), or (4) maximum intensity projection (MIP). These strategies will help to identify the arteries and veins according to their

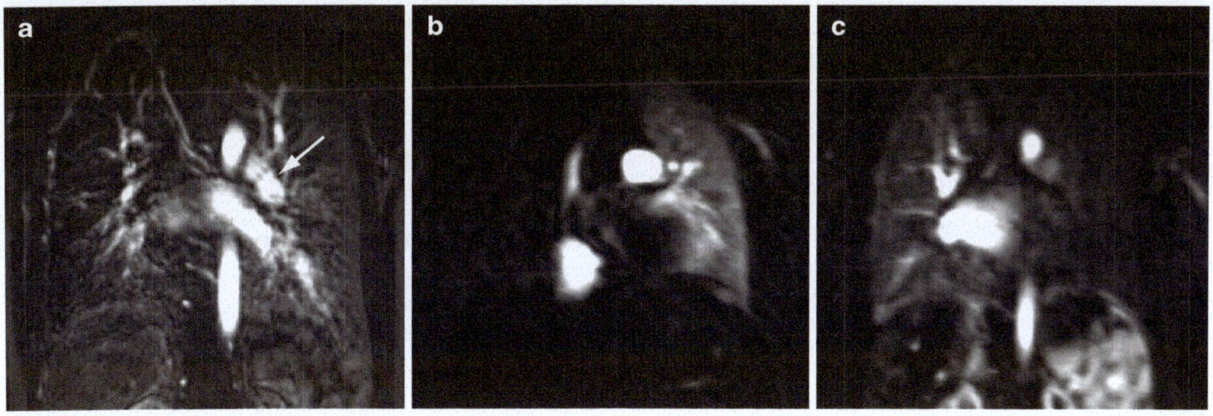

Fig. 9.1 Agenesis of the right pulmonary artery. (**a**) MR angiogram showing a normal pulmonary artery on the left (*arrow*), while the right pulmonary artery is missing. (**b**) MR perfusion early phase showing regular perfusion of the left lung, while there is no perfusion on the right side; (**c**) MR perfusion delayed phase showing perfusion of the right lung via major systemic collaterals

particular anatomical course (arteries have a steeper course, whereas veins have a more horizontal course within the chest).

An alternative approach is to optimize the sequence for high temporal resolution and perform a multiphasic acquisition. In time-resolved MRA, the scan time for an individual 3D data set is reduced to less than 5 s. The rationale is threefold. First, patients with severe respiratory disease and very limited breath-hold capabilities can be examined. Second, the arterial-venous discrimination is improved. Thus, more or less selective pulmonary arteriograms and venograms can be generated after subtraction of the data sets. This allows for characterization of vascular territories, especially in anomalies and shunts (Fig. 9.1). Finally, time-resolved multiphase CEMRA is independent from the bolus timing, since contrast injection and the MR sequence are started simultaneously.

9.2.4 Pulmonary Perfusion

MR perfusion imaging can be accomplished using either contrast-enhanced perfusion MRI or nonenhanced pulmonary arterial spin labeling (ASL) based on spin tagging.

The basic principle of contrast-enhanced perfusion MRI is a dynamic MR image acquisition following an intravenous bolus injection of a paramagnetic contrast agent. Perfusion MRI of the lung requires a high temporal resolution in order to visualize the peak enhancement of the lung parenchyma. Consequently, contrast-enhanced perfusion MRI uses T1-W ultrashort TR and TE gradient echo MRI. Depending on the spatial resolution, gradient hardware, and pulse sequence design, both 2D and 3D perfusion MRI techniques have been described.

The advantage of 2D perfusion MRI is the excellent temporal resolution of up to 0.3 s per image; however, there is limited anatomic coverage and insufficient spatial resolution in the *z*-axis. Fortunately, with the introduction of parallel imaging techniques, 3D perfusion imaging with a high spatial and temporal resolution as well as an improved anatomic coverage and *z*-axis resolution can now be achieved and should be preferred in clinical practice. Various injection protocols have been described for contrast-enhanced perfusion MRI. However, only few studies have assessed the influence of the contrast agent dose and injection rate on the degree and duration of pulmonary enhancement. High injection rates (i.e., faster than 3 mL/s) and low injection volumes will improve the separation of pulmonary and systemic circulation, while higher contrast agent doses will increase the peak enhancement of the lung.

There are several ways of processing contrast-enhanced perfusion MRI data. For a better visualization of the perfusion signal, contrast-enhanced 3D perfusion MRI is usually processed by subtraction of a mask image data acquired before contrast bolus arrival (Fig. 9.1). A rather simple approach for a semi-quantitative analysis of contrast-enhanced perfusion MRI data consists of the calculation of signal time curves, SNR, and contrast-to-noise ratios (CNR) using region-of-interest (ROI) analysis of the signal of the lung tissue. In addition, MR perfusion can be quantified by using the indicator dilution principle. However, a linear relationship between the signal intensity of perfusion MR images and the concentration of the contrast agent is assumed when obtaining these measurements. The quantitative indices, such as relative regional transit time, blood volume, and blood flow, are derived from the time intensity curve, defined by the dynamic series of perfusion MR images.

Besides contrast-enhanced pulmonary perfusion MRI, nonenhanced perfusion MRI has also been evaluated. ASL uses the moving red blood cells as magnetic particles. Thus, the inflowing red blood cells can be visualized, providing information of lung perfusion. Although the effectiveness of ASL for the assessment of pulmonary perfusion has been demonstrated in a number of studies, this technique has not entered the stage of a clinical application in patients with respiratory diseases. Among the reasons for this are the more complex MRI technique, higher artifact susceptibility, and lower SNR compared to contrast-enhanced pulmonary perfusion MRI.

9.3 Lung and Pleura

9.3.1 Anatomy

The airways are made up of large central airways, which contain cartilage in their walls. These airways subsequently branch down to three lobes on the right and two lobes on the left. Following these lobar divisions, the lobes are further divided in segments and continue to divide down to the 16th order, which is the alveolar space itself. The airways are surrounded by connective tissue, and there are distinct neurovascular, lymphatic, and airway bundles within this lung structure.

The lung is surrounded by the visceral pleura, which has areas of invagination to give rise to the interlobar fissures. The chest wall is covered by the parietal pleura. Between the pleural surfaces, a small amount of fluid allows for smooth sliding of the lung during in- and expiration.

Proton MRI is capable of visualizing the central tracheobronchial tree, the pleura, and the interlobar fissures. Furthermore, the respiratory motion during inspiration and expiration can be visualized. More distal airways and the alveolar space can be visualized using different technologies for ventilation imaging, such as hyperpolarized He-3 MRI.

9.3.2 Pathology

9.3.2.1 Bronchogenic Carcinoma and Nodules

Bronchogenic Carcinoma

Imaging techniques have to detect, characterize, and stage malignant masses. Staging is based on the tumor, nodes, metastases (TNM) classification (Table 9.2). MRI seems more or less equivalent to CT in the staging of bronchogenic carcinoma. The primary tumor will appear hypo- to isointense as compared with paravertebral muscle. After the administration of Gd, a strong enhancement is observed (Figs. 9.2 and 9.3). It will be homogeneous in tumors smaller than 3 cm in diameter (T1 tumors) (Fig. 9.2), whereas larger carcinomas will also exhibit central necrosis (Fig. 9.3). T2 tumors (>3 cm in diameter) are easily depicted by MRI, as they are on both chest radiography and CT, when they are located in the periphery of the lungs. Delineation and staging are affected in case of poststenotic atelectasis. Here, MRI has some clear advantages (see below). Other particular advantages of MRI include the assessment of infiltration of adjacent structures, such as mediastinum,

Table 9.2 New TNM classification of bronchogenic carcinoma (short version)

T1	≤3 cm in greatest dimension
T2	>3 but ≤ 7 cm in greatest dimension; or involvement of the main brochures ≥ 2 cm distal to the carina, invasion of the visceral pleura, or atelectasis extending to the hilum but not involving the whole lung
T3	> 7 cm in greatest dimension; or invasion of the chest wall, diaphragm, mediastinal pleura, or pericardium, etc.; involvement of the main bronchus ≤ 2 cm distal to the carina; atelectasis of the complete lung; or separate tumor nodules in the same lobe
T4	Invasion of the mediastinum, heart, great vessels, trachea, oesophagus, etc.; or separate tumor nodules in a different ipsilateral lobe
N1	Metastasis to peribronchial or ipsilateral hilar lymph nodes
N2	Metastasis to ipsilateral mediastinal lymph nodes
N3	Metastasis to contralateral mediastinal lymph nodes

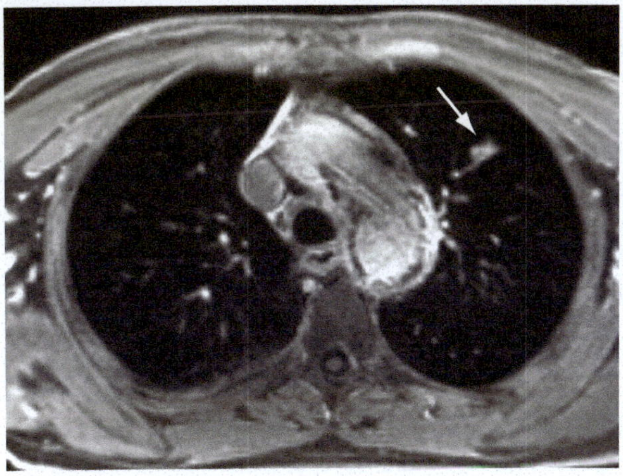

Fig. 9.2 Peripheral neuroendocrine bronchogenic carcinoma (T1). T1-WI after contrast showing a small nodule in the left upper lobe with a strong enhancement (*arrow*)

chest wall, and great vessels, which is relevant for staging (T3 and T4). The infiltration of the parietal pleura is one of the criteria for a T3 tumor. T2-W images in coronal or sagittal orientation yield best results in the evaluation of pleural thickening, extent of contact between tumor and pleura, and differentiation between visceral and parietal pleura. The high signal intensity of the tumor on T2-W images is in clear contrast to the muscles of the chest wall. MRI is well suited to study the direct infiltration of the mediastinum (T3 or T4 tumor). The expectation that MRI might be superior to CT has not been proven. Although changes within the mediastinal fat are easily depicted due to the high contrast resolution, the cause of these changes, whether malignant or inflammatory, frequently remains unclear. Obviously, broad infiltrations are easily delineated whereas small infiltrations are more difficult. The direct contact between tumor and mediastinum is not a reliable sign of infiltration. Additionally, the loss of the regular fatty demarcation is not specific. Signs for resectable infiltrations of the mediastinum are (1) contact between tumor and mediastinum <3 cm, (2) contact with the aorta <90° of the circumference, and (3) visible fat layer between tumor and adjacent structures. Definitive signs for non-resectability of large tumors (T4) are more difficult to define, as the management is dependent on the surgeon and the individual circumstances of the patient. The use of contrast does not seem to improve the evaluation. The direct acquisition of coronal or sagittal sections facilitates the delineation of infiltrations of the aorto-pulmonary window and the subcarinal space. This is also valid for the evaluation of a direct infiltration of the carina and the main bronchi, which requires distance measurements between the tumor and the carina.

MRI has some inherent advantages in the evaluation of the infiltrations of the chest wall. Definite proof, however, can only be derived from osseous destruction of a huge soft-tissue mass invading the chest wall. In addition, pain is a very specific sign. The loss of the extrapleural fat layer is often caused by reactive fibrotic or inflammatory changes. They can lead to false-positive results. The more extensive the changes are, the more likely the infiltration. On the other hand, the presence of a fat layer is a good indicator that no infiltration is present. Compared to CT, MRI seems to be at least equal if not superior in the evaluation of an infiltration of the chest wall with a sensitivity going up to 90% and an accuracy of 88%. T1-W images pre- and postcontrast will show the best resolution and a clear delineation. Tumor-identical changes within the extrapleural fat have a sensitivity of 85% and a specificity of 100% for an infiltration of the chest wall.

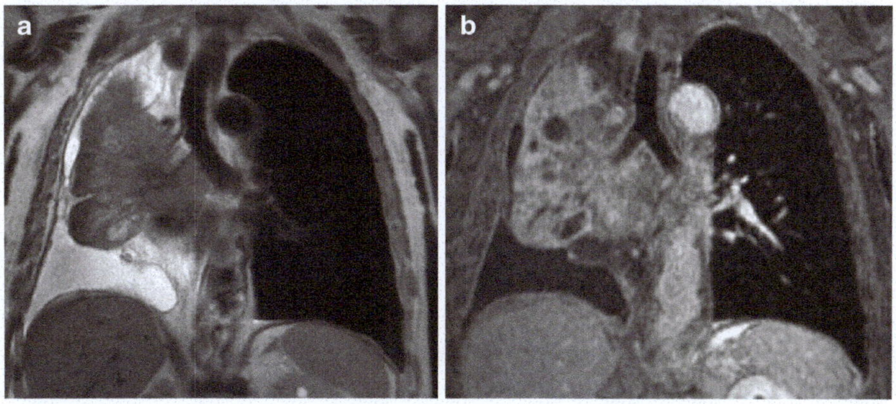

Fig. 9.3 Bronchogenic carcinoma of the right lung. (**a**) T2-WI showing a lobulated mass and a large pleural effusion; (**b**) T1-WI post contrast demonstrating tumor heterogeneity and mediastinal infiltration

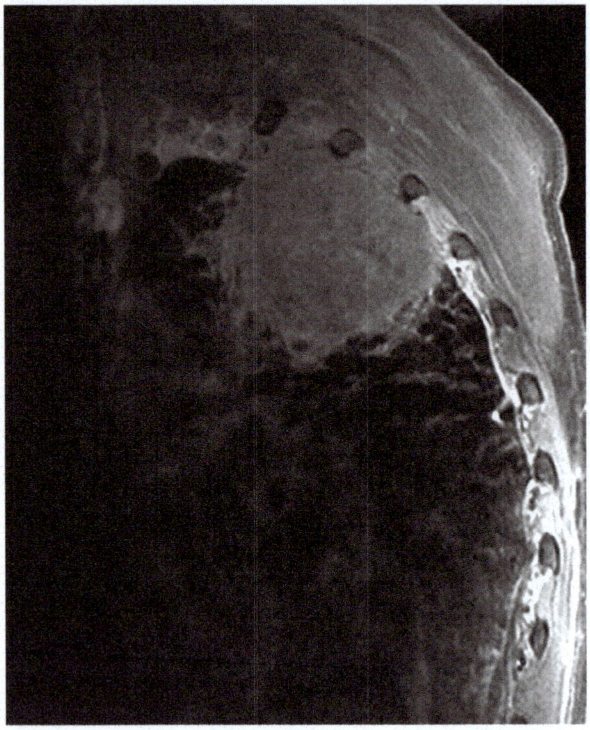

Fig. 9.4 Pancoast tumor with infiltration of the chest wall and cervico-thoracic junction. Fat-suppressed T1-WI after contrast showing a mass with infiltration of the pleura and soft tissue

MRI is regarded as the modality of choice for the investigation of superior sulcus (Pancoast) tumors. Direct coronal and sagittal acquisitions using fat suppression and T1-W imaging after contrast are recommended (Fig. 9.4). Infiltration through the lung apex is diagnosed on the basis of direct extension of the tumor into the extrapleural fat and the cervico-thoracic junction. These direct infiltrations and an involvement of the main blood vessels and the brachial plexus are far better observed on MRI than on CT.

At CT, the great vessels can only be evaluated after the application of a contrast agent. If there are contraindications for iodinated contrast, MRI (in spite of recent identification of side effects) remains the method of choice. Involvement of the great vessels can even be assessed using nonenhanced MR images with high contrast between the flow void within the vessels and the tumors exhibiting relatively high signal. Alternatively, MR contrast agent is much better tolerated than iodinated contrast media. The involvement of central pulmonary artery branches by tumor can be accurately evaluated using CEMRA, with a sensitivity of 80% and a specificity of 95%. Source images and MIP are used to recognize irregularities of the vascular wall or lumen as well as cut-offs of peripheral vessels. MRI is also superior to CT for the demonstration of endoluminal tumor spread within the superior vena cava, the pulmonary veins, and the heart chambers. Cine images are useful to separate slow-flowing blood from tumor infiltrations.

In summary, MRI and CT are equivalent in the T-staging of bronchogenic carcinoma with regard to a surgical or conservative therapeutic approach, with the sensitivity ranging between 43–63% for CT and 52–81% for MRI and the specificity between 94–97% for CT and 80–96% for MRI, respectively. For superior sulcus tumors, MRI is superior and should be the preferred modality.

Pulmonary Nodules

High contrast between nodules and underlying parenchyma is an inherent advantage of MRI, which might compensate for the relatively low spatial resolution (Fig. 9.2). Different techniques are available for the detection of pulmonary nodules. In general, the joined assessment of signal intensities and contrast enhancement is used to categorize nodules as malignant or benign. T2-W TSE images detected pulmonary metastases with an overall sensitivity of 84% as compared to CT, which served as the gold standard. The sensitivity is clearly size dependent. It was as low as 36% for tiny nodules (<5 mm) and increased steadily to 100% for nodules >15 mm. The combination of T1-W and T2*-W Turbo FLASH sequences without using contrast yielded similar results: sensitivity 82%, specificity 67%. A wide variety of different sequences have been applied in the detection of pulmonary nodules. Generally, fat-suppressed short tau inversion recovery (STIR), T2-W SE or GRE, such as ultra-fast TSE, and T1-W GRE, such as FLASH, pre- and postcontrast should be applied. The precontrast images are generally sufficient for detection of nodules. Dynamic acquisitions during and after the administration of contrast are advised for the characterization of the nodules. Malignant nodules are characterized by a fast increase in signal intensity during the first pass of the contrast agent. When smaller than 3 cm, they show a strong and homogeneous enhancement without significant necrosis. Granulomas, however, exhibit a significantly lower enhancement. Cysts typically do not enhance and follow fluid characteristics (low signal T1 and high signal T2).

9.3.2.2 Atelectasis and Pneumonia

Atelectasis

MRI is successful in the differentiation of different types of atelectasis as well as separation of central tumors from poststenotic atelectasis. Nonenhanced T1-W images show nearly identical low signal intensity from tumor and atelectasis. On T2-W imaging, obstructive atelectasis exhibits high signal, whereas nonobstructive atelectasis is hypointense. This is explained by the accumulation of secretions and fluid in obstructive atelectasis. For the same reason, poststenotic atelectasis in lung cancer also appears hyperintense on T2-W images and can be separated from central tumor, which appears hypointense. Contrast-enhanced T1-W images are also helpful. In most cases, the tumor will only enhance moderately together with a strong enhancement within the atelectasis. The tumor will be iso- or hyperintense with regards to the poststenotic changes after contrast administration in only a minority of cases. As in the characterization of pulmonary nodules, dynamic investigations are helpful in the differentiation. The poststenotic atelectasis will exhibit a fast enhancement (within the first 3 min) with a slow decrease thereafter, whereas the lung cancer will show a slow enhancement with a peak after about 10 min followed by a slow decrease of signal intensity.

Pneumonia

In inflammatory changes of lung parenchyma, the local increase in tissue fluid and cell infiltration results in much higher proton density and higher signal intensity. This leads to a high sensitivity of signs and patterns of specific diseases and septal, reticular, or nodular patterns can be more easily observed. Consolidation and ground-glass changes become even more pronounced, because the fluid increase affects the whole lung parenchyma and not only small structures. Accompanying atelectasis or effusions are likewise easy to be identified. Pneumonia will be isointense in T1- and hyperintense in T2-WIs (Fig. 9.5). Following contrast administration, there is usually a bright enhancement (Fig. 9.5). Likewise, bronchial wall thickening and mucus plugging result in increased signal intensity. MRI may also be used for the detection and characterization of inflammatory pulmonary infiltrates, particularly in immunocompromized patients. Invasive pulmonary aspergillosis (IPA) belongs to the most dangerous complications in these patients. Early detection and diagnosis of IPA are of great importance to introduce or continue antifungal therapy. In the early stages, IPA infections exhibit nodular or patchy infiltrates in the upper lobes. Enlargement of the infiltrates and/or development of segmental/lobar consolidations are typical for later stages, when they show their characteristic signs: (1) target sign on T1-WI with peripheral high signal due to hemorrhage and a hypointense center caused by central necrosis. After contrast administration, a strong rim enhancement reflecting active inflammation and central necrosis is seen. (2) hyperintense angiotropic consolidations on T1-WI indicating

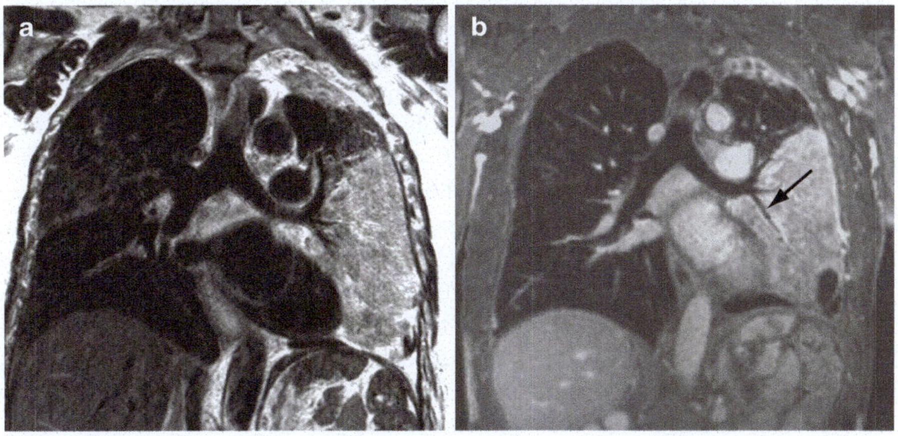

Fig. 9.5 Consolidating aspiration pneumonia in the left lung. (**a**) T2-WI showing a homogeneous infiltration with high signal intensity and a concomitant pleural effusion; (**b**) T1-WI after contrast showing a homogeneous infiltration with strong enhancement and positive bronchoaerograms (*arrow*)

hemorrhagic infarcts due to vascular invasion. (3) reverse target sign on T2-WI with high signal intensity in the centre indicating necrosis and a peripheral rim with low signal intensity. MRI is at least as sensitive as conventional chest X-ray in the detection of round infiltrates and possibly more specific than CT in the characterization of IPA and the depiction of central necrosis and pulmonary abscesses in different settings of pneumonia.

Lipoid pneumonia is a rather rare condition, induced by mineral oil aspiration in most cases. MRI has a high sensitivity on the detection of fat, which will exhibit high signal intensity on both T1- and T2-WIs, which is characteristic for lipoid pneumonia.

Infarcts due to PE are either of triangular or nodular shape. Nodular infarcts are often seen as a sessile mass on the pleura and appear as humps. They often exhibit high signal intensity on T1-W images due to hemorrhage. The high signal is attributed to methemoglobin formation in subacute hemorrhage. This appearance is also present in different diseases with pulmonary hemorrhage, such as Goodpasture's syndrome or IPA. Thus, MRI will differentiate infarctions and hemorrhage from pneumonia or atelectasis without hemorrhage more easily than CT. Detection and characterization of infarction is included in the work-up protocol for PE.

9.3.2.3 Fibrosis and Alveolitis

Fibrotic lung disease is much better diagnosed using CT. The disease itself is associated with an increase in spin density and a reduction of susceptibility artifacts. This increase in signal intensity is highly unspecific, and is not successful in the differentiation of various causes of airspace disease, because there is considerable overlap in the measured T1 and T2 values between different underlying diseases. The extent and distribution of fibrotic lung disease is represented by parenchymal bands and reticulation, nodules, and interlobular septal thickening. Concomitant alveolitis (active inflammation) is represented by higher signal intensity on T1-W and T2-W than fibrosis. Signal intensity is related to clinical severity of disease and a potential indicator for the response to therapy. Due to the active inflammatory process, it also shows marked enhancement after contrast administration. Subsequently, successful anti-inflammatory treatment, which reduces the activity of alveolitis and the development of fibrosis, is associated with a marked decrease in signal intensity. This has been demonstrated for radiation pneumonitis in patients with bronchogenic carcinoma and in bleomycin-induced lung damage. Again, the reduction of active inflammation can be observed either on T2- or on T1-WIs after contrast administration.

In areas of progressive massive fibrosis in silicosis and silicotuberculosis, marked contrast enhancement of the inflammatory process within may be observed by MRI. It is hypointense on T2-W images compared to skeletal muscle with some high signal areas centrally. These areas most likely correspond to (liquefactive) necrosis. Before contrast, the consolidations are isointense to skeletal muscle in 70% of cases. After contrast, about 50% of the consolidations show rim enhancement with nonenhancing central areas. Since signal intensities are different in fibrotic and neoplastic tissue, lung cancer can be differentiated as a lesion with high signal on T2-W imaging.

The findings encountered in Wegener's granulomatosis, which is characterized by solid and cavitated intrapulmonary nodules, are similar to progressive massive fibrosis. The walls of larger nodules show marked enhancement after contrast administration, whereas the central, necrotic areas do not enhance.

9.3.2.4 Airway Diseases and Emphysema

The tissue loss in emphysema renders proton imaging incompatible for internal structure analysis. However, there is high contrast with the chest wall, and segmentation to determine lung volumes are easily performed. Dynamic T1-W sequences are capable of demonstrating the respiratory pump mechanism of the diaphragm in chest wall. These parameters may be important in the preoperative work-up and postoperative follow-up of patients who are candidates for, or have undergone, lung volume reduction surgery for emphysema. Airway disease with bronchial wall thickening and mucus plugging, such as in cystic fibrosis and other bronchiectatic diseases can be visualized by MRI. The direct visualization of the bronchial wall is inferior to CT, but mucus and inflammatory changes are shown with high signal and sensitivity. In cystic fibrosis, bronchi with thickened walls can be visualized down to the sub pleural space. The T2-W signal of the bronchial walls shows a huge variety between high and low intensity, most likely reflecting different amounts of fluid and inflammatory activity. Mucus

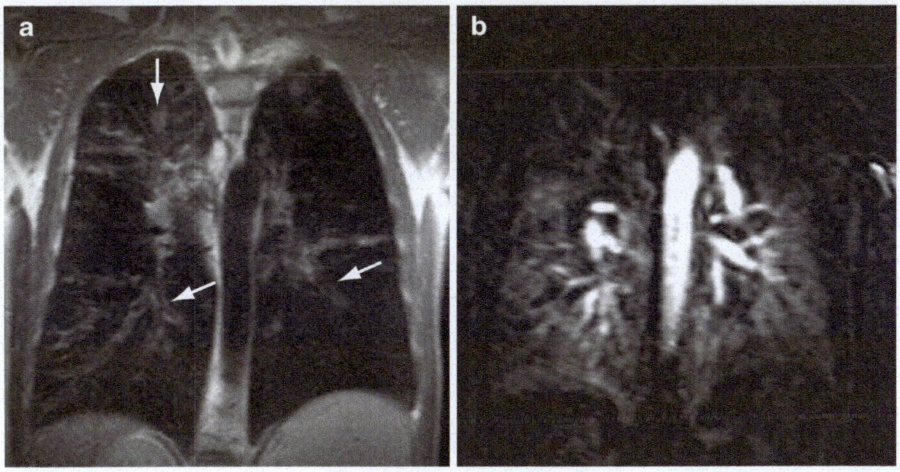

Fig. 9.6 Cystic fibrosis. (**a**) Coronal T2-WI showing bronchiectasis and bronchial wall thickening in both lungs (*arrows*). (**b**) Corresponding coronal MR perfusion shows perfusion defects in the upper lobes which are most severely affected

plugging is very well visualized with high T2-W signal because of the huge proton density of the fluid (Fig. 9.6). The appearance of central and peripheral mucus plugging has to be differentiated. In central mucus plugging, there is high T2-W signal filling the bronchus within its course, partly or completely. Peripheral mucus plugging shows a grape-like appearance of small T2-W high intensity areas, almost like the "tree in bud" sign known from HRCT. Air fluid levels occur in saccular or varicose bronchiectasis and are visible on MRI due to the huge fluid proton density on T2-W images. With progression of cystic fibrosis, complete destruction of lung segments or lobes can occur, which is easily appreciated on MRI. Bronchial obstruction leads to hypoxic vasoconstriction, which is easily assessed by defects observed on a MR perfusion series (Fig. 9.6).

He-3 MRI demonstrates severe localized and diffuse, nodular or wedge-shaped signal heterogeneities in airway diseases, such as in cystic fibrosis, chronic obstructive pulmonary disease (COPD), asthma, bronchiectasis, and emphysema (Figs. 9.7 and 9.8). The different findings are attributed to airway obstructions or increased size of airspaces at different levels. Obviously, He-3 MRI is a highly sensitive modality for the detection and visualization of airway disease. The various sequences are also capable of demonstrating microstructural and dynamic airflow changes and may also be able to detect changes in oxygen uptake by the lungs. However, the low specificity still has to be improved, and quantitation and interpretation of the findings need further improvements before this technology can be widely advocated.

9.3.2.5 Pleural Disease

Pleural Effusion

Pleural effusion is easily depicted by MRI, showing low signal intensity on T1-WI and high signal intensity on T2-W images as expected for fluid (Fig. 9.2).

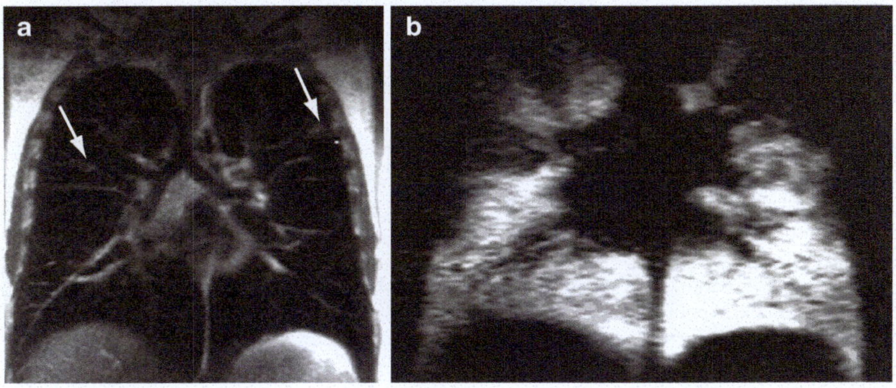

Fig. 9.7 Cystic fibrosis: (**a**) Coronal T2-WI showing moderate airway pathology in both lungs (*arrows*). (**b**) Coronal He-3 MRI showing multiple wedge-shaped ventilation defects in both upper lobes

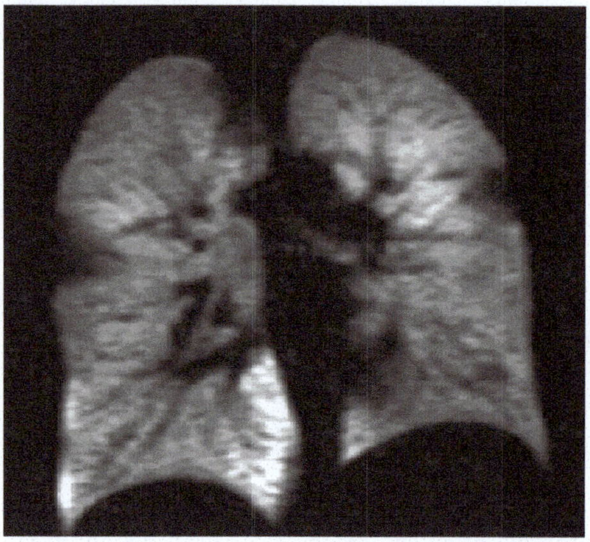

Fig. 9.8 Chronic obstructive pulmonary disease (COPD): coronal He-3 MRI showing peripheral wedge-shaped ventilation defects in a smoker

Compared to conventional chest radiography, MRI is more sensitive in the detection of pleural fluid collections. Although equally sensitive to CT, MRI may be able to better distinguish exudates from transudates based on higher signal intensity on T1-W and T2-W of exudates. Septae are also more easily demonstrated on T2-W imaging. Subacute or chronic hemorrhages exhibit characteristic signal intensity based on the age of clot, with methemoglobin having higher signal compared to hemosiderin (signal void). Although differentiation between benign and malignant effusions is not possible, pleural effusions are strong indicator for poor prognosis in patients with bronchogenic carcinoma.

Benign Masses

Benign masses of the pleura include lipoma, fibroma, and round atelectasis. Lipoma typically shows the signal characteristics of subcutaneous fat on all sequences. Pleural fibromas are isointense to muscle on T1-W and iso- to hyperintense on T2-W images, and enhance following Gadolinium contrast.

Rounded atelectasis has a typical morphological appearance: the classical comet-tail sign, which describes the course of the vessels and bronchi into the ovoid or wedge-shaped mass. They have similar signal characteristics to fibroma.

Malignant Masses

The primary malignancy of the pleura is the mesothelioma, which is frequently associated with pleural effusion. Many are related to previous asbestos exposure, and calcified (often anterior) pleural plaques are a hallmark of this etiology. MRI is less sensitive than CT for the demonstration of these calcifications. Generally, mesothelioma is a diffuse pleural process with the signal intensity slightly increased on T1-W and moderately increased on T2-W imaging (Fig. 9.9). Most mesotheliomas will enhance after the administration of contrast (Fig. 9.9). MRI is superior to CT in the assessment of the extension of multiple pleural foci and infiltration of chest wall, diaphragm, and peritoneum. Pleural metastases secondary to carcinomas of the breast, lung, stomach, kidneys, and ovaries are far more common. They often appear as diffuse nodular pleural thickening or as a large solid mass with pulmonary encasement and effusion mimicking mesothelioma.

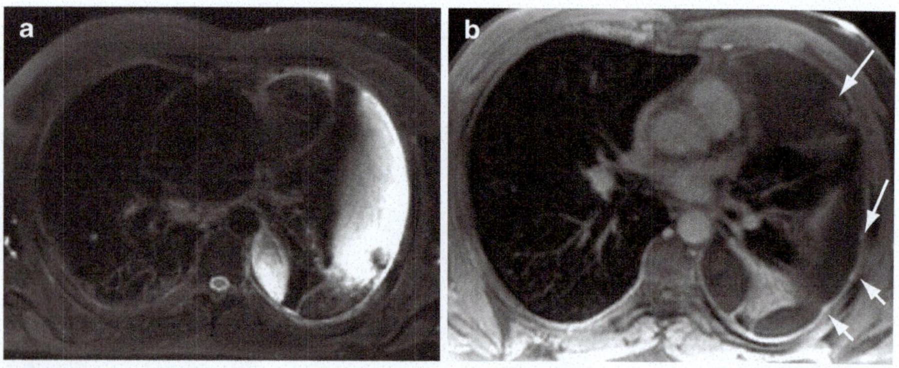

Fig. 9.9 Pleural mesothelioma. (**a**) T2-WI hypointense pleural nodules within the hyperintense pleural effusion. (**b**) T1-WI showing multiple, small enhancing pleural nodules within the hypointense pleural effusion (*arrows*)

9.4 Mediastinum

9.4.1 Anatomy

The mediastinum consists of fatty tissue. Apart from the heart, it contains multiple different anatomical structures: arteries, veins, nerves, and lymphatics, as well as the esophagus belonging to the gastrointestinal tract and the tracheobronchial tree belonging to the respiratory tract and finally a primary mediastinal organ, the thymus. All of them can be the origin for disease spreading throughout the mediastinum and involving the other structures. Additionally, adjacent structures, such as lungs, pleura, pericardium, thyroid, or spine, can afflict the mediastinum by means of continuous infiltration. We will not deal with the heart and pericardium, as this is described elsewhere. The thymus is a particularly relevant structure, as it changes appearances from childhood to adulthood. Normally, it will demonstrate progressive involution and fatty degeneration, but there is great variability in these appearances.

9.4.2 Pathology

Mediastinal masses are differentiated into primary and secondary tumors, which also include lymphadenopathy. Additionally, benign diseases arising from one of the numerous structures within the mediastinum, e.g., aortic aneurysm, have to be differentiated. The location of masses often indicates the type of tumor one can encounter (Table 9.3). MRI plays an important role in the delineation and characterization of mediastinal tumors, wherein localization, tissue composition, growth pattern, as well as patient's age and tumor markers are important for the differential diagnosis. Because of its superiority in tissue characterization with regard to CT, and the high number of young people affected by mediastinal tumors, MRI should be regarded as the first-line imaging modality in this population. Nonenhanced MRI can benefit from black-blood techniques, which reduce flow artifacts. It allows for identification of vessel walls and better differentiation to lymph nodes, but at the price of diminished signal intensity. ECG-triggered sequences provide excellent detail of structures close to the heart. Navigator or respiratory belt-triggered sequences do not enhance image quality sufficiently enough to justify the significant higher acquisition time. One of the preferred fast methods is the application of black blood-prepared HASTE. Identification and classification of mediastinal processes is possible by using unsaturated and fat saturated native 3D gradient echo sequences and repeating the latter after contrast administration. With an inplane resolution of 1.6 mm, even very small lymph nodes can be detected. It is imperative to apply fat saturation to contrast-enhanced images so as not to obscure enhanced lymph nodes within the signal of the surrounding fatty tissue.

9.4.2.1 Primary Mediastinal Tumors

Thymus

Thymus masses are among the most frequent primary tumors in the mediastinum. The majority of thymus masses are benign, including thymoma, thymolipoma, and (reactive) hyperplasia. More infrequently, malignant tumors may arise in the thymus, and this is almost invariably thymic carcinoma (although up to 30% of thymomas may invade surrounding structures). Thymoma is typically a well-defined, rounded, or lobulated mass that is mostly homogeneous and isointense on T1-W images, low enhancement postcontrast, and hyperintense on T2-W imaging. There may be inhomogeneous signal on T2-W images (which favors a benign nature), and cysts may also be present. Encapsulated thymomas exhibit a complete tumor capsule on MRI, whereas invasive thymomas will penetrate the capsule and diffusely infiltrate the mediastinal fat and the adjacent structures, e.g., pericardium, great vessels. Furthermore, invasive thymomas more commonly show multinodularity with low intensity fibrous septa.

Thymolipoma is a relatively rare mass, showing high amounts of fat, but also some thymic tissue. This is easily demonstrated on T1-W sequences. The mass may arise from the thymus or be connected by a pedicle, and can often be large with compression of surrounding structures.

Thymus hyperplasia is indistinguishable from normal signal intensities. The thymus will be enlarged, however. Rebound thymus hyperplasia has to be suspected in those patients who are undergoing treatment for lymphoma or leukemia.

Table 9.3 Typical appearance of mediastinal tumors of MRI

Origin	Type	Typical location	Features Morphology	T1-W	Enhancement	T2-W
Thymus	Thymoma	Anterior	Encapsulated, inhomogeneous invasive, lobulated, septae	Low		High
	Thymolipoma	Anterior	Large	High		Intermediate
	Hyperplasia	Anterior	Homogeneous, large	Intermediate		High
	Carcinoma	Anterior	Inhomogeneous	Intermediate	Strong	High
Germ cell tumors	Teratoma	Anterior	Inhomogeneous, cystic & solid, fat-fluid levels		Strong	
	Seminoma	Anterior	Large, lobulated, inhomogeneous			
	Non-seminoma	Anterior	Large, irregular, Inhomogeneous			
Thyroid	Grave's disease	Anterior	Band-like	High		High
	Goiter	Anterior	Multinodular, inhomogeneous Hemorrhage Cystic	Low high low	Strong	High
Neurogenic tumors	Nerve sheath benign	Posterior	Sharply marginated spherical lobular	Variable	Uniform	Periphery High centre low target sign
	Nerve sheath malignant	Posterior	Large, inhomogeneous	Low	Inhomogeneous	High
	Sympathetic ganglia, ganglioneuroma, neuroblastoma	Posterior	Well-marginated, homogeneous Irregular, inhomogeneous	Intermediate variable	Inhomogeneous	Intermediate variable
Lymphatics	Lymphoma	Anywhere				
	Untreated		Homogeneous	Low	Strong	High
	Early response phase		Inhomogeneous	Low	Variable	Variable
	Complete response		Inhomogeneous	Variable	Minor	Variable
	Inactive residual fibrosis		Homogeneous	Low	None	Low
	Metastatic disease	Anywhere	Homogeneous	Low	Strong	Intermediate
	Infectious disease	Anywhere	Homogeneous	Low	Variable	Intermediate
Mediastinal Cysts	Thymic	Anterior	Well-circumscribed	Low	None	High
	Bronchogenic	Middle	Well-circumscribed	Low	None	High
	Esophageal	Posterior	Well-circumscribed	Low	None	High
	Neurenteric	Posterior	Well-circumscribed	Low	None	High
	Pericardial	Middle	Well-circumscribed	Low	None	High

Thymic carcinoma is less common than thymoma. It shows high signal intensity on both T1- and T2-W images, and may exhibit inhomogeneity due to necrosis, cyst formation, or hemorrhage. Although MRI is not capable to differentiate invasive thymoma from thymic carcinoma, it has been suggested that invasive thymoma is more frequently lobulated.

Germ Cell

Germ cells tumors also have a predilection for the anterior mediastinum. They account for approximately 15% of mediastinal masses. These masses are benign in 80%, and these are mainly teratomas. Teratoma may consist of different types of tissue, which is reflected in the signal intensity pattern. Thus, fat tissue, cysts, and solid component may all be demonstrated, and fat-fluid levels are thought to be highly pathognomonic. Different classifications exist according to maturity of differentiation, with most mature teratomas presenting early in life.

Malignant germ cell tumors are almost exclusively seen in men, with seminoma as the most common type. These masses are usually very large at presentation, and may be inhomogenous due to necrosis and hemorrhage.

9.4.2.2 Secondary Mediastinal Tumors

Goiter

The most frequently encountered secondary mediastinal tumor is the goiter extending through the cervicothoracic junction into the mediastinum. Mainly, the anterior mediastinum is affected with the goiter extending into the retrosternal supra-aortic space. However, different ways are also possible, and include the middle mediastinum, with the thyroid tissue extended in between the trachea and the esophagus as well as in the posterior mediastinum.

The normal thyroid gland is isointense with muscle on T1-W and hyperintense on T2-W imaging. Multinodular goiter shows a relatively low signal on T1-W and inhomogeneous high signal on T2-W imaging due to hemorrhage, necrosis, and cyst formation. In patients with hypothyroidism (Graves' disease), the features change and signal intensity is high on both T1 and T2-W images. Furthermore, there are the appearances of band-like structures and dilated vascular structures throughout the thyroid gland.

Neurogenic Tumors

Neurogenic tumors are typically positioned in the posterior mediastinum. There is a close relationship with the vertebral column and frequently there is a relationship with the nerve root canal. Three main subgroups can be distinguished: peripheral nerve tumors (neurofibroma and Schwannoma), malignant nerve sheath tumors (malignant neurofibroma, malignant Schwannoma, and neurofibrosarcoma), and tumors arising from the sympathetic ganglia (ganglioneuroma, ganglioneuroblastoma, neuroblastoma, and paraganglioma). The benign tumors arising from the nerve sheath present themselves as well-defined, spherical, or lobulated masses (Fig. 9.10). They invariably show variable T1-W signal and high signal on T2-W imaging, characteristically with low central T2-W signal as a result of fibrosis ("target sign"). The malignant nerve sheath tumors present themselves as large masses with inhomogeneous signal due to hemorrhage and necrosis. Finally, ganglioneuromas and ganglioneuroblastomas, which take their origin from the sympathetic ganglia, present as well-demarcated, homogeneous masses of intermediate signal intensity on T1-W and T2-W imaging. Paragangliomas are also well demarcated, but might be inhomogeneous and hyperintense on T2-W images and with an intermediate enhancement on T1-W images (Fig. 9.10). Conversely, neuroblastomas show inhomogeneous signal regardless of sequence due to hemorrhage, necrosis, cystic generation, and calcium deposition. Neuroblastoma shows inhomogeneous enhancement following Gd. Malignant neuroblastomas usually present early in childhood. The level of malignancy is often reflected in the amount of necrosis and hemorrhage. In this setting, MRI is clearly the imaging modality of choice and superior to CT since MRI can much better illustrate the relationship of the tumor with regard to neural foramina, spinal chord, and bone.

Esophagus

Esophageal tumors are the second most encountered masses in the posterior mediastinum. However, MRI

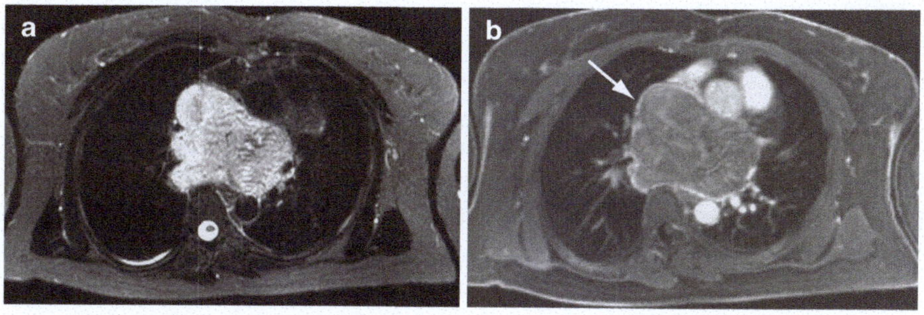

Fig. 9.10 Paraganglioma originating from the posterior mediastinum. (**a**) Fat-suppressed T2-WI showing a well-demarcated, slightly inhomogeneous hyperintense mass; (**b**) T1-WI post contrast showing an inhomogeneous enhancement (*arrow*)

plays an insignificant role in the staging and diagnosis of these malignancies since it does not offer any essential advantages over CT.

9.4.2.3 Lymphatic Tissues

Lymphadenopathy is a common feature of both benign and malignant diseases. MRI is capable of demonstrating lymph nodes with accuracy, and is also able to show the effects of lymph node enlargement on adjacent structures. T1-GRE and T2-HASTE are limited in the detection of metastastic mediastinal lymph nodes. Principally, spectral fat saturation does enhance the visibility of lymph nodes on T2-W images such as HASTE, but particularly in the mediastinum, it is often inhomogeneous and incomplete. Therefore, short inversion recovery sequences (STIR or TIRM) are recommended for the detection and follow-up of mediastinal lymph nodes in a multiple breath-hold acquisition technique. MRI is less capable of demonstrating calcification than CT, although a decrease in signal on T2-W imaging may be appreciated.

Lymphoma

Malignant lymphoma is the most common primary mediastinal neoplasm (Fig. 9.11). Mediastinal manifestations occur either in isolation or as a part of generalized disease. Hodgkin's disease is the most common, and often presents as a huge mediastinal bulk. NHL is more prone to extra nodular involvement while HD often affects the thymus. Although MRI is superior to CT in displaying the extent of the mass, it does not lead to a change in clinical management. MRI can be employed in monitoring treatment effects in patients with lymphoma. Four different signal patterns can be defined, which may help (to some extent) to determine these effects:

(a) Homogeneous, hyperintense pattern of untreated lymphoma, which shows low signal T1-W and high signal T2-W imaging. This is never encountered in inactive residual masses.
(b) Heterogeneous, active pattern of posttreatment response phase, which exhibits homogeneous low signal on T1-W and inhomogeneous high and low signal on T2-W images. This pattern can also be present in untreated nodular sclerosing Hodgkin's disease.

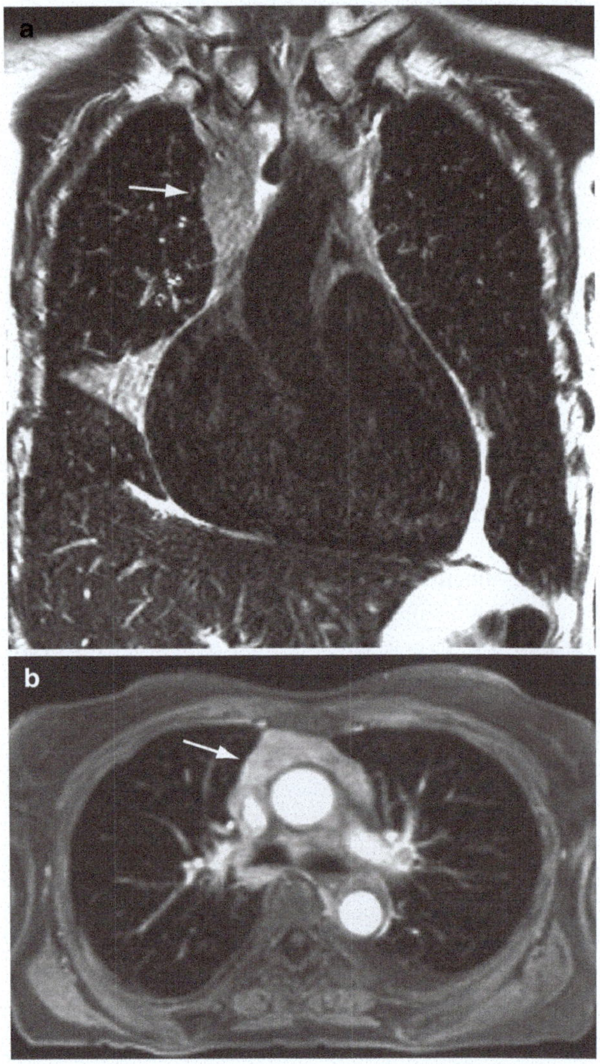

Fig. 9.11 Non-Hodgkin lymphoma (NHL) in the anterior mediastinum. (**a**) T2-WI showing a well-demarcated mass in the anterior mediastinum with intermediate signal intensity (*arrow*); (**b**) Fat-suppressed T1-WI post contrast showing a strong and homogeneous enhancement (*arrow*)

(c) Heterogeneous, inactive pattern of early complete response phase. During this phase, there is mixed high and low intensity on both T1-W and T2-W imaging.
(d) Homogeneous, hypointense pattern of inactive residual fibrosis, which shows low signal on both T1-W and T2-W imaging.

However, the potential of MRI to separate vital from nonvital lymphoma tissue is not reliable enough to provide conclusive prognostic information or to detect recurrent disease early. Thus, it has not been generally established as the first-line imaging modality in mediastinal lymphoma instead of CT. Positron emission tomography (PET) offers clear advantages over both technologies, as it is more sensitive in detecting metabolically active cells.

Metastatic Disease

Malignant involvement of lymph nodes is mainly determined by size (Fig. 9.12). Similarly to CT, a short axis diameter of more than 1 cm is generally considered as suggestive for malignancy, which carries a negative predictive value of approximately 85%. Lymph node size should also be regarded with respect to the anatomical location, e.g., lymph nodes in the paratracheal region are often bigger without being malignant. Thus, comparing lymph nodes size between right and left side might be helpful, with a difference of more than 5 mm suggesting malignancy. Calcifications, which are an important sign of benign lymphadenopathy are difficult to appreciate on MRI. The differentiation between lymph nodes and blood vessels is straight forward – even on nonenhanced scans – if fast-flowing blood leads to a flow void. In case of slow-flowing blood or turbulence, the differentiation can be difficult. The addition of CEMRA or bright blood techniques may offer useful information in this setting.

Although some early indications suggested that differences in signal intensities could differentiate between benign and malignant, this has not proven to be clinically useful. However, current ongoing clinical trials are evaluating new contrast agents with a main focus on lymphography and decreased uptake of contrast in malignant lymph nodes. MR lymphography is based on T2 and T2* W GRE images 24–48 h after intravenous administration of ultrasmall superparamagnetic iron particles (USPIO). The effect is based on the fact that macrophages take up iron oxide much more avidly than tumor cells. Thus, normal lymph nodes will show a decrease in signal intensity, whereas the contrast effect is absent or less pronounced in neoplastic nodes. In preliminary clinical studies, MR lymphography in patients with bronchogenic carcinoma yielded a sensitivity of 100%, and a specificity of 38%.

In clinical routine, CT and MRI are more or less equivalent regarding the N-staging (see Table 9.2), especially N2. Both can be used to stratify patient for invasive procedures, such as mediastinoscopy or thoracotomy with mediastinal lymph node dissection. Advantages and disadvantages of CT and MRI in this context are given in Table 9.4. Although MRI seems to have some capability to distinguish between normal and invaded lymph nodes, PET seems to have greater diagnostic accuracy for the identification of mediastinal metastatic lymph nodes.

Table 9.4 Advantages and disadvantages of MRI vs. CT

Criteria	MRI	CT
Independence from motion artifacts	–	+
Spatial resolution	+	++
Detection of calcifications	–	++
Cost	+	+
Need for contrast agents	+	–
Multiplanar capabilities	++	+
Soft-tissue contrast	++	–
Tissue characterization	++	+
Vascular studies	++	+

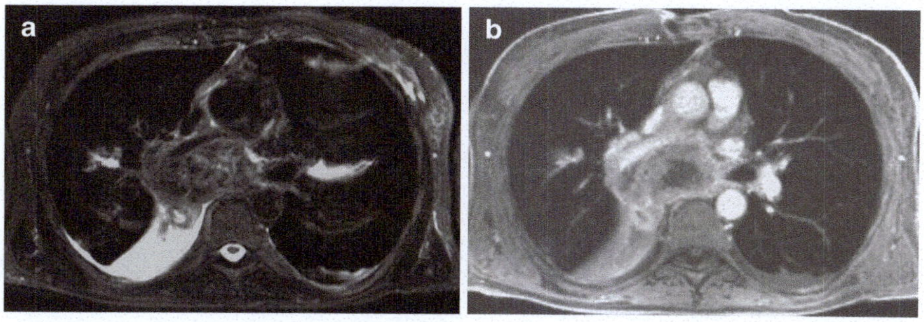

Fig. 9.12 Mediastinal lymphadenopathy due to bronchogenic carcinoma. (**a**) Fat-suppressed T2-WI showing a large inhomogeneous subcarinal mass low signal intensity and pleural effusion; (**b**) Fat-suppressed T1-WI post contrast showing a strong and inhomogeneous enhancement

Benign Disease

A wide range of benign causes of lymphadenopathy exists and differentiation between these is very difficult. Some etiologies more commonly give rise to calcifications, which will result in more inhomogeneous signal (especially on T2-W imaging). The poor spatial resolution can lead to blending together of numerous small lymph nodes and the suggestion of a single enlarged lymph node resulting in a false-positive finding.

9.4.2.4 Mediastinal Cysts

Five different types of cystic masses can be identified, and these are usually classified based on their primary location. Thus, thymic cysts are found in the anterior mediastinum, bronchogenic cysts and pericardial cysts are mainly present in the middle mediastinum (Fig. 9.13), while esophageal duplication cysts and neurogenic cysts are found in the posterior mediastinum. All cysts have characteristically well-defined margins and show low signal on T1-W and high signal on T2-W imaging. Typically, no enhancement is observed after the administration of contrast. In case of multiple cysts and the presence of cysts below the diaphragm, pancreatic pseudocysts or hydatid disease is likely the differential diagnosis.

9.5 Pulmonary Arteries

9.5.1 Anatomy

Using state-of-the-art techniques (see above) and breath-holding, the central and lobar arteries can be completely visualized on a routine basis (Fig. 9.14). Furthermore, more than 90% of segmental arteries and more than 80% of subsegmental fourth order arteries can be depicted routinely. Some of the congenital abnormalities of the heart also involve the pulmonary arteries, but these are dealt with elsewhere.

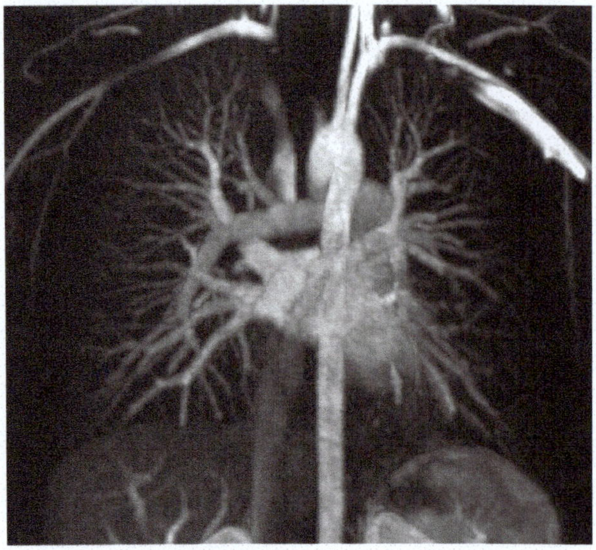

Fig. 9.14 Normal pulmonary MR angiogram (maximum intensity projection)

9.5.2 Pathology

9.5.2.1 Pulmonary Embolism

PE is an extremely common and potentially life-threatening disorder. Its clinical signs, history, clinical examination, and chest radiograph are generally unspecific. Pulmonary angiography is generally regarded as the gold standard modality, but is invasive. Therefore, accurate,

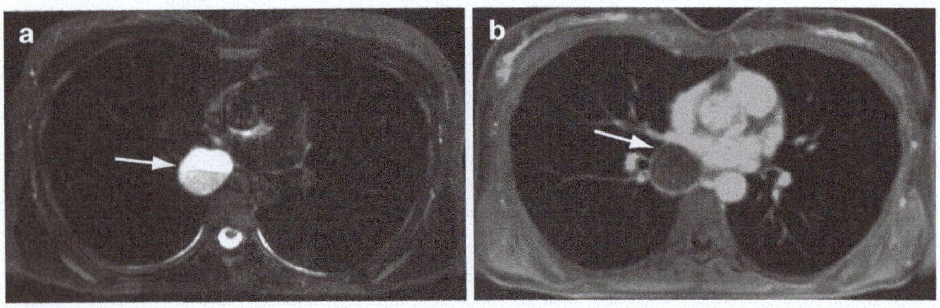

Fig. 9.13 Bronchogenic cyst. (**a**) Fat-suppressed T2-WI showing a large well-defined homogeneous lesion with some sedimented debris (*arrow*); (**b**) Fat-suppressed T1-WI post contrast showing no enhancement (*arrow*)

Table 9.5 Criteria for the MRI diagnosis of pulmonary embolism

Criteria	Acute embolism	Chronic thromboembolic pulmonary hypertension (CTEPH)
Direct – filling defects	Central, intraluminal, convex Lack of opacification	Wall-adherent, concave Lack of opacification Intraluminal webs
Direct – vascular wall		Irregular wall thickening Abnormal proximal-to-distal tapering Variations in size of segmental vessel Absence of segmental vessels (cut-off)
Indirect – parenchyma	Infarction Pleural-based, round Pleural effusion	Infarction Mosaic perfusion Pleural effusion
Indirect – pulmonary hypertension	Cardiomegaly Paradoxical movement of interventricular septum	Cardiomegaly Negative axis of interventricular septum Dilation of central pulmonary arteries Pericardial effusion, ascites

highly sensitive, highly specific, easy and fast to perform, cost-effective, and widely available noninvasive alternatives are required. Spiral CT meets most of these expectations with an average sensitivity >90% and specificity >90%. In parallel, encouraging results have been observed using CEMRA, which may be a competitive alternative in the future. Several findings can indicate the presence of acute PE (Table 9.5). In CEMRA, homogeneous intravascular high signal intensity is reliably obtained. Slow or turbulent flow does no longer mimic PE, which is diagnosed as a constant intraluminal filling defect (Fig. 9.15) or an abrupt vascular cut-off. Multiplanar reformats are frequently used to depict wall-adherent, segmental, or subsegmental emboli with a high level of confidence. From the beginning, CEMRA was superior to nonenhanced MRA for the central pulmonary artery branches. Using state-of the art techniques (see above), CEMRA achieves a sensitivity >85%, a specificity >95% for the diagnosis of PE on a per-patient basis. On a per-embolus basis, the sensitivity is >65%. Furthermore, isolated subsegmental emboli cannot be reliably excluded; a problem largely solved by 16-slice and 64-slice CT pulmonary angiography. Secondary signs of PE may include pleural effusions and lung consolidation (including pulmonary infarction) as well as hyperlucency. These are usually easily identifiable on MRI, as discussed above, as this will result in high signal on T2-W imaging. Hemorrhagic infarction will also show high signal on T1-W imaging. Unilateral hyperlucent lung can either be caused by central PE, Swyer-James syndrome, or agenesis of a pulmonary artery (Fig. 9.1), which can be easily differentiated by MRI.

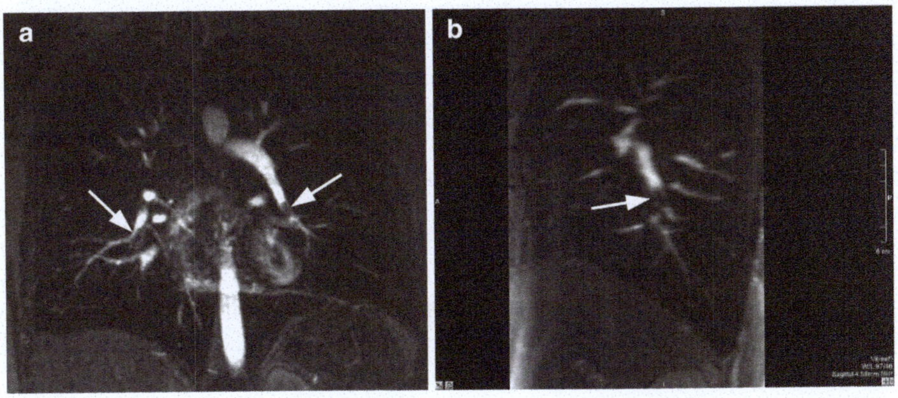

Fig. 9.15 Acute pulmonary embolism. (**a**) Coronal MR angiogram showing filling defect in both lower lobe arteries (*arrows*); (**b**) Sagittal MR angiogram illustrating the filling defect in the left lower lobe artery (*arrow*)

Perfusion MRI also provides important information in patients with suspected PE by showing perfusion defects in addition to the visualization of thrombotic material in the pulmonary arteries by CEMRA. When compared to the nuclear medicine gold standard (V/Q scintigraphy), perfusion MRI shows a comparably high sensitivity and specificity for the detection of perfusion defects with high interobserver agreement. Perfusion MRI is also helpful in the differential diagnosis between PE, pneumonia, and chronic obstructive lung disease.

Using MR phlebography, the entire venous system can be assessed for thrombosis in the same imaging session without using ionizing radiation. In indirect MR phlebography, the venous system is imaged after the contrast agent bolus has passed the arterial system and capillary bed, whereas direct or ascending MR phlebography refers to an enhancement of the veins of the lower extremity after peripheral injection into the veins of the foot. Additionally, ventilation MRI might be used allowing for a differentiation of perfusion changes caused by hypoxic vasoconstriction. Finally, the right heart function, which is important for the prognosis of the patient, may be assessed by CINE MRI and phase-contrast MR flow measurements.

9.5.2.2 Chronic Thromboembolic Pulmonary Hypertension (CTEPH)

CTEPH is a long-term outcome following acute PE in approximately 3–7% of patients. Although this represents a minority of patients with acute PE, it is being diagnosed with an increasing frequency. The differentiation between acute or chronic PE is possible by CEMRA in most patients (Table 9.5). A diagnosis of CTEPH can be confidently made, when using the following criteria: dilated central pulmonary arteries, direct visualization of wall-adherent thrombotic material and thickening of the vessel wall, absence of segmental vessels (cut-off), abnormal proximal-to-distal tapering of pulmonary vessels, variations in size of segmental vessel, intraluminal webs, and heterogeneous contrast enhancement within the lung parenchyma. In addition, the effects on the right ventricle may be observed: hypertrophy, dilatation, and left bulging of the interventricular septum. Several studies have shown a high accuracy of MRA for the visualization of thrombotic material in CTEPH compared to conventional angiography or CT. The main differential diagnosis of CTEPH is primary pulmonary hypertension (PPH). This disorder gives similar findings in general, but without the signs of (previous) PE. More than 90% of patients with PPH can be differentiated from those with CTEPH and normal subjects on the basis of CEMRA.

9.5.2.3 Primary and Metastatic Tumors Involving the Pulmonary Arteries

Tumors involving the pulmonary artery (sarcomas or metastases) are depicted as filling defects at CEMRA. In patients who are suspected for a mass involving the pulmonary arteries, delayed scans after contrast administration are advised to demonstrate enhancement, indicating neoplasms instead of PE. Care has to be taken since neoplasms have different degrees of vascularity, and they may be associated with secondary thrombus formation or necrosis. MRI can also be used for the evaluation of central pulmonary arterial and venous involvement in lung cancer. Besides conventional SE and TSE MRI, which have the advantage of a high contrast between the vascular lumen, wall, and surrounding tissue, contrast-enhanced 3D MRA has been demonstrated to be effective for the evaluation of vascular infiltration by bronchogenic carcinoma. In patients with central lung tumors, the combination of the angiographic and perfusion information of contrast-enhanced perfusion MRI allows an accurate classification of vascular involvement when compared to DSA or perfusion scintigraphy.

9.5.2.4 Pulmonary Artery Aneurysms

Aneurysms of the pulmonary arteries are rare and may be associated with a wide variety of conditions, such as congenital heart disease, hereditary telangiectasia, and trauma. Multiple aneurysms may be observed in patients with Behcet's disease or Hughes-Stovin syndrome. Noninvasive diagnosis, which is particularly important in these patients, is easily obtained by CEMRA. The imaging data can be used as the basis for surgical planning. Finally, false aneurysms can be caused by interventions, such as the introduction of Swan Ganz catheters.

9.5.2.5 Pulmonary Arteriovenous Malformations

They consist of a racemose convolute of vascular structures. Flow within the malformation can be highly variable. Patent vessels will show flow void; whereas slow flow will exhibit low signal and thrombosed vessels and hemorrhage will show by high signal. After contrast administration, malformations are strongly enhancing, while high caliber feeding arteries and draining veins are easily depicted at CEMRA. CEMRA and pulmonary perfusion MRI are well suited to be used for the management of pulmonary arteriovenous malformations, including planning of embolotherapy and follow-up. Differentiation of arteriovenous malformations from other pulmonary nodules or masses is obvious.

9.5.2.6 Pulmonary Sequestrations

These consist of nonfunctioning lung tissue, which is not in continuity with the tracheobronchial tree. They contain mucus, inflammatory, granulomatous, and fibrotic tissue, and they exhibit high signal intensity on T2-WI and intermediate to high signal on nonenhanced T1-WI. After contrast administration, the lesion demonstrates strong enhancement. The atypical systemic arteries arise from the descending or abdominal aorta in most cases. They are visualized by MRI, including CEMRA, with a high degree of confidence, thus avoiding conventional angiography in most cases.

9.5.2.7 Anomalous Pulmonary Venous Return

MRI and MRA can be successfully used for accurate identification of pulmonary venous confluence and total or partial anomalous pulmonary venous return, such as seen in Scimitar syndrome (Fig. 9.16). Additional information of concomitant bronchial and visceral abnormalities can be obtained. Flow measurements will allow for quantitation of shunt volumes. Limitations of echocardiography and invasiveness of angiography make CEMRA the modality of choice for the assessment of anomalies of the pulmonary veins.

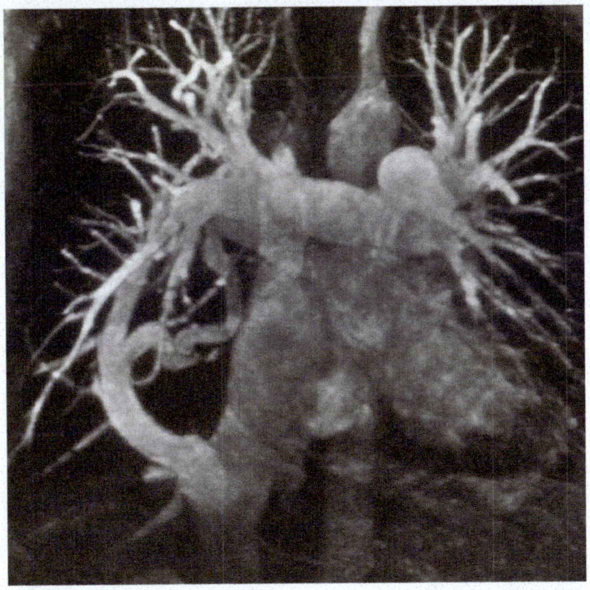

Fig. 9.16 Scimitar Syndrome. Coronal maximum intensity projection showing an anomalous venous drainage of the right lower lobe into the inferior vena cava

9.6 Future Prospects

MRI of the chest is increasingly used for a variety of disorders. The introduction of fast and ultrafast sequences, allowing breath-hold techniques, has paved the way for improved visualization of the main structures in the chest. Thus, MRI of the mediastinum, chest wall, and superior sulcus is now commonly regarded as the modality of choice. CEMRA is now routinely employed in the assessment of vascular pathology, and progress is being made in the assessment of patients with suspected acute PE, where niche applications (such as pregnancy) are now widely accepted. Airway imaging is becoming available by the application of fast imaging techniques in the presence of pathological changes in the lung parenchyma, such as consolidations and masses. Finally, dynamic processes of the lung, including airway dynamics and oxygen exchange mechanisms are currently being investigated.

9.7 Key Issues

During the past decade, significant developments have been achieved in the field of MRI of the chest, enabling it to enter the clinical arena on a broad scale. Standard protocols are now implemented on up-to-date scanners, allowing MRI to be used as a first-line imaging modality for various lung diseases, including cystic fibrosis, pulmonary hypertension, and even lung cancer. The diagnostic benefits of MRI of the chest consist in the visualization of changes in lung structure while simultaneously imaging different aspects of lung function, such as perfusion, respiratory motion, ventilation, and gas exchange. This book provides a comprehensive overview of how to use MRI for imaging of lung disease and reviews the most frequent findings and differential diagnoses.

Further Reading

Altes TA, Eichinger M, Puderbach M (2007) Magnetic resonance imaging of the lung in cystic fibrosis. Proc Am Thorac Soc 4:321–327

Benamore RE, O'Doherty MJ, Entwisle JJ (2005) Use of imaging in the management of malignant pleural mesothelioma. Clin Radiol 60:1237–1247

Erasmus JJ, Truong MT, Munden RF (2005) CT, MR, and PET imaging in staging of nonsmall-cell lung cancer. Semin Roentgenol 40:126–142

Fain SB, Korosec FR, Holmes JH, O'Halloran R, Sorkness RL, Grist TM (2007) Functional lung imaging using hyperpolarized gas MRI. J Magn Reson Imaging 25:910–923

Fink C, Ley S, Schoenberg SO, Reiser MF, Kauczor HU (2007) Magnetic resonance imaging of acute pulmonary embolism. Eur Radiol 17;2546–2553

Fujimoto K (2008) Usefulness of contrast-enhanced magnetic resonance imaging for evaluating solitary pulmonary nodules. Cancer Imaging 3:36–44

Ginsberg MS, Grewal RK, Heelan RT (2007) Lung cancer. Radiol Clin North Am 45:21–43

Gotway M (2008) Chest MR. Magn Reson Imag Clin North Am 16:137–384

Hirsch W, Sorge I, Krohmer S, Weber D, Meier K, Till H (2008) MRI of the lungs in children. Eur J Radiol 68:278–288

Kauczor HU (2004) Pulmonary ventilation imaged by magnetic resonance. Eur Resp Monogr 30:325–342

Kovacs G, Reiter G, Reiter U, Rienmüller R, Peacock A, Olschewski H (2008) The emerging role of magnetic resonance imaging in the diagnosis and management of pulmonary hypertension. Respiration 76:458–470

Laurent F, Montaudon M, Corneloup O (2006) CT and MRI of Lung Cancer. Respiration 73:133–142

Ley S, Kreitner KF, Fink C, Heussel CP, Borst MM, Kauczor HU (2004) Assessment of pulmonary hypertension by CT and MR imaging. Eur Radiol 14:359–368

Möller HE, Chen XJ, Saam B, Hagspiel KD, Johnson GA, Altes TA, de Lange EE, Kauczor HU (2002) MRI of the lungs using hyperpolarized Noble Gases. Magn Reson Med 47:1029–1051

Mosbah K, Ruiz-Cabello J, Berthezène Y, Crémillieux Y (2008) Aerosols and gaseous contrast agents for magnetic resonance imaging of the lung. Contrast Media Mol Imaging 3:173–190

Pedersen MR, Fisher MT, van Beek EJ (2006) MR imaging of the pulmonary vasculature–an update. Eur Radiol 16:1374–1386

Puderbach M, Hintze C, Ley S, Eichinger M, Kauczor HU, Biederer J (2007) MR imaging of the chest: a practical approach at 1.5T. Eur J Radiol 64:345–355

Van Beek EJR, Wild JM, Fink C, Moody AR, Kauczor HU, Oudkerk M (2003) MRI for the diagnosis of pulmonary embolism. J Magn Reson Imaging 18:627–640

Van Beek EJR, Wild JM, Schreiber W, Kauczor HU, Mugler III J, de Lange EE (2004) Functional MRI of the lung using hyperpolarized 3-helium gas. J Magn Reson Imaging 20:540–554

Van Beek EJ, Hoffman EA (2008) Functional imaging: CT and MRI. Clin Chest Med 29:195–216

White CS (2000) MR imaging of the thorax. Magn Reson Imaging Clin N Am 8:1–219

Heart

10

James F. M. Meaney and John Sheehan

Contents

J. F. M. Meaney (✉)
MRI Department, St. James's Hospital, St. James's Street, Dublin 8, Ireland
e-mail: jmeaney@meaneys.com

10.1 Introduction

Over the last 100 years, cardiac disease has dramatically increased in incidence, now accounting for approximately 30% of all causes of death worldwide compared to approximately 10% 100 years ago. It is predicted that within the next 50 years, cardiovascular disease will become the most common killer disease globally. However, the fact that many of the manifestations of cardiovascular disease are treatable, presents an epidemiological challenge in terms of unraveling the complex interactions between interdependent risk factors, their control and subsequent treatment, and also an enormous challenge in terms of refining the exact nature and distribution of the abnormality with imaging.

Since the introduction of cardiac triggering, breath-hold imaging and other fast imaging techniques, electrocardiographically gated cardiac MRI (CMR) has become a valuable tool for detailed evaluation of cardiac morphology and function in both congenital and acquired heart disease (Figs. 10.1–10.38). Recent improvements in hardware and software, for example reliable T1-W first-pass imaging, improved steady-state imaging, and the introduction of parallel imaging techniques have brought greatly improved reliability and results. The future introduction of coronary magnetic resonance angiography (MRA) into clinical practice will pave the way for a comprehensive "one-stop-shop" evaluation with CMR that will compete with the information provided by a multimodality combination of coronary CTA, echocardiography, nuclear scanning, and catheter arteriography.

P. Reimer et al. (eds.), *Clinical MR Imaging*,
DOI: 10.1007/978-3-540-74504-4_10, © Springer-Verlag Berlin Heidelberg 2010

High quality CMR now offers the following:

- Anatomic imaging for chamber morphology.
- Tissue characterization (high signal from fatty tumors and arrhythmogenic right ventricular cardiomyopathy (ARVD) and definition of myocardial scarring).
- Myocardial perfusion in ischemic heart disease.
- Flow quantification (valvular lesions and shunts).

MR imaging is contraindicated in patients with an implanted cardiac device such as a pacemaker, defibrillator, or other electrical device. Mediastinal clips, coronary intravascular stents, and most cardiac prostheses may produce artifacts and may limit diagnostic accuracy, but do not contraindicate the examination.

To address the criticism that growth in CV imaging sometimes occurs in the absence of an evidence base to support its use, eight international scientific organizations (American College of Cardiology Foundation, American College of Radiology, Society of Cardiovascular Computed Tomography, Society for Cardiovascular Magnetic Resonance, American Society of Nuclear Cardiology, North American Society for Cardiac Imaging, Society for Cardiovascular Angiography and Interventions, and Society of Interventional Radiology) embarked on a process, whereby 33 indications for CMR were reviewed by an international panel which rated indications based on a maximum 9 point score as appropriate (7–9), unsure (4–6), or inappropriate (1–3). Briefly, their findings supported CMR as appropriate (score 7 or higher) for the following indications:

- Ventricular and valvular function
- Specific cardiomyopathies
- ARVD
- LV function post MI
- LV function when results of other tests are discordant
- Myocarditis or myocardial infarction with normal coronary arteries
- Detection of myocardial scarring and viability
- Cardiac valve function
- Cardiac masses
- Pericardial disease
- Pulmonary vein geometry for mapping purposes
- Patients with chest pain and uninterpretable ECG or those unable to exercise
- Anomalous coronary artery origins

10.1.1 Preparation

As CMR is usually the last of a series of cardiac investigations, communication between the referring physician and the radiologist is essential as much of the information required to direct appropriate treatment may already be available from a combination of other modalities. Although a comprehensive CMR takes up to 1 h, studies targeted to a specific clinical question (e.g., HOCM/ARVD/scarring) can be easily performed in less than 30 min, and the examination, where possible, should be targeted to a specific clinical question. Because of potentially long scan times, patients should empty the bladder immediately before the examination. If patients require sedation, the dose must be accurately titrated so that the patient may comply with breathing instructions.

Cardiac images free from motion artifact are possible by a combination of ECG triggering (to compensate for cardiac motion) and either respiratory triggering/navigator echoes to eliminate breathing artifact. For breath-hold sequences, the patient should be instructed carefully prior to initiating scanning to guarantee high image quality. To ensure consistency of slice position between multiple breath-holds, most experts advocate data acquisition at end-expiration rather than end-inspiration.

10.1.2 ECG Gating and Respiratory Triggering

Uncompensated cardiac motion adversely affects MR image quality, thus rendering untriggered images of the heart virtually useless. The successful synchronization of data acquisition with different phases of the cardiac cycle by ECG gating and implementation of methods to compensate for or eliminate motion related to changes in diaphragmatic position with breathing have together been the critical developments that have allowed generation of high quality CMR images.

10.1.3 Addressing Cardiac Motion

Using ECG gating, each successive phase-encoded line is acquired at the same part of the cardiac cycle. Multislice imaging is possible, although each slice is acquired at a different phase of the cardiac cycle. Traditional methods of ECG gating by placing three monitoring electrodes on the anterior or posterior chest wall in close proximity to the heart were plagued with inconsistencies in triggering and much time was wasted in attempting to secure optimal electrode placement.

The more recent development of vector gating (VCG), which monitors two leads simultaneously has resulted in higher accuracy of detection of the R wave and improved image quality. VCG lead placement virtually eliminates the requirement for the multiple electrode repositioning which was characteristic of earlier methods and allows for more efficient use of scanner time.

Disposable electrodes, which are precoated with electrode jelly, assure good contact with the patient's skin, which should be cleaned and shaved if necessary.

In occasional patients, adequate gating may not be obtained, and in these patients, peripheral pulse gating may be helpful although image quality is usually severely compromised.

10.1.4 Addressing Respiratory Motion

Without compensation for changes in the position of the heart with respiration, any improvements in image quality provided by ECG triggering alone would be useless. As (successful) breath-holding completely eliminates respiratory motion artifact, it offers advantages over competing techniques, but suffers from several limitations including short breath-holding ability, varying position between consecutive breath-holds and cranial migration of diaphragmatic position during long breath-holds even in patients with excellent breath-hold capability. The patient should be instructed carefully prior to initiating scanning to guarantee high image quality.

Another competing technique, known as Navigator Imaging, has gained widespread acceptance as an excellent technique to eliminate motion artifact, particularly for coronary MRA. Using this technique, cranio-caudad motion of the diaphragm is monitored by a 2D sequence in real-time, which feeds back diaphragmatic (and therefore cardiac) position to the host computer.

10.1.5 Coil Selection

In high-field MR systems, the body is the predominant source of noise. Careful selection of radiofrequency (RF) coils that are optimized for imaging specific anatomical structures allow the detector to be as near as possible to the region of interest and have, therefore, proven very beneficial. Today, most manufacturers provide dedicated multichannel cardiac surface coils although other coil combinations (e.g., a spine coil placed across the chest) may be used. Phased-array coils provide high image quality, excellent signal-to-noise ratio, adequate spatial resolution, and sufficient contrast resolution.

Infants and small children may be scanned within a head-imaging coil which gives adequate coverage, good signal-to-noise, and excellent spatial resolution.

10.1.6 Image Plane Construction

A great advantage of MR imaging is the ability to select and image in any plane. By convention, images must be acquired in standardized planes including long- and short-axis orientation, which allows for comparison of the MR images with the information obtained using other cross-sectional techniques, such as echocardiography and angiocardiography. To obtain these axes, a series of low-resolution, ungated, gradient-echo (GRE) scout images (localizers) are acquired as follows:

1. Coronal images, through the middle third of the chest to provide cranial and caudal landmarks.
2. Axial images to define the interventricular septum and chamber morphology.
3. Oblique images, parallel to the ventricular septum.

10.2 Sequence Protocols

10.2.1 Localizer/Scout

The fast imaging with steady precession (FISP), two-dimensional (2D) sequence is a standard scout protocol used with nonbreath-hold imaging techniques. Multiple acquisitions may be used to reduce respiratory and cardiac motion artifacts. The turbo fast low-angle shot sequence (FLASH) combines a dark-blood single-shot sequence which freezes respiratory motion.

10.2.2 Morphology

10.2.2.1 Dark-Blood Imaging

Spin-echo (SE) sequences generate excellent anatomical details and provide the basis of black-blood multislice cardiac imaging. They have the drawbacks of long scan times and sensitivity to respiratory motion. They are routinely employed for multislice demonstration of myocardial and pericardial morphology, but otherwise are used less frequently because of the availability of faster, improved sequences that demonstrate both morphology and function. Great improvement in black-blood imaging has been achieved by double or triple-inversion techniques which yield heavily T1-W studies. By combining this approach with single-slice breath-hold imaging, excellent contrast between flowing blood (dark) and cardiac muscle (intermediate) is generated.

10.2.3 Function

Several methods are available including "cine" imaging, myocardial tagging, and flow quantification with phase-contrast methods. Perfusion imaging also gives an indirect assessment of function.

10.2.3.1 Bright Blood Imaging: Gradient Echo (GRE) and Balanced (SSFP) Imaging

Standard Gradient echo imaging is a rapid imaging technique that generates high signal from flowing blood due to the use of short TRs and short TEs which "freeze" cardiac motion as a result of data collection (image readout) before excited spins have had time to exit the slice. Multiple slices triggered to the ECG can be viewed in a continuous cine loop thus giving the impression of dynamic imaging throughout the cardiac cycle. Because of artifacts and nonuniform signal from flowing blood, standard GRE sequences have now given way to "balanced" sequences (steady-state free precession or fast imaging with steady-state precession (SSFP/FISP)), so called because images with a rather unique weighting (reflecting the ratio of T2/T1) are produced. With the most widely used "balanced" sequences, uniform bright signal is visualized from normally flowing blood, as SSFP images are inherently insensitive to in-plane flow. However, dark signal is generated from rapidly flowing turbulent blood which enters the slice in the short interval between scan excitation and data collection. This finding of linear dark signal within otherwise uniform flowing blood indicates turbulence related to stenosis, regurgitation, and shunting (which can be quantified using a phase-contrast technique – see below). Cine imaging can also be exploited to accurately determine cardiac output, either manually or with an automated or semiautomated contouring methods which determine cross-sectional area for each location at end systole and end diastole from a comprehensive set of short-axis images acquired from base to apex in several minutes.

10.2.3.2 Myocardial Tagging

Myocardial tagging (grid or stripe tagging) is an MR imaging method that applies RF pulses perpendicular to the imaging plane to presaturate part of the myocardium prior to data collection. Tags can be applied solely parallel to one another ("stripes") or in two orthogonal directions ("grids"). These grids or stripes persist in the myocardium throughout most or all of the cardiac cycle and indicate the degree of myocardial contractility depending on how much they deform. For example, if a grid pattern of tagging is used, progressive deformation of the regular square grid pattern throughout systole indicates good contractility, whereas persistence of the "square" pattern (i.e., failure to deform) indicates poor contraction. As tags fade progressively throughout the cardiac cycle, they are applied just after the "R" wave to image systolic function and in late diastole to image diastolic function. Numerous postprocessing algorithms are now available, which generate accurate estimates of tag displacement/deformation and therefore an indication of segmental dyskinesia or hypokinesis.

10.2.3.3 Phase-Contrast Techniques

Phase-contrast techniques can be used not only to generate angiograms but also to assess blood-flow velocities. Phase-contrast images (generated by subtracting images acquired with opposite flow encoding gradients) demonstrate flowing blood as bright and background tissues as dark (absence of phase shift ensures complete nulling of background). In general, phase shifts are proportional to flow velocity in the presence of a flow encoding gradient. By collecting multiple ECG synchronized images, a time resolved velocity profile can be generated, which, along with knowledge of the cross-sectional area can be exploited to give volumetric flow rates. This approach can be used to quantify regurgitatant jets and intracardiac shunts.

10.2.3.4 Angiography

Although MRA, particularly contrast-enhanced MRA is in widespread clinical use for virtually all vascular territories, the main remaining limitation is in imaging the coronary arteries. The reasons for this include small artery size, tortuosity, complex anatomy, and artifacts related to cardiac and diaphragmatic motion. Although each of these limitations has been addressed at least in part their complex interaction in the coronary vasculature presents a unique challenge that is yet to be overcome. Despite improvements in technique, currently only broad categorization of stenosis diameter is possible and a sufficiently comprehensive analysis to allow for accurate surgical planning is not possible in most instances. As a result, despite enormous advances and widespread acceptance of CMR, coronary MR in the era of widely available and high quality coronary CTA is routinely advocated only for determining the position of the coronary artery ostia in patients with suspected anomalous origins.

2D approaches during breath-holding have now given way to ECG-triggered segmented k-space 3D approaches that now form the basis for all current coronary artery MR methods. Numerous k-space lines are acquired during the quiet part of consecutive cardiac cycles (middiastole), a process that is repeated over as many heartbeats as is necessary until the full k-space data-set is covered, during either breath-holding or free breathing. Breath-holding allows only limited anatomical coverage and multiple breath-holds are required for each coronary artery. With free breathing, a real-time navigator echo detects diaphragm position and updates the superior-to-inferior motion of the right hemidiaphragm thus allowing high in-plane acquisition matrix with good SNR albeit at the expense of prolonged scan time. With this approach, whole-heart coverage is feasible, optimally using a three-dimensional approach.

SSFP Method

The high SNR and blood-myocardial contrast generated with this technique allow clear definition of the coronary arteries. Although Gadolinium-based contrast agents offer potential benefit with this technique, their short blood half-life limits their use owing to dramatic changes in intravascular T1 values throughout the (long – 10–15 min) acquisition time. The use of blood-pool agents such as Gadofosveset Trisodium (ablavar), which persists in the blood pool for a very long time (therefore minimal change in blood T1, if any, over the acquisition period), may offer benefit in this regard.

10.2.3.5 Perfusion

Assessment of myocardial perfusion by increase in myocardial signal on T1-W GRE images following injection of paramagnetic contrast agent is a widely practiced technique that gives information similar to, but at a much higher resolution than nuclear techniques such as cardiac SPECT and positron emission tomography (PET). Currently, myocardial perfusion is carried out following injection of an extracellular contrast agent, despite significant (30–50%) leakage of these agents into the interstitial tissues on first pass. Therefore, in order to quantify myocardial perfusion, modeling of tissue extraction must be performed. The newly introduced blood-pool (intravascular) contrast agents at least in theory simplify this task as increases in myocardial T1 values reflect only tissue perfusion as there is no extravascular contrast leakage. As a result, improved parameters of myocardial perfusion may be anticipated with this new generation of contrast agents although this is as yet unproven. Perfusion can be evaluated under the following conditions:

At rest: This is only moderately sensitive for significant steno-occlusive coronary artery lesions. However, detection of perfusion abnormalities at rest in the early post-acute infarct phase correlates with LV functional impairment and remodeling.

Stress perfusion: This can be performed with physical exercise, which is extremely difficult to enact within the MR environment or by delivery of pharmacological stress (e.g., Dipyridamole or preferably Adenosine due to its superior safety profile and more reliable course of action) via an infusion pump.

Numerous studies report high accuracy of stress perfusion compared to SPECT/PET for significant CAD.

10.2.4 Contrast Agents

Paramagnetic contrast agents in clinical studies are for the most part gadolinium chelates. Contrast agents are required for only some cardiac examinations – specifically, evaluation of masses, assessment of myocardial blood flow and viability, and possibly for whole-heart coronary MRA. In the normal myocardium, water passes freely through the capillary wall and cellular membrane and the standard extracellular low-molecular gadolinium chelates are free to equilibrate throughout the interstitium, but they do not enter the cells. In contrast, macromolecular contrast agents (intravascular or blood-pool agents) do not exit the blood pool into the interstitial spaces. This advantage of blood pool over extracellular agents can potentially be exploited to generate superior quality perfusion studies and also improved whole-heart coronary MRA with SSFP imaging.

10.3 Clinical Applications of Cardiac MR Imaging

10.3.1 Ischemic Heart Disease

Ischemic heart disease remains a leading cause of morbidity and mortality in industrial nations. The clinical use of MR imaging techniques in ischemic heart disease is gaining momentum as MR imaging offers a comprehensive, noninvasive evaluation of cardiac morphology, function, and perfusion (Figs. 10.1–10.9).

Determining the presence, size, and location of acute myocardial infarctions and differentiating between acute and chronic myocardial infarctions is now possible. MR imaging may reveal complications associated with myocardial infarctions and may allow for the assessment of global and regional myocardial function, cardiac morphology, and blood flow through native coronary arteries and bypass grafts. Moreover, the application of contrast agents may allow for the evaluation of regional myocardial perfusion at different stages of ischemic heart disease, including characterizing occlusive and reperfused myocardial infarctions and determining the presence of stunned and hibernating myocardium in regions being considered for revascularization. The one major remaining limitation of suboptimal depiction of the coronary arteries is at least partially compensated for by the fact that cardiac perfusion imaging (at rest and/or stress) effectively assesses the coronary microvasculature and arguably gives superior information than that obtained from depiction of the coronary arteries with CTA or catheter angiography, which demonstrate only the degree of stenosis and give no indication of the tissue effect of the stenosis.

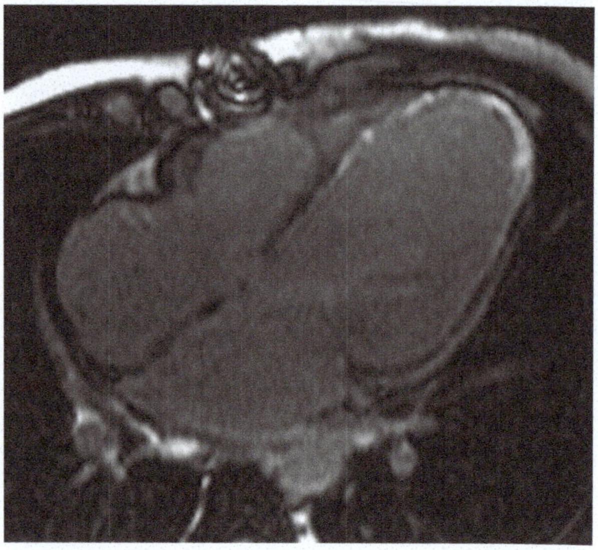

Fig. 10.1 Dilated ischemic cardiomyopathy in a 75-year-old female. The single-shot inversion-recovery sequence, 4-chamber view demonstrates enlargement of the left ventricle and atrium. There is diffuse, predominantly nonviable late gadolinium enhancement in the LAD territory

Many clinicians now believe that MR will soon offer a comprehensive "one-stop-shop" modality for the evaluation of patients with chest pain and suspected myocardial ischemia.

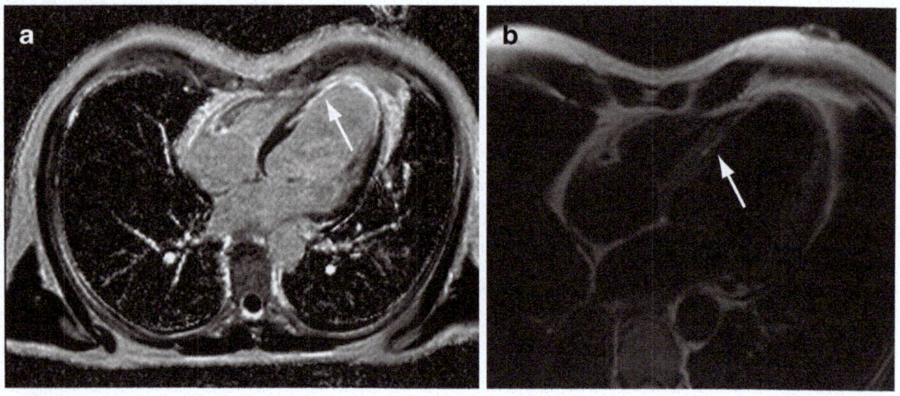

Fig. 10.2 Fibro-fatty LAD infarct in a 55-year-old male. The single-shot inversion-recovery sequence, 4-chamber view (**a**) demonstrates transmural late gadolinium enhancement which is nonviable in the mid and distal LAD territory. The dark blood, HASTE (**b**), sequence reveals fat within the infarcted septal wall

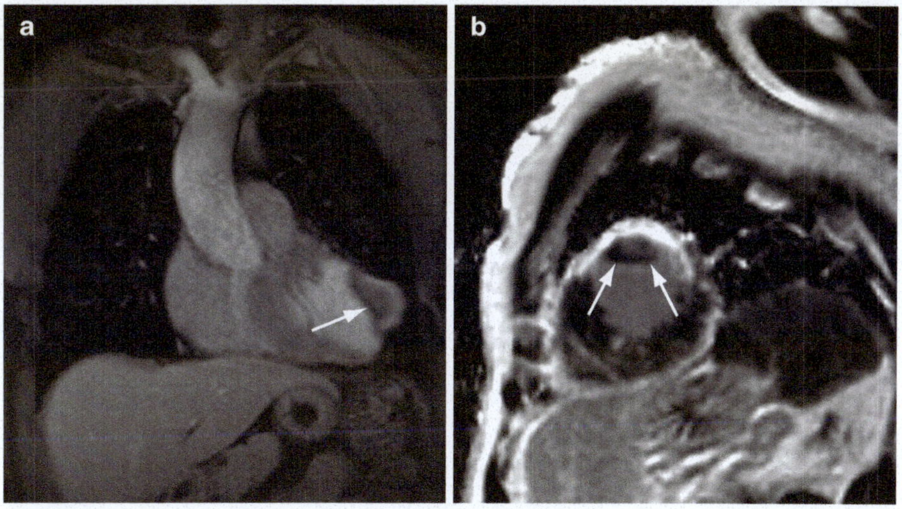

Fig. 10.3 A 58-year-old male patient who presents with a cryptogenic stroke. The coronal T1-W fat-saturation sequence (**a**) reveals a left ventricular aneurysm containing a thrombus. The phase-sensitive inversion-recovery TurboFLASH, short-axis sequence (**b**) demonstrates the thrombus lying adjacent to transmurally infarcted left ventricular aneurysm

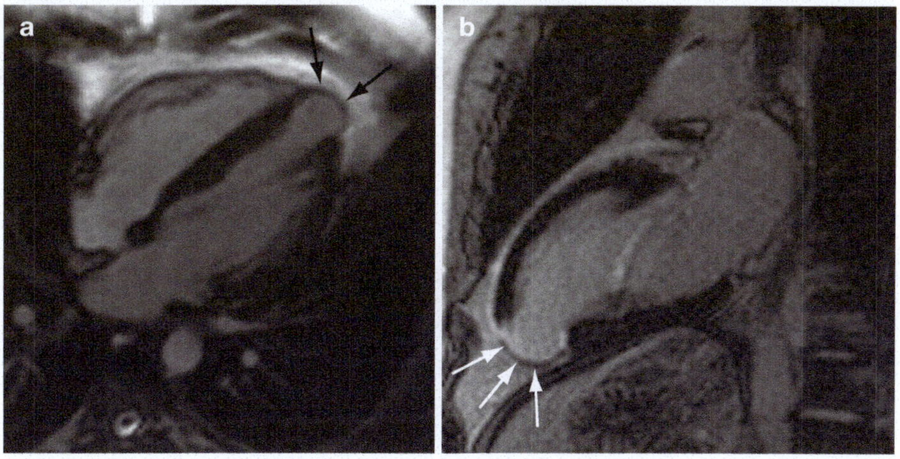

Fig. 10.4 Left ventricular apical aneurysm in a 70-year-old male with a history of a recent myocardial infarction. The 4-chamber cine trueFISP sequence (**a**) demonstrates the focal aneurysm. The single-shot inversion-recovery sequence (**b**) demonstrates thinning and out pouching of the apical wall with transmural late gadolinium enhancement

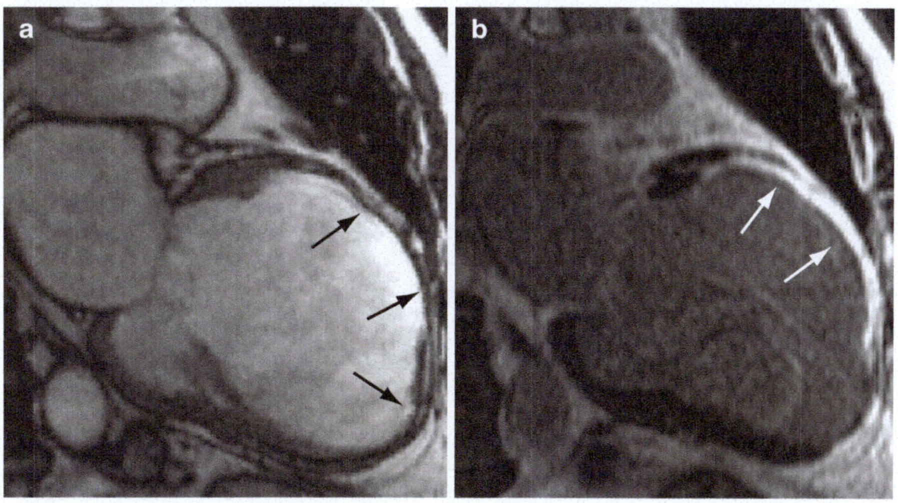

Fig. 10.5 (**a**, **b**) Dilated ischemic cardiomyopathy in a 67-year-old male patient. The 2-chamber cine trueFISP sequence (**a**) demonstrates the markedly enlarged left ventricle and anterior wall thinning. The single-shot inversion-recovery sequence demonstrates transmural late gadolinium enhancement of the anterior wall in the LAD territory. Images courtesy of James Carr, Northwestern Memorial Hospital, Chicago, IL

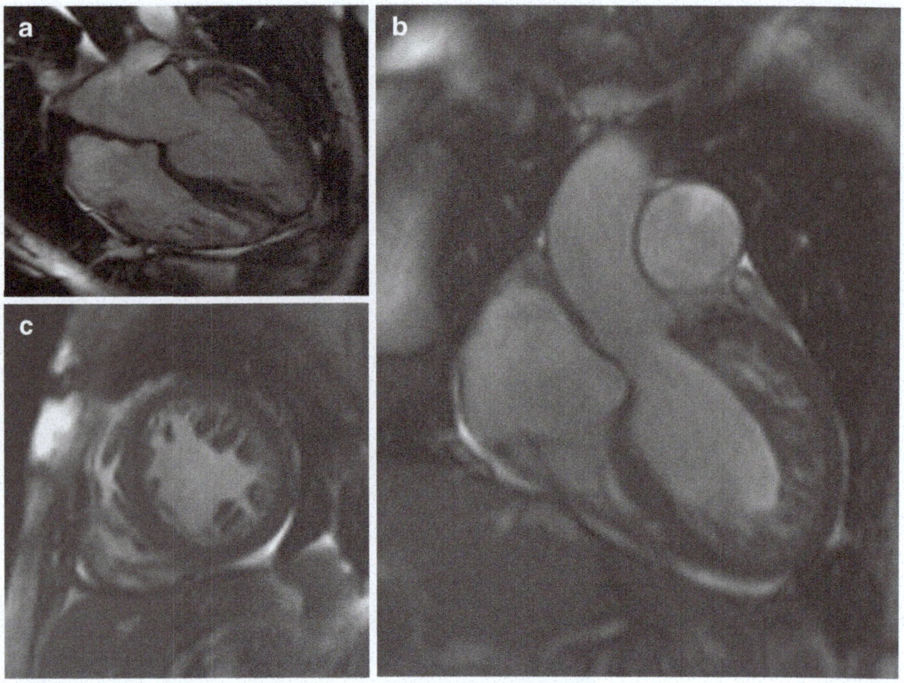

Fig. 10.6 Left ventricular noncompaction in a 35-year-old male. The various cine trueFISP sequences (**a–c**) demonstrate an increased ratio (>2.3) of the noncompacted to the compacted myocardium involving the lateral and apical walls of the left ventricle

10.3.1.1 MR Imaging Protocol

For MR studies in patients with ischemic heart disease, a comprehensive protocol with morphological and functional studies and evaluation of perfusion and viability is recommended.

Morphology

In acute myocardial infarction, ECG-gated T2-W MR images show high signal intensity. This is consistent with myocardial edema and the pattern of contrast change that occurs with increasing echo time (TE). Animal studies have revealed a significant prolongation of the T2-relaxation time as early as 4 h after myocardial ischemia is induced by coronary occlusion. Initial hypoperfusion, followed by evolving edema in the infarct and the surrounding region, plays a role in producing transient changes in T1- and T2-relaxation times. The size of the infarcted region can be determined very accurately with MR imaging.

Even though changes in T1 and T2 due to infarction and edema provide excellent MR contrast, infarcted regions can be better distinguished from normal myocardium using contrast-enhanced MR imaging. Old myocardial infarctions do not show enhancement by gadolinium, because the ischemic myocardium is replaced by scar tissue (Figs. 10.1, 10.4, 10.5, 10.9). Regional wall thinning also occurs in patients with old myocardial infarction.

Myocardial infarctions involving the left ventricle often produce aneurysms and mural thrombi (Fig. 10.3). Aneurysms are frequently located in the apex or the antero-lateral region and are recognized as severe wall thinning and diastolic bulging of the left ventricular wall (Figs. 10.3, 10.4). Mural thrombi are recognized as a mass adhering to the myocardium or as filling defects within an aneurysm sac. The signal intensity of mural thrombi varies, depending on age. In subacute cases, the thrombus shows an intermediate or high signal intensity on T1-WI and a high signal intensity on T2-WI. The signal decreases with increasing age, and an organized thrombus has a low signal intensity on both T1 and T2 weighted images. It is difficult to differentiate a thrombus from slow-flowing blood on SE images (nonbreath-holding) in some cases. However, on the cine-mode images, the thrombus produces low signal intensity and is contrasted against the high signal of the left ventricular blood pool.

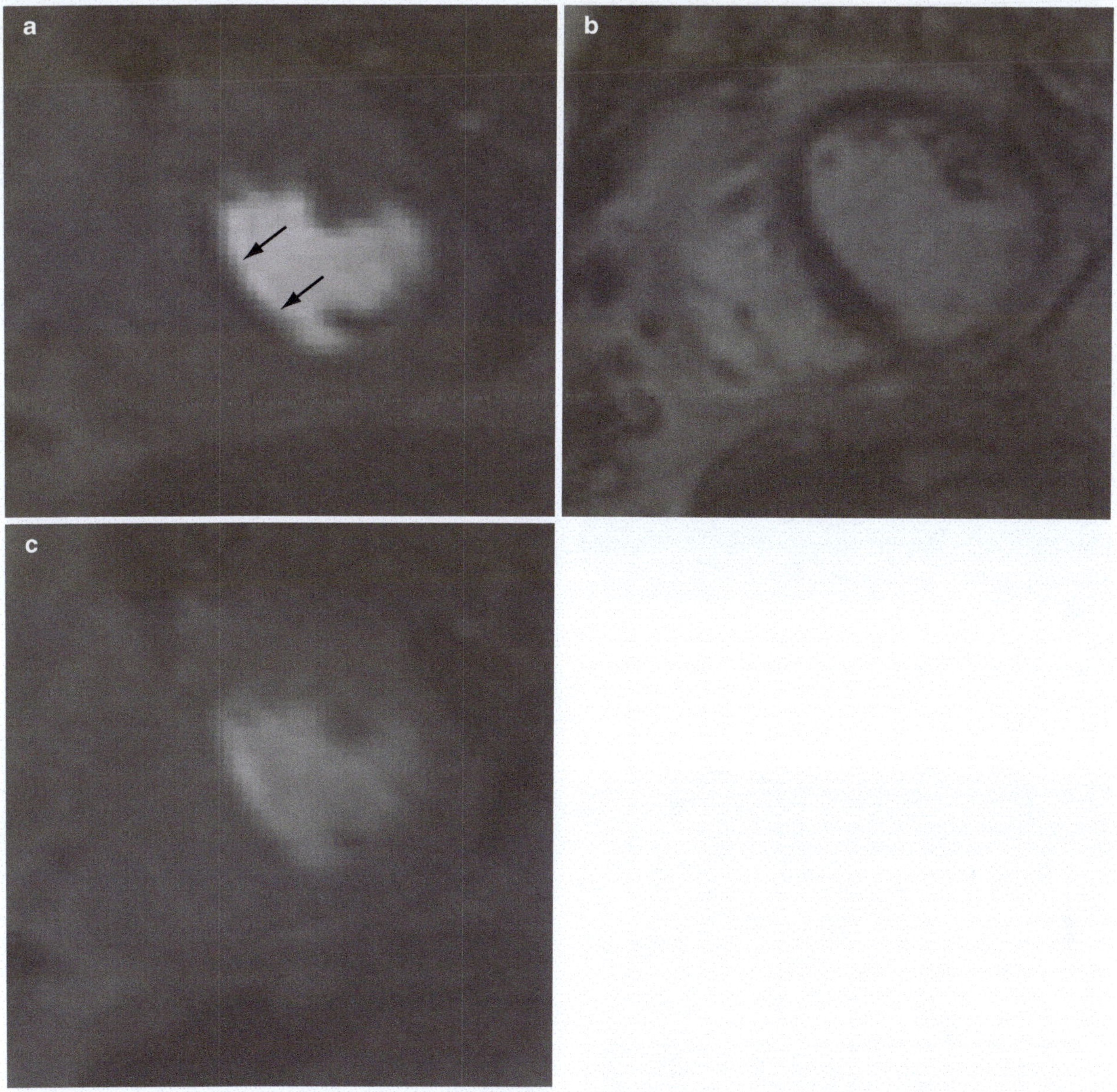

Fig. 10.7 (**a–c**) First pass myocardial perfusion imaging performed in a 56-year-old male with angina. The adenosine stress perfusion short-axis image (**a**) demonstrates a subendocardial perfusion defect in the distribution of the LAD and RCA, which reverses on the rest image (**b**). The single-shot inversion-recovery sequence (**c**) demonstrates no late gadolinium enhancement

10.3.1.2 Functional Assessment of Ischemia

Myocardial function is determined by a combination of Cine MR imaging and tagging techniques. Cine imaging is useful for defining focal areas of myocardial dyskinesia and for demonstrating valvular dysfunction, which may either contribute to or be caused by myocardial ischemia. Normal thickening is about 60% over baseline (end diastole). At sites of myocardial infarction, thinning of the wall at end diastole occurs, the LV thickness in the infarcted area is less, and wall contractility, as determined by cine images and tagging techniques is impaired. In severe cases, there is paradoxical wall motion leading to LV aneurysm formation (Figs. 10.3 and 10.4). Comparative studies of fluorodeoxyglucose (FDG), PET, and cine MR imaging have concluded that

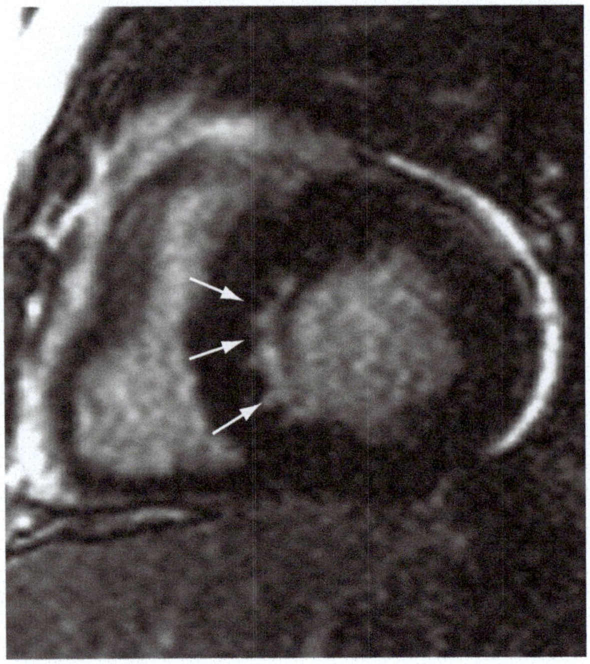

Fig. 10.8 2D single-shot inversion-recovery, short-axis, viability sequence demonstrates 25% subendocardial enhancement of the septal wall in the mid chamber consistent with a viable LAD territory infarct

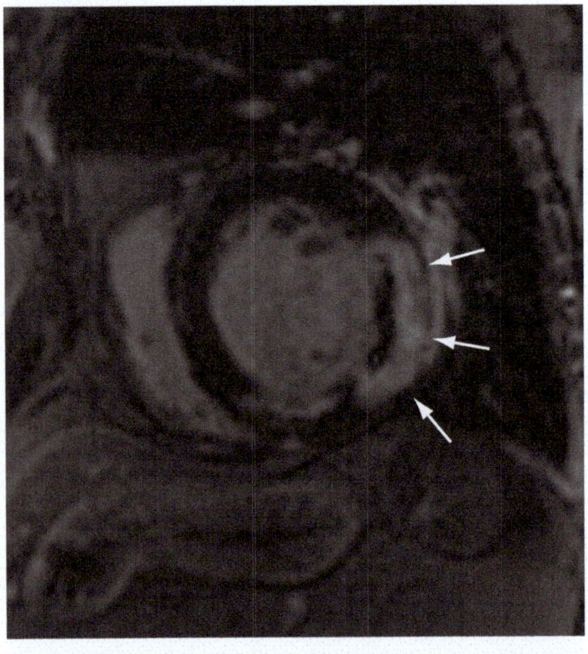

Fig. 10.9 Acute left circumflex infarct with microvascular obstruction in a 59-year-old male. The single-shot inversion-recovery sequence short axis at the mid chamber level demonstrates transmural late gadolinium enhancement with a zone of no reflow within the subendocardium

wall thickness and systolic wall thickening provide reliable evidence that regions with a moderate reduction in FDG activity represent viable myocardium. Absence of systolic wall thickening may be present both in hibernating and nonviable myocardium; however, the combination of severely reduced or absent FDG activity associated with significant wall thinning and no systolic wall thickening indicates nonviable myocardium, which can be confirmed by late gadolinium enhancement (LGE) (see below) (Figs. 10.1, 10.4–6, 10.8, 10.9). Using cine and tagged MR imaging, regional wall thinning in ischemic cardiomyopathy can be distinguished from uniform wall thinning in patients with idiopathic congestive dilated cardiomyopathy (Fig. 10.10).

10.3.1.3 Perfusion and Viability

With the development of ultrafast imaging techniques, it has become possible to visualize regional myocardial perfusion by monitoring first-pass passage of standard, extracellular contrast media. An inversion-recovery technique is recommended to improve the contrast between normal and abnormal areas. Although little gadolinium enters the interstitial spaces of the myocardium under normal circumstances due to the myocytes being tightly packed together, nonetheless there is an early and progressive increase in signal intensity within the myocardium following gadolinium injection reflecting a small amount of contrast agent leakage added to by the presence of intravascular contrast agent within the microvasculature. However, in areas of absent blood flow (i.e., infarcted), there is a progressive accumulation of gadolinium within the infarcted areas as a result of cellular disruption and expansion of the interstitial component (Figs. 10.1–10.4, 10.8, 10.9). These observations can be exploited to generate information regarding myocardial perfusion as follows. A normally perfused myocardial region demonstrates T1-shortening effect, with an increase in signal intensity, followed by washout from the tissue after intravenous bolus administration of contrast agent. Ischemic (hypoperfused) but viable myocardium demonstrates reduced signal intensity compared with normal myocardium, (which may only be visible on stress imaging – see below) (Fig. 10.7). In infarcted (nonviable) areas, there is progressive accumulation of gadolinium in areas of scarring (Figs. 10.1, 10.8, 10.9). Although this observation appears to fly in the face of accepted

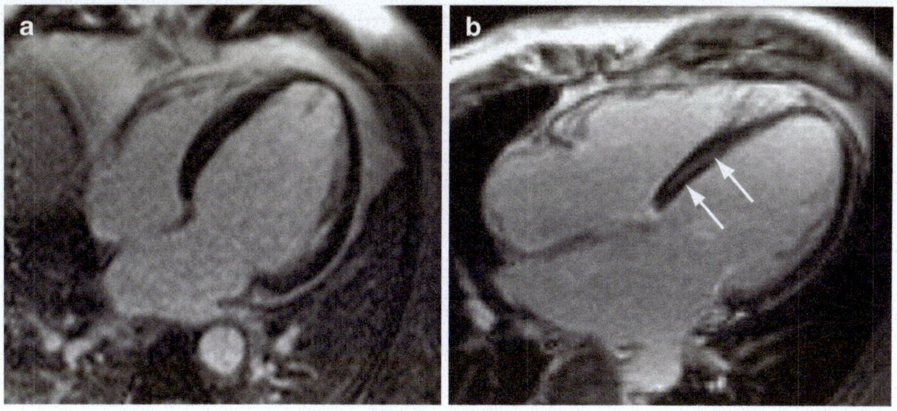

Fig. 10.10 Nonischemic cardiomyopathy in two patients. The first patient (**a**) has a mildly dilated cardiomyopathy with no late gadolinium enhancement. The second patient (**b**) has dilated cardiomyopathy with mid myocardial late gadolinium enhancement of the septal wall which may represent left ventricular strain secondary to hypertension

dogma (i.e., bright on postcontrast imaging = perfused), in the case of CMR, bright appearance on late postcontrast imaging (LGE) reflects expansion of the extracellular interstitial space in infarcted tissue. Imaging for LGE is best performed at least 10 min postcontrast injection and in order to accentuate this hyperenhancement in the presence of otherwise normally enhancing myocardium, an inversion-recovery pulse is applied which nulls the normal myocardium, thus accentuating the brightly enhancing nonviable myocardium. In general, an inversion time of 200–300 ms is optimal; however, this should be tailored specifically for each patient by performing a single slice through the myocardium employing multiple inversion times and then choosing that inversion time that optimally suppresses the myocardium for definitive multislice imaging from base to apex.

Although 99mTc sestamibi SPECT scanning and cardiac PET scanning were previously regarded as the gold standard for the assessment of myocardial perfusion, the spatial and temporal resolution of these techniques is greatly exceeded by CMR, and Gadolinium-enhanced CMR has become the defacto gold standard for the assessment of myocardial perfusion. In particular, in has been shown in both animal and human studies that perfusion imaging with MR accurately demonstrates subendocardial infarction (i.e. less than transmural) which is frequently missed by scintigraphic techniques.

Interpretation of the large number of images generated and subtle differences between areas will be simplified by automated pixel-based programs and the creation of perfusion maps.

10.3.1.4 Stress MR Imaging

MR imaging during dynamic exercise, as in an ECG laboratory, is currently not feasible within conventional magnets because of the constrained MR environment and motion-related artifacts. Patients who have coronary artery disease with normal left ventricular function and normal myocardial perfusion at rest can have stress-induced wall motion or wall-thickening abnormalities indicating ischemic myocardium (Fig. 10.7). Pharmacological stress MR with dipyridamole, Dobutamine or, because of improved safety profile, Adenosine, is reproducible, accurate, and suitable for patients in whom stress echocardiography cannot be performed. Dipyridamole stress MR imaging for hemodynamically significant stenoses associated with major coronary arteries has a sensitivity of 85% and specificity of 90%. Dobutamine stress MR imaging, using the analysis of ventricular wall segment thickening, gives up to 100% sensitivity for three-vessel disease. With dobutamine stress MR imaging, wall motion abnormalities can be induced in myocardial areas fed by coronary arteries with hemodynamically significant and subcritical stenoses (insufficient coronary reserve). Cine MR imaging with dobutamine stress testing correlates well with the results of myocardial stress scintigraphy, but has demonstrated higher sensitivity and specificity than dobutamine stress echocardiography, attributed to consistently superior image quality coupled with the ability to detect subtle wall motion abnormalities with tissue tagging.

10.3.1.5 Coronary Artery Mapping in Ischemia

Results in clinical practice have been less than that achieved with CTA, and clinical acceptance of coronary MRA poor. Improved results are anticipated with whole-heart coronary MRA possibly with the use of blood-pool agents.

10.3.2 Cardiomyopathies

10.3.2.1 Introduction

Cardiomyopathies are disorders of the heart muscle that result from a myriad of insults (Figs. 10.10–10.14). They are classified into five subcategories as follows; (1) dilated, (2) hypertrophic, (3) restrictive, (4) ARVD, and (5) unclassified. Echocardiography has traditionally been the primary technique used for the evaluation of cardiomyopathies; however, MR imaging offers similar information to Echo in many cases, superior information in others, and in some instances demonstrates findings that cannot be elucidated by other approaches. MR imaging demonstrates not only the phenotypic abnormalities associated with these diseases, but also gives functional information, assessment of perfusion, and viability. Cine MR and tagged imaging studies demonstrate global and regional systolic and diastolic ventricular function, which can be accurately quantified, both prior to and in response to drug treatment in patients with congestive cardiomyopathy.

Congestive (dilated) cardiomyopathy is a pathophysiological, not an etiological classification; it is characterized by ventricular dilatation, systolic dysfunction, and congestive heart failure (Fig. 10.10). Alcohol, peripartum cardiomyopathy, various toxins, ischemia, diabetes, hypertension, obesity, viral disease, and hereditary factors may all lead to a dilated left ventricle with reduced function and heart failure. This disease is the most common of the forms of cardiomyopathy.

Hypertrophic cardiomyopathy (HCM) is probably a genetic disorder, characterized by inappropriate left ventricular hypertrophy, often with left ventricular outflow tract obstruction and myocardial cellular disorganization (Fig. 10.11). Restrictive cardiomyopathy is also a pathophysiological and not an etiological classification; it is characterized by impaired ventricular diastolic filling due to myocardial disease. It is a relatively rare condition.

10.3.2.2 Congestive (Dilated) Cardiomyopathy

In patients with congestive cardiomyopathy, the left ventricle is grossly dilated and may be globular in shape, with a smooth endocardial surface (Fig. 10.10). The left ventricular wall thickness is usually within the normal range, but is sometimes surprisingly hypertrophied, thus resulting in a substantial overall increase in the left ventricular mass (up to 1,000 g). Even with hypertrophy, the ventricular walls are often thinned, but the thickness is uniform around the circumference of the left ventricle. Patients with ischemic cardiomyopathy

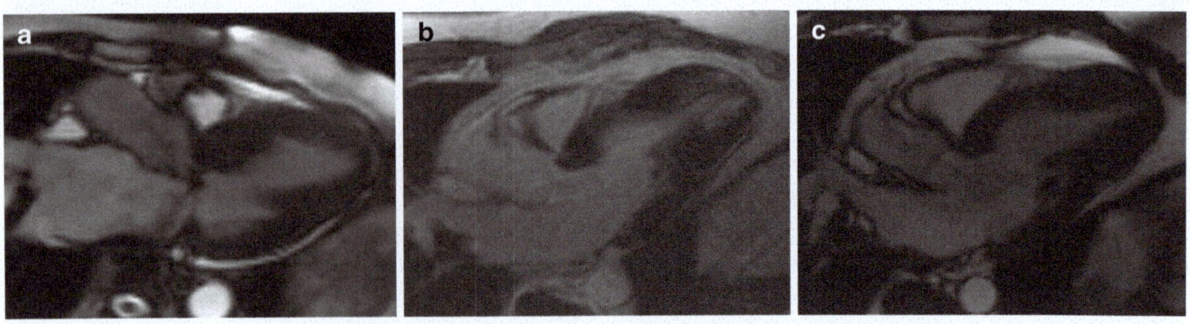

Fig. 10.11 Hypertrophic cardiomyopathy in two patients. The first patient (**a**) has asymmetric basal septal hypertrophy, which results in left ventricular outflow tract obstruction and systolic anterior motion (SAM) of the mitral valve, with resultant mitral regurgitation. The second patient (**b**) has apical hypertrophic cardiomyopathy with patchy subendocardial and mid myocardial late gadolinium enhancement (**c**)

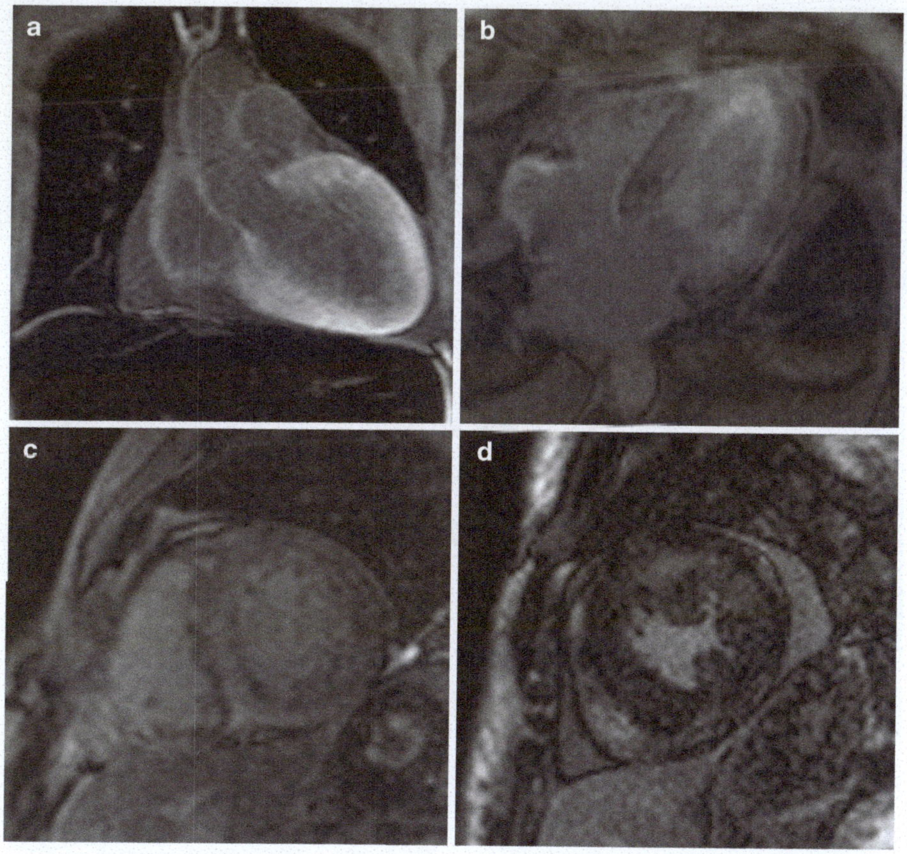

Fig. 10.12 Amyloid-related infiltrative cardiomyopathy. The coronal T1-W fat-saturation sequence (**a**) reveals diffuse significant increased signal intensity of the hypertrophied left ventricular myocardium. The single-shot inversion recovery 4-chamber sequence (**b**) demonstrates the classical diffuse circumferential subendocardial late gadolinium enhancement. Another patient (**c**) has predominantly mid myocardial regional enhancement of the inferomedial walls. (**d**) The final patient has a focal area of mid myocardial enhancement of the anterior wall at the mid chamber level

generally show a nonuniform pattern. Regions of wall thinning exist in these patients as a consequence of myocardial infarction (Fig. 10.5).

The primary value of morphological MR imaging in patients with congestive cardiomyopathy lies in the exclusion of other pathological causes of the dilatation, such as infarction or the formation of local aneurysms. MR imaging can differentiate these causes from the global dilatation of congestive cardiomyopathy. Patients with congestive heart failure frequently present with mural thrombi in the left ventricular cavity (mass adhering to the ventricular wall), usually located at the septum or apex of the ventricle.

Cine MR imaging can provide functional information about the left ventricular cavity that is useful in the diagnosis and management of patients with congestive cardiomyopathy. It may be used to demonstrate left ventricular wall thickening during the cardiac cycle (Fig. 10.6) and to calculate the stroke volume and ejection fraction. The ejection fraction is the most commonly used clinical parameter in these patients, and changes of the ejection fraction give the most reliable information about the therapeutic response or nonresponse. Furthermore, the presence of valvular regurgitation may be evaluated. Valvular regurgitation presents as a signal void, e.g., retrogradely projecting into the left atrium during ventricular systole in patients with mitral regurgitation.

10.3.2.3 Hypertrophic Cardiomyopathy

HCM is a relatively common autosomal dominant disorder that is characterized by a grossly thickened left ventricle in the absence of another predisposing cause (such as valvular heart disease, hypertension or ischemia) (Fig. 10.11). Pathologically, the condition is characterized by bizzarely shaped, swollen myocytes, which are arranged in a disorganized fashion. HCM is a cause of sudden cardiac death with an incidence of up to 0.2% of the population. The disorder is more commonly referred to as HOCM; however, left ventricular outflow

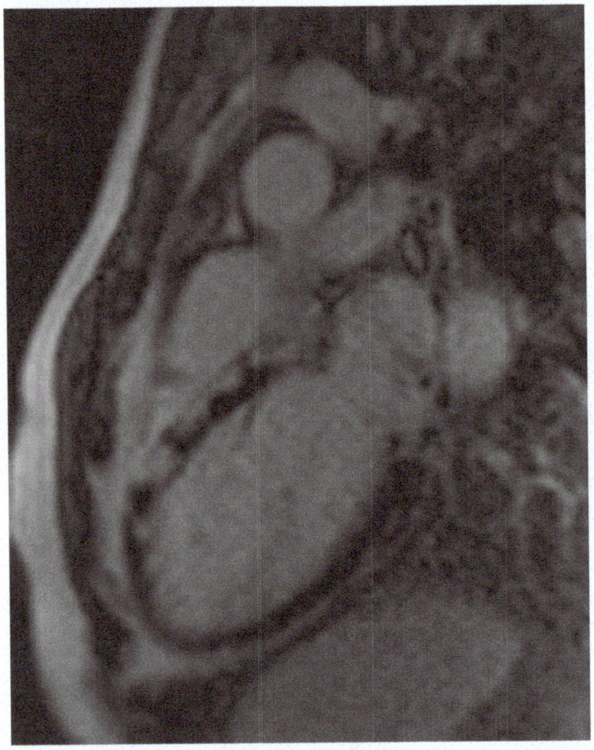

Fig. 10.13 Infiltrative myocardial sarcoidosis in a 35-year-old female. The 2-chamber single-shot inversion-recovery sequence demonstrates multifocal, predominantly midmyocardial and subepicardial late gadolinium enhancement of the anterior wall

tract obstruction, although common, is not ubiquitous or necessary for the diagnosis, hence the more correct all embracing term HCM. Obstruction is present at rest or can be induced by exercise in at least 50%. Other names include muscular subaortic stenosis (MSS) and idiopathic hypertrophic sub aortic stenosis (IHSS).

Imaging Findings

As patients with HCM have increased cardiac mass without LV dilatation, a characteristic finding is ventricular hypertrophy with narrowing of the LV cavity (Fig. 10.11). Hypertrophy can affect any part of the LV, the best known pattern being asymmetric hypertrophy of the interventricular septum, usually at the base (i.e., closest to the mitral valve) (Fig. 10.11a). However, any pattern of hypertrophy in the correct setting (i.e., no other cause) can be associated with and is consistent with HCM. Hypertrophy can be easily visualized on spin-echo images; however, cine MR imaging gives optimal

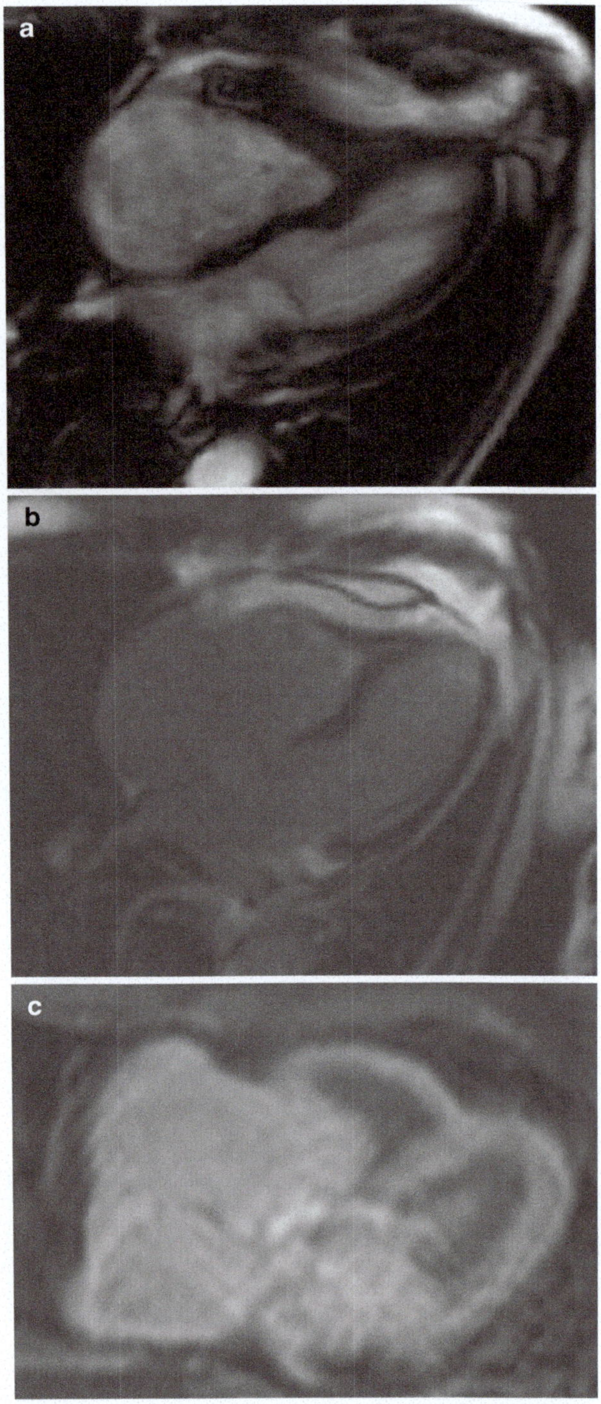

Fig. 10.14 A 74-year-old female present with shortness of breath and a history of hypereosinophilia. The 4-chamber cine trueFISP sequence (**a**) demonstrates an enlarged right atrium and a small right ventricle which has contracted toward its apical region. The single-shot inversion-recovery sequence (**b**) demonstrates subendocardial enhancement of the right ventricular apex, consistent with endomyocardial fibrosis. Another patient (**c**) has involvement of both ventricles with subendocardial thrombus formation evident on the postcontrast T1 fat-saturation sequence

definition of the degree of location and degree of septal thickening, and also optimally demonstrates outflow obstruction which may be visualised in late systole only. In some patients HCM mainly or exclusively affects the area around the apex (Fig. 10.11b). Associated abnormalities of the mitral valve are also commonly present, on echo cardiography or MRI where anterior motion of the mitral valve during systole is characteristic. Although the cause of this finding remains uncertain, it is believed to be secondary to a combination of a Venturi effect, which draws the mitral leaflet toward the septum as a result of the high velocity jet of blood directed along the septum toward the aortic valve and also a "drag" effect of flow directed along the leaflet. Despite deformity of the mitral valve, any resultant mitral regurgitation is usually mild; indeed, in the presence of significant mitral regurgitation another cause should be considered.

Myocardial fibrosis, which may reflect secondary myocardial ischemia as a result of inadequate capillary density relative to the increased LV mass, is identified as an area of increased signal intensity on delayed contrast-enhanced MR images (Fig. 10.11c).

In active athletes, increased LV mass can occur in response to long-term athletic conditioning ("athletes heart"). Although absolute increases in LV wall thickness are usually mild, differentiation of athletes heart from mild HCM can be problematic in some patients especially if the only finding on MR is mild generalized hypertrophy. Clear differentiation between the two conditions can be difficult or impossible on MRI, especially when the only finding is "generalized" LVH. In the absence of clear-cut indicators of HCM (e.g., "asymmetric" septal hypertrophy), other factors such as genetic testing, family history of HCM, impaired diastolic filling, and LVED dimension less than 45 mm must be taken into account.

10.3.2.4 Restrictive Cardiomyopathy

Restrictive cardiomyopathy is characterized by a restriction of diastolic ventricular filling due to abnormalities of the endocardium and/or the myocardium itself. MR imaging is of little use in the diagnosis of restrictive cardiomyopathy, but may demonstrate anatomical changes associated with infiltrative myocardial disease (Figs. 10.12–10.15). The characteristics of restrictive cardiomyopathy are enlargement of the atria combined with relatively normal-sized ventricles and prominent intracavity signal caused by stasis and slow movement of the blood through the chambers. It is helpful to use MR imaging to discriminate between restrictive cardiomyopathy and constrictive pericarditis, especially given that the treatment of constrictive pericarditis is surgical. These two entities show essentially the same clinical picture, but the treatment differs. Typical findings of constrictive pericarditis are a thickened pericardium with right ventricular narrowing, a disproportionally dilated right atrium and caval veins, and pericardial calcification.

10.3.2.5 Arrhythmogenic Right Ventricular Dysplasia/Cardiomyopathy (ARVD)

ARVD is a cardiomyopathy that almost exclusively involves the right side of heart and occurs in sporadic or familial (autosomal dominant) form. There is a

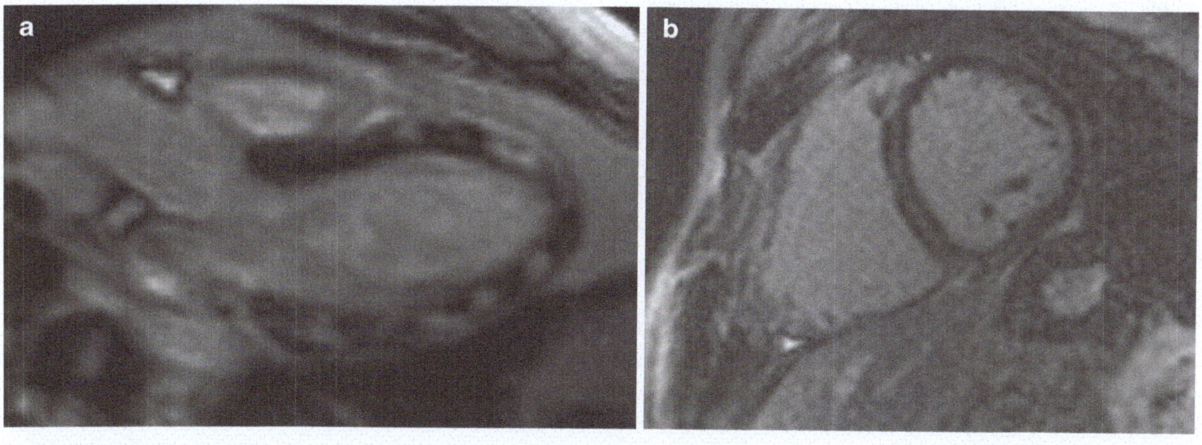

Fig. 10.15 (**a**, **b**) Myocarditis in a 29-year-old female. The 3-chamber single-shot inversion-recovery sequence (**a**) demonstrates diffuse multifocal predominantly midmyocardial and subepicardial late gadolinium

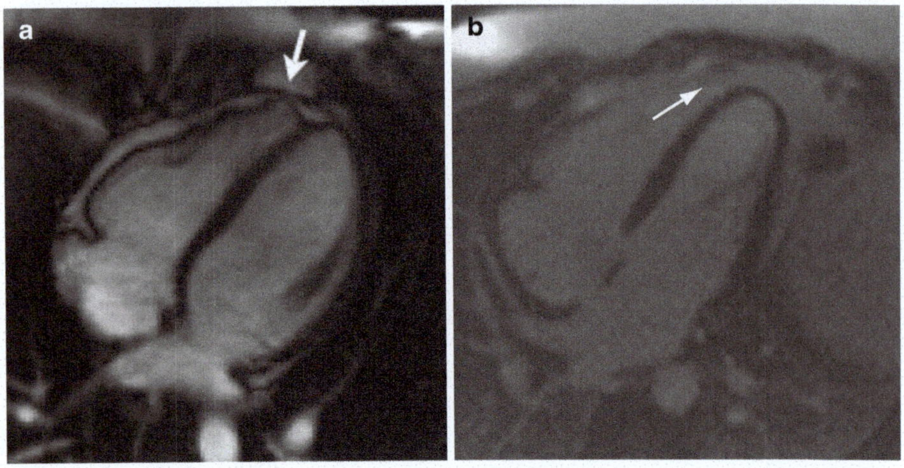

Fig. 10.16 Arrhythmogenic right ventricular dysplasia in a 35-year-old male. The 4-chamber cine trueFISP sequence (**a**) demonstrates a small focal aneurysm of the right ventricular free wall in the apical region (*arrow*). The delayed enhanced imaging (**b**) reveals diffuse enhancement of the free wall. Another patient (**b**) demonstrates subtle mid myocardial enhancement of the septal wall

strong association with malignant ventricular arrhythmia resulting in sudden death in young individuals. Morphologically, it is characterized by progressive RV dilatation and dysfunction, and histologically by fatty infiltration of the myocardium (Fig. 10.16). Although the disease almost invariably affects the RV, there are rare reports of LV involvement. Previously, the disorder could only be confirmed with certainty at autopsy; however, MRI is now regarded as the most reliable modality for imaging of the RV, and accurate depiction of the right cardiac chambers coupled with the characteristic appearance of fat on MRI images allows the diagnosis to be established noninvasively in many instances.

The prevalence is thought to be approximately 200 cases per million of population (1:5,000). It is thought to account for 2.5–5% of all cases of sudden cardiac death (SCD) and up to 25% of all exercise-induced cases as a result of ventricular arrhythmia. Once the diagnosis is established, there is approximately a 2.5% risk of SCD per year. This factor leads to the insertion of implanted defibrillators in almost all affected patients.

The majority of patients presenting with this disorder have evidence of left bundle branch block on ECG.

Diagnosis of ARVD

Because of the complexities in determining the significance of various laboratory and imaging tests, a task force which reported in 1994 suggested that the diagnosis be based on a set of major and minor diagnostic criteria given below. In order for the diagnosis of ARVD to be made with confidence, there must be two major criteria, one major and two minor criteria or four minor criteria.

Abnormalities in ARVD are defined as functional or morphological, as follows:

Functional abnormalities

- RV dilatation and hypokinesis in the presence of normal LV function.
- RV aneurysms

Morphological abnormalities

- Fatty infiltration of the RV wall
- Focal thinning
- Aneurysm formation
- RVH, increased RV trabeculation, and moderator band hypertrophy

Of these RV aneurysms, severe global or segmental dilatation and global systolic dysfunction are considered major criteria.

More recently, it has been reported that delayed enhancement following injection of gadolinium-based contrast agents is a marker for fibrofatty replacement in ARVD and that fibrous replacement (as defined by late enhancement) may be more arrhythmogenic than fat alone.

Histological Diagnosis of ARVD

In many patients the diagnosis is established at autopsy only. In patients in whom the diagnosis is suspected, RV endomyocardial biopsy demonstrates fatty infiltration, fiber disarray, and fibrosis.

Criteria for diagnosis of ARVD (McKenna et al. 1994):

1. Global and/or regional dysfunction and structural alterations[1]

- Major

  Severe dilatation and reduction of right ventricular ejection fraction with no (or only mild) left ventricular impairment
  Localized right ventricular aneurysms (akinetic or dyskinetic areas with diastolic bulging)
  Severe segmental dilatation of the right ventricle

- Minor

  Mild global right ventricular dilatation and/or ejection fraction reduction with normal left ventricle
  Mild segmental dilatation of the right ventricle
  Regional right ventricular hypokinesia

2. Tissue characterization of Wall

- Major

  Fibrofatty replacement of myocardium on endomyocardial biopsy

3. Repolarization abnormalities

- Minor

  Inverted T waves in right precordial leads (V2 and V3) in people aged >12 years, in absence of right bundle branch block

4. Depolarization/conduction abnormalities

- Major

  Epsilon waves or localized prolongation (>110 ms) of the QRS complex in right precordial leads (V1–V3)

- Minor

  Late potentials (signal-averaged ECG)

5. Arrhythmias

- Minor

  Left bundle branch block type ventricular tachycardia (sustained and nonsustained) by ECG, Holter or exercise testing
  Frequent ventricular extrasystoles (>1,000/24 h) by Holter

6. Family history

- Major

  Familial disease confirmed at necropsy or surgery

- Minor

  Family history of premature sudden death (<35 years) due to suspected right ventricular dysplasia
  Familial history (clinical diagnosis based on present criteria)

The diagnosis of ARVD would be fulfilled by the presence of two major, or one major plus two minor criteria or four minor criteria from different groups.

Cardiac MR Imaging in ARVD

CMR has emerged as the optimal modality for imaging of ARVD (Fig. 10.16). It offers clear visualization of the RV in all orientations, demonstrates regional and global RV dyskinesis, and can confirm high signal areas within the RV wall as fatty infiltration by use of fat suppression.

Another disease affecting the right cardiac chambers, pulmonary hypertension (Fig. 10.17), is discussed in the following chapter (Chap. 11).

10.3.3 *Cardiac Tumors and Tumor-Like Conditions*

10.3.3.1 Introduction

Although most emphasis is placed on diagnosis of primary cardiac tumors (Figs. 10.18–10.20), secondary involvement of the heart is at least 20 times more common (Fig. 10.21). Approximately 75% of all primary cardiac tumors are benign (mostly myxomas). Sarcomas are the most common malignant cardiac tumors, followed by lymphoma.

Regardless of etiology, cardiac tumors can be responsible for a myriad of clinical presentations including syncope, arrhythmias, chest pain, pericardial effusion, heart failure, and systemic embolization.

[1]Detected by echocardiography, angiography, magnetic resonance imaging, or radionuclide scintigraphy.

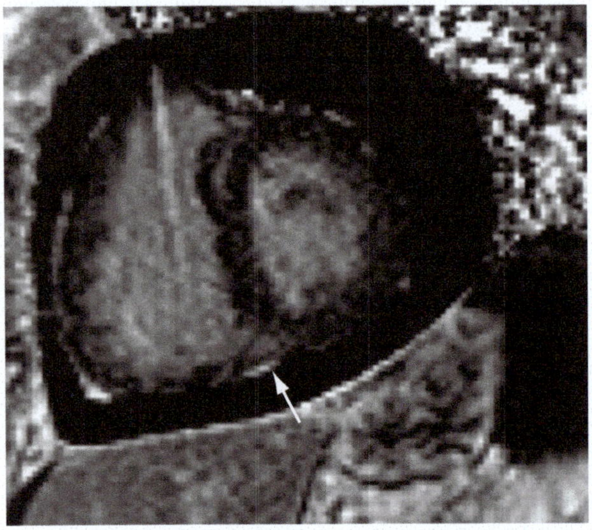

Fig. 10.17 A 45-year-old female patient with pulmonary arterial hypertension (PAH). The short-axis phase-sensitive inversion-recovery TurboFLASH sequence demonstrates a pericardial effusion and mid myocardial late gadolinium enhancement of left ventricle at the right ventricular insertion points, which is often seen in patients with PAH

10.3.3.2 Tumor-Like Lesions

Intracardiac thrombi are relatively common and can occur in any chamber. Most commonly, they occur within the LV adherent to a segment of wall rendered hypokinetic as a result of prior myocardial infarction (Fig. 10.3). Left atrial thrombi are most commonly associated with mitral valve disease, usually in patients with mitral stenosis, the majority of whom have atrial fibrillation. Right-sided thrombi are usually associated with an underlying condition, for example, blood disorders with a predisposition to abnormal clotting such as antiphospholipid syndrome. Isolated RV clot is extremely rare; occasionally, it can be observed as a transient phenomenon in patients with pulmonary embolism.

10.3.3.3 Secondary Cardiac Tumors

In most instances, secondary involvement of the heart by malignancy is a manifestation of either an inoperable

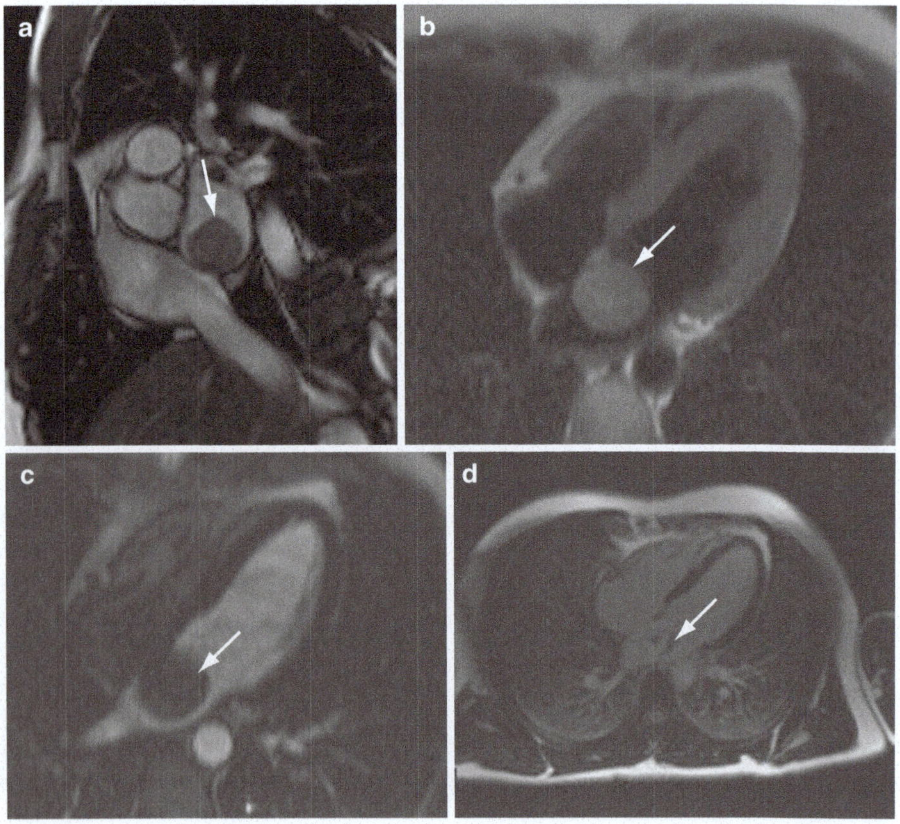

Fig. 10.18 (**a–d**) Left atrial myxoma in a 50-year-female. The short-axis cine trueFISP sequence (**a**) and dark-blood T1-W sequence (**b**) demonstrates a well-defined round lesion in the left atrium arising from the interatrial septum. The first pass inversion-recovery trueFISP (**c**) demonstrates no immediate enhancement. The single-shot inversion-recovery sequence demonstrates patchy late gadolinium enhancement

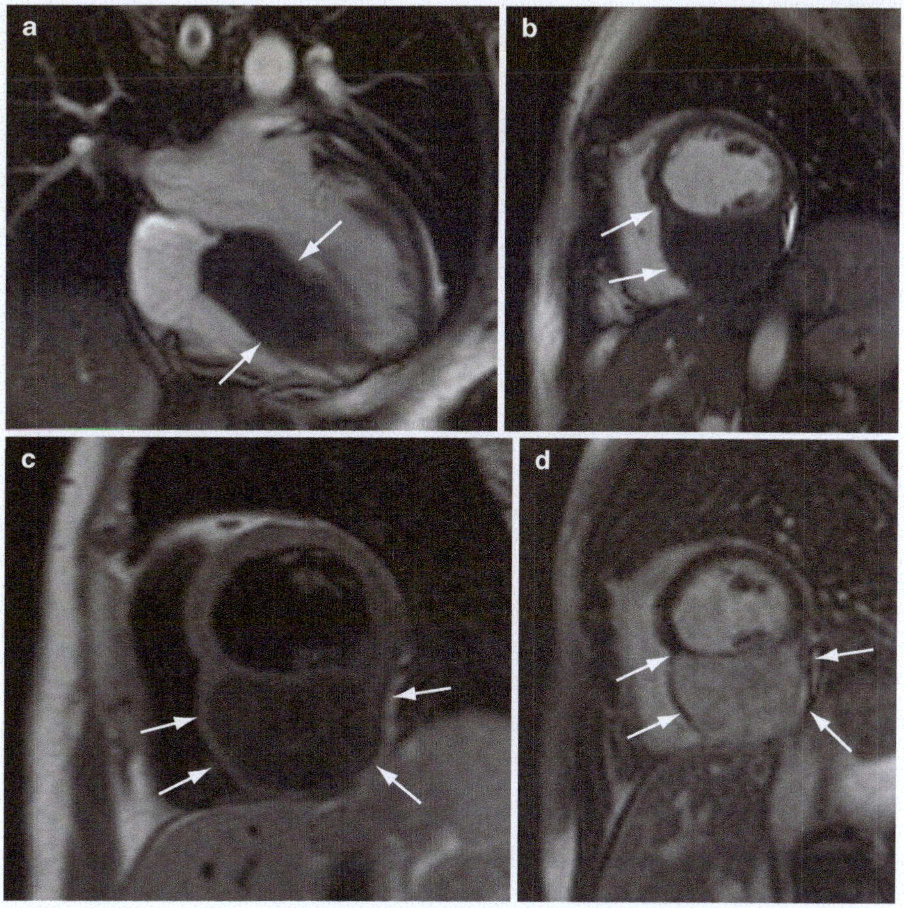

Fig. 10.19 (**a–d**) Intramyocardial fibroma in 45-year-old female patient. The bright blood trueFISP 4-chamber and 2-chamber views (**a, b**) demonstrate a smooth, well-demarcated intramyocardial mass of low signal intensity arising from the inferior septum with mass effect on the right ventricle. The mass is low signal intensity on the dark-blood T1-W sequence (**c**) and demonstrates diffuse late gadolinium enhancement

lung cancer which directly invades the heart, or a widespread systemic spread of a malignant tumor (Fig. 10.21). In patients with lung cancer, tumor can reach the heart by direct invasion through the pericardium or alternatively by extension along a pulmonary vein into the left atrium. Both findings indicate locally advanced disease (TNM staging T4). Extrathoracic tumors can also reach the heart by direct extension along the IVC, most commonly from a renal cell carcinoma in adults and Wilm's tumor in children. Other examples include hepatocellular carcinoma extension to the right atrium via the hepatic veins and adrenal carcinoma via the suprarenal vein, renal vein and IVC. Occasionally thyroid carcinoma can extend along the brachiocephalic vein and SVC to the right atrium. Involvement of the IVC and right atrium does not make a renal tumor inoperable as the tumor is usually mobile and removable at surgery, but does indicate inoperability in hepatocellular and adrenal carcinoma.

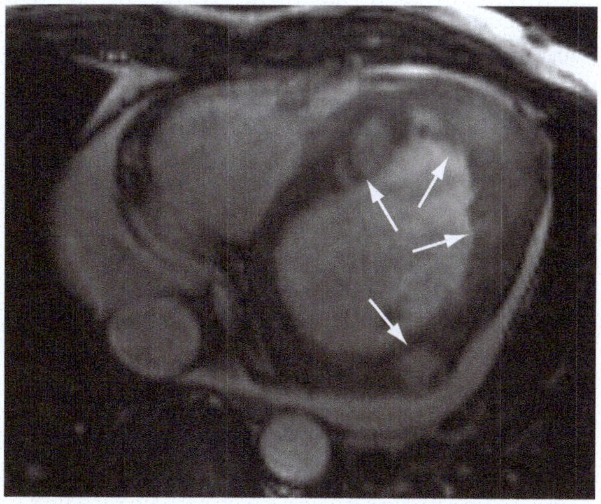

Fig. 10.20 Primary synovial cell sarcoma in 46-year-old female. The postcontrast axial trueFISP demonstrates multifocal enhancing lesions within the left ventricle

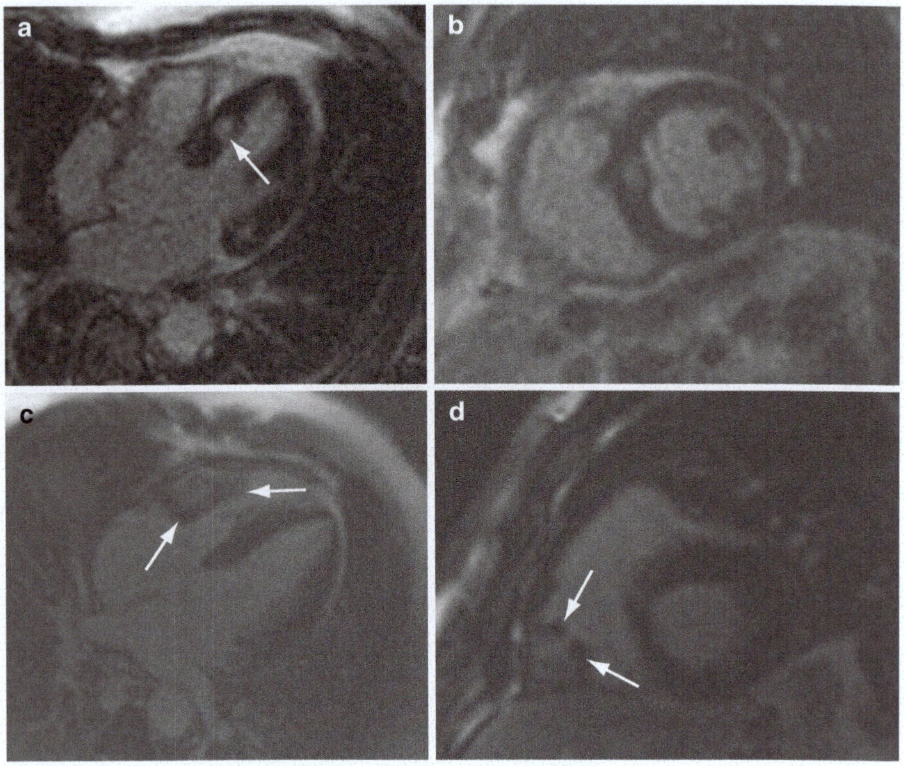

Fig. 10.21 Intramyocardial metastases in two patients. The first patient has renal cell carcinoma and demonstrates enhancing intramyocardial lesions on delayed enhanced imaging (**a**, **b**). The second patient has an angiosarcoma and demonstrates an enhancing intramyocardial lesion involving the right ventricular free wall on delayed enhanced imaging (**c**, **d**)

10.3.3.4 Primary Cardiac Tumors

10.3.3.5 Atrial Myxomas

These account for at least 50% of benign cardiac tumors that occur most commonly in the left atrium (> 80%), approximately 10% in the right atrium, and a minority within the ventricles (left much more common than right) (Fig. 10.18). The tumor has its highest incidence in the sixth decade, with a predominance in women (up to 70%). Morphologically, they present as pedunculated masses typically with a site of attachment to the fossa ovalis. These features lead to the characteristic appearance of a highly mobile mass on MR imaging, which often shows the tumor better than echocardiography. Atrial myxomas are characterized by intermediate signal intensity on T1-W and T2-W SE images. Contrast-enhanced studies may show an intermediate tumor enhancement (Fig. 10.18d).

10.3.3.6 Other Benign Tumors

Cardiac lipomas, similar to those elsewhere throughout the body are benign encapsulated fatty tumors which are easily diagnosed on MRI because of the unique signal characteristics associated with fat. Most are asymptomatic and diagnosed incidentally. They typically arise in a subendocardial location and like myxomas usually present as a mobile mass, albeit one with different signal characteristics to myxomas.

Lipomatous hypertrophy of the interatrial septum (LHAS) is a poorly understood condition but appears to represent an accumulation of nonencapsulated fat within the interatrial septum (Fig. 10.22). Despite its name, it represents hyperplasia rather than a true tumor and might be more accurately referred to as lipomatous hyperplasia. It is more common with increasing age and obesity. It is postulated to arise because of trapping of mesenchymal cells (which can develop into adipocytes with an appropriate stimulus) within the interatrial septum during fetal development which is formed by fusion of the septum primum and secundum.

Virtually all cases of LHAS are asymptomatic with the diagnosis being discovered incidentally on imaging or at autopsy.

Papillary fibroelastomas are tumor-like lesions involving the heart, but it is uncertain as to whether they represent a true neoplasm or reactive or hamartomatous lesions. They most commonly arise on the

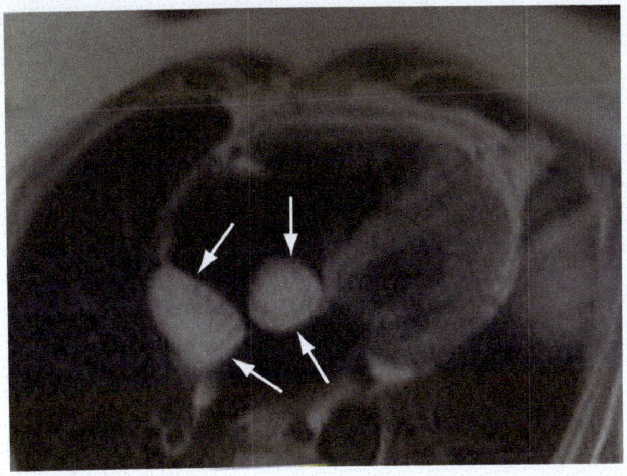

Fig. 10.22 Lipomatous hypertrophy of the interatrial septum. The dark-blood T1-W sequence demonstrates the typical dumb-bell pattern of hypertrophy and fat signal characteristics

valvular endothelium (particularly the aortic valve) but can involve any valve or occasionally the atrial or ventricular endothelium. Approximately 50% are asymptomatic. Patients with left-sided lesions may present with embolic symptoms, most commonly TIA or stroke. Pulmonary embolism has also been reported with right-sided lesions.

Rhabdomyoma, a hamartomatous lesion rarely diagnosed after 1 year of age, is the most common pediatric tumor and is associated with tuberous sclerosis in 50% of cases. The tumors are often multiple and intramural and are usually isointense to the myocardium on non-contrast T1-WI and T2-WI. They are therefore difficult to diagnose unless they deform the myocardial wall but are well demonstrated on contrast-enhanced images as a result of enhancement which is greater than normal myocardium.

Lymphangiomas, hemangiomas, fibromas, and hamartomas are other benign tumors that occasionally involve the heart. There are no distinguishing imaging features.

10.3.3.7 Malignant Tumors

10.3.3.8 Cardiac Sarcomas

These are sub classified as angiosarcoma, endomyocardial sarcoma, and rhabdomyosarcomas (Fig. 10.20). Angiosarcomas, which peak in the fourth decade most commonly arise within the right atrium around the AV groove and may demonstrate a "sun-ray" pattern of enhancement on post gadolinium imaging. A hemorrhagic pericardial effusion strongly points toward this diagnosis. Prognosis is extremely poor as most patients have lung and liver metastases at presentation.

Endomyocardial sarcomas (which have been subclassified as malignant fibrous histiocytomas, osteosarcoma, leiomyosarcoma, and fibro/myxofibrosarcoma) are most commonly found in the left atrium.

Rhabdomyosarcoma, a rare (1–5% of cardiac sarcomas) but particularly well-known variety of sarcoma is associated with tuberous sclerosis.

10.3.3.9 Cardiac Lymphoma

Cardiac lymphoma presents most commonly as a manifestation of widespread lymphoma but occasionally as primary cardiac lymphoma. Ten to twenty percent of patients who die with widespread lymphoma have cardiac involvement at autopsy. Cases of primary cardiac lymphoma are reported in both immunocompetent and immunosuppressed patients, but primary cardiac lymphoma, although rare, is increasing in incidence in HIV patients. An increasing incidence is also reported in post-transplant candidates, related to Ebstein Barr infection and immunosuppression. Primary cardiac lymphoma, although rare, has a better prognosis than lymphomatous involvement of the heart as a result of systemic lymphoma.

Cardiac lymphoma typically occurs in the atrial wall but can involve any chamber and is poorly defined and widely infiltrating on imaging.

10.3.3.10 MR Imaging of Cardiac Tumors

A combination of spin-echo and cine MR imaging is recommended to evaluate cardiac tumors (Figs. 10.18–10.22). Fat suppression is required for all masses that demonstrate high signal on T1-W images to investigate the presence of fat (Fig. 10.22). Contrast-enhanced imaging is also routinely used.

Most cardiac masses present intermediate or low signal on T1-W images and present as low signal within the bright blood on cine images. High signal on T1-W images raises the possibility of thrombus or a lipoma, which can be distinguished by fat-saturation techniques.

10.3.4 Valvular Diseases

10.3.4.1 Introduction

CMR imaging is useful for depicting and evaluating the severity of valvular disease, but in the overwhelming majority of cases where an adequate Doppler signal can be obtained, the relevant information can be provided without recourse to MRI. However, when Echo is inadequate CMR offers significant benefit (Figs. 10.23–10.30). Although cardiac valves are quite thin and therefore suboptimally demonstrated when normal, they are almost invariably thickened when abnormal and easily visualized, provided the patient can breath-hold. Valvular regurgitation is present when a linear dark signal passes retrogradely through a valve during systole or diastole depending on the location of the valve (Figs. 10.26, 10.27, 10.29); valvular stenosis when a dark signal passes antegradely through a narrowed valve (Figs. 10.25, 10.30). Calcification on the valve could potentially exaggerate valve cross-section area, although this is unlikely as calcification is mainly located on the annulus. Valve opening and closing is well demonstrated on SSFP images acquired in the plane of the valve (Figs. 10.23, 10.24]. Using flow-encoded MR imaging, it is possible to quantify the severity of valvular regurgitation and to monitor the effects of therapeutic interventions. Qualitative assessment of the severity of valvular stenosis is more challenging.

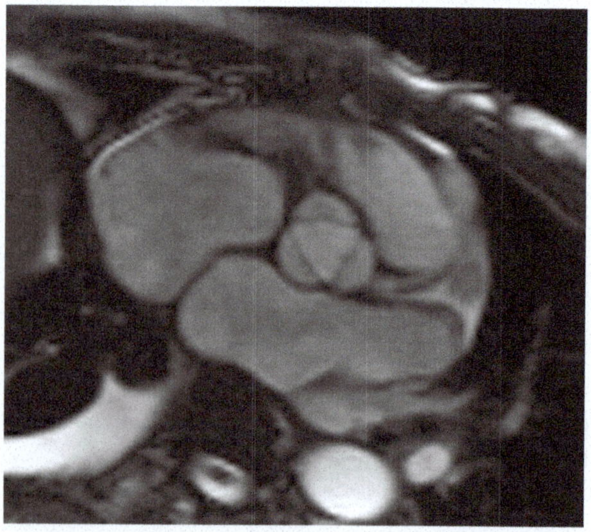

Fig. 10.23 Normal trileaflet aortic valve. A through plane view on trueFISP demonstrates a normal trileaflet aortic valve configuration while open during systole

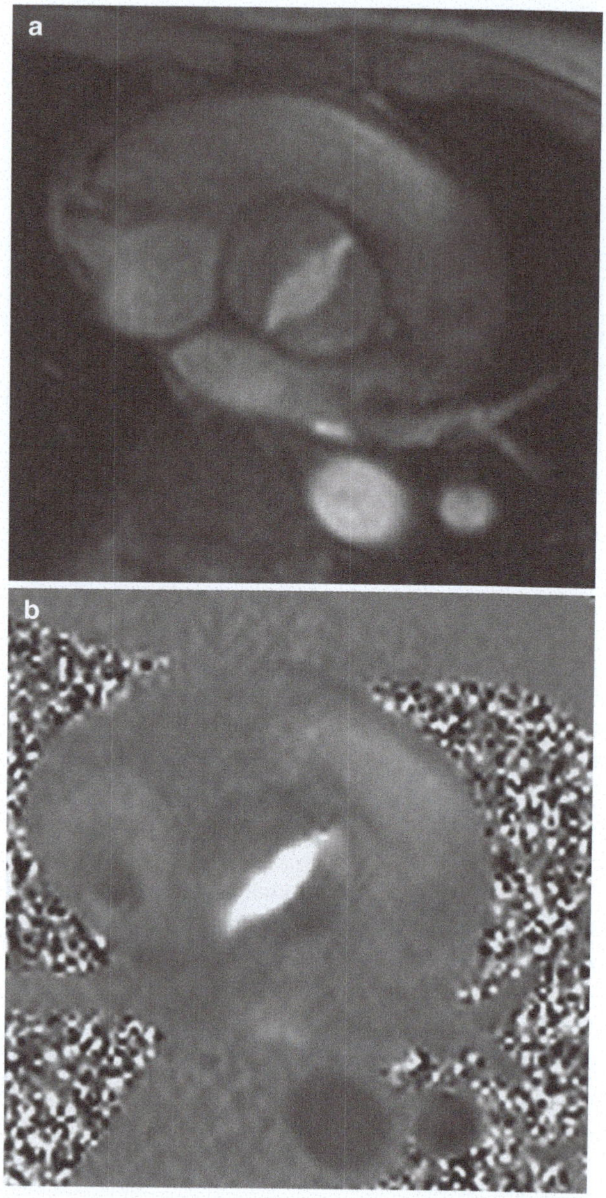

Fig. 10.24 (**a**, **b**) A 34-year-old male with a congenitally bicuspid aortic valve. The through plane magnitude phase-contrast image (**a**) demonstrates fusion of the right and noncoronary cusps. The phase-contrast image during systole demonstrates forward flow through the valve without evidence of stenosis

Evaluation of valvular heart diseases is incomplete without an assessment of the degree of left ventricular dysfunction. Therefore, it is necessary to acquire short-axis cine MR imaging from the base to the apex. This data set is used to measure left ventricular volumes (end-systolic and end-diastolic), ejection fraction, stroke volume, and ventricular mass. In patients undergoing

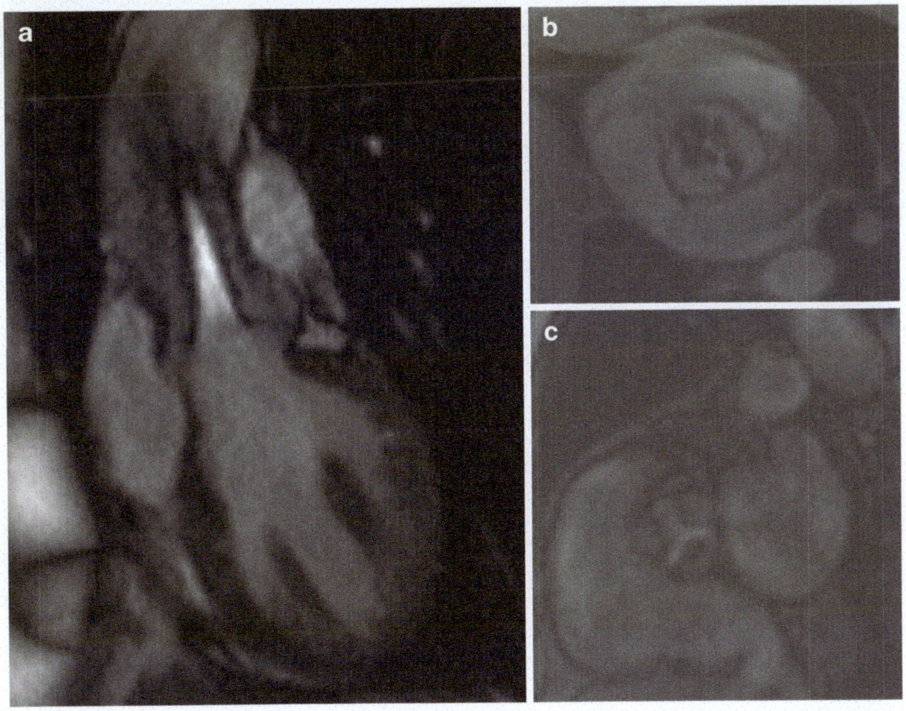

Fig. 10.25 (**a–c**) Aortic valve stenosis. The cine trueFISP left ventricular outflow tract view (**a**) demonstrates flow acceleration through the aortic valve. The through plane view (**b**) reveals moderate to severe stenosis of a trileaflet valve. Another patient with fusion of the left and right coronary cusps demonstrates severe calcified aortic stenosis

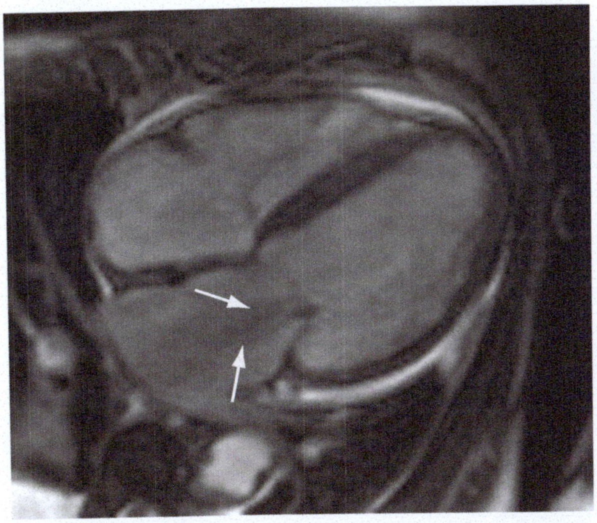

Fig. 10.26 Mitral regurgitation in a 50-year-old female. A 4-chamber cine trueFISP sequence demonstrates moderate mitral regurgitation during ventricular systole

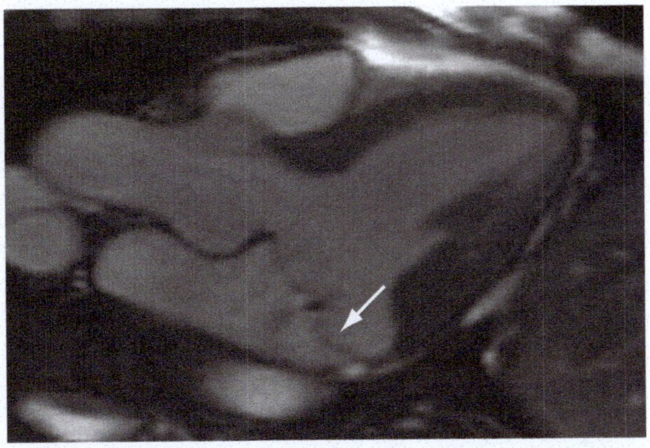

Fig. 10.27 Mitral valve prolapse in a 30-year-old male. The 3-chamber cine trueFISP sequence reveals prolapse of the posterior leaflet of the mitral valve

valve replacement, assessment of myocardial perfusion and viability is also advisable, especially if coronary bypass grafting is also being considered.

Imaging of virtually all implanted valves is safe at 1.5 T, although specific details must be sought from the manufacturer prior to scanning patients with prosthetic valves.

10.3.4.2 MR Findings

Both antegrade and retrograde flow through normal and diseased valves is well demonstrated on MRI.

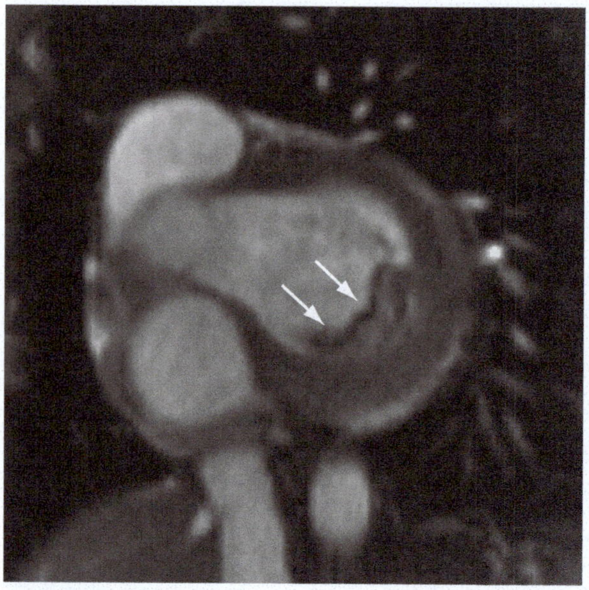

Fig. 10.28 Mitral valve endocarditis in 33-year-old male. The short-axis cine trueFISP sequence demonstrates a thickening and irregularity of the posterior leaflet of the mitral valve

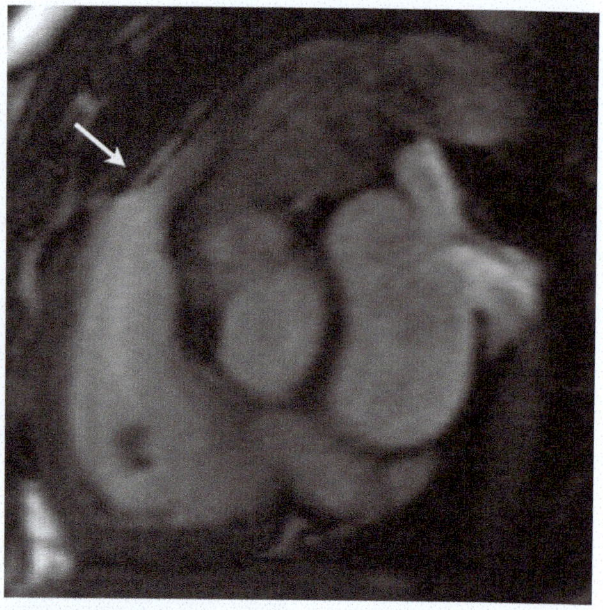

Fig. 10.30 Pulmonary stenosis in 35-year-old male. The right ventricular outflow tract, phase-contrast magnitude image demonstrates a flow acceleration gradient across the pulmonary valve

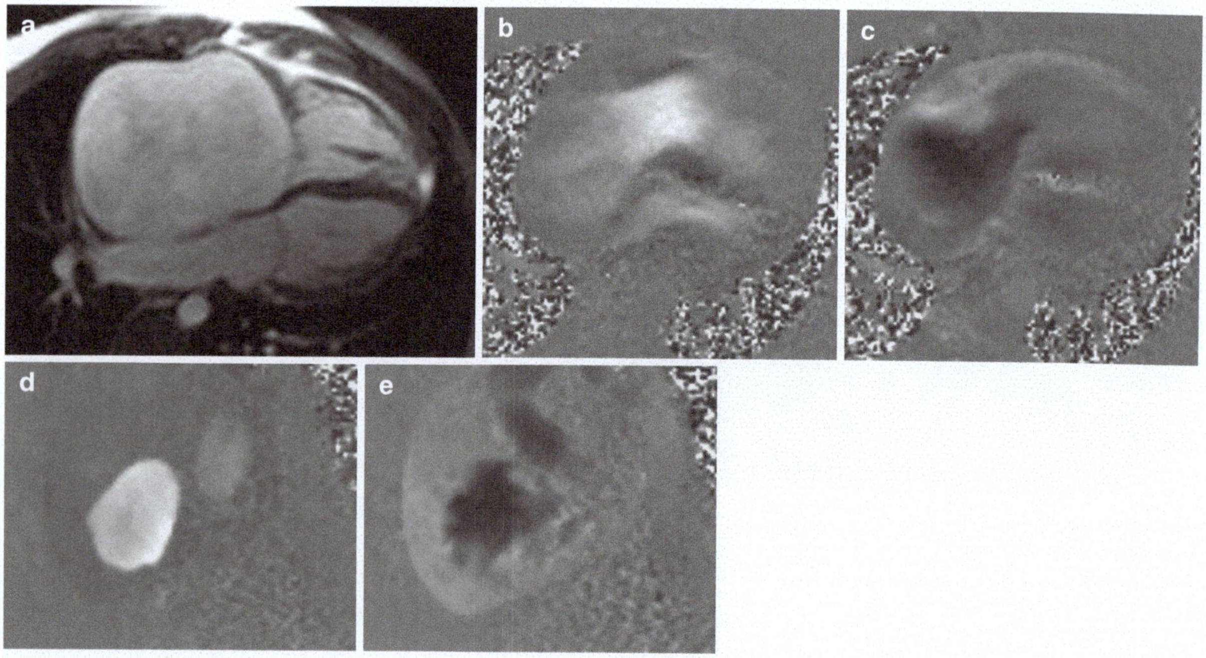

Fig. 10.29 Severe tricuspid regurgitation in a 56-year-old female. The 4-chamber cine trueFISP sequence (**a**) demonstrates severe right atrial enlargement. The phase-contrast flow imaging 4-chamber view in ventricular diastole demonstrates the filling of the ventricle (**b**) During systole (**c**) the severe reversal of flow (dark signal) back into the right atrium is seen. The findings are confirmed on the through plane phase-contrast images in diastole (**d**) and systole (**e**)

Specific MR findings in valvular regurgitation and stenosis follows.

10.3.4.3 Regurgitation

Quantitative assessment can be performed by either of the two methods as follows:

1. As the output from both ventricles, by definition, is equal, by directly measuring the cardiac output of both LV and RV using a short-axis cine imaging stack, the degree of regurgitation is given by the difference in output of the two ventricles assuming that single valvular lesion exists. If single valves on both sides of the heart are involved a similar approach normalized for great vessel (aorta and pulmonary trunk) flow can be performed.
2. A phase-sensitive flow-encoded sequence is used to measure both forward flow and retrograde flow after closure of the valve. A regurgitant fraction, derived by dividing forward by regurgitant flow is reproducible and potentially useful for longitudinal and posttreatment follow-up.

10.3.4.4 Stenosis

Accurate measurement of cross-sectional area of the aortic valve, which correlates with severity of stenosis can be performed by imaging in the plane of the valve. In order to directly measure the severity of stenosis with MR, restoration of signal within the core of the jet is required, possible only with use of an ultrashort TE sequence.

10.3.5 Pericardial Diseases

10.3.5.1 Introduction

The pericardium is a fibro-serous structure that consists of internal serous and external fibrous components. The serous component includes visceral and parietal layers. The fibrous component adheres to the diaphragm, and adipose tissue separates the outer pericardium from the sternum anteriorly. The pericardial space normally contains 15–50 mL of fluid.

10.3.5.2 MR Findings

10.3.5.3 Normal Pericardium

The normal pericardium appears as a curvilinear line of low signal intensity between the high or medium signal intensity of the external pericardial fat and the internal epicardial fat. Its normal thickness ranges from 1 to 2 mm but occasionally up to 4 mm. Some parts of the pericardium may not be visible because of a lack of adjacent epicardial fat in some regions.

10.3.5.4 Pericardial Effusion

Common causes of pericardial effusion are viral or idiopathic pericarditis, neoplasia, uremia, trauma, collagen vascular diseases, postpericardectomy or postinfarction (Dressler) syndromes, and acquired immunodeficiency syndrome (AIDS). The distribution of pericardial fluid is frequently asymmetrical. The signal characteristics are fluid-like with low signal intensity on T1W imaging and high signal intensity on T2W imaging (Figs. 10.31 and 10.32). In cases of hemorrhagic or proteinaceous pericardial effusion, T1W imaging often shows areas of intermediate or high signal intensity.

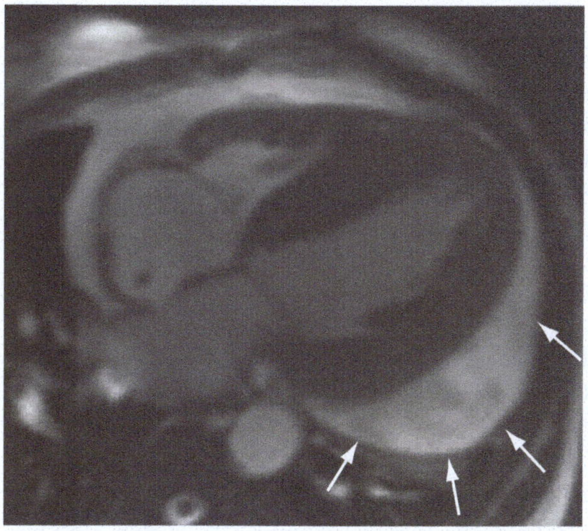

Fig. 10.31 Pericardial effusion in 43-year-old female. The 4-chamber trueFISP sequence demonstrates a large pericardial effusion without signs of tamponade

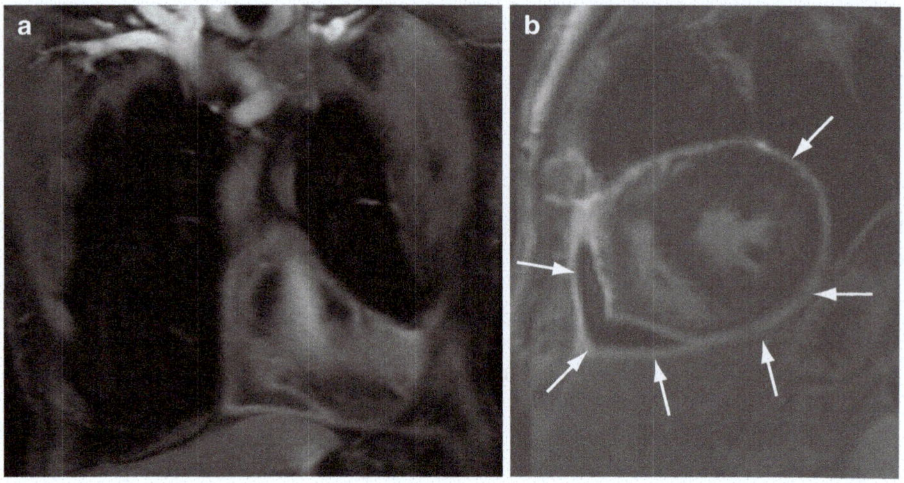

Fig. 10.32 Pericarditis in a 56-year-old female. The postcontrast coronal T1-W fat-saturation sequence (**a**) demonstrates a pericardial effusion. The visceral and parietal pericardium is also thickened and enhances on the phase-sensitive inversion-recovery TurboFLASH short-axis view (**b**)

10.3.5.5 Constrictive Pericarditis

Constrictive pericarditis limits diastolic filling of the heart due to thickening and fibrosis of the pericardium. Presenting symptoms are often similar to those of restrictive cardiomyopathy, but the differentiation between these two conditions is essential, because the treatment of choice for patients with constrictive pericarditis is surgical pericardectomy.

MR imaging effectively demonstrates pericardial thickening (greater than 4 mm). Patients with a history of cardiac surgery or postpericardectomy syndrome may have significant pericardial thickening without underlying constrictive pericarditis. Other MR imaging findings include narrow, tubular-shaped ventricles, dilatation of the right atrium, inferior vena cava, and hepatic veins. Ascites and pleural effusion may be present.

10.3.5.6 Pericardial Cyst

Pericardial cysts are benign but uncommon developmental lesions formed within the embryonic pericardium. Most cysts are well-marginated and contain clear fluid. They are typically located in the right anterior cardiophrenic angle and occur less often in the left cardiophrenic angle. Most patients are asymptomatic. The cysts typically have a round or ovoid appearance and demonstrate low signal intensity on T1W imaging and high signal intensity on T2W imaging. This may be different for complicated cysts (hemorrhagic or proteinaceous).

10.3.5.7 Neoplastic Pericardial Disease

Primary neoplasms are very rare; secondary involvement is much more frequent and commonly results from lung and breast carcinoma, melanoma, lymphoma, and leukemia. Neoplastic pericardial involvement may present different signal characteristics on MR imaging. It may demonstrate pericardial effusion and regional pericardial thickening.

10.3.6 Congenital Heart Disease

10.3.6.1 Introduction

Congenital cardiac malformations which occur in approximately 0.8% of livebirths can be a direct or indirect result of genetic disorders, related to toxins (alcohol, thalidomide), infection (Rubella), or excess radiation exposure, but in many cases are sporadic. MR datasets are highly effective in mapping structural abnormalities which can then be assessed by a functional study and are less operator dependent than echocardiography [10.33–10.40]. The combination of transesophageal cardiac echo and CMR has virtually eliminated the requirement for invasive cardiac catheterization in most instances. Although sedation is usually required for CMR in neonates and young children, this is also true for TOE. CMR is also ideally suited to the evaluation of long-term survivors with congenital heart disease, many

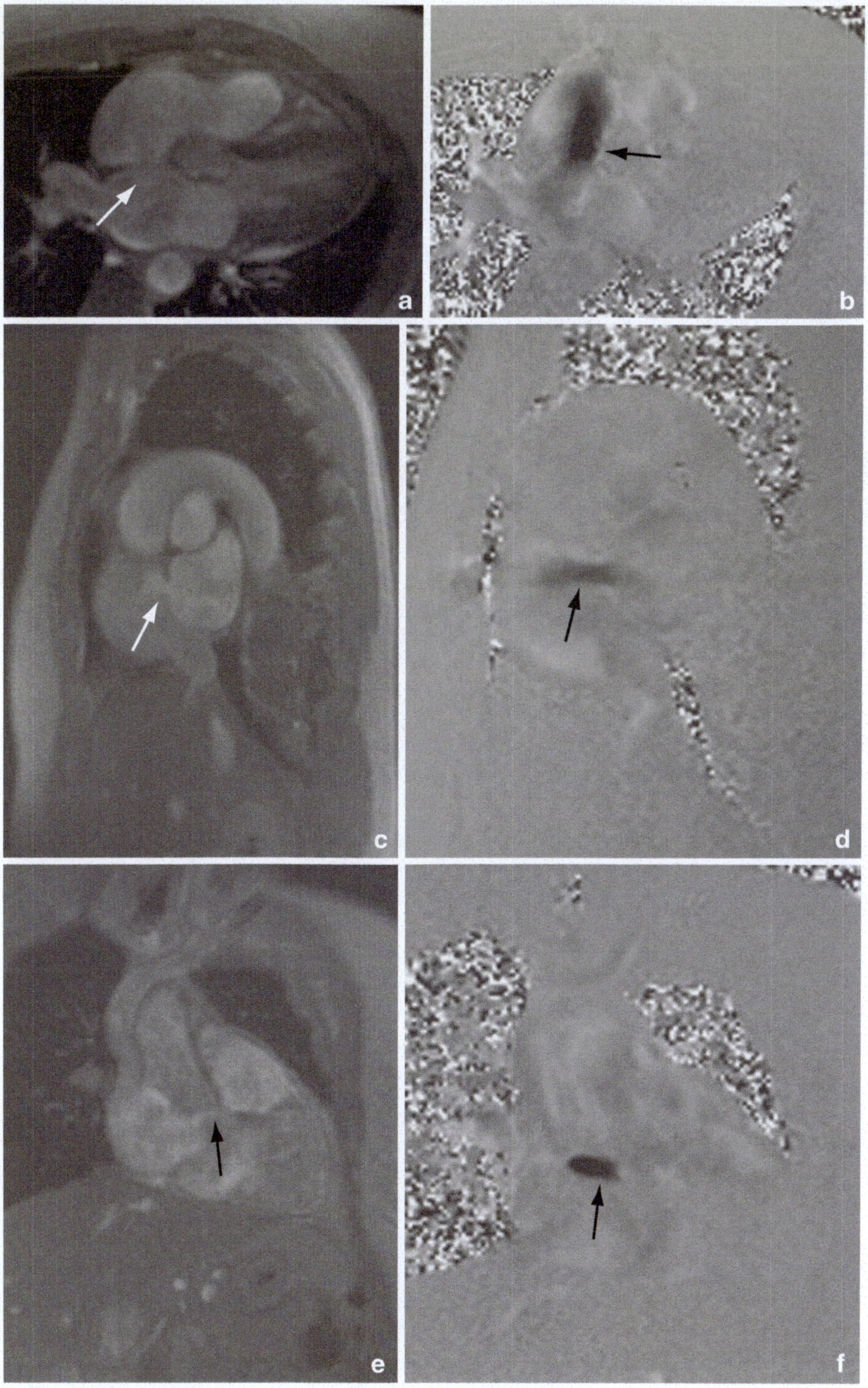

Fig. 10.33 Atrial septal defect in a 45-year-old female. Phase-contrast imaging: magnitude 4-chamber (**a**), phase 4-chamber (**b**), magnitude short axis (**c**), phase short axis (**d**), magnitude through plane (**e**) and phase through plane (**f**) demonstrate an atrial septal defect with a right to left shunt (*arrows*). The *oval shaped* defect is adjacent to the superior vena cava and is located in the posterior aspect of the interatrial septum suggesting the presence of a sinus venosus defect

of whom would have had complex surgery, the details of which might have been lost over time. Also, the ability to detect myocardial scar tissue in addition to the fact that postsurgical scar tissue within the thorax does not interfere with CMR performance or interpretation also favors MR for long-term follow-up. Multi-planar ECG-gated SE and ultra-fast TSE sequences are very useful in the evaluation of the complex anatomy of these patients.

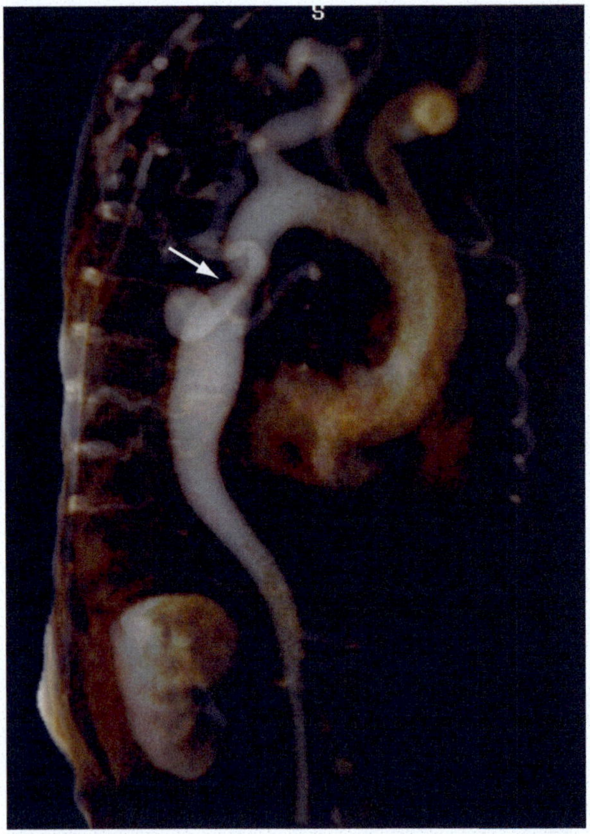

Fig. 10.34 Aortic coarctation in a 33-year-old male. The volume rendered, high resolution static MR angiogram reveals a severe postductal aortic coarctation with significantly increased size of the inter-costal and mammary arteries

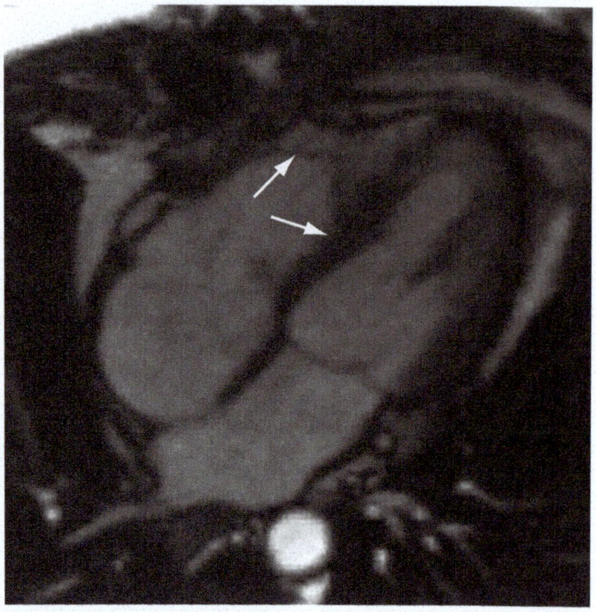

Fig. 10.36 Ebstein's anomaly in a young female patient. The 4-chamber cine trueFISP sequence demonstrates downward displacement of the septal and posterior leaflets of the tricuspid valve and right atrial enlargement

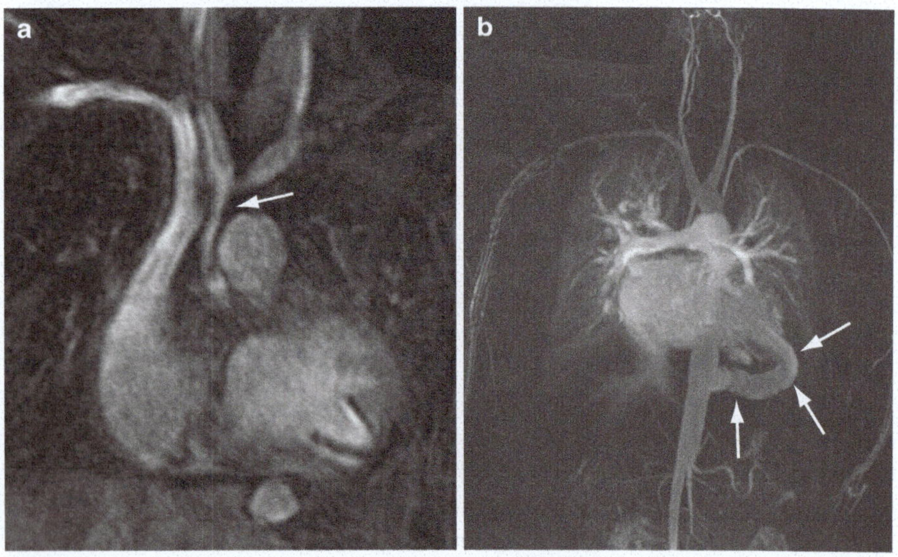

Fig. 10.35 Aortic atresia and bypass graft in a young male. The static MR angiogram (**a**) in the coronal plane demonstrates severe atresia of the ascending aorta. There is a surgical defect in the left ventricular apex to which a graft is fixed. The MIP of the MRA (**b**) redemonstrates the atretic ascending aorta and clearly shows the bypass graft arising from the left ventricular apex, anatomizing with the distal descending thoracic aorta

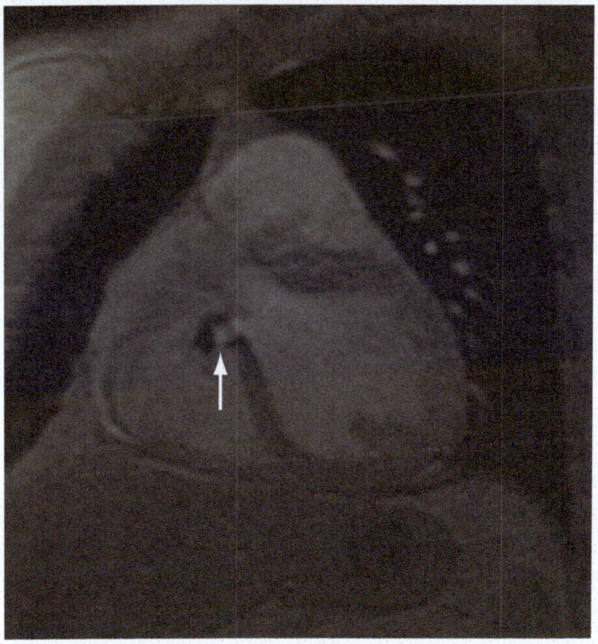

Fig. 10.37 Membranous ventricular septal defect in a young male patient. The magnitude phase-contrast sequence demonstrates a perimembranous ventricular septal defect, with gradient flow acceleration seen on the right ventricular side, suggestive of a left-to-right shunt

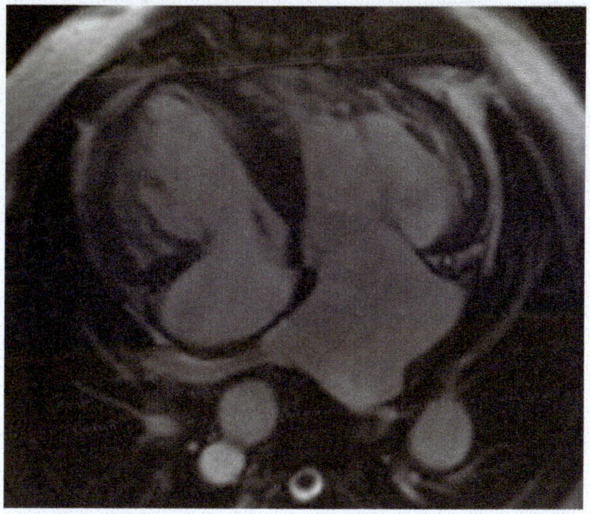

Fig. 10.39 Transposition of the great arteries. A 4-chamber trueFISP sequence demonstrates a subpulmonic left ventricle and mitral valve on the right side and a systemic right ventricle and tricuspid valve on the left side consistent with a TGA

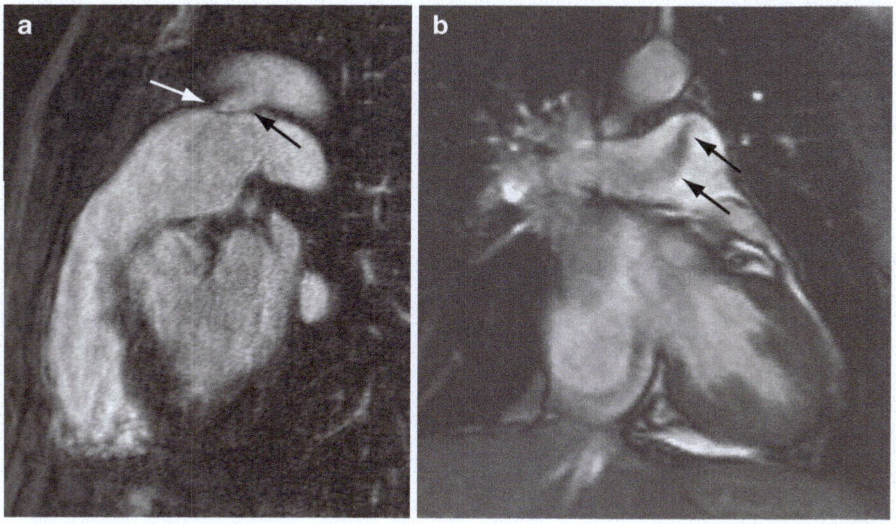

Fig. 10.38 Patent ductus arteriosus in a 25-year-old male. The saggital oblique reconstructed, static high resolution MRA (**a**) reveals a persistent arterial duct from the proximal descending aorta and the main pulmonary artery. (**b**) The coronal cine trueFISP sequence reveals an acceleration flow jet directed toward the right pulmonary artery

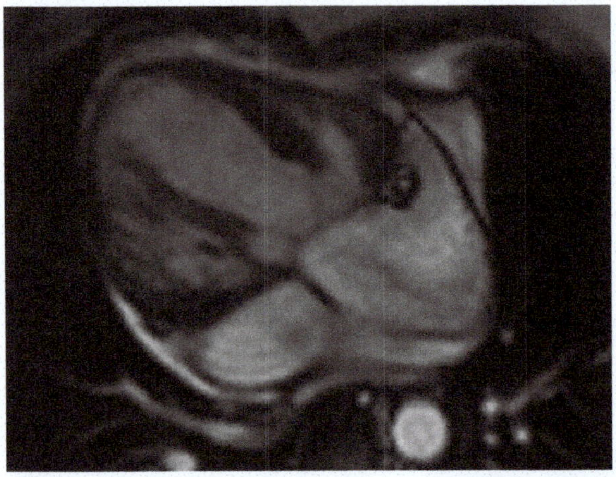

Fig. 10.40 Single ventricle defect in a young female. The 4-chamber, trueFISP sequence reveals a small right ventricle, absent tricuspid valve, atrial septal defect, and a ventricular septal defect

Cine studies (SSFP images) are applied to detect stenosis, regurgitation, and left-to-right shunts and to visualize surgical anastomoses and conduits following treatment. With multisection cine-mode MR imaging, it is possible to measure global left and right ventricular function. MR velocity-encoded GRE techniques measure peak blood-flow velocities and are therefore useful for the quantitative assessment of hemodynamics. These combined possibilities make MR imaging a useful comprehensive tool for initial evaluation and follow-up of congenital heart disease.

10.3.6.2 MR Findings

Analysis of complex anatomical relationships in patients with congenital heart disease and complex cardiovascular malformation is best done using step-by-step analysis of cardiac segmental anatomy, based on the premise that the three cardiac segments (atria, ventricles, and great arteries) develop independently of one another. Initial analysis includes the assessment of atrial situs, ventricular morphology, atrioventricular connections, position and morphology of the great vessels, ventriculoarterial connections, associated defects and surgically created shunts and complications (Figs. 10.33–10.40).

Normal atrial situs (atrial situs solitus) exists when the morphological left atrium is located on the left side of the patient; the morphological right atrium is located on the right side. The morphological right atrium receives the hepatic venous drainage and the vena cava. It contains an appendage with a triangular configuration and has a wide base of implantation into the atrial chamber. The left atrium receives the pulmonary veins and contains an appendage that is usually longer and thinner than the right atrium appendage. In atrial situs inversus, there is a mirror-image of the normal morphological connections.

The morphological right and left ventricles are distinguished in MR images by their different characteristics. Short-axis MR images usually reveal a landmark moderator band in the morphological right ventricle which passes from the distal septum to the anterior wall near the apex. The right ventricle demonstrates a coarse trabecular pattern compared to the smooth left ventricular interior. The septal attachment of the atrioventricular valve is closer to the apex in the right ventricle. An important morphological difference between the two sides relates to the presence of an infundibulum in the right ventricle that separates the tricuspid and pulmonary valves – in the left ventricle no infundibulum exists and there is fibrous continuity in a figure of "8" pattern between the mitral and aortic valve.

Atrioventricular concordance (i.e., the normal situation) exists when blood flows from the morphological right atrium through the tricuspid valve into the right ventricle, and from the morphological left atrium through the mitral valve into the left ventricle. Ventriculo-arterial concordance exists when the right ventriclar outflow is to the pulmonary artery via the pulmonary valve, and the left ventricular outflow is through the aortic valve into the aorta. Ventriculo-arterial discordance (transposition of the great arteries) is easily identified on MR images and occurs in two important forms, D-transposition and congenitally corrected transposition of the great arteries.

The aorta and pulmonary artery are defined by their usual branching pattern. Anomalies of the aortic arch are common, and the most common symptomatic congenital lesion is coarctation (Fig. 10.34). This is defined as a constriction of the aorta, most commonly near the junction of the ductus arteriosus and the aortic arch. In aortic coarctation, MR velocity-encoded GRE images may show the functional significance of this anomaly.

MR imaging is useful for detecting pulmonary artery malformations. The pulmonary valve is normally supported by the right ventricular infundibulum and lies anterior, superior, and to the left of the aortic arch. Pulmonary arterial abnormalities, including pulmonary artery sling and origin from the ductus arteriosus, can be demonstrated directly. Marked dilatation of the pulmonary artery may be seen in patients with valvular stenosis or in pulmonary insufficiency.

An important step in MR imaging is to identify and characterize any associated defect (e.g., atrial or ventricular septal defects) and also to identify associated extracardiac anomalies such as spinal defects and liver/spleen anomalies, etc.

Further Reading

1. Pai VM, Axel L (2006) Advances in MRI tagging techniques for determining regional myocardial strain. Curr Cardiol Rep 8:53
2. Grothues F, Moon JC, Bellenger NG et al (2004) Interstudy reproducibility of right ventricular volumes, function, and mass with cardiovascular magnetic resonance. Am Heart J 147:218
3. Elliott MD, Kim RJ (2005) Late gadolinium cardiovascular magnetic resonance in the assessment of myocardial viability. Coron Artery Dis 16:365
4. Syed MA, Paterson DI, Ingkanisorn WP et al (2005) Reproducibility and inter-observer variability of dobutamine stress CMR in patients with severe coronary disease: implications for clinical research. J Cardiovasc Magn Reson 7:763
5. Muehling OM, Jerosch-Herold M, Panse P et al (2004) Regional heterogeneity of myocardial perfusion in healthy human myocardium: assessment with magnetic resonance perfusion imaging. J Cardiovasc Magn Reson 6:499
6. Appelbaum E, Botnar RM, Yeon SB, Manning WJ (2005) Coronary magnetic resonance imaging: current state-of-the-art. Coron Artery Dis 16:345
7. Kim WY, Danias PG, Stuber M et al (2001) Coronary magnetic resonance angiography for the detection of coronary stenosis. N Engl J Med 345:1863
8. Terashima M, Meyer CH, Keeffe BG et al (2005) Noninvasive assessment of coronary vasodilation using magnetic resonance angiography. J Am Coll Cardiol 45:104
9. Assomull RG, Prasad SK, Lyne J et al (2006) Cardiovascular magnetic resonance, fibrosis, and prognosis in dilated cardiomyopathy. J Am Coll Cardiol 48:1977
10. Moon JC, Reed E, Sheppard MN et al (2004) The histologic basis of late gadolinium enhancement cardiovascular magnetic resonance in hypertrophic cardiomyopathy. J Am Coll Cardiol 43:2260
11. Moon JC, McKenna Caruthers SD, Lin SJ, Brown P et al (2003) Practical value of cardiac magnetic resonance imaging for clinical quantification of aortic valve stenosis: comparison with echocardiography. Circulation 108: 2236
12. Prasad SK, Soukias N, Hornung T et al (2004) Role of magnetic resonance angiography in the diagnosis of major aortopulmonary collateral arteries and partial anomalous pulmonary venous drainage. Circulation 109:207
13. Maron BJ (2003) Sudden death in young athletes. N Engl J Med 349:1064
14. Maron BJ (2002) Hypertrophic cardiomyopathy: a systematic review. JAMA 287:1308
15. Magnani JW, Dec GW (2006) Myocarditis: current trends in diagnosis and treatment. Circulation 113:876
16. Taylor AM, Dymarkowski S, Verbeken EK, Bogaert J (2006) Detection of pericardial inflammation with late-enhancement cardiac magnetic resonance imaging: initial results. Eur Radiol 16:569
17. Maceira AM, Joshi J, Prasad SK et al (2005) Cardiovascular magnetic resonance in cardiac amyloidosis. Circulation 111:186–193
18. Nazarian S, Bluemke DA, Lardo AC et al (2005) Magnetic resonance assessment of the substrate for inducible ventricular tachycardia in nonischemic cardiomyopathy. Circulation 112:2821–2825
19. McKenna WJ et al Diagnosis of Arrhythmogenic Right Ventricular Dysplasia/cardiomyopathy. Br Heart J 1994;71: 215-218

MR Angiography

11

James F. M. Meaney, John Sheehan, and Mathias Boos

Contents

J. F. M. Meaney (✉)
MRI Department, St. James's Hospital, St. James's Street, Dublin 8, Ireland
e-mail: jmeaney@meaneys.com

11.1 Introduction

Magnetic resonance angiography (MRA) is a noninvasive method that provides images similar to those obtained by X-ray digital subtraction angiography (DSA). Blood motion causes two phenomena that change longitudinal and transverse spin magnetization, both of which can be exploited to generate angiographic images. First, time of flight (TOF) effects arise from the movement of longitudinal magnetization during a relatively long period. Second, a flow phenomenon occurs when transverse magnetization moves in the direction of a magnetic field gradient. These effects can be exploited to generate "time of flight" and "phase contrast" angiographic images, respectively, without

P. Reimer et al. (eds.), *Clinical MR Imaging*,
DOI: 10.1007/978-3-540-74504-4_11,

the use of contrast medium (CM), and their use in clinical practice reflects the state-of-the-art technology available at the time (see also Chap. 1).

Noncontrast techniques, although accurate in clinical practice for many indications, have many limitations such as intravoxel dephasing, saturation effects, high reliance on appropriate choice of the velocity encoding (Venc) gradient, and long scan times. Contrast-enhanced techniques overcome most of the problems associated with noncontrast techniques. Although intracranial MRA still relies heavily on noncontrast techniques, contrast-enhanced techniques have supplanted noncontrast techniques for almost all applications within the body since their introduction by Prince in 1994 due to their high spatial resolution, high contrast-to-noise ratios, ease of performance, and short scan times.

11.1.1 Patient Preparation for MRA

No special patient preparation or positioning is necessary for MRA. If echocardiogram (ECG) gating is used for two-dimensional (2D) PC-MRA or sequential (2D) TOF-MRA, electrodes must be appropriately placed on the patient. For thoracic and abdominal imaging where breath-holding is required, the patient should be instructed and coached in breath-holding. Use of oxygen via nasal prongs, and hyperventilation prior to the breath-hold scan may be appropriate, especially for contrast-enhanced MRA. It is helpful to exercise breath-holding with the patient using slight hyperventilation prior to a moderate inspiration.

11.1.2 Coils

All available coils are suitable for MRA. The integral body coil is used for signal transmission, and either the standard body, or preferably, phased-array (wrap-around) coils are used for signal reception. Dedicated neck and peripheral coils are useful for selective MR angiograms of the carotid arteries and peripheral arteries, respectively.

11.2 MRA Techniques

11.2.1 Time of Flight MRA

For neuro-MRA applications, the most widely employed method of performing TOF angiograms is a 3D acquisition, mainly used to visualize the intracranial vessels and carotid bifurcation (Figs. 11.1–11.4). A significant advantage of the 3D technique is that thin slices can be acquired. This results in diminished intravoxel phase dispersions and fewer signal voids. In addition, 3D acquisitions give high resolution and sufficient signal-to-noise ratio (SNR), ideal for visualizing the small peripheral intracranial vessels. Finally, because of thick slab excitation, radiofrequency (RF) pulses of short duration can be used, thus allowing shorter echo times (TE), with resultant less dephasing. In comparison with 3D techniques, 2D (sequential-slice) techniques are more useful for visualizing slow flow (e.g., the venous circulation) and for acquiring data over a long segment where 3D techniques are suboptimal due to progressive saturation within the imaging slab as a result of the flowing spins experiencing multiple excitations during the 3D acquisition. Therefore, the 2D technique and not the 3D technique can be applied to imaging of vessels over large distances (such as the complete carotid arteries and peripheral arteries).

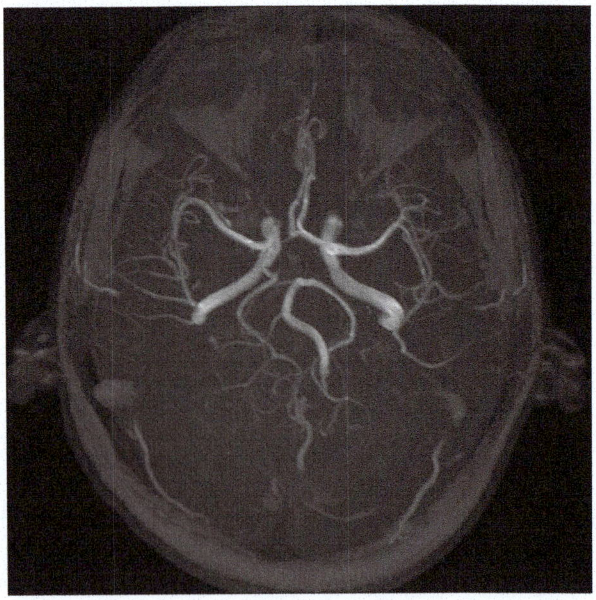

Fig. 11.1 Time of flight MRA demonstrating a hypoplastic right vertebral, right A1, and right P2 cerebral arteries

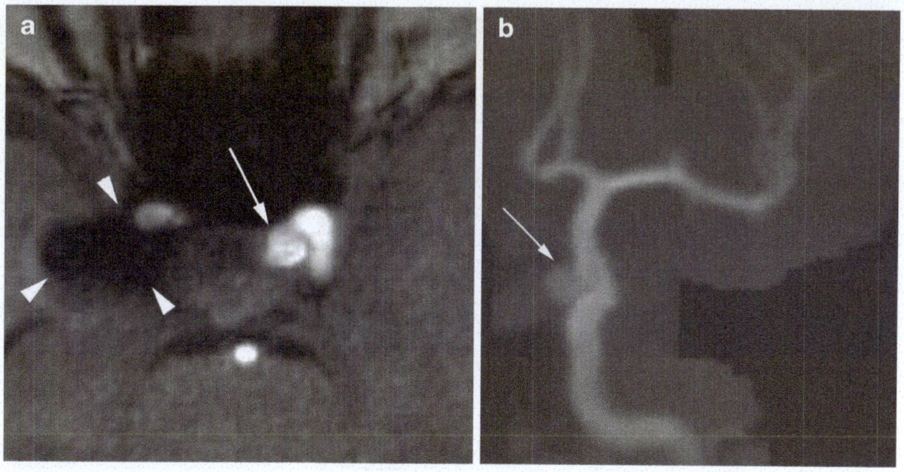

Fig. 11.2 Time of flight-MRA MIP (**a**) depicts the superior hypophyseal aneurysm. The source image axial slice (**b**) through left superior hypophyseal aneurysm (*arrow*) demonstrates metallic artifact on right (*arrowheads*) due to previously clipped right paraclinoid aneurysm. Images courtesy of Michael Hurley, Northwestern Memorial Hospital, Chicago, IL

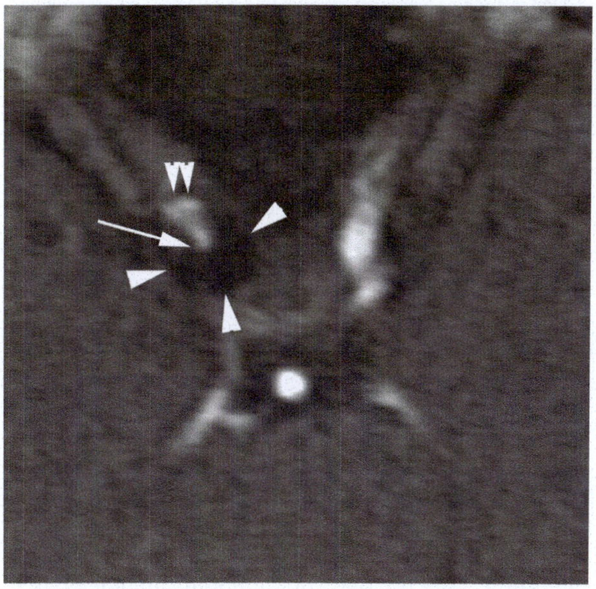

Fig. 11.3 Time of flight MRA axial source through previously coiled right ophthalmic artery aneurysm shows lack of blooming artifact from inert platinum coils (*arrowheads*). The residual neck (*arrow*) is well demonstrated arising from the ICA (*double-arrowheads*). Image courtesy of Michael Hurley, Northwestern Memorial Hospital, Chicago, IL

Prior to introduction of contrast-enhanced MRA, the 2D sequential-slice MRA technique was the most commonly used technique for the evaluation of the large vessels of the abdomen, thorax, and peripheries. The larger voxel size (2D slices are typically 2–4 mm thick compared with the effective slice thickness of 1 mm or less for 3D volumes) combined with a longer TE results in an increased intravoxel phase dispersion, and as a result, saturation effects with diminished intravascular signal. In severe cases, signal voids lead to exaggeration of the degree of stenosis and artifactual stenosis and occlusions. These are most marked in tortuous vessels and those with slow flow.

Flow voids and artifacts also occur due to the pulsatile nature of flow, an effect which is particularly marked in the peripheral arteries, where reversal of flow during diastole is frequent in patients with severe arterio-occlusive disease. This effect can be partially overcome by the use of ECG synchronization, however, one of the main disadvantages of the 2D-TOF technique is the long scan time of about 40–60 min to screen the pelvis and lower extremities, which is prolonged further by ECG triggering. Bone marrow and subcutaneous fat present a relatively bright signal intensity on TOF-MRA. This can be addressed by the use of fat-saturation techniques, although this incurs a further time penalty. Because of the relatively long TE (relative to CEMRA), severe intravascular signal loss is encountered around prosthetic hip and knee replacements, an effect that cannot be easily minimized (less artifact with CEMRA because of the shorter TE). Despite the many limitations of 2D TOF-MRA, it remains widely available and is used for selective indications. For example, more patent pedal vessels can be shown with TOF-MRA compared with conventional angiography, because of its exquisite sensitivity to slow flow. But, because of the long scan times, this technique is restricted to niche indications where CEMRA is not possible or advisable.

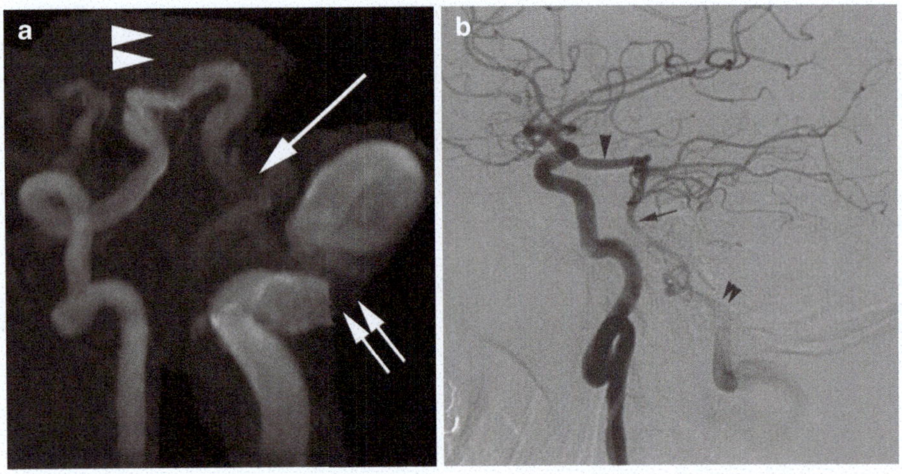

Fig. 11.4 Time of flight MRA MIP (**a**) of vertebrobasilar junction in a patient with a high flow left C1/C2 vertebral arteriovenous fistula demonstrates hypertrophied left vertebral artery with cropping artifact (*double arrows*). Reversed flow in the distal left vertebral artery down to AVF (*arrow*) with associated signal drop off (saturation). There is absent signal in basilar artery (*arrowheads*) due to reversed flow (supplied by right PCOM artery as seen on corresponding DSA (**b**) *arrowhead* posterior communicating artery, *arrow* – Basilar artery, *double-arrowheads* – Left VA). Images courtesy of Michael Hurley, Northwestern Memorial Hospital, Chicago, IL

11.2.2 Optimization Strategies in Time of Flight MRA

Flow-related enhancement can be improved by using gradient-motion rephasing (GMR or flow compensation), in which an additional gradient pulse is used to eliminate flow-related phase shifts. Use of gadolinium (Gd)-chelates improves visualization of distal vessels within the brain, but at the expense of increased overlay of venous structures and higher signal from surrounding tissue. An appropriate balance between repetition time (TR) and flip-angle is necessary to decrease the relative signal intensity of stationary tissue, and conversely, increase the signal intensities of flowing blood. A reasonable compromise is to use a moderate flip-angle (30–60°) in conjunction with a shorter TR in instances where vessel orientation ensures good through-plane flow, and a somewhat longer TR and smaller flip-angle for vessels where slow flow or in-plane flow is anticipated.

In conclusion, the following modifications reduce saturation effects and increase the inflow-related signal intensity in TOF-MRA (Table 11.1):

1. Ensure that images are acquired orthogonal to the direction of flow
2. Increase TR
3. Decrease the flip-angle
4. For intracranial TOF-MRA, use multiple, overlapping, thin-slab acquisition (MOTSA)
5. Implement tilted, optimized, nonsaturating excitation (TONE)
6. Use CM (not commonly implemented for TOF-MRA because of increased venous signal)
7. Remember that TOF-MRA is substantially improved at 3.0 T.

Quality of TOF-MRA can be further optimized by reducing pixel size (improves resolution and reduces saturation effects) and by applying magnetization transfer (MT) pulses. MT works by applying an RF pulse (shifted 1,500 Hz from water), which results in saturation of protons bound to macromolecules. The bound protons transfer the saturation to nearby water, resulting in improved suppression of the background (e.g., brain or muscle) signal.

MOTSA (Multiple Overlapping Thin Slice Acquisition) aims to combine the benefits of higher spatial resolution and more accurate grading of stenosis of 3D-TOF techniques with the superior spatial coverage offered by 2D TOF-MRA. In order to reduce the saturation effects associated with a thick slab 3D slab, multiple thinner 3D slabs are used, each of which overlaps the adjacent volume by approximately 30%. As each individual 3D volume is smaller, MOTSA technique allows the use of higher flip-angles, bringing

Table 11.1 Effect of changing various sequence parameters

Parameter Change	Action	2D TOF-MRA Effect		Parameter Change	Action	3D TOF-MRA Effect	
TE	Decrease	Dephasing, flow voids	Less	TE	Decrease	Dephasing (higher order motion)	Decrease
TR	Decrease	Background suppression, measurement time	Less	TR	Decrease	Intraluminal signal, measurement time	Increase Decrease
FA	Increase	Intraluminal signal, background suppression	Increased	FA	Increase	Inflow saturation, background suppression	Decrease Increase
Slice thickness	Decrease	Intraluminal signal (slow flow)	Increased	Slice thickness	Decrease	Resolution dephasing	Increase Decrease
Number of slices	Increase	FOV in flow direction	Increased	No. of slices	Increase	Resolution, measurement time	Increase Increase
FOV	Decrease	Resolution dephasing	Increase Decrease	FOV	Decrease	Resolution dephasing	Increase Decrease

TOF time of flight; *D* dimension; *MRA* magnetic resonance angiography; *TE* echo time; *TR* repetition time; *FOV* field-of-view

the benefits of both higher intravascular signal intensities and improved background suppression. The final MIP image generated from the processed MOTSA imaging volume is created by discarding slices at the top and bottom of the volume (which are more affected by saturation effects). The main drawback of this technique is the "Venetian-blind" artifact due to differences in signal intensity between adjacent 3D volumes at the points where the slabs overlap; however, this can be minimized by processing algorithms.

For TOF-MRA, progressive saturation of intraluminal signal occurs as the blood flows through the imaging slab. By applying a specially designed ramped RF pulse (TONE), these saturation effects can be minimized, as the flip-angle progressively increases from the entry to the exit slice. This affords better visualization of distal vessels and those with slow flow.

Overestimation of stenosis: A pitfall of TOF-MRA

It is well-known that stenosis can be overestimated by MRA. The main reasons for this are listed in Table 11.2, along with some features that reduce this effect.

Table 11.2 Tools to reduce the effects causing stenosis overestimation on MRA images

Stenosis overestimation by	Effects	Reduce the effects by
Flow acceleration	Dephasing during TE	Decrease TE (TOF)
Turbulent flow		Increase VENC (PC)
Vortex flow		
Stream separation distal to stenosis		Increase resolution, dose (CEMRA)
Vessel tortuosity	Dose	CEMRA
Overlay of vessels within one voxel (PC-MRA)	Dephasing Æ signal loss	Small volume TOF or CEMRA

CE contrast-enhanced; *PC* phase contrast; *VENC* velocity encoding gradient determining the sensitivity to flow velocity; *TOF* time of flight; *MRA* magnetic resonance angiography; *TE* echo time

11.2.3 Black-Blood MRA

"Black-blood MRA" refers to the observation that (fast flowing) blood presents a signal void on spin-echo images, an effect best maximized on T1-W images. It is not a photo negative of bright-blood MRA. On spin-echo imaging, rapidly flowing blood (arterial flow) demonstrates flow-related signal loss, whereas slow-flowing blood (venous flow) has a higher signal intensity. This black-blood "washout" effect can be maximized by using a longer TE (20–30 ms) than that used with standard T1-W imaging. The TE used for black-blood MRA is similar to the TR used for TOF-MRA, as both techniques rely on the same phenomenon of movement of excited protons out of the imaging volume. Various presaturation and dephasing pulses can be employed in this technique to null blood signal and therefore optimize the black-blood effect.

The advantages of this method include the absence of any dephasing artifact (this is the goal of black-blood MRA), which leads to less overestimation of the degree of stenosis. However, a significant disadvantage is that calcified plaques and other black materials may also be isointense with flowing blood, thus leading to underestimation of the degree of stenosis. Also, it is inherently much more difficult to reproject dark vessels than bright vessels into a 3D display.

11.2.4 Phase Contrast MRA

PC-MRA is widely available with sequences allowing the visualization of a particular range of flow velocities, with both 2D and 3D techniques. A thick slab is typically acquired with 2D PC-MRA and displayed as a projection, while 3D PC-MRA offers all of the advantages of a volumetric technique, including video display and subvolume reformatting.

Flow-related signal occurs when transverse magnetization moves in the direction of a magnetic field gradient, resulting in phase shifts. These phase shifts can be compensated for by applying a second gradient pulse of equal duration but opposite polarity. If the protons move during the interval between these two gradient pulses, a movement or flow-related phase shift will occur. This phase shift is directly proportional to the flow velocity and can be displayed in an angiographic image where pixel brightness is proportional to blood flow velocity. Using this approach, the amplitude and duration of the flow-velocity encoding gradient determine the sensitivity to flow velocity (*Venc*). In the case of phase shifts larger than 180°, aliasing occurs, and the MR signal does not reflect real velocity information. For this reason, the expected maximum velocity either has to be estimated before the measurement is started or set by prior knowledge of the range of velocities that typically exist in the vessel-of-interest. All PCA methods require the acquisition of a flow-compensated data set and then additional flow-encoded data sets in different directions. The differences of these two data sets are used to calculate angiographic images. For 3D PCA, the scan times are very long as four measurements must be made: a flow-compensated image, and additionally, a flow-encoded image acquired in each of the three orthogonal planes.

PC methods can be applied with both small and large fields-of-view (FOVs) and typically provide complete suppression of signals from stationary tissue. Unlike inflow (TOF) techniques, PC methods directly measure flow and thus are not hindered by the artificial appearance of tissues having short T1, such as fresh thrombi. This ability to measure flow directly can be exploited to determine flow rates (FRs) within individual arteries, using a 2D ECG-triggered technique.

2D PCAs are comparable to the projections achieved with intraarterial (i.a.) DSA. Compared with sequential inflow MRA, this technique is more efficient; nonetheless, it has some disadvantages: (1) a *Venc* parameter has to be prospectively selected for the acquisition, (2) the necessity for the subtraction of flow-compensated from flow-encoded image sets can result in artifacts from pulsatile flow, (3) breathing and peristalsis within the abdomen and pelvis impair image quality, (4) the highly anisotropic image voxel of this projection technique may result in destructive phase interference in the case of overlapping vessels. For these reasons, PCA is not widely used within the thorax and abdomen, and although accurate for evaluating the peripheral arteries, has few proponents (primarily due to the success of CEMRA). However, the ability to measure flow within individual vessels, e.g., renal arteries in patients with renal artery stenosis (see later), may stimulate further interest in this technique in the future.

11.2.5 Postprocessing of MRA Datasets

For all angiographic data, regardless of the acquisition technique, inspection of the source data is crucial. For black-blood MRA, reprojection techniques are rarely used and interrogation of the images relies solely on evaluation of the source images. For all bright-blood techniques, reprojection techniques are used to create a (pseudo) 3D image of the vascular tree.

11.2.6 Postprocessing of the 3D Time of Flight MRA Data Set

The maximum-intensity projection (MIP), in conjunction with operator-defined multiplanar reformats (MPRs), is the standard-bearer for postprocessing techniques for bright-blood MRA. The MIP technique employs a computer algorithm that extracts all voxels from the image which demonstrates signal intensity significantly above a certain threshold (all bright blood

MRA techniques strive to make the arteries the brightest structures on the image). However, MIP has substantial drawbacks. Areas of diminished flow, including the edges of blood vessels and small vessels with slow flow, have diminished signal and thus may be poorly represented or absent from the reprojected image. Whole vessels or vessel segments may be obscured by overlap of brighter stationary tissue, particularly marked, for example, where vessels are surrounded by fat, or run close to or overlap fat rich medullary cavities of bone. These effects can be minimized by using fat saturation to eliminate fat or by using closely targeted selective MIPs. As a result, the apparent vessel lumen may be falsely narrowed and stenoses exaggerated. Also, the nonselective MIP reprojects other objects into the final image if sufficiently bright. Therefore, fresh extraluminal blood that appears bright on TOF-MRA due to its short T1 (e.g., in patients with intraparenchymal brain hemorrhage) may obscure details of vessels, for example, in patients with intracranial aneurysm rupture. In such cases, however, the bright methemoglobin may be useful in pointing to the site of rupture even if the aneurysm cannot be seen. Clearly this is not a limitation for PC-MRA as all stationary tissue including haematoma appears dark.

Other methods such as surface rendering, volume rendering, and virtual intraluminal endoscopy may be used as appropriate.

11.3 Contrast-Enhanced MRA

11.3.1 Basics and System Requirements

CEMRA is based on the principle of a 10- to 25-fold shortening of the blood T1-relaxation time by injection of a paramagnetic CM. This results in large signal-intensity differences between background tissues (the brightest of which is fat which has a T1 of approximately 200 ms) and contrast-enriched arteries (blood T1 < 50 ms after injection of an appropriate volume of contrast agent) (Figs. 11.5–11.37). Image acquisition is performed with a heavily T1-W sequence. Because intravascular vessel contrast depends on the T1 shortening

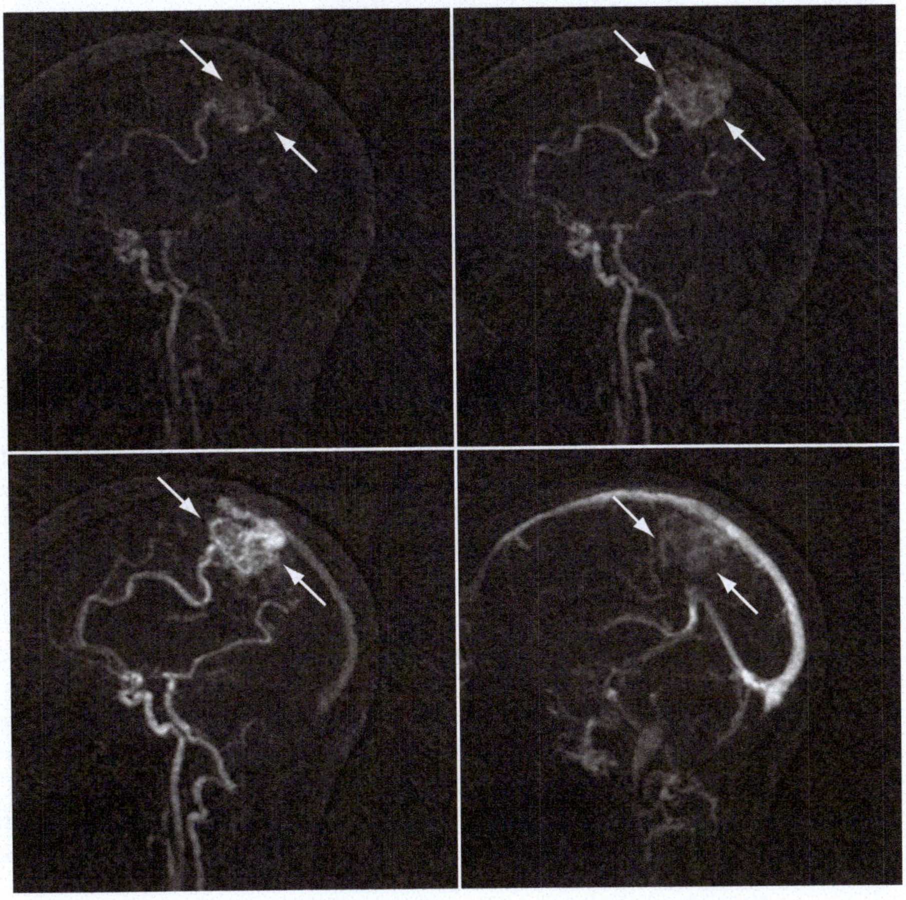

Fig. 11.5 Time-resolved MRA of a parietal hemispheric AVM using overlapping radial sliding window k-space sampling and sliding subtraction. Separate arterial, nidal, early, and late venous phases are defined. Image courtesy of Michael Hurley, Northwestern Memorial Hospital, Chicago, IL

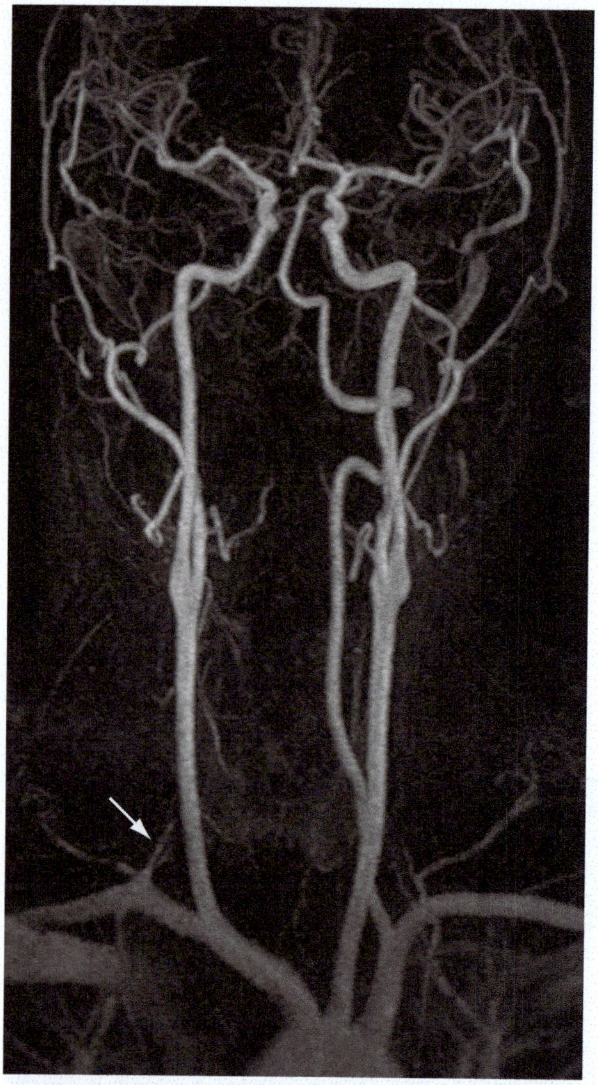

Fig. 11.6 Time-resolved MRA of neck demonstrates a hypoplastic right vertebral artery

effect of a contrast agent injection and not on inherent flow effects, the images are said to be "flow-independent." Therefore, data acquisition can be performed in whatever plane best suits the anatomy, without consideration for inflow or other flow-related effects. SNR limitations are not prevalent, and in any case, anticipated SNR limitations can be addressed by increasing the contrast injection rate for improved T1 shortening.

Because intravenously injected contrast agent eventually reaches arteries and veins, selective arteriogram's must be acquired *during* the relatively short "arteriovenous window" (defined as that time interval between the onset of peak arterial enhancement and that of venous enhancement). Therefore, a fast or ultrafast gradient-echo (GRE) sequence is used. The resultant 3D data has excellent contrast-to-noise ratios and can be easily postprocessed using both MIP and MPR format to allow different projections of the vessels.

11.3.2 System Requirements

In order to generate a sufficiently high-resolution 3D data set within either the arteriovenous transit time or the breath-hold capability of the patient (for thoracic and abdominal vasculature), CEMRA is best performed on a high-performance MR system with short TR and TE. Strong gradients (≥20 mT/m) with short rise times (≤600 ms/mT/m) offered by state-of-the-art 1.0 T field strength or greater are best. Although most CEMRA studies were initially validated at 1.5 T, high image quality can also be achieved at lower field strength (especially 1.0 T). 3 T imaging, because SNR increases linearly with field strength offers significant benefit for CEMRA.

11.3.3 Vessel Contrast and K-Space

Using the most basic "linear" k-space filling strategy, k-space is filled line by line following the basic format of starting at one periphery of k-space, progressing in an incremental linear fashion through the center, and ending with the last line at the other edge of k-space. However, k-space lines can be filled in any order, a unique characteristics of data acquisition on MR that can be exploited to improve the quality of CEMRA. The reason is that the higher k-space frequencies, which determine the spatial resolution of the resulting image, are represented by the outer lines of k-space, whereas the center 20% or so of k-space (low spatial frequencies, central lines) determine the image contrast. Therefore, for selective arterial imaging (i.e., optimal depiction of arteries but no veins), it is essential to acquire the central k-space lines at the start of the scan ("centric") coincident with the arterial peak and prior to the onset of venous enhancement. If this condition is met, higher spatial resolution than otherwise might be possible can be achieved by continuing acquisition of peripheral k-space data into the venous phase, providing synchronization of the contrast bolus (see later) with the central lines of k-space (acquired at the start of the 3D

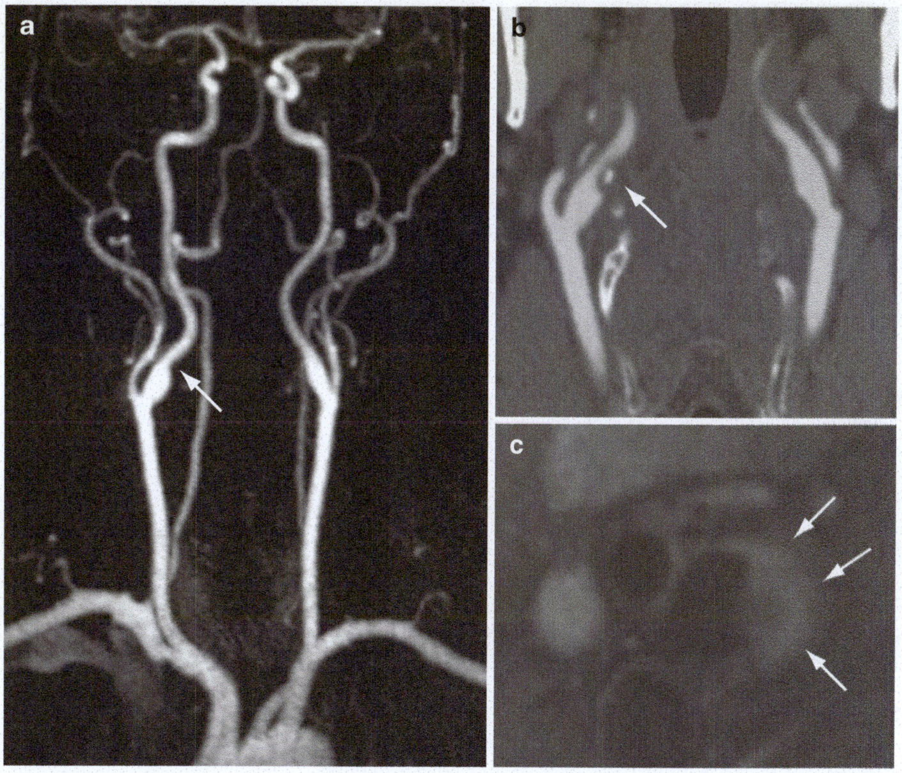

Fig. 11.7 (**a–c**) Time-resolved MRA (**a**) of the neck demonstrates mild stenosis of the proximal internal carotid artery secondary to a calcified mixed plaque disease seen on CT (**b**) and 2D T2-W dark blood imaging

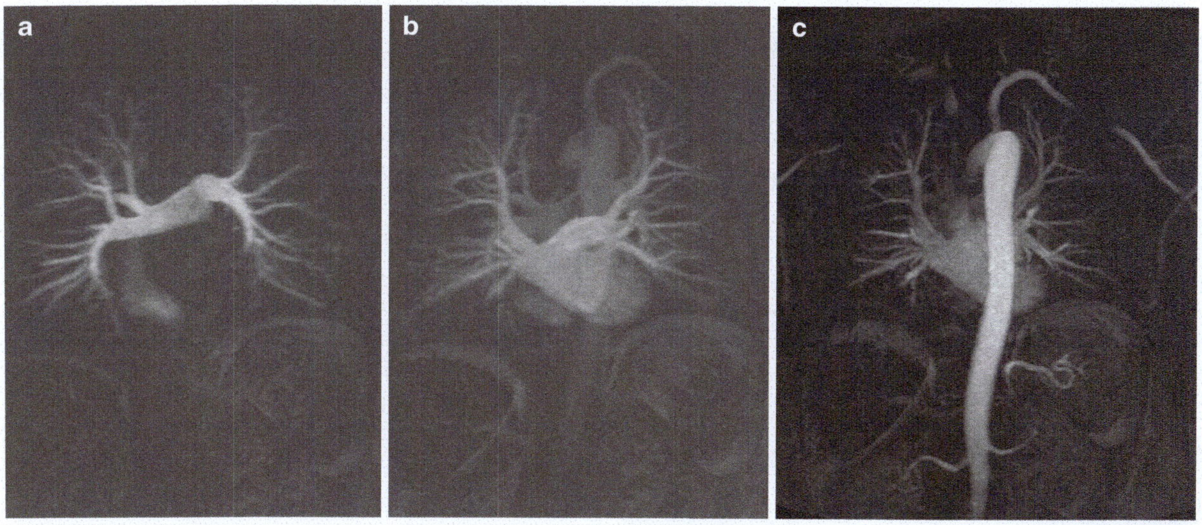

Fig. 11.8 (**a–c**) Normal time-resolved thoracic MRA. After administration of 0.05 mmol/kg dose of Gd-DTPA at 5 cc/s, a time-resolved coronal 3D MRA with a temporal resolution of 3.5 s was acquired. The coronal 3D MRA sequence demonstrates the pulmonary arterial system (**a**), pulmonary venous system (**b**), and the systemic arterial system

acquisition) can be assured. This emphasises the requirement for a robust method for the detection of contrast agent within the artery to be imaged ("bolus detection"). This "centric" acquisition approach coupled with accurate bolus detection offers advantages at all anatomical sites, but particularly where high resolution is required in the face of an extremely short arteriovenous circulation e.g., carotid and infrapopliteal arteries.

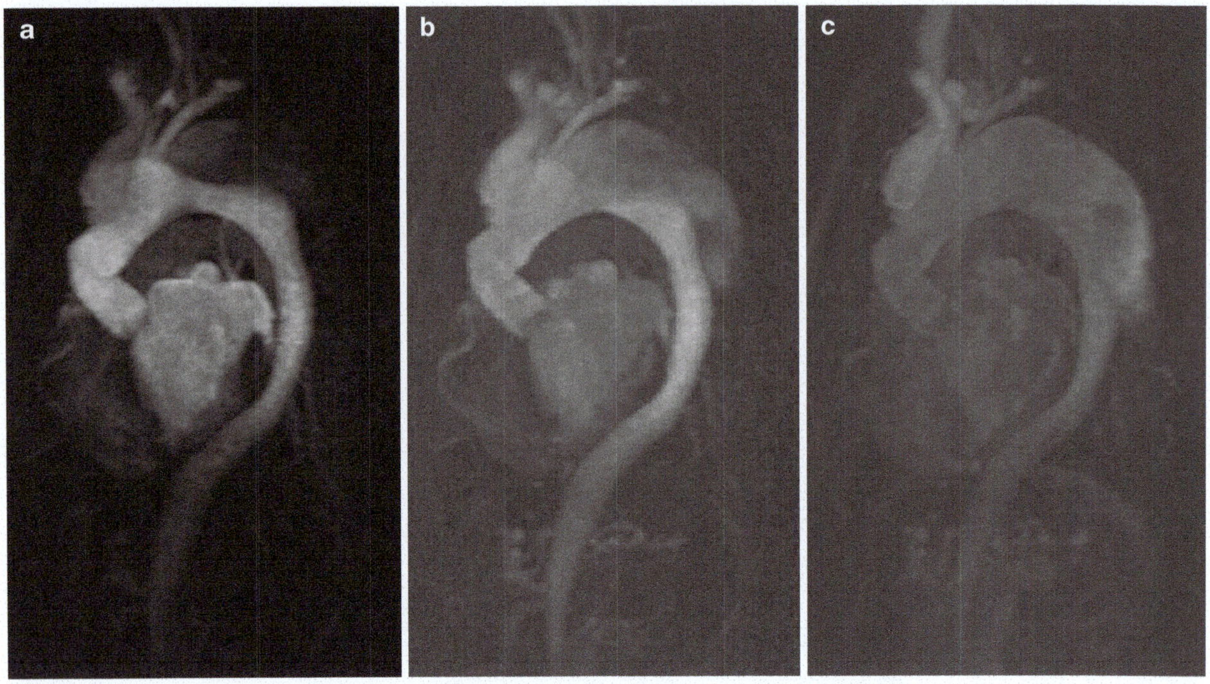

Fig. 11.9 Type A aortic dissection in a 55-year-old male. A time-resolved, saggital oblique MRA (**a–c**) using 0.05 mmol/kg dose of Gd-DTPA administered at 5 cc/s with a temporal resolution of 3.5 s demonstrates a dissection starting in the aortic arch and extending into the brachiocephalic and descending thoracic aorta

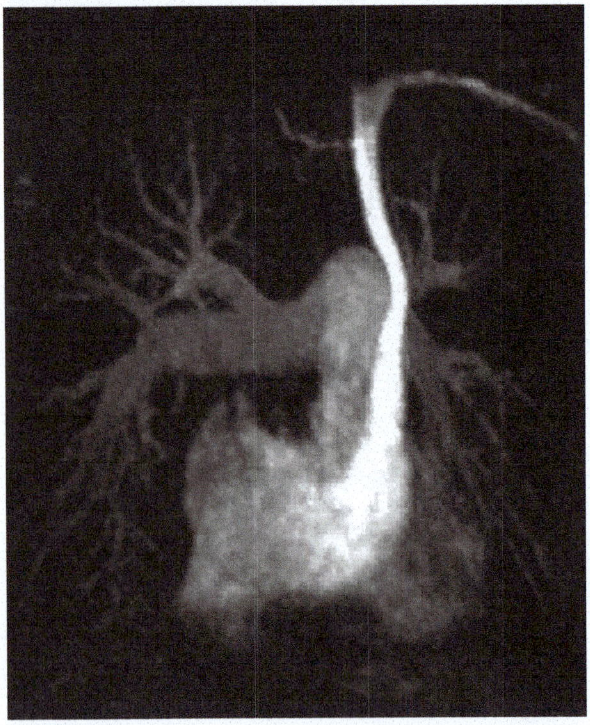

Fig. 11.10 Left-sided SVC. A time-resolved coronal MRA of the thorax demonstrates a left-sided SVC draining into an enlarged coronary sinus

11.3.4 Measurement Parameters

For CEMRA, any scan plane is possible and the acquisition volume can be tailored to the region-of-interest. This offers substantial benefit, in that redundant tissue coverage can be avoided and best resolution maintained. The coronal plane is most commonly chosen due to optimal coverage for any combination of field-of-view, slice thickness, and slab depth. The measurement parameters are tailored to cover the entire region of interest (ROI) related to the clinical requirement but in order to ensure the shortest possible scan time, in-plane and through-plane resolution must be balanced against scan time. The shortest TR possible is used and wider bandwidths which afford a slightly shorter scan time over narrower bandwidths (albeit at the expense of a usually insignificant SNR penalty) owing to the inherent high SNR. The use of such short TRs (typically <5 ms) would eliminate intravascular signal for TOF-MRA, but are is essential for CEMRA to ensure short scan times. In order to minimize dephasing, the shortest TE possible should be used. To maximize spatial resolution, whenever possible 512 resolution is used in the read

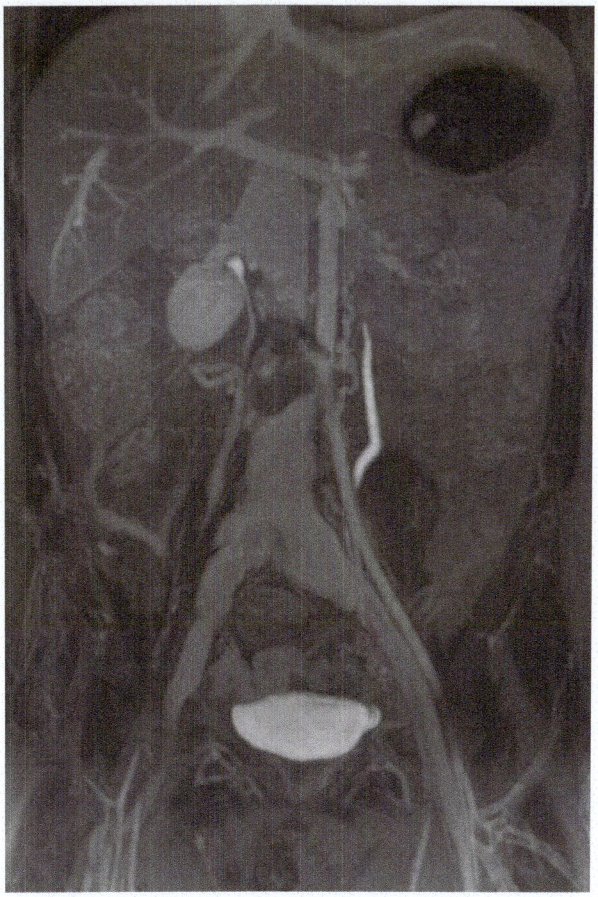

Fig. 11.11 IVC thrombus. The MIP of the 3D high-resolution MRA in the venous phase demonstrates a large filling defect in the juxtra-renal IVC consistent with a thrombus

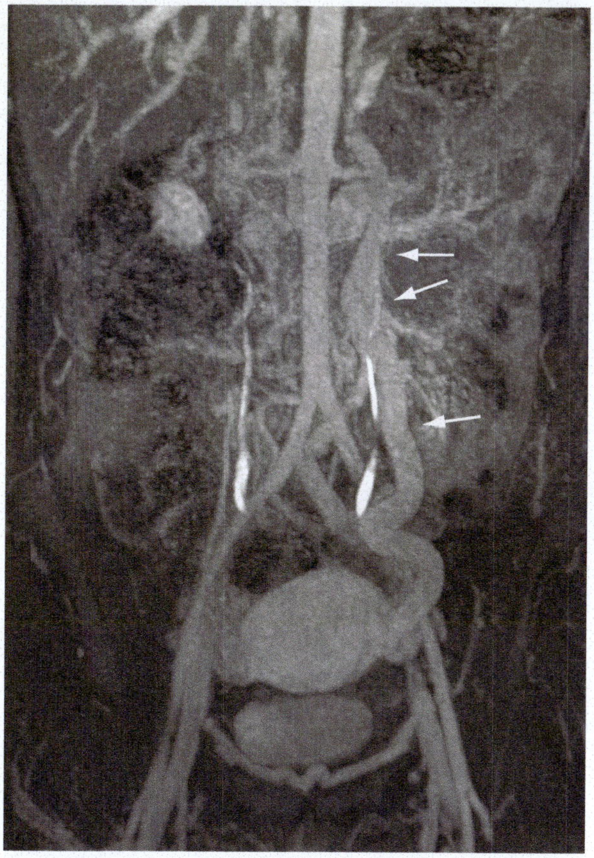

Fig. 11.12 Absent inferior vena cava. The MIP of the 3D high-resolution MRA in the venous phase demonstrates absence of the IVC. The blood is returning via numerous collaterals including a significantly enlarged left gonadal vein (*arrows*)

(frequency-encoding) direction (no time penalty), the slight disadvantages of reduced SNR (smaller voxel size) and slightly increased TE (more dephasing) being acceptable. Higher resolution in the phase-encode and slice-select directions can be achieved by adding more phase-encoding steps and thinner slices respectively, both of which lengthen the scan time. The scan time is limited by either the AV window, or more commonly, by the breath-holding capability of the patient for imaging within the thorax and abdomen. It is important to appreciate that a lower resolution breath-hold scan may be superior to a higher resolution nonbreath-hold scan for imaging of the aortic branches which usually move with respiration. Therefore, the best resolution possible within the breath-hold capability of the patient is used to ensure accurate stenosis grading. The choice of flip-angle is not critical but should be as close as possible to the range of 35–50°.

Because of the unique, symmetric, structure of k-space, it is not always essential to acquire all lines of k-space. If more than half (including the central lines) of k-space lines are measured, the remainder (40% or so) can be reconstructed from the measured data, a technique referred to as partial Fourier imaging. This gives a reduction in scan time proportional to the amount of data that is reconstructed rather than measured, a huge benefit considering the stringent requirement for a short scan time.

Currently, sufficiently short scan times with adequate resolution are possible with most modern scanners. However, shorter scan times can also be achieved by using lower in-plane resolution and lower spatial resolution in the slice select direction (thicker slices). Slice interpolation, a widely exploited technique to improve the visual quality of MIP images does not overcome this problem because the calculated resolution cannot be considered as real spatial resolution.

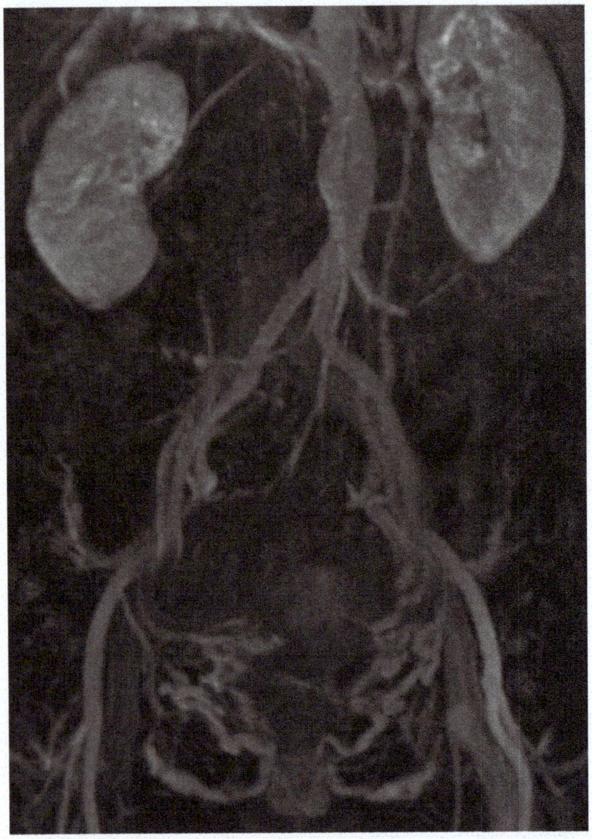

Fig. 11.13 Pelvic congestion syndrome. The MIP of the 3D high-resolution MRA in the venous phase demonstrates multiple, bilateral enlarged pelvic veins and a visible left gonadal vein

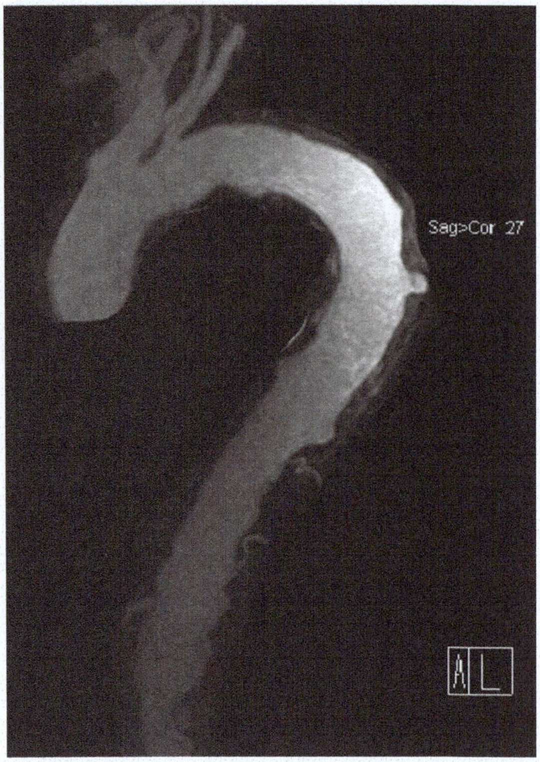

Fig. 11.15 Multiple thoracic aortic penetrating ulcers. A MIP reconstruction of a static saggital oblique, high-resolution MRA of the aorta demonstrates multiple small focal penetrating ulcers involving the aortic arch and descending thoracic aorta. Image courtesy of James Carr, Northwestern Memorial Hospital, Chicago, IL

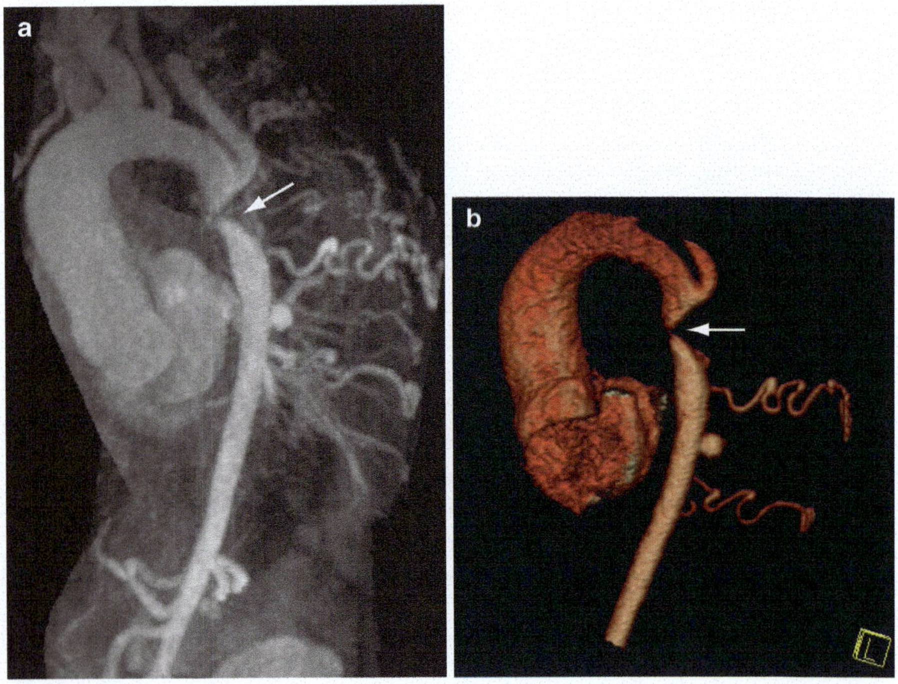

Fig. 11.14 Aortic coarctation in a 26-year-old female. A static saggital oblique, high-resolution MRA of the aorta demonstrates a severe postductal coarctation with extensive collateralization through the intercostal arteries seen on the MIP (**a**) and volume rendered (**b**) reconstructions

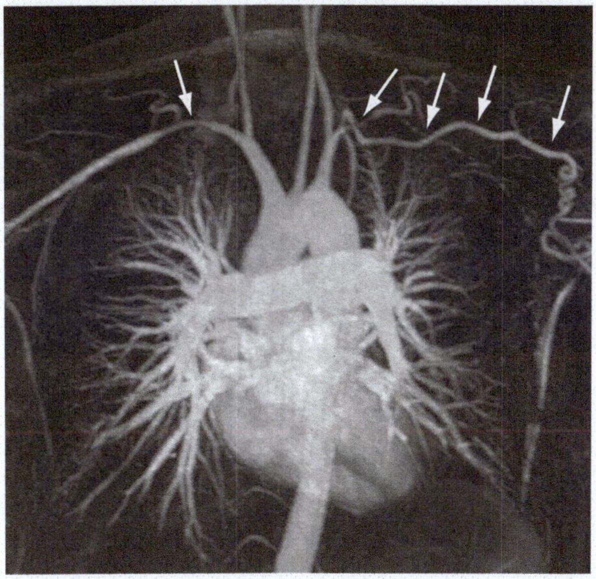

Fig. 11.16 Takaysau's arteritis in a 36-year-old female. A MIP reconstruction of a static coronal, high-resolution MRA of the thorax demonstrates a segmental moderate to severe stenosis of the right subclavian artery (*single arrow*). The left subclavian artery is occluded beyond its origin. A large collateral arising from the region of the thyrocervical trunk provides arterial flow to the upper limb (*short arrows*)

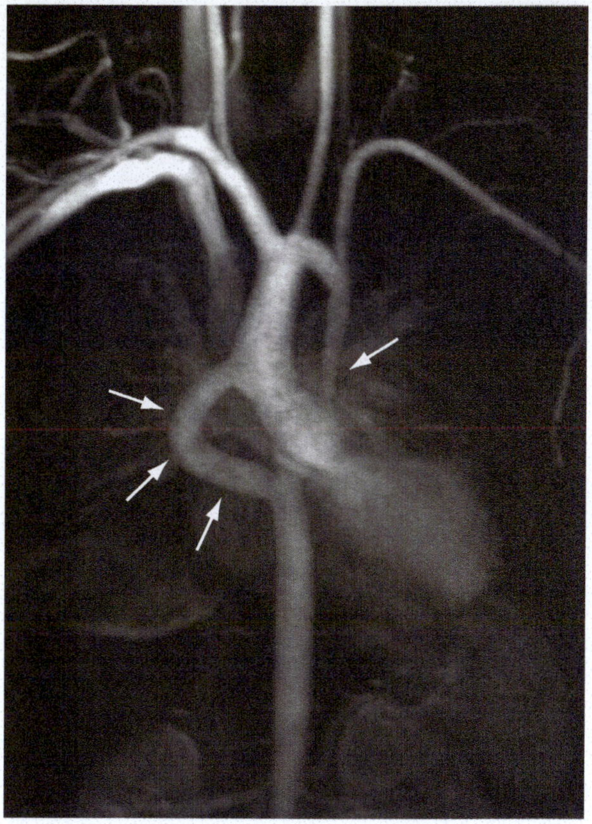

Fig. 11.17 Thoracic aortic stenosis and bypass. A MIP reconstruction of a coronal static high-resolution MRA of the thorax demonstrates severe stenosis of the descending thoracic aorta (*single long arrow*). The patient had a bypass graft placed between the ascending thoracic aorta and the distal descending thoracic aorta (*3 short arrows*). Image courtesy of James Carr, Northwestern Memorial Hospital, Chicago, IL

11.3.5 Are All Contrast Agents for CEMRA the Same? Relaxivity and Safety Issues

Until recently all CEMRA was performed as a first-pass imaging technique with the same extracellular contrast agents introduced into clinical practice for all other contrast-enhanced applications. More recently, a dedicated contrast agent, Gadofosveset trisodium has been introduced, which remains in the blood pool for significantly longer than extracellular contrast agents and offers some benefit.

The previously widely held belief that gadolinium-based contrast agents were almost identical in their efficacy and safety as contrast agents for MRA can no longer be supported due to differences in relaxivity, protein binding, and formulation strength. Also, the assertion that gadolinium agents were almost entirely safe has now been tempered by the recognition of nephrogenic systemic fibrosis (NSF) as a rare but potentially catastrophic consequence of gadolinium injection. These factors now weigh on contrast agent choice for MRA.

11.3.6 Relaxivity and T1 Shortening for First-Pass MRA

Reductions in blood T1 achieved by gadolinium injection depend primarily on three factors; first, the injection rate, second, the total volume injected, and third, the relaxivity of the agent. The relaxivity, which is given by the R1 value, is a physical constant for each agent. For many years, it was assumed that blood T1 shortening varied little between the "traditionally" available MR contrast agents as they were all formulated at 0.5 M and had similar R1 values. However, one of the "traditional" contrast agents (Gadobenate Dimeglumine®, Bracco SpA) offers superior blood T1 shortening as a result of weak protein binding. Also,

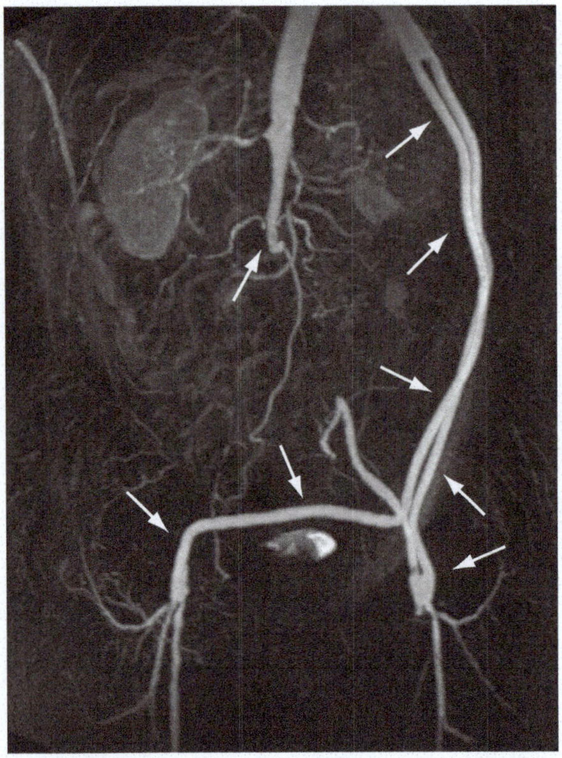

Fig. 11.18 Thoracic aorto-bifemoral artery bypass. The MIP of the 3D high-resolution MRA demonstrates occlusion of the distal aorta (*long arrow*) and iliac vessels with reconstitution of the common femoral arteries via a bifurcated graft (*short arrows*) arising from the descending thoracic aorta with the distal limbs anatomizing with the common femoral arteries bilaterally. Image courtesy of James Carr, Northwestern Memorial Hospital, Chicago, IL

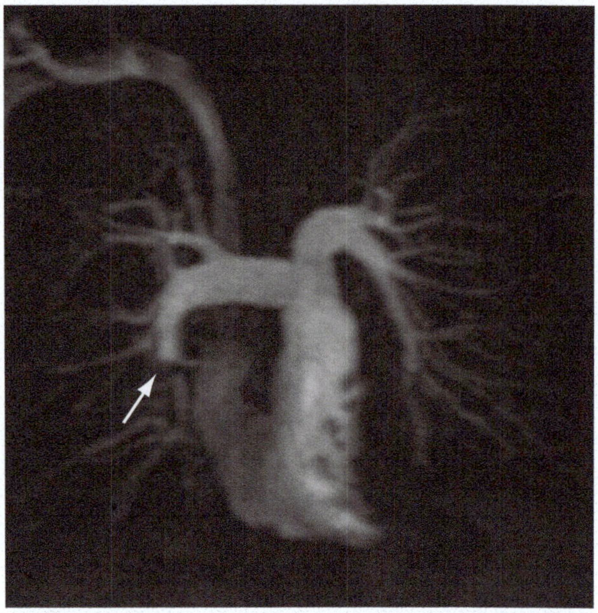

Fig. 11.19 Time-resolved MRA demonstrating a right lower lobe pulmonary embolus (*arrow*). After administration of 0.05 mmol/kg dose of Gd-DTPA at 5 cc/s, a time-resolved coronal 3D MRA with a temporal resolution of 3.5 s was acquired. The MIP demonstrates a filling defect in the right lower lobe pulmonary artery consistent with an acute pulmonary embolus

there is now an agent formulated at 1.0 M (Gadoteridol®, Schering), which on a volume basis offers approximately twice the T1 shortening of 0.5 M agents.

Blood pool agents: A single contrast agent, Gadofosveset has received regulatory approval in many countries. Although introduced primarily as a blood pool agent for delayed imaging, its' superior T1 shortening properties make it ideal for first pass imaging also. Therefore, a potential use of this agent is as a first-pass imaging agent with the potential for delayed imaging at higher resolution. Delayed or blood pool imaging with this agent is performed after an equilibrium has been reached between the injected contrast agent and the blood pool (usually at least 20 min after contrast injection). Therefore, images are acquired without the need for bolus timing which facilitates higher resolution imaging than otherwise might be possible, but at

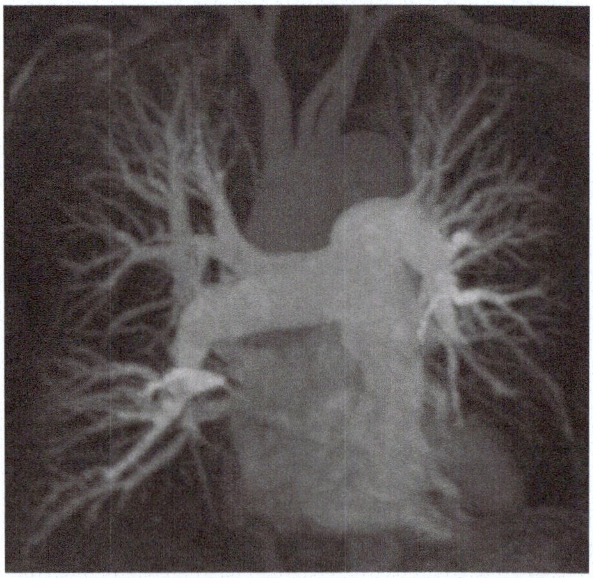

Fig. 11.20 Pulmonary arterial hypertension secondary to chronic pulmonary emboli. After administration of 0.05 mmol/kg dose of Gd-DTPA at 5 cc/s, a time resolved coronal 3D MRA with a temporal resolution of 3.5 s was acquired, demonstrating significant enlargement of the central pulmonary arterial system

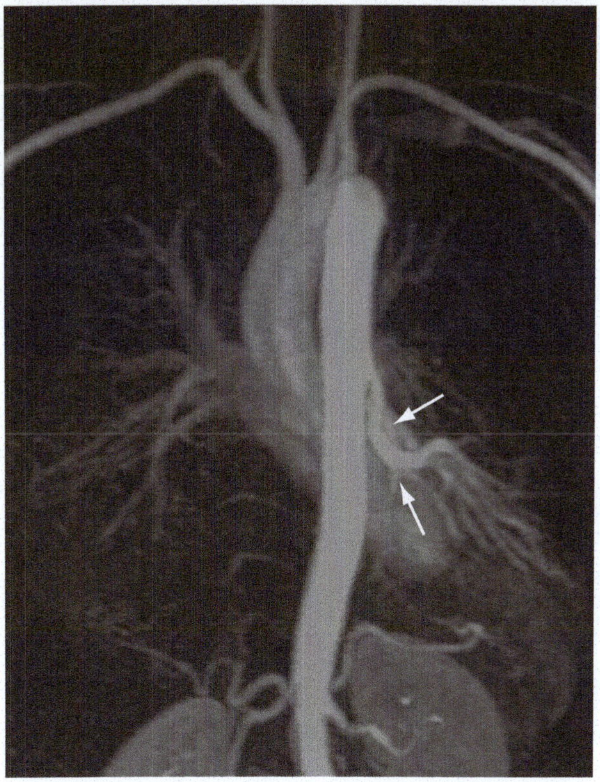

Fig. 11.21 Left lower lobe pulmonary sequestration. A MIP reconstruction of a coronal, static high-resolution MRA of the thorax demonstrates systemic arterial supply to the left lower lobe, arising from the descending thoracic aorta (*arrows*). Image courtesy of David Tuite and James Carr, Northwestern Memorial Hospital, Chicago, IL

the expense of nonselective images which demonstrate arteries and veins equally. An evolving approach to bloodpool CEMRA is to acquire a "standard" CEMRA during first pass with Gadofosveset (using the same technique as used for CEMRA with standard (extracellular) contrast agents) and to either perform dedicated imaging at high resolution >20 min later in all patients once the steady state is reached or alternatively to reserve blood-pool phase imaging for areas not fully evaluated or identified as abnormal on first-pass imaging.

Regardless of which agent is used, the aim is to obtain the highest concentration in the arteries of interest during the acquisition of the central lines of k-space for all first pass imaging (as described above). The bolus geometry depends on the parameters of the i.v. bolus injection [flow rate (FR), CM dose, and NaCl flush volume] and additionally on individual physiological and pathophysiological parameters such as flow rates within individual vessels, total blood volume, and physiological status (e.g., impaired cardiac output, anxiety, etc.).

Studies have demonstrated that for any given volume, improved vascular contrast may be achieved by increasing the FR from 1ml/s to 2ml/sec. Faster injections will shorten the bolus, and although increased contrast is anticipated, image quality may be unchanged or even get worse if the bolus is so short that contrast is not present throughout the whole of the acquisition. Prolongation of the saline flush volume causes a lengthening of the contrast bolus by wash-out of contrast that otherwise might remain within the brachial and subclavian veins due to stasis. The bolus is progressively diluted by CM passage through the heart and lungs, but a susceptibility effect can be seen in the subclavian and brachiocephalic arteries on the side of injection due to the extremely high concentration of contrast agent within the adjacent vein. CM bolus dilution effects are similar for all undiseased systemic vessels (Table 11.11), but despite this, some vessels may be less conspicuous due to increased bolus dilution factors (Table 11.11), resolution constraints, proximity to overlap of subcutaneous or bone-marrow fat, if fat is not eliminated by subtraction or saturation effects and motion. Additionally, segments distal to severe stenosis or distal segments reconstituted via collaterals may be poorly visible due to delayed arrival of CM.

However, it does not make sense to prescribe a high resolution scan if the bolus duration is not long enough to be present during acquisition of the high spatial frequencies at the outer k-space edge (at the end of the scan) which define image resolution. Therefore, the bolus geometry must be tailored to the scan duration, and a frequently employed approach to address these concerns (which results in a lower total injected dose) is to decrease the injection rate for the latter part of the scan. Using this approach, the bolus length is increased thus ensuring that contrast agent is present during acquisition of the detail-defining high spatial frequencies, albeit at a lower concentration.

11.3.7 Bolus Timing and Contrast Medium Considerations for Contrast-Enhanced MRA

For CEMRA, spatial resolution is dictated not only by the traditional mathematical calculation of voxel size

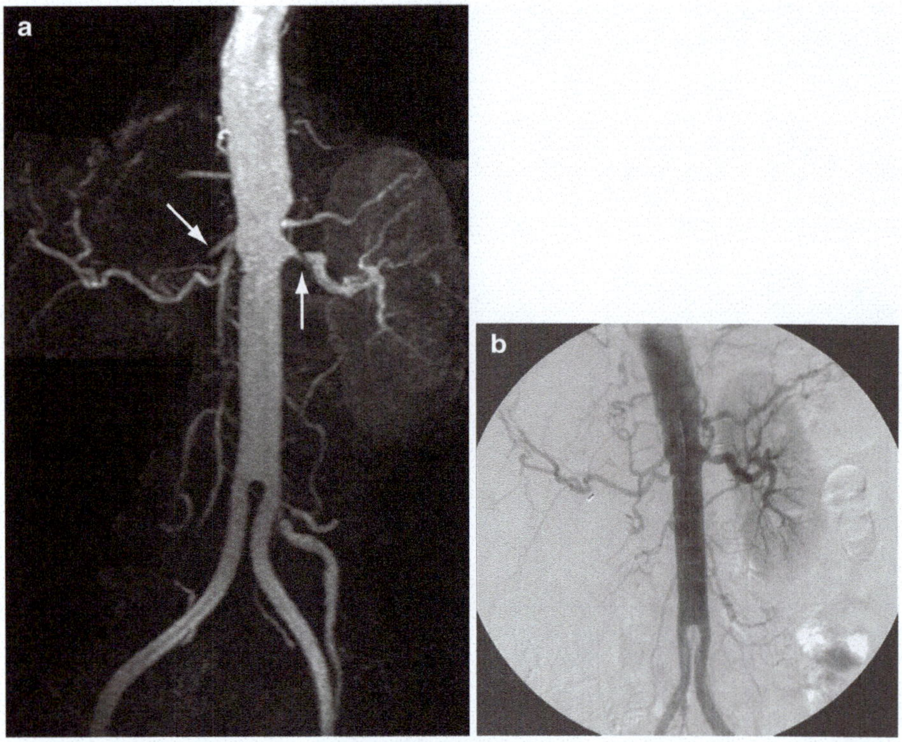

Fig. 11.22 Renal artery stenosis. The MIP of the 3D high-resolution MRA (**a**) demonstrates an aorto-bifemoral artery trouser graft, occlusion of the right renal artery (*short arrow*), and a severe stenosis of the left renal artery (*long arrow*) beyond the ostia. The conventional angiogram (**b**) demonstrates the vascular lesions. Images courtesy of James Carr, Northwestern Memorial Hospital, Chicago, IL

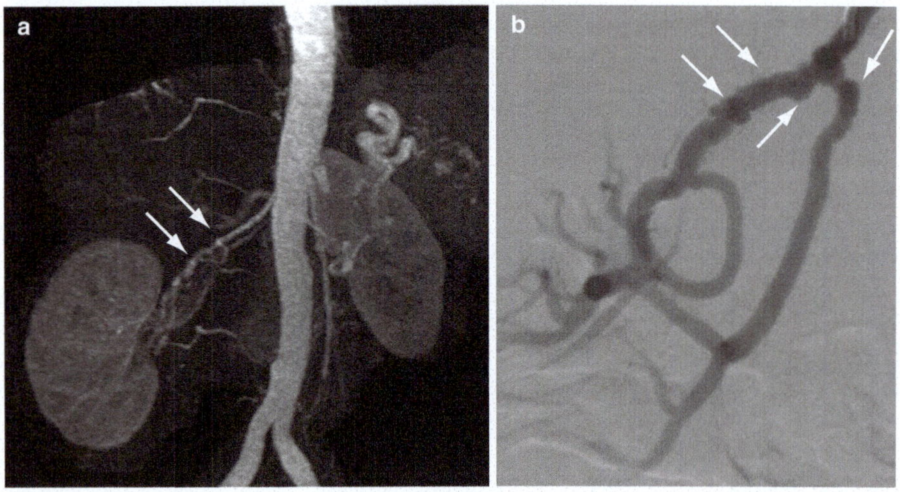

Fig. 11.23 Renal artery fibromuscular dysplasia. The MIP of the 3D high-resolution MRA (**a**) demonstrates long segment of alternating areas of focal stenosis and aneurysmal dilatation of the mid and distal right renal artery, which was confirmed on conventional angiography (**b**) prior to therapeutic balloon angioplasty. Images courtesy of James Carr, MD., Northwestern Memorial Hospital, Chicago, IL, USA

(FOV in each direction divided by the number of samples), but also by the intravascular concentration of gadolinium during data acquisition. For example, diagnostic quality renal MRAs can be acquired using either a single dose [0.1 mmol/kg] or double dose [0.2 mmol/kg] using the same FR. However, if the same CEMRA sequence parameters are used, the double-dose technique yields better resolution (edge detail) and superior depiction of small branches than the single-dose examination (Table 11.10.)

Although CEMRA is "flow-independent" (i.e., little or no dependence on "inflow" or "phase" effects), achieving optimal image quality relies on data acquisition (specifically, the central k-space lines) during peak arterial enhancement. Once contrast agent is delivered into a peripheral vein, the widely varying circulation time from injection site into a peripheral vein to artery-of-interest emphasizes that the scan delay time (time from start of infusion to start of scanning) must be carefully selected. Although this interval can be set

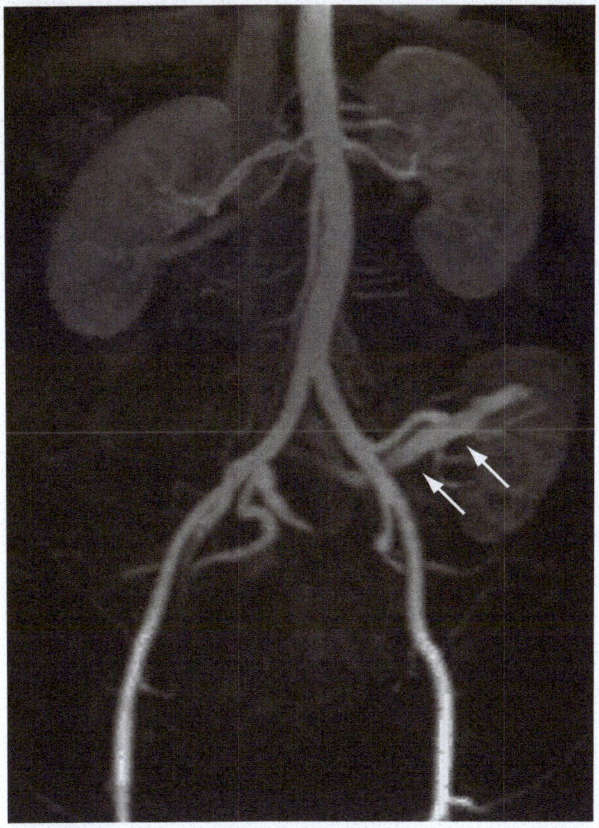

Fig. 11.24 Renal transplant arterial-venous malformation. The MIP of the 3D high-resolution MRA demonstrates early filling of the transplanted kidney renal vein secondary to a fistulous connection with the transplanted renal artery. Images courtesy of James Carr, MD., Northwestern Memorial Hospital, Chicago, IL, USA

empirically, based on the fact that the circulation time is affected by such parameters as age, cardiovascular and pulmonary status, in order to eliminate uncertainty automated or semiautomated methods have been developed as follows:

1. Use of a timing bolus to determine circulation time: Bolus arrival time (BAT) is measured prior to the 3D CEMRA being performed by dynamically scanning over the ROI following injection of a (test) dose of 1–2 mL CM, followed by a 20–30cc saline chaser. A time-resolved single-slice (2D GRE) imaging with a temporal resolution of 1 image/s is sufficient to visualize the arrival of the bolus. The scan delay (T_{sd}) of the subsequent 3D CEMRA can then be calculated using the following formula (provided that a linear phase-encoding table is applied):

   $$T_{sd} = BAT - (1/2MT - [MT/10]).$$

   (MT = measurement time).

2. Automated Bolus Detection. Two methods are used:
   (a) “Black-box” detection (SMARTPREP): a tracker volume is placed within the region-of-interest, and the signal intensity within the voxel is measured continuously. Increase in the signal intensity above a certain threshold signifies arrival of the contrast agent, and the 3D scan is “triggered.” The disadvantage of this method is that the operator has no control over when the 3D scan commences.
   (b) Fluoroscopic detection (CAREBOLUS, BOLUSTRAK, FLUOROPREP): A 2D single-slice (see below) with a temporal resolution of 1 image/s is dynamically acquired and reconstructed in real-time on the scan monitor. Slice thickness usually encompasses the entire imaging volume (e.g., 50–100 mm) thus giving excellent visualization of the temporal pattern of vessel filling. A software modification implemented with bolus detection packages allows immediate commencement of the 3D scan once the operator visualizes contrast within the ROI on the 2D scan (allowing for a breath-hold if necessary).
3. *Multiphase MRA.* This approach does not use a timing sequence; rather several short 3D data sets are acquired in rapid succession, and the appropriate data set is chosen. The disadvantage of this technique is the requirement for very high performance gradients and the need for several breath-holds, which precludes its use in many patients. It may be implemented in association with TRICKS (time resolved imaging of contrast kinetics – see later).

11.3.8 Spatial and Temporal Resolution for CEMRA

There is an inverse relationship between spatial and temporal resolution, i.e., the greater the spatial resolution the worse the spatial resolution and vice versa. For many indications, a single high resolution data set can be assured without venous enhancement by adhering to the above principles. However, in some instances, “dynamic” type information is required and the acquisition time of a 3D scan is too long to facilitate this. In such instances, the following approaches can be used:

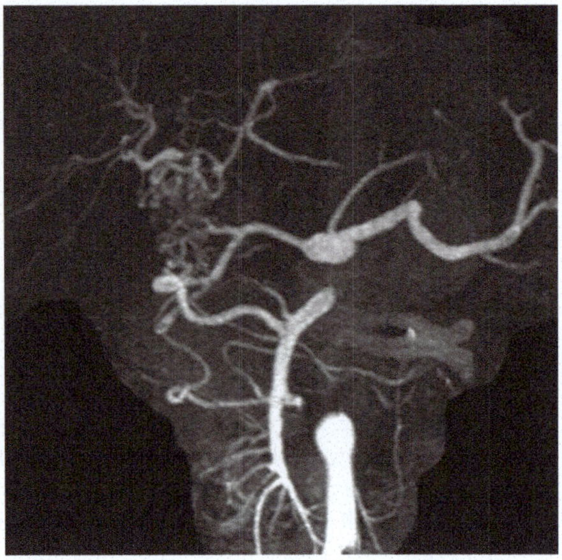

Fig. 11.25 Hepatic artery occlusion. The MIP of the 3D high-resolution MRA demonstrates occlusion of the proper hepatic artery with reconstitution of the branch vessels via collaterals. Image courtesy of James Carr, Northwestern Memorial Hospital, Chicago, IL

- 2D scanning: A single thick slice is prescribed over the ROI, with a slice thickness that encompasses the relevant anatomy (Fig. 11.5). Although through-plane resolution is extremely poor, with this technique the temporal pattern of vessel filling can be identified and patent arterial segments that fill later via collaterals can be visualized which might be missed on 3D scanning. This is particularly useful for imaging of the distal run-off (infrapolpiteal and pedal) vessels. A good precontrast mask is required to optimize vessel contrast for this approach.
- TRICKS: This k-space sampling algorithm repetitively samples low and high spatial frequencies in an interleaved, asymmetrical fashion. Central k-space data (low spatial frequency) is updated at a much faster rate than the peripheral (high spatial frequency) lines. The peripheral k-space data (which varies little during the passage of the bolus) is combined with the rapidly updated central k-space data and the resultant reconstructed data sets yield time resolved information, the temporal resolution of which is determined by the rate of central k-space sampling. Images also benefit from high spatial resolution.
- Ultrafast 3D MRA (another form of time resolved imaging): The T1 pulse sequence is optimized for extremely rapid scan time (Figs. 11.5–11.9). Ultrashort TRs (1–2 ms) and high parallel imaging factors are required; however, this technique which potentially generates subsecond 3D MRAs is possible only on the most modern ultrafast gradient scanners.

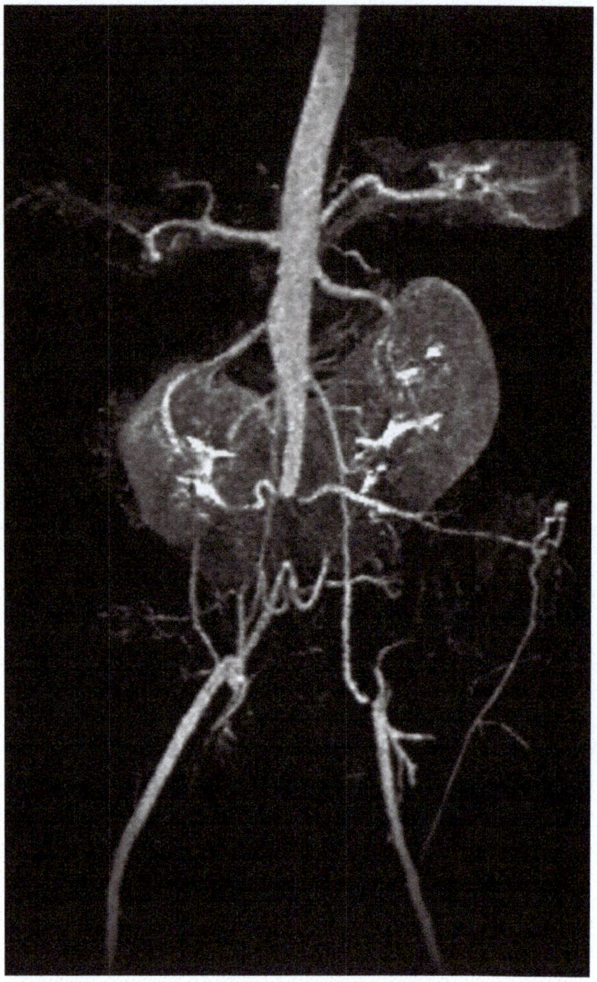

Fig. 11.26 Aorto-iliac occlusion in 64-year-old male. The MIP of the 3D high-resolution MRA demonstrates occlusion of the distal aorta with reconstitution of the common femoral arteries via a variety of lumbar collaterals. Image courtesy of James Carr, Northwestern Memorial Hospital, Chicago, IL

11.3.9 3T Imaging: Role in MRA?

Signal to noise increases almost linearly with field strength. Thus, an approximate doubling of SNR is anticipated at 3 T over 1.5 T. For TOF-MRA, improved vessel conspicuity results not only from improved SNR but also from shorter TEs which reduce both susceptibility and flow-related artifacts and T1 prolongation of

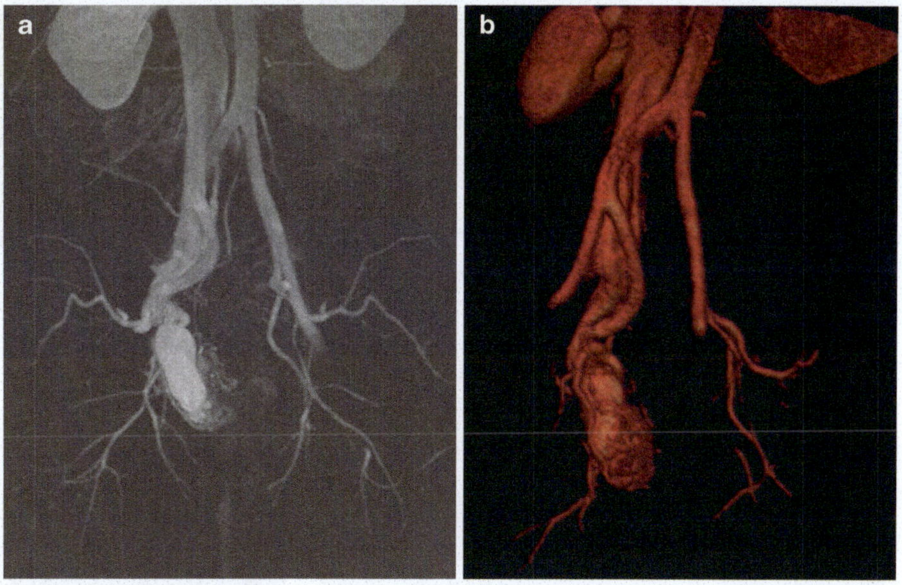

Fig. 11.27 Internal iliac artery arterial-venous malformation. The MIP (**a**) and volume rendered image (**b**) demonstrates an enlarged arterialized right internal iliac vein, which is filling via the adjacent internal iliac artery

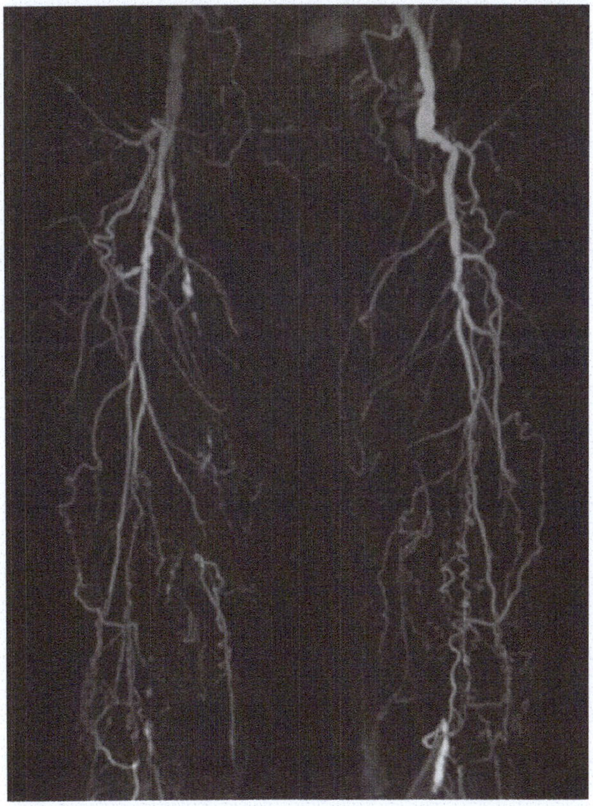

Fig. 11.28 Severe bilateral peripheral arterial disease in a 58-year-old male. After a single dose of Gd-BOPTA a three station static high-resolution MRA at 3T was performed. The thigh demonstrates bilateral superficial artery occlusion along with impressive collateralization

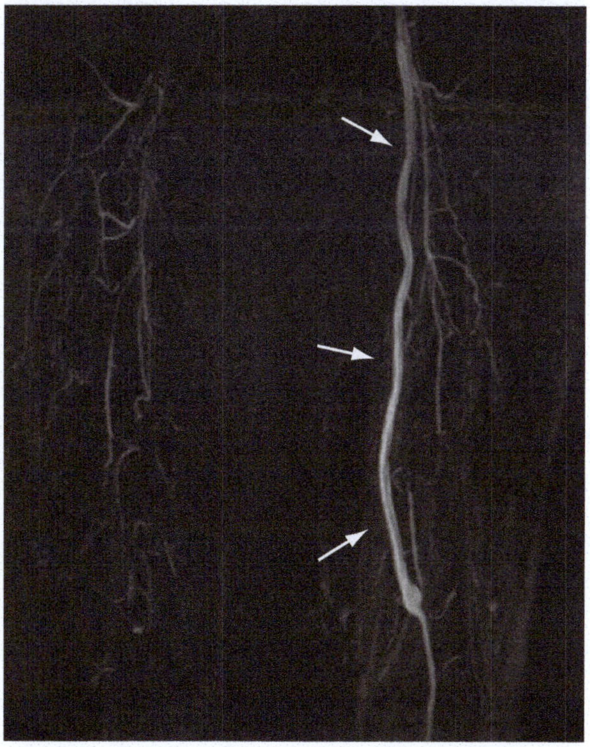

Fig. 11.29 Femoral-popliteal artery by-pass. The MIP image of the thigh MRA demonstrates occlusion of the right femoral-popliteal artery by-pass. The graft on the left is patent (*arrows*)

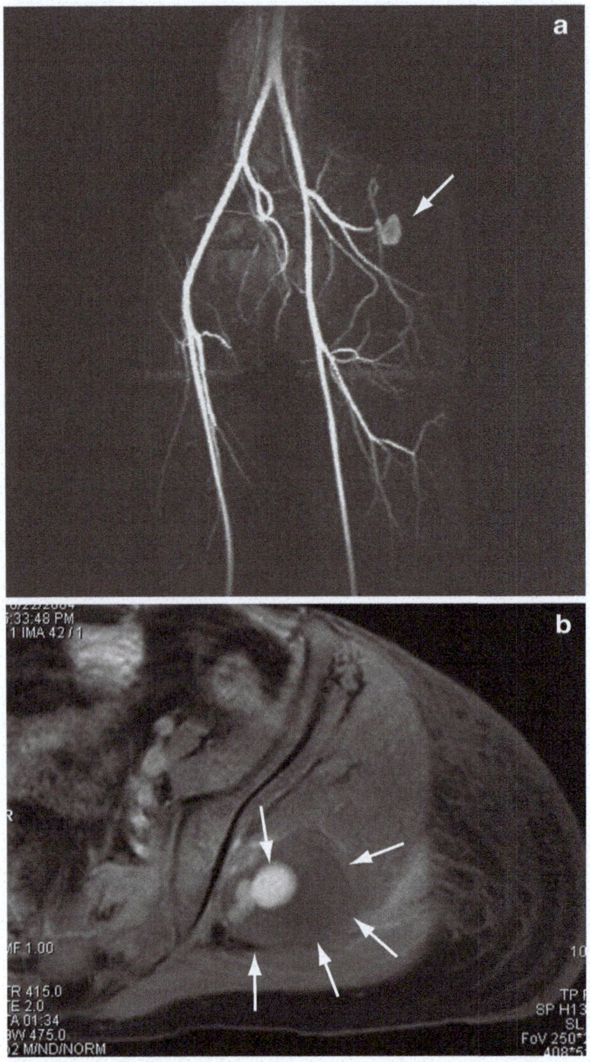

Fig. 11.30 Gluteal artery aneurysm. The MIP of the 3D high-resolution MRA (**a**) in the arterial phase demonstrates an aneurysm of the left gluteal artery(arrow). The postcontrast fat saturation axially acquired sequence (**b**) show the aneurysm within the left gluteus medius (long arrow), surrounded by a contained hematoma (short arrows). Images courtesy of James Carr, Northwestern Memorial Hospital, Chicago, IL

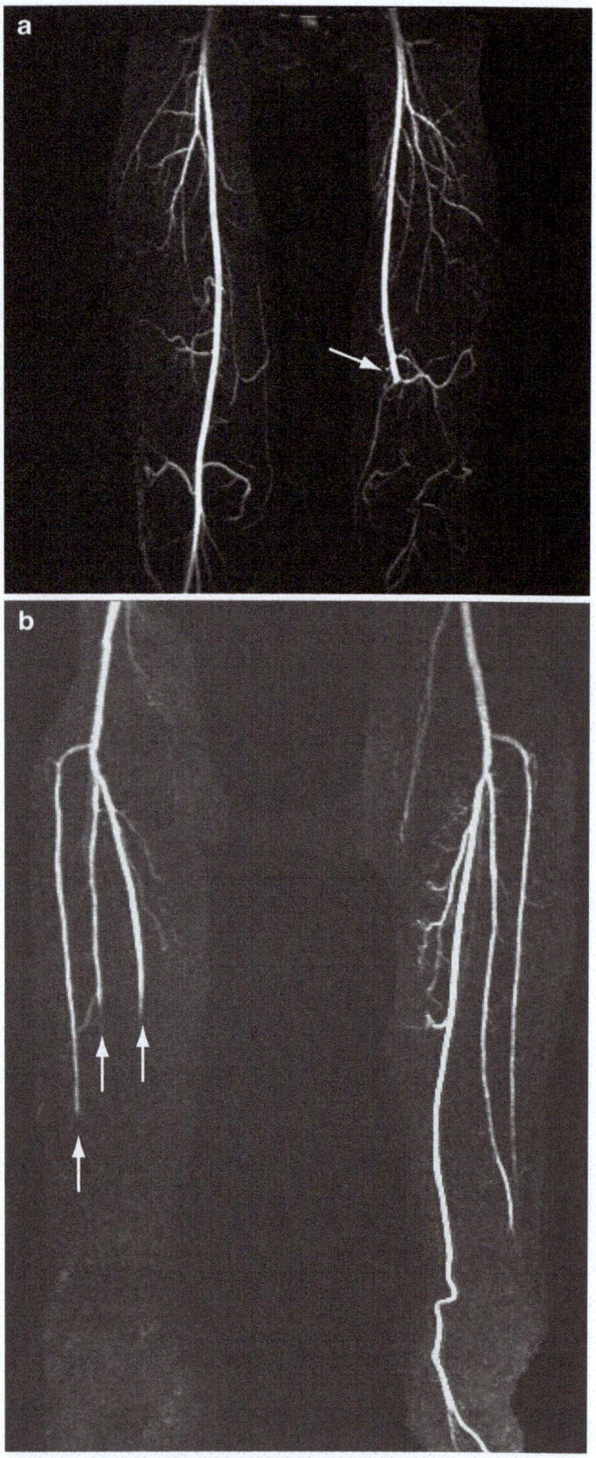

Fig. 11.31 Lower extremity emboli. The MIP image of the thigh MRA (**a**) demonstrates an abrupt occlusion of the distal left superficial femoral artery (*arrow*)secondary to an embolus in a patient with atrial fibrillation. Another patient (**b**) has occluded the right anterior tibial, peroneal, and posterior tibial arteries secondary to emboli (*arrows*)

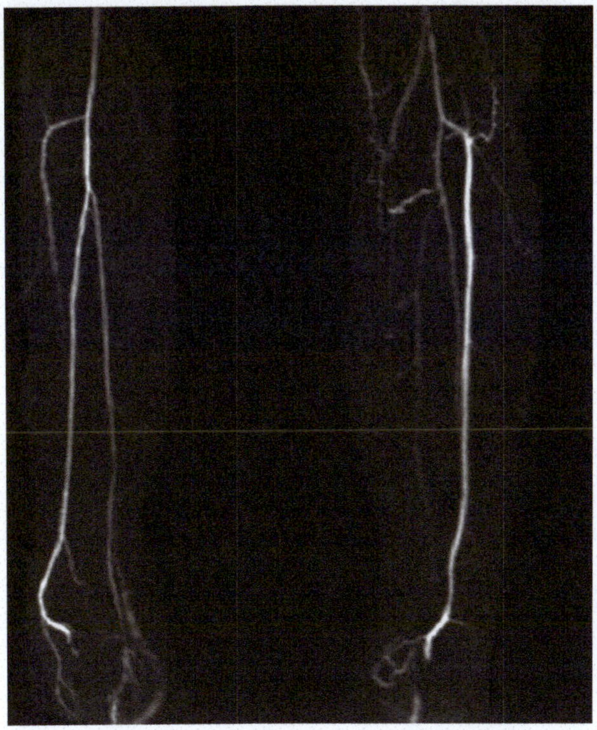

Fig. 11.32 Peroneus magnus. A time resolved calf MRA demonstrates a congenitally hypoplastic right anterior tibial artery and an associated peroneus magnus

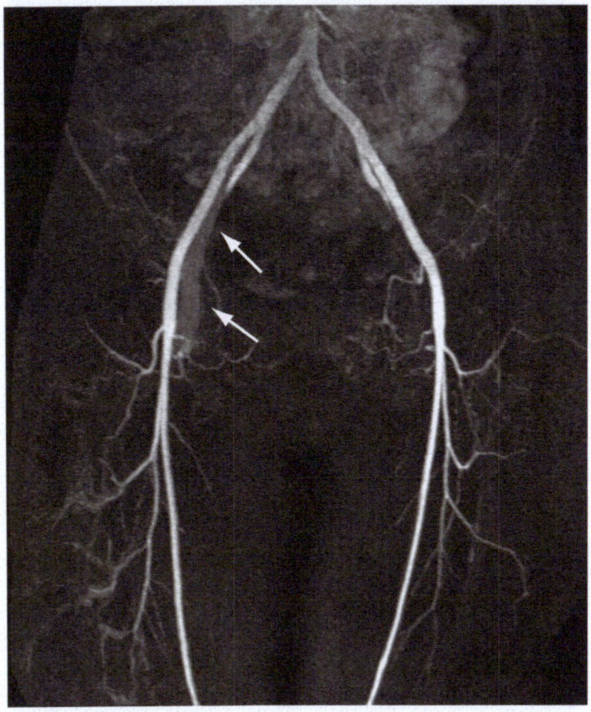

Fig. 11.33 Common femoral artery arterio-venous fistula. The MIP of the 3D MRA demonstrates early filling of the right common femoral vein secondary to a fistulous connection between the common femoral artery and vein

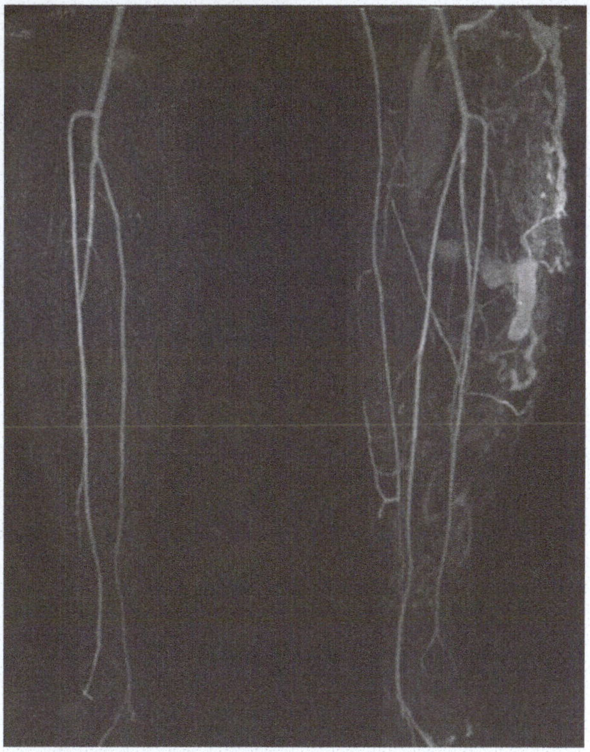

Fig. 11.34 Kippel-Trenaunay syndrome. A MIP of a calf station MRA demonstrates hypertrophy of the left calf, numerous varicosities and arteriovenous fistulae

stationary tissues which affords improved background suppression over 1.5 T. Improved TOF-MRA at 3T is particularly suited to the imaging of the intracranial arteries. Parallel imaging can also be used to maintain reasonable scan times and high spatial resolution.

11.3.10 Contrast-Enhanced MRA: Tips and Tricks

- Use a dedicated phase-array coil if possible.
- Use parallel imaging to reduce scan time/increase resolution or both.
- Practice breath-holding with the patient and use oxygen via nasal prongs if necessary.
- Use an automated mechanical injection pump to standardize the CM administration.
- Optimize dose (and agent used) of CM according to the clinical question and NSF risk.
- Acquire a noncontrast 3D-MRA data set ("mask") for subtraction purposes before administration of CM.

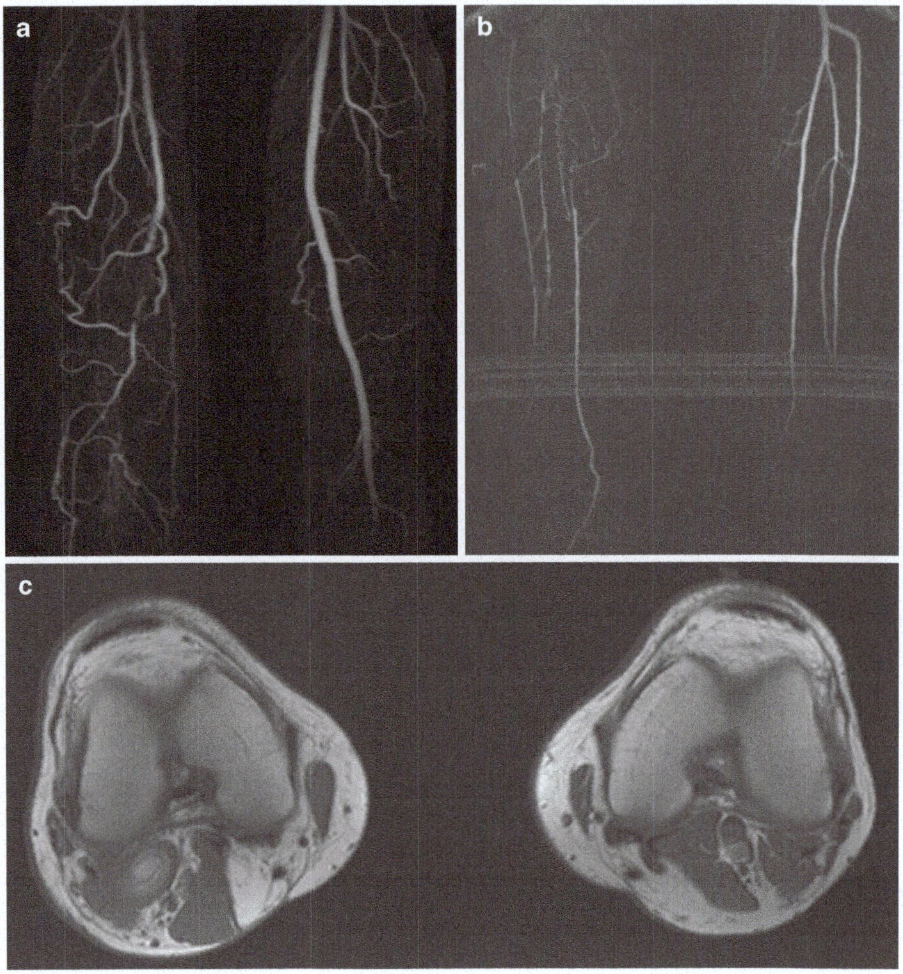

Fig. 11.35 Popliteal artery entrapment. The thigh MRA (**a**) demonstrates thrombosis of the right superficial femoral and popliteal arteries. The calf station (**b**) demonstrates thrombosis of the proximal right anterior tibial, peroneal, and posterior tibial arteries. The axial T1-W image (**c**) demonstrates thrombosis and enlargement of the right popliteal artery, which is entrapped in the medial head of gastrocnemius. Images courtesy of James Carr, Northwestern Memorial Hospital, Chicago, IL

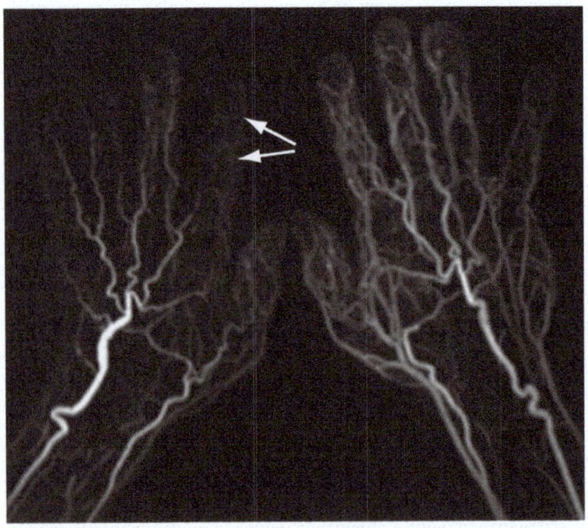

Fig. 11.36 Raynauds disease. A static high-resolution MRA of the hands demonstrates occlusion of the digital arteries of the left forefinger in a patient with suspected Raynaud's disease

11.4 Summary of Basic Advantages and Disadvantages Associated with Different MRA Techniques

All MRA methods suffer from limitations and artifacts, some of which are summarized in Table 11.3. With each new generation of software and hardware, many of the limitations are satisfactorily addressed. Direct comparison of different MRA techniques demonstrates that CEMRA, which is still evolving at a breath-taking pace, offers substantial benefit over other techniques in terms of temporal and spatial resolution and freedom from artifacts. The obvious disadvantage of requiring gadolinium contrast agent injection for CEMRA was regarded as an acceptable consequence of acquiring such high quality MR angiograms, because of the traditional perception that these agents

Table 11.3 Advantages, disadvantages, and special features of various MRA techniques

Technique Advantages	Disadvantages	Special features	
2D TOF	Increase flow/background contrast Improved visualization of slow flow Low saturation effects Reduced measurement time	Reduced SNR Reduced visualization of in-plane flow Sensitive to short T1 species Flow voids due to diastolic back flow	ECG-gating: improves inflow signal during systole
3D TOF	Increased SNR Increased resolution	Slow flow saturation Less background suppression Sensitive to short T1 species	MOTSA TONE MT-saturation
2D PC	Reduced measurement time Improved background suppression Reduced saturation effects intensive to short T1 species sensitive to slow flow	Projection technique (single thick slice) Dephasing artifacts due to vessel overlap Aliasing (VENC to low) Requires experience in interpretation and input by the operator	ECG-gating Flow measurement Different flow images within cardiac cycle (diastolic and systolic images) Multiple VENC along main flow direction Use as fast vessel localizer
3D PC	Reduced dephasing artifacts Improved SNR Improved background suppression Insensitive to short T1 species Improved resolution	Longer measurement time Aliasing (VENC to low) Requires experiences in interpretation and input by the operator	
3D CE	Improved SNR Improved resolution, FOV Reduced measurement time (breath-hold is possible) Relative flow independent Relative robust technique	Bolus timing is necessary Dephasing artifacts occur Contrast agents have to be applied	Time-resolved technique Digital subtraction (measure native and CE) Future special coils, blood pool agents

PC phase contrast; *CE* contrast-enhanced; *FOV* flied-of-fiew; *D* dimension; *TOF* time of flight; *ECG* electrocardiogram; *SNR* sound-to-noise ratio; *MOTSA* multiple overlapping thin-slab acquisition; *TONE* tilted optimized nonsaturating excitation; *VENC* velocity encoding gradient determining the sensitivity to flow velocity

were almost completely devoid of serious side effects. However, the well-known axiom that the benefits of contrast-enhanced imaging over noncontrast methods must be carefully weighed, regardless of modality, came sharply into focus with the realization that gadolinium contrast agent injection, particularly when used in high dose and/or in patients with impaired renal function, was associated with NSF. Unfortunately, the previously stated dogma of the safety of MR contrast agents over iodinated contrast agents in patients with renal impairment can no longer go unchallenged.

11.5 Nephrogenic Systemic Fibrosis: Observations and Strategy for Avoiding or Eliminating this Serious Disorder

NSF is a debilitating and potentially fatal disorder characterized, amongst others, by skin rashes, dermal thickening, joint contractures, and reduced mobility. Prior to the documented association between gadolinium injection and NSF, it was widely believed that MR

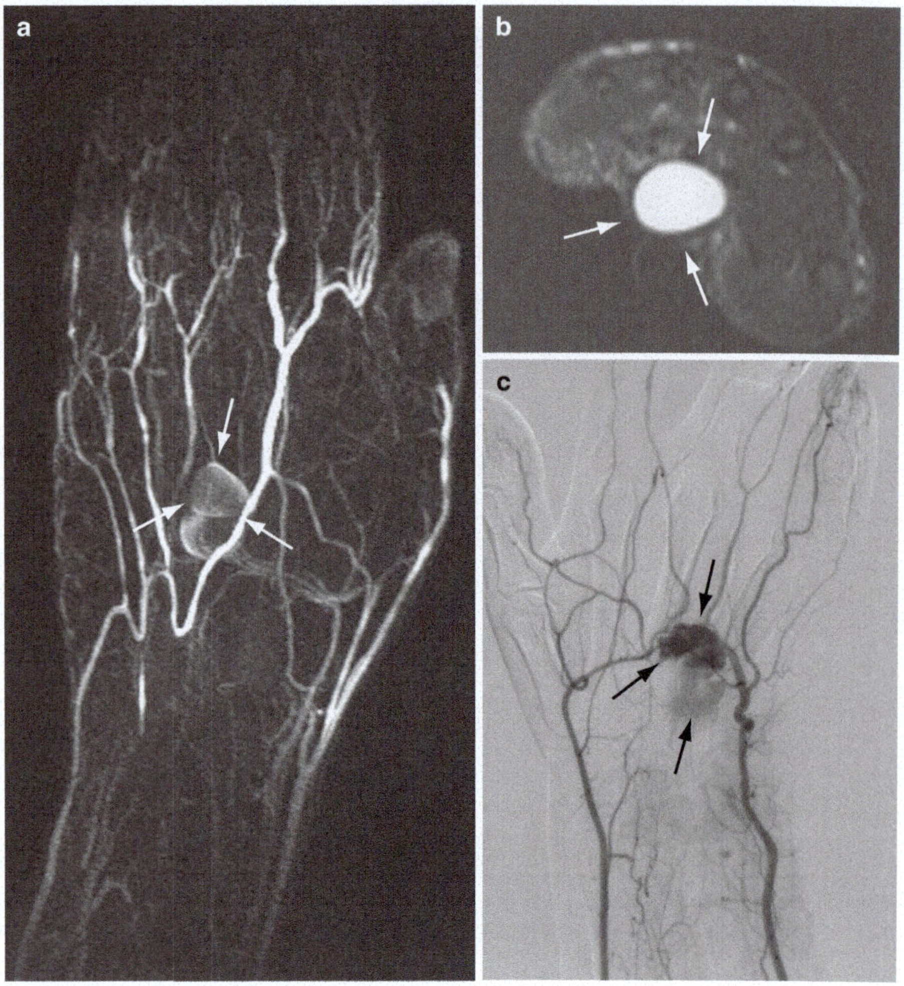

Fig. 11.37 Hypothenar hammer syndrome. A static high-resolution MRA (**a**) of the hands demonstrates an aneurysm of the superficial palmar arch (*arrows*) supplied by the ulnar artery. The axial T1-W sequence (**b**) demonstrates the vascular lesion on the volar aspect of the hand (*arrows*). The conventional digital subtraction angiogram demonstrates the aneurysm (*arrows*), fed by the ulnar artery. Images courtesy of James Carr, Northwestern Memorial Hospital, Chicago, IL

contrast agents were largely devoid of side effects or at least had a safety profile that was superior to almost all other injectable agents used in medical practice. Some early confusion about the disorder has led to greater clarity about MR contrast agent use, which, following exhaustive efforts have been vindicated as being almost completely safe in most instances. The following statements can be made regarding NSF:

- NSF is virtually unknown in patients with normal renal function.
- NSF is virtually unknown in patients with undocumented renal function who present for outpatient imaging (i.e., assumed that renal function is normal).
- NSF is virtually unknown in patients receiving a single dose of CM.
- Risk of NSF is related to creatinine clearance.
- Risk of NSF is low in patients with chronic renal failure who are undergoing dialysis.
- There is a high risk of NSF in patients with acute renal failure whose creatinine is rising and who do not undergo dialysis for at least 2 days after contrast injection.
- NSF is more common in patients with proinflammatory events.
- Not all MR contrast agents are associated with NSF and the reported risk varies greatly between those agents that have been implicated. Further details are available at http://www. fda.gov.

Remember, however, that if a single dose of gadolinium is used, the risk of NSF is less than the risk of death related to iodinated contrast material used for CT.

Recommendations for CM use to reduce or eliminate the risk of NSF:

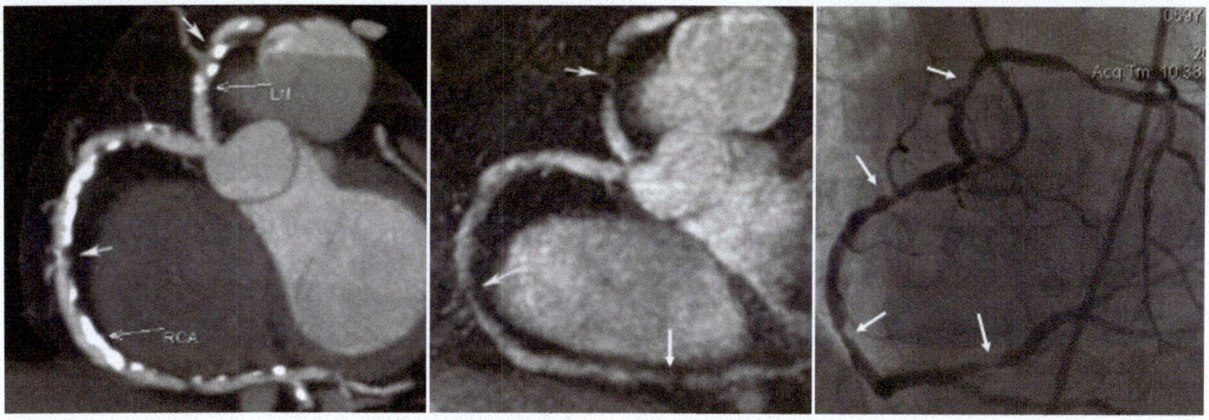

Fig. 11.38 Coronary MRA. This 65-year-old male patient had a CT angiogram (*left*), MR angiogram (*middle*), and invasive coronary angiogram (*right*). The Left main and the RCA share a common ostia arising from the right coronary cusp. The patient has multifocal moderate and severe complex plaque throughout. The degree of stenosis on the segments of the arterial tree is difficult to assess on the CT due to blooming artifact. The coronary MRA is useful to evaluate the degree of stenosis in heavily calcified proximal and mid coronary vessels. Images courtesy of Xin Liu and James Carr, Northwestern Memorial Hospital, Chicago, IL

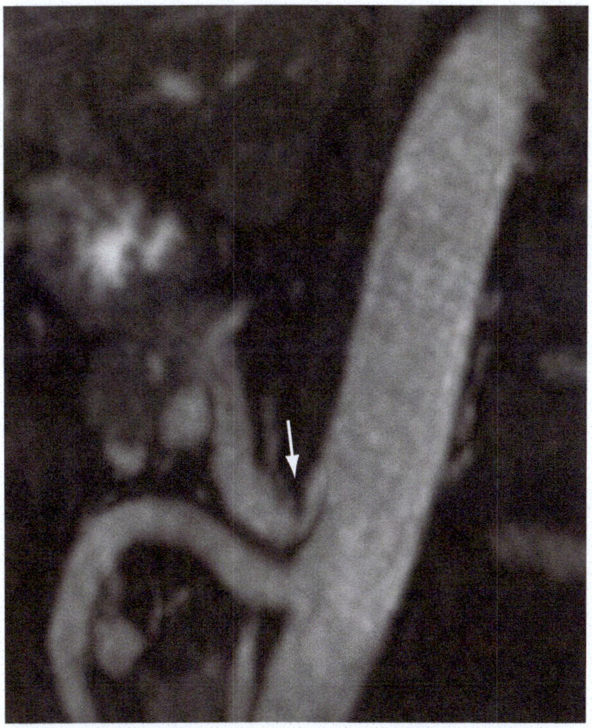

Fig. 11.39 Median arcuate ligament syndrome. A noncontrast 3D steady state free precession sequence reconstructed in the saggital plane demonstrates severe proximal stenosis of the celiac artery with mild poststenotic dilatation

- Screen all patients for history of dialysis or renal impairment.
- Consider using a noncontrast method (Figs. 11.38 and 11.39) in patients, especially those with eGFR<30 mL/min.
- Avoid contrast agent injection in patients with acute renal failure with rising creatinine who are not on dialysis.
- If gadolinium injection is required in patients with renal impairment, use a single dose.
- Use an agent that has fewer reported cases of NSF.
- If patients with impaired renal function are to undergo gadolinium injection, dialysis should follow at the earliest possible opportunity and the hemodialysis personnel should be informed that gadolinium contrast agent has been injected to allow the use of an optimal dialysis regimen for eliminating gadolinium. Despite definitive evidence to support this approach, the ACR adopts the prudent approach of recommending initiation of hemodialysis within 2 h of contrast agent injection in patients already on dialysis.
- Carefully monitor the examination to ensure that a diagnostic scan is obtained, so that repeat injection can be avoided.

11.6 MR Venography (MRV)

Both noncontrast and contrast-enhanced methods are used for MRV.

11.6.1 Noncontrast MR Venography

All MR images can be used to demonstrate filling defects within veins, and/or absence of signal voids in vessels with complete thrombosis.

- TOF images, acquired without saturation pulses or with pre-saturation of arterial flow, generate high quality MR venograms.
- Phase contrast MRV is typically employed to generate MRVs of the major intracranial venous sinuses.
- Balanced sequences (e.g., Balanced FFE/TrueFISP/Fiesta sequences) give reasonable T2 weighting and accurately demonstrate the filling defects of venous thrombosis as dark structures within bright vessels.

11.6.2 Contrast-Enhanced MR Venography

As for contrast-enhanced MR arteriography, CE-MRV gives excellent depiction of venous thrombosis. Two fundamentally different approaches are employed for CEMRV based on the observation that intravenously injected commercially available contrast agent shortens not only the T1 of the contrast-enriched blood, but also T2*, resulting in susceptibility. This causes severe signal dropout within the veins on the side of the injection of undiluted gadolinium contrast in first pass (because the T2* value is close to the TE), which precludes routine acquisition of contrast-enhanced MR venograms with undiluted contrast. However, brightly enhancing arteries result from intravenous injection of CM as a result of dilution of the injected contrast volume during passage through the heart and pulmonary circulation, which prolongs the T2*, thus minimizing or eliminating the artifact. This consideration gives rise to two different ways to perform contrast-enhanced MRV as follows:

11.6.3 Direct MRV

Technique: CM is diluted with saline (e.g., 3 cc 0.5 M Gadolinium in 50 cc saline = 6% dilution effect) prior to injection and MR venograms acquired during the first pass (Fig. 11.10). This approach can only be used in territories where CM can be injected "upstream" of the region-of-interest (e.g., evaluation of the superior vena cava following injection into both upper extremities).

11.6.4 "Indirect" MRV

After completion of arterial phase imaging, delayed images are acquired during the "venous" phase (Figs. 11.11–11.13). This approach can be used for any venous territory. Common indications include splenoportal patency, renal vein involvement in renal cell carcinoma, and pulmonary vein geometry in patients being evaluated for radiofrequency ablation. Blood pool contrast agents, because of their long intravascular half-life, are ideally suited for this type of venous imaging.

11.7 Sequence Protocols and Clinical Application

11.7.1 Intracranial Vessels

3D TOF-MRA is traditionally the most commonly used technique for imaging of the intracranial arteries (Tables 11.1–11.4) (Figs. 11.1–11.4). Stenoses of the primary branches of the circle of Willis are well depicted. Unfortunately, the technique is less reliable

Table 11.4 Magnetic resonance (MR) angiography protocol recommendations for intracranial vessels

Sequence	WI	Plane	TR (ms)	TE (ms)	Flip-angle	Slice thickness (mm)	No part	Effth	Matrix	FOV	recFOV (%)	BW	Acq.	Acq. Time (min:s)
3D GRE	T1	Tra	40–60	5–6	20–30	56	64	0,8–1	512	200	62,5	390	1	8
2D GRE	T1	Tra	30	5–9	60	2	50		256	180	75	195	1	5:40

WI weighted image; *TR* repetition time; *TI* inversion time; *TE* echo time; *No part* number of partitions; *Effth* effective thickness (mm); *Matrix* matrix (phase ¥ frequency matrix); *FOV* field of view (mm); *recFOV %* rectangular field of view, *BW* bandwidth (Hz); *Acq* number of acquisitions

Table 11.5 Magnetic resonance angiography sequence parameters recommendations for extracranial carotid vessels

Sequence	WI	Plane	TR (ms)	TE (ms)	Flip-angle	Slice thickness (mm)	No part	Effth	Matrix	FOV	recFOV (%)	BW	Acq.	Acq. Time (min:s)
3D GRE (CE)	T1	Cor	4.2	1.9	35	50	50	1	256	260	50	390	1	0:25
3D GRE	T1	Ax	30	6	25	132	132	1	256	220	75	390	1	12:40
MOTSA	T1	Ax	30	6	25	132	20 x 4-8	1	256	220	75	390	1	14:00

WI weighted image; *TR* repetition time; *TI* inversion time; *TE* echo time; *No part* number of partitions; *Effth* effective thickness (mm); *Matrix* matrix (phase ¥ frequency matrix); *FOV* field of view (mm); *recFOV %* rectangular field of view; *BW* bandwidth (Hz); *Acq* number of acquisitions

for evaluating small, distal vessels. The use of Gd-chelates may improve the visualization of smaller vessels, but at the cost of increased venous enhancement (Fig. 11.5). Collateral flow can be determined using specially placed presaturation pulses that suppress signal within the vascular territory supplied by the presaturated vessel. Grading of vertebrobasilar stenoses is reliable, thereby influencing treatment strategies (anticoagulation). Anatomic variations such as the termination of the vertebral artery at the posterior inferior cerebellar artery or hypoplastic vessels (fetal or hypoplastic posterior cerebral artery) are well visualized (Fig. 11.1).

3D TOF-MRA high-resolution imaging provides a high accuracy for the detection of small (>3 mm) aneurysms. The source images of the 3D data set should be carefully evaluated. MIP reconstruction of subvolumes (targeted MIP) is also helpful to eliminate the overlay of several different vessels. This technique can also be used to determine a persistent nidus after radiosurgery in the case of intracranial vascular malformations but cannot substitute for conventional catheter angiography in defining feeder vessels and shunting. Sometimes, 3D or 2D PC-MRA may improve the visualization of such vessel structures. There is growing support for use of high resolution whole brain CEMRA for all intracranial vascular applications including depiction of aneurysms and vascular malformations (Fig. 11.5).

Intracranial MRV can be obtained by several means, including 2D TOF with arterial presaturation, 2D and 3D phase contrast approaches and contrast-enhanced techniques. Thrombosis involving the major venous sinuses can be depicted by all methods; however, contrast-enhanced MRV is now the technique of choice due to clear visualization of filling defects within the veins and absence of artifacts.

11.7.2 Carotid Arteries

Traditional noncontrast MRA sequences are 2D TOF or MOTSA 3D TOF of the whole carotid artery, or 3D TOF of the bifurcation only (Table 11.5) (Figs. 11.1–11.4). Because of its sensitivity to slow flow, 2D TOF-MRA is more accurate for differentiating near from complete occlusion than 3D TOF-MRA; however, detection of the “string” sign on CEMRA is the most reliable method of all. Signal loss in areas of turbulence may occur with both 2D and 3D techniques, but 3D techniques give superior evaluation of the carotid bifurcation than 2D techniques for both severity and length of stenosis. MOTSA techniques overcome many of the limitations of 3D TOF-MRA, but suffer from movement artifacts due to the long acquisition times (10–12 min) compared with 3D CEMRA (~10–40 s).

The entire region of the carotids and the vertebral system can easily be depicted by CEMRA, which has supplanted other methods in most institutions (Figs. 11.6, 11.7). Comprehensive high quality images can be acquired from the aortic arch to the base of the skull using a phase-array neck coil. Since the normal mean ICA diameter measures approximately 8 mm, accurate visualization of a residual diameter of approximately 2.4 mm is necessary to allow the detection of stenosis at the 70% cut-off. Therefore, high spatial resolution that increases the scan time substantially beyond the normally short cerebral AV window must be used. This is achieved by combining fluoroscopic bolus detection with “centric” imaging which allows acquisition of central k-space imaging during the arterial peak prior to the onset of jugular venous enhancement, despite the fact that the AV transit time is typically 8–12 s only. Using state-of-the-art technology, isotropic

Table 11.6 Magnetic resonance angiography sequence parameters recommendations for aorta, subclavian, and brachial arteries

Sequence	WI	Plane	TR (ms)	TE (ms)	Flip-angle	Slice thickness (mm)	No part	Effth	Matrix	FOV	recFOV (%)	BW	Acq.	Acq. Time (min:s)
3D GRE	T1	Par-sag	3.85	1.5	35	90	58	1.55	256	400	75	650	1	0:43
3D GRE	T1	Par-sag	4.6	1.8	35	100	32 (64)	3.12 (2.3)	256	400	75	390	1	0:28

WI weighted image; *TR* repetition time; *TI* inversion time; *TE* echo time; *No part* number of partitions; *Effth* effective thickness (mm); *Matrix* matrix (phase ¥ frequency matrix); *FOV* field of view (mm); *recFOV %* rectangular field of view; *BW* bandwidth (Hz); *Acq* number of acquisitions

less than 1 mm resolution can easily be achieved, but further improvements in spatial resolution will bring additional benefit within the carotid system. Assuming no contraindication (e.g., impaired renal function), optimal vessel contrast is achieved by a double-dose of gadolinium contrast agent injected at a rate of 1–2 mL/s. Breath-hold acquisitions may improve visualization of the aortic arch vessels.

Artifacts caused by swallowing can be avoided by instructing the patient not to swallow during the 3D MRA (typically less than 40 s duration).

11.7.2.1 Imaging of the Vessel Wall: Plaque Imaging and Detection of Vessel Dissection

Currently, high resolution imaging of the carotid and vertebral lumen from aortic arch to circle of Willis is possible. Most attention focuses on the carotid bifurcation in patients with atherosclerosis; however, imaging of the vessel wall for differentiation of stable from unstable plaque remains elusive (Fig. 11.7c). Despite the fact that useful information regarding plaque within the vessel wall cannot be routinely obtained currently from MR images, this is not the case for the dissection of the vertebral or carotid arteries where demonstration of concentric intramural hyperintensity on fat-saturated spin-echo T1-W and T2-W images confirms the diagnosis.

11.7.3 Thoracic and Abdominal Aorta, Subclavian and Brachial Arteries

Congenital and acquired diseases of aortic arch vessels, thoracic and abdominal aorta can lead to aneurysm formation, stenosis, and occlusion (Figs. 11.14–11.18). Diverse etiologies such as atherosclerosis, trauma, infection, radiation, connective tissue disorders, fibrodysplasia, and dissection may be encountered. All of these pathologies, including treatment planning and follow-up, are well depicted by CEMRA. The measurement time should be tailored to breath-holding, and parallel imaging should be used to improve resolution (Table 11.6). To supplement information from the CE scan, it may be appropriate to orientate the timing sequence or 2D fluoroscopic technique in a sagittal plane in order to obtain information such as the differential blood supply to the two lumina in case of aortic dissection.

The evaluation of steno-occlusive disease in the subclavian or brachial region, such as thoracic outlet syndrome, is possible by CEMRA by performing two measurements in normal and abducted arm positions. Because of contrast-induced susceptibility, contrast agent should always be injected on the asymptomatic side to avoid overinterpretation due to artifactual stenosis where the subclavian artery and vein lie adjacent to one another; in patients with bilateral symptoms, the right side should be used due to the more favorable anatomy. A better, but rarely used approach is to inject a lower extremity vein that avoids the possibility of susceptibility-induced signal drop off in the region of the subclavian artery. The subclavian and proximal brachial arteries require a moderately thick volume of approximately 60–90 (FOV = 350–400) during breath-holding, which dictates the use of moderate resolution (voxel size = $0.7 \times 1.5 \times 1.7$ mm^3). A phased-array body coil is preferred because of the improved SNR. When performing selective CEMRA of subclavian and brachial arteries, a flexible wrap-around coil (FOV = 300, double-dose technique, FR 2 mL/s) or an eccentrically placed body phased-array coil can be used.

MRA is particularly useful for diagnosis of subclavian steal syndrome (SSS). Because of the high spatial coverage and high in-plane spatial resolution requirements of head and neck MRA, 3D scan times of 10–40 s clearly preclude the identification of the temporal pattern of retrograde flow within the vertebral arteries in SSS, one of which has antegrade flow, the other retrograde flow which supplies the subclavian artery beyond the stenosis. Prior to the 3D acquisition, a time-resolved study with high temporal resolution (<500 ms/image) can be acquired following injection of a small volume (1–2 cc) of contrast agent. However, this consideration is only relevant in those cases where the diagnosis is suspected prior to carotid MRA, and in our experience, SSS is unsuspected in the majority of cases. However, in most institutions, the localizer initially performed to allow careful placement of the subsequent 3D imaging volume consists of a low-resolution MR angiogram acquired with an inflow (TOF) technique which employs a superior saturation pulse to eliminate venous flow from the head. The saturation volume, however, is "unselective" and saturates all the blood flowing in a caudad direction. In normal circumstances, the only blood flowing inferiorly from the head towards the heart is venous blood, but in patients with SSS, the retrogradely flowing blood within the vertebral artery is also saturated by the presaturation pulse. For CEMRA, vascular signal solely depends on the presence of blood with T1 shortening the blood within the vessel of interest and is completely independent of how it got there; hence there are no differentiating features between antegrade and retrograde flow on CEMRA. This observation of the absence of vertebral artery signal on the TOF localizer in the presence of a normal appearing artery on the subsequent CEMRA is referred to as the "localizer" sign and is pathognomic of SSS.

Aneurysm assessment: Endovascular aortic aneurysm repair (EVAR), a technique whereby a covered stent graft is percutaneously sited within the aneurysm sac to act as a conduit for blood flow is now the treatment of choice for many thoracic and abdominal aortic aneurysms. Unlike open repair, careful preintervention determination of the size, location, and configuration of the aneurysm is essential to allow selection of an appropriate graft size. Stent evaluation, long considered as the preserve of CTA (due to its ability to visualize vessel wall calcification) is also optimally performed with MRA. Dimensions of the aneurysm sac, location and integrity of side branches in relation to the aneurysm sac, and optimal route for accessing the relevant area can easily be determined.

Post EVAR, lifetime follow-up that is essential to disclose complications such as endoleaks (blood flow within the aneurysm sac but outside the stent-graft), which develops in up to 25% of cases, is also more commonly performed with CTA. However, MRA lends itself ideally to endoleak evaluation (no confusion from calcification and no considerations of radiation dose which reduces the acceptability of dynamic scanning) in patients with Nitinol stents. Elginoy stents are also well evaluated but the artifact associated with stainless steel stent-grafts essentially precludes MRA use in this patient group. Fast dynamic imaging with ultrafast MRA/TRICKS may be beneficial. Blood pool agent imaging may potentially offer additional benefit over first pass agents.

11.7.4 Pulmonary Arteries

11.7.4.1 CEMRA

CEMRA gives high CNR between brightly enhancing, contrast-enriched blood and emboli which appear dark (Fig. 11.19). Although fifth- to seventh-order branches of the pulmonary artery can be visualized, a reliable diagnosis of acute pulmonary embolism can be made to the fourth order (segmental arteries) only. This technique is also suitable for treatment planning and follow-up studies in chronic pulmonary embolic disease. Although MIP provides a complete overview of the pulmonary vasculature (Figs. 11.19, 11.20), partially occluding emboli may be completely masked. These emboli are better visualized by viewing the individual slices and performing subvolume MIP and MPR images. At the subsegmental level, MIPs may improve the review process.

Because of the limited breath-hold capability of most patients with suspected pulmonary embolism, it may be necessary to sacrifice spatial resolution in favor of a shorter scan time that is within the patient's breath-hold capability (Table 11.7). This, however, impairs the ability to diagnose small subsegmental emboli, although the significance of such emboli remains uncertain. Both the lungs can be evaluated in a single acquisition in the coronal plane, but scan times are relatively long. In order to shorten the acquisition, each lung can be evaluated separately in the sagittal plane, which shortens scan time, with the use of separate injections. Alternatively, in patients with reasonable breath-hold capability, images

Table 11.7 Magnetic resonance angiography sequence parameters recommendations for pulmonary vessels

Sequence	WI	Plane	TR (ms)	TE (ms)	Flip-angle	3D Slice thickness (mm)	No part	Effth	Matrix	FOV	recFOV (%)	BW	Acq.	Acq. Time (min:s)
3D GRE	T1	Cor	3.85	1.5	40	96	48	2	256	350	75	650	1	0:35

WI weighted image; *TR* repetition time; *TI* inversion time; *TE* echo time; *No part* number of partitions; *Effth* effective thickness (mm); *Matrix* matrix (phase ¥ frequency matrix); *FOV* field of view (mm); *recFOV* % rectangular field of view; *BW* bandwidth (Hz); *Acq* number of acquisitions

with increased resolution can be acquired by employing the sagittal plane. The use of a body phased-array coil is preferable to boost SNR within small peripheral vessels where resolution constraints are most marked. With parallel imaging, sufficiently short scan times that can be easily tolerated by the patient but which nonetheless generate sufficiently high-resolution images to depict smaller vessels can now be routinely acquired.

Another promising approach is to extend the examination beyond the thorax and to evaluate the lower extremity veins (using a moving table approach) following the pulmonary MRA study for sources of pulmonary embolism, emulating current CT practice. This "one-stop-shop" MRI approach for PE and DVT detects more cases of thromboembolism when compared with separate examinations. Some authorities advocate that MRI should be considered not only as a second-line technique in patients with contraindications to CT but also as a primary comprehensive stand-alone technique for diagnosing thromboembolism. Although initial results are encouraging, data is keenly awaited on the role of blood-pool contrast agents, which are ideally suited in the assessment of deep venous thrombosis and pulmonary embolism. Blood-pool contrast agents offer the potential both for first-pass breath-hold MRA in addition to high-resolution targeted equilibrium-phase pulmonary MRA during multiple breath-holds and lung perfusion.

11.7.4.2 Noncontrast Pulmonary MRA

Balanced sequences: These promising techniques that do not require injection of contrast material hold promise for the detection of both DVT and PE and may be of particular use in pregnancy and in patients with renal function impairment. TrueFISP imaging, a "balanced" technique, depicts vessels as bright structures, and shows promise for diagnosis of both DVT and PE. Images can be acquired in any plane, and although breath-holding is essential, small imaging volumes tailored to the breath-hold capability can be acquired.

Direct thrombus imaging: Direct thrombus imaging is based on the principle that reproducible changes in blood clot appearance on MR occur with time. Specifically, methemoglobin, one of the intermediate products of clot evolution, presents a characteristic appearance on MRI due to significant T1 value reduction, which can be highlighted with a heavily T1-W sequence.

11.7.5 Pulmonary Hypertension

In patients predisposed to recurrent PE, chronic thrombo-embolic pulmonary hypertension (CTEPH) occurs when approximately 60% of the pulmonary vascular bed is affected and 5-year survival is approximately 30%. Surgical thrombo-endarterectomy of organized thrombi offers the potential for cure in these patients but can be performed only if large (lobar and segmental) arteries are involved. Catheter pulmonary angiography has been supplanted by CTA and MRA, both of which can depict these large arterial segments (Fig. 11.20). MR has the additional benefit of allowing evaluation of pulmonary perfusion and myocardial dysfunction. Functional RV assessment demonstrates impaired right ventricular ejection fraction, paradoxical septal motion, normal left ventricular ejection fraction, and differences in flow rates through the pulmonary trunk and ascending aorta. Follow-up MRI/MRA also allowed comprehensive study of the morphology and functional characteristics in patients who have undergone surgery.

11.7.6 Miscellaneous Disorders of the Pulmonary Circulation

Anomalous pulmonary venous drainage, arteriovenous malformations, pulmonary sequestration (Fig. 11.21) and pulmonary artery involvement in primary bronchogenic carcinoma and pulmonary artery sarcoma can be performed with MRA (Fig. 11.21). Although there is little data on its use in clinical practice, CEMRA can also directly visualize the bronchial arteries.

11.7.7 Renal and Mesenteric Arteries

Breath-hold 3D CEMRA of the medium-sized renal arteries has been one of the enormous success stories of the last decade (Table 11.8) (Figs. 11.22–11.25). In institutions with access to high-quality CEMRA, catheter arteriography has now been completely supplanted for screening patients with suspected renal artery stenosis. Using a fast scanner and parallel imaging, high spatial resolution can be achieved in a short measurement time, with a resulting isotropic voxel size of approximately 1 mm^3. In many instances where coexistent cardiopulmonary disease limits the breath-hold capability, slightly lower resolution may be accepted to facilitate a successful breath-hold scan. The short renal artery to renal veins transit time (approximately 4–5 s), and signal superposition caused by renal veins (especially on the left) can be avoided by exact bolus timing and the use of short breath-hold scans. In order to boost SNR, a body phased-array coil is superior to the standard body coil. Assuming normal renal function, a double dose (0.2 mmol/kg) is superior to a single-dose. If optimal image quality is achieved, small accessory renal arteries can be depicted, which is important for surgery treatment planning. Intrarenal arteries are poorly visualized due to a combination of resolution constraints, venous overlap, and brightly enhancing renal parenchyma.

Numerous studies attest to the accuracy of this technique for the detection of renovascular disease, with sensitivities and specificities over 90% in almost all studies. Few patients with fibromuscular dysplasia have been included in reported studies, and the exclusion value for FMD is uncertain, although likely to be high, especially with protocols using parallel imaging (Fig. 11.23). Although the severity of renal artery stenosis is usually assessed visually, secondary signs such as reduction in the intensity of the contrast nephrogram and shrunken kidneys are valuable secondary signs. Evaluation of flow rates within the renal arteries using a cardiac-triggered 2D PC acquisition offers enormous promise for determining both the appropriateness of revascularization and response to treatment. A somewhat cruder method of determining the functional significance is given by a 3D PCA acquisition where the severity and length of signal drop-off within the renal artery distal to the stenosis correlates with increasingly severe grades of stenosis.

Although conventional renal artery stents give extensive susceptibility artifact that precludes evaluation of the in-stent lumen, stents manufactured from platinum which give little artifact are currently under investigation. Use of minimum TE and extremely high flip-angles (70°) are necessary in such cases.

The mesenteric arteries are also medium-sized arteries that are ideally evaluated with CEMRA (Fig. 11.25). Although subclinical stenosis within any of the three mesenteric arteries is common, symptomatic chronic mesenteric ischemia which occurs only with severe stenosis or occlusion of at least two of the three mesenteric arteries is rare. CEMRA is now the investigation of choice for the evaluation of patients with suspected chronic mesenteric ischemia (Table 11.8).

11.7.7.1 Miscellaneous Disorders of the Renal and Mesenteric Vasculature

MRA/V can diagnose visceral artery aneurysms, arteriovenous malformations, visceral thrombosis, and involvement by thrombus of the renal veins and inferior vena cava in nephrotic syndrome and involvement by renal carcinoma and retroperitoneal sarcomas.

Table 11.8 Magnetic resonance (MR) angiography sequence parameters recommendations for renal and mesenteric arteries

Sequence	WI	Plane	TR (ms)	TE (ms)	Flip-angle	3D Slice thickness (mm)	No part	Effth	Matrix	FOV	recFOV (%)	BW	Acq.	Acq. Time (min:s)
3D GRE	T1	Cor	3.85	1.5	35	70	56	1.25	256	320	75	650	1	0:40

WI weighted image; *TR* repetition time; *TI* inversion time; *TE* echo time; *No part* number of partitions; *Effth* effective thickness (mm); *Matrix* matrix (phase ¥ frequency matrix); *FOV* field of view (mm); *recFOV %* rectangular field of view; *BW* bandwidth (Hz); *Acq* number of acquisitions

11.7.8 Vessels of Lower Extremities (Arteries of the Pelvis, Thigh, Leg, and Foot)

11.7.8.1 TOF-MRA

Although CEMRA has supplanted TOF-MRA for most applications, TOF-MRA is an accurate technique for the evaluation of the lower extremity arteries (Table 11.9). Better results have been achieved within the relatively straight arteries of the thighs and legs where the sensitivity of TOF-MRA to slow flow offers advantages, than for the somewhat more tortuous aorto-iliac segments where in-plane saturation effects can lead to artifact. Although scan times for CEMRA continue to improve with faster gradient technology and improved parallel imaging techniques, a rapid scanning approach cannot be implemented for TOF-MRA for two main reasons both related to the need to maximize inflow effects – first, the requirement to maintain a relatively long TR (optimally >30 ms), second, the need to orientate the acquisition slice orthogonal to the direction of flow. Therefore, the limitation of poor scan time efficiency is a physical constraint related to the physiology of flow which cannot easily be overcome, and as a result TOF-MRA is usually reserved for situations where CEMRA cannot be employed.

11.7.8.2 PC-MRA

Although 3D PCA scan times are long, a single flow-encoding gradient (rather than the customary three) can be applied in the head–foot direction due to the predominant craniocaudal direction of flow within the peripheral arteries, which substantially reduces the scan time (2D technique). However, as several velocities may be encountered within the imaging field, multiple *Venc* gradients must be applied for optimal imaging. Although this technique is reasonably accurate, there are few proponents of the approach; firstly; due to difficulties in appropriately selecting the *Venc*, and secondly; due to the success of competing MRA techniques.

11.7.8.3 Fresh-Blood Imaging (FBI)

This is a 3D half-Fourier fast-spin-echo technique which does not require contrast agent injection. Although FSE images usually demonstrate blood vessels as signal voids (black blood technique), FBI generates a bright-blood "angiographic" effect as a result of several factors as follows. First, the reduction in the echo train spacing length in half Fourier FSE reduces the single shot acquisition time which minimizes motion-related artifacts and susceptibility artifacts. Second, the fact that "centric" k-space ordering is known to reduce flow voids in the phase encode minimizes artifacts. Finally, species with short T2 such as blood show blurring in the phase encode direction in FSE sequences, resulting in the blood signal being dispersed over several slices. However, by matching the phase-encode direction with the direction of flow, enhancement of vascular signal is obtained from the overlapping T2 signal blurring between the adjacent pixels, which maximizes the bright-blood effect. This approach and a related

Table 11.9 Magnetic resonance angiography sequence parameters recommendations for iliac, femoral, and lower leg arteries

Sequence	WI	Plane	TR (ms)	TE (ms)	Flip-angle	Slice thickness (mm)	No part	Effth	Matrix	FOV	recFOV (%)	BW	Acq.	Acq. time (min:s)
3D GRE LR	T1	Cor	3.85	1.5	35	90 3D	58	1.55	256	350	75	650	1	0:43
3D GRE HR	T1	Cor	4.57	1.95	35	70 3D	70	1	512	400	75	650	1	1:07
2D FL PC	Ph	Cor	83	9	11	80 3D	–	–	512	400	75		1	2:30
2D FL TOF	T1	Ax	8	5	30	3	160	2	256	270	75		1	5

WI weighted image; *TR* repetition time; *TI* inversion time; *TE* echo time; *No part* number of partitions; *Effth* effective thickness (mm); *Matrix* matrix (phase ¥ frequency matrix); *FOV* field of view (mm); *recFOV %* rectangular field of view; *BW* bandwidth (Hz); *Acq* number of acquisitions; *LR* low resolution; *HR* high resolution technique called contrast inflow angiography (CIA) have been proposed as alternatives to CEMRA for some indications, e.g., patients with severe renal failure who may be at risk of developing NSF.

11.7.8.4 CEMRA

CEMRA can be performed as a single location examination (as dictated by the clinical scenario); consecutive scans can be acquired at different imaging locations using separate injections for each location, or a moving table approach can be used that allows imaging at successive locations during a single injection (Figs. 11.26–11.35).

Single-Location MRA

Using CEMRA, high-resolution images with high SNR can be acquired. Images over a 40–50 cm FOV, targeted to the anatomically relevant area, can be acquired using a standard approach. The scan delay time can be determined using either a timing bolus, or preferably, a fluoroscopic technique. Use of parallel imaging facilitates increased resolution and reduced scan time.

Multilocation, Multiinjection MRA

The limitation of poor spatial coverage in the head–foot direction (requirement of a distance of more than 100 cm for coverage compared with a maximum permissible FOV of <50 cm on all commercially available systems) was initially overcome by performing successive imaging of the arteries of the pelvis, thighs, and legs with separate injections. However, background and venous signal from earlier injections hampered evaluation of successive locations. Using this approach, the traditional recommendation was to use 0.1 mmol/kg for each of the three measurements, with the body phased-array coil if possible (the coil position has to be changed twice) as it gives higher SNR for all regions. Either the pelvic arteries or the tibial vessels should be evaluated first; otherwise, overlay by the bladder and other enhancing structures may complicate image evaluation. However, awareness of the risks of NSF posed by high dose imaging in conjunction with improved moving table techniques which require a lower dose and troublesome venous enhancement for the last location renders this technique less attractive in clinical practice.

One way of addressing the issue of the triple dose (i.e., single dose × 3), an approach that also addresses the issue of excessive background contrast from the earlier two injections, is to evaluate the more distal run-off in the foot with a TOF-MRA acquired prior to a 2 station CEMRA. This limits the cumulative dose to a double dose. Evaluation of the foot arteries may not be necessary in all patients, but it is important in cases where distal bypass surgery is considered.

Moving Table MRA

The spatial limitation of head–foot coverage greater than a single FOV has been overcome by using a moving-table approach for patients with peripheral MRA with rapid table translation between successive scans centered over the pelvis, thighs, and legs in association with a single contrast injection. Because the scan time for three consecutive 3D scans is relatively long compared to the transit time from aorta to leg arteries and veins, careful tailoring of imaging parameters and use of shortest scan times possible must be implemented to ensure completion of imaging prior to the onset of venous enhancement within the second and third stations. For example, high contrast injection rates that boost intravascular signal may lead to earlier venous enhancement; therefore injection rate must be tailored accordingly. Lower infusion rates also serve to lower total dose, a factor of increasing importance in the face of concerns of NSF. Dedicated phase-array coils that boost SNR should be used whenever possible. A precontrast mask can overcome some of the limitations of the lower infusion rate by eliminating fat from the image after digital subtraction of the precontrast mask. Some manufacturers implement automatic mask subtraction and generate a composite image of all three locations stitched together..

Although breath-holding is not necessary for the evaluation of the arteries below the aortic bifurcation, the frequent (20–45%) association of renal artery stenosis with peripheral vascular disease indicates that a breath-hold acquisition for the first imaging location to allow visualization of the renal arteries is preferable. Relatively thick 3D volumes (approximately 60–100 mm) in coronal orientation are required for the aorto-iliac region because of the tortuosity of the vessels included in this imaging volume. The partition thickness must optimally be reduced to 1.5 mm or less. In our experience, isotropic resolution of 1.5 mm is sufficient to estimate the therapeutic relevance of iliac artery stenosis using a 256 (frequency-encoding direction) matrix. However, use of a 512 matrix doubles the resolution in the head–foot direction without increasing the scan time, with the minor penalties of reduced SNR and slightly increased TE.

For evaluation of the second and third locations, progressively higher resolution is necessary at each location because of the stepwise decrease in artery size from femoral to pedal artery. Additionally, although the scan volume in the AP plane is relatively small for the femoro-popliteal arteries, it is much larger for the infrapopliteal arteries if the pedal arch is to be included in the images which should be the case. In order to address these issues, many manufacturers have introduced flexible imaging parameters for each location.

11.7.8.5 "Spatial" vs. "Temporal" Resolution Issue for Moving Table Peripheral CEMRA: Relevance to Venous Contamination in the Legs

A minimum spatial resolution requirement for accurate grading of stenosis is dictated by the size of the artery in question. For moving-table MRA (MT-MRA), the spatial requirement increases from first-to-third location as the arteries progressively decrease in size from aorta to pedal arch. MT CEMRA requires central k-space data collection coincident with the arterial peak for all three locations and completion of central k-space data prior to the onset of venous enhancement. For the first location, this is virtually guaranteed by triggering 3D data collection once contrast is visualized by the bolus "detection" technique. As data collection for the second location follows relatively quickly, images for this (femoro-popliteal) location are rarely degraded by venous enhancement despite the fact that the arterial phase has commenced at least several seconds prior to commencement of data collection. However, central k-space data collection at the third location is significantly delayed after contrast arrival in the infrapopliteal arteries, by the sum of the first two scan acquisition times plus the time required for two table movements and venous contamination of the infrapopliteal segments occurs when the combined imaging time for the first two locations plus two table movements is greater than the circulation time from aorta to calf vein. Reports indicate, on average, a transit time from CFA to popliteal artery of 5 s, with an additional 7 s required to reach the ankle arteries. However, it is not the arterial transit time from one location to another per se that dictates venous enhancement; rather, it is the arterial transit time plus the arteriovenous transit time within the third location that governs venous enhancement.

What steps can be instituted to reduce or eliminate the risk of venous enhancement within the calf?

1. Use bolus detection to signal arrival of contrast at the first location.
2. *Optimized k-space filling strategies:* "Centric" k-space filling strategies reduce the likelihood of venous enhancement at all locations, and additionally facilitate higher resolution imaging of the (smaller) leg arteries by allowing acquisition of resolution-defining peripheral k-space mapping to continue into the venous phase.
3. *Tailor the 3D scans to the anatomy and use individually tailored scan parameters for each ROI.* The goal of arterial phase imaging over three consecutive locations can be achieved only if the smallest possible imaging volume per location can be prescribed, indicating the need for high quality localizers to allow the operator the opportunity to prescribe the minimum scan volume so that all of the arteries of interest are enclosed within the FOV while avoiding redundancy. While isotropic voxels are ideal, spatial resolution must be sacrificed in favor of better temporal resolution especially for the first two locations. In-plane resolution of 1.2–1.6 mm and through-plane resolution of 3–4 mm (slices reconstructed to 1.5–2 mm by interpolation or zero-padding) for the aorto-iliac and thigh arteries may be sufficient. For the third location, higher in-plane and through-plane resolution is required (ideally 1 mm^3).
4. Parallel imaging: Parallel imaging has been a huge breakthrough for CEMRA and offers an ideal method for maintaining or improving both spatial and/or temporal resolution, albeit with a small SNR penalty (proportional to the square root of the time saving – i.e., halving the scan time gives an SNR penalty of $\sqrt{1/2} = 30\%$). If implemented in MT-MRA

for the first and/or second locations, imaging times can be reduced to levels that virtually eliminate the risk of venous enhancement within the third location and isotropic 1 mm resolution (or close) can be achieved. This approach gives increased acquisition speed by utilization of multiple phase-array coils with known sensitivities.

5. *Hybrid approaches for peripheral MRA:* Even using a highly optimized approach for MT CEMRA, venous enhancement still occurs in the calf in some patients, leading some investigators to propose alternative approaches, all aimed at improving acquisition speed, as follows:
   (a) *Time-resolved imaging:* Time-resolved imaging can be performed with either a 2D single thick slice with high in-plane resolution or a 3D (TRICKS) approach.
   (b) *2D and Hybrid 3D/2D approaches:* Single thick slice 2D imaging (with a slice thickness appropriate to the anatomy – typically 6–8 cm) with complex subtraction and high in-plane spatial resolution but poor through-plane resolution can be achieved in a short scan time (<3 s). The best use of 2D imaging therefore is as part of a hybrid technique that uses 3D acquisitions for the aorto-iliac location, 2D for the thighs, and 2D or 3D for the legs and feet to keep up with the bolus. Some investigators advocate 2D imaging of the infrapopliteal arteries PRIOR to a moving-table approach of the first two or three locations.

6. *Delay the onset of venous enhancement by the use of venous compression techniques:* An alternative approach to faster scanning is to delay the onset of venous enhancement, which therefore increases the amount of time available for arterial phase imaging. Compression of the thigh with tourniquets inflated to a value intermediate between arterial and venous pressure (~60 mmHg) significantly reduces the incidence of venous enhancement in moving-table peripheral MRA without costly hardware or software upgrades. An additional benefit is that it also facilitates higher-spatial-resolution imaging due to the prolongation of the arterio-venous window. Thigh compression during time-resolved MR angiography increases contrast travel time from the common femoral artery to the popliteal artery by 62% when elastic tourniquets were used, but this increased to 94% with the application of a dedicated thigh blood pressure cuff specifically contoured for the local anatomy. Improved sharing of the contrast bolus between stations may result in better synchronization of peak arterial enhancement with acquisition of the center of k-space with corresponding increase in the arterial signal-to-noise ratio. Although the mechanism remains unproven, it is suggested that reduced venous enhancement is due to engorgement of the veins with blood before the injection of gadolinium, so that when the contrast material eventually arrives in peripheral veins, it is rapidly diluted.

11.7.9 MRA of the Hands

Because of the small vessel size, high spatial resolution is necessary (Figs. 11.36, 11.37). The resultant long acquisition time is partially offset by the small imaging volume required (Figs. 11.36 and 11.37). Because of the relatively short AV transit time, a modification of the tourniquet compression technique called timed arterial compression ("T.A.C. MRA"), is used. This technique employs supraarterial pressure tourniquet compression (~200 mmHg) to "freeze" the circulation once contrast has been detected in the hand arteries, and prevents passage of contrast into the veins. This level of tourniquet compression, which is well tolerated in the upper extremities, may be unacceptable to patients with lower extremity peripheral arterio-occlusive disease due to already compromised arterial blood supply.

11.7.10 Whole-Body MRA

Whole-Body MRA is a promising extension of the moving-table approach and typically employs four or five rather than three imaging stations. The initial implementation of a 5-station study with identical imaging parameters for each location in 72 s has been superseded by techniques offering improved resolution, "tailored" to each individual ROI. The challenges and limitations of moving-table CEMRA are amplified in a 5-station approach; however, the ultimate goal of "optimized" imaging at each location may be possible using very fast scanners, highly-accelerated parallel imaging and tourniquet compression.

11.7.11 Future Prospects

MRA is a dynamically evolving modality, with improvements in image quality occurring at a rapid rate. All arteries apart from the coronary arteries can currently be evaluated (Fig. 11.38). In-depth knowledge of contrast dynamics, approximate contrast arrival times, AV transit times, k-space filling order, parameter choice, image resolution, and SNR is necessary to ensure the highest standard of practice.

Improvements in pulse sequences design (including non-contrast (Fig. 11.38) and parallel imaging techniques), improved contrast agents, more efficient k-space filling algorithms, better coil design, improved fat suppression techniques, and better postprocessing will further enhance MRA, especially CEMRA, which promises to revolutionize noninvasive imaging of patients with suspected vascular disease without the use of ionizing radiation, arterial puncture, or nephrotoxic contrast agents. A robust whole-body MRA, tailored to each individual region-of-interest, which will provide information about all vascular territories from skull base to pedal arch, is within reach in the next 5 years. Physicians managing patients with vascular disease would then enjoy delineation of the entire burden of atherosclerosis, regardless of which vascular territory led to the patient's presentation.

Table 11.10 Different spatial resolution of images can be obtained using various coils, Gd dosage, and slab volume thickness

Spatial resolution	Coil	Dose	Slab-volume thickness (mm)
Low	Standard body	0.1 mmol Gd/kg bw	70–120
Moderate	Standard body	0.1 mmol Gd/kg bw	70–90
Moderate	Body phased-array	0.1 mmol Gd/kg bw	70–120
High	Body phased-array	0.2 mmol Gd/kg bw	70–120
High	Body phased-array	0.3 mmol Gd/kg bw	120–170

Table 11.11 Vessel regions and bolus dilution factor

Vessel region	BDF
Renal arteries	2.0
Iliac arteries	2.1
Femoral arteries	2.4
Tibial arteries	2.7
Feet arteries	3.0

Further Reading

Anderson CM, Edelman RR, Turski PA (1993) Clinical MRA. Raven, New York

Arlart IP, Bongartz GM, Marchal G (2001) MRA. Springer, Berlin

Fraser DGW, Moody AR, Morgan PS, Martel AL, Davidson I (2002) Diagnosis of lower-limb deep venous thrombosis: a prospective blinded study of magnetic resonance direct thrombus imaging. Ann Intern Med 136:89–98

Graves MJ (1997) MRA. Br J Radiol 70:6–28

Hashemi RH, Bradley WG Jr (1997) MRI: the basics. Williams and Wilkins, Baltimore

Hendrick RE, Russ PD, Simon JH (1993) MRI: principles and artifacts. In: Lufkin RB (ed) The Raven MRI teaching file. Raven, New York

Huston J et al (2001) Carotid artery: elliptic centric contrast-enhanced MR angiography compared with conventional angiography. Radiology 218:138

Ho KY, Leiner T, de Haan MW, Kessels AG, Kitslaar PJ, van Engelshoven JM (1998) Peripheral vascular tree stenoses: evaluation with moving-bed infusion-tracking MR angiography. Radiology 206:683–692

Lee HM et al (1998) Distal lower extremity arteries: evaluation with two-dimensional MR digital subtraction angiography. Radiology 207:505

Ley S, Kreitner KF, Fink C, Heussel CP, Borst MM, Kauczor HU (2004) Assessment of pulmonary hypertension by CT and MR imaging. Eur Radiol 14(3):359–368.

Meaney JFM, Prince MR, Nostrant TT, Stanley JC (1997a) Gadolinium-enhanced MR angiography of visceral arteries in patients with suspected chronic mesenteric ischemia. J Magn Reson Imaging 7:171–176

Meaney JFM, Weg JG, Chenevert TL, Stafford-Johnson D, Hamilton BH, Prince MR (1997b) Diagnosis of pulmonary embolism with MRA. N Engl J Med 336:1422–1427

Meaney FM, Ridgway JP, Chakraverty S, Robertson I, Kessel D, Radjenovic A, Kouwenhoven M, Kasner A, Smith MA (1999) Stepping-table gadolinium-enhanced digital substraction MR angiography of the Aorta and lower

extremity arteries: preliminary experience. Radiology 211: 59–67
Moody AR, Pollock JG, O'Connor AR, Bagnall M (1998) Lower-limb deep venous thrombosis direct MR imaging of the thrombus. Radiology 209:349–355
Nael K, Ruehm SG, Michaely HJ, Saleh R, Lee M, Laub G, Finn JP (2007) Multistation whole-body high-spatial-resolution MR angiography using a 32-channel MR system. Am J Roentgenol 188(2):529–539
Nelemans PJ, Leiner T, de Vet HCW, van Engelshoven JMA (2000) Peripheral arterial disease: meta-analysis of the diagnostic performence of MR Angiography. Radiology 217:105–114
Oudkerk M, Edelman RR (1997) High-power gradient MR-imaging. Advances in MRI II. Blackwell Science, Oxford
Oudkerk M, van Beek EJ, Wielopolski P, van Ooijen PM, Brouwers-Kuyper EM, Bongaerts AH, Berghout A (2002) Comparison of contrast-enhanced magnetic resonance angiography and conventional pulmonary angiography for the diagnosis of pulmonary embolism: a prospective study. Lancet 359(9318):1643–1647
Owen RS, Carpenter JP, Baum RA et al (1992) Magnetic resonance imaging of angiographically occult runoff vessels in peripheral arterial occlusive disease. N Engl J Med 326:157–1581
Prince MR (1998) Contrast-enhanced MR angiography: theory and optimisation. MRI Clin North Am 6:257
Prince MR, Grist TM, Debatin JF (1997a) 3D contrast MR angiography. Springer, Berlin
Prince MR et al (1997b) Hemodynamically significant atherosclerotic renal artery stenosis: MR angiographic features. Radiology 205:128
Reimer P, Boos M (1999) Phase-contrast MR angiography of peripheral arteries: technique and clinical application. Eur Radiol 9:122
Rofsky NM, Johnson G, Adelman MA, Rosen RJ, Krinsky GA, Weinreb JC (1997) Peripheral vascular disease evaluated with reduced-dose gadolinium-enhanced MR angiography. Radiology 205:163–169
Ruehm SG, Goyen M, Barkhausen J, Kroger K, Bosk S, Ladd ME, Debatin JF (2001) Rapid magnetic resonance angiography for detection of atherosclerosis. Lancet 357(9262): 1086–1091
Wallner B (1993) MR angiography. Thieme, Stuttgart
Weiger M, Pruessmann KP, Kassner A, Rodite G, Reid A, Boesiger P (2000) Contrast-enhanced 3D MRA using SENSE. J Magn Reson Imaging 12:671–677
Wentz KU, Frohlich JM, von Weymarn C, Patak MA, Jenelten R, Zollikofer CL (2003) High-resolution magnetic resonance angiography of hands with timed arterial compression (tac-MRA). Lancet 361(9351):49–50

MRI of the Breast

12

Uwe Fischer

Contents

U. Fischer
Diagnostisches Brustzentrum Göttingen, Bahnhofsallee 1d, 37081 Göttingen, Germany
e-mail: uwfisch@web.de

12.1 Tumorangiogenesis

Probably all invasive breast cancer and many of the intraductal carcinomas are associated with increased vascularization due to tumor neoangiogenesis. MRI allows the visualization of breast cancer because these tumors are associated with signal enhancement after peripheral administration of a contrast material. Thus, MRI gives information on hemodynamic as well as morphologic aspects of a tumor. The provision of hemodynamic information by MRI of the breast is the relevant difference in comparison to X-ray mammography and ultrasonography, which give primary information on the morphologic changes based on radiation absorption and ultrasound reflection, respectively.

12.2 Technique and Methods

Indispensable equipment for MRI of the breast is a magnetic resonance tomography diagnostic unit and a dedicated bilateral breast surface coil. For performing a MRI of the breast, a field strength of 1.5 T or more is recommended. The breast surface coil should be open bilaterally to allow MR-guided interventions such as a percutaneous biopsy or pretherapeutic localization. Moreover, dedicated tools are available to perform an examination at a high comfort level for the patient. A dedicated headrest is helpful to place the patient's head and neck in a comfortable position (Fig. 12.1). For MR-guided interventions, special MR-compatible equipment is necessary to calculate the required coordinates of unclear findings. Usually, these tools are integrated into the lateral parts of an open surface coil (Fig. 12.2).

P. Reimer et al. (eds.), *Clinical MR Imaging*,
DOI: 10.1007/978-3-540-74504-4_12, © Springer-Verlag Berlin Heidelberg 2010

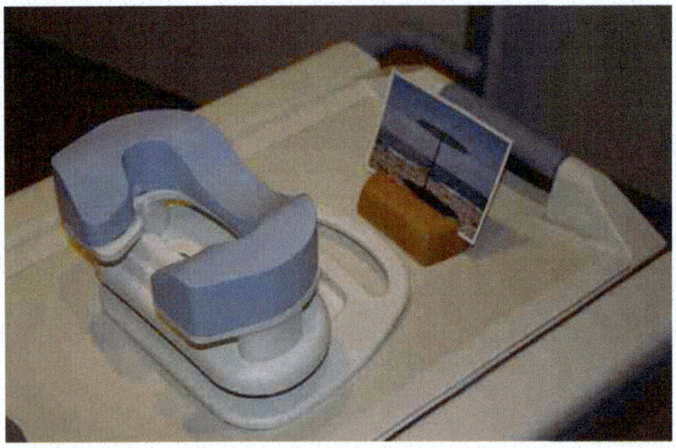

Fig. 12.1 Devices for the comfortable positioning of the patient during MRI of the breast. A dedicated headrest with an integrated mirror allows the patient to look out, e.g., at a postcard or a picture of her own choice

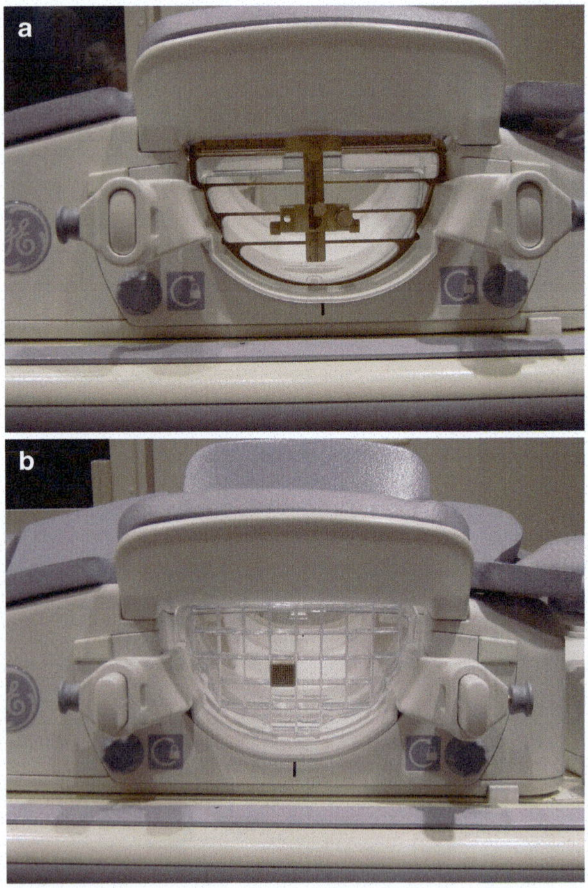

Fig. 12.2 Compression devices for MR-guided interventions. Two different systems available for use in open breast surface coils for the performance of percutaneous biopsy or wire localization. Post-and-pillar system (**a**) and grid system with a puncture cube (**b**)

The patient history must be collected before beginning MRI. Special questions that should be asked are

- Personal history, especially with respect to previous breast cancer (type, stage, age at diagnosis, treatment) or biopsies with benign histology
- Family history of breast or ovarian cancer (degree of relationship, age at diagnosis)
- Abnormalities, suspicion of malignancy (e.g., palpable mass, skin retraction, nipple discharge)
- Hormonal status (e.g., premenstrual/menopausal/postmenopausal, hormonal-replacement therapy)
- Previous allergic reaction after administration of MR contrast material

Moreover, previous imaging studies such as mammography and/or sonography, and their findings should be available.

Before starting the MRI, the patient must be informed about the general conditions during MRI of the breast and the requirements made of her. These include the following aspects:

- MR study is accompanied by unpleasant, loud noises.
- Patient movement must be prevented during the entire examination.
- Measurements are announced by the radiographer.
- An announcement will be made before application of the contrast material.
- Measurement will be stopped immediately if the patient indicates indisposition. (In this case, however, the study cannot be repeated on the same day.)

For application of the contrast material, a venous line (18–20 G) must be inserted, preferably in the antecubital vein, before starting the examination. Use of peripheral veins (e.g., on the back of the hand) should be avoided because the inflow time of the contrast material will be lengthened significantly. An extension tube of 2–2.5 m is used to connect the patient with the injector while the patient is positioned in the MRI system.

MRI must be performed with the patient in the prone position. It is recommended that the arms be placed alongside the body. It is helpful to use something like a bathrobe in order to fix the arms to the body with the belt raising the arms up above the head runs the risk of the breast partially slipping out from the surface coil. Moreover, the inflow of the contrast material could be impeded.

In the past, two different philosophies existed concerning the performance of MRI of the breast: either high temporal resolution with measurement times of less than 1 min per sequence, or high spatial resolution with voxels of 1–2 mm^3 or less were preferred. Modern high-performance MR systems today allow the imaging of the breast with a high temporal as well as a high spatial resolution. If there is spare capacity to modify the examination further, an increase in spatial resolution is recommended.

The most relevant prerequisite for attaining a high-quality MRI of the breast is patient comfort. To achieve this, the patient must be sufficiently informed about the conditions expected during the performance of the examination. This includes information about the prone positioning, the necessity of breast compression, and the possible reactions to the application of contrast material. In this context, practical experience of the personnel is as relevant as the surrounding conditions such as room temperature and music. The best imaging technique will not result in a high-quality MRI of the breast if patient comfort is absent.

For 1.5 T systems, the following image parameters are adequate: transversal (alternative: coronal, sagittal), T1-W 3D (alternative: 2D), gradient-echo (GRE) pulse sequences once before and repetitively 4–6 times after bolus injection of 0.1 mmol/kg gadopentetate dimeglumine. In our protocol, we use TR/TE/FA 8.4 ms/4.1 ms/10° with a non-interpolated 512 x 512 imaging matrix. Depending on the field strength, TE is selected so that in-phase settings of fat and water resonance frequencies are warranted. The field of view (FoV) typically ranges from 280 to 320 mm, depending on the breast size. The slice thickness should be 3 mm or less, and without gaps. With these parameter settings, about 30 slices are needed to visualize the entire breast parenchyma. With this protocol, 40–50 slices should be acquired within an examination time of 2 min per dynamic scan. There is no need for higher temporal resolution. If there is more scanner capacity, it should be used for better spatial resolution, i.e., a slice thickness of 2 mm. It could be demonstrated that MRI of the breast is feasible on a 3.0 T system, whereas 0.5 and 1.0 T systems are no longer recommended.

Today, technical developments allow an examination of both breasts in axial, coronal, or sagittal angulation with a high temporal and spatial resolution. Therefore, the angulation of MRI of the breast depends on the user's preference. Many users prefer the axial orientation because radiologists are accustomed to this view from CT examinations. Moreover, it allows a better assessment of the retroareolar as well as the prepectoral regions, and it allows a reduction of the slice thickness when cranio-caudal compression devices are used.

In all protocols for breast MRI, the signal from fatty tissue must be suppressed to improve the detection and delineation of contrast-enhancing lesions. Fat suppression can be effectively achieved by two different approaches: (1) active fat saturation using a frequency- or spectral-selective prepulse (American way) or (2) passive subtraction of pre and postcontrast images (European way). Notably, it is also possible to use the passive subtraction method on active fat-saturation images to allow better differentiation between signal-intense parenchymal tissue and enhancing lesions. When using the European method of fat suppression, it is recommended that the precontrast images be subtracted from the second postcontrast measurement images ("early subtraction"). If the parenchyma shows a strong contrast enhancement in the early subtraction, an additional "earliest subtraction," that is, the subtraction of the precontrast images from the first postcontrast measurement images, may be performed. There is no need for a later subtraction.

After image subtraction, it is useful to obtain a maximum intensity projection (MIP) of the early postcontrast subtraction images. This makes it easier to assess the topographic aspects of a breast lesion. Moreover, diffusely enhancing structures, such as an intraductal tumor component (EIC), are sometimes better visualized in the MIP image.

Prior to T1-WIs, the recommended practice is to obtain water-sensitive T2-w images using T2-w turbo spin-echo (TSE) or T2-w inversion recovery (IR) sequences with geometric parameters (thickness, slice position) equivalent to those of the dynamic contrast-enhanced series. T2-w images are helpful to better characterize solid enhancing masses. Moreover, it improves the detection of interstitial edema (e.g., radiation therapy, diffuse inflammatory disease, lymphangiosis).

MRI of the breast using a dedicated breast surface coil is usually not adequate for the staging of the locoregional lymph nodes. Occasionally, however, enlarged axillary or internal mammary lymph nodes can be depicted on precontrast T1-W, as well as on T2-w images, and assessed to be suspicious for metastases.

For documentation and communication purposes, the recommended practice is to present the complete data set of precontrast T1-weighted, early postcontrast subtraction images, and earliest postcontrast subtraction images, if calculated. In addition, prepared signal-to-time intensity curves and selected T2-weighted images should be documented together with the corresponding lesion.

12.3 Evaluation

The evaluation criteria for MRI of the breast take into account information presented in the precontrast, postcontrast, and T2-w images. Some specific findings may already be seen on the precontrast T1 images, for example lymph nodes with a fatty hilus, macrocalcifications in regressive fibroadenomas, and sanguineous or protein-rich content of complicated cysts. The detection of, especially, a fat-equivalent signal within an unclear mass should be assessed as a sign of benignity.

The contrast uptake of the breast parenchyma should be described to define the reliability of the individual examination. In analogy to the BI-RADS reporting system for X-ray mammography, four categories are differentiated (MRM-density types I-IV). MRM-density type I is associated with a high sensitivity for the detection of breast cancer. MRM-density type IV is associated with a highly limited sensitivity. In this case, an earliest image subtraction (1. postcontrast – precontrast) should be performed in addition to the routinely performed early image subtraction (2. postcontrast – precontrast) (Table 12.1).

The extent of motion artifacts is another aspect that should be included in the written report. Usually, there are four categories for image quality, ranging from MRM artifact category I to artifact category IV. MRI with artifact category I has the highest sensitivity for the detection of breast cancer. Accuracy is reduced with increasing artifacts. MRI with artifact category IV is insufficient, and should be repeated after correcting the causes of bad quality (Table 12.2).

Table 12.1 Density types in MRI of the breast

MRM density	Description	Sensitivity
Type I	No enhancement	Excellent
Type II	Spotty enhancement	Good
Type III	Patchy enhancement	Moderate
Type IV	Strong diffuse enhancement	Poor

Table 12.2 Artifact categories in MRI of the breast and the corresponding sensitivity for the detection of breast cancer

MRM artifacts	Description	Sensitivity
Category I	No artifacts	Excellent
Category II	Little artifacts	Good
Category III	Moderate artifacts	Moderate
Category IV	Unacceptable artifacts	Poor

According to the BI-RADS Lexicon of the American College of Radiology, enhancing areas in the breast are differentiated into focus/foci, masses, and non-mass-like lesions. Moreover, associated findings are described. A *focus* is a small isolated spot of enhancement, generally less than 5 mm in size, that is so tiny that no definitive morphologic descriptors can be applied. Foci describe several such tiny spots, separated widely by normal tissue. Although commonly a normal finding, a very small carcinoma can appear as a focus. A *mass* is a three-dimensional space-occupying lesion that may or may not displace or otherwise affect the surrounding normal tissue. For the evaluation of masses, different criteria are described. The so-called Fischer score (Table 12.3) contains morphologic and dynamic criteria for a multimodal analysis of enhancing masses in the breast. Criteria include shape, border, endotumoral type of contrast material distribution, and the initial and post-initial signal behavior in relation to the precontrast signal. Other authors describe defined types of signal curves. Apart from the above named criteria, other "signs" on MRI of the breast are recognized. *Non-mass-like lesions* on MRI of the breast are enhancing areas that are neither a focus nor a mass. Depending on the distribution of the enhancement, it can be described as a focal area, linear, ductal, segmental, regional, multiple regions, or diffuse. Additionally, internal characteristics of the enhancing area, like homogeneous, heterogeneous, stippled/punctuate, clumped, or reticular/dendritic, can be evaluated. Typically, non-mass-like lesions are associated with normal findings, mastitis, ductal carcinoma in situ (DCIS), and invasive lobular carcinomas (Fig. 12.3).

Information from T2 images is important if there are unclear enhancing lesions seen on T1 images. In this case, the T2 signal is helpful to increase the specificity of MRI. High endotumoral signal in a solid mass, for example, is often associated with benign lesions,

Table 12.3 Fischer score for evaluation of masses in MRI. The total number of points defines the score and the MRM-BI-RADS category (MRM-BI-RADS 1: 0 points, MRM-BI-RADS 1: 1 point, MRM-BI-RADS 2: 2 points, MRM-BI-RADS 3: 3 points, MRM-BI-RADS 4: 4–5 points, MRM-BI-RADS 5: 6–8 points)

Criteria	Points		
	0	1	2
Shape	Round, oval	Irregular	–
Border	Well-defined	Ill-defined	–
CM distribution	Homogeneous	Inhomogeneous	Rim sign
Initial signal increase (%)	<50	50–100	>100
Postinitial signal	Continuous increase	Plateau	Washout

while malignant tumors usually have low water content. This is, however, not a reliable criterion, because mucinous tumors as well as other carcinomas may also be associated with a high T2 signal. Moreover, T2 images are helpful in recognizing endotumoral dark septations, which are sometimes better visualized on water-weighted images than on postcontrast images. Uncomplicated cysts also have a high signal on T2 images, as expected.

12.4 BI-RADS for MRI of the Breast

In 2003, the American College of Radiology defined a Breast Imaging MRI Lexicon and a Reporting System including seven categories for findings of the breast on MRI. While the category MRM-BI-RADS 0 describes an incomplete assessment and the category MRM-BI-RADS 6 is given to a histological verified breast carcinoma, the other five categories give a practical assessment of MRI findings:

Category MRM-BI-RADS 1: "negative"

No abnormal enhancement is found, and routine follow-up is advised.

Category MRM-BI-RADS 2: "benign"

MRI shows a benign finding, for example a hyalinized nonenhancing fibroadenoma, cysts, and old nonenhancing scars, fat-containing lesions such as oil cysts, lipomas, galactoceles, or mixed-density hamartomas.

Category MRM-BI-RADS 3: "probably benign"

Changes that are highly unlikely to be malignant, i.e., those that have a very high probability of being benign, are placed in this category. The consequences resulting for a finding in this category will likely undergo modifications in the future.

Category MRM-BI-RADS 4: "suspicious"

These are lesions that do not have the characteristic morphology of breast carcinoma, but do have a definite low to moderate probability of being malignant. Biopsy should be considered for these lesions.

Category MRM-BI-RADS 5: "highly suggestive of malignancy"

Lesions categorized as MRM-BI-RADS 5 have a high probability of being cancerous. They show the typical findings of a malignant breast tumor, and appropriate action should be taken.

12.5 Normal Findings

Enhancement of normal breast tissue after i.v. administration of contrast material depends especially on the hormonal stimulation of the parenchyma. As a consequence, significant intraindividual and interindividual variability may be seen. For premenopausal women, the contrast material uptake is usually stronger in the premenstrual than in the postmenstrual phase. For this reason, a highly recommended practice is to perform a MRI examination of the breast in the second (or third) week of the cycle, while the first and fourth week should be avoided. For postmenopausal women, there is usually a stronger parenchymal enhancement in patients with hormonal replacement therapy than in women without hormonal substitution (Fig. 12.4). An extremely high uptake of the contrast material is found during lactation.

In contrast to the hormonal stimulation, the breast parenchymal density on X-ray mammography does not correlate with enhancement after administration of contrast material. Even very dense breast tissue (i.e., ACR type IV) is often associated with absent or very low enhancement (Fig. 12.5).

12.6 Benign Findings

A *fibroadenoma* is the most common breast tumor found in young women. The presentation in MRI varies strongly, and depends essentially on the tumor age and the degree of fibrosis. A myxoid fibroadenoma in a young patient is usually characterized as a round or oval mass, with well-defined borders. Myxoid fibroadenomas frequently show a very strong initial enhancement – often stronger than in breast cancer – and a post-initial plateau (Fig. 12.7). A washout phenomenon is rare and should be a cause to reconsider the diagnosis. If there is any doubt, percutaneous biopsy is recommended to confirm the diagnosis. Myxoid fibroadenomas typically have a high signal on T2 images due to their gelatinous matrix. They often show endotumoral dark lines on subtraction and/or T2 images, corresponding to small fibrotic septations. Some authors assess endotumoral dark septations as pathognomonic for a fibroadenoma. The differential diagnoses for a myxoid fibroadenoma include the phyllodes tumor, papilloma, and mucinous carcinoma. Within increasing tumor age, a fibroadenoma becomes increasingly sclerotic. This is characterized by decreasing enhancement after administration of contrast material and decreasing signal intensity in the T2 images. A completely sclerotic fibroadenoma shows no enhancement on subtraction images and is hypointense on water-sensitive T2 images. In this stage, diagnosis is clear, and there is no differential diagnosis for a sclerotic fibroadenoma.

A *cyst* is a fluid-filled lesion and characteristically shows a high signal on T2 images and a low signal on precontrast T1 images. It is typically round and well-defined (Fig. 12.6). Sometimes, the cyst wall is inflamed, and a corresponding enhancement of the thin wall after contrast material administration is seen. In the case of a *complicated cyst*, intracystic proliferation with increased enhancement is seen on the postcontrast image.

Inflammatory changes of the breast are characterized by non-mass-like enhancement in the area of increased vascularization. Sometimes, skin thickening, increased edema of the subcutaneous area, and enlarged axillary lymph nodes are seen. MRI, however, does not allow a reliable differentiation between nonpuerperal mastitis and inflammatory breast cancer.

Postoperative scars typically show spiculated or ill-defined signal alterations on T1-WIs. Normally, there is no more increased enhancement in the scar area 6 months after open biopsy (Fig. 12.8). However, unspecific uptake of the contrast material will be visible if there are granulomatous inflammatory changes accompanying the scarring. In patients with postoperative radiation therapy after breast conserving therapy (BCT), a minimum interval of 12 months is recommended before performing a MRI of the breast.

12.7 Borderline Lesions

Borderline lesions are defined as benign findings with an increased risk of malignant transformation or coincidence with a malignant tumor. Borderline lesions of the breast include papillomas, radial scars, and lobular intraepithelial neoplasia (LIN).

Papillomas are benign proliferative epithelial breast lesions with a papillary architecture. They may occur at any site in the ductal and lobular system, from the nipple to the terminal ductal-lobular unit. Solitary (central) papillomas are distinguished from multiple (peripheral) papillomas. The risk for malignant transformation is as high as 30% for peripheral papillomas, while it is rare in central papillomas. MRI shows round or oval foci or masses, with increased uptake of contrast material and unspecific signal-time curves. Typical for papillomatos is a linear or segmental distribution of tumors.

A *radial scar* is a variant of sclerosing adenosis and has a coincidence with breast cancer ranging from 5 to 30%. In MRI, it is usually most conspicous on precontrast T1 images, presenting as a stellate hypointense lesion with a defined central area. Enhancement after administration of contrast material is unspecific, sometimes missing (Fig. 12.10).

The generic term "lobular intraepithelial neoplasia" refers to the entire spectrum of noninvasive, atypical epithelial proliferations of the lobular type. LIN is associated with an increased relative risk of developing invasive breast cancer in either breast. Usually, there is no corresponding lesion in mammography and ultrasound. MRI sometimes demonstrates a small focus or foci, with a signal increase after administration of contrast material. Signal-to-time curves are unspecific.

12.8 Malignant Findings

Malignant tumors of the breast are differentiated into intraductal carcinomas and invasive breast cancer. While DCIS is considered a localized disease within the breast ducts, invasive tumors have the potential for systemic tumor dissemination (systemic disease). In the diagnostic MRI of the breast, the criteria used for recognizing invasive breast cancer may not be transferred to the diagnosis of DCIS.

In the past, DCIS was usually detected on the basis of ductal microcalcifications on mammography. Clinical and ultrasound examinations show a very low sensitivity for the detection of intraductal proliferative processes. There is also enough evidence confirming that microcalcifications are not directly visible on MRI. Nevertheless, there are reports in the current literature stating that DCIS can be seen on high resolution MRI examinations more reliably than on mammography. This is especially true for lesions with a high tumor grade. Study data suggest that low grade DCIS is associated with a lower angiogenetic potential and a stronger disposition for developing intraductal microcalcifications. High grade DCIS, on the other hand, seems to have a stronger angiogenetic activity and is therefore better visualized on MRI.

For detection of DCIS, the typical tumor growth within the intramammary ducts and the anatomy of the ductal system of the breast must be taken into account. In analogy to the distribution of microcalcifications on mammography, the enhancement pattern on MRI is usually characterized as a non-mass like lesion with linear, dendritic, or segmental uptake of contrast material. In order to detect such enhancement patterns, a high spatial resolution with a noninterpolated matrix of a least 512 x 512 is a prerequisite. For the reliable detection of small DCIS lesions, a high spatial resolution is much more important than kinetic aspects such as initial signal increase or post-initial signal behavior (Fig. 12.11; 12.12). Multimodal evaluation protocols including dynamic criteria are, therefore, not helpful in the analysis of ductal enhancement patterns. In a few cases, DCIS may present as a focal lesion with strong and rapid enhancement, with or without washout phenomenon, indistinguishable from an invasive breast cancer.

Recent study data show that the sensitivity for the detection of DCIS by mammography ranges from 52 to 56%, while state-of-the-art high resolution contrast-enhanced MRI depicted 89–92% of all DCIS, especially high grade tumors. DCIS was missed by breast MRI in approximately 10–15% of all detected cases. For this reason, a recent state-of-the-art mammogram must be available when a breast MR study is performed. Moreover, a negative breast MR study cannot, at the current state of experience, negate the necessity for biopsy if a mammogram shows suspicious microcalcifications.

There are many different histopathologic subtypes of *invasive breast cancer*: ductal invasive cancers, not otherwise specified (NOS; approximately 80% of invasive cancers), lobular invasive cancers (10–15%), and rare invasive cancers (e.g., medullary, mucinous, or tubular cancers).

The typical appearance of *ductal invasive breast cancer* on MRI is a focal mass with irregular morphology, indistinct margins, and an inhomogeneous internal architecture. These morphologic criteria are, as expected, equivalent to those that have been found useful in mammography and ultrasonography. In addition, peripheral tumor enhancement (ring-enhancement, rim sign) is almost pathognomonic for breast cancer. The rim corresponds to the growing tumor periphery, while the central tumor areas of fibrosis or necrosis show less or no uptake of the contrast material. The dynamic characteristics typically shown by ductal invasive carcinoma are a moderate to strong initial signal increase and a post-initial plateau or washout. When a rim sign is observed, a centripetal enhancement spread is especially suspicious of malignancy. The T2 signal of breast cancer is unspecific. Invasive ductal carcinoma, however, often shows an intermediate or hypointense signal in comparison to the adjacent parenchyma (Fig. 12.9; 12.14; 12.15; 12.16; 12.17).

The growth pattern of *lobular breast cancers* effects a typically non-mass, non-space-occupying enhancement pattern on MRI. This type of tumor grows more or less diffusely, with displacement of the surrounding breast parenchyma. Lobular carcinoma is an important differential diagnosis for non-mass-like lesions (beside other changes, like DCIS, radial scar, mastitis, or circumscribed areas of adenosis). Most invasive carcinomas show typical signal-to-time curves, with strong initial enhancement followed by a plateau or washout (Fig. 12.13). Some lobular cancers, however, may differ and show a gradual and/or low enhancement.

Medullary breast cancer is typically characterized as a hypervascularized, well-circumscribed lesion with microlobulated borders, and an increased signal intensity on T2-WIs. This tumor entity is more frequent in patients with a strong family history of breast cancer and in BRCA1 or BRCA2 mutation carriers.

In contrast to ductal or lobular type of breast carcinoma, high signal intensity on T2-WIs is also seen in *mucinous cancer*. This tumor type is histopathologically characterized by small islands of tumor cells within large mucus-filled areas. Mucinous tumors are usually round and well-circumscribed.

Another histopathologically well-differentiated malignant tumor of the breast is the *tubular breast cancer*. MRI typically shows a spiculated tumor with increased contrast enhancement. T2 signal is low and signal-to-time curves are unspecific.

Inflammatory breast cancer is characterized by the clinical trio of swelling, erythema, and pain. Imaging demonstrates cutaneous edema and hypervascularization. MRI typically shows enhancement of the thickened skin. The associated intramammary lymphangiosis often shows low or no uptake of the contrast material. If there is an underlying cancer, a strong enhancement will usually be detectable within solid tumor manifestations. MRI cannot, however, distinguish puerperal or nonpuerperal mastitis from inflammatory breast cancer.

12.9 Indications

Appropriate indications for breast MRI are:

Preoperative staging in breast cancer	In patients with a proven breast carcinoma, MRI is superior to all other imaging modalities in the depiction of additional intramammary tumor lesions, e.g., peritumoral extensive intraductal component (EIC), multifocality, multicentricity, and contralateral tumor manifestations
Follow-up after BCT	MRI allows the differentiation between scar and tumor relapse, with a high degree of reliability. Postoperative scar tissue usually demonstrates no or very low perfusion and shows no contrast enhancement. In contrast, a tumor relapse is typically associated with a strong uptake of contrast material. In the case of accompanying inflammatory changes, a postoperative scar may demonstrate an unspecific enhancement pattern
Screening in high-risk women	A high-risk profile for the development of breast cancer is defined as an increased lifetime risk of ≥30%. Women with such a high-risk profile include those with a positive test for a BRCA gene mutation, or increased number of young relatives with breast or ovarian cancer. The mean age of these women at the time of breast cancer diagnosis is approximately 40 years. Several studies have shown that for this group of young women, MRI is the most sensitive method for the detection of breast cancer
Monitoring of neoadjuvant chemotherapy	The tumor response in patients with breast cancer primarily undergoing chemotherapy can be monitored reliably by MRI. Criteria for evaluation of the effectiveness of the neoadjuvant therapy are a reduction of tumor size and a decrease in vascularization
Search for primary in CUP syndrome	MRI is indicated to search for the primary tumor in patients with a histopathologically proven metastasis of an axillary lymph node if mammography and ultrasound are inconspicious. In this constellation, even semi-suspicious findings on MRI should be evaluated by percutaneous biopsy
Diagnostic evaluation of breast implants	In women with breast implants, MRI is the method of choice to rule out or detect complications like herniation, migration, gel bleeding, and intra- or extracapsular rupture. For this indication, special exam protocols, with selective presentation of saline- and silicone signal, are recommended

12.9.1 Optimized Imaging Concept for Early Detection of Breast Cancer (Optipack-Concept)

The combination of digital full-field mammography in the MLO-view with contrast-enhanced high resolution MRI of the breast is currently the best concept for the early detection of breast cancer. It offers the highest sensitivity for the detection of breast carcinoma, using the lowest radiation dosage. In this combination, mammography allows the detection of microcalcifications with very high reliability, while MRI depicts noncalcifying breast cancer., MRI, especially within dense parenchyma, shows a higher sensitivity in detecting such tumors by visualizing pathologic tumor neoangiogenesis that is found in many high grade intraductal tumors and all invasive breast cancers. This combination of digital 1-view mammography and MRI was introduced as the so-called Göttinger Optipack in 2003.

12.9.2 Breast Cancer Screening with MRI

Summarizing all data on the sensitivity and specificity of MRI of the breast in the detection of breast cancer, this method seems to be the perfect tool for breast cancer screening: Its high sensitivity is superior to that of all other imaging modalities. The specificity is acceptable and equivalent to that of mammography and ultrasonography. Moreover, there is no radiation exposure in MRI. Considering only these medical aspects, MRI should be the method of choice for screening (Fig. 12.20). Unfortunately, however, there are still problems with image quality, especially concerning motion artifacts and spatial resolution. Moreover, costs are generally too high to perform a population-based screening with MRI.

12.10 MR-Guided Interventions

MR-guided interventions are indicated for the histologic work-up of lesions classified as MRM-BI-RADS 4 and 5 that have no corresponding findings in mammography or ultrasound. A targeted ultrasound examination (second-look US) should always be performed in knowledge of the exact localization and size of the suspicious lesion on MRI.

In comparison to US-guided or stereotactic interventions, there are some additional specific aspects to be considered when performing a MR-guided biopsy or localization. First, the equipment must be compatible with a strong magnetic field. Second, the target of intervention is usually visible for only a short period of time, lasting 3–5 min. This is due to the washout of contrast material from the tumor and the increasing signal of the surrounding breast tissue in postcontrast imaging.

Another prerequisite for MR-guided interventions is an open dedicated breast surface coil, and additional perforated compression plates or post-and-pillar tools to access the breast from the lateral and/or medial aspect after the calculation of appropriate coordinates of the lesion. For MRI-guided percutaneous biopsy of unclear findings, vacuum biopsy in coaxial technique is recommended. Six to twelve specimens should be acquired, depending on the gauge of the needle. Available needle sizes range from 12 to 8 gauge (Figs. 12.18 and 12.19).

For MR-guided vacuum biopsy, hand-held-systems that have to be removed after acquisition of each specimen (e.g., VACORA), as well as systems that remain at the biopsy site during the excision of the specimens (i.e., ATEC, MAMMOTOME), are available. After termination of the percutaneous vacuum biopsy, it is possible to place a small marker coil or clip within the resection cavity for later identification.

Findings seen only on MRI should be localized preoperatively, using a wire or coil/clip technique. The assortment of localization wires ranges from permanent hook and double hook types to repositionable j-like configurations and threaded hooks.

Study data demonstrate that MR-guided interventions can be performed in an acceptable time, with high reliability (Table 12.4).

12.11 MRI Summary and Perspectives

All current data document that contrast-enhanced MRI of the breast is the most sensitive method for the detection of intraductal as well as invasive breast cancer. In all studies published in the last 10 years, MRI is shown to be superior to other imaging modalities. The specificity of MRI is within the range of that attained by mammography and ultrasonography. MRI is thus the best diagnostic tool for the detection of breast cancer at all stages if a high technical standard, appropriate methodical strategy, and a high level of experience on the part of the performing radiologist prevail. Further improvements should aim to optimize the examination protocols by reducing the study to the basic essentials and decreasing the examination costs.

Table 12.4 MR-guided vacuum biopsies. Results, time required, and complication rates in different working groups

Author	Liberman	Perlet	Orel	Kuhl	Fischer
Number of biopsies	112	538	85	316	389
Malignant findings (%)	25	27	61	43	27
Borderline lesions (%)	20	3	21	5	13
Benign findings (%)	52	70	18	52	60
Accuracy (%)	97	96	98	99	99
Time required (min)	33	38	30–60	34	39
Complication rate (%)	5	<1	0	3	<1

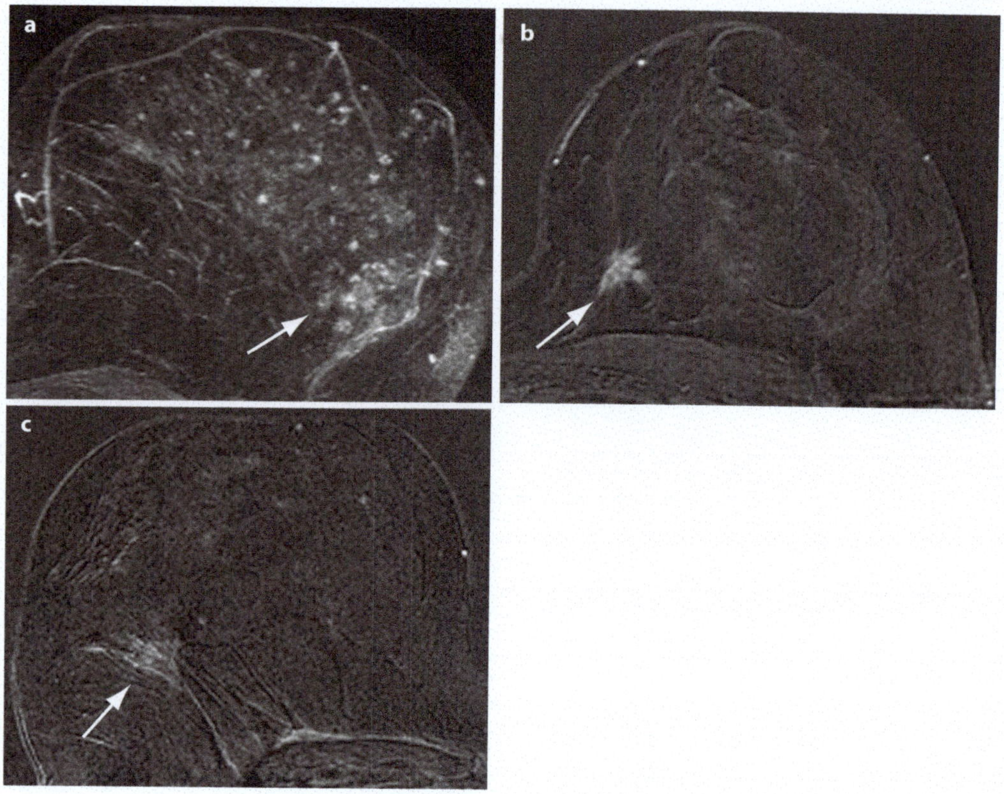

Fig. 12.3 Focus, mass, and non-mass-like lesion. Types of enhancement after administration of contrast material in MRI of the breast: multiple foci, each under 5 mm in size (**a**), enhancing mass (**b**), and non-space-occupying non-mass-like lesion (**c**) (*arrows*)

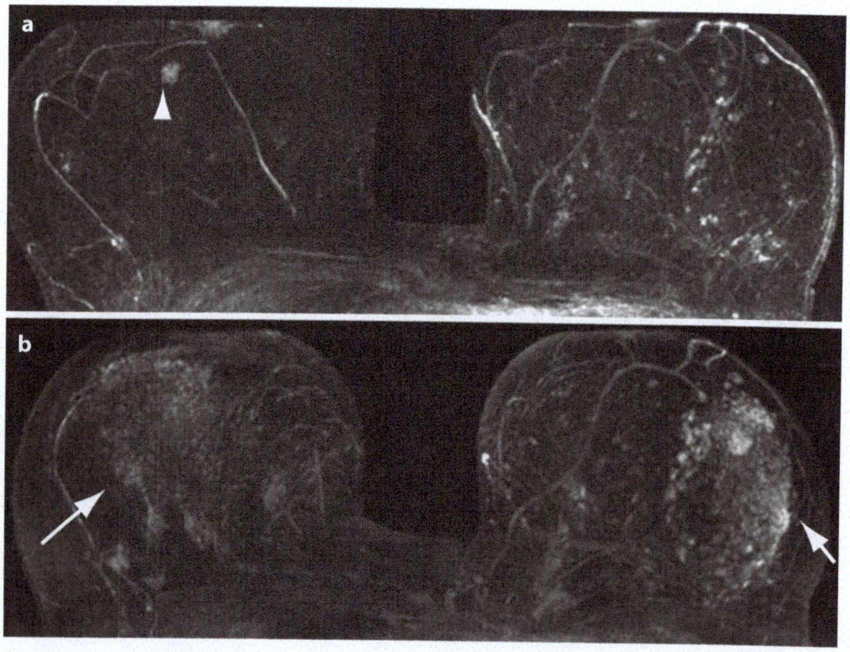

Fig. 12.4 Intraindividual variability of enhancement in a premenopausal woman. MIP of subtraction images in a 38-year-old woman. Low uptake of the contrast material 7 days after the beginning of the menstrual cycle (**a**). Stronger enhancement 1 year later, on the 11th day of menstrual cycle (*arrows*) (**b**). Accompanying finding: hypervascularized fibroadenoma behind the nipple of the right breast (*arrowhead*)

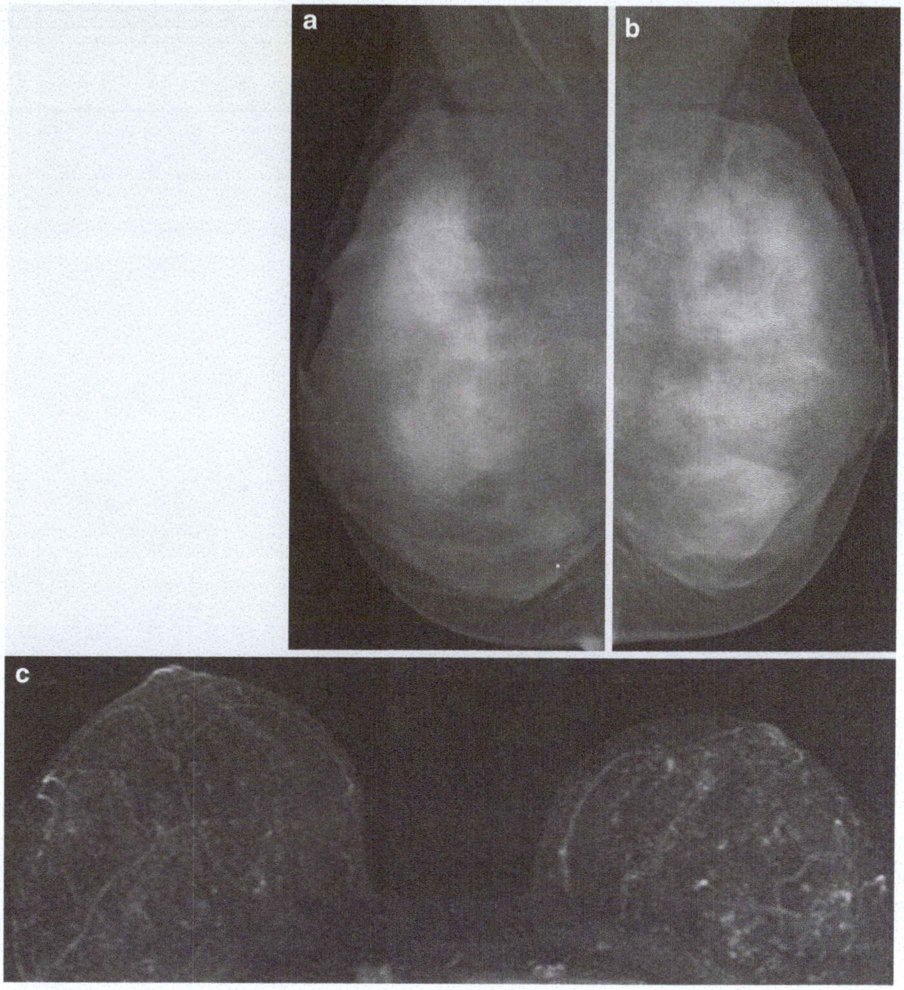

Fig. 12.5 High parenchymal density in digital mammography in comparison to CE-MRI of the breast. Digital mammography in MLO view demonstrates high parenchymal density type IV according to the American College of Radiology (**a+b**). MRI after administration of contrast material shows high transparency of the parenchyma (MIP; MRI-density type I) (**c**)

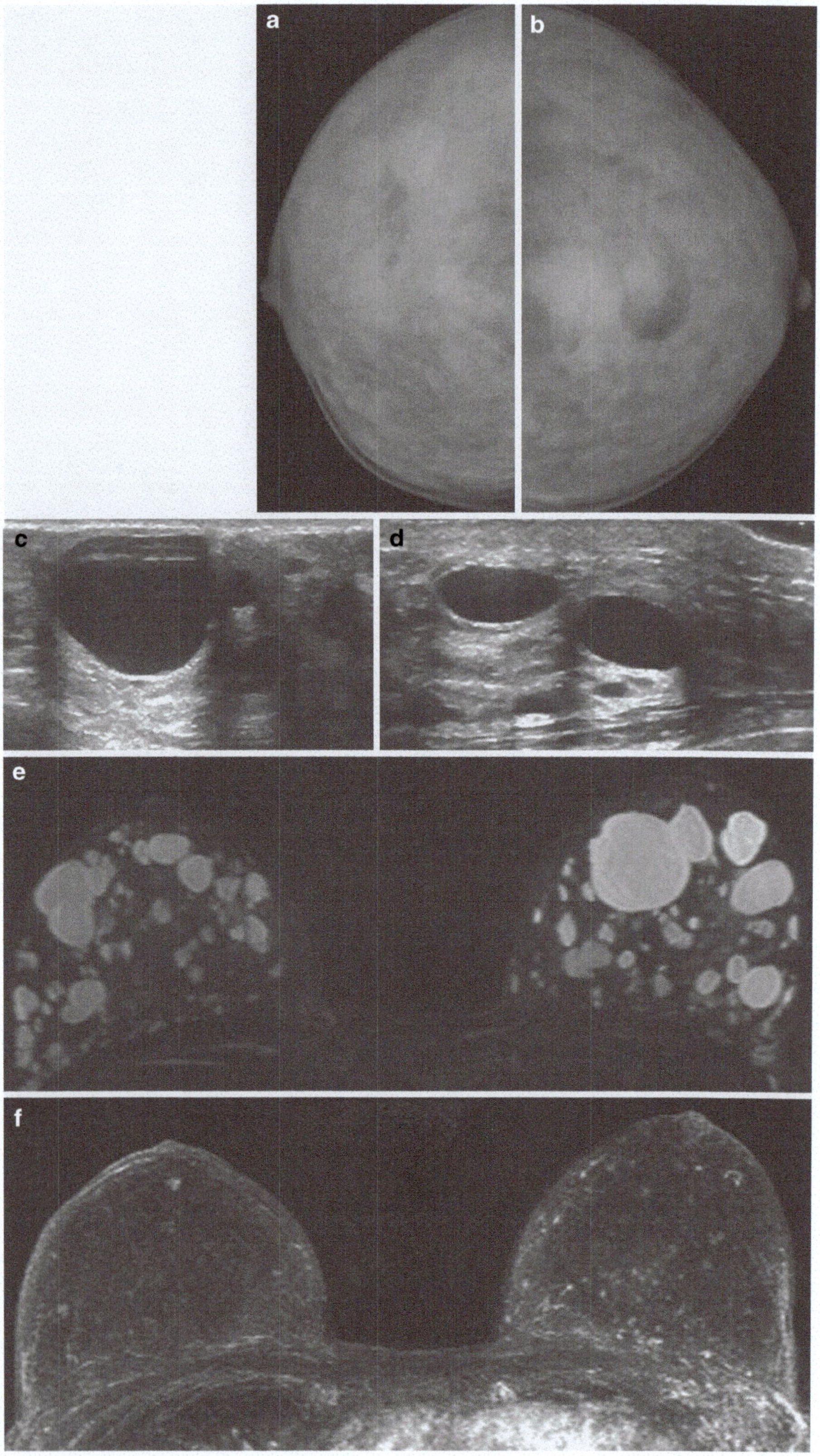

Fig. 12.6 MRI in a patient with extreme fibrocystic changes. Digital mammography in CC view shows extremely high density type IV according to the American College of Radiology and clearly reduced sensitivity (**a**, **b**). Multiple micro- and macro-cysts in both breasts on ultrasound (**c**: right breast, **d**: left breast). Demonstration of the multitude of cysts in both breasts in the MIP presentation of water-sensitive IR images (**e**). High reliability for the detection of breast cancer in the MIP of the MRI subtraction images (**f**). Demonstrating only few small foci (MRM-density type I)

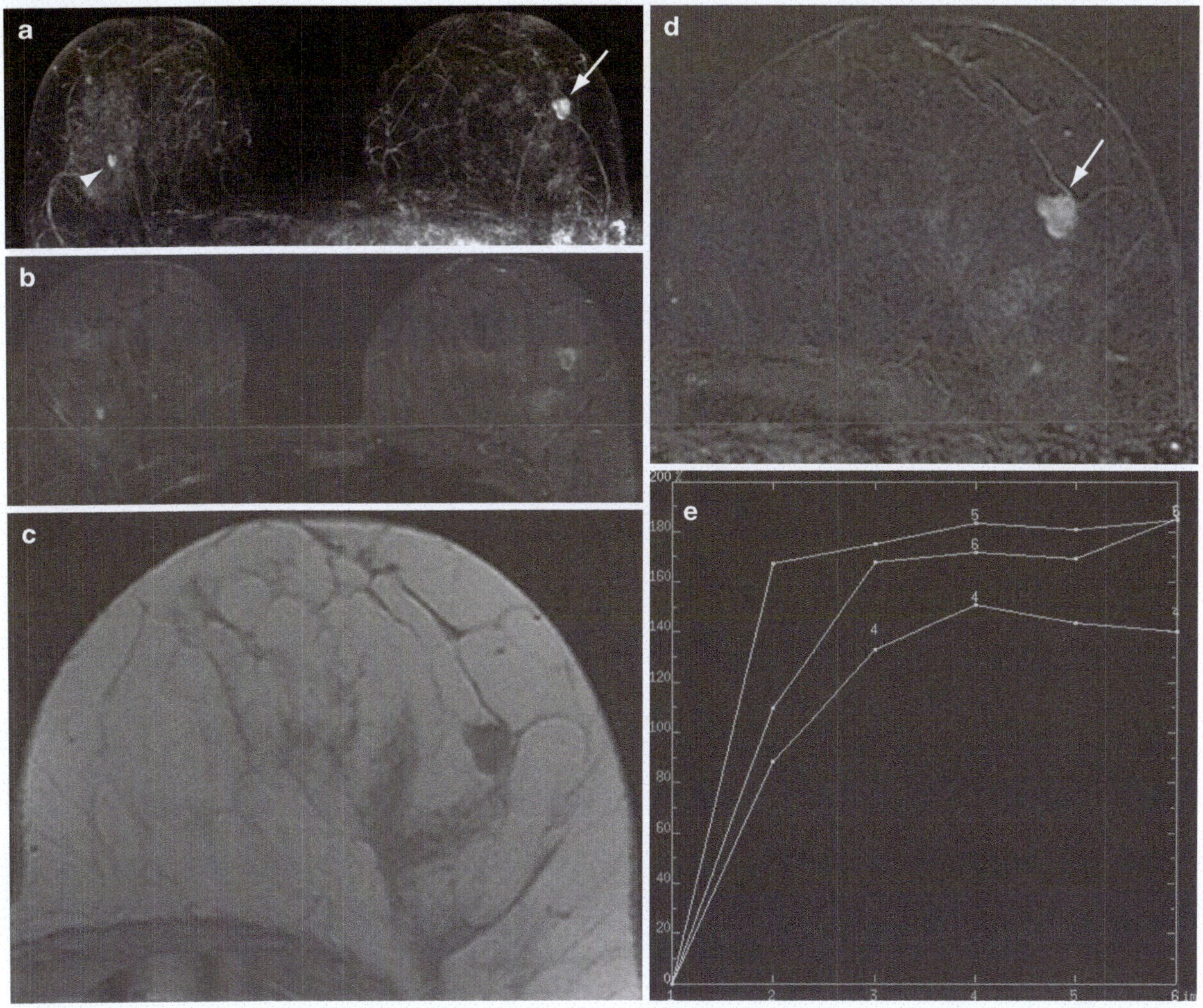

Fig. 12.7 Myxoid fibroadenoma (*arrows*) of the breast on MRI. Lobulated, well-defined mass with endotumoral septation in the lateral aspect of the left breast. Additional small tumor with similar signal behavior in the center of the right breast (*arrowhead*). Presentation in MIP technique (**a**). High water content of both tumors in T2-IR single slice with improved visualization of the endotumoral septations (**b**). Left tumor in precontrast T1-WI (**c**) and in single slice subtraction image (**d**). Signal-to-time curve in the tumor, with strong initial increase (>160%) and post-initial plateau (**e**). Histology after percutaneous core biopsy: myxoid fibroadenoma

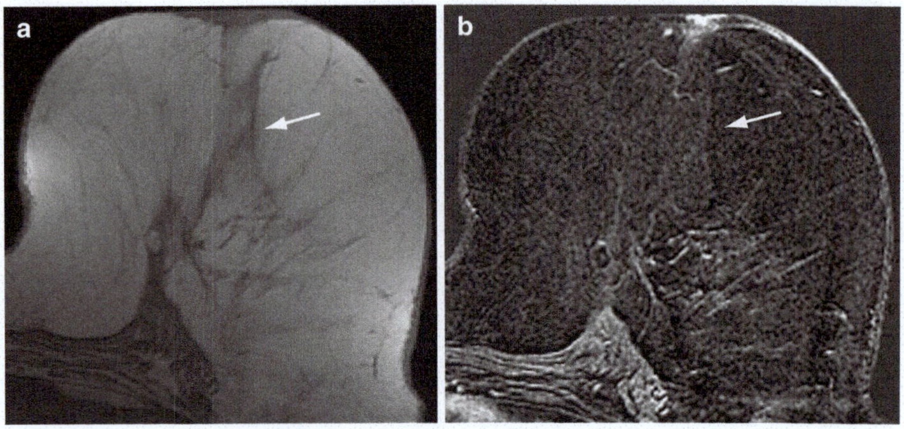

Fig. 12.8 Postoperative scarring (*arrows*) in MRI. MRI after breast conserving therapy in a patient with a history of a small breast cancer 3 years ago. The T1-W precontrast image showed a scar with an architectural distortion accompanied by a fat necrosis (**a**). Subtraction image after administration of contrast material demonstrated no enhancement within the scar (**b**). Follow up over more than 2 years confirmed the diagnosis of a postoperative scar

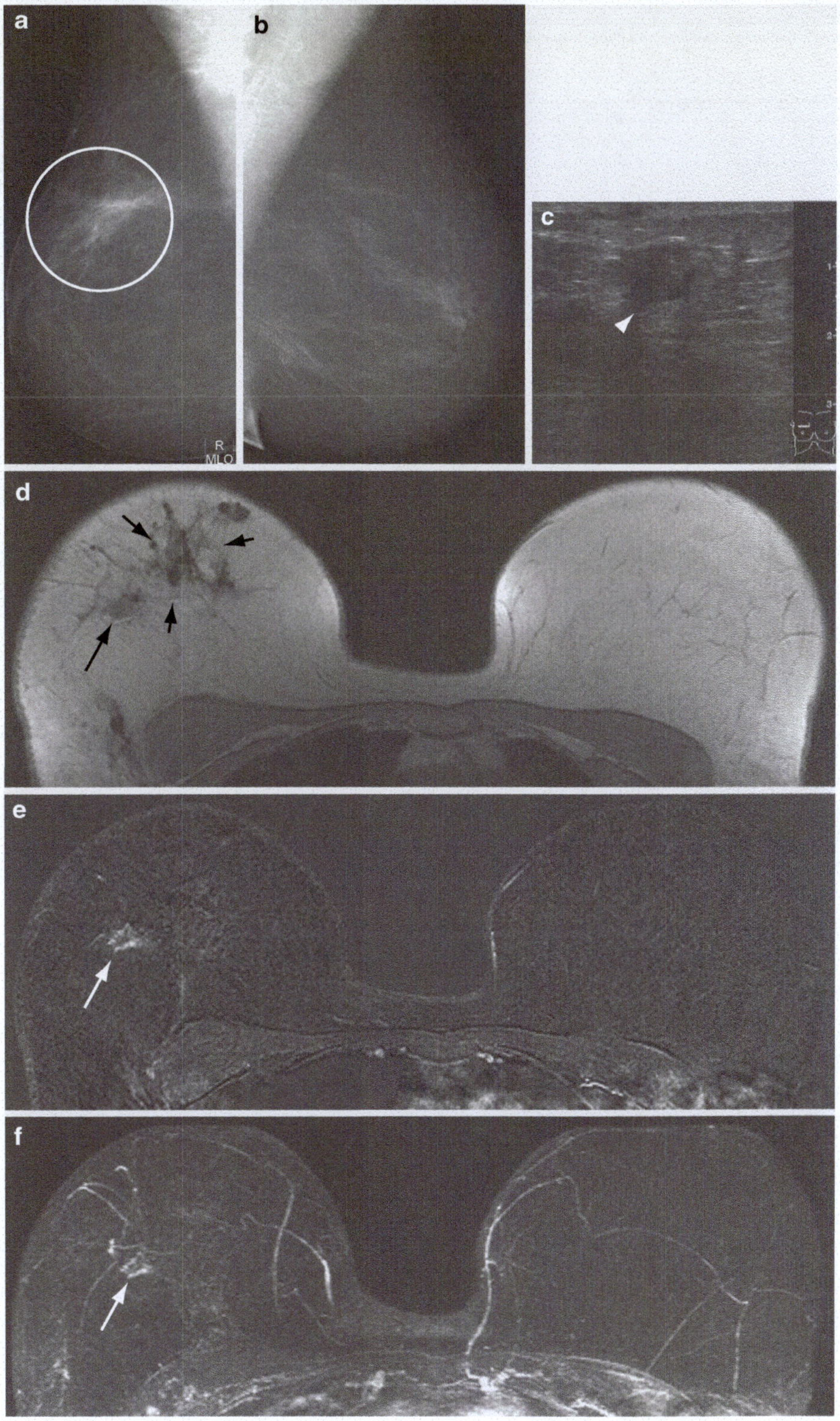

Fig. 12.9 Tumor relapse after breast conserving therapy (BCT). Digital mammography of both breasts in MLO view 3 years after BCT on the right side (**a, b**). Architectural distortion in the right breast compatible with a postoperative scar (*circle*) (**a**). Ultrasound in the region of tumorectomy demonstrates a circumscribed signal alteration compatible with fat necrosis (**c**) (*arrowhead*). The precontrast T1-W GE sequence shows multiple susceptibility artifacts due to electro-cautering during surgery (**d**) (*short arrows*). The single slice subtraction image demonstrates an irregular enhancement within the scar region (**e**). Presentation of the non-mass-like enhancement in MIP technique (**f**). Histology after MR-guided vacuum biopsy revealed invasive ductal carcinoma (tumor recurrence) (*long arrows*)

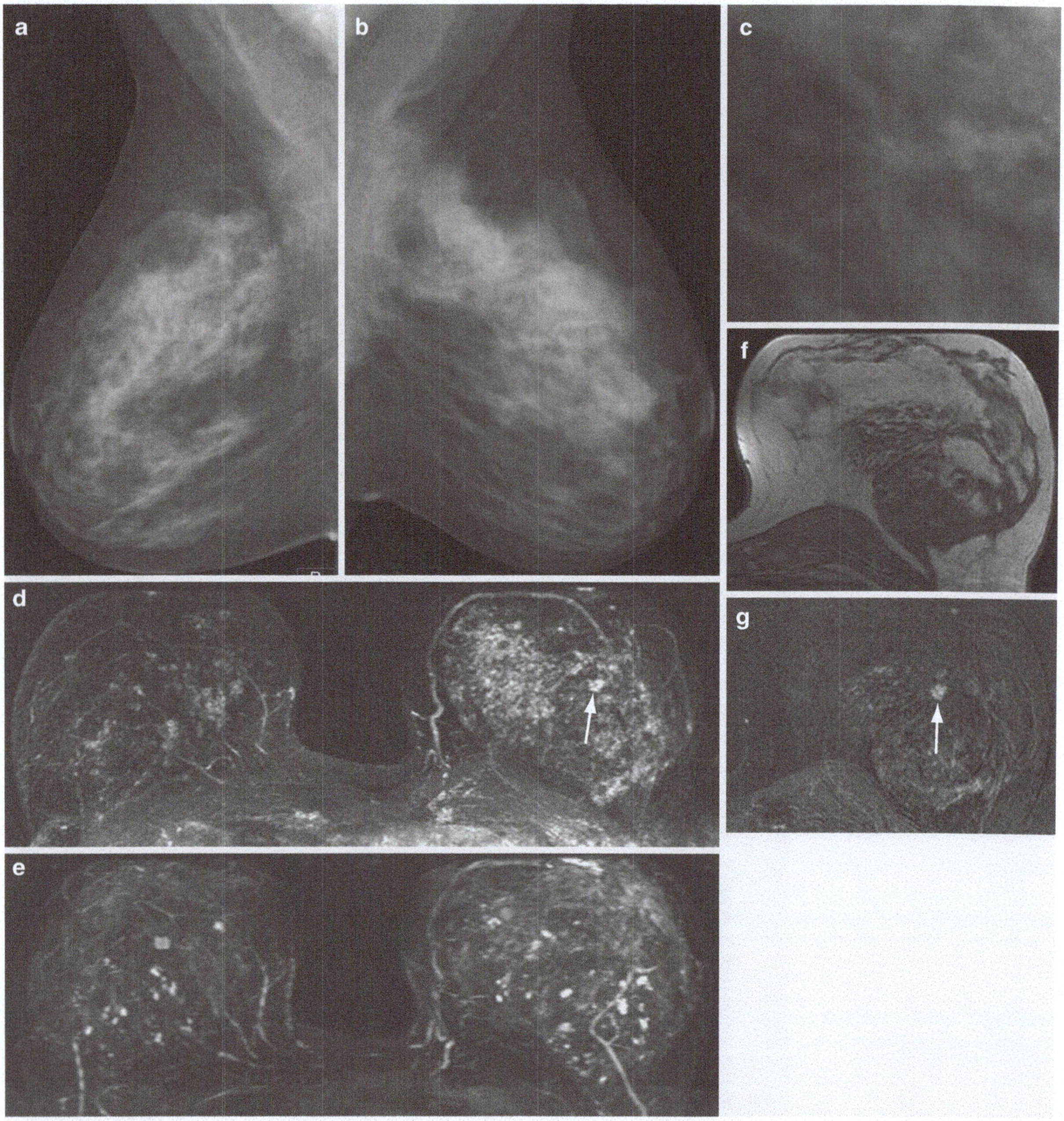

Fig. 12.10 Radial scar with associated small breast cancer. Digital mammography in MLO projection (**a**, **b**). Density type ACR IV. Architectural distortion in the center of the left breast (**b**), better seen on magnification mammogram (**c**). MRI demonstrates asymmetric uptake of the contrast material (left > right). Small hypervascularized nodule in the center of the left breast (**d**), without water signal on T2 IR image (**e**, MIP technique). Reproducibility of the architectural distortion on precontrast T1-W gradient echo sequence (**f**), with the enhancing ill-defined lesion in the center of the distortion (**g**, single slice subtraction image) (*arrows*). Histology after MR-guided vacuum biopsy: 3 mm invasive ductal carcinoma within a radial scar

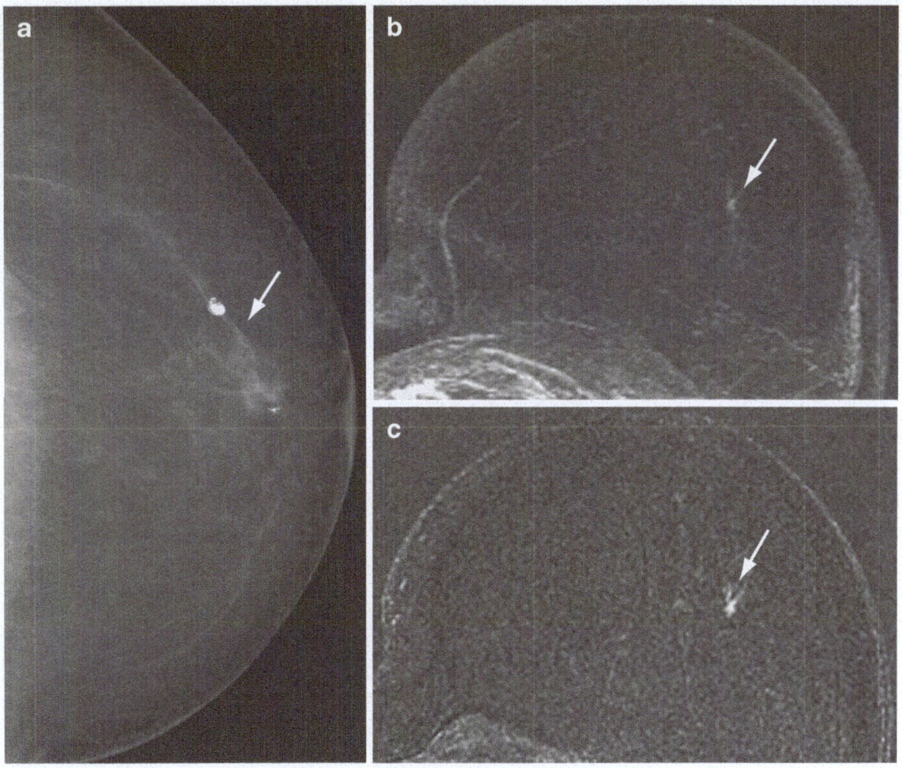

Fig. 12.11 Small high-grade DCIS in MRI. Digital mammography of the left breast in CC view. No suspicious findings. Macrocalcification (**a**). Small dendritic enhancement (non-mass-like lesion) in the lateral part of the left breast in MIP technique (**b**) and on single slice subtraction image (**c**). Histology after preoperative MR-guided needle localization: high-grade DCIS of 24 mm size (*arrows*)

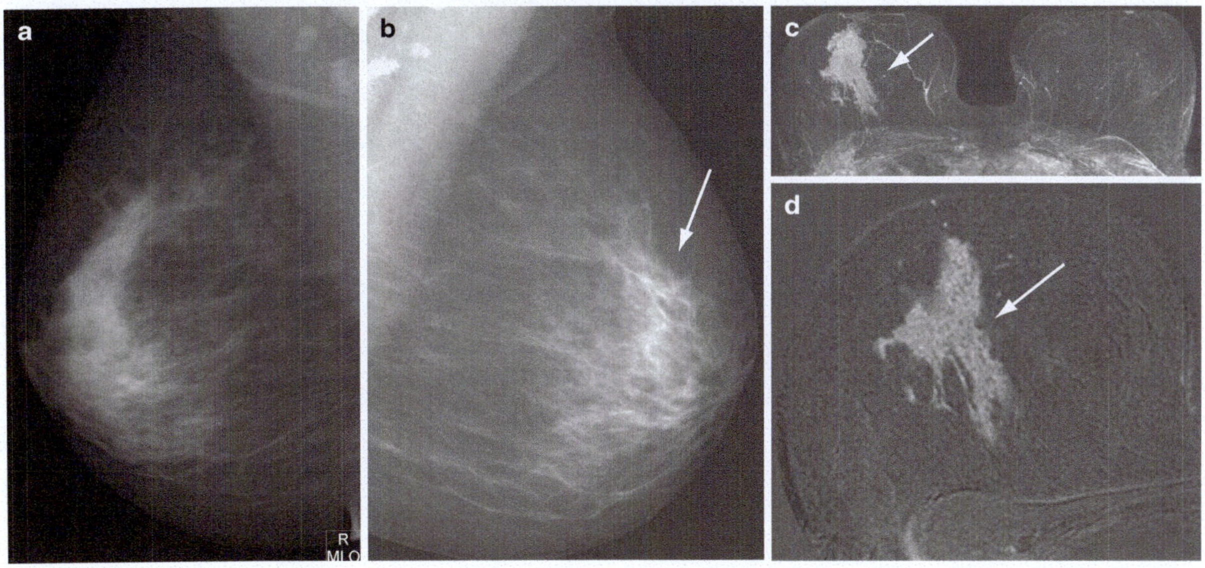

Fig. 12.12 Large high-grade DCIS in MRI. Digital mammography of both breasts in medio-lateral view. Shrinking sign of the parenchymal structures of the right breast without any associated microcalcifications (**a**, **b**). Large non-mass-like enhancement in the center of the right breast in MIP technique (**c**) and on single slice subtraction image (**d**). Histology after open biopsy (mastectomy): high-grade DCIS size (*arrows*)

Fig. 12.13 Small invasive lobular breast carcinoma in mammographically dense breasts. Digital mammography of both breasts demonstrates normal findings. Density ACR type III. BI-RADS right 1, left 1 (**a**, **b**). Demonstration of an 11 mm lesion in the center of the left breast. MR-density type I. Histology after MR-guided vacuum biopsy and open biopsy: ILC, pT1b, pN0, G2, R0 (*arrow*) (**c**)

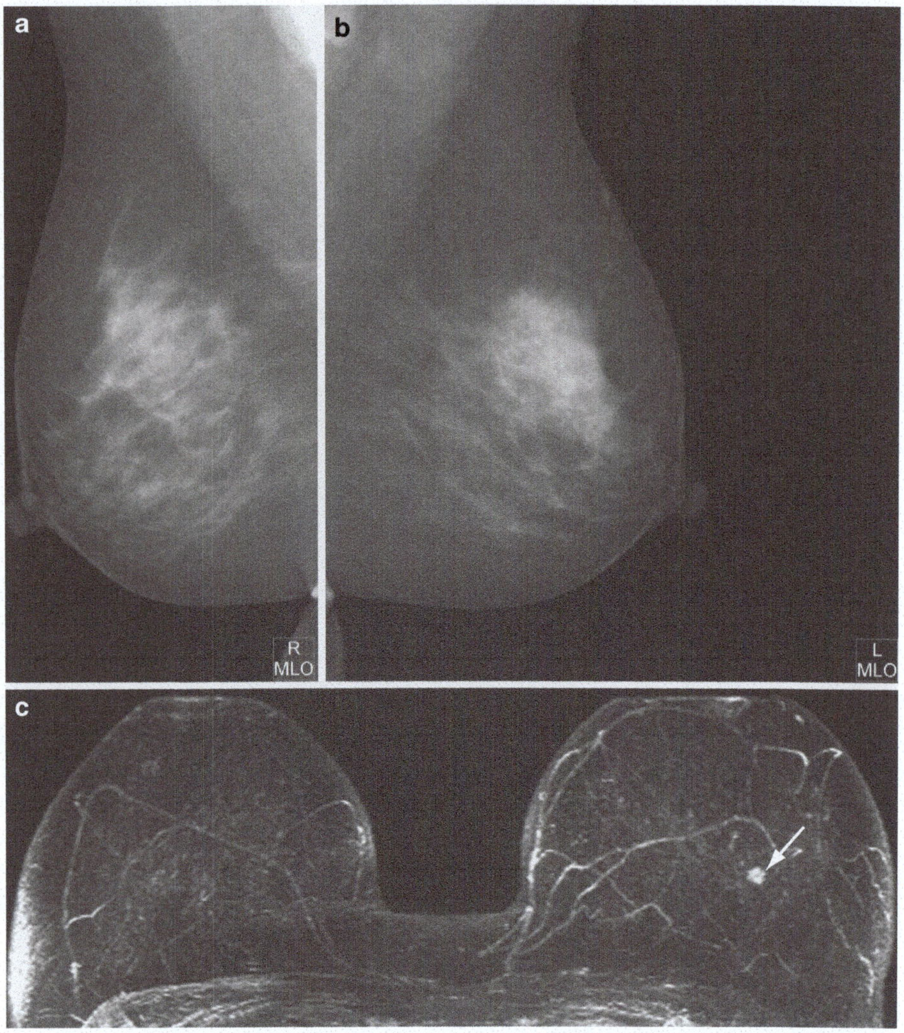

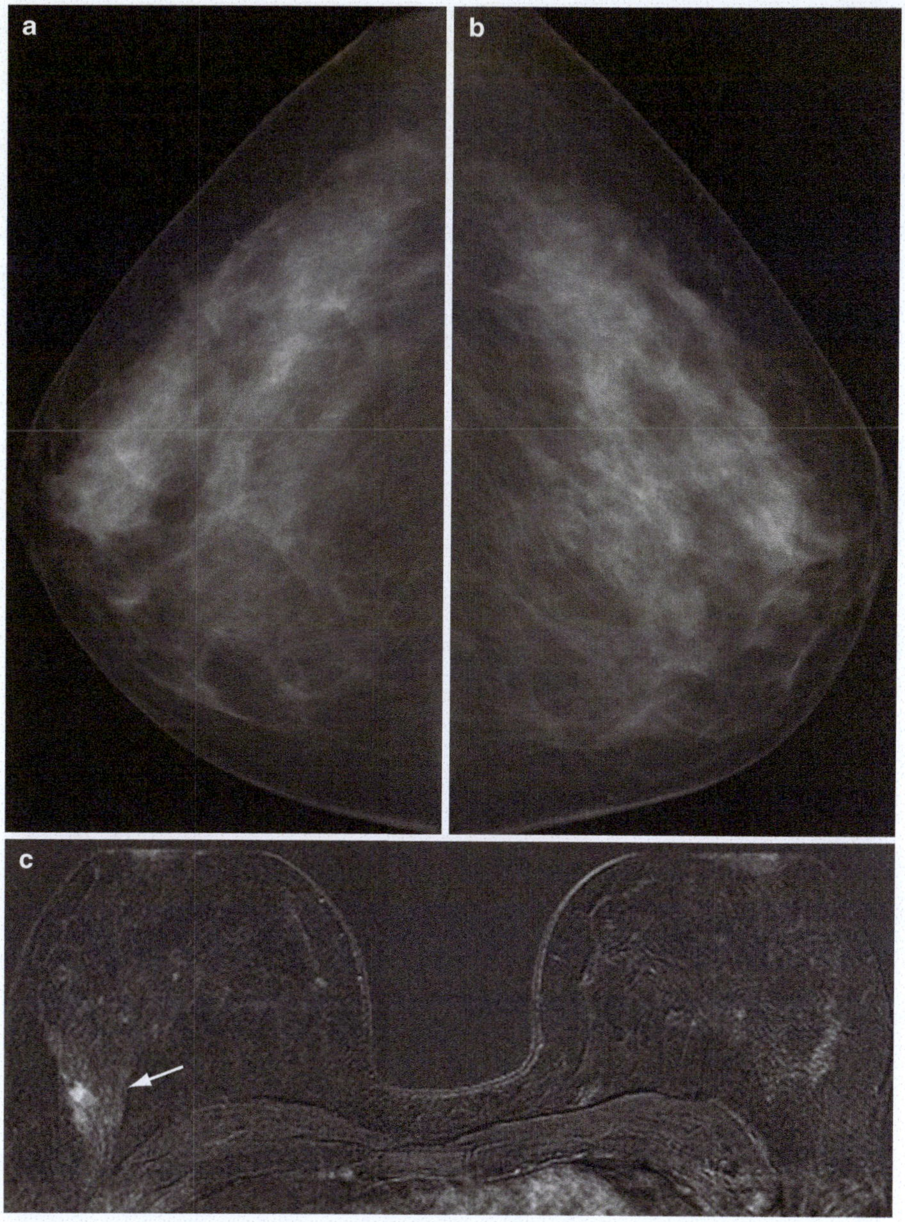

Fig. 12.14 Small invasive ductal breast carcinoma in mammographically dense breasts. Digital mammography of both breasts demonstrates normal findings. Density ACR type III. BI-RADS right 1, left 1 (**a**, **b**). Depiction of an 8 mm invasive ductal breast cancer in the lateral parts of the left breast with surrounding non-mass-like enhancement, suspicious for extensive intraductal component (EIC). MR-density type I. Histology after US-guided core biopsy (second-look) and open biopsy: IDC, pT1b, pN0, G2, R0 (*arrow*) (**c**)

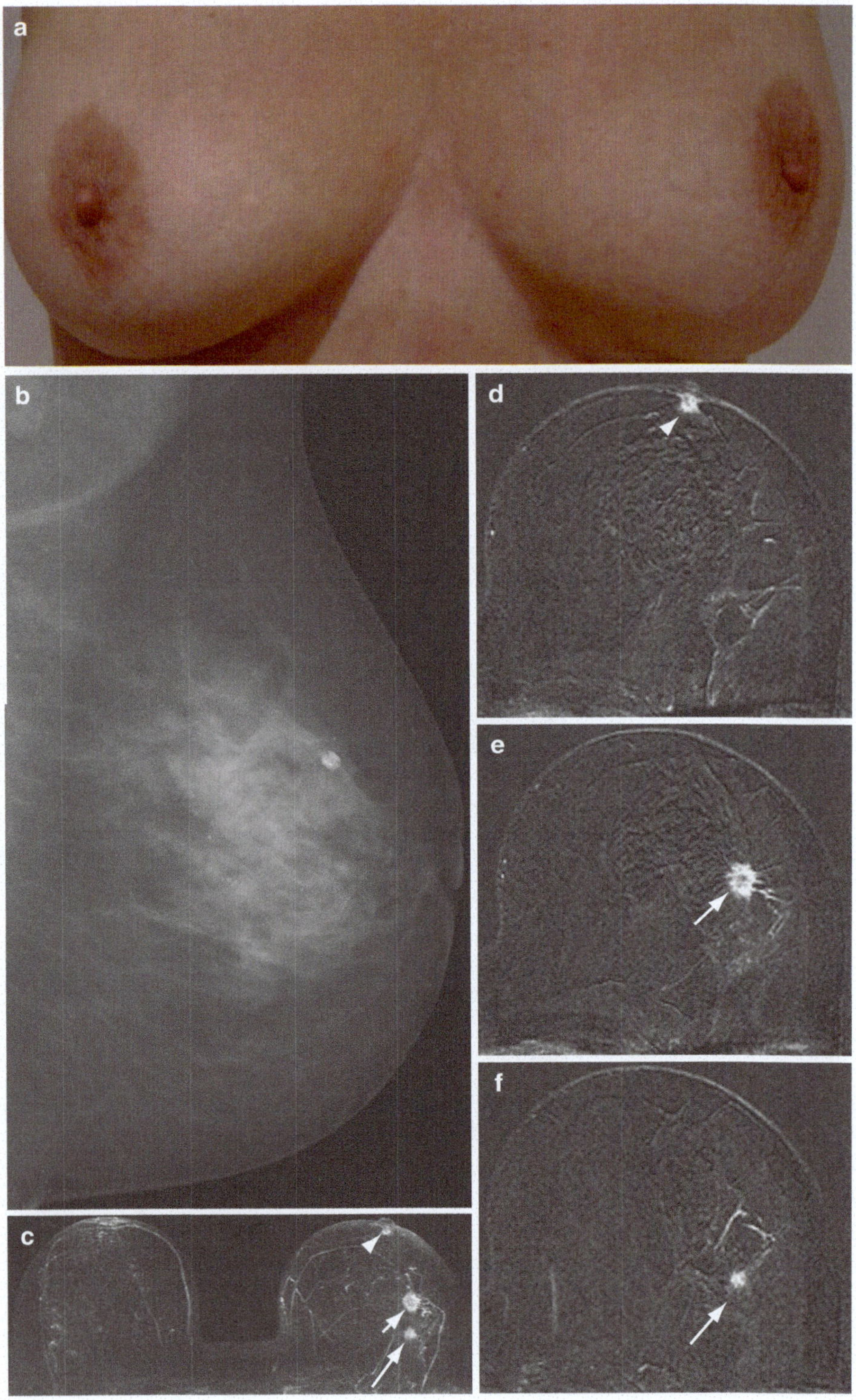

Fig. 12.15 Preoperative local staging in a patient with a trifocal breast cancer. Digital mammogram of a patient with left-sided nipple retraction (**a**) demonstrates dense parenchymal tissue (ACR type IV), unsuspicious diffuse calcifications, and nipple retraction (**b**). MRI depicted a small enhancing lesion directly behind the left nipple (**d**), the index tumor in the lateral part of the left breast (also seen on ultrasound, **e**), and a third enhancing nodule in the lower outer quadrant (**f**). Visualization of all three tumors in MIP technique (**c**). Histology revealed invasive ductal carcinoma of 13 mm (index tumor), and further cancer manifestations in the retromamillary region (6 mm) and in the lower outer quadrant (12 mm; pT1c, pN1a, G2) (*different arrows*)

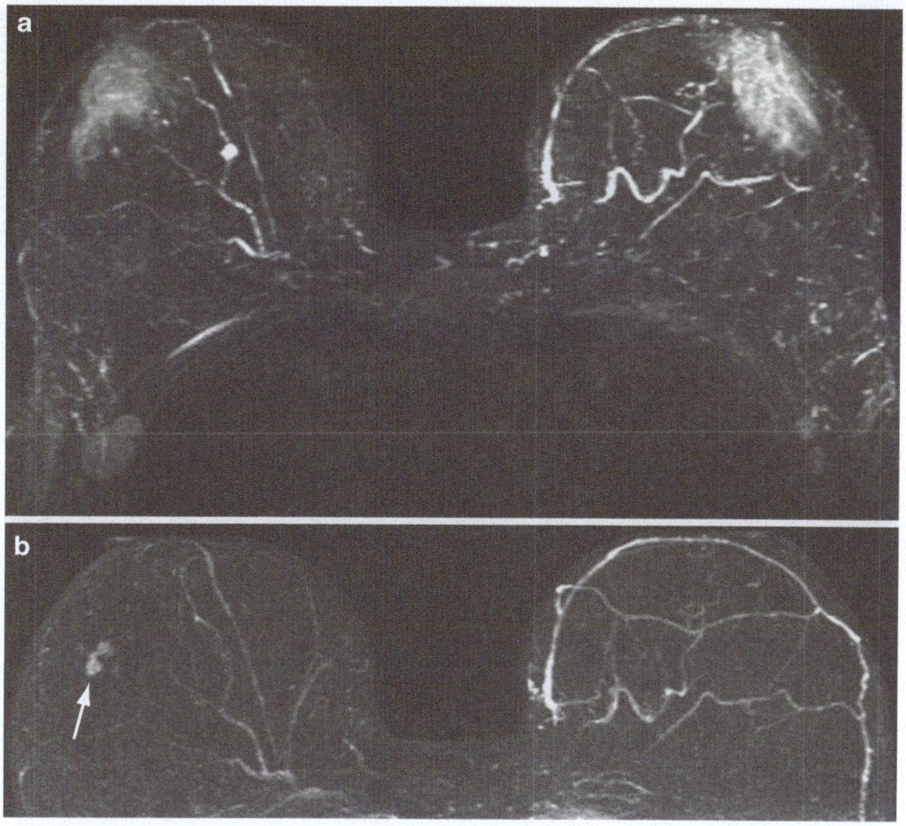

Fig. 12.16 MRI in patient with CUP syndrome (carcinoma of unknown primary). Pathologic enlargement of a lymph node in the right axilla was noticed by this patient. Histopathology after US-guided core biopsy revealed a metastasis of an adenocarcinoma. Mammography and ultrasound did not show any suspicious lesion. T2-W MR imaging demonstrated lymph node metastasis in the right axilla (**a**, MIP of T2 images). MIP of subtraction images depicted the primary carcinoma of 8 mm size in the lateral parts of the right breast (*arrow*) (**b**). Open biopsy after needle localization confirmed this diagnosis (IDC, pT1b, pN2)

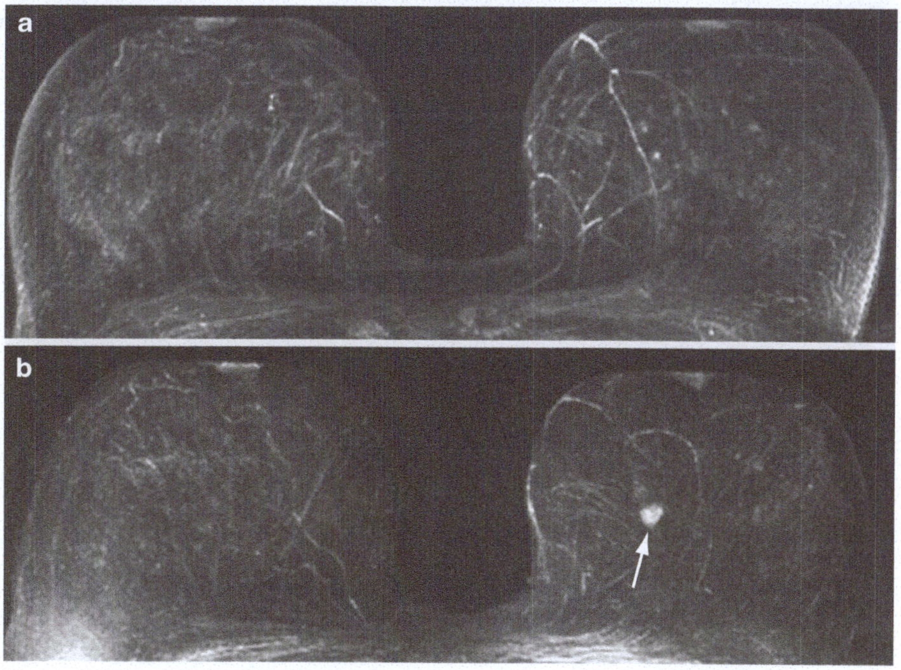

Fig. 12.17 Goettinger Optipack – follow–up. MRI in a woman with high familial risk profile. MIP of subtraction images demonstrates several foci in both breasts (**a**). No suspicious findings were diagnosed (MRM BI-RADS 1). Eighteen months later, MRI depicts an 8 mm enhancing mass in the center of the left breast (**b**). This lesion was occult in mammography and ultrasound. MR-guided vacuum biopsy verified an invasive ductal carcinoma (pT1c, pN0) (*arrow*)

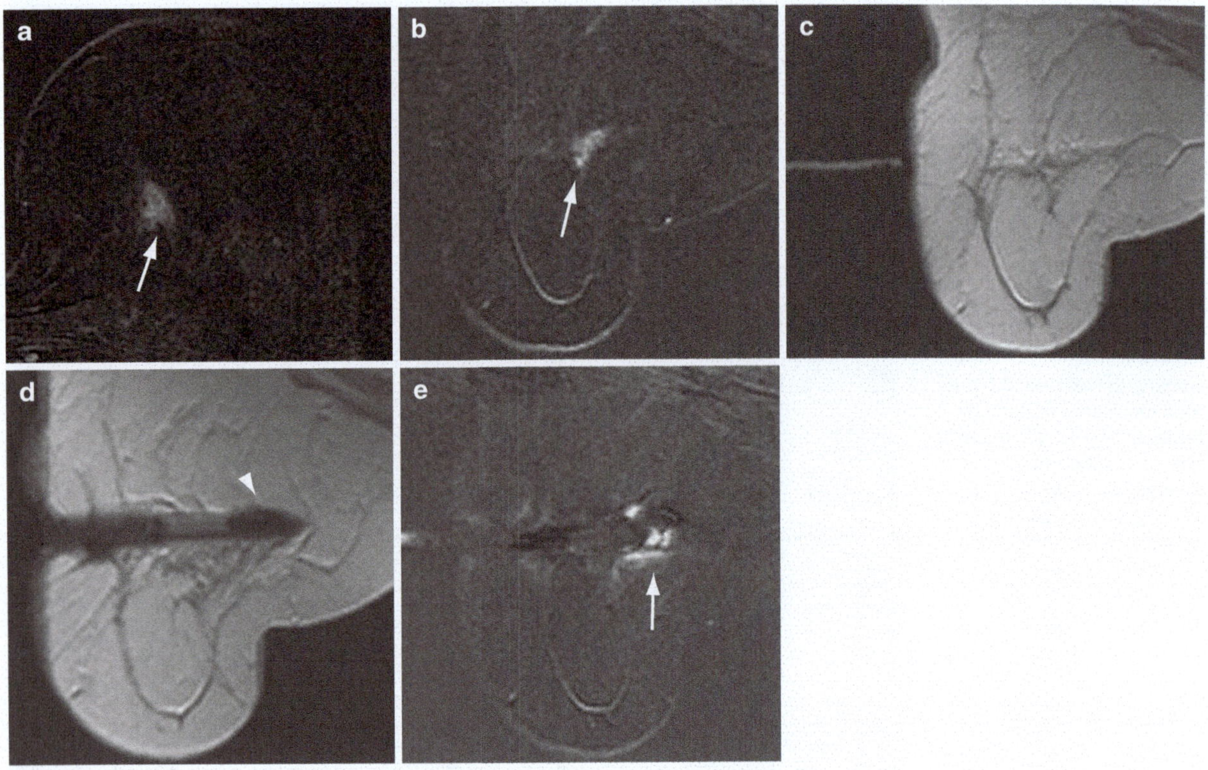

Fig. 12.18 MR-guided vacuum biopsy of the breast. Suspicious non-mass-like lesion on diagnostic MRI of the breast, categorized as MRM-BI-RADS IV (**a**; single slice subtraction image). Reproduction of the enhancing lesion during the MR-guided interventional procedure (*arrowhead*) (**b**). Confirmation of the correct needle position after calculation of appropriate coordinates (**c**). Documentation of the coaxial cannula with the notch in the center of the lesion (**d**). Final documentation of the successful biopsy after renewed application of contrast material and subtraction image (**e**). Histology revealed a radial scar without associated carcinoma (*arrows*)

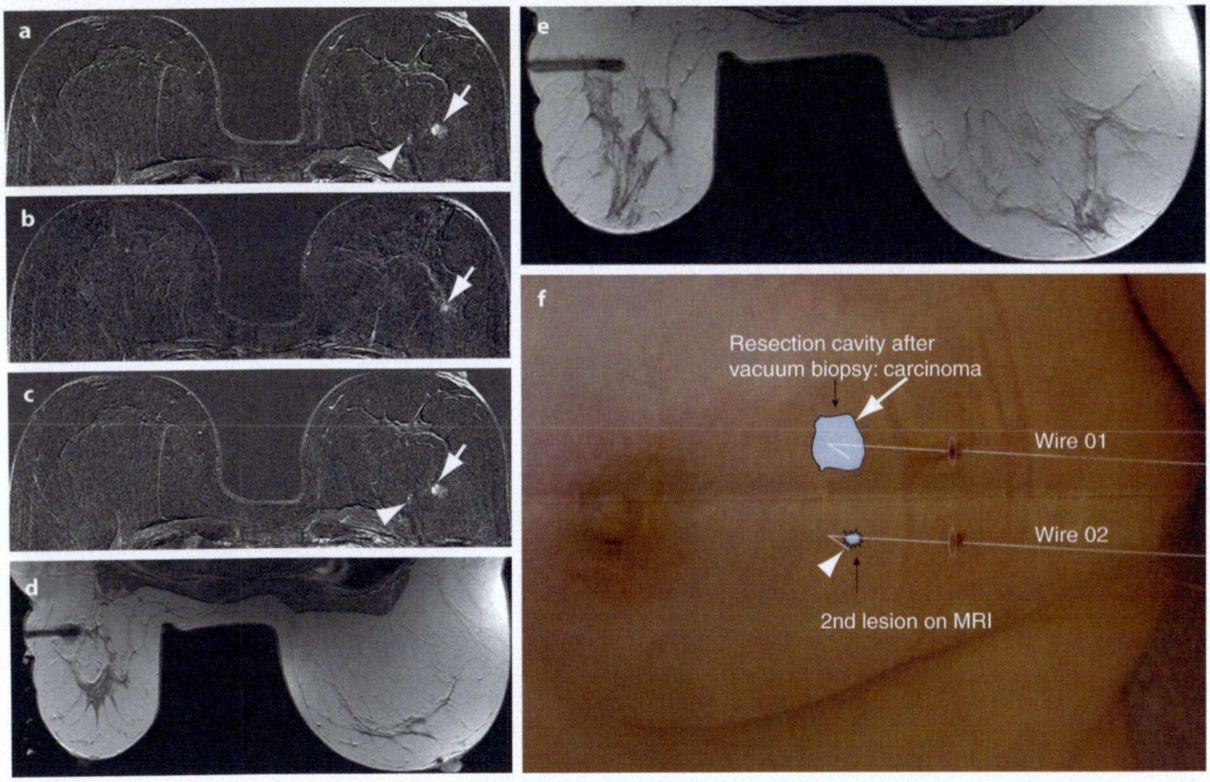

Fig. 12.19 MR-guided preoperative wire localization of two lesions. Diagnostic contrast-enhanced MRI of the breast with an enhancing mass (index tumor) in the outer upper quadrant of the left breast (*arrows*) (**a**) and another enhancing focus 2 cm caudally from the first (*arrowheads*) (**b**). Demonstration of both findings in MIP projection (**c**). Histology of the index tumor after percutaneous vacuum biopsy: invasive lobular breast cancer. Precise preoperative wire localization of the cavity after vacuum biopsy (**d**) and the second lesion (**e**). Photo documentation after intervention with presentation of the wire positions. Final histology: invasive lobular carcinoma pT1b, pN0 (index tumor); lobular carcinoma in situ (second lesion)

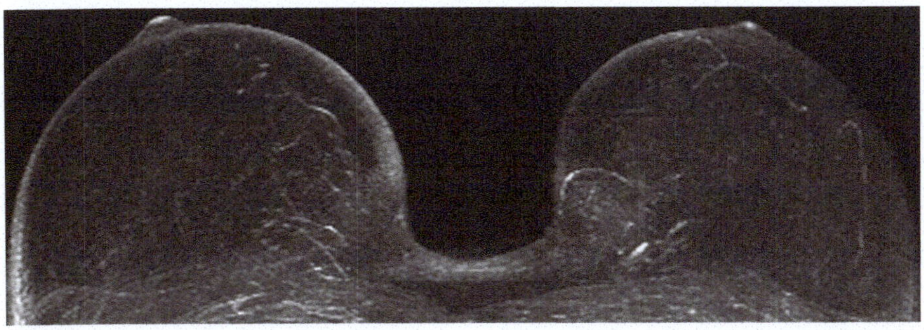

Fig. 12.20 MRM-BI-RADS 1 in superior quality MRI – do we need more diagnostics? High resolution MRI of the breast without any motion artifact (MRI artifact type I) demonstrating no parenchymal enhancement after administration of contrast material (MRI density type I) and no enhancing lesion (MRI-BI-RADS 1). In this situation, a relevant breast tumor can be excluded with extremely high reliability. In this constellation, two questions are important: Can additional mammography give more information than MRI has already given? Is it ethical to perform an additional mammography, considering the radiation exposure?

Further Reading

Berg W et al (2004) Diagnostic accuracy of mammography, clinical examination, US, and MR imaging in preoperative assessment of breast cancer. Radiology 233:830–849

Fischer U (1999) Lehratlas der MR-mammographie. Thieme, Stuttgart. ISBN 3131185813

Fischer U et al (2006) Preoperative MR imaging in patients with breast cancer: preoperative staging, effects on recurrence rates, and outcome analysis. Magn Reson Imaging Clin N Am 14:11–12

Fischer U et al (2008) MR-gesteuerte interventionen. In: Interventionen der Mamma. Thieme, Stuttgart, pp 86–126

Ikeda D et al. ACR-imaging and reporting system - magnetic resonance imaging? illustrated BI-RADS?-MRI?. American College of Radiology, Reston, VA (in press)

Kriege M et al (2004) Efficacy of MRI and mammography for breast-cancer screening in women with a familial or genetic predisposition. NEJM 352:427–437

Kuhl CK (2007a) The current status of breast MR imaging. Part I: choice of technique, image interpretation, diagnostic accuracy, and transfer to clinical practice. Radiology 244: 356–378

Kuhl CK (2007b) The current status of breast MR imaging. Part II: clinical applications. Radiology 244:672–691

Kuhl CK et al (2007) MRI for diagnosis of pure ductal carcinoma in situ: a prospective observation study. Lancet 370:485–492

Orel SG (2001) MR imaging of the breast. Magn Reson Imaging Clin N Am 9:273–288

Sardanelli F (2004) Sensitivity of MRI versus mammography for detecting foci of multifocal, multicentric breast cancer in fatty and dense breasts using the whole-breast pathologic examination as a gold standard. AJR 183:1149–1157

Magnetic Resonance Imaging of Pediatric Patients

13

Birgit Kammer, Hermann Helmberger, Claudia M. Keser, Eva Coppenrath, and Karl Schneider

Contents

13.1 General Considerations and Remarks for MRI of Pediatric Patients

The lack of radiation exposure, the possibility of multiplanar imaging, and the wide range of tissue contrast have made magnetic resonance imaging (MRI) an important tool in the evaluation of pediatric diseases. Unfortunately, majority of the radiologists are not as familiar as necessary with normal variations, developmental anomalies, and the variety of illnesses that are often unique in children. Therefore, a spectrum of uneasiness or discomfort to frank anxiety is encountered when it comes to pediatric radiology. The purpose of this chapter is to provide some basic information about the most common pediatric entities that differ from diseases in the adult population and will be sent to MRI for evaluation. There may be some overlap between this chapter and others in this book, but it is worthwhile to study the information given from different authors. In pediatric radiology, imaging studies like ultrasonography, conventional radiography, and fluoroscopy remain the primary imaging modalities for the majority of clinical requests. If there is a need for further evaluation and the diagnostic information from both CT and MRI is comparable,

B. Kammer (✉)
Pediatric Radiology, Dr. von Haunersches Kinderspital, LMU-University of Munich, Innenstadt Campus, Lindwurmstrasse 4, 80337 Munich, Germany
e-mail: Birgit.Kammer@med.uni-muenchen.de

P. Reimer et al. (eds.), *Clinical MR Imaging*,
DOI: 10.1007/978-3-540-74504-4_13, © Springer-Verlag Berlin Heidelberg 2010

then MRI should be the next step, to avoid radiation exposure. However, CT is a widely available and comparably quick method to evaluate a variety of diseases in a superb manner. A good quality CT may provide more information than a substandard MRI study. A good deal of a pediatric radiologist's daily work consists of reviewing imaging studies from different referral centers and deciding whether these studies are good enough to base clinical decisions on them. A poor CT or MRI study may have to be repeated, which leads to increasing costs, unnecessary radiation exposure, or additional sedation or general anesthesia. Therefore, it is of vital interest for pediatric radiologists to share their knowledge with other radiologists. In many institutions, majority of the children with diseases involving the airways and chest are evaluated by CT. Some diseases of the chest (i.e., tumors) occurring in other locations that require an MRI evaluation are covered in the abdominal and musculoskeletal section of this chapter. This chapter mainly focuses on brain, spine, abdominal, and musculoskeletal diseases in children. Some information about congenital heart disease is provided in Chap. 10.

13.1.1 Patient Preparation, Sedation, and Monitoring

It is essential for any successful pediatric examination to achieve sufficient immobilization of the frequently uncooperative patients during the long acquisition times. In the first 3 months of life, an examination after feeding and immobilization by wrapping in blankets may be sufficient. The age group between 3 months and 5 years requires sedation or even general anesthesia, thus necessitating the assistance of anesthesiologists. By the age of 5 years, a simple explanation of the examination and the attendance of the parents or nursing staff often enable a successful examination. If administration of intravenous paramagnetic contrast is necessary or planned, the referring colleagues should place a peripheral line in advance, to avoid excitement immediately before the examination.

Numerous protocols for sedation and general anesthesia have been developed in different hospitals; the choice of the protocol strongly depends on the radiologist's training and the availability of anesthesiologists. In our institution, the common practice includes monitored conscious sedation, deep sedation, or general anesthesia. For any sedation procedure, children should not eat or drink anything for at least 4 h prior to the examination. Monitoring of vital functions is fundamental, and easily achieved by the use of a pulse oximeter. A nurse remains in the procedure area for the imaging time and periodically records vital signs (oxygenation, ventilation, circulation, and temperature). When conscious sedation is the method selected, the physician applying sedative drugs should be familiar with those agents, aware of their possible complications, and must have some training in pediatric advanced life support. Drugs for conscious sedation include: (1) chlorprothixene 1–2 mg/kg orally, (2) chloral hydrate 50–100 mg/kg rectally, or (3) diazepam 0.2–0.5 mg/kg rectally. Alternatively, children can receive oral midazolam 0.2–0.5 mg/kg in a specially flavored preparation. Sufficient time should be allowed for drug administration before the onset of the procedure (0.5–1.5 h). For optimal sedation, it is often helpful to move the child and parents into a dark, quiet room after drug administration and wait until the patient is asleep. Monitored conscious sedation is most appropriate for healthy children and short diagnostic examinations. If deeper levels of sedation are necessary, a pediatric anesthesiologist must be in charge of the intravenous drug administration and monitoring. One intravenous regimen in our institution includes midazolam 0.1–0.15 mg/kg, supplemented with small doses of thiopental, if necessary. Another efficient sedation method for children is the titrated intravenous application of propofol 0.5–1.5 mg/kg until the child is asleep. Sedation is maintained by a continuous infusion of propofol 3–5 mg/kg/h during imaging time. After the procedure is completed, all sedated children should be transferred to a recovery room close to the examination area. Monitoring should be continued until the patient is alert and able to drink. For many examinations, general anesthesia with tracheal intubation is the best choice.

13.1.2 Contrast Media

Administration of paramagnetic contrast is necessary in many clinical requests. For children, 0.2 mL/kg of gadolinium chelates is used for intravenous application.

Oral contrast media and organ-specific contrast agents are not approved for use in children on a regular basis.

13.2 Pediatric Brain Imaging

13.2.1 Technique

13.2.1.1 Coils and Patient Positioning

The standard head coil, recently available as multichannel phased array coil, is used for the majority of examinations of the pediatric brain. If available, dedicated pediatric head and/or spine coils offer better spatial resolution and signal-to-noise ratio, especially in very small infants. Optimal positioning in the center of the coil, and immobilization with vacuum beds, sponges, sand bags, and blankets are mandatory for the patients.

13.2.1.2 Sequence Protocol

Sequences used in pediatric brain imaging are spin-echo (SE) or fast spin-echo (FSE), and also gradient-echo (GRE) sequences if available. In addition, inversion recovery (IR) sequences and diffusion-weighted imaging (DWI) are used.

SE sequences are still commonly used because of their accurate anatomical depiction of brain tissue and representation of tissue characteristics based on T1- and T2-relaxation. Frequently used parameters are repetition times (TR) of 500–600 ms and echo times (TE) of 10–15 for T1-WI. For T2-WI, a differentiation of the parameters according to the age of the patient is recommended. To maximize T2 differences between the normal unmyelinated brain tissue and abnormal tissue in the first 18 months of life, it is necessary to use longer TR. A repetition time of at least 3,000 ms and an echo time of 120 ms should be chosen in children from birth to 3 months of age. TR of 3,000 ms and TE of 100 ms are recommended in children from 3 to 6 months. For children older than 6 months, TR of at least 2,500 ms and TE of 100 ms should be used.

IR sequences are most commonly used for one of two reasons: to improve T1 contrast or to eliminate the signal from one tissue. IR sequences significantly improve T1-weighted (T1-W) contrast by doubling the distance that spins have to recover. Thus, these sequences are ideal to evaluate myelination and subtle lesions such as cortical dysplasia. Fluid attenuated IR (FLAIR) sequences eliminate the signal from cerebrospinal fluid (CSF) by using a T1 around 2,000 ms, and allow images of the brain with no fluid signal for heavily T2-W.

A three-dimensional (3D) GRE can also be used to obtain T1-WIs with excellent gray/white matter differentiation. This technique also has the ability to acquire very thin contiguous images (<1 mm), and can be reformatted in any plane due to isotropic image matrices. These sequences are specially recommended for the evaluation of complex malformations, tumors, and subtle lesions.

For studies of the intracranial vasculature, 3D time of flight (TOF), multislice 2D phase contrast (PC), 2D TOF or contrast-enhanced 3D-GRE sequences should also be performed. To quantify cerebrospinal fluid (CSF) flow, a 3D PC sequence can be used.

DWI or high-resolution DWI is commonly applied in all patients, due to very short acquisition time and its potential to detect very early pathologic findings. Further applications are diffusion tensor imaging modalities. In special cases, MR spectroscopy, if available, is a useful tool.

In addition to the transverse plane, a sagittal plane is mandatory for the evaluation of the corpus callosum, midline structural development, and tumors. In elucidation of schizencephaly, holoprosencephaly, septo-optic dysplasia, and periventricular leukomalacia, coronal planes are helpful. Furthermore, in patients with seizures, evaluation of the hippocampus in the coronal plane in thin slices is necessary. Another important thing to keep in mind is that the examination must be performed within the time frame of either allowable sedation or patience of the little patients. The order of sequences should be chosen so that the essential information is acquired first.

13.2.2 Developmental Anomalies

The development of the brain is a complex process, beginning with the closure of the neural tube during the fourth week of gestation. Classification systems for malformations of the cerebrum, cerebellum, and brainstem are constantly revised according to newer insights delivered by scientific research. It is beyond the scope of this chapter to cover this very special neuroradiological knowledge, and therefore I will stay with the old traditional concept. In a simplified manner, developmental abnormalities can be classified into two main types. The first category consists of disorders of organogenesis in which genetic defects or any ischemic, metabolic, toxic, or infectious insult to the developing brain can cause malformation. These malformations result from abnormal neuronal and glial proliferation and from anomalies of neuronal migration and/or cortical organization. They may be supra- and/or infratentorial and/or may involve gray and white matter. When dealing with these kinds of abnormalities, the examiner should keep in mind that as soon as one anomaly is found, expanded scrutiny of the whole brain for further anomalies is required. The second category of congenital brain abnormalities is disorders of histogenesis, which result from abnormal cell differentiation with a relatively normal brain appearance. The neurocutaneous abnormalities (phakomatosis) fall into this group.

13.2.2.1 Anomalies of Organogenesis

Anomalies of the Corpus Callosum

Formation of the corpus callosum occurs during weeks 8–20 of gestational age. It is composed of four sections: the rostrum, the genu, the body, and the splenium. Anteriorly, the corpus callosum forms from the genu, progressing posteriorly through the body to the splenium. The rostrum (anterior) forms last. The normal corpus callosum appears thin at birth and thickens as myelination of its fibers occurs, a process that develops from posterior to anterior. Any insult occurring during formation always affects the posterior aspect of the corpus callosum and the rostrum, which results in partial agenesis. If insult occurs very early, complete agenesis may be the result. The sagittal images clearly show the exact extent of callosal dysgenesis. Loss of the supporting function of the corpus callosum leads to a high riding third ventricle, occasionally extending between the interhemispheric fissure to form an interhemispheric cyst. Axons usually crossing the interhemispheric fissure within the corpus callosum instead extend medially to the medial walls of the lateral ventricles, parallel to the interhemispheric fissure. These so-called bundles of Probst invaginate the medial borders of the lateral ventricles to give them a crescent shape in the coronal plane (Fig. 13.1). The anterior commissure is usually present, whereas the hippocampal commissure is usually absent or hypoplastic. A further consequence of an absent corpus callosum is an everted cingulate gyrus and an absent cingulate sulcus, as normal inversion of the cingulate gyrus and consecutive formation of the cingulate sulcus do not take place. As a result, the mesial hemispheric sulci course uninterrupted, in a radial manner, into the third ventricle (Fig. 13.2). The shape and the size of the normal ventricular system, especially posteriorly, are maintained by the presence of an intact corpus callosum. When the genu is absent, the frontal horns are prominent and are laterally convex instead of concave. In case of an absent body, the lateral ventricles are straight and parallel. If the splenium is missing, the trigones and the occipital horns dilate more and may be strikingly distended, a condition referred to as colpocephaly. The associated anomalies are Arnold-Chiari II, neuronal migration disorders, Dandy-Walker complex, and interhemispheric lipoma. Most patients have mental retardation, seizures, or a large head; only a small proportion remains asymptomatic.

Cephaloceles

The term cephaloceles refers to a defect in the skull and dura, with extension of intracranial structures. Cephaloceles are divided into four types: *meningoencephaloceles* (Fig. 13.3) are herniations of brain tissue, CSF, and meninges through a skull defect; *meningoceles* consist of meninges and CSF; *atretic cephaloceles* are formes fruste of cephaloceles consisting of dura, fibrous tissue, and degenerated brain tissue; *glioceles* refers to herniation of a glial-lined cyst containing CSF. The cause of cephaloceles is still under debate; some authors argue that this condition is due to failure of neurulation, while others claim that cephaloceles are not a result of brain maldevelopment, but rather a calvarial defect, which allows extracranial herniation of the brain and the meninges. However, it is most likely that cephaloceles are the result of several developmental disorders. Cephaloceles may be occipital, frontoethmoidal, and, rarely, parietal or sphenoidal. Atretic cephaloceles are located in the midline parietal and present as sub-scalp masses, which are connected by a fibrous tract to the dura via the cranium bifidum. The sagittal venous sinus is divided by this tract (Fig. 13.4), and very often a persistent falcine vein points to cephalocele. MRI, MRA, and CECT are complementary tools in the evaluation

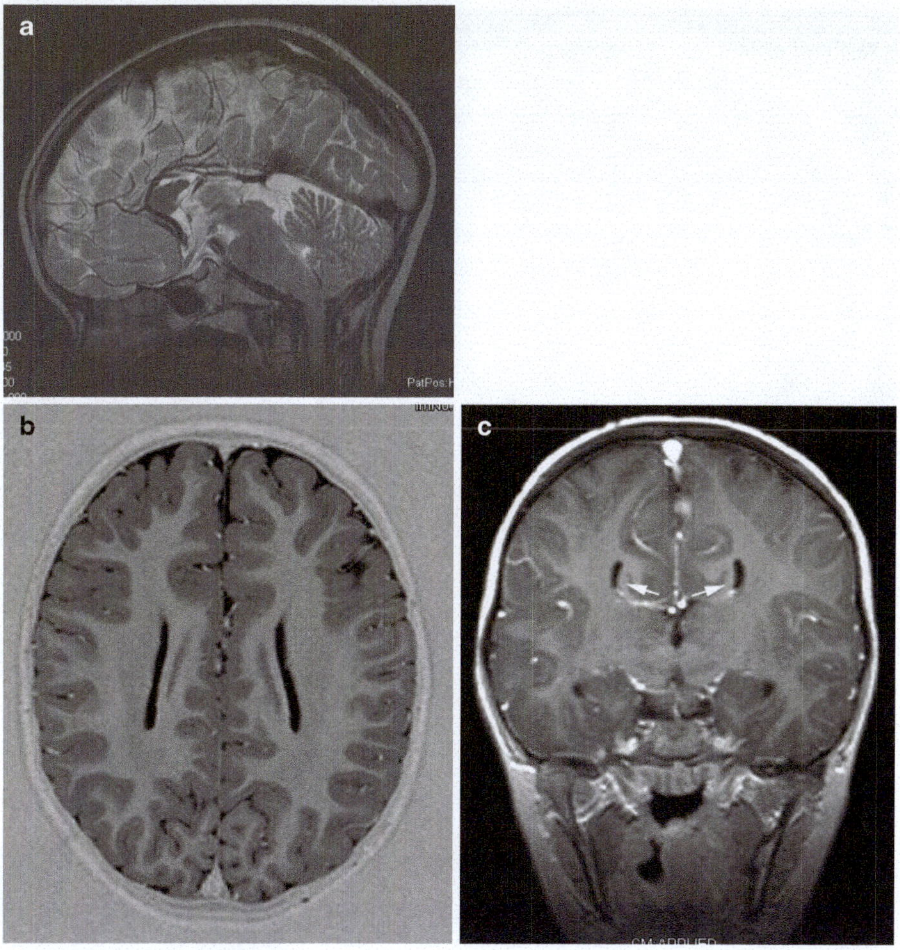

Fig. 13.1 Callosal dysgenesis. Sagittal T2-WI (**a**) shows a part of the genu of corpus callosum, transverse inversion recovery image (**b**) demonstrates parallel, widely-spaced lateral venticles, and contrast-enhanced coronal T1-WI (**c**) shows crescentic lateral ventricles compressed by Probst bundles (*arrows*)

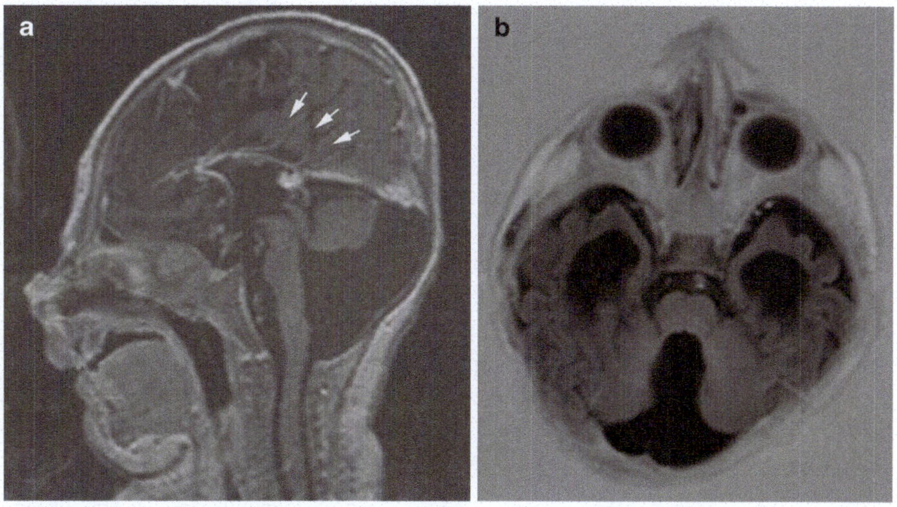

Fig. 13.2 Agenesis of the corpus callosum. Sagittal contrast-enhanced T1-WI (**a**) and transverse inversion recovery image (**b**) show complete agenesis of the corpus callosum and a radial array of gyri "pointing" (*arrow*) to the third ventricle in concert with Dandy–Walker malformation

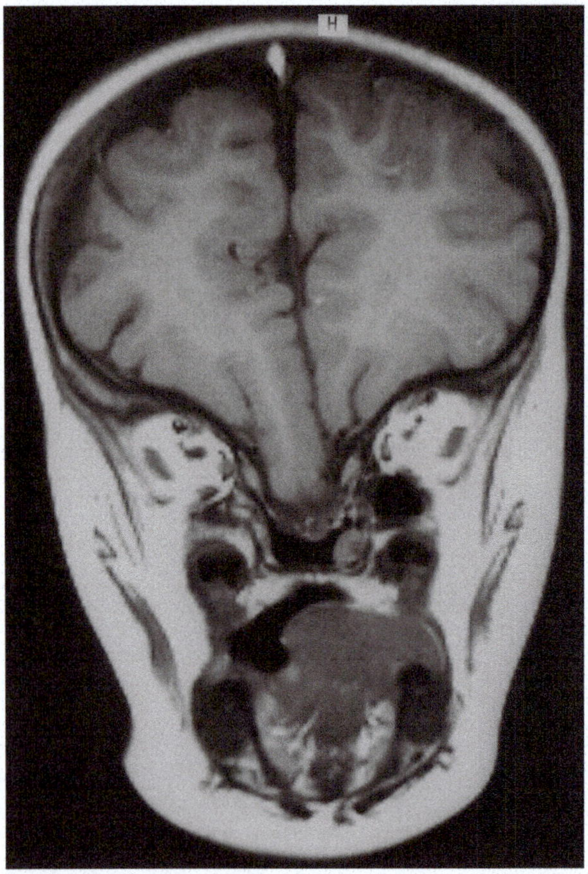

Fig. 13.3 Fronto-ethmoidal meningoencephalocele. Coronal T1-WI shows extension of brain tissue and CSF through a defect in the skull base in the region of the cribriform plate and crista galli

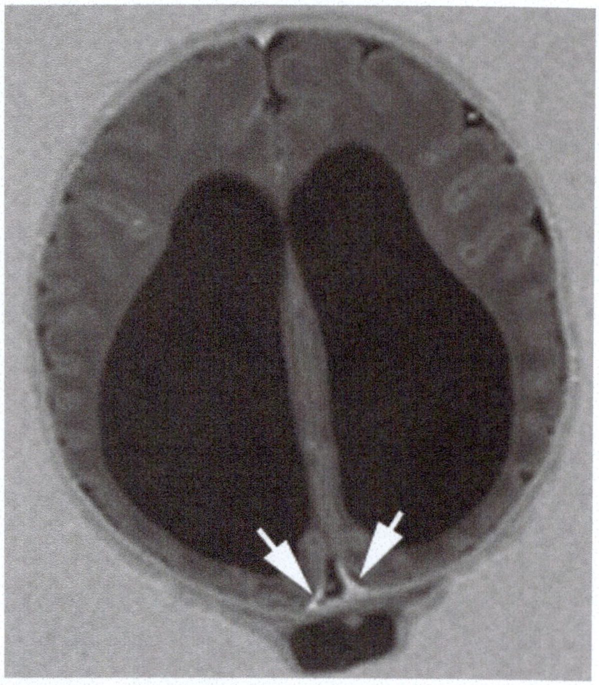

Fig. 13.4 Atretic cephalocele. Transverse inversion recovery image shows a midline sub-scalp atretic cephalocele. The superior sagittal sinus is duplicated at the site of herniation (*arrows*)

of cephaloceles and atretic cephaloceles, and help to differentiate these entities from sinus pericranii and to diagnose concomitant anomalies of associated intracranial venous anomalies.

Gray Matter Heterotopia

Normal gray matter in an abnormal location other than the cortex is defined as gray matter heterotopia. An insult to the germinal matrix during neuronal migration can cause migrational arrest, resulting in heterotopic gray matter. Heterotopia can be divided into subependymal, focal subcortical, and band heterotopia (double cortex) (Fig. 13.6). The latter condition is now thought to belong to the spectrum of lissencephalies. Subependymal heterotopias are usually seen along the lateral ventricles, either subependymal or within the periventricular white matter (Fig. 13.5). Because they represent foci of normal

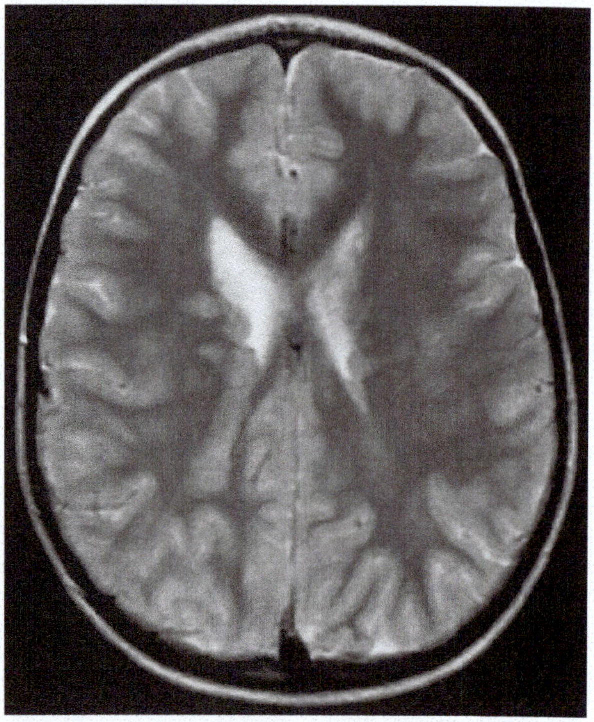

Fig. 13.5 Gray matter heterotopia. Transverse T2-WI shows multiple nodular gray matter heterotopia along the borders of the lateral ventricles

gray matter, they will be isointense with gray matter on all sequences, and will not enhance with contrast. The major differential diagnostic consideration is tuberous sclerosis; however, in the latter condition, the subependymal hamartomas are typically isointense with white matter rather than gray matter. Focal subcortical heterotopias appear as multinodular or swirling, curvilinear gray matter masses, and the overlying cortex is thin with shallow sulci. Band heterotopias are uncommon, and present as a band of gray matter between the cortex and the periventricular white matter. Patients with heterotopic gray matter usually have seizures.

Lissencephaly and Pachygyria

In these conditions, the neuronal migration is subcortically stopped, involving a large area of the brain. In lissencephaly (agyria), the brain shows a smooth surface with no sulcations and the so-called "figure-of-eight" brain configuration with shallow sylvian fissures (Fig. 13.6). In pachygyria, there are some cortical sulci present (Fig. 13.7). In both conditions, imaging reveals thickened gray matter and enlargement of the ventricular trigones and occipital horns. The brainstem often appears hypoplastic. The cerebellum is only rarely involved. Clinically, patients present with hypotonia at birth and develop spasticity, seizures, and mental retardation.

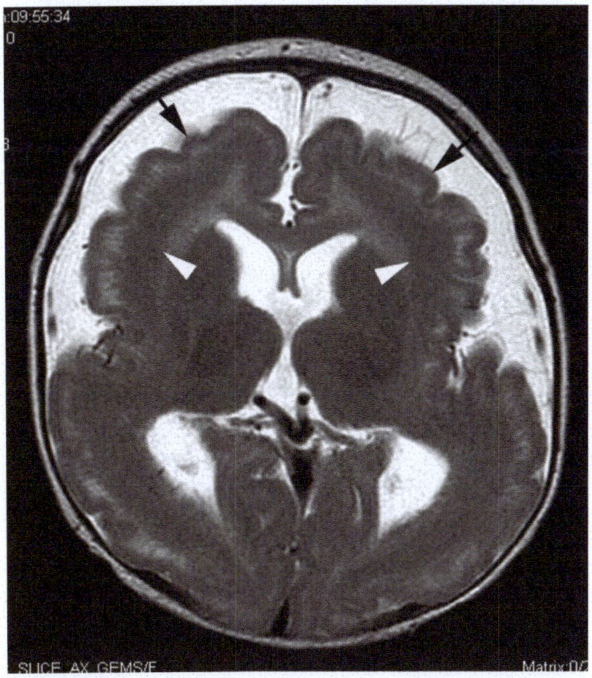

Fig. 13.6 Lissencephaly type 1. Transverse T2-WI shows thin, smooth cortical ribbon (*black arrows*) and thick inner band of gray matter (*white arrowheads*). Primitive sylvian fissures give the brain a "figure-of-eight" configuration

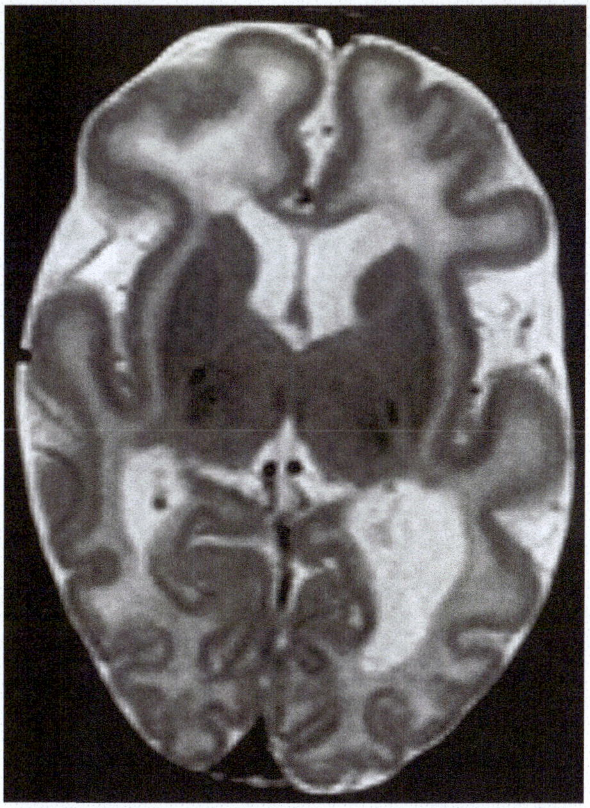

Fig. 13.7 Pachygyria. Transverse T2-WI shows some cortical sulci, thickened cortex, and widened sylvian fissures

Polymicrogyria (Sometimes Referred to as Cortical Dysplasia)

Polymicrogyria (PMG) is defined as a malformation due to abnormality in late neuronal migration and cortical organization. Therefore, PMG belongs to the malformations of cortical development (Table 13.1). Two imaging patterns can be distinguished, which are influenced by the degree of myelination. In children younger than 12 months, the cortex appears fine and undulating, with normal thickness (2–3 mm). In children older than 18 months, the cortex is thick and bumpy (5–8 mm), and hypomyelination and cortical

Table 13.1 Malformations of cortical development (Adapted from Barkovich 2005)

Malformation due to abnormal neural and glial proliferation or apoptosis
Decreased proliferation/increased apoptosis – microcephalies
Microcephaly with normal to thin cortex
Microlissencephaly (extreme microcephaly with thick cortex)
Microcephaly with polymicrogyria/cortical dysplasia
Increased proliferation/decreased apoptosis (normal cell types) – megaloencephalies
Abnormal proliferation (abnormal cell types)
Nonneoplastic
Cortical hamartomas of tuberous sclerosis
Cortical dysplasia with balloon cells
Hemimegalencephaly
Neoplastic (associated with disordered cortex)
DNET (dysembroyoplastic neuroepithelial tumor)
Ganglioglioma
Gangliocytoma
Malformation due to abnormal neural migration
Lissencephaly/subcortical band heterotropia spectrum
Cobblestone complex
Congenital muscular dystrophy syndrome
Syndromes with no involvement of muscle
Heterotropia
Subependymal (periventricular)
Subcortical (other than band heterotopia)
Marginal glioneural
Malformation due to abnormal cortical organization (including late neural migration)
Polymicrogyria and schizencephaly
Bilateral polymicrogyria syndromes
Schizencephaly (polymicrogyria with clefts)
Polymicrogyrai with other brain malformations or abnormalities
Polymicrogyria or schizencephaly as part of multiple congenital anomaly/mental retardation syndrome
Cortical dyplasia without balloon cells
Microdysgenesis
Malformation of cortical development, not otherwise classified
Malformations secondary to inborn errors of metabolism
Mitochondrial and pyruvate metabolic disorder
Peroxisomal disorders
Other unclassified malformations
Sublobar disorder
Others

infolding may be associated (Fig. 13.8). In PMG, the cortical-white matter junction is always irregular and sulci are always abnormal, being shallow or absent. The dysplastic cortex is isointense to the normal cortex, but in 20–25% of the patients, the MRI shows an abnormally high signal intensity of the underlying white matter on T2-W and FLAIR sequences, probably reflecting demyelination and/or gliosis. In addition,

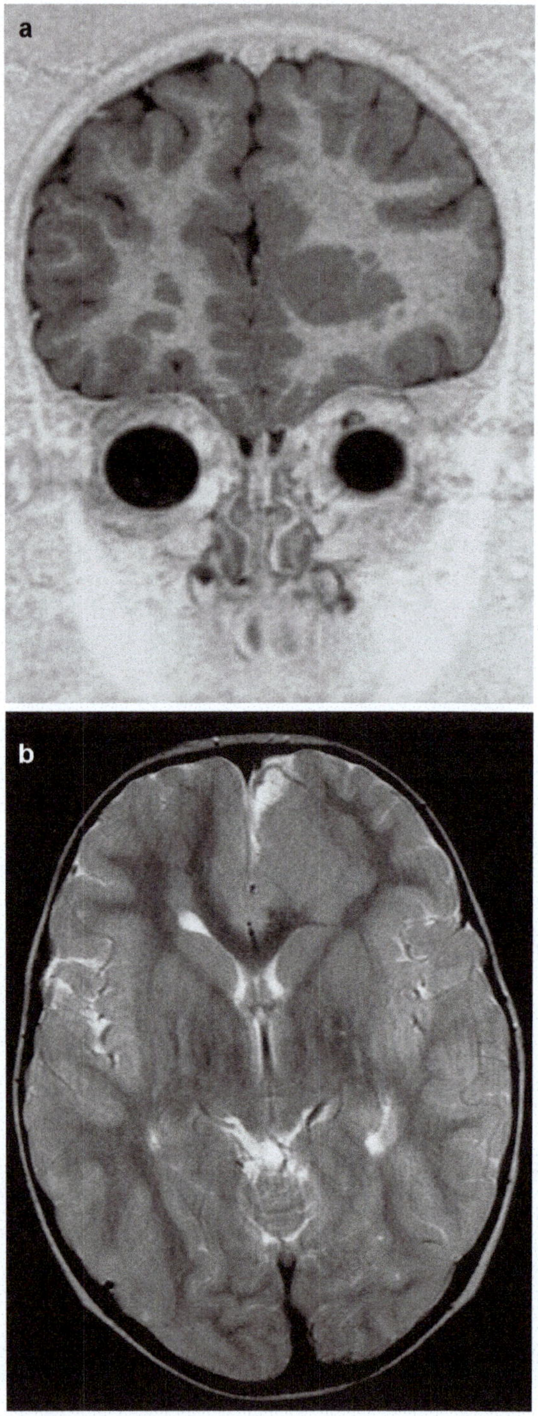

Fig. 13.8 Polymicrogyria/cortical dysplasia. Coronal inversion recovery image (**a**) and transverse T2-WI (**b**) show thickened gray matter in the left frontal lobe

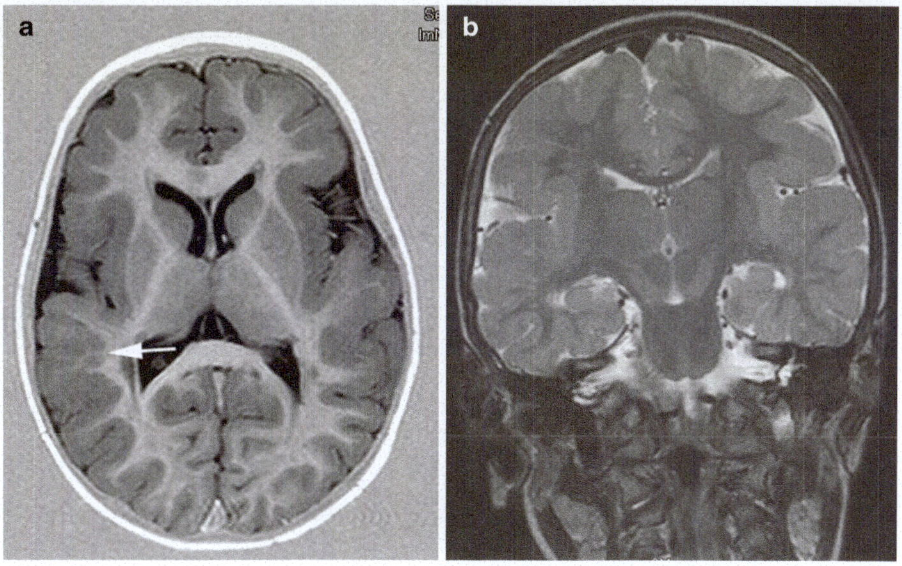

Fig. 13.9 Congenital bilateral perisylvian polymicrogyria. Transverse inversion recovery image (**a**) and coronal T2-WI (**b**) show thickened insular, frontal, and parietal cortex on both sides. The cortical white matter junction looks smooth on both sequences, with the exception of an irregularity at the right parietal cortex (*arrow*)

persistent embryonic veins overlying the abnormal cortex may be present in approximately 50% of the patients, helping to differentiate this condition from pachygyria. As PMG may be overt or subtle, techniques that accentuate cortical-white matter interface, such as IR sequences with 2 mm slice thickness or volume 3D gradient-echo acquisitions with thin partition size (1.5 mm or less) and evaluation in three planes are recommendable. Small or large portions of the hemispheres can be involved, with the perisylvian region being the most common location. Bilateral perisylvian involvement is very often syndromic (Fig. 13.9). In addition, PMG is a common manifestation of congenital cytomegalovirus (CMV) infection, and therefore noncontrast-enhanced CT (NECT) should be performed to detect calcifications in suspected infection. Seizures are the most common clinical manifestation of PMG, but, depending on extend of malformation, patients suffer from faciopharyngoglossomasticatory diplegia, developmental delay, hemiparesis, or hemiplegia.

Holoprosencephaly

Holoprosencephalies are a group of disorders with a failure of diverticulation and cleavage of the prosencephalon, and represent a continuum of forebrain malformations. Facial dysmorphism, such as hypotelorism and midline facial clefts, is seen in severe forms. This spectrum of congenital forebrain malformations is characterized by lack of formation of midline structures. DeMyer has divided holoprosencephaly into three subgroups: alobar, semilobar, and lobar holoprosencephaly.

The alobar form is the severest type, and presents with an anteriorly located pancake of brain tissue with fused thalami and a huge monoventricle leading into a large dorsal cyst. No septum pellucidum, falx cerebri, or interhemispheric fissure can be delineated. These patients are rarely imaged, as they are stillborn or have a very short life span.

The semilobar form (Fig. 13.10) presents with underdeveloped and fused frontal regions of the brain, fused caudate heads in midline, a monoventricle, which shows rudimentary occipital and temporal horns, and an absence of the septum pellucidum. A small third ventricle can be recognized because the thalami are partially separated. The falx cerebri and the interhemispheric fissure are usually partially formed posteriorly. The callosal splenium is present without the body or genu in many patients with holoprosencephaly. Therefore, holoprosencephaly is the only disorder in which the posterior corpus callosum forms in the absence of the anterior corpus callosum.

In lobar holoprosencephaly, the frontal lobes and the frontal horns are hypoplastic, and the septum pellucidum is absent. The third ventricle is fully formed, and the thalami are normal. The falx cerebri and the interhemispheric fissure extend into the frontal area of the brain, with the anterior falx and anterior fissure being formed to a varying degree. The genu can be either

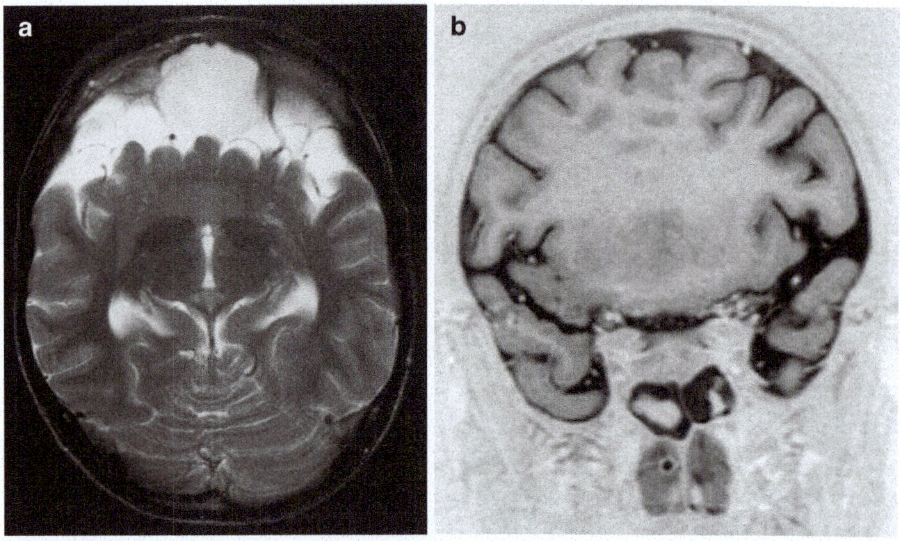

Fig. 13.10 Semilobar holoprosencephaly. Transverse T2-WI (**a**) and coronal inversion recovery image (**b**) show fused frontal lobes with abnormal gyral configuration

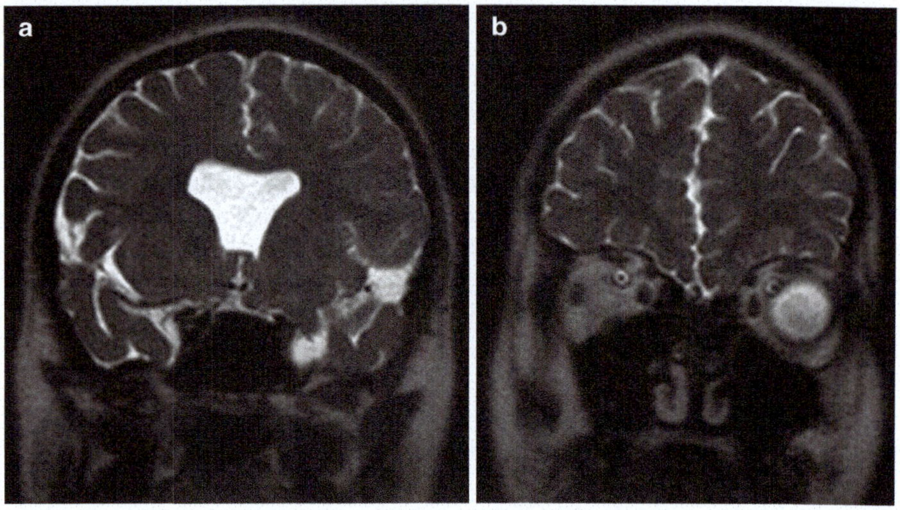

Fig. 13.11 Septo-optic dysplasia. Coronal T2-WI (**a, b**) show absence of septum pellucidum and hypoplastic optic nerves

absent or hypoplastic. Patients with lobar holoprosencephaly present with visual problems, mild to moderate developmental delay, and hypothalamic-pituitary dysfunction. The mild form of lobar holoprosencephaly may be indistinguishable from septo-optic dysplasia, as these entities present a continuum of developmental abnormalities.

Septo-Optic Dysplasia

Septo-optic dysplasia is a heterogeneous disorder characterized by an absent or hypoplastic septum pellucidum and by hypoplastic anterior optic pathways, and (usually) hypothalamic-pituitary dysfunction (Fig. 13.11). Hypoplasia of the optic chiasm and the hypothalamus often results in dilatation of the anterior recess of the third ventricle and a large suprasellar cistern. Mild hypoplasia of the optic tract may be difficult to recognize. Clinical presentations of patients with septo-optic dysplasia are variable, but the main symptoms are visual problems and hypothalamic-pituitary dysfunction. There are at least three subsets of patients with septo-optic dysplasia, which can be distinguished by MRI. One group has schizencephaly, gray-matter heterotopia, a remnant of the septum pellucidum, an almost normal visual apparatus, and classically suffers from seizures. A second subset of patients presents with hypoplasia of white matter, consecutive enlarged ventricles, and an absent septum pellucidum, but otherwise normal cortex. This form is believed to be a mild form of lobar holoprosencephaly. The third subset of patients demonstrates a hypoplastic or absent septum pellucidum along with a sometimes mild hypoplasia of the optic nerves, and suffers from endocrine dysfunction secondary to either hypoplastic or ectopic pituitary gland.

Aplasia/Hypoplasia of the Pituitary Gland

The pituitary gland develops between 28 and 48 days of embryonic life. The posterior lobe forms from a downward extension of the embryonic hypothalamus, known as the neurohypophysis, whereas the anterior lobe and pars intermedia form from Rathke's pouch, which appears on the roof of the foregut and grows dorsally toward the infundibulum. Rathke's pouch detaches from the buccal cavity and becomes associated with the developing posterior pituitary lobe.

The normal appearance of the pituitary gland in a newborn is convex, with a uniform high signal on T1-WI (Fig. 13.60). By the age of 2 months, the adenohypophysis loses its high SI, while the neurohypophysis still shows a high signal on T1-WI. During infancy and childhood, the superior margin flattens, and the gland grows normally, showing a height between 2 and 6 mm in the sagittal plane. During puberty, the gland increases dramatically in size in girls, and demonstrates an upward convexity with a height up to 10 mm. The normal height of the gland in boys during puberty is 7–8 mm. After puberty, the pituitary gland diminishes slightly in size, evolving to adult appearance.

Patients with aplasia or hypoplasia of the pituitary gland suffer from growth failure due to growth hormone deficiency (GHD) and/or symptoms of anterior pituitary hormone deficiencies (multiple pituitary hormone deficiencies - MPHD). Imaging findings consist of one or more of the following: small shallow sella, small anterior pituitary gland, absence of the usually high SI from the posterior pituitary gland, absence or hypoplasia of the distal pituitary stalk, and an anomalous high signal area in the proximal pituitary stalk. Three patterns are frequently encountered: one subset of patients presents with posterior lobe ectopia (high signal area in the proximal pituitary stalk), aplasia of the stalk, aplasia or hypoplasia of the anterior lobe (small sella), and almost always suffers from MPHD (Fig. 13.12). The second subset of patients demonstrates only anterior lobe hypoplasia (small sella and loss of high signal in the posterior pituitary gland) and suffers from GHD. The third subset of patients clinically presents only with mild endocrine dysfunction and has a normal-appearing pituitary gland. These anomalies are often associated with other midline anomalies, and both developmental anomalies and

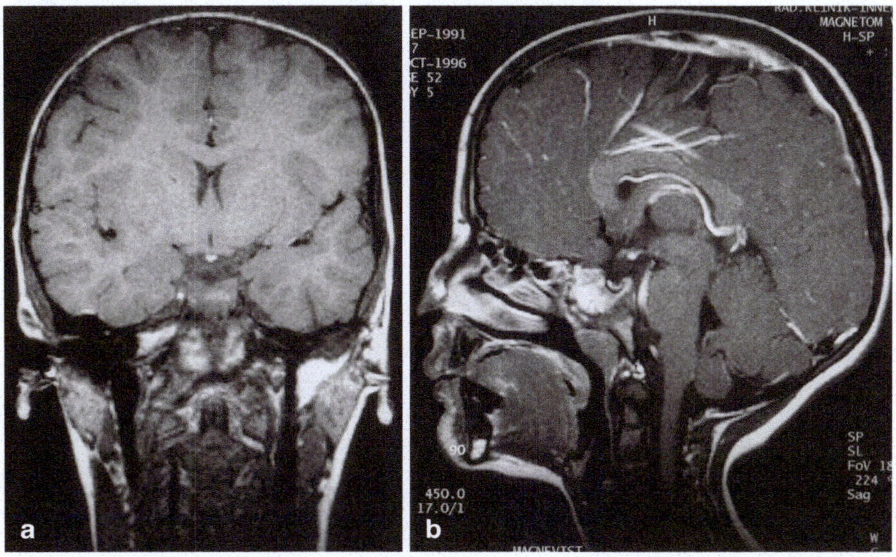

Fig. 13.12 Growth hormone-deficient dwarfism. Coronal T1-WI precontrast (**a**) and contrast-enhanced sagittal T1-WI (**b**) demonstrate aplasia of the pituitary stalk and hypoplasia of the anterior lobe in a small sella, in concert with a focal area of high signal intensity at the proximal infundibulum, demarcating the ectopic location of the posterior pituitary lobe

"trauma" secondary to breech delivery have been accused of being responsible for this entity.

Unilateral Megalencephaly (Hemimegalencephaly)

Unilateral megalencephaly is defined as a localized or complete hamartomatous overgrowth of one hemisphere due to defects in neuronal proliferation, migration, and organization. Pathologically, the affected hemisphere contains areas of polymicrogyria, pachygyria, heterotopia, dyslamination, enlarged neurons, balloon cells, and astrogliosis of the underlying white matter. The affected hemisphere is enlarged on imaging studies, with the sulci appearing shallow and the gyri broad. The dysplastic cortex appears thickened, and is often hypointense on T2-WI. The margin between the cortex and the underlying white matter may be indistinct. Areas of gliosis in the white matter show high signal on T2-WI and low signal on T1-WI (Fig. 13.13). Size and signal intensity of the affected hemisphere can change due to progression of myelination, development of calcifications, and volume loss secondary to seizures. There is a characteristic appearance of the enlarged lateral ventricle on the affected side, with a straight, superiorly and anteriorly pointing frontal horn. However, the changes can be subtler, and the cerebrum appears grossly normal. Patients with this anomaly usually present with intractable seizures, often starting within the first month of life, as well as developmental delay and hemiplegia. There are indications for partial or complete resection of the affected hemisphere in selected cases, if the other hemisphere is definitively normal. Unilateral megalencephaly is associated with neurofibromatosis type 1 (NF-1), tuberous sclerosis, Klippel-Trenaunay-Weber syndrome, Proteus syndrome, epidermal nevus syndrome, congenital infiltrating lipomatosis, incontinentia pigmenti, and unilateral hypomelanosis of Ito. A condition referred to as total hemimegalencephaly is defined by an associated enlargement and dysplasia of the ipsilateral cerebellar hemisphere and brainstem.

Schizencephaly

Schizencephaly is defined as a cleft extending from the lateral ventricles to the cortical surface lined by dysplastic gray matter (polymigrogyria) (Fig. 13.14). Schizencephaly is divided into clefts with open and fused lips. In open-lip schizencephaly (Fig. 13.15), the cleft contains CSF, and in closed-lip schizencephaly, the walls of the cleft are in apposition to each other and therefore may be difficult to detect. The dimple usually seen in the wall of the lateral ventricle, and the linear hyperintense signal intensity representing the pial and arachnoid lining of the cleft in T2-WI are helpful signs in depicting this condition. Bilateral clefts are not uncommon, and in approximately half of the patients there are other

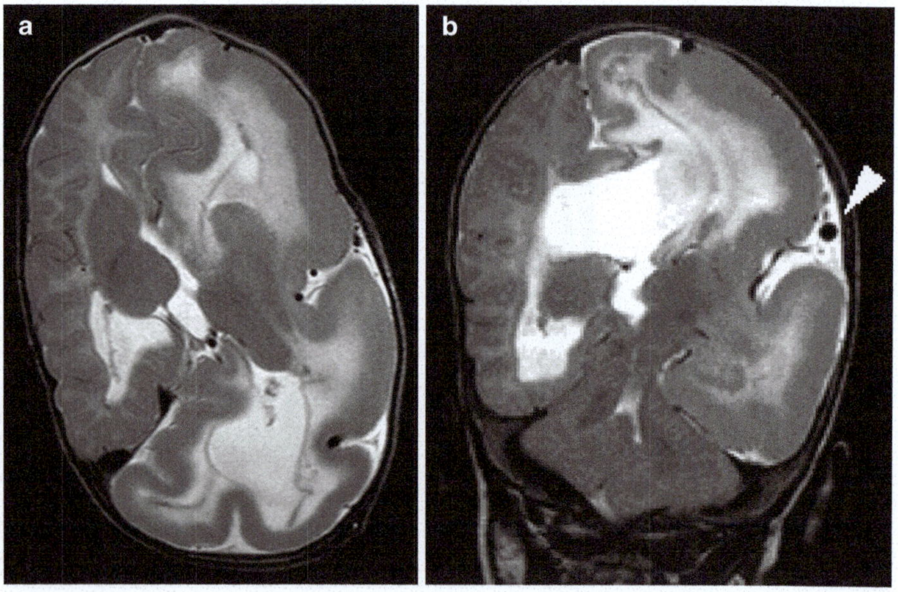

Fig. 13.13 Hemimegalencephaly. Transverse (**a**) and coronal (**b**) T2-WI show overgrowth of the left cerebral hemisphere, with excess of white matter, flattened gyri, cortical dysplasia, and primitive veins in the enlarged sylvian fissure (*arrowhead*)

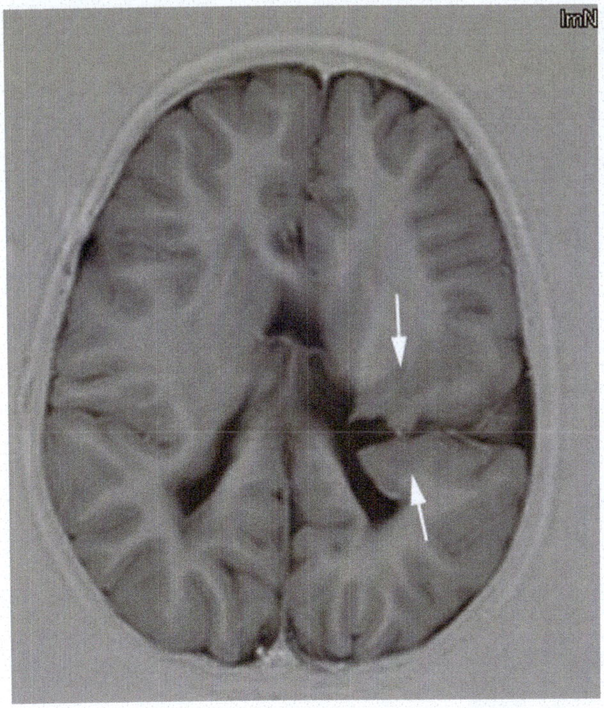

Fig. 13.14 Unilateral schizencephaly. Transverse inversion recovery image shows unilateral small open-lip schizencephaly. Thickened gray matter (polymicrogyria) (*arrows*) lines the cleft

neuronal migration anomalies. The septum pellucidum is absent in 70% of the patients with schizencephaly. Clinical symptoms, usually seizures and hemiparesis, are proportional to the size of the clefts.

Arnold-Chiari Malformations

The Arnold-Chiari I malformation is more often found in adults than in children, and is defined as displacement of ≥5 mm or more of the elongated pointed cerebellar tonsils below the foramen magnum. Displacement of the tonsils between 3 and 6 mm is indeterminate; in the age group between 5 and 15 years, displacement of 6 mm in asymptomatic patients should not be considered pathological. When the cerebellar tonsils extend more than 5–6 mm below the foramen magnum, clinical symptoms such as occipital or posterior headaches, lower cranial nerve palsies, otoneurologic disturbances and nystagmus are more likely to occur. Midline sagittal MR images reveal peglike cerebellar tonsils displaced inferiorly to the foramen magnum, and sometimes an elongated but normally located fourth ventricle. Concurrent findings are hydrocephalus, syringohydromyelia, osseous malformations of the craniocervical junction, or acquired deformities of the foramen magnum. In patients with a typical clinical history or borderline imaging findings, CSF flow studies may be helpful in further evaluation.

The Arnold-Chiari II malformation is always associated with a meningomyelocele (Fig. 13.16), inferior tentorial attachment, and small posterior fossa. The cerebellar tonsils, and often both the vermis and medulla, are displaced inferiorly into the cervical canal, frequently causing a cervicomedullary kink. The cerebellar hemispheres may extend anterolaterally,

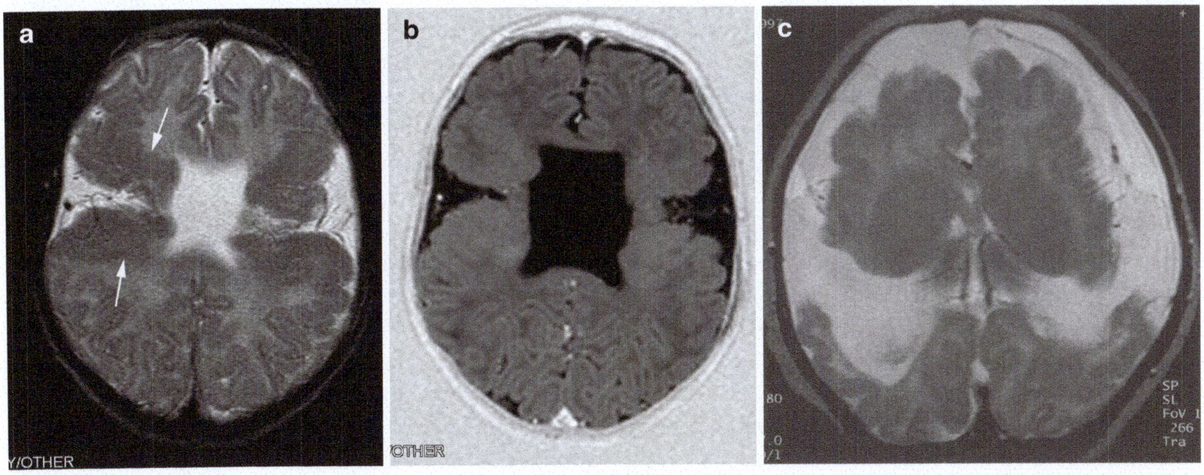

Fig. 13.15 Bilateral schizencephaly. Transverse T2-WI (**a**) and inversion recovery image (**b**) show bilateral small open-lip schizencephaly. Thickened gray matter (polymicrogyria) (*arrows*) lines the clefts. The septum pellucidum is absent. Transverse T2-WI (**c**) of another patient shows huge bilateral open-lip schizencephaly

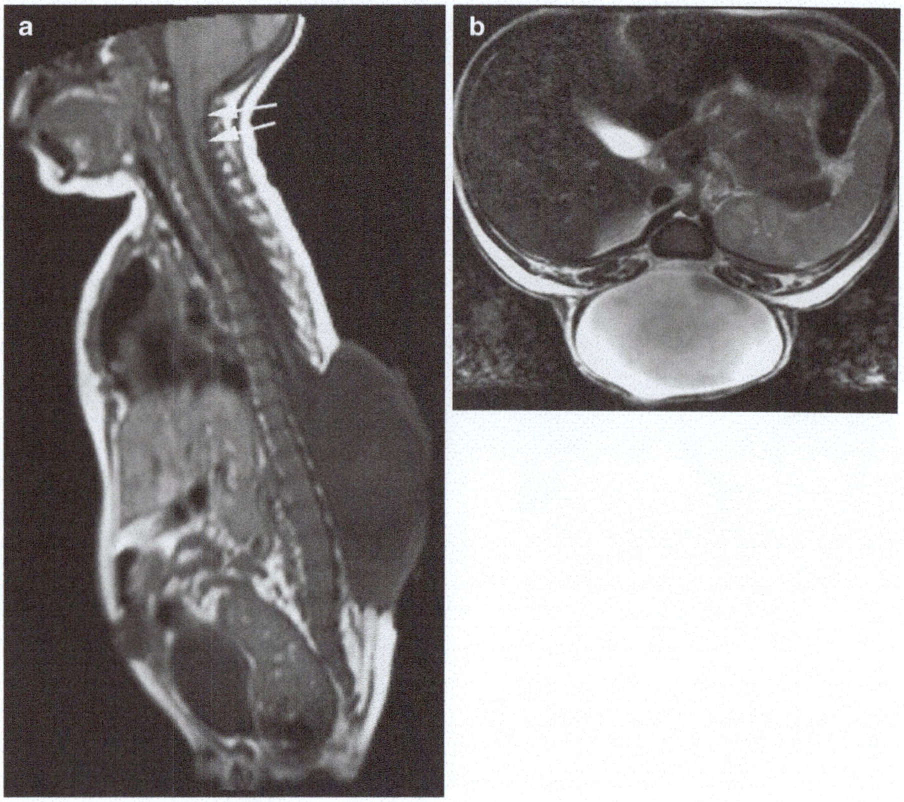

Fig. 13.16 Arnold-Chiari Malformation II. Sagittal T1-WI (**a**) and transverse T2-WI (**b**) show herniation of the cerebellar vermis into the cervical spinal canal (*arrows*), and a large myelomeningocele

wrapping around the brainstem. The fourth ventricle is narrow and low in position, and beaking of the tectum occurs. Supratentorially, callosal dysgenesis and, subsequently, colpocephaly is seen in 80–90% of the patients. The falx is hypoplastic, often fenestrated, and interdigitation of the gyri occurs. A large massa intermedia is usually present. Most patients show further anomalies, such as stenogyria, which is defined as an abnormal pattern in the medial aspect of the occipital lobes due to dysplasia, resembling multiple small gyri. Approximately 90% of patients have concurrent hydrocephalus and/or spinal-cord cysts. Segmentation anomalies of the upper cervical spine are seen in 10% of cases.

The Arnold-Chiari III malformation is an extremely rare malformation, which combines the intracranial features of Arnold-Chiari II with a herniation of the posterior fossa contents through a posterior spina bifida C1-C2. This encephalocele may contain the cerebellum, and sometimes the brainstem and aberrant venous structures. Spinal-cord cysts may be present. According to Barkovich, this condition should preferably be considered as a high cervical myelocystocele.

The Dandy–Walker Complex

The Dandy–Walker complex represents a spectrum of malformations, classically being divided into the Dandy–Walker malformation, the Dandy–Walker variant, and the mega cisterna magna. The classic Dandy–Walker malformation (Fig. 13.17) is characterized by a superior attachment of the tentorium, resulting in a large posterior fossa, a cystic dilatation of the fourth ventricle filling the posterior fossa, and concurrent hypoplasia or aplasia of the cerebellar vermis. The cerebellar hemispheres are almost always hypoplastic. Hydrocephalus develops in 75% of patients by the age of 3 months; there are associations with corpus callosum agenesis, neuronal migration anomalies, and occipital cephaloceles.

The term Dandy–Walker variant has different meanings and is under debate. Some authors define unilateral or bilateral hypoplasia of the cerebellar hemispheres, mild hypoplasia of the vermis, and a slightly enlarged fourth ventricle in a normal or near normal posterior fossa as a Dandy–Walker variant, whereas others use this term for a Dandy–Walker type malformation in which one or more of the fourth ventricular outflow

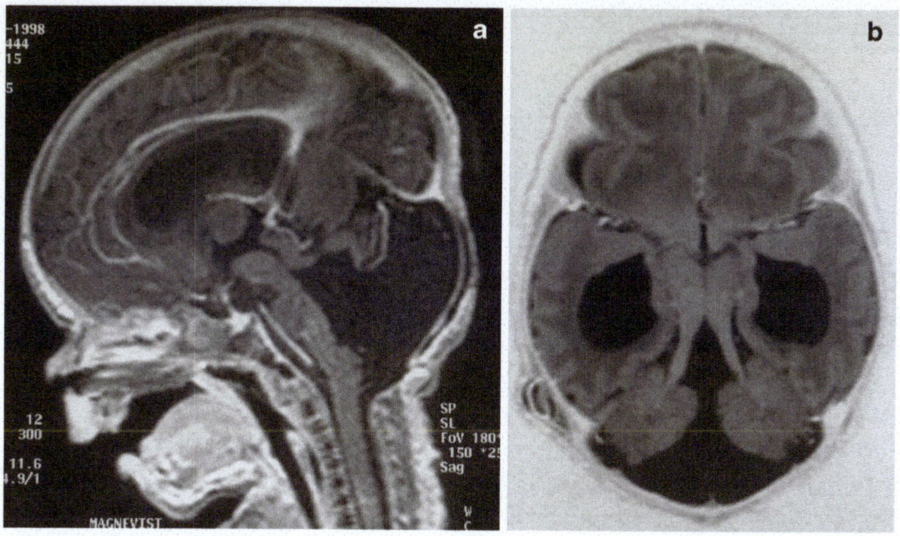

Fig. 13.17 Dandy–Walker malformation. Contrast-enhanced sagittal T1-WI (**a**) and transverse inversion recovery image (**b**) show dilatation of the fourth ventricle, expanded posterior fossa, high insertion of venous torcular, and absence of the inferior vermis

foramina are patent. According to Barkovich, the first setting should better be considered as cerebellar hypoplasia. Hydrocephalus may develop during infancy or early childhood.

Mega cisterna magna is characterized by expansion of the cisterna magna, leading to an enlarged posterior fossa and both a morphological normal vermis and fourth ventricle. Whether this entity represents a true malformation or a normal variant is subject to debate. In addition, it is important to mention that in patients with a hypoplastic vermis the cisterna magna may appear big.

Patients with these anomalies may present with developmental delay and enlarged head circumference, due to hydrocephalus or mass effect by the enlarged fourth ventricle sometimes scalloping the inner table. The degree of developmental delay correlates with the extent of supratentorial anomalies and the level of control of the hydrocephalus.

Blake's Pouch Cyst

Blake's pouch cyst is an arachnoid cyst of the posterior fossa and an important differential diagnosis to the aforementioned posterior fossa malformations. The cyst is located posterior to the inferior vermis. Arachnoid cysts are benign lesions developing between the layers of the arachnoid membrane and do not communicate freely with the subarachnoid or ventricular spaces. Depending on the location and size of Blake's pouch cyst, children may develop hydrocephalus and present with an increased head circumference and signs of increased intracranial pressure. MR imaging demonstrates a well marginated, mostly unilocular, nonenhancing lesion compressing adjacent structures, with CSF signal characteristics on all sequences. Due to mass effect, there may be scalloping of the inner table (Fig. 13.18).

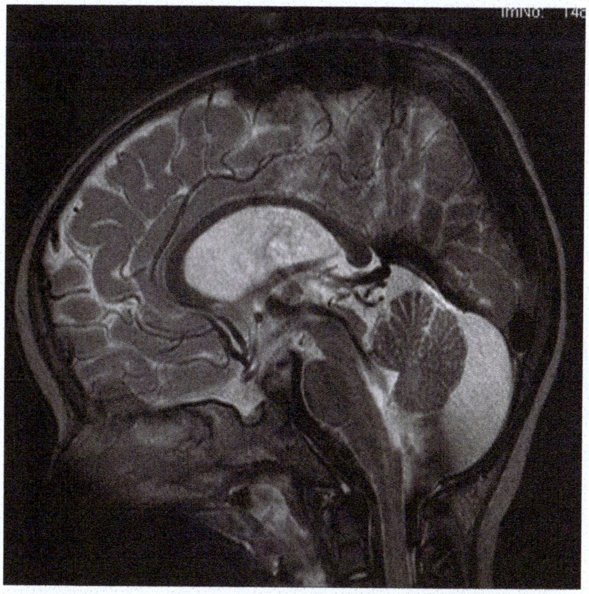

Fig. 13.18 Blake's Pouch Cyst. Sagittal T2-WI shows a retrocerebellar cyst with subtle scalloping of the occipital bone

13.2.2.2 Anomalies of Histogenesis: Phakomatoses

Neurofibromatosis Type 1

NF is an autosomal dominant disorder and is classified as type 1 (NF-1) and type 2 (NF-2). NF-1 (incidence 1:3,000–5,000) is ten times more common than NF-2 (incidence 1:50,000) and inherited via a genetic defect located on chromosome 17q12. The NF gene product is neurofibromin, which seems to be a tumor suppressor gene that is inactivated, a circumstance serving as an explanation for tumor development in these patients. Furthermore, neurofibromin appears to be necessary for normal myelination by Schwann cells. In addition, the gene for oligodendrocyte myelin glycoprotein, a myelin protein, is embedded within the NF-1 gene. The former and the latter findings are currently thought to be responsible for the white matter abnormalities in NF-1. Clinically, the most reliable diagnostic criteria are the demonstration of six or more "cafe-au-lait" spots of 1.5 cm in size, Lisch spots (pigmented hamartomas of the iris), and a family history. Central nervous system (CNS) abnormalities include true neoplasms, usually optic nerve (bilateral in 10–20%) and parenchymal gliomas, as well as dysplastic, hamartomatous lesions, and multifocal signal changes with bright signal on T2-WI. In children, optic gliomas and white matter lesions are the most frequent findings. The characteristically multiple white matter lesions are typically located in the brainstem, midbrain, cerebellar white matter, globus pallidus, and splenium. They represent regions of myelin vacuolization, and begin to appear at the age of 3 years. They increase in number and size until puberty, and subsequently decrease and disappear in adolescence. On MRI, these lesions are hyperintense on T2-WI, cannot be detected on T1-WI, show no mass effect or associated edema, and do not enhance with paramagnetic contrast. However, one exception to this rule are the lesions in the globus pallidus, which demonstrate abnormally high signal on T1-WI in more than 50% of the affected patients, and are often associated with mild mass effect (Fig. 13.19). However, as always, the true nature of small nonenhancing lesions with T2 prolongation can not be predicted. If these lesions show contrast enhancement and mass effect on follow-up examinations, they have to be considered as low-grade gliomas (Fig. 13.20b)

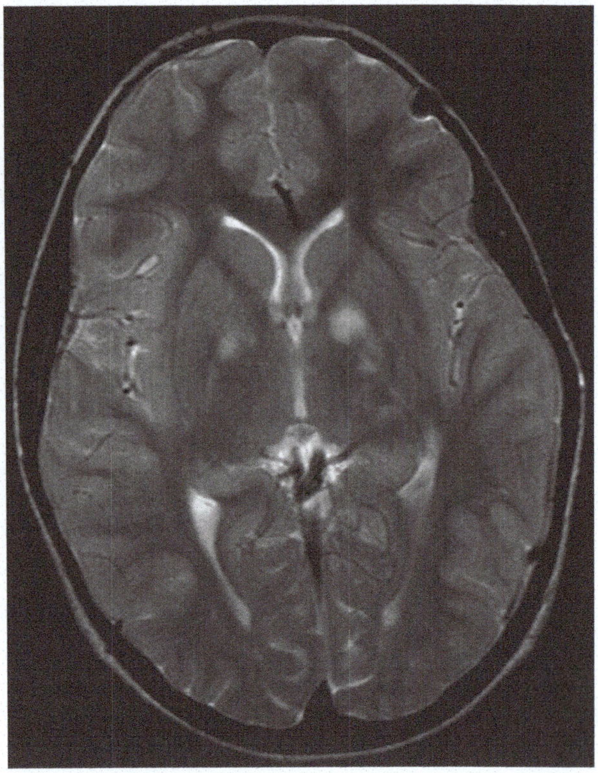

Fig. 13.19 Neurofibromatosis type 1. Axial T2-WI (**a**) shows bright signal changes in the pallidum and posterior thalami on both sides, consistent with myelin vacuolization or hamartomatous change

The gliomas are usually pilocytic astrocytomas (but low-grade and higher grade tumors also occur), and extend from the optic nerves (Fig. 13.20c) along the optic pathway, or primarily arise from the optic chiasm, hypothalamus, thalamus, basal ganglia, occipital lobe, or brainstem. Gliomas are hyperintense on T2-WI, isointense or hyperintense to gray or white matter on T1-WI, and enhance after administration of contrast. It is worthwhile mentioning that two different forms of optic nerve involvement can be distinguished. The first is a diffuse expansion of the optic nerve itself, without subarachnoid tumor; the second is a predominant infiltration of the subarachnoid space, generating a rim of tumor around the relatively untouched nerve. These two forms can be differentiated using T1-W fat saturation sequences after contrast administration, the former showing an enhancing tumor within the optic nerve sheath, the latter exhibiting a rim of enhancing tumor around the nerve. In addition, the biological behavior of brainstem, mesencephalic, and pons tumors in NF-1

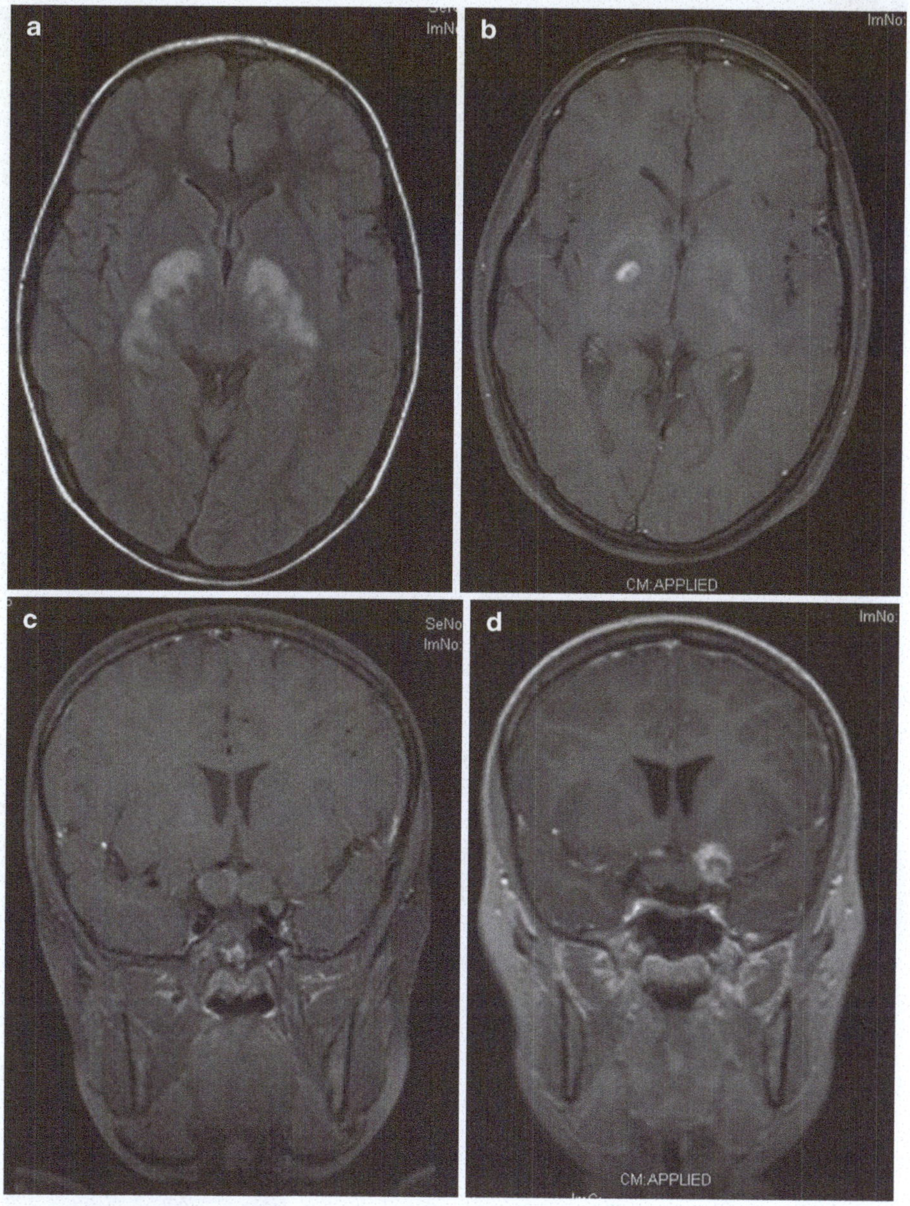

Fig. 13.20 Neurofibromatosis type 1. Transverse FLAIR image (**a**) shows hyperintense bilateral lesions in the globi pallidi. Transverse contrast-enhanced fat-saturated T1-WI (**b**) demonstrates enhancement in the right globus pallidus. Coronal contrast-enhanced T1-WI (**c**) shows bilateral optic nerve gliomas. Coronal contrast-enhanced fat-saturated T1-WI (**d**) of the same patient acquired 4 years later shows development of a considerably enhancing lesion next to the left optic nerve glioma

patients is different compared to those in the general population, as they may regress, especially in the tectum, or have a better outcome with respect to the other locations. Common locations of astrocytomas are, in addition, the cerebral hemispheres and the cerebellum.

In one third of patients with NF-1, there will be neurofibromas affecting the intraorbital and facial branches of the cranial nerves III-VI and/or diffuse plexiform neurofibromas of the face and the eyelids (Fig. 13.21). Plexiform neurofibromas are hyperintense on T2-WI and hypointense or heterogeneous on T1-WI, and demonstrate a variable enhancement. In 5–10% of the patients, there is a proptosis of the globe because of dehiscence and dysplasia of the sphenoid bone. Dysplasia of the greater wing of sphenoid is a diagnostic feature for NF-1.

Vascular dysplasia of the proximal cerebral vessels can also occur, and can lead to moya-moya syndrome.

Hydrocephalus occurs in NF-1 due to aqueduct stenosis or secondary to mass effects by hamartomatous or

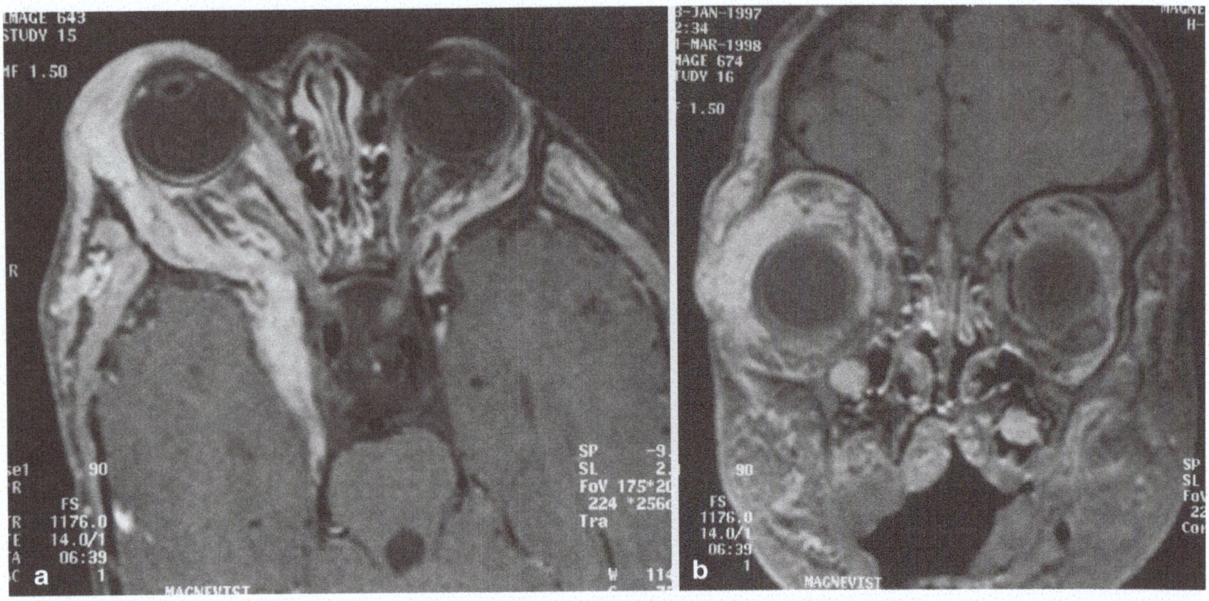

Fig. 13.21 Neurofibromatosis type 1. Transverse (**a**) and coronal (**b**) fat-saturated contrast-enhanced T1-WI show plexiform neurofibromas of the cranial nerves (N III-IV), eyelids, and face

neoplastic lesions. Spine abnormalities are present in more than 60% of NF-1 patients, and consist of acute angle kyphoscoliosis, expansion of neuroforamina, and widening of the spinal canal due to neurofibromas arising from the spinal and paraspinal nerves, or due to arachnoid cysts, dural ectasia, or dysplastic neuronal foramina. Whether malignant neurofibrosarcomas develop de novo or are a result of malignant degeneration is still under debate. Additionally, lateral thoracic meningoceles are strongly suggestive of NF-1.

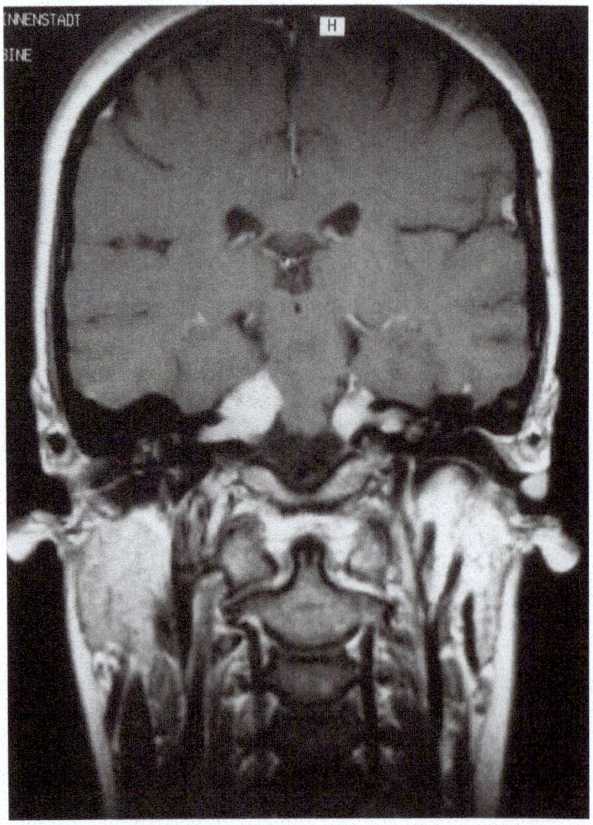

Fig. 13.22 Neurofibromatosis type 2. Coronal T1-WI shows bilateral enhancing vestibular nerve schwannomas

Neurofibromatosis Type 2

NF-2 is an autosomal dominant disease, with the abnormality located on chromosome 22q12. The product of the NF-2 gene is merlin. Mutated merlin inhibits cell adhesion, which is important in regulating cell growth, and leads to an unstable cytoskeleton. The diagnostic criteria for NF-2 are unilateral or bilateral presence of vestibular nerve schwannomas (Fig. 13.22), plus two of the following: neurofibroma or schwannoma in other locations, meningioma, glioma, juvenile posterior subcapsular lens opacity, or a first-degree relative with NF-2. Therefore, a meningioma in a child should always raise suspicion of NF-2. Cutaneous lesions in NF-2 are rare. Patients with NF-2 develop multiple schwannomas of the cranial and spinal nerves (Fig. 13.81), meningiomas occurring in atypical locations, and spinal cord ependymomas. On MRI, schwannomas show high signal on T2-WI and low signal on T1-WI, with prominent enhancement after the administration of contrast media (CM). As they enlarge and age, schwannomas tend to become heterogeneous masses with heterogeneous enhancement because of cystic degeneration and hemorrhage.

Tuberous Sclerosis

Tuberous sclerosis is an autosomal dominant disorder and related to abnormalities in chromosomes 9 and 16. The TSC1 gene is localized to chromosome 9q34 and codes for the protein hamartin, whereas the TSC2 gene is localized to chromosome 16p13.3 and codes for the protein tuberin. These two proteins interact physically in vivo and are thought to be involved in regulating cell proliferation and differentiation. The classic triad includes facial angiofibromas, seizures, and mental retardation, although recent examinations have shown that only 75% of affected patients have epilepsy, and 50% of affected patients have normal intelligence. Nevertheless, the diagnosis of tuberous sclerosis should be considered in any child with infantile spasms and seizures. The estimated incidence was revised from approximately 1 in 100,000 to 1 in 6,000 live births. Depigmented nevi occurring on the trunk and the extremities are often present at birth and are as common as angiofibromas, which appear between the ages of 1 and 5 years. The retinal hamartomas may not be present at birth, but usually develop during infancy.

Approximately 95% of patients present with hamartomas, with and without calcifications, which occur in the periventricular regions, the subependymal region, or anywhere in the white matter or cortex. Cerebellar lesions are occasionally seen. The cortical hamartomas (Fig. 13.23a) flatten the gyri, giving them a more pachygyric appearance. Gross calcification within these hamartomas is extremely rare in infants, but can be commonly seen in children 2 years and older, and in adults. Hamartomas can be solitary or multiple; they are isointense or hypointense on T1-WI, and hyperintense on T2-WI. Subependymal hamartomas (Fig. 13.23b) most commonly occur at the head of the caudate nucleus and/or the lateral bodies of the ventricles. They are usually multiple and bilateral, and contain calcification more often than cortical or white-matter hamartomas. They are usually hyperintense on T2-WI and isointense with, or slightly hyperintense to, gray matter on T1-WI, and show a variable enhancement after administration of CM. Although MRI lacks sensitivity and specificity for the detection of calcifications, large calcium deposits may be seen as hypointensity or hyperintensity on T1-WI and hypointensity on T2-WI. Hamartomas can degenerate to giant-cell astrocytomas. Most commonly, subependymal hamartomas at the level of the foramen of

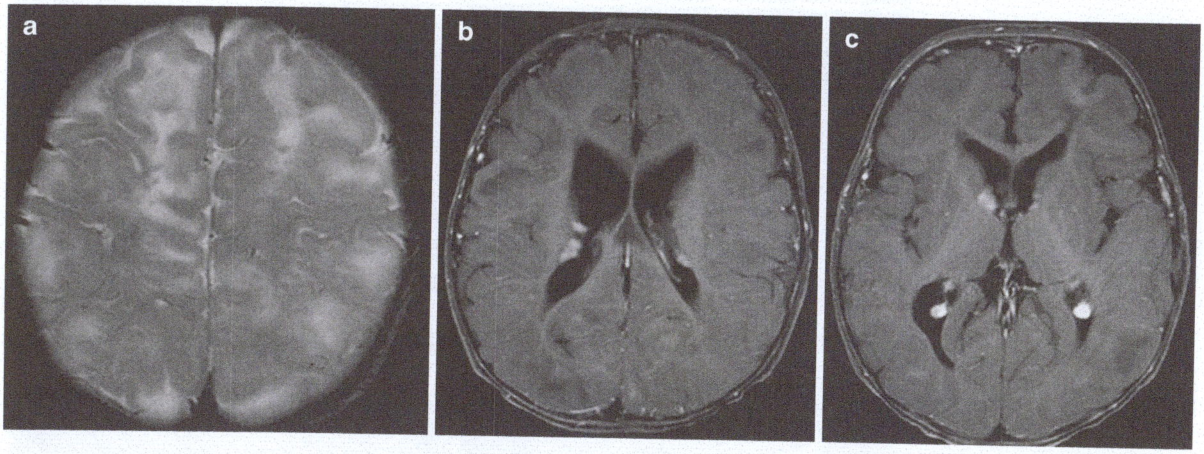

Fig. 13.23 Tuberous sclerosis. Transverse T2-WI (**a**) shows multiple hyperintense cortical tubers. Transverse contrast-enhanced T1-WI demonstrate multiple subependymal hamartomas at the lateral bodies of the ventricles (**b**) and at the foramen of Monro (**c**) on both sides, which enhance after administration of contrast

Monro (Fig. 13.23c) degenerate to subependymal giant-cell astrocytomas. These lesions do grow slowly on sequential studies, lead to unilateral and/or bilateral dilatation of the lateral ventricles, and show contrast enhancement. In addition, white matter lesions along the lines of neuronal migration consistent with tubers and cyst-like white matter lesions compatible with cystoid brain degeneration are typical MR findings in tuberous sclerosis. Extracranial manifestations of tuberous sclerosis can affect almost any organ of the body (angiomyolipoma and cysts in the kidneys (Fig. 13.126), cardial rhabdomyomas, cystic lymphangiomyomatosis and fibrosis of the lung, adenomas and leiomyomas in solid organs).

Sturge–Weber Syndrome

The Sturge–Weber syndrome is characterized by angiomatous malformation of the skin, eyes, and brain. It is defined as a sporadic congenital, but not inherited malformation, with abnormal development of the fetal cortical veins. Although patients are normal at birth, more than 90% develop seizures, dementia, hemiparesis, hemianopsia, and glaucoma during their lifetime. The main manifestation consists of a port-wine nevi in a trigeminal nerve distribution, and there is angiomatosis of the pia mater in the ipsilateral occipitoparietal region. However, angiomatosis of the pia mater can also be located anywhere in the cerebrum, and can be bilateral. Cortical veins do not develop in the area of the pial angioma, leading to blood stasis and therefore chronic ischemia with secondary calcification of the cortex. After contrast administration, the pial angioma may be clearly delineated by MRI (Fig. 13.24). The white matter subjacent to the affected cortex is hyperintense on T2-WI and FLAIR images, probably reflecting gliosis, whereas calcified cortex is hypointense on T2-WI. Calcifications

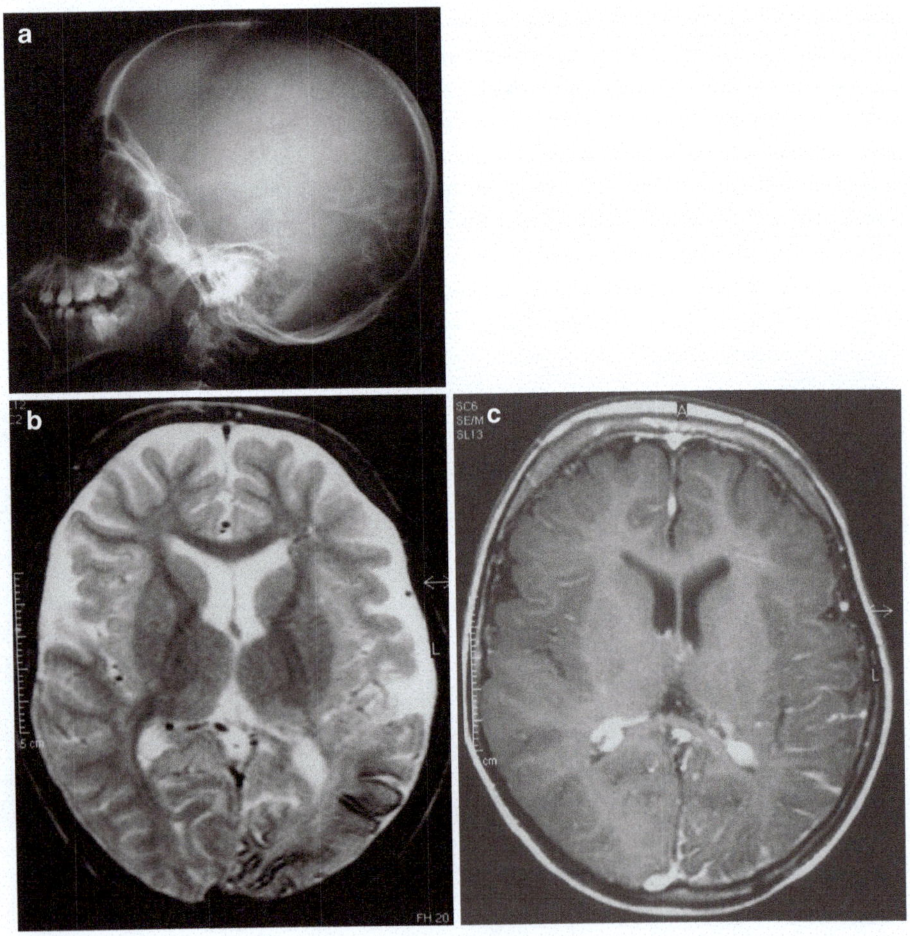

Fig. 13.24 Sturge-Weber syndrome. Lateral skull film (**a**) and transverse T2-WI (**b**) demonstrate calcification of left occipital cortex. Transverse contrast-enhanced T1-WI (**c**) reveals marked pial enhancement, representing pial angioma involving the left parieto-occipital region (Courtesy of W. Michl)

are better visualized using T2*-WI, but NECT remains the best modality to document full extent. Another important finding is an enlarged ipsilateral choroid plexus with vivid enhancement due to increased venous blood flow of the affected hemisphere. In children, the extent of plexal enlargement shows a positive correlation with size of leptomeningeal angioma and therefore degree of parenchymal involvement. Frequently, the involved cortex or hemisphere becomes atrophic.

Von Hippel–Lindau Syndrome

Von Hippel–Lindau syndrome (VHL) is an autosomal dominant disorder, and is linked to a defect at chromosome 3p25–26. Both alleles of VHL tumor suppressor gene are inactivated; therefore cell cycle regulation and angiogenesis are disturbed. Incidence is 1:35–50,000, and VHL typically presents in young adults during the third decade of life. The association of angiomatous retinal tumors and angiomatous tumors of the CNS characterizes this syndrome. Approximately 50% of hemangioblastomas are located in the spinal cord, 38% in the cerebellum, 10% in the brainstem, and 2% in the cerebrum. Approximately 20–40% are solid, but the majority are typically cystic, with a mural nodule. Contrast-enhanced MRI of brain and spine is recommended to detect small solid tumors that are often ill-defined. In a lesion with associated cyst, the tumor nodule enhances strongly after contrast administration, whereas the cyst wall does not. Retinal angiomas leading to retinal detachment and vitreous hemorrhages are present in half of the patients, and are the only prepubertal manifestation. In 7% of the patients, papillary cystadenomas of the endolymphatic sac occur. These patients typically present with hearing loss, disequilibrium, or aural fullness. Other VHL-associated tumors are pheochromocytomas (mean age of manifestation 30 years), angiomas of the liver and kidneys, and renal cell carcinomas (mean age of manifestation 33 years).

13.2.3 Myelination

Familiarity with the normal process and appearance of myelination is important in pediatric MRI of the brain. The appearance of myelination varies with magnet field strength and imaging sequence used. Myelination changes seem to appear earlier at lower field strengths and on IR sequences.

Myelination begins in utero and continues after birth. By the age of 2 years, the degree of myelination is close to that of an adult. The process of deposition of myelin, which is a hydrophobic glycolipoprotein, can be followed by MRI. On one hand, deposition of myelin can be followed in T1-WI, as fat is hyperintense on T1-WI. The accumulating lipid content results in a relatively increased signal in the white matter. This change is greatest on T1 in the first 6 months of life. On the other hand, deposition of myelin results in a decrease of the water content of the white matter. A transition on T2-WI from hyperintense, unmyelinated white matter to hypointense, myelinated white matter can be seen with the development of myelination. T1-WI demonstrates signal change related to the presence of myelin approximately 2 months prior to T2-WI, because the quantity of myelin deposition required to change SI is smaller in T1-WI than in T2-WI. However, the final assembly of myelin is better reflected on T2-WI. Therefore, to study the process of myelination, the recommended practice is to use T1-WI in children under 6 months of age, and to use T2-WI subsequently.

In general, myelination progresses from caudal to cranial and from posterior to anterior. Central structures are myelinated first, with more peripheral areas following. Central sensory pathways tend to myelinate before the central motor pathways. It is therefore possible to establish a series of milestones in myelination. At 40 weeks' gestational age, myelin can be seen on T1-WI in the medulla oblongata, the middle cerebellar peduncle, the tegmentum pontis, and especially the medial lemniscus and the colliculus inferior. Additionally, myelination is seen in the central tegmental part of the mesencephalon, the optic tracts, the posterior limb of the capsula interna, the white-matter tracts in each of the basal ganglia, the ascending tracts towards the postrolandic gyrus, and the primary sensory cortex.

By 3 months of age, high SI (myelination) should appear in the anterior limbs of the internal capsule and should extend distally from the deep cerebellar white matter into the cerebral folia. By the age of 4 months, the splenium of the corpus callosum should be of moderately high SI. By the age of 6 months, the genu of the corpus callosum should be of high SI. As stated earlier, after the age of 6 months, T2-WI is recommended to assess normal brain maturation. On T2-WI, the splenium of the corpus callosum should be of low SI by 6 months, like the genu of the corpus callosum by 8 months and the anterior limb of the internal capsule by 11 months of age. By the age of 14 months, the deep frontal white matter should be of low SI, with the temporal lobes being the last to myelinate. By 18 months, the entire brain should have an adult appearance, except for the most peripheral arcuate fibers (Fig. 13.25 and Table 13.2).

However, persistent areas of high signal intensity on T2-WI in the white matter dorsal and superior to the ventricular trigones and lateral to the bodies of the lateral ventricles are a frequent finding in the age group from 16 months to 10 (sometimes 20) years, and probably result from delayed myelination. In addition, large perivascular spaces contribute to the high signal. These so-called terminal zones have to be differentiated from white matter injury in periventricular leukomalacia (PVL) or toxic or metabolic brain disorders. In contrast to PVL (see under cerebrovascular disease), normal immature periventricular white matter is not accompanied by any loss of white matter, and a layer of myelinated white matter is present between the trigone of the ventricle and the terminal zones in normal patients.

A delayed or abnormal myelination pattern is an important finding in the pediatric brain. It may reflect failure in myelin formation or dysmyelination; it may be a consequence of white-matter injury in utero or at the

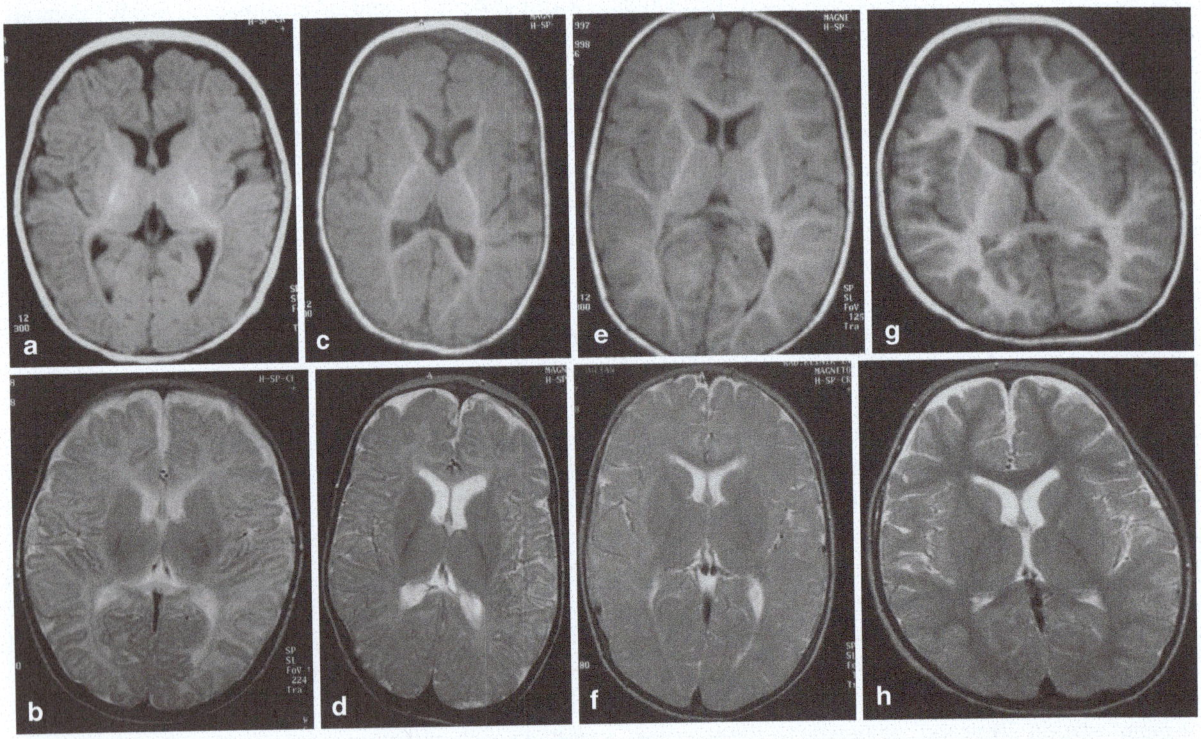

Fig. 13.25 Normal myelination according to age. Transverse T1-W (**a**) and T2-W (**b**) images of a 2-month-old infant. Unmyelinated deep white matter tracts are hypointense on T1-W and hyperintense on T2-W. Myelination of the posterior horns of the internal capsule is seen on both T1-WI and T2-WI. Transverse T1-W (**c**) and T2-W (**d**) images of a 6-month-old infant. Myelination of the deep white-matter tracts has further progressed. Both the splenium and the genu of the corpus callosum are of high signal intensity on T1-WI. On T2-WI, the splenium of the corpus callosum is of low signal intensity. Transverse T1-W and T2-W images of a 10-month-old infant. T1-WI (**e**) shows myelination of the external capsule, and the hyperintensity extends far more peripherally into a branching pattern in the occipital, parietal, and frontal lobes. T2-WI (**f**) shows decreasing signal intensity of the white matter throughout the brain. The cortex and the underlying white matter are isointense throughout most of the brain. The anterior limbs of the internal capsule are hypointense compared with the surrounding structures in essentially all patients of this age. Compare this with the mature brain of a 2.5-year-old child (**g, h**)

Table 13.2 Normal myelination of the brain (Adapted from Barkovich 2005)

Anatomic region	Myelination changes with age in months	
	T1-WI bright signal	T2-WI dark signal
Middle cerebellar peduncle	0	0–2
Cerebellar white matter	0–4	3–5
Posterior limb of internal capsule		
Anterior portion	1	4–7
Posterior portion	36 Gestational weeks	40 Gestational weeks
Anterior limb internal capsule	2–3	7–11
Genu of corpus callosum	4–6	5–8
Splenium corpus callosum	3–4	4–6
Occipital white matter		
Central	3–5	9–14
Peripheral	4–7	11–15
Frontal white matter		
Central	3–6	11–16
Peripheral	7–11	14–18
Centrum semiovale	2–4	7–11

WI weighted image

time of birth; or it may simply be seen in children with delayed development without obvious cause. Sometimes an abnormal myelination pattern is found in asymptomatic children, or occasionally both clinical development and myelination fall behind expected milestones and show a later recovery to normal in both parameters.

13.2.4 Metabolic and Neurodegenerative Disorders and Disorders with Abnormal Myelination

Normal brain maturation can be severely disturbed by alterations in the cellular metabolism, which can primarily affect either gray matter, white matter, or both. The principal effect of neurodegeneration and altered cellular metabolism in gray matter is the loss of the neuron, whereas metabolic anomalies affecting the white matter mainly involve the formation and structure of myelin. When both gray matter and white matter are involved, the primary injury may be to the gray matter, with secondary degeneration of the axons in the white matter, or vice versa. The diagnosis of metabolic and neurodegenerative disorders and disorders with abnormal myelination is often based on the clinical history, symptoms, and subsequent metabolic and pathologic testing. Patients with affection of the deep gray matter clinically present with athetosis, chorea, and dystonia, whereas those with involvement of the cortical gray matter suffer from seizures, visual loss, and dementia. In contrast, patients with white matter disorders present with ataxia, hyperreflexia, and spasticity. If an imaging study is to have a role in the diagnosis of these entities, the study should be performed early in the course of the disease, as most disorders have a similar imaging appearance in the late stages of the disease. By proper analysis of the early pattern of brain involvement, many disorders may be diagnosed or excluded. Symmetry, spread pattern, involvement of the subcortical or the deep white matter, the basal ganglia, the brainstem, and associated cortical infarctions are clues to the diagnosis. For the following, all common entities are listed in two tables using the cellular organelle classification, and important diseases are elucidated (Tables 13.3 and 13.4).

13.2.4.1 Metachromatic Leukodystrophy

Metachromatic leukodystrophy (MLD) is inherited as a recessive disorder, with a deficiency of arylsulfatase A, resulting in the accumulation of sulfatides that are toxic to white matter. Three clinical forms are differentiated: the infantile (most common), the juvenile, and the adult form (uncommon). Most patients will present between 14 months and 4 years of life with gait disturbances, ataxia, spasticity of the lower limbs, strabismus, dysarthria, and mental retardation. Death usually occurs 1–4 years after the onset of symptoms. Imaging studies show diffuse “butterfly-shaped” white matter disease with high SI on T2-WI and FLAIR images,

Table 13.3 Common metabolic disorders based on involved organelle (Adapted from Ball 1997)

Disorders of the lysosome Predominant white matter involvement
Metachromatic leukodystrophy[a]
Krabbe disease (Globoid cell leukodystrophy)[a]
Predominant gray matter involvement
GM_1-Gangliosidosis
Neuronal ceroid lipofuscinosis
Mucolipidosis
Both gray and white matter involvement
GM_2-Gangliosidosis
Mucopolysaccharidosis
Mannosidosis
Disorders of the peroxisome Predominant white matter involvement
Zellweger's syndrome
Pseudo-Zellweger's syndrome
Neonatal adrenoleukodystrophy[a]
X-linked (classic) adrenoleukodystrophy[a]
Adrenomyeloneuropathy
Infantile Refsum's disease
Disorders of the mitochondria
Leigh disease (subacute necrotizing encephalopathy)[a]
MELAS (myopathy, encephalopathy, lactat acidosis, stroke)[a]
MERRF (myopathy, encephalopathy with ragged red fibers)
Kearns–Sayre syndrome
Alper's disease

[a]Diseases discussed in the text

Table 13.4 Common metabolic disorders without specific organelle involved (Adapted from Ball 1997)

Disorders of amino acid metabolism
Lowe's disease (Oculocerebral syndrome)
Phenylketonuria
Maple syrup urine disease
Homocystinuria
Nonketotic hypoerglycinemia
Urea acid cycle defects
Organic acidurias
Methylmelonic aciduria
Proprionic aciduria
Glutaric aciduria type I[a]
Primary disorders in myelin formation
Cockayne's syndrome
Pelizaeus-Merzbacher disease[a]
Trichothiodystrophy
Disorders with macrocrania
Canavan disease[a]
Alexander disease[a]
Hepatic disorders with neurodegeneration
Wilson's disease
Galactosemia
Chronic hepatic encephalopathy
Carnitine deficiency
Miscellaneous disorders
Neuroaxonal dystrophy
Hallervorden-Spatz disease
Seitelberger's disease
Neuronal ceroid lipofuscinosis
Congenital muscular dystrophy with white matter changes
Encephalitis disseminata

[a]Disease discussed in the text

with sparing of subcortical U-fibers in early disease. Another important sign is the so-called "radial stripes," which are hypointense linear areas extending from ventricular wall to cerebral cortex on T2-WI. In late disease, progressive involvement of U-fibers, corpus callosum, descending pyramidal tracts, and internal capsules develops. The cerebellum may be involved as well. On T1-WI after contrast administration, no enhancement of white matter can be observed. The endstage of the disease shows generalized cerebral and spinal cord atrophy.

13.2.4.2 Globoid Cell Leukodystrophy: Krabbe Disease

Krabbe disease is an autosomal recessive disorder characterized by a deficiency of the enzyme galactocerebroside β-galactosidase. This lysosomal enzyme degrades cerebroside to galactose and ceramide; thus, the globoid cells found within the white matter contain cerebroside. The brain may be initially enlarged, but later becomes atrophic. Onset of symptoms occurs between 3 and 6 months of life, with irritability, intermittent fever, feeding problems, and progressive stiffness, in conjunction with opisthotonic spasms, depressed deep tendon reflexes, and seizures. Hyperacusis and optic atrophy often develop in this rapidly progressive and fatal disease. MRI shows nonspecific patchy white-matter hyperintensity in T2-WI, especially in the periventricular regions and in the deep cerebellar nuclei and white matter (Fig. 13.26). Later in the course of the disease, the deep cerebral white matter, especially the parietal lobes, the splenium, and the posterior limb of the internal capsule, are affected. Evidence of thalamic involvement is seen rather late in the course of disease, and therefore NECT can be very helpful in the early stage of the disease, as bilateral hyperdensities, probably reflecting microcalcifications that resolve with progressing disease, can be depicted in the thalami, and sometimes in the caudate nuclei, corona radiata, and cerebellar dentate nuclei. In addition, optic nerve enlargement due to accumulation of globoid cells is a typical finding.

13.2.4.3 X-Linked Adrenoleukodystrophy

X-linked Adrenoleukodystrophy (X-ALD) is a peroxisomal disorder, causing an impaired capacity to degrade very-long-chain fatty acids, due to a mutation of the ALD gene, which codes for a peroximal membrane protein. To date, more than 300 different mutations of this gene, located at Xq28, have been described. Besides the classic childhood cerebral X-ALD (CCALD), at least six other variants exist: presymptomatic X-ALD, adolescent cerebral Adrenoleukodystrophy (AdolCALD), adult cerebral Adrenoleukodystrophy (ACALD), Adrenomyeloneuropathy (AMN), Addison only, and symptomatic female carriers. X-ALD and AMN account for 80% of cases. A severe inflammatory demyelination in the cerebral white matter and an axonal degeneration that predominates in the posterior fossa and spinal cord are the two hallmarks of this entity. The CCALD is characterized by the inflammatory demyelination of the cerebrum with involvement of peritrigonal white matter and the splenium of the corpus callosum in early disease. Therefore, T2 prolongation is seen bilateral and symmetrical peritrigonal, in the splenium, the corticospinal

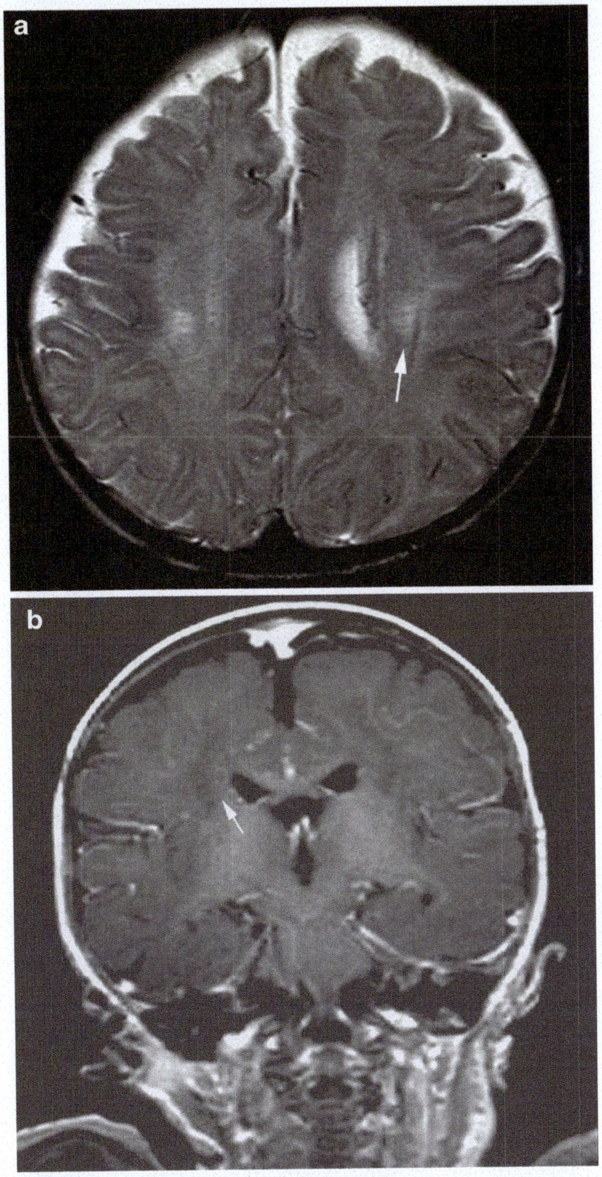

Fig. 13.26 Globoid cell leukodystrophy. Transverse T2-WI (**a**) and contrast-enhanced coronal T1-WI (**b**) of a 6-month-old child show a stripe-like pattern (*arrows*) in the periventricular area, indicating disappearance of myelin that had already been formed

tracts, the fornix, and the visual and auditory pathways. After contrast administration, an enhancing margin (leading edge) at the front of inflammatory demyelination can be depicted on T1-WI (Fig. 13.27). Patients with CCALD are boys, typically presenting between 3 and 10 years of age, with visual disturbance, behavioral changes, progressing gait disturbances, and slight intellectual impairment. Symptoms of adrenal insufficiency

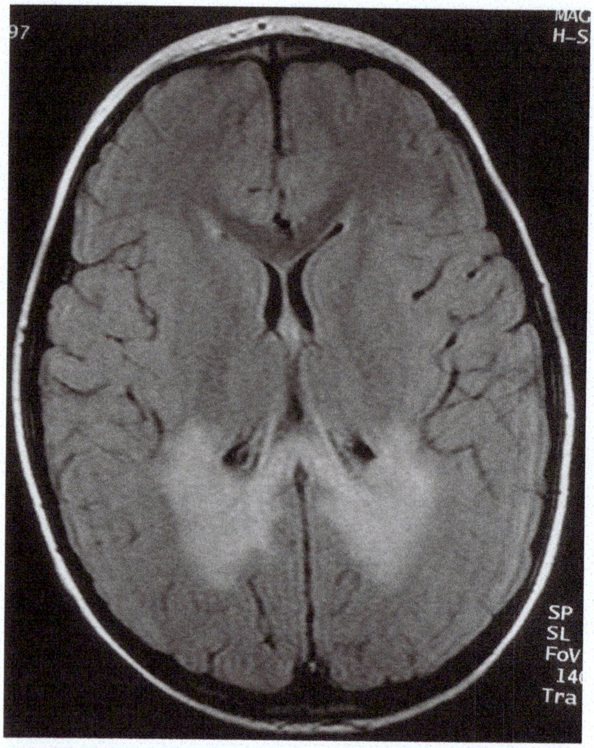

Fig. 13.27 Adrenoleukodystrophy. Transverse fluid-attenuated inversion recovery image shows high signal intensity in the occipital white matter

(skin bronzing, fatigue, nausea and vomiting) may precede neurological manifestations of disease or may not occur at all. A smaller percentage of children present with acute adrenal crisis, seizures, acute encephalopathy, or coma. A vegetative state or death usually occurs 2 years after the onset of symptoms. In contrast, AMN typically presents in young adults, and is mainly characterized by axonal degeneration in the brainstem and spinal cord (corticospinal tracts). However, brain involvement is present in up to 50% of patients. In addition, several other patterns of CNS involvement in this disease have been described, but it is beyond the scope of this chapter to cover them all.

13.2.4.4 Leigh Syndrome

Leigh syndrome is a genetically heterogeneous mitochondrial disorder characterized by progressive neurodegeneration, which seems to be the result of impaired energy production due to defective terminal oxidative metabolism. To date, four main groups are thought to be responsible for the majority of cases: defects of the pyruvate dehydrogenase complex, cytochrome *c* oxidase deficiency, mutations of the adenosine triphosphatase 6 gene, and complex I deficiency. Therefore, it is not surprising that different patterns of brain involvement are encountered. In pyrovate dehydrogenase complex deficiency corpus striatum, and in infants, thalami are involved. In addition, white matter cavitations are observed. In cytochrome *c* oxidase deficiency with *SURF1* mutation subthalamic nuclei, periaqueductal gray matter, central tegmental tract, cerebellar nuclei, cerebellar peduncles, and inferior olivary nuclei show high signal on T2-WI and FLAIR sequences. In Complex V deficiency with ATP*ase 6* mutation, anterior putamina, globi pallidi, dorsal mesencephalon and pons are involved (Fig. 13.28). The exact pattern in complex I deficiency has not yet been clarified. In some patients, elevation of lactate and pyruvate in the blood and CSF are observed. The clinical presentation of Leigh disease is that of a

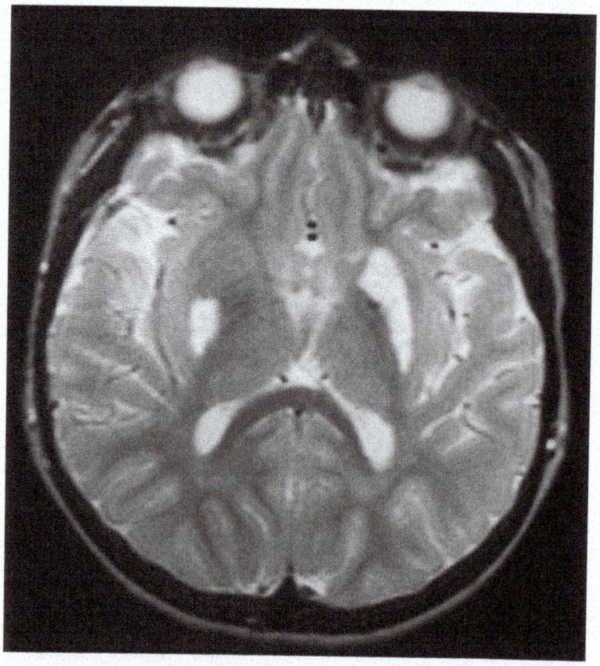

Fig. 13.28 Leigh disease. Transverse T2-WI demonstrates increased signal intensity in the putamina

multisystemic disorder dominated by the signs of CNS dysfunction, such as hypotonia, psychomotor deterioration, ophthalmoplegia, and respiratory and/or swallowing problems. The disease typically starts toward the end of the first year of life and leads to death within months or years.

13.2.4.5 Mitochondrial Encephalomyopathy with Lactic Acidosis and Stroke

In mitochondrial encephalomyopathy with lactic acidosis and stroke (MELAS), patients most commonly present as older children, or in the second decade of life, with headache, permanent or reversible stroke-like events, and episodes of nausea and vomiting. Typical imaging findings include calcium deposits in the globus pallidus and the caudate nucleus, due to basal ganglia involvement, and are more easily depicted on CT than MRI. Interestingly, these infarcts do not follow vascular border zones, and usually affect the cortex of the parietal and occipital lobes more severely than the underlying white matter. The “shifting spread” with migrating infarcts is the typical finding, and may help to differentiate this disease from embolic or thrombembolic infarction or vasculitis. In the acute phase, cortex and subjacent white matter show high signal on T2-WI and FLAIR images (Fig. 13.29). In the chronic phase, multifocal hyperintensities in the basal ganglia and deep white matter are present on T2-WI and FLAIR images. In addition, elevated lactate in CSF in a normal-appearing brain on MRS and a lactate double peak at 1.3 ppm are other imaging clues. Finally, progressive atrophy results.

13.2.4.6 Glutaric Aciduria Type 1

Glutaric aciduria type 1 is an autosomal recessive aminoacidopathy resulting from a defect in mitochondrial glutaryl-CoA dehydrogenase. Patients present with macrocephaly, acute encephalopathy, hypotonia, progressive dystonia, and tetraplegia, usually beginning in the first year of life. MR imaging reveals delayed myelination, degeneration of the basal ganglia with low SI on T1-WI, high SI on T2-WI and FLAIR images, and frontotemporal atrophy with widening of the sylvian fissure (“bat wing” sign) (Fig. 13.30). Glutaric aciduria type 1 is a child abuse mimic, probably due to the fact that wide subarachnoid spaces predispose development of subdural hematomas from relatively minor trauma.

13.2.4.7 Pelizaeus-Merzbacher Disease

Pelizaeus-Merzbacher disease belongs to a group of sudanophilic leukodystrophies, and most authors distinguish between two types: the classic form, which is an X-linked recessive disorder, and the connatal form, which is either autosomal or X-linked recessive inherited; girls can therefore also be affected. The classic form presents in young boys, with pendular eye movements, failure to develop normal head control, spasticity, choreoathetoid movements, cerebellar ataxia, and mental retardation, and has a progressive course, with death ensuing in the second or third decade of life. The rapidly fatal connatal form presents at birth or in infancy, with nystagmoid eye movements, extrapyramidal hyperkinesia, spasticity, and seizures. Currently, both types are thought to result from a defective *PLP1* gene coding for proteolipid protein 1 and its isoform, two components of myelin. Depending on the exact type of gene defect, myelin can be formed to a variable degree or not at all. The impaired function of oligodendrocytes leads to hypomyelination. The lack of mature myelin manifests as diffuse high SI on T2-WI, involving both cerebral and cerebellar hemispheres as well as the long white-matter fiber tracts of the brainstem and spinal cord. Therefore, the brain appears like the brain of a newborn. Later in the course of disease, existing myelination and white matter is continuously diminished, and atrophy ensues.

13.2.4.8 Canavan Disease

Canavan disease is an autosomal recessive disorder characterized by a deficiency of *N*-acetylaspartylase, and is also referred to as spongyform leukodystrophy of the CNS. The most common infantile type appears within the first 6 months of life. Patients present with

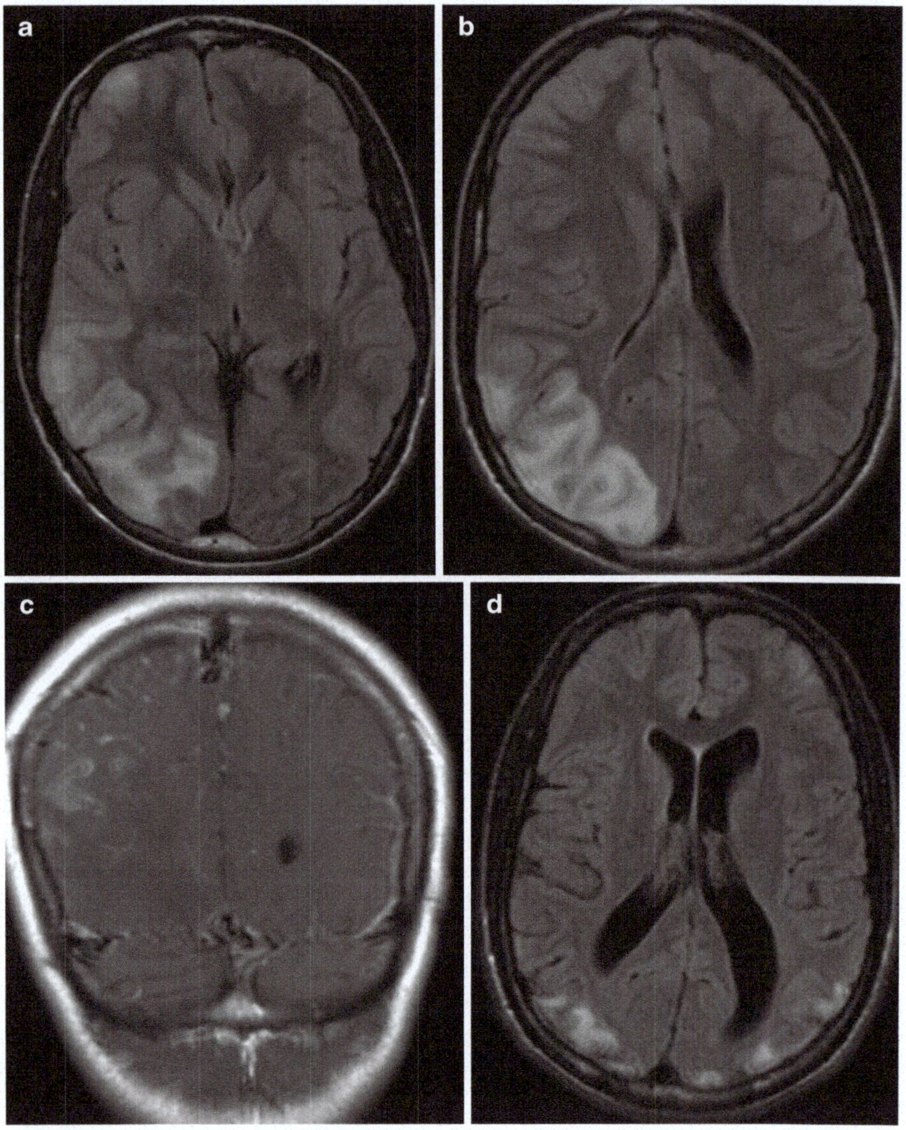

Fig. 13.29 Mitochondrial encephalopathy with lactic acidosis and stroke-like episodes (MELAS). Transverse FLAIR images (**a, b**) show swelling and hyperintense lesions in the right occipital lobe and in the right frontal lobe. Notice that the right occipital lesion crosses vascular boundaries. Contrast-enhanced T1-WI (**c**) shows enhancement of the lesion in the right occipital lobe. Transverse FLAIR image (**d**) obtained several weeks later show atrophy and T2 prolongation of both occipital lobes and enlargement of both ventricles, and a smaller lesion in the left frontal lobe

hypotonia, spasticity, blindness, myoclonic seizures, irritability, and enlarging head size. The disease usually has a rapid and fatal course. Demyelination typically begins in the peripheral subcortical U-fibers, and only involves all white matter of the brain in the later stages, causing atrophy. In addition, symmetric involvement of the striatum can be depicted. Therefore, MRI demonstrates low SI on T1-WI and high SI on T2-WI of the white matter and striatum (Fig. 13.31). Usually, proton MR spectroscopy shows a large *N*-acetylaspartate peak.

13.2.4.9 Alexander Disease

Alexander disease is also known as fibrinoid leukodystrophy. Three clinical types exist: infantile, juvenile, and adult. The infantile type is the most common, with symptoms starting from birth, with developmental delay, pyramidal tract signs, seizures, and progressive macrocephaly. Death occurs 2–3 years after birth. Both the juvenile and the adult forms present with bulbar or pseudobulbar signs and ataxia; additionally, spasticity and developmental regression are present in

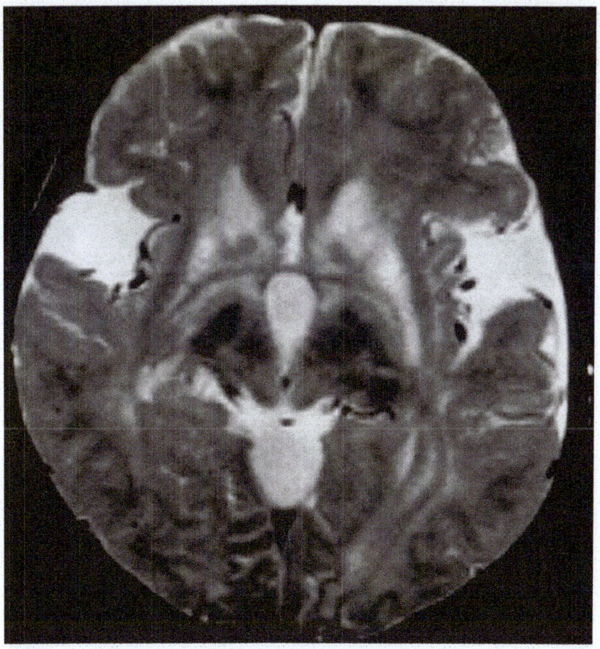

Fig. 13.30 Glutaric aciduria type 1. Transverse T2-WI shows abnormal hyperintensity in the putamina, with widening of the sylvian fissures due to atrophy

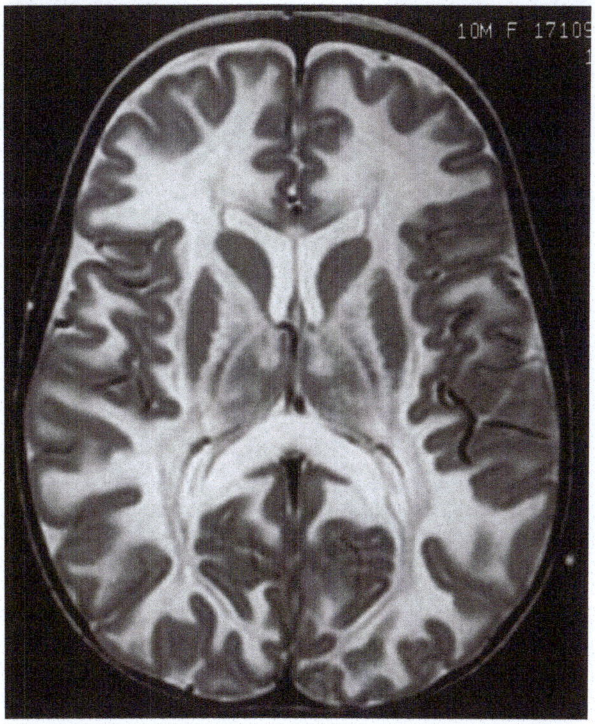

Fig. 13.31 Canavan disease. Transverse T2-WI shows hyperintense signal intensity in the white matter, with involvement of the internal and external capsules and the subcortical U-fibers

the juvenile type. Macrocephaly results from increased astrocytic eosinophilic Rosenthal's fibers within the white matter, leading to increased weight and size of the brain. Recent findings suggest that mutations of the gene for glial fibrillary acidic protein (GFAP) lead to an aggregation of the protein in the cytoplasm, consistent with those inclusions seen in Rosenthal's fibers. Therefore, brain biopsy is no longer necessary, as diagnosis can be made by clinical and typical imaging findings in concert with genetic testing. Most commonly, the disease shows high SI on T2-WI, occurring in the periventricular region of the frontal lobes and later extending to entire cerebral hemispheres, due to demyelination. Frequently, a periventricular rim can be depicted with low signal on T2-WI and high signal on T1-WI. This rim enhances after contrast administration, as does the frontal white matter, especially in early disease in the infantile form. Additionally, there is involvement of the basal ganglia, thalami, brain stem, dentate nuclei, fornix, optic chiasm, and spinal cord (Fig. 13.32).

13.2.5 Infections and Inflammation

13.2.5.1 Congenital Infections

Congenital infections of the CNS are most commonly due to toxoplasma, rubella, CMV, and herpes simplex organisms (TORCH), human immunodeficiency virus (HIV), and bacteria. The developing fetal brain and the immature fetal immune system have a limited ability to respond to an inflammatory insult. Depending on the time point of infection, in utero infections can cause either developmental brain anomalies (hydranencephaly, schizencephaly, neuronal proliferation alterations) or focal or multifocal destructive changes (necrotizing encephalitis, vasculitis, and meningitis).

Toxoplasmosis

Toxoplasmosis is the second most common congenital CNS infection after CMV infection. The principal CNS findings are bilateral chorioretinitis (85% of the patients), seizures, hydrocephalus, microcephaly, and

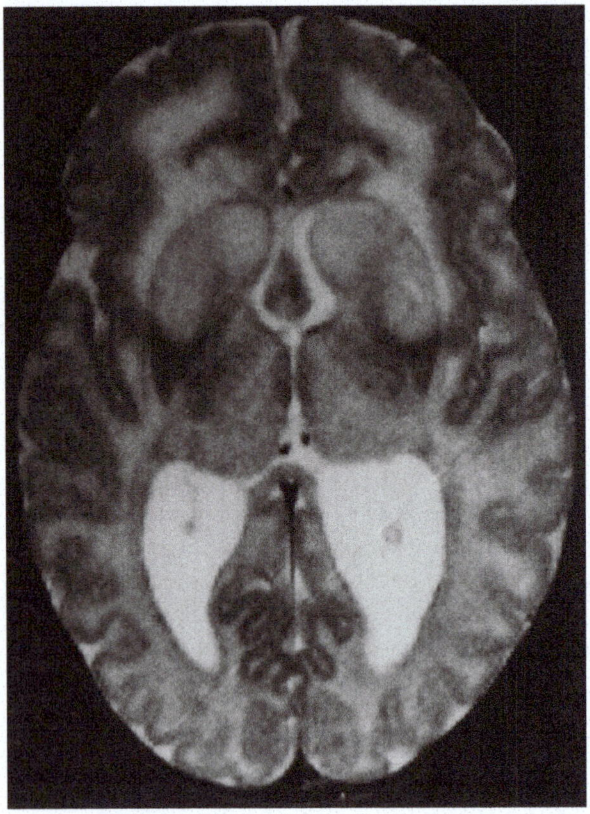

Fig. 13.32 Alexander disease. Transverse T2-WI shows high signal intensity in the frontal white matter involving the U-fibers and extending posteriorly into the external capsules, and affection of the head of the caudate nuclei and putamina

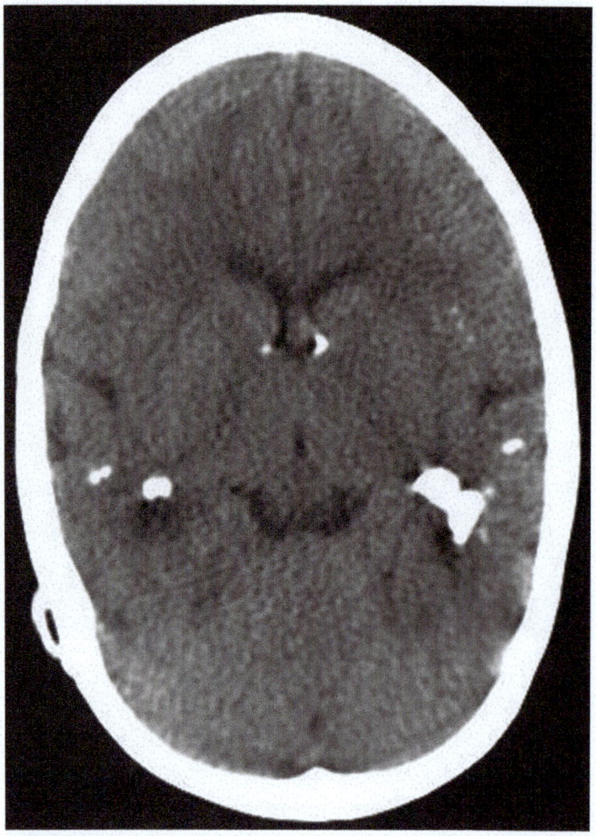

Fig. 13.33 Toxoplasmosis. CT shows multiple calcifications in a periventricular, basal-ganglia, and subcortical location in a patient with a shunt-tube

intracranial calcifications. The calcifications vary with the extent of disease, and typically occur in a periventricular or basal-ganglia distribution (Fig. 13.33), but may involve the cerebral cortex in severe cases with near-total destruction. Hydrocephalus is due to ependymitis, leading to aqueductal stenosis. Severity of disease seems to depend on the time point of infection. Infections before 20 weeks are more serious, and usually result in ventricular dilation, porencephaly, extensive calcifications, and microcephaly. By contrast, infections after the 30th week are rarely accompanied by ventricular dilation and show less calcifications. An important differentiating feature is the absence of cortical malformations, which is a common finding in congenital CMV infection. CT is the best modality to depict calcifications, whereas MRI is primarily performed to prove the absence of cortical dysplasia.

Cytomegalovirus

CMV is the most common congenital infection among newborns. The most common clinical features of symptomatic CMV infection include hepatosplenomegaly, jaundice, chorioretinitis, microcephaly, impaired hearing, and optic atrophy. Approximately 10–15% of infected infants develop neurological and developmental deficits in the first year of life. Patients infected in the beginning of the second trimester have complete lissencephaly, with a thin cortex, hypoplastic cerebellum,

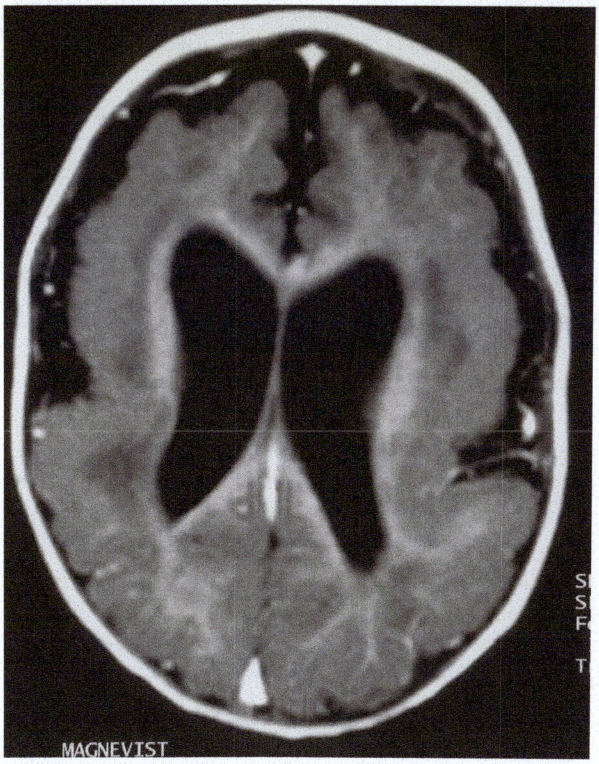

Fig. 13.34 Congenital cytomegalovirus infection. Transverse T1-WI shows pachygyria with cortical thickening and irregularity of the gray-matter/white-matter border

delayed myelination, ventriculomegaly, and significant periventricular calcifications. Those infected later will present with polymicrogyria, less ventricular dilatation, and less cerebellar hypoplasia. Patients infected perinatally have normal gyral patterns, mild atrophy due to damaged white matter, periventricular calcifications, and hemorrhage. CT is the best modality to evaluate calcifications, whereas MRI best demonstrates polymicrogyria, myelination delay, and gliosis (Fig. 13.34).

Herpes Simplex Virus

Approximately 75–90% of congenital herpes simplex infections are caused by type 2. In the vast majority of cases, infection is transmitted during vaginal delivery. If transplacental infection occurs in the first trimester, it may produce microcephaly, atrophy, hydranencephaly, and intracranial calcifications. Perinatally infected newborns present with meningoencephalitis, seizures, and fever, as well as respiratory distress, cyanosis, and jaundice. Patchy areas of low SI on T1-WI and high SI on T2-WI in the white matter can be delineated on MRI examinations. Meningeal contrast enhancement may be observed, as well as areas of hemorrhagic infarction. Cortical gray matter is involved with progressing disease. The end stage of severe herpes simplex virus (HSV) infection is cystic encephalomalacia and atrophy. Dystrophic calcifications in a periventricular and basal-ganglia distribution or in the cortex are more easily evaluated by CT.

Human Immunodeficiency Virus

Vertical HIV infection happens either in utero or at delivery, or by breastfeeding. In untreated mothers, maternal transmission of HIV occurs in up to 30% of cases. Fortunately, the rate of infection can be reduced to 2% by adequate therapy for the mother with antiretroviral drugs and delivery by cesarian section. The manifestation of neurological symptoms in children with congenital acquired immunodeficiency syndrome (AIDS) generally occurs between the ages of 2 months and 5 years. Typical imaging findings are bilateral symmetrical calcifications of the basal ganglia and subcortical white matter, most commonly in the frontal lobes, as well as atrophy, mineralizing microangiopathy, and microcephaly. Extracranial manifestations are lymphadenopathy and benign lymphoepithelial parotid cysts.

13.2.5.2 Postnatal Infections

Meningitis

Meningitis is the most common CNS infection in children, and may be either bacterial or viral. It is most commonly caused by hematogenous spread, and primarily diagnosed by clinical symptoms and lumbar puncture. Neuroimaging is only performed prior to lumbar puncture to rule out hydrocephalus or abscess, and especially if the diagnosis is unclear or if complications such as focal neurologic deficits, persistent seizures, or signs of increased intracranial pressure occur. Cerebral infections can have severe sequelae in newborns, due to the immature immune system. Intense contrast enhancement of the ependyma and meninges, reflecting ventriculitis and arachnoiditis, is observed; the latter two frequently lead to hydrocephalus. Abscess formation is relatively rare. In addition, meningitis can be complicated by arterial infarctions due to arteritis and venous thrombosis due to coexisting dehydration, followed by venous infarction. Consequently, imaging reveals edema with or without ischemic or hemorrhagic infarction due to vessel occlusion.

Imaging is often negative in older children in the acute stage. Later stages present similar imaging findings, although, more often, subdural effusions, dilated subarachnoid spaces, and ventricular enlargement are present with contrast-enhancing meninges.

Cerebritis, Abscess, and Empyema

Bacterial infection of the brain produces cerebritis and meningitis and, if not sufficiently treated, abscess or empyema. It usually results from hematogenous spread, penetrating trauma, postoperatively, or from contiguous spread of mastoiditis and sinusitis. In newborns and small infants, the most common organisms involved are *Escherichia coli, Proteus, Klebsiella*, followed by group B-streptococci, *Pseudomonas, Listeria*, and occasionally *Citrobacter* (Fig. 13.35). In infants and older children, *Meningococcus* and *Pneumococcus* prevail. In early cerebritis, edema may be present, demonstrating low SI on T1-WI, high SI on T2-WI, and patchy contrast enhancement. When abscess formation develops, the center of the abscess and the surrounding edema are hypointense on T1-WI and hyperintense on T2-WI. The rim of an abscess is isointense on T1-WI and hypointense on T2-WI, and will enhance with paramagnetic contrast. Subdural and epidural empyemas occur more frequently in adolescents, and usually follow sinusitis. Imaging reveals crescent- or lens-shaped extracerebral fluid accumulations with peripheral contrast enhancement.

Lyme Disease

Children are frequently affected by this multisystemic disorder, which is a tick-borne disease caused by *Borrelia burgdorferi*. In children, the typical triphasic course, comparable to that of lues, is not always observed. In 15–22% of cases, a neurologic involvement with lymphocytic meningitis, meningoencephalitis, facial palsy, or palsy of other cranial nerves, or a pseudotumor cerebri-like syndrome is present. Although MRI is often negative, leptomeningeal enhancement, with or without enhancement of the affected cranial nerve, may be found in patients with cranial neuropathy. Furthermore, focal lesions of the cerebral white matter may be detected, with high SI on T2-WI and enhancement after paramagnetic contrast on T1-WI.

Encephalitis

Encephalitis is a nonsuppurative inflammation of the brain, sometimes accompanied by meningitis. The vast majority of encephalitides are caused by viral infections. A smaller percentage is due to autoimmune processes or other pathogens.

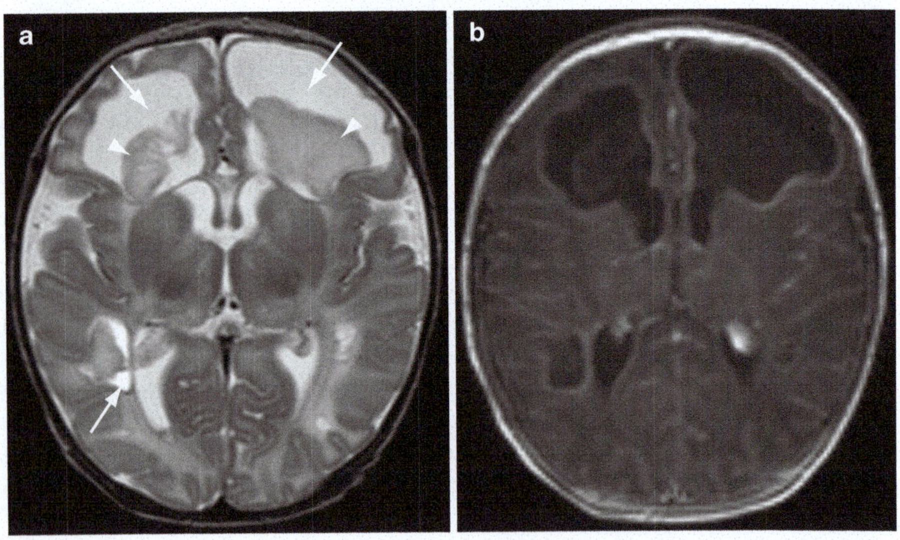

Fig. 13.35 *Citrobacter* cerebritis. Transverse T2-WI (**a**) shows multiple cavities (*arrows*) in the cerebral hemispheres on both sides, some filled with necrotic brain parenchyma (*arrowheads*). Contrast-enhanced fat-saturated T1-WI (**b**) shows irregular enhancement in the periphery of the cavities, consistent with neonatal abscess due to the immature immune system

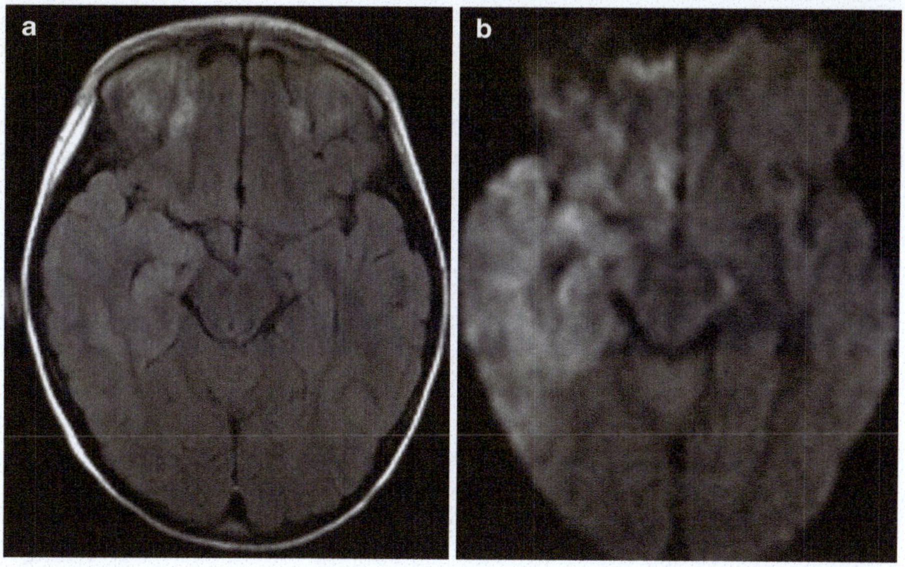

Fig. 13.36 Herpes simplex I. Transverse FLAIR image (**a**) shows swelling and hyperintense SI in the right temporal lobe. Diffusion-weighted image (**b**) demonstrates restricted diffusion in the same area, involving the cortex and the subcortical white matter

Herpes Simplex I

In older children, herpes simplex type 1 produces a more focal, localized meningoencephalitis, with swelling and mass effect involving the frontal and temporal lobes, displaying low SI on T1-WI and high SI on T2-WI (Fig. 13.36). However, in children younger than 10 years of age, a generalized involvement of the brain is typically encountered. As the virus has a predilection for the limbic system, the hippocampus and the amygdala are frequently involved. Encephalitis may be bilateral but asymmetric, and hemorrhage or hemorrhagic infarction may occur. Gyriform enhancement after administration of paramagnetic contrast may be present by the end of the first week. Calcifications occur as late sequelae in the following weeks. End-stage findings include volume loss and cystic encephalomalacia.

Progressive Multifocal Leukencephalopathy

Progressive multifocal leukencephalopathy is an inflammation caused, in immunocompromised patients, by the JC polyomavirus, belonging to the family of papovaviruses. The disease has a fatal course, with death occurring within 1 year after onset of symptoms, which commonly consist of progressive mental deterioration, sensory deficits, ataxia, hemiparesis, and visual impairment. On MRI, initially multifocal lesions, later in the course confluent lesions in the periventricular and/or subcortical white matter are detected, with increased SI on T2-WI, most commonly in the frontal and parieto-occipital regions. Mass effect is uncommon, and contrast enhancement is usually not seen.

Subacute Sclerosing Panencephalitis

Subacute sclerosing panencephalitis is probably the result of a progressive, reactivated measles infection, typically affecting those children between the ages of 5 and 15 years, who had clinical measles before the age of 2–3 years. There is a relentless progression of the disease, with death occurring within 2–6 years. In the first 3–4 months after onset of clinical symptoms such as behavioral changes, myoclonus, ataxia, seizures, and mental deterioration, MRI may be normal. Later in the course of disease, MRI shows nonspecific imaging findings of leukencephalopathy with atrophy and diffuse asymmetrically bilateral areas of increased SI on T2-WI in the periventricular white matter and basal ganglia, with extension in the corpus callosum; these will not enhance with paramagnetic contrast or show mass effect. Occasionally, MRI will demonstrate involvement of the cerebellar white matter, midbrain, and pons.

Rasmussen Encephalitis

Rasmussen encephalitis or chronic focal encephalitis is a progressive, relentless inflammation of the brain, of uncertain etiology, typically affecting one hemisphere, and can only be diagnosed by brain biopsy or postmortem. The disease usually starts in childhood, between 18 months and 14 years, with intractable focal seizures. Other clinical symptoms are progressive hemiplegia and psychomotor deterioration. Initial MRI examinations may be normal. In the course of the disease, MRI demonstrates areas of increased SI on T2-WI in the cerebral cortex and subcortical white matter, and with frequent affection of frontal and temporal lobes, with swollen gyri. In 65% of cases, the basal ganglia (early occurring caudate atrophy) are additionally involved. On follow-up studies, progressive focal or hemispheric atrophy is revealed. Therefore, Rasmussen encephalitis is an important differential diagnosis of atrophies affecting one hemisphere, including congenital aplasia of the common carotid artery, MELAS, and atrophy secondary to infarction or perinatal infection.

Acute Disseminated Encephalomyelitis

Acute disseminated encephalitis (ADEM) is defined as an autoimmune-mediated demyelination late in the course of a viral infection or after vaccination, with involvement of the brain and spinal cord. It is assumed that precipitating illness induces a host-antibody response against a central-nervous antigen. Common clinical presentations are seizures and focal neurologic signs 4–7 days after the clinical onset of the viral infection. Less severe cases present with headache, fever, and myelopathy. The neurological symptoms resolve over a period of weeks, although 10–30% of patients will have some permanent neurological damage. ADEM is typically monophasic and, to date, multiphasic or relapsing ADEM is supposed to be a variant of multiple sclerosis (MS). On MRI, the lesions presenting inflammation and demyelination are often multifocal, asymmetric hyperintensities on T2-WI in the subcortical white matter, either unilateral or bilateral, with no mass effect, and may show occasional enhancement with paramagnetic contrast on T1-WI (Fig. 13.37). Cortical and deep gray matter, particularly the thalami, may be involved. The brainstem, spinal cord, and the cerebellar white matter may also be affected. Acute hemorrhagic leukencephalitis (AHEM) is currently considered to be a subtype of ADEM, characterized by larger lesions, with more mass effect and hemorrhage.

Multiple Sclerosis: Encephalitis Disseminata

MS is usually considered an adult disease, but occasionally manifests in childhood. MS is indistinguishable from ADEM by imaging findings, and differentiation therefore depends on lack of remittance, labor findings, clinical history, and follow-up examinations. Imaging findings in children with MS do not differ from those in adults (Fig. 13.38).

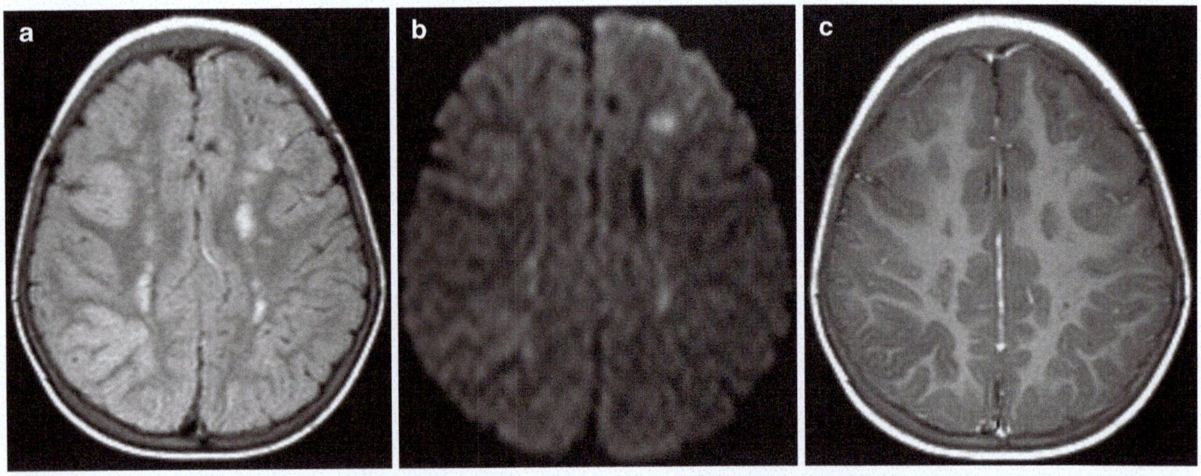

Fig. 13.37 Acute disseminated encephalitis. Transverse FLAIR image (**a**) reveals multiple hyperintense lesions in a periventricular location as well as lesions in the subcortical white matter. Diffusion-weighted image (**b**) shows restricted diffusion of the lesions. On contrast-enhanced (single dose) T1-WI (**c**) none of the lesions is enhancing

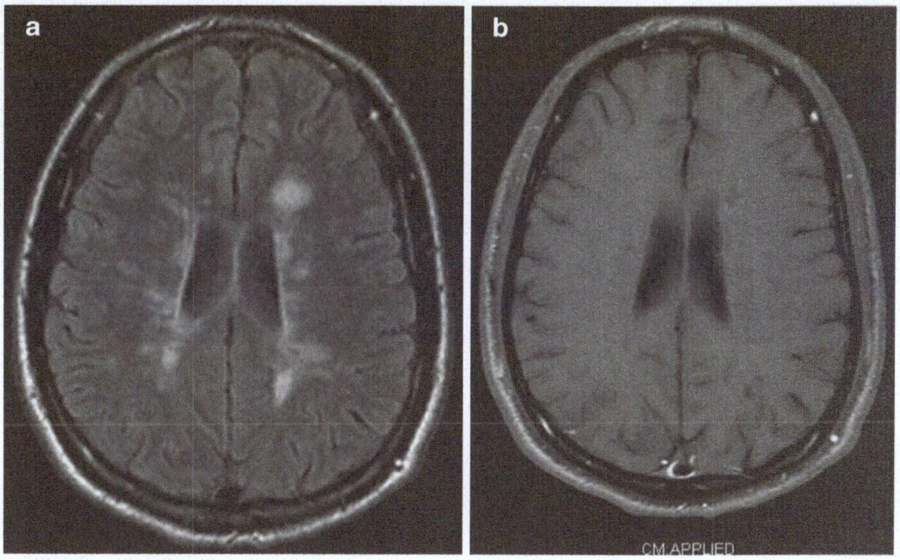

Fig. 13.38 Multiple sclerosis. Transverse FLAIR image (**a**) shows multiple hyperintense lesions in a periventricular location with perpendicular orientation as well as lesions in the subcortical white matter. On fat-saturated contrast-enhanced (single dose) T1-WI (**b**) some of the lesions in the left cerebral hemisphere next to the ventricle display a faint (rim) enhancement

Tuberculosis

Tuberculosis is an infection with *Mycobacterium tuberculosis*, which typically causes basal meningitis, with marked contrast enhancement of the basal leptomeninges (Fig. 13.39). Basal meningitis is very often complicated by hydrocephalus, and may cause vasculitis of the lenticulostriate and thalamoperforate vessels, leading to infarctions of the basal ganglia and thalami, displaying low SI on T1-WI and high SI on T2-WI. Parenchymal tuberculomas will present as nodular (noncaseating) or ring-enhancing (caseating) lesions, often located at the gray/white matter junction, and may calcify.

Fungal Infections

Fungal diseases of the CNS are less common in children than in adults. The most common fungi involved are *Cryptococcus neoformans, Candida, Aspergillus* (Fig. 13.40), *Coccidioides immitis, Histoplasma capsulatum,* and

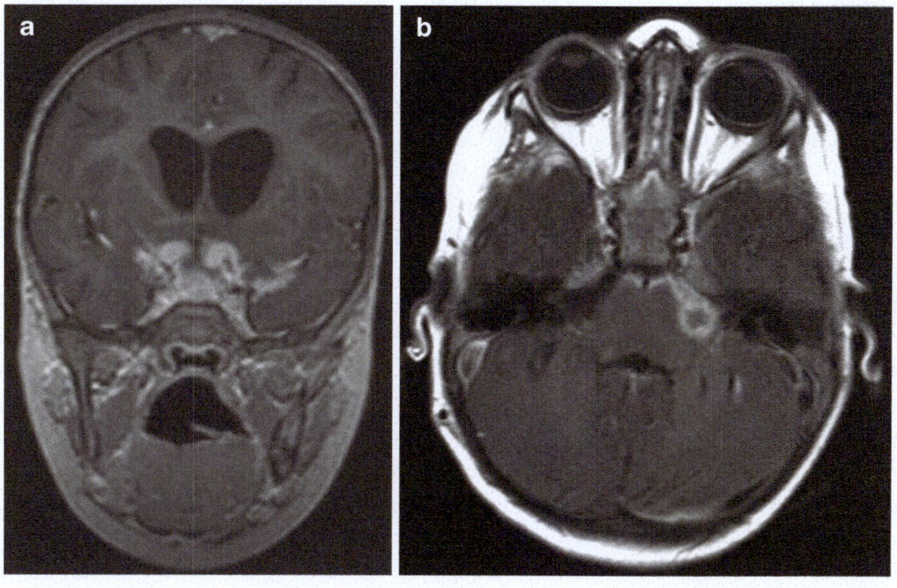

Fig. 13.39 Tuberculosis. Coronal contrast-enhanced fat-saturated T1-WI (**a**) shows basal meningitis. Transverse contrast-enhanced T1-WI (**b**) reveals a tuberculoma in the left cerebellopontine angle

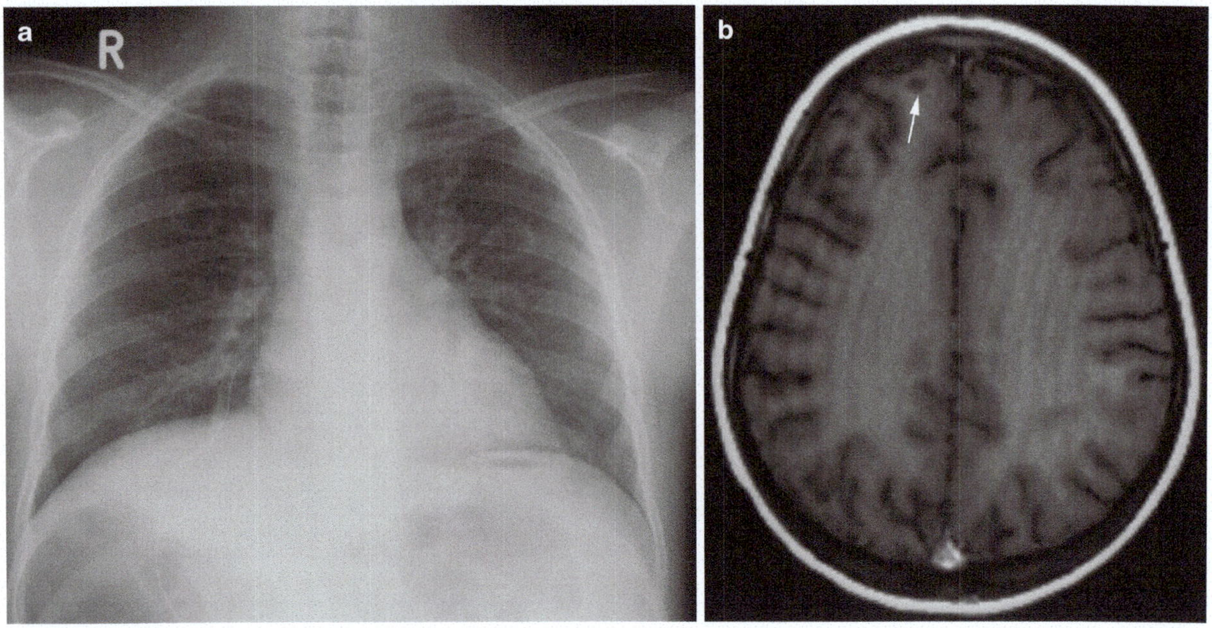

Fig. 13.40 Aspergillosis. Chest X-ray (**a**) shows multiple bilateral cavitating lesions, consistent with aspergillosis, in a 14-year-old girl with autoimmune hepatitis after steroid therapy. Transverse contrast-enhanced T1-WI (**b**) shows a lesion with rim enhancement in the right frontal lobe (*arrow*)

Mucor. They typically produce granulomatous basal meningitis similar to that seen in tuberculosis. Parenchymal abscesses, granulomas, and infarction due to vasculitis may also be present, depending on the species of fungi.

Neurocysticercosis

Neurocysticercosis is caused by a parasitic infection of the pork tapeworm *Taenia solium,* and is the most common parasitic infection in the world. Man can either be the intermediate or definitive host, and is infected by ingestion of eggs from contaminated food or water, or larval cysts from uncooked pork. From the gastrointestinal (GI) tract, oncopheres spread into the CNS and skeletal muscle, where they develop into cysticerci. Patients typically present with seizures, headaches, hydrocephalus, and learning disabilities. Four pathologic stages are distinguished: vesicular, colloidal vesicular, granular nodular, and nodular calcified (Fig. 13.41). In the vesicular stage, cystic lesions on MRI are isointense to CSF, both on T1-WI and T2-WI. After contrast administration, a mild enhancement with a discrete eccentric dot (viable larva) may be seen. The colloidal stage is characterized by a cystic lesion, which is mildly hyperintense to CSF on T1-WI and T2-WI, with surrounding edema showing a thick enhancing cyst wall on T1-WI. In the granular stage, a thickened retracting cyst wall with decreasing edema can be depicted and, after contrast administration, the wall can show either nodular or ring-enhancement. In the calcified nodular stage, the lesion may be difficult to detect on T1-WI and T2-WI and, after administration of contrast media, a minimal enhancement may be shown. In addition, lesions can be present in cisterns, parenchyma, and ventricles, with the subarachnoid spaces of the convexity being the most frequent location. Parenchymal cysts are often located at the gray-white matter junction, and in the basal cisterns cysts may be racemose (multiple, grape-like).

13.2.6 Brain Tumors in Childhood

CNS neoplasms during childhood are the second most common pediatric tumors, being exceeded only by leukemia (Fig. 13.42). Overall infratentorial and supratentorial tumors occur with almost the same frequency. In the first 2–3 years of life, supratentorial tumors predominate, whereas infratentorial tumors are in the majority in the age group from 4 to 10 years. An equal distribution is found in children older than 10 years. In general, the most common tumors in the pediatric age group are gliomas, ependymomas,

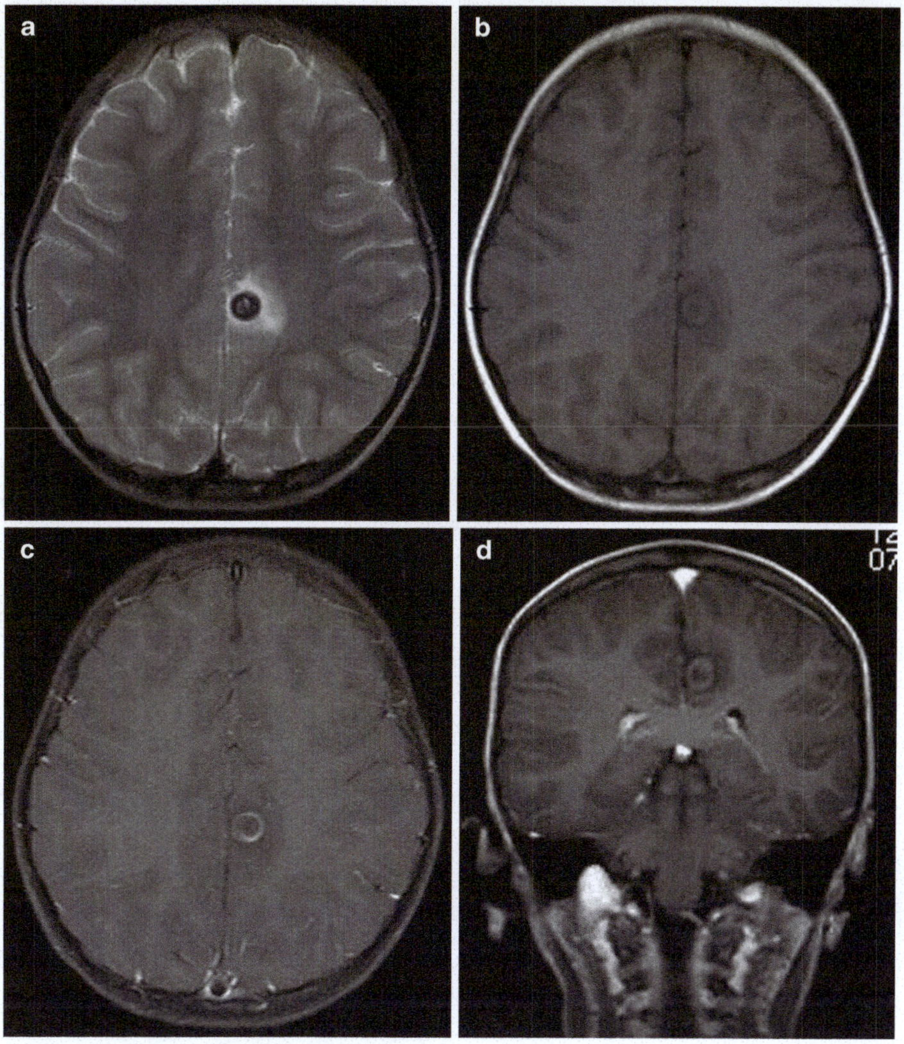

Fig. 13.41 Neurocysticercosis. Transverse T2-WI (**a**) shows a hypointense lesion in the left cingulum that was calcified on CT (not shown), with perifocal edema. Transverse T1-WI (**b**) pre- and transverse fat-saturated T1-WI (**c**), and coronal T1-WI (**d**) postcontrast reveal ring enhancement

medulloblastomas (PNETs), craniopharyngiomas, and pinealomas (Fig. 13.43).

For MR imaging of CNS neoplasms, T2-WI, FLAIR sequences, DWI, and T1-WI should be obtained in two planes, before and after the administration of paramagnetic contrast, preoperatively and postoperatively, to analyze the neoplasm and its possible recurrence. Early postoperative imaging (in the first 72 h) is important, as the surgically-induced contrast enhancement at the operative margins directly increases postoperatively. It will decrease on sequential exams after approximately 6 weeks, and will generally disappear within 12 months. Meningeal enhancement is almost always seen on follow-up examinations and may persist, especially in patients with shunt tubes or subdural hygromas (Fig. 13.44). However, to date, realistically, CT is almost certainly the initial imaging modality used in many cases. Therefore, it is reasonable to perform an examination pre- and postcontrast administration and reformate coronal and sagittal images. As a matter of fact, CT can add valuable information concerning differentiation of tumors. A focus on the most common infratentorial and supratentorial tumors in children follows.

13.2.6.1 Intra-Axial Infratentorial Tumors

The most common tumors encountered in the posterior fossa in children are medulloblastomas, astrocytomas of the cerebellum and brainstem, atypical teratoid/rhabdoid tumors, and ependymomas. Due to the fact that brainstem tumors have different prognoses with respect to their sites of origination, they are now separated into different groups.

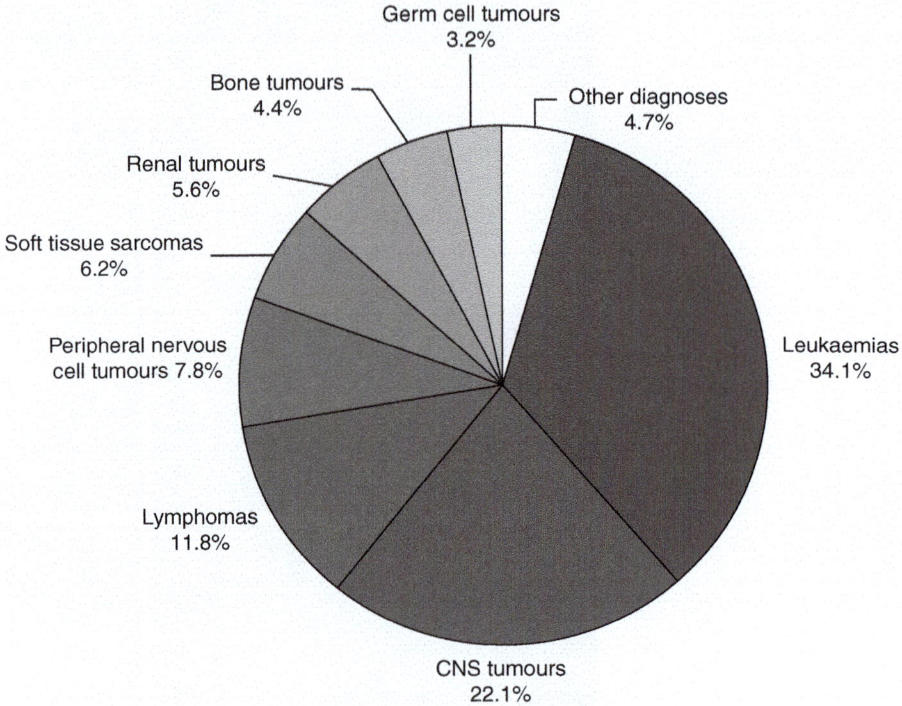

Fig. 13.42 Relative frequencies of the registered patients aged under 15 years in Germany according to the most common main ICCC-3 diagnosis groups (1997–2006) (n = 18,283) (Adapted from Kaatsch et al. 2000)

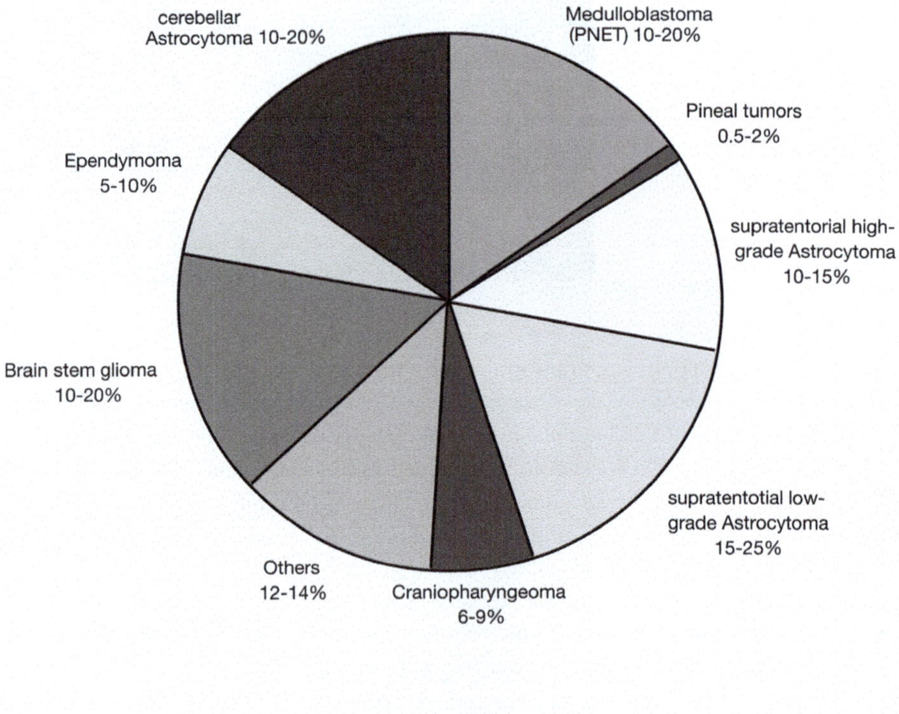

Fig. 13.43 Approximate incidence of common central nervous system tumors in children (Adapted from Pizzo and Poplack 2006)

Medulloblastomas: Primitive Neuroectodermal Tumors (PNETs)

Medulloblastomas (PNETs) are highly malignant tumors composed of very primitive, undifferentiated, small, round cells, and account for approximately 20% of CNS tumors and for 30–40% of posterior fossa neoplasms in children (Fig. 13.43). They are the most common tumor in the 6–11-year age group, and patients typically present with nausea, vomiting,

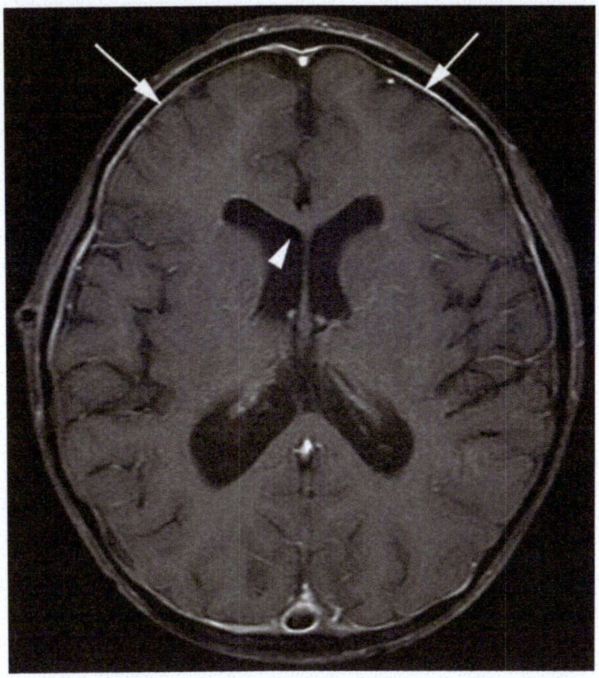

Fig. 13.44 Persistence of meningeal enhancement (*arrows*) in a patient with a shunt tube in the right ventricle (*arrowhead*) after surgical resection of a medulloblastoma

ataxia, and headaches. Classically, medulloblastomas present as round or lobulated fourth ventricle masses arising from the vermis. They are isointense to gray matter on T1-WI, and show variable contrast-enhancement pattern, ranging from homogeneous to patchy. On T2-WI, medulloblastomas appear heterogeneously hypointense or isointense compared with gray matter. Cystic components may be present in up to 80% of medulloblastomas. Because of the location of this lesion, consecutive hydrocephalus is often observed. Medulloblastomas readily spread via CSF pathways, infratentorially and supratentorially, and develop subarachnoid metastasis, which may reinvade brain parenchyma. At initial diagnosis, approximately 30–40% of patients have spinal metastasis, which imparts a poorer prognosis. Therefore, precontrast and postcontrast studies of the brain and spine in two separate examinations are recommended before surgery and for follow-up (Figs. 13.45 and 13.82; Table 13.5).

Astrocytomas

Overall, astrocytomas are the most common brain tumors in children (40–50%). Cerebellar astrocytomas account for 10–20% of common CNS tumors in children (Fig. 13.43). Approximately 60% of astrocytomas are located in the posterior fossa (40% in the cerebellum, 20% in the brainstem). Astrocytomas are glial

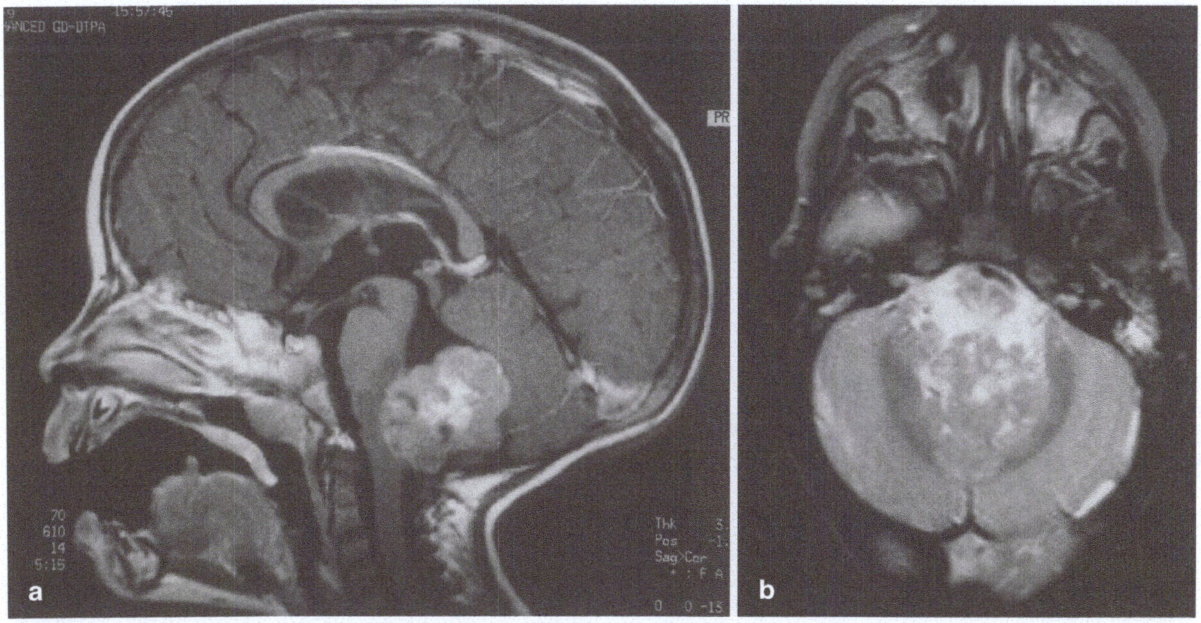

Fig. 13.45 Medulloblastoma (primitive neuroepithelial tumor). Sagittal contrast-enhanced T1-WI (**a**) shows an inhomogeneously enhancing mass sitting in the fourth ventricle. Transverse T2-WI (**b**) shows the tumor to be of slightly mixed signal intensity, probably reflecting necrosis and solid tumor

Table 13.5 Posterior fossa tumors in childhood (Adapted from Atlas 1996)

	JPA	Medulloblastoma (PNET)	Ependymoma	Brainstem astrocytoma
SI characteristics on T2	Cystic, sharply demarcated	Homogenous, low to moderate SI	Markedly heterogenous	Ill-defined, high SI
Contrast enhancement	Common in solid portion	Common, dense	Common, irregular	Common
Calcification	Uncommon	Uncommon	Common	Rare
Hemorrhage	Rare	Uncommon	Common	Uncommon
Tendency to seed via CSF	Extremely low	High	Low to moderate	Low
Prognosis (estimated survival)	>90% 10-year survival	50% 5-year survival	50% 5-year survival	20% 5-year survival

PNET primitive neuroepithelial tumors; *JPA* juvenile pilocytic astrocytoma; *SI* signal intensity; *CSF* cerebrospinal fluid

tumors that arise from astrocytes, and can be divided into two major groups: the infiltrative or diffuse astrocytomas and the localized, noninfiltrative astrocytomas (Table 13.6). In children, 85% of cerebellar astrocytomas are juvenile pilocytic astrocytomas (JPAs), which are of the localized type and considered relatively benign, with a 94% survival rate at 10 years after total resection. Approximately 15% of cerebellar astrocytomas are of the infiltrating type, similar to cerebral astrocytomas in adults. The peak incidence of these tumors is from birth to 9 years of age. Clinically, patients present with early morning headache, vomiting, and ataxia. Usually, the MR appearance of JPAs is virtually diagnostic. JPAs appear as well-demarcated cysts arising either from the vermis or one cerebellar hemisphere, with a contrast-enhancing mural nodule (Fig. 13.46) on T1-WI after contrast administration. On T1-WI, the cystic component is usually hypointense, but may be isointense to hyperintense due to hemorrhage or proteinaceous content. The infiltrating astrocytomas are solid lesions, frequently associated with hemorrhage and necrosis, with variable presentation on MR imaging (Table 13.5).

Table 13.6 Classification of astrocytic brain tumors (Adapted from Atlas 1996)

Diffuse or infiltrative type	Localized or non-infiltrative type
Astrocytoma	Pilocytic astrocytoma
Anaplastic astrocytoma	Pleomorpohic xanthoastrocytoma
Glioblastoma multiforme	Subependymal giant cell astrocytoma

Ependymomas

Ependymomas account for 8–12% of pediatric brain tumors, and for 8–15% of posterior fossa tumors. They are more commonly infratentorial (70%) than supratentorial (30%), and originate either from ependymal cells lining the fourth ventricle, extending into the foramina of Luschka, or from ependymal rest cells found far from ventricular linings within the cerebral hemispheres. The peak incidence of these tumors is between 1 and 9 years in childhood. Clinically, patients present with nausea, vomiting, hydrocephalus, and ataxia. Infratentorial ependymomas present as intraventricular masses, which are frequently calcified (50%). On T2-WI, MRI reveals foci of high intensity (necrotic areas and cysts) and low intensity (calcifications or hemorrhage) within the tumors. On T1-WI, they may present as iso- to hypointense masses with foci of marked hypointensity, with the solid portion of the tumors showing either a homogeneous or inhomogeneous enhancement after the administration of CM. However, ependymomas may be homogeneous on all imaging sequences; therefore, the pattern of growth is a major hint to the diagnosis. Ependymomas grow directly along an ependymal surface, particularly through the foramen of Luschka into the cerebellopontine angles and the foramen of Magendie into the upper cervical canal (Fig. 13.47). In addition, they are the

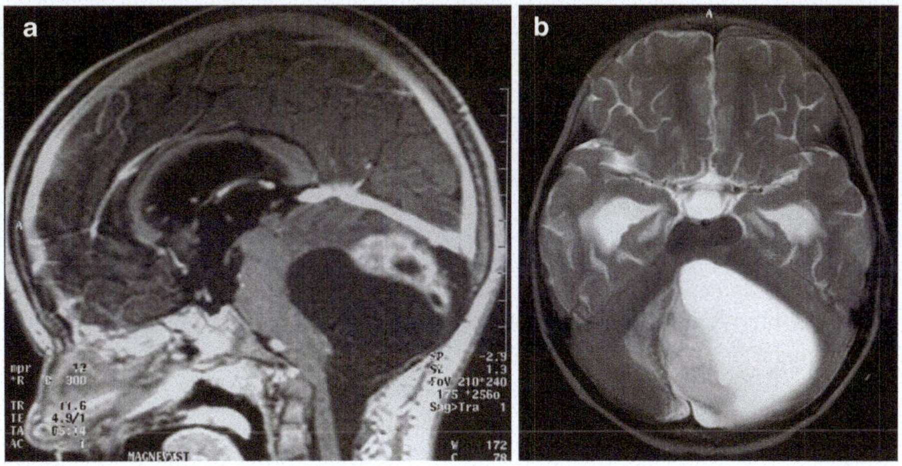

Fig. 13.46 Juvenile pilocytic astrocytoma. Sagittal T1-W contrast-enhanced image (**a**) and transverse T2-WI (**b**) show the typical cystic lesion with a contrast-enhancing mural nodule

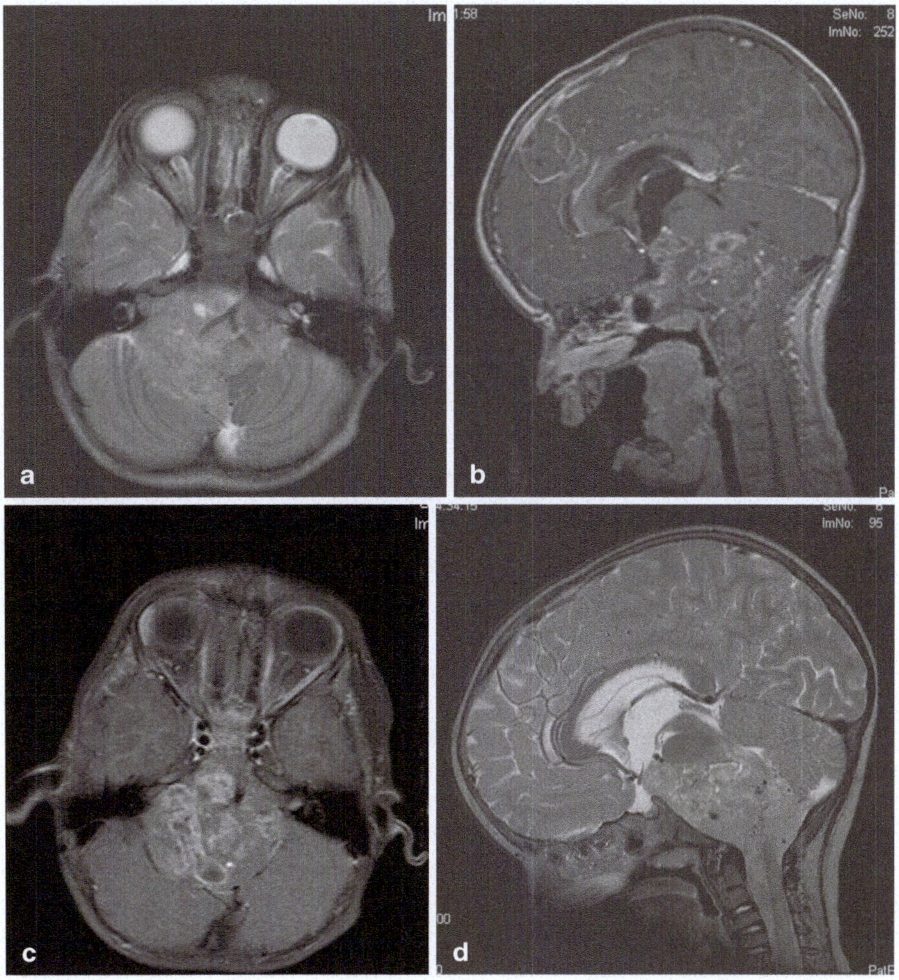

Fig. 13.47 Ependymoma. Transverse (**a**) and sagittal T2-WI (**b**) demonstrate heterogeneous enhancement (**c**) and sagittal T1-WI (**d**) and show a huge mass within the fourth ventricle extending down below the foramen magnum into the spinal canal and extending up into the infundibular recess. Contrast-enhanced transverse

second most common brain tumor to metastasize outside the CNS; medulloblastomas are the most common (Table 13.5).

Brainstem Gliomas

Brainstem gliomas account for 15% of all CNS tumors in childhood, and are can be separated into at least four subgroups: mesencephalic tumors, pontine tumors, medullary tumors, and tumors associated with neurofibromatosis type 1 (NF-1). Furthermore, diffuse lesions are distinguished from focal lesions.

Mesencephalic Tumors

The midbrain is the second most common site of brainstem tumors, and focal tumors prevail. Patients with diffuse tumors present with blurred vision or double vision and, sometimes, motor weakness. Clinically, presentation of focal tumors includes headache, vomiting, diplopia, and sometimes hemiparesis and upward gaze paresis. Tectal tumors present with signs and symptoms of hydrocephalus.

Diffuse midbrain tumors are uncommon tumors extending into the cerebral hemisphere and pons, and are treated with chemotherapy and radiation. They are characterized by a modest local mass effect, and exhibit minimal enhancement after administration of contrast.

Focal midbrain tumors are usually pilocytic astrocytomas (WHO-grade-I-tumors), but in contrast to tectal gliomas they grow, and therefore they have to be treated surgically and/or by a combination of chemotherapy and radiotherapy. They are typically sharply marginated masses in midline, or eccentric within the cerebral peduncle that may extend superiorly into the thalami or inferiorly into the pons, showing T1 and T2 prolongation. In addition, hemorrhage or cysts are present in 25% of focal midbrain tumors. After administration of contrast, ring enhancement can be depicted in small tumors, and homogeneous or heterogeneous enhancement can be seen in larger tumors.

Tumors of the quadrigeminal plate (tectal gliomas) are usually pilocytic astrocytomas (WHO-grade-I-tumors) and extremely benign. However, even small tectal gliomas may lead to hydrocephalus due to obstruction of the aquaeduct, and therefore CSF diversion is necessary. Usually, tumor growth is unusual, but sequential MRI should be obtained to monitor the tumor. Tectal gliomas are hyperintense on T2-WI, may be calcified and are occasionally hyperintense on T1-WI, and show variable enhancement (Fig. 13.48a, b).

Pontine Tumors

Pontine tumors are the most frequently encountered brainstem tumors in childhood. Patients typically present with cranial nerve palsies, pyramidal tract signs, ataxia, and nystagmus.

Diffuse pontine tumors are usually fibrillary astrocytomas (WHO-grade-II-, III-, or IV-tumors.) and therefore have a poor prognosis. They are often large, infiltrative tumors, which are poorly circumscribed, extending to midbrain and medulla, sometimes engulfing the basilar artery. Diffuse pontine tumors are hyperintense on T2-WI and FLAIR images and hypointense on T1-WI. Enhancement after administration of contrast is rarely seen (Fig. 13.48c, d).

Focal pontine tumors are relatively uncommon (<5% of brainstem tumors) and by definition occupy less than 50% of the transverse area of the pons, and may be sharply or poorly marginated, exhibit T1 and T2 prolongation, and typically enhance heterogeneously. When they originate in the periphery of the pons, they may grow exophytically into the fourth ventricle or cerebellopontine angle. They have a much better prognosis than diffuse pontine tumors.

Medullary Tumors

Medullary Tumors typically present in children with signs and symptoms of increased intracranial pressure, difficulties in swallowing, and sometimes hemiparesis or quadriparesis. Medullary tumors can be differentiated into three major categories: focal dorsal exophytic tumors, diffuse tumors, and small focal medullary tumors, usually seen in patients with NF-1.

Focal dorsal exophytic medullary tumors are typically pilocytic astrocytomas (WHO-grade-I-tumors) growing exophytically into the fourth ventricle, and therefore may lead to hydrocephalus. On T2-WI, they are very bright, and show a variable enhancement after administration of contrast on T1-WI.

Diffuse medullary tumors have a less favorable prognosis, because they are more infiltrative tumors and are difficult to resect. On MRI, the medulla is diffusely enlarged, with the tumor extending cranially to

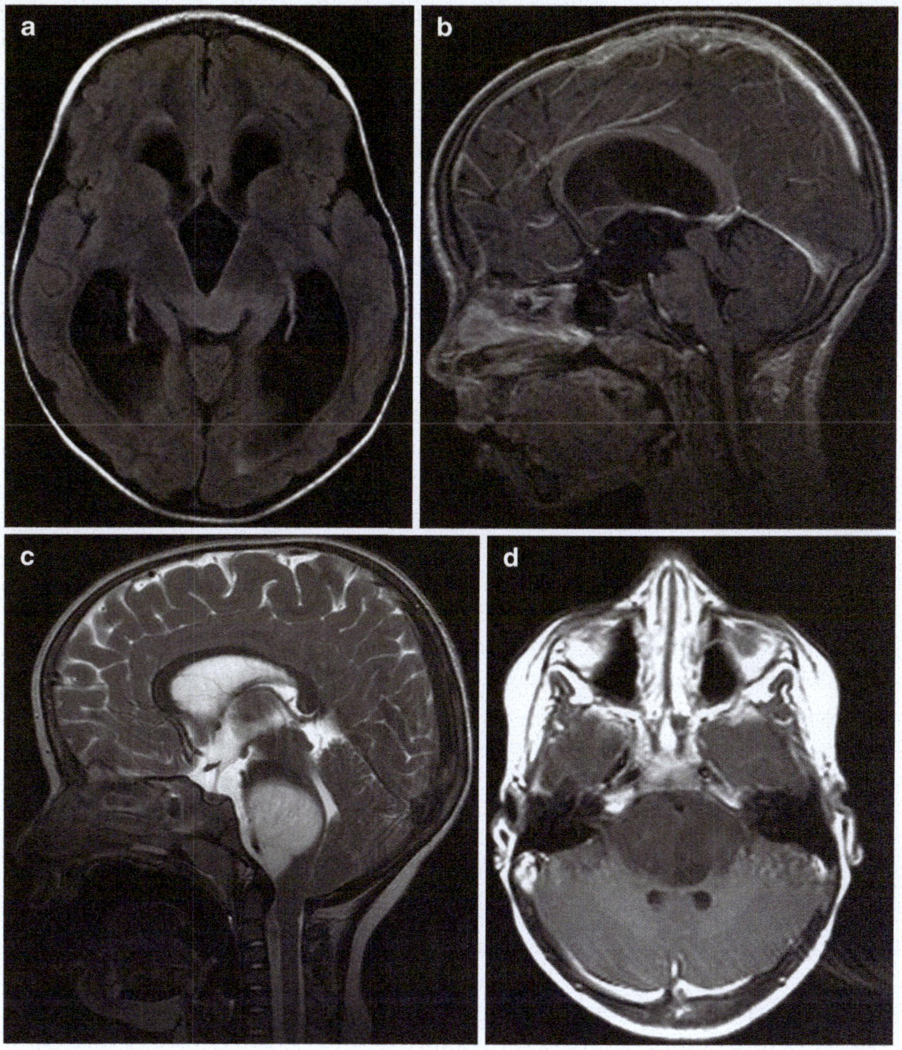

Fig. 13.48 Two examples of brainstem gliomas. Transverse FLAIR image (**a**) and contrast-enhanced sagittal T1-WI (**b**) show a nonenhancing mass in the quadrigeminal plate, consistent with tectal glioma and resultant hydrocephalus. Sagittal T2-WI image (**c**) and transverse contrast-enhanced T1-WI (**d**) of another patient show a large nonenhancing diffuse pontine tumor

the pons and caudally to the spinal cord. On T2-WI, and especially on FLAIR images, hyperintense tumor can be most precisely delineated. On T1-WI, these tumors are hypointense and show a variable enhancement after administration of contrast.

In contrast, *focal medullary tumors* grow very slowly, and appear as focal expansions of the dorsal medulla, exhibiting T1 and T2 prolongation. Enhancement after administration of contrast is uncommon. In addition, these tumors are frequently encountered in patients with NF-1. Interestingly, in patients with NF-1, brainstem tumors generally exhibit a different biological behavior than in children without predisposing disease. Many of these tumors do not enlarge or enlarge minimally over time, and cause either no symptoms at all or show relatively benign clinical courses, and may even regress. Therefore, a policy of wait-and-see is adopted.

13.2.6.2 Intra-Axial Supratentorial Tumors

Astrocytomas

Supratentorial astrocytomas account for 25–40% of brain tumors in children (Fig. 16.24). As already stated, astrocytomas can be divided into two major groups: the infiltrative or diffuse forms and the localized, non-infiltrative forms (Table 13.6). Of the latter, the pilocytic type arises in the optic chiasm and hypothalamus and is seen with a higher frequency in patients with

NF-1. Pleomorphic xanthoastrocytomas are most often located on the surface of the temporal (50%) and parietal (15–20%) lobes, and are typically well-circumscribed peripherically located tumors. Subependymal giant-cell astrocytomas are lateral ventricular masses, particularly in young adults with tuberous sclerosis. Presently, the most widely accepted approach to grading of infiltrating astrocytomas derives from the World Health Organization's (WHO) classification of brain tumors, which separates these tumors into astrocytoma, anaplastic astrocytoma, and glioblastoma multiforme. These infiltrating lesions can arise in any part of the hemispheres, as well as in the infratentorial locations. On MR imaging, astrocytomas have very variable imaging features, and the tumors may be solid, cystic, or both. The absence or presence and pattern of contrast enhancement, surrounding edema, and heterogeneity are key factors in evaluating the grade of astrocytoma. With the exception of JPAs, most low-grade astrocytomas show little or no contrast enhancement, whereas higher grade tumors tend to show enhancement after administration of paramagnetic contrast, inhomogeneous signal intensities on T1-WI and T2-WI, and edema.

Gangliogliomas and Gangliocytomas

Gangliogliomas and gangliocytomas (also called ganglioneuromas) are relatively benign tumors, and account for 3% of brain tumors in children. They typically arise in the supratentorial space within the cerebral hemispheres. Frequent locations are the temporal lobes and the frontoparietal region, but the basal ganglia, the thalamus, or hypothalamus and optic pathways also may be involved. These slow-growing tumors are important because they are almost always associated with a long history of seizures without other neurologic findings, due to their site of occurrence in the region between the frontal and parietal lobes, and may be found in concert with, and are suspected to cause, mesial temporal sclerosis. Therefore, resection is necessary for symptomatic relief. Gangliogliomas and gangliocytomas are hypodense on CT in 38% of cases; approximately one third appear cystic, one third contain calcifications, and half of the tumors show contrast enhancement. The tumor signal is therefore variable on MRI. The solid tumors are usual hypointense on T1-WI and hyperintense on T2-WI. Cystic areas are higher in signal than surrounding CSF, and calcifications may cause mixed SI on T1-WI and hypointense signal on T2-WI.

Dysembryoplastic Neuroepithelial Tumors

Dysembryoplastic neuroepithelial tumors (DNETs) are relatively common benign cortical tumors that typically cause longstanding medically refractory partial complex seizures in children or young adults. The most frequent locations are the temporal lobe (60%) and the frontal lobe (30%), but DNETs can occur in the other lobes, in the deep cerebral nuclei, and even infratentorially. Cortical dysplasia is frequently encountered adjacent to DNETs, hence they are thought to result from developmental defects or stem cell disorders. On MRI, DNETs show a very variable appearance. However, a well-demarcated, wedge-shaped micro- or macrolobular intracortical tumor, located in the temporal lobe, with minimal or no mass effect, which may have lead to scalloping of the inner table of skull, is prototypical.

Desmoplastic Infantile Gangliogliomas

Desmoplastic infantile gangliogliomas (DIGs) and Desmoplastic infantile astrocytomas (DIAs) are very similar tumors that are grouped together as desmoplastic neuroepithelial tumors. Infants typically present with macrocephaly and seizures. These tumors are composed of astrocytic and gangliocytic cells in a desmoplastic stroma, showing areas of mitotically active cells, which may lead to diagnosis of a malignant tumor. Therefore, imaging and suggestion of a DIG or DIA play an important role in patient management, as these tumors are curable by complete resection, without the need for chemotherapy or radiation. On MRI, DIGs or DIAs have a fairly characteristic appearance. They are located in the hemisphere, more often in the frontal lobes, as in the parietal or in the temporal lobes, and present as a large cyst with a cortical-based nodular or plaque-like solid tumor. After administration of contrast, the solid tumor and the adjacent leptomeninges and dura typically enhance, while the cyst walls do not.

Supratentorial Ependymomas

Supratentorial ependymomas account for approximately 30% of childhood ependymomas, and are traditionally thought to arise from ependymal cells or ependymal rests at the angle of lateral ventricles. However, as 80% of supraventricular ependymomas arise within the parenchyma and do not relate to ventricles, some authors suggest that they derive from radial glia. Ependymomas are WHO-grade-II- or WHO-grade-III-tumors, and occur in the frontal, the temporal, and the parietal lobes. Like their infratentorial counterparts, their appearance on MRI and CT is very variable. MRI reveals well-demarcated, spherical or multilocular heterogeneous masses, with foci of high intensity (necrotic areas and cysts) and low intensity (calcifications or hemorrhage) within the tumors on T2-WI. On T1-WI, they may present as iso- to hypointense masses, with foci of marked hypointensity, with the solid portion of the tumors showing either a homogeneous or inhomogeneous enhancement after the administration of CM. However, supratentorial ependymomas may be homogeneous on all imaging sequences. In addition, they may erode overlying calvarium.

Supratentorial Primitive Neuroectodermal Tumors

Supratentorial primitive neuroectodermal tumors (sPNETs) are embryonal tumors composed of more than 90% of undifferentiated or poorly differentiated neuroepithelial cells, and are histologically very similar to medulloblastomas, peripheral neuroblastomas, pineoblastomas, and atypical teratoid/rhabdoid tumors. In the WHO classification of 2000, neuroblastomas and ganglioneuroblastomas are listed as variants of sPNET. sPNETs typically occur in children under 5 years of age, and account for less than 5% of supratentorial tumors in children. They can occur everywhere in the hemispheres and in the pineal or suprasellar region. sPNETs are usually quite large at the time of presentation, and have an extraordinary variability. MR appearance ranges from homogeneous to markedly heterogeneous to a rim of solid tumor surrounding a central necrosis. Calcifications occur in 50–70%, and may be apparent as foci of low SI. Cystic areas may present with or without hemorrhage. After administration of CM, there is always some enhancement, which varies from homogeneous to inhomogeneous, or may be ring-like, depending on the size and number of cysts and necrotic areas. On magnetic resonance spectroscopy, they show taurine elevation. When a large, sharply marginated, and markedly heterogeneous mass inducing only minimal edema is seen in a young child, the diagnosis of sPNET should be made (Fig. 13.49). Seeding of tumor through the CSF pathways and metastases to the spinal cord are often present at time of presentation, and MRI of the spinal canal should therefore be performed. Additionally, spread of tumor in lungs, liver, and bone marrow has been reported.

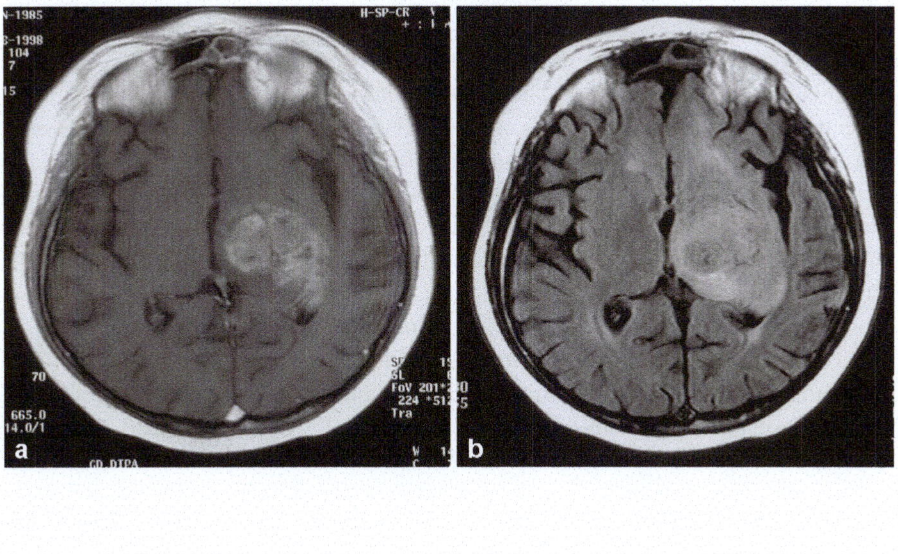

Fig. 13.49 Primitive neuroepithelial tumor. Transverse T1-W contrast-enhanced image (**a**) and transverse fluid-attenuated inversion recovery image (**b**) show heterogeneous enhancement of a large thalamic mass

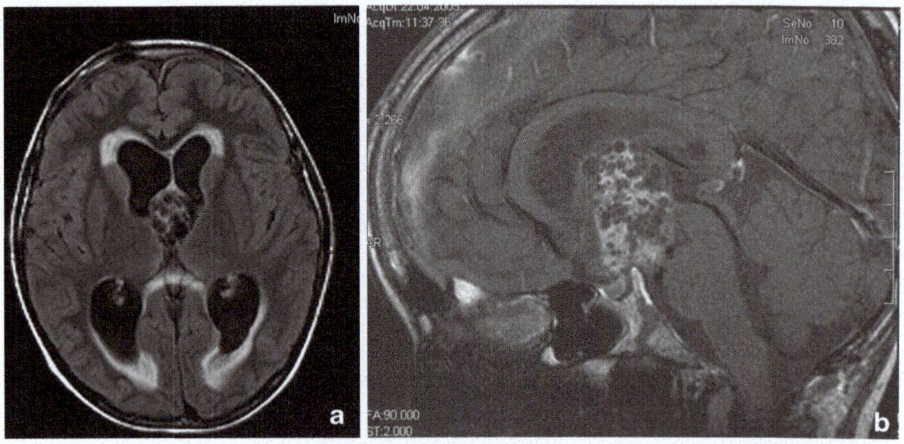

Fig. 13.50 Immature teratoma (grade 2–3). Transverse FLAIR image (**a**) and sagittal contrast-enhanced T1-WI (**b**) show a large suprasellar heterogeneously enhancing mass, with multiple cysts and resultant hydrocephalus

Germ-Cell Tumors

Approximately two-thirds of germ-cell tumors (65%) are germinomas, 26% are nongerminomatous (16% teratomas, 6% endodermal sinus tumors or embryonal carcinomas, 4% choriocarcinomas), and 9% are mixed. Approximately 30–40% of germ-cell tumors arise from the pineal region and 50–60% from the suprasellar/hypothalamic region (Fig. 13.50). The remainder occur in the basal ganglia, cerebellopontine angle, cerebellum, corpus callosum, and spinal cord. Patients with tumors in the pineal region typically present with signs and symptoms of hydrocephalus resulting from compression of the aqueduct, Parinaud sign or diplopia, while patients with suprasellar/hypothalamic tumors suffer from diabetes insipidus, visual disturbances, or amenorrhea. In general, it is important to realize that in patients with diabetes insipidus, which results from dysfunction of supraoptic or paraventricular nuclei of the hypothalamus, a negative MRI examination does not exclude presence or absence of disease, as infiltration of the aforementioned nuclei may be present and the infundibulum still looks normal. These patients have to be reevaluated at least twice, at 3–6 month intervals, to rule out lymphocytic hypophisitis, granuloma, or tumor. Germ-cell tumors often secrete tumor markers in serum and CSF, a circumstance faciliating diagnosis and monitoring of patients. Placental alkaline phosphatise (PLAP) is secreted primarily by germinomas, β-human chorionic gonadotrophin (β-HCG) by choriocarcinomas, α-feto-protein (AFP) by endodermal sinus tumors, and both β-HCG and AFP by embryonal cell tumors. With the exception of mature teratomas, all germ-cell tumors are classified as malignant tumors and possibly seed along CSF pathways. Germinomas are well-marginated, round or lobulated tumors demonstrating variable SI, ranging from hypointense to isointense to gray matter on T1-WI and isointense to hyperintense to gray matter on T2-WI. A strong, sometimes "speckled" contrast enhancement is seen after injection of CM. If a pineal lesion is discovered in concert with a suprasellar lesion in a child, the diagnosis of germinoma (Fig. 13.51) is practically assured. Whether this results from the spread of the tumor from the pineal region via CSF or multifocality of the tumor is still under debate.

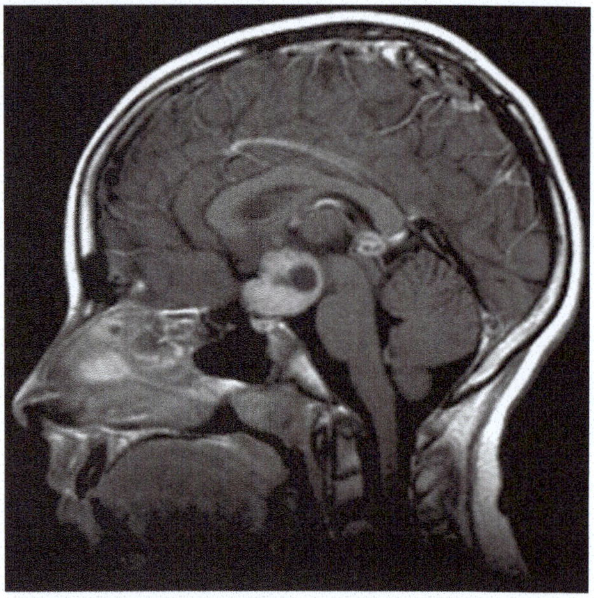

Fig. 13.51 Germinoma. T1-W contrast-enhanced image shows a pineal lesion in concert with a suprasellar lesion (Courtesy of A. Heuck, MD)

Embryonal cell carcinomas and endodermal sinus tumors are usually heterogeneous masses, and cannot be differentiated by MRI.

Choriocarcinomas may be differentiated from the other tumors by their tendency to hemorrhage.

Teratomas contain a mixture of differentiated tissue derived from all three embryonic germ layers and may be immature or mature. These tumors are usually sharply marginated, lobulated heterogeneous masses composed of solid tissue, cysts, fat, calcification, bone, or teeth. Less sharply defined margins, surrounding edema, and contrast enhancement after administration of contrast are suggestive of malignant teratomas.

Pinealomas

Pineal parenchymal tumors include pineoblastomas and pineocytomas. Pineoblastomas, also referred to as primitive neuroectodermal tumors (PNETs) of the pinal gland, are highly malignant tumors, readily metastasizing via CSF. Usually, they are large lobulated masses, demonstrating iso- to hyperintense signal on T2-WI and hypo- to isointense signal on T1-WI. Pineoblastomas contain calcifications and will show prominent enhancement in the solid portions, with paramagnetic contrast. There is almost always ventricular enlargement due to obstruction. Pineocytomas are uncommon in children, and indistinguishable from pineoblastomas by CT and MRI.

13.2.6.3 Extra-Axial Supratentorial Tumors

Craniopharyngiomas

Craniopharyngiomas are benign epithelial tumors arising from squamous rests along the involuted craniopharyngeal duct, and account for 6–9% of childhood intracranial tumors and for 50% of suprasellar tumors in children. Children with craniopharyngiomas will present with headache, nausea, vomiting, visual symptoms, and, in one third of cases, endocrinological disturbances. Craniopharyngiomas may be entirely cystic or entirely solid, but most commonly are a combination of both. Calcifications are seen on CT in more than 90% of the cases, but are less obvious on MRI; CT may therefore be necessary to prove their presence. The heterogeneous nature of craniopharyngiomas results in a variety of appearances on MR imaging. Solid tumors are usually isointense on T1-WI and hyperintense on T2-WI, but may be inhomogeneous due to tumor hemorrhage and/or calcifications. Cystic tumors are hyperintense on T2-WI and may be hypo-, iso-, or even hyperintense on T1-WI, depending on the presence of free methemoglobin or protein in the cysts (Fig. 13.52). Therefore, it is difficult to distinguish the cystic component from solid portions of the tumor without the administration of contrast. Cysts and solid portions of the tumor will enhance in 90% of cases. Furthermore, craniopharyngiomas are separated

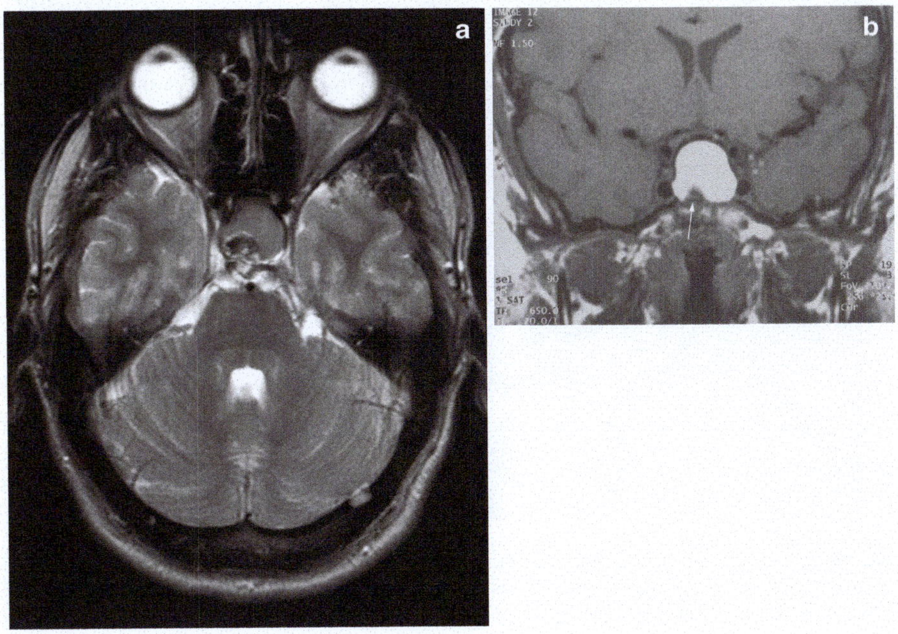

Fig. 13.52 Craniopharyngioma. Transverse T2-WI (**a**) and coronal T1-WI (**b**) show a tumor with a smaller heterogeneous hypointense solid portion, probably reflecting calcification (*arrow*), and a larger portion that is isointense to brain tissue on T2-WI and hyperintense on T1-WI, consistent with a hemorrhagic cyst

into sellar, prechiasmatic, and retrochiasmatic lesions, as this plays an important role for the neurosurgical approach.

Hamartomas of the Tuber Cinereum

Hypothalamic hamartomas are congenital malformations composed of heterotopic neurons and glia, and arise between the tuber cinerum and the mamillary bodies. Children with hamartomas of the tuber cinereum will present with luteinizing hormone-releasing hormone (LHRH)-dependent central precocious puberty and, more pathognomonically, with gelastic seizures characterized by fits of laughter-like outbursts. These either pedunculated or sessile (presenting as a mass within the hypothalamus) lesions demonstrate isointense SI to gray matter on T1-WI and isointense or slightly hyperintense SI on T2-WI. Hamartomas do not enhance after administration of CM (Fig. 13.53).

Choroid Plexus Papillomas and Carcinomas

Choroid plexus papillomas and carcinomas arise from the epithelium of the choroid plexus, and account for 5% of supratentorial tumors in children. Most of these lesions are discovered within the first 5 years of life. Papillomas are most often found in the first year of life, due to the resultant hydrocephalus. The most common sites of these lesions are the lateral ventricles, with the glomus being a frequent location. The diagnosis of papillomas is easily made on CT because of the location, punctate calcifications, and a homogeneous contrast enhancement after administration of contrast (Fig. 13.54). On MRI, choroid plexus papillomas are lobulated intraventricular masses, mostly isointense in T1-WI, with uniform intense enhancement after the administration of CM. On T2-WI, these lesions are somewhat hypointense compared with gray matter.

Choroid plexus carcinomas have a more heterogeneous appearance, and invade the surrounding brain parenchyma. Due to hemorrhage and necrotic and cystic components, they often present with areas of high and low SI on T1-WI and T2-WI (Fig. 13.55). These lesions have a poor prognosis because of their tendency to metastasize via the CSF.

However, it is important to know that choroid plexus papillomas and carcinomas can only be differentiated by histology. Some benign-looking tumors may finally turn out to be carcinomas and, vice versa, more aggressive- and invasive-looking tumors may end up with the diagnosis of anaplastic papillomas.

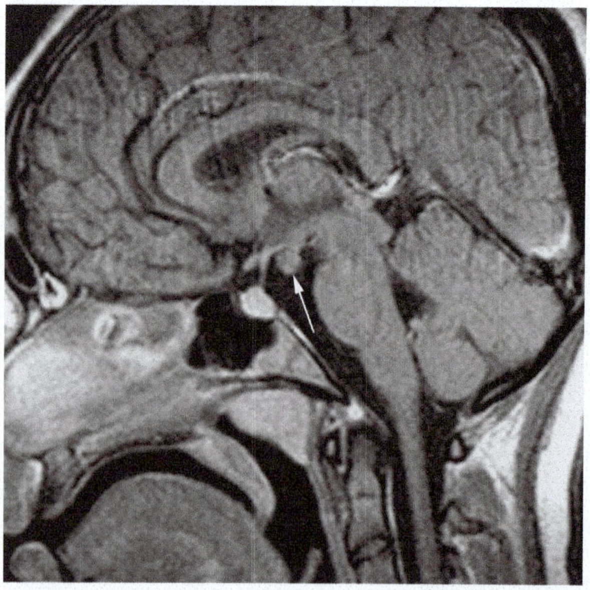

Fig. 13.53 Hamartoma of the tuber cinereum. T1-W sagittal contrast-enhanced image shows a sessile lesion (*arrow*) originating from the tuber cinereum posterior to the stalk

13.2.7 Cerebrovascular Disease

Cerebrovascular disease in children is far more common than generally recognized. Cerebral infarctions, developmental vascular anomalies (persistent primitive arteries, hypoplasia/aplasia of the carotid arteries), fistulas, intracerebral vascular malformations, intracranial aneurysms, and the moyamoya syndrome are encountered in children.

As in adults, cerebral infarction can occur from intraluminal arterial or venous occlusion (thrombosis), or vasospasm induced by hypoxia or infection. Basically, imaging findings of basal-ganglia infarctions, arterial infarctions restricted to a typical territory, watershed, and venous infarctions do not differ from those encountered in adults. Approximately 55% of strokes in children are ischemic, and 45% are hemorrhagic. Ischemic infarction may progress to a hemorrhagic stroke, or hemorrhagic infarction may be

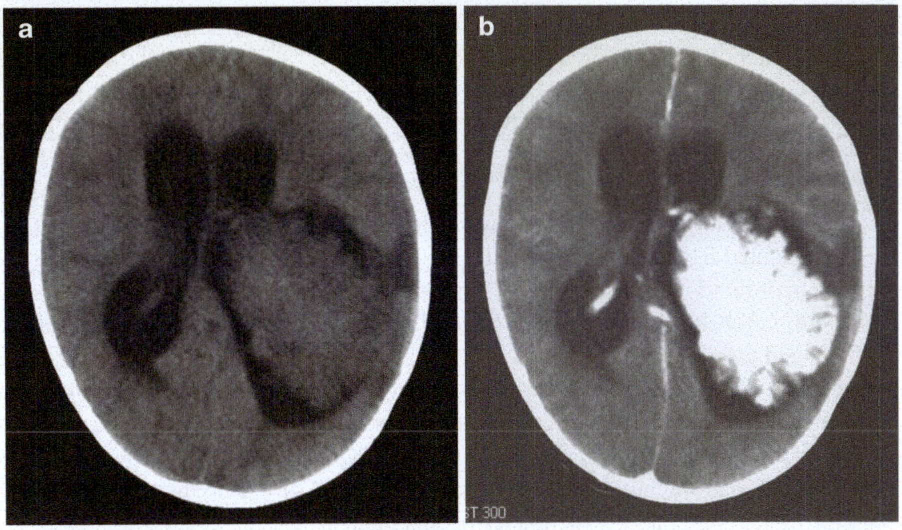

Fig. 13.54 Choroid plexus papilloma. Transverse precontrast (**a**) and postcontrast CT (**b**) show a uniformly enhancing tumor in the left ventricle, with enlargement of both ventricles, and a perifocal edema in the left hemisphere

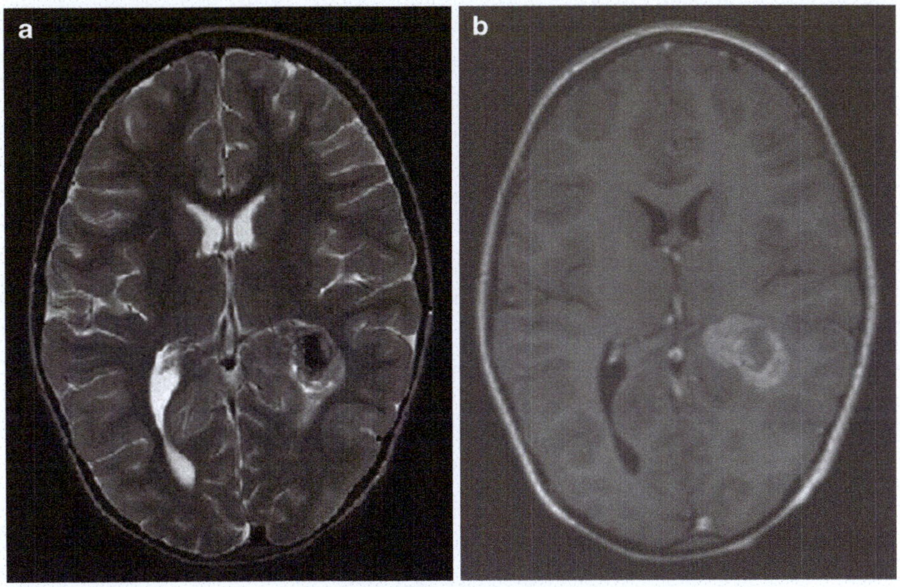

Fig. 13.55 Choroid plexus carcinoma. Transverse T2-WI (**a**) and contrast-enhanced T1-WI (**b**) show an inhomogeneous tumor located in the left ventricle, with a hypointense center on T1- and T2-WI, reflecting calcification or haemorrhage

the initial presentation. Common causes for ischemic infarctions in children include cardiac disease, trauma, disorders of coagulation, primary dyslipoproteinemia, CNS infection, vascular disease associated with syndromes, primary or secondary CNS vasculitis, collagen-vascular disease, hemoglobinopathies, inborn errors of cerebral metabolism, and drug/irradiation-induced injury to the CNS. Hemorrhagic infarctions in children are frequently secondary to superficial and/or deep venous sinus occlusion. MR angiography should be additionally included in the sequence protocol for the evaluation of cerebrovascular disease in children.

13.2.7.1 Hypoxic-Ischemic Brain Injury in Preterm and Term Infants

Perinatal asphyxia is the most important cause of hypoxic-ischemic encephalopathy (HIE). HIE is one of the most common causes of cerebral palsy and other severe neurologic deficits in children, affecting 0.2–0.9 of 1,000 live births. The exact pathophysiology of HIE is not completely understood, but the lack of sufficient blood flow in concert with decreased oxygen content in the blood leads to loss of cerebral autoregulation and diffuse brain injury. Prolonged periods of hypoxia or anoxia result in severe damage to the brain, and the pattern of destruction depends on three different factors:

1. Severity of hypotension
2. Duration of the event
3. Maturity of the brain

In case of mild to moderate reduction of blood flow, blood is shunted from the anterior to the posterior circulation in order to maintain sufficient perfusion of the brainstem, cerebellum, and basal ganglia. Therefore, the damaged areas are limited to vascular border zones between the major arterial territories. In profound hypotension with complete or near-complete cessation of blood flow, the deep cerebral nuclei (thalami and basal ganglia) and the brainstem are initially affected. Damage to the cortex and white matter occurs later in the course of the hypotensive episode. The extent of the damage additionally depends on the duration of the event. Patients with relatively short arrests (10–15 min) have damage limited to the ventrolateral thalami, globus pallidus, posterior putamen, sensorimotor cortex, and sometimes the hippocampi. With longer arrests (15–25 min), the superior vermis, the optic radiations, and the calcarine cortex are additionally affected. Finally, when arrest extends into the 25–30-min range, nearly all of the gray matter is injured, and the child is left with diffuse multicystic encephalomalacia and shrunken basal ganglia (Fig. 13.56).

The regions of the brain that are most susceptible to hypoxic-ischemic injury change with the postconceptional age of the child because, on the one hand, the vascular system is still under development and, on the other hand, the relative energy requirements of various portions of the brain vary with the state of maturity (Table 13.7). There is no consensus regarding the gestational age demarcation at which an infant is considered preterm or term. The majority of authors describe a pattern of injury in neonates who are at less than 36 weeks of gestation that is distinct from the pattern in neonates at 36 weeks or older. Thus, it is reasonable to define a preterm neonate as being one who is at less than 36 weeks of gestation. Therefore, although some overlapping exists, the four distinct patterns of brain injury that will be described herein are mild to moderate hypotension in preterm infants, severe hypotension in preterm infants, mild to moderate hypotension in term infants, and severe hypotension in term infants.

Table 13.7 Patterns of hypoxic-ischemic brain injury (Adapted from Barkovich 2000)

Age of child	Mild to moderate hypotension	Profound hypotension
Preterm newborn (<34–36 weeks postconception)	Periventricular white-matter injury	Thalamic, basal ganglia, and brainstem injury
Term newborn (~36–56 weeks postconception)	Parasagittal watershed injury	Dorsal brainstem, thalamic, basal ganglia, and perirolandic cortex injury
Older child (> ~6 months postnatally)	Parasagittal watershed injury	Basal ganglia and diffuse cortical injury

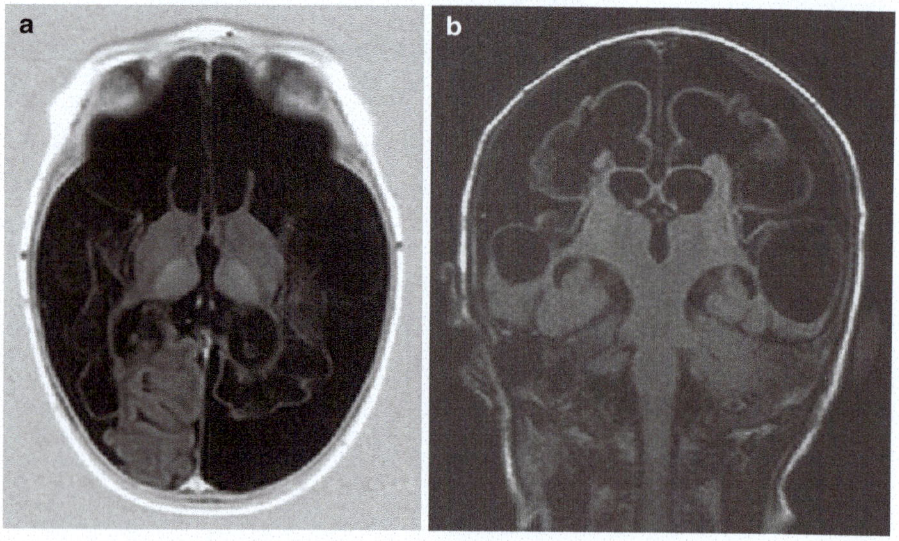

Fig. 13.56 Multicystic encephalomalacia. Transverse inversion recovery image (**a**) and coronal T1-WI image (**b**) show enlargement of the lateral ventricles with multicystic encephalomalacia involving the hemispheric white matter, and thinning of the cerebral cortex, with preservation of the deep gray matter, and a part of the right occipital lobe

In the preterm infant, most ischemic injury leads to germinal matrix bleeding, intraventricular hemorrhage, and periventricular leukomalacia (PVL). Prior to 35–36 weeks of gestational age, the border zone or watershed area between the major arterial territories (posterior choroidal branches and middle cerebral arteries) is in a periventricular location. Ischemic injury to the periventricular region produces necrosis of white matter, resulting in PVL and subsequent cystic degeneration. The two most common locations for PVL are the white matter adjacent to the foramen of Monro and the posterior periventricular white matter adjacent to the lateral aspect of the trigone of the lateral ventricles.

In severe hypotension, the thalami, brainstem, and cerebellum are additionally affected, as these regions are the most metabolically active in the immature brain. MRI does not play a major role in the early diagnosis of PVL, as these sick premature neonates are primarily diagnosed and monitored by ultrasound (US) in the neonatal intensive care unit. If they are imaged, MR images reveal areas of T1 hyperintensities consistent with hemorrhage within larger areas of T2 hyperintensities, and restricted diffusion in the involved structures. However, MRI examinations play a very important role in determining the extent of damage in severely affected patients at a later time. MR findings of end-stage PVL (Fig. 13.57) are:

1. Abnormally increased SI in the periventricular white matter on T2-WI, most commonly bilaterally observed in the peritrigonal regions
2. Ventriculomegaly with irregular outline of the body and trigone of the lateral ventricles
3. Reduced quantity of periventricular white matter, always at the trigones, but involving the whole centrum semiovale in severe cases
4. Deep, prominent sulci that abut or nearly abut the ventricles, with little or no interposed white matter
5. Delayed myelination
6. Thinning of the corpus callosum, most commonly the posterior body and splenium, and in case of severe hypotension
7. Small, shrunken, often calcified thalami
8. Small brainstem and cerebellum
9. Small or absent basal ganglia (especially in patients injured prior to 30 weeks of gestation)

Four important points to keep in mind are:

1. The finding of periventricular hyperintensity and volume loss on T2-WI and FLAIR images is not specific for white matter injury of prematurity, but can also be a sequela of ventriculitis, inborn errors of metabolism, hydrocephalus, and in utero events.
2. The pattern of brain damage seen in infants who have suffered in utero injury is identical to that seen in postnatal infants of the same gestational age.

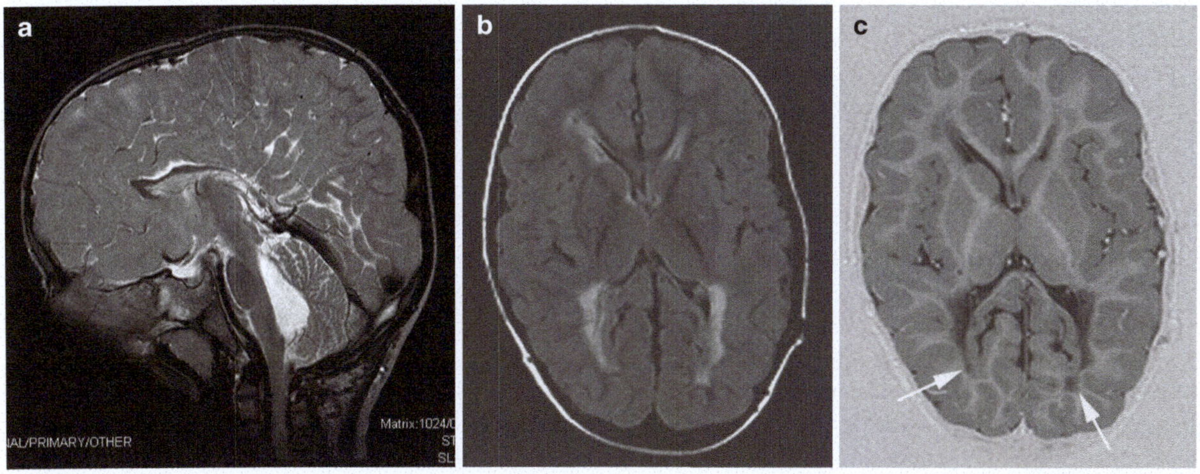

Fig. 13.57 End-stage periventricular leukomalacia. Sagittal T2-WI (**a**) shows a thin callosum and an enlarged fourth ventricle. Transverse FLAIR image (**b**) and inversion recovery image (**c**) demonstrate ventricles with irregular borders and severe periventricular gliosis. The cerebral cortex nearly abuts the ventricular surface because of the diminished volume of white matter (*arrows*)

3. Prior to the 30th gestational week, damage to the brain parenchyma results in liquefaction and resorption of parenchyma, whereas damage after the 30th week leads to reactive astrogliosis.
4. Typical periventricular leukomalcia may occur in full-terms with HIE and sepsis.

In term infants, the severity of an insult compared with that in a preterm infant must be significantly greater to lead to morphologic changes. In term infants, the most metabolically active regions are the lateral thalami, globus pallidus, posterior putamina, hippocampi, brainstem, corticospinal tracts (because of increasing myelination), and sensimotor cortex. In addition, the vascular border zones are typically in a parasagittal location high over the cerebral convexities between the anterior and middle cerebral arteries and the middle and posterior arteries. These border regions lie within the cortical mantle and the underlying white matter. In mild to moderate hypotension, sometimes subtle hyperintense T2 signal and restricted diffusion in both the cortex and the underlying white matter are observed and, if performed, MR spectroscopy shows increased lactate concentration in the intervascular zone compared with the deep gray matter. In severe hypotension, abnormal T1 hyperintensity and variable T2 hyper- or hypointensity can be depicted in the lateral thalami, globus pallidus, posterior putamina, hippocampi, brainstem, and sensimotor cortex. However, DWI is more sensitive, and shows restricted diffusion in the affected areas. In addition, MR spectroscopy reveals an elevation of lactate concentration in the basal ganglia and thalami. Consequently, asphyxia in a term infant produces a pattern referred to as ulegyria (mushroom-shaped gyri), with shrunken gyri and enlarged sulci. In the chronic phase, encephalomalacia is noted in the parasagittal regions (Figs. 13.56 and 13.58).

13.2.7.2 Arterial Infarctions in Preterm and Term Infants

Based on autopsy data, arterial infarctions in the term infant are far more common (17% of cases) than in the preterm infant (3–5% of cases). Due to the normal appearance of the unmyelinated brain, it may be difficult to detect subtle edema and/or hypoperfusion of the involved brain. Cortical infarctions are best identified on T1-WI as areas of hypointensity, while adjacent white matter becomes slightly hyperintense. The gyri may be minimally hyperintense and appear swollen on T2-WI. There is a loss in the ability to distinguish between white and gray matter (missing cortex sign). DWI is more sensitive and shows restricted diffusion in the affected areas. Gyral enhancement with paramagnetic contrast is common within 5–10 days of the acute event (Fig. 13.58).

13.2.7.3 Venous Thrombosis

Superficial and/or deep venous sinus occlusion in children is frequently secondary to prematurity and germinal-matrix hemorrhage, dehydration, hypercoagulable states, infection, or trauma (Figs. 13.59 and 13.60). Hemorrhagic infarctions not corresponding to an arterial vascular territory should suggest venous thrombosis. Deep venous system occlusion is more common in children than in adults, and presents with infarction and hemorrhage of the deep gray-matter nuclei and the thalami. The combination of infarction and hemorrhage of the thalamus associated with intraventricular bleeding should raise the suspicion of underlying deep-vein thrombosis, especially in full-term neonates (Fig. 13.61).

13.2.7.4 Vein of Galen Aneurysm

A vein of Galen aneurysm is a rare congenital-vascular malformation demonstrating single or multiple fistulas between cerebral arteries and the vein of Galen. It is classified into choroidal and mural types. The choroidal type is more common (90%), usually presenting in the neonate with congestive heart failure, intracranial bruit, and/or hydrocephalus (Fig. 13.62). The mural type of Galenic malformation presents later in infancy, with developmental delay, seizures, and hydrocephalus. These two conditions must be differentiated from a parenchymal arteriovenous malformation (AVM) in the midbrain or thalamus with drainage into the deep venous system, including the vein of Galen and the straight sinus. These AVMs frequently present with hemorrhage in older children and adults. MR imaging of a vein of Galen aneurysm demonstrates a huge, rounded lesion, dorsally located in the midline, which displays no signal on both T1-WI and T2-WI, due to flow void. Concurrent thrombosis can be depicted by T1-W sequences before contrast and by MR angiography. A 3D PC MR angiography should be

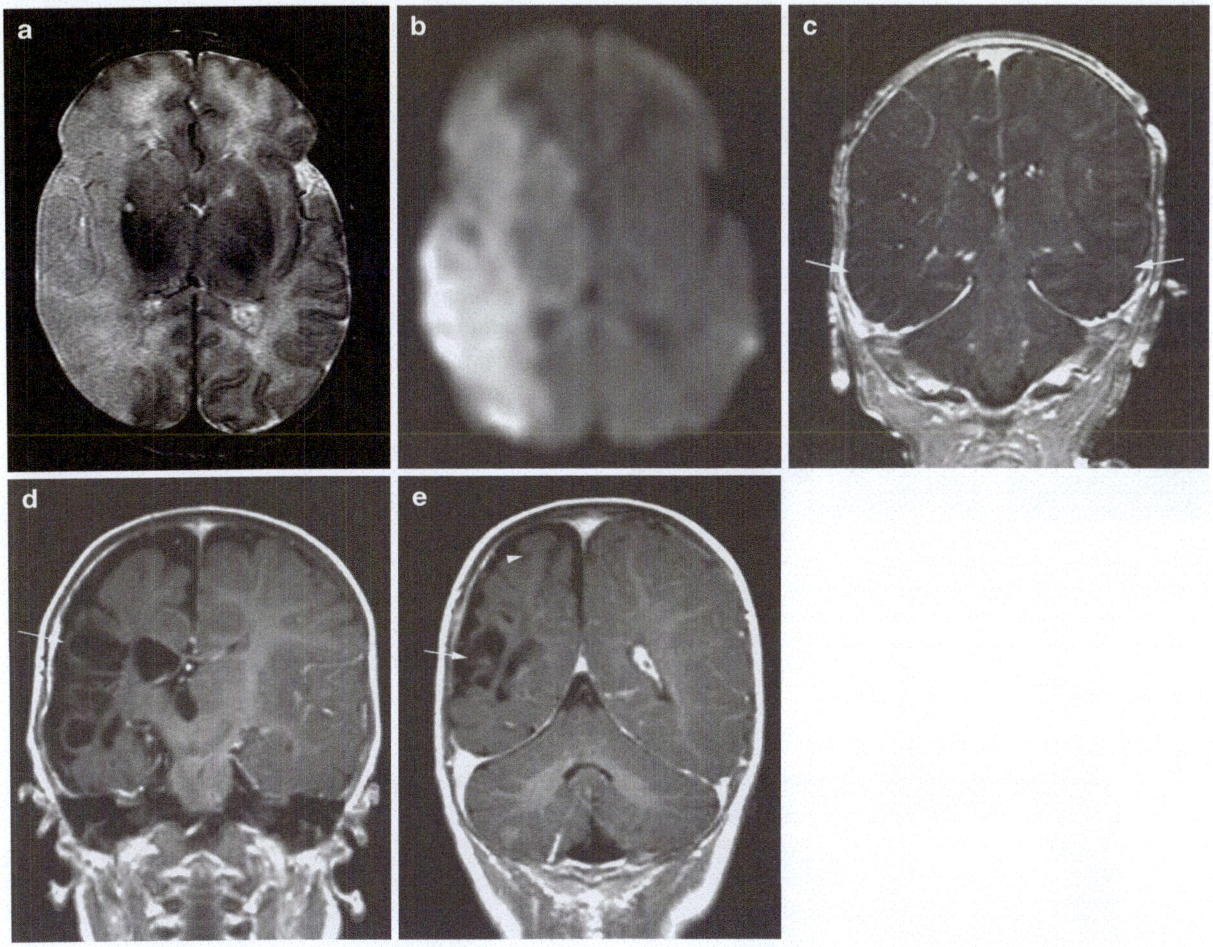

Fig. 13.58 Arterial infarction in a mature 3-day-old boy. Transverse T2-WI (**a**) and diffusion-weighted image (**b**) show hyperintensity in the right cerebral hemisphere, with restricted diffusion in the territory of the middle cerebral artery. Coronal fat-saturated contrast-enhanced T1-WI (**c**) demonstrates no contrast enhancement in the acute phase. Note that the cortical ribbon of gray matter can neither be delineated on T2- nor on T1-WI ("missing cortex sign" *arrows*). Coronal contrast-enhanced T1-WI (**d, e**) acquired 7 months later shows cystic encephalomalacia (*arrows*) and ulegyria (*arrowhead*)

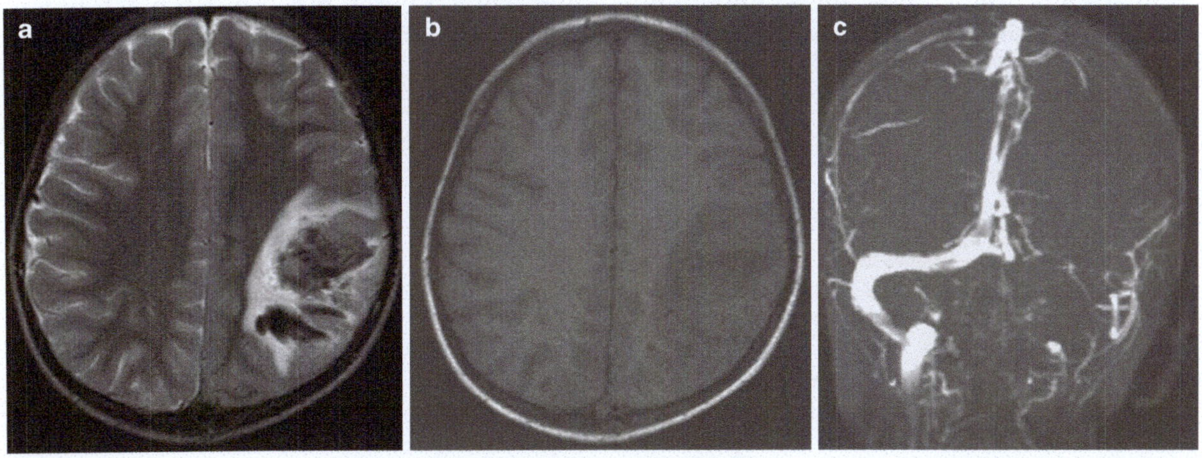

Fig. 13.59 Venous infarction. Transverse T2-WI (**a**), T1-WI (**b**) and time-of-flight venography (**c**) show hemorrhagic venous infarction in the left parietal lobe, secondary to thrombosis of transverse and sigmoid sinus

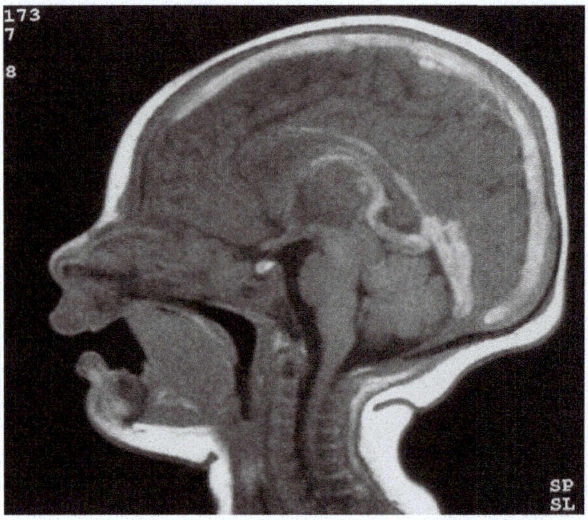

Fig. 13.60 Venous thrombosis. Sagittal T1-WI demonstrates high signal intensity in the superior sagittal sinus, straight sinus, inferior sagittal sinus, vein of Galen, and internal cerebral vein. Note that the pituitary gland is convex and demonstrates a uniform high signal; this is the normal appearance of the pituitary gland in newborns (Courtesy of W. Michl)

performed to display feeding vessels and venous drainage of this lesion.

13.2.7.5 Moyamoya Disease

Moyamoya disease is a primary arterial disorder leading to occlusion of the intracranial internal carotid artery, accompanied by the development of collaterals. It is mainly encountered in Japan. Moyamoya is Japanese and means "hazy, like a puff or cloud of smoke," and describes the angiographic appearance of this condition. Furthermore, the same radiographic pattern has been described in children with sickle-cell anemia, collagen-vascular disorders, NF-1, Down syndrome, as well as after radiation therapy. This condition is referred to as the moyamoya syndrome by some authors. MRI reveals infarcts in up to 80% of cases and multiple flow voids corresponding to enlarged basal collateral arteries at the level of the middle cerebral artery and the basal ganglia (Fig. 13.63).

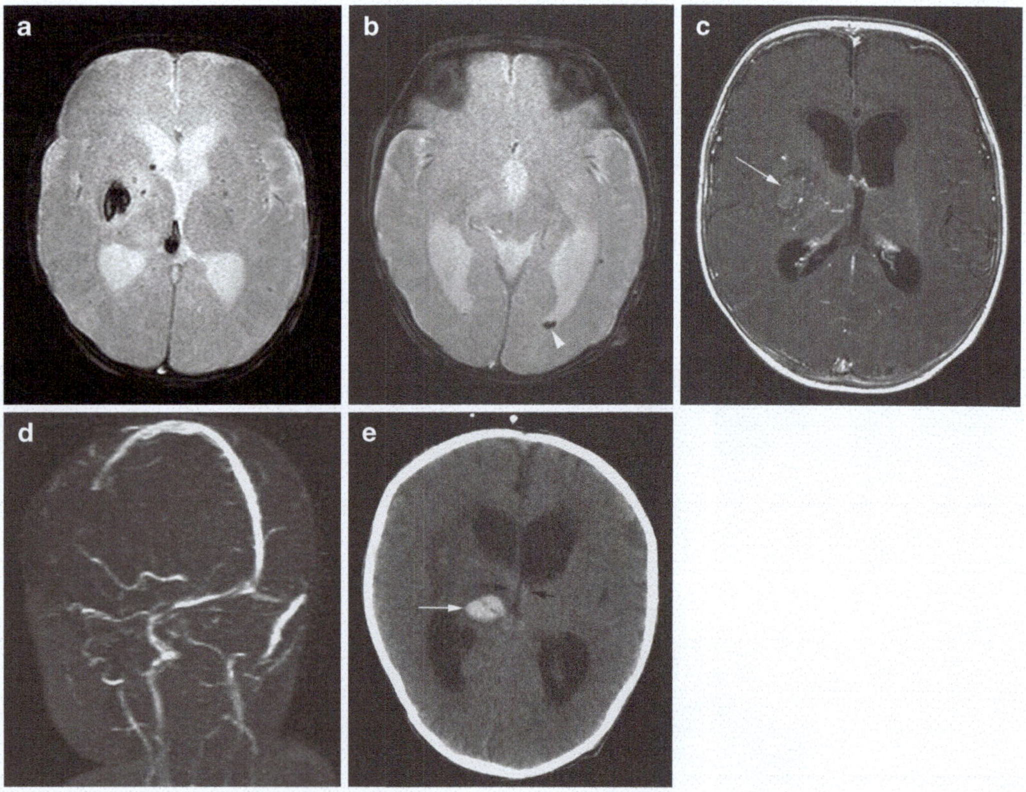

Fig. 13.61 Deep-vein thrombosis. Transverse T2*-WI (**a, b**), contrast-enhanced T1-WI (**c**), and CT (**e**) show the typical combination of infarction and hemorrhage of the deep gray-matter nuclei and thalamus on the right side (*white arrows*), associated with intraventricular bleeding (*arrowhead*). In addition, enlargement of both ventricles and periventricular edema is present. MRV (**d**) does not show deep veins. Note that on CT (**e**) hyperdense thrombi are present in the internal cerebral veins (*black arrows*)

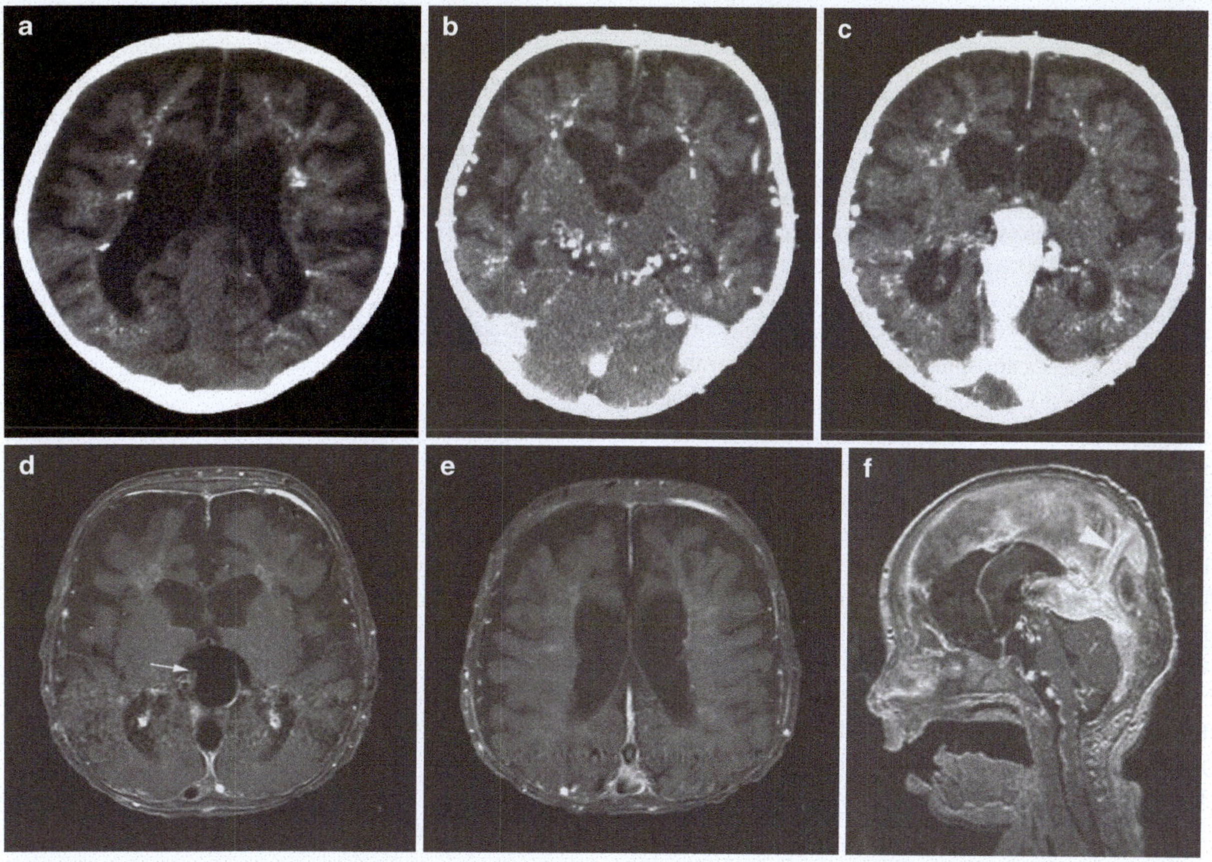

Fig. 13.62 Vein of Galen aneurysm. Unenhanced CT (**a**) shows multiple calcifications and cerebral atrophy in a 5-month-old boy with cranial bruit. Enhanced CT (**b, c**) and fat-saturated contrast-enhanced transverse (**d, e**) and sagittal (**f**) T1-WI demonstrate a huge choroid type of the vein of Galen aneurysm, with hypertrophy of the choroid arteries and flow-void (*arrow*) in the dilated vein of Galen. Note persistent falcine vein (*arrowhead*)

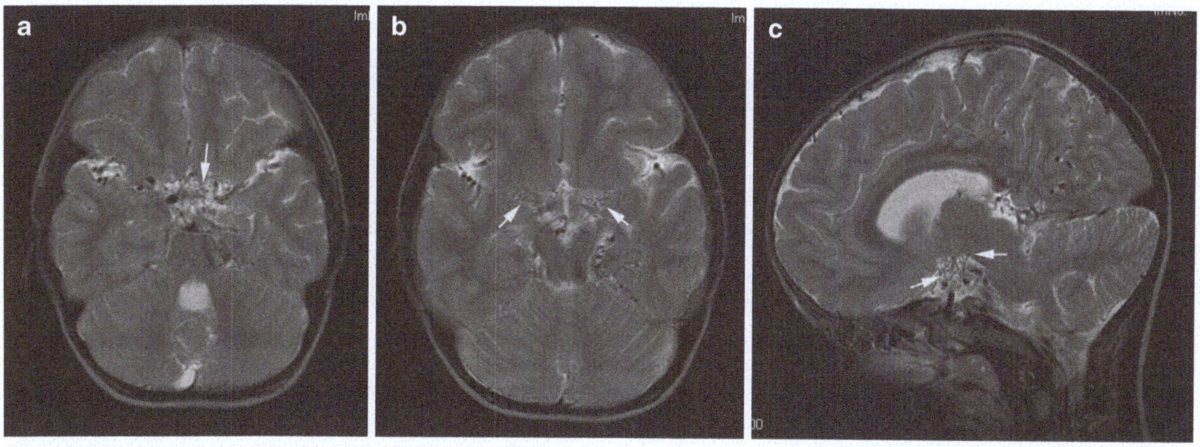

Fig. 13.63 Moyamoya syndrome. Transverse and sagittal T2-WI (**a–c**) show multiple dot-like flow-voids in the suprasellar cistern and the basal ganglia, consistent with collaterals (*arrows*) due to progressive occlusion of the distal ICA on both sides, in a patient with trisomy 21

13.2.8 Non-Accidential Head Injury

Intracranial injury is the main reason for death and disability in cases of child abuse. If an inconclusive history is given for an injury in a young child or injuries of varying ages are present, child abuse should be considered. Approximately 40% of physically abused children are infants, and 80% of children are less than 5 years of age. Child abuse is the most common reason to cause brain injury deaths in children <2 years. Signs of child abuse in the CNS are spread sutures and bilateral skull fractures (Fig. 13.64), subdural and subarachnoid hemorrhages, petechial hemorrhages of the parenchyma, shearing injuries, cortical contusions, cerebral edema, infarctions, and retinal hemorrhages. Intrahemispheric subdural hematoma (shaken-impact injury) and subdural hematoma associated with hypoxic-ischemic injury or infarction (strangulation/suffocation injury) make one particularly suspicious of child abuse. Noncontrast CT depicts acute hemorrhage with high sensitivity and remains the best modality for initial evaluation. Furthermore, contrast-enhanced MRI, including DWI, for assessment of parenchymal injury should be performed. Timing of CNS injuries is an extremely challenging task, as blood loses density based upon multiple factors, and one should be aware that it is impossible to precisely determine age of bleeding by one study alone and that it is still remains difficult even with a follow-up study. In addition, child abuse mimics such as Menkes syndrome, glutaric acidurias, other mitochondrial encephalopathies, and differential diagnoses such as benign macrocrania, subdural empyema, and accidental trauma should be taken into consideration. It is important to keep in mind that Menkes syndrome, glutaric aciduria type 1, and Hermansky-Pudlak syndrome can cause both subdural hematomas and retinal hemorrhages. Furthermore, concomitant spine injury and posttraumatic pseudoaneurys should be ruled out.

13.3 Pediatric Spine Imaging

13.3.1 Technique

13.3.1.1 Coils and Patient Positioning

The standard spine coil should be used for imaging of the spine in children. Optionally, an adapted phased array surface coil can be utilized. Optimal positioning in the center of the coil and immobilization with vacuum beds, sponges, sand bags, and blankets are mandatory for patients.

13.3.1.2 Sequence Protocol

The standard protocol for evaluation of the spine should include T2-WI, STIR sequence, and T1-WI in a sagittal plane and a transverse plane through the region of interest. For the evaluation of associated tumors in spinal dysraphism, tumors, infections, and

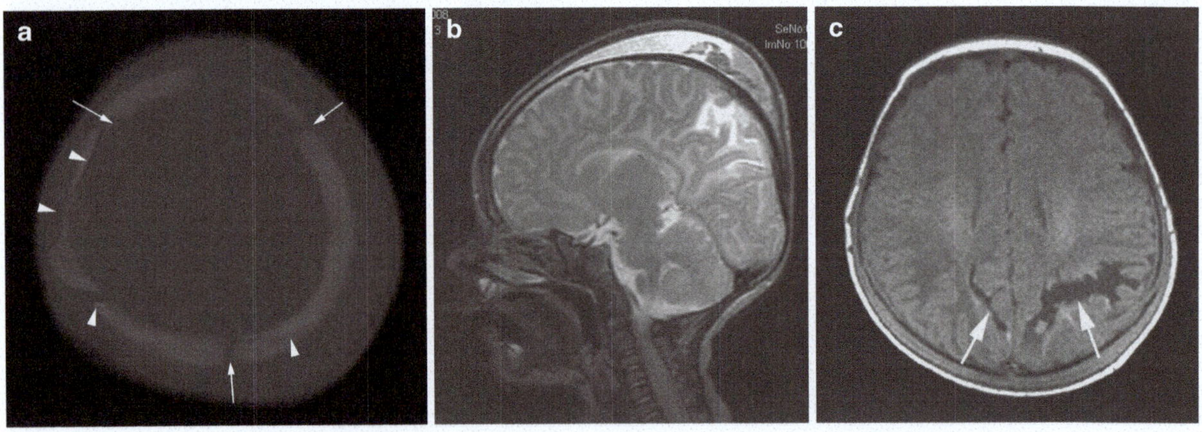

Fig. 13.64 Non-accidental head injury. CT (**a**) shows normal width of skull sutures (*arrows*) and bilateral skull fractures (*arrowheads*) in an 8-week-old girl. Sagittal T2-WI (**b**) and transverse T1-WI (**c**) demonstrate subgaleal hemorrhage and bilateral parenchymal lacerations in the parietal and occipital lobes (*arrows*) (Courtesy of H. Schmidt)

inflammations, paramagnetic contrast agents should be administered, and FS T1-WI in sagittal and transverse planes should be additionally obtained. Coronal planes are useful in the evaluation of patients with paraspinal masses (NF, neuroblastoma), scoliosis, and split-cord malformation.

13.3.2 Appearance of the Spine in the Neonate

The normal appearance of the spine can be difficult to interpret, especially in newborns and young infants. From birth to 1 month of age, T1-WI show hypointense ossified vertebral bodies adjacent to hyperintense nonossified cartilage, with small hypointense disks. T2-WI are easier to interpret, as ossified and nonossified parts of the vertebrae are hypointense, while the disks are hyperintense (Fig. 13.65). From 1 to 6 months, conversion of the vertebrae start, from the periphery to the center. Therefore, the periphery of the vertebrae is hyperintense on T1-WI, with the center of the vertebrae and the disks remaining hypointense. Appearance on T2-WI remains the same. From 7 months on, vertebrae are hyperintense and disks hypointense on T1-WI. T2-WI remain the same and are easy to interpret.

13.3.3 Developmental Anomalies

During the fourth week after gestation, the conversion of the neural plate into the neural tube takes place by a process called neurulation (Fig. 13.66a–f). Neurulation

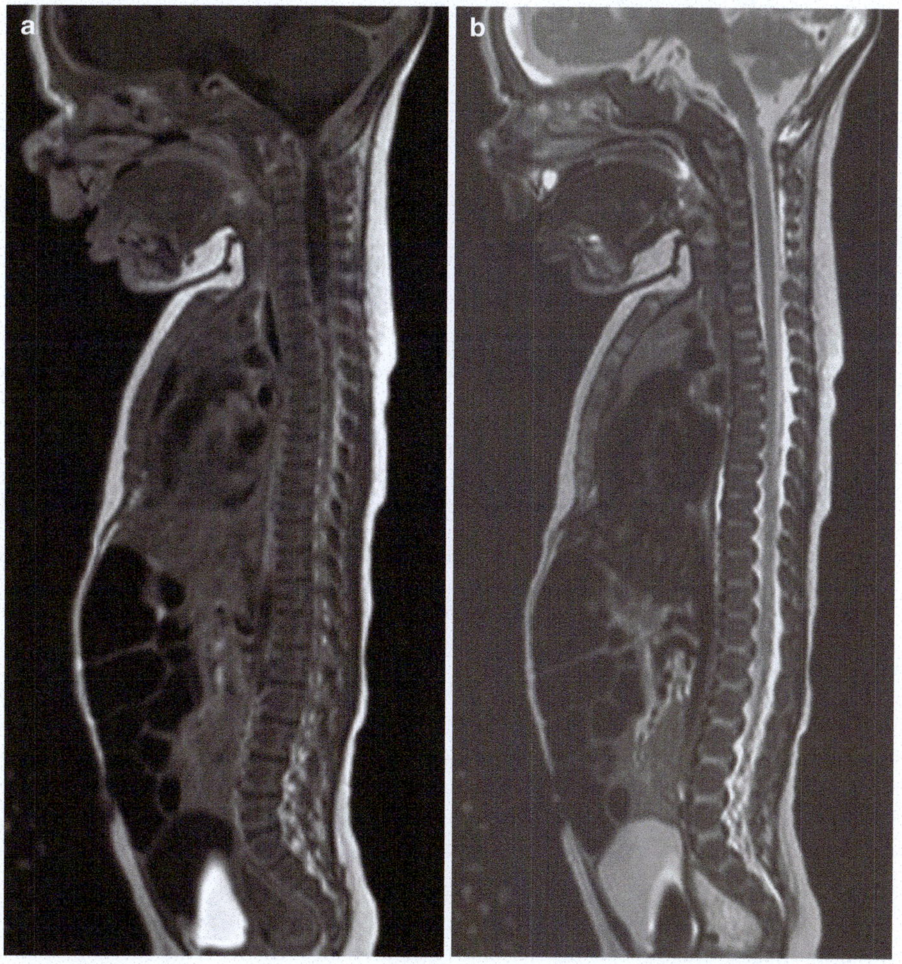

Fig. 13.65 Normal appearance of the vertebral bodies and disks from birth to 3 months of age. Sagittal T1-WI (**a**) of a 3-month-old infant reveals the hypointense ossified vertebrae with the hyperintense, nonossified cartilage on each end. The hyperintense endplates of the vertebral bodies are separated by a thin, hypointense structure that represents the intervertebral disk. Sagittal T2-WI (**b**) demonstrates ossified and nonossified parts of the vertebrae as hypointense, while the disks are hyperintense

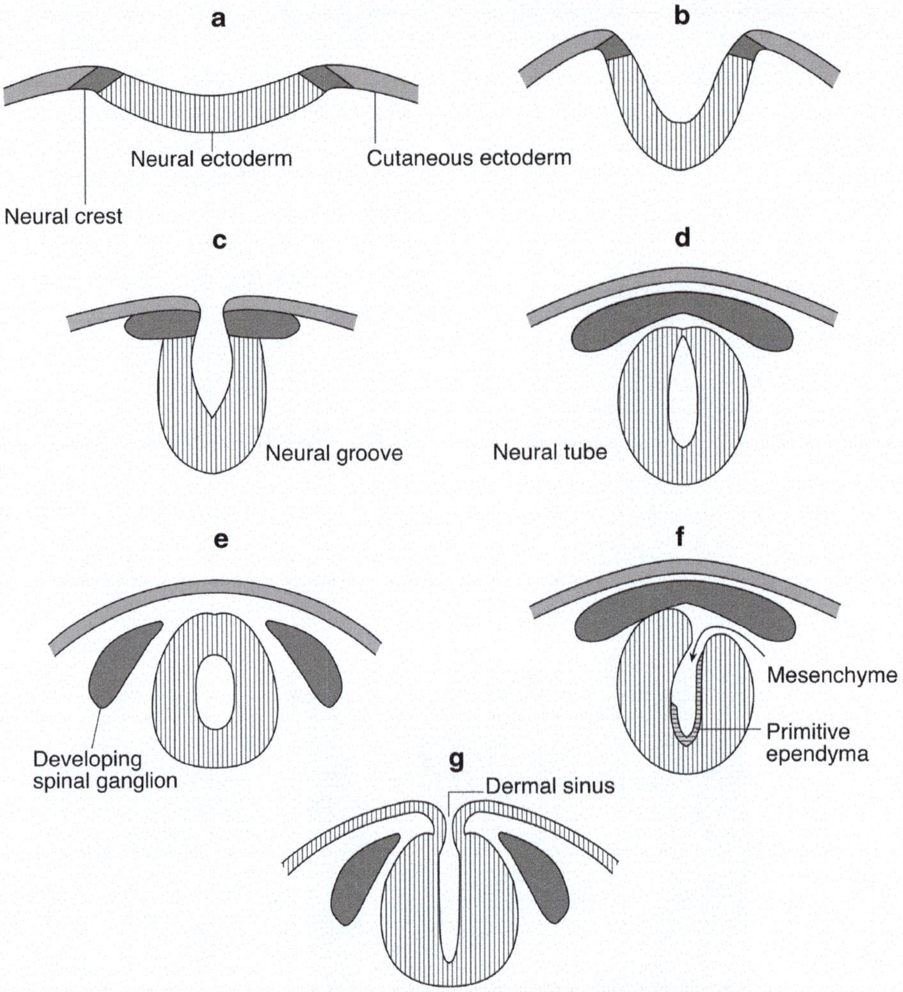

Fig. 13.66 Normal and abnormal neurulation. (**a–e**) Normal neurulation. The neural plate is composed of neural ectoderm, neural crest, and cutaneous ectoderm. (**b**) During the third week of gestation, the neural plate begins to thicken and fold. (**c**) The neural plate invaginates along its central axis and forms the median neural groove. (**d**) Neurulation (closure of the neural tube) begins when the neural folds meet in the midline. The overlying ectoderm separates from the neural tissue and fuses in the midline and becomes continuous over the neural tube. At the same time, the neural crest cells migrate ventrolaterally and form a transient structure immediately dorsal to the tube. (**e**) The neural crest then separates into right and left parts and migrates to form root ganglia and multiple other structures. (**f, g**) Abnormal neurulation. (**f**) In case of premature dysjunction of the neural ectoderm from the cutaneous ectoderm, the surrounding mesenchyme gains access to the inner surface of the neural tube and evolves to fat. This process is postulated to give rise to spinal lipomas. Complete nondysjunction of cutaneous ectoderm from neural ectoderm results in the formation of myelomeningoceles. (**g**) Focal nondysjunction results in the formation of a dorsal dermal sinus (Adapted from Barkovich 2000)

begins in the occipitocervical region as the neural plate invaginates along its central axis to form a longitudinal median neural groove that has neural folds on both sides. The lateral edges of the neural folds meet in the midline and fuse, while simultaneously separating from the surface ectoderm. The free edges of the surface ectoderm then fuse with each other, so that this layer becomes continuous over the neural tube. At the same time, the neural crest cells migrate ventrolaterally on each side of the neural tube and form a flattened mass, called the neural crest. The neural crest then separates into right and left parts, and begins to migrate and give rise to dorsal-root ganglia, ganglia of the autonomic nervous system, and some other structures. Disturbance of this process may result in severe anomalies. In the case of premature separation of neural ectoderm from cutaneous ectoderm, mesenchyme cells gain access to the inner surface of the neural tube. Mesenchyme cells are believed to evolve into fat when mingling with primitive ependyma, thus giving rise to spinal lipomas. Complete nondysjunction of cutaneous ectoderm from neural ectoderm results in the formation of myelomeningoceles, whereas focal nondysjunction results in the formation of a dermal sinus. Furthermore, multiple spine anomalies can be present in the same patient. A patient with myelomeningocele may have diastematomyelia, a tight filum terminale, and a dorsal sinus as well. Consequently, it is important to image the whole spine as soon as a cutaneous or vertebral body anomaly is discovered.

13.3.3.1 Spinal Dysraphism

Spinal dysraphism is a group of spinal column and neuroaxis disorders in which there is a defective midline closure of the neural, bony, and other mesenchymal tissues. In almost all cases of spinal dysraphism, there are vertebral body anomalies indicating the level of the lesion. The term spina bifida refers to incomplete posterior closure of the bony elements of the spine. Spina bifida aperta refers to an open neurulation defect, in which the neural tissue is exposed through a spina bifida without skin covering. Meningoceles, myelomeningoceles, and myeloceles belong to this group. Occult spinal dysraphism, in which the myelodysplasia lies beneath intact skin, includes lesions such as dermal sinus, spinal lipoma, lipomyelomeningoceles, myelocystoceles, tight filum terminale syndrome, diastematomyelia, and caudal-regression syndrome. Patients with occult spinal dysraphism almost always have cutaneous stigmata, such as a hairy patch, a nevus, a hemangioma, or a sinus tract.

13.3.3.2 Myelocele, Meningocele, and Myelomeningocele

Myelocele, meningocele, and myelomeningocele result from a lack of closure of the neural tube. In a myelocele, the neural tissue cannot separate from the cutaneous ectoderm, and therefore the placode of reddish neural tissue is seen in the middle of the back. Myelomeningocele is almost identical to myelocele, with the exception that there is an expansion of the ventral subarachnoid space, which posteriorly displaces the placode. A meningocele is characterized by the frequent presence of a complete skin covering and herniation of distended spinal meninges, but not neural tissue, through the dysraphic spine (Fig. 13.67). The Arnold Chiari II malformation is rarely present in patients with meningocele, but is essentially always associated with myelomeningocele and myelocele (Fig. 13.16). Due to the risk of infection, these entities are rarely imaged and are operated on within the first 24–48 h of life.

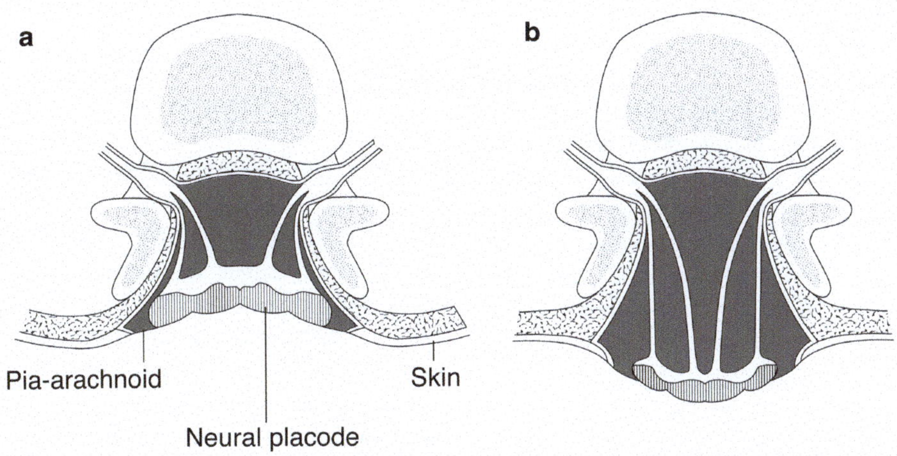

Fig. 13.67 Myelocele and myelomeningocele. (**a**) Myelocele. The neural placode is a flat plaque of neural tissue that is exposed to air. The dura is deficient posteriorly, and the ventral surface of the placode and dura is lined by the pia and arachnoid, forming an arachnoid sac. Both the dorsal and ventral roots arise from the ventral surface of the placode. (**b**) Myelomeningocele. In this similar entity, the placode is posteriorly displaced due to expansion of the ventral subarachnoid space (Adapted from Barkovich 2000)

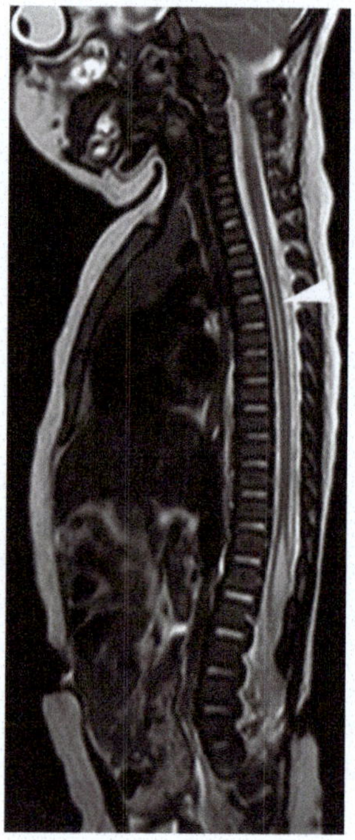

Fig. 13.68 Sagittal T2-WI shows syringohydromyelia (*arrowhead*) in a newborn with Arnold Chiari II malformation

13.3.3.3 Hydrosyringomyelia/ Syringohydromyelia

By definition, hydromyelia is the accumulation of fluid in the enlarged, ependymal-lined central canal of the spinal cord. Syringomyelia and syrinx are defined as diverticulation of the central canal with associated dissection of CSF into the cord parenchyma, resulting in glial-lined cysts, which may or may not communicate with the central canal. Because these two are difficult to distinguish by imaging, the terms hydrosyringomyelia or syringohydromyelia are used to describe these findings (Fig. 13.68). Hydrosyringomyelia or syringohydromyelia are observed in multiple congenital anomalies, such as Arnold Chiari I and II, lipomyelomeningocele, myelomeningocele, diastematomyelia, Dandy-Walker cysts, or may occur secondary to intramedullary or extramedullary tumors, ischemia, inflammation, and trauma.

13.3.3.4 Congenital Dermal Sinus

Congenital dermal sinus is an epithelium-lined channel that extends from the skin to the spinal canal, and may either reach the dura or pass through it (Fig. 13.66g). If the sinus tract passes the dura, it may end in or traverse the subarachnoid space and terminate within the conus medullaris, the filum terminale, a nerve root, or an epidermoid/dermoid cyst.

13.3.3.5 Lipomyelocele, Lipomyelomeningocele, Myelocystocele

Lipomyelocele and lipomyelomeningocele are very similar to myelocele and myelomeningocele, with the following additional features: a symmetrical or asymmetrical lipoma is attached to the dorsal surface of the placode, which is continuous with the subcutaneous fat and covered by an intact layer of skin (Figs. 13.69–13.71).

13.3.3.6 Intradural Lipoma

Intradural lipomas are a group of fatty tumors lying almost entirely within the bony spinal canal. They are typically subpial-juxtamedullary dorsal lesions, with the lipoma located between the central canal and the pia. Most commonly, intradural lipomas are found in the cervical or thoracic spine. The imaging characteristics of intradural lipomas are similar to those of subcutaneous fat (Figs. 13.69 and 13.72).

13.3.3.7 Tight Filum Terminale and Tethered Cord

Tethered cord may occur alone or in association with other lower spinal anomalies, and is defined as an abnormal low position of the conus terminalis. This tethering may either be primary, due to a tight filum terminale, or secondary to other dysraphic entities, such as diastematomyelia, lipo/myelomeningoceles, or after meningomyelocele repair. Patients will present with neurologic symptoms (bowel or bladder dysfunction, gait disturbances, weakness), orthopedic symptoms (scoliosis, foot deformities, back pain), or urologic symptoms (urinary incontinence, recurrent urinary-tract infections). The definitive diagnosis is made by demonstration of the conus medullaris below

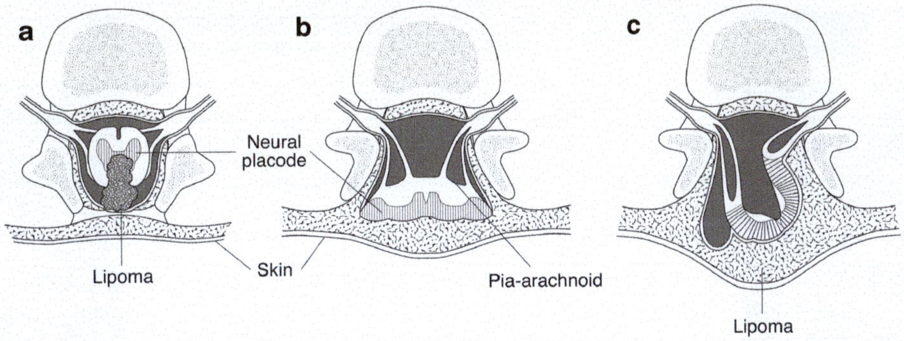

Fig. 13.69 Illustration of spinal lipomas, lipomyelocele, and lipomyelomeningocele. (**a**) Intradural (subpial-juxtamedullary) lipoma. The spinal cord is open in the midline dorsally, with the lipoma located between the unapposed lips of the placode. (**b**) Lipomyelocele. This lesion is very similar to a myelocele, with two additional features: the lipoma is situated dorsally and attached to the surface of the placode. It is continuous with subcutaneous fat and covered by skin. (**c**) Lipomyelomeningocele with rotation of the neural placode. When the lipoma is asymmetric, it extends into the spinal canal and causes the ventral meningocele to herniate posteriorly and the dorsal surface of the placode to rotate to the side of the lipoma (Adapted from Barkovich 2000)

the L2/L3 interspace, associated with a short and thickened filum terminale, or termination of the conus or filum in a dysraphic lesion, such as a lipomyelocele (Fig. 13.70) or other developmental tumors, such as epidermoids/dermoids or lipomas (Fig. 13.72).

13.3.3.8 Diastematomyelia

Diastematomyelia is the most common anomaly of the split notochord syndrome spectrum. A bony or fibrous band coursing from the posterior elements

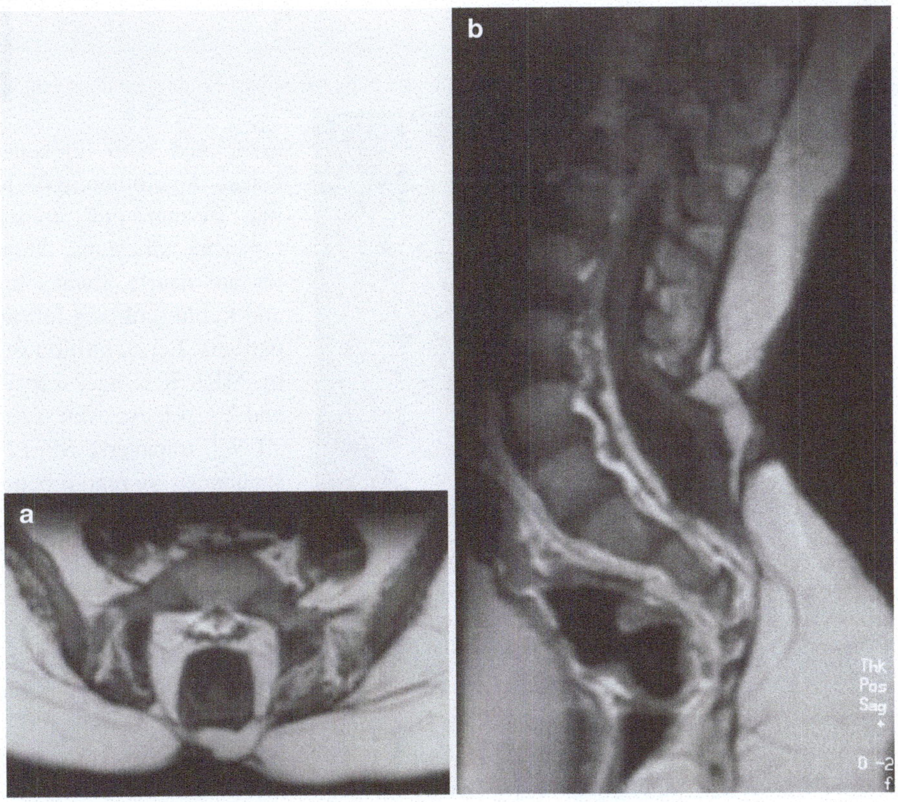

Fig. 13.70 Lipomyelocele. Transverse (**a**) and sagittal (**b**) T1-WI display a typical example of a lipomyelocele with tethered cord. Compare with Fig. 13.69b

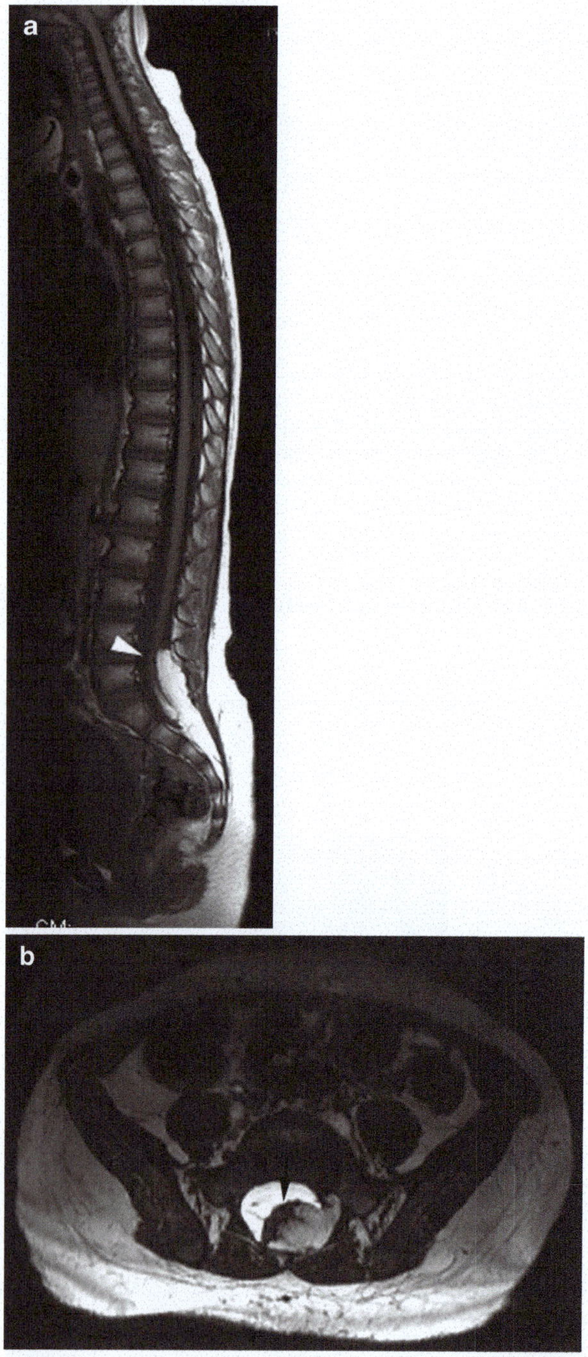

Fig. 13.71 Lipomyelomeningocele. Sagittal T1-WI (**a**) and transverse CISS image (**b**) show an asymmetric lipoma extending into the spinal canal, with rotation of the neural placode (*black arrow*) and tethered cord (*arrowhead*). Compare with Fig. 13.69c

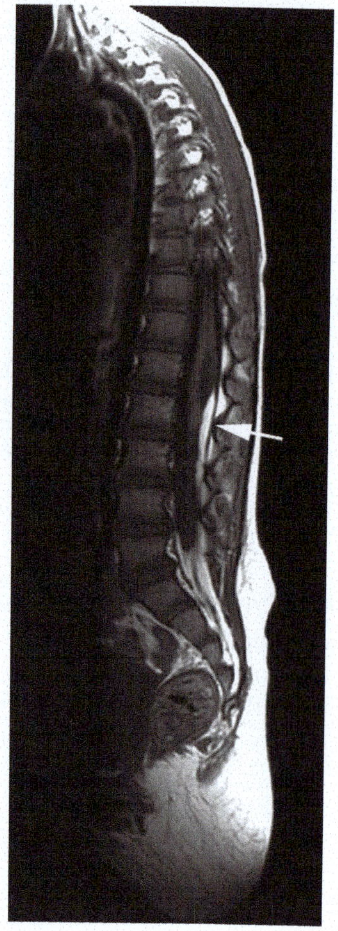

Fig. 13.72 Intradural lipoma. Sagittal T1-WI demonstrates a hyperintense mass (*arrow*) within the lumbar spinal canal and tethered cord

to the vertebral body splits the spinal cord sagittally into two symmetric or asymmetric hemicords, each having the ventral and dorsal nerve roots for that side (Fig. 13.73). Diastematomyelia is commonly associated with thickened filum terminale, myeloceles, myelomeningoceles, hemimyeloceles, lipomas, dermal sinus, epidermoid/dermoid tumors, and tethering adhesions. Anomalies of the vertebral bodies are nearly always present in diastematomyelia, and kyphoscoliosis follows in more than 50% of the patients. For definition of the bony or fibrous septum by MRI, it is necessary to obtain transverse T1-WI and T2-WI. As even osseous spurs can be missed on T1-WI, transverse SE T2-W or transverse T2* GRE sequences are recommended. The spur is hypointense compared with CSF on T1-WI if nonossified, and hyperintense if ossified. On T2-WI, the spur is hypointense, whether it is bony, cartilaginous, or fibrous.

13.3.3.9 Hemimyelocele

In 31–46% of patients with myelomeningocele or myelocele, there is an association with diastematomyelia. In some patients, only one of the hemicords

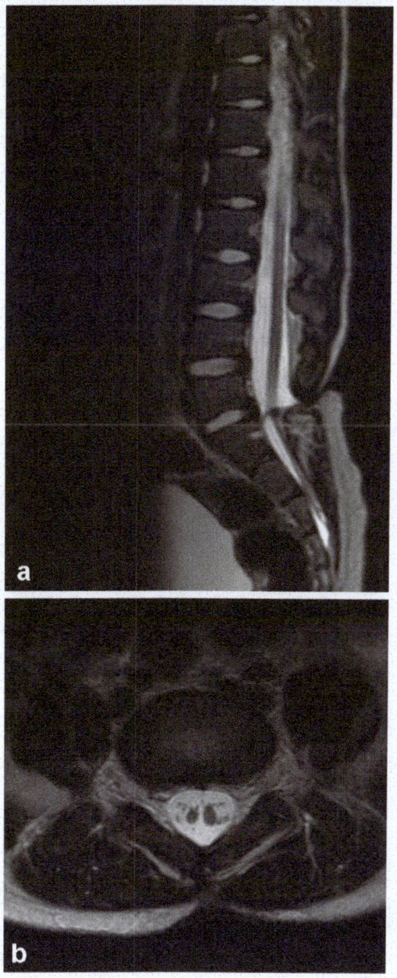

Fig. 13.73 Diastematomyelia. Sagittal T2-WI (**a**) shows a tethered-cord syndrome in concert with a spur. Transverse T2-WI (**b**) displays diastematomyelia with two hemicords, each having the ventral and dorsal nerve roots for that side

is combined with a myelomeningocele. The term hemimyelocele is used to describe this anomaly. The other hemicord most commonly terminates in the filum terminale within the spinal canal, and may or may not be associated with either a second small myelomeningocele at a lower level and/or tethered cord.

13.3.3.10 Caudal-Regression Syndrome

Caudal-regression syndrome is a part of the caudal-dysplasia spectrum, and consists of one or more of the following: partial or total agenesis of the lumbar and sacral vertebrae, anal atresia, malformation of genitalia, renal abnormalities, pulmonary hypoplasia, and, rarely, fusion of the lower extremities (sirenomelia). Most patients present with neurogenic bladder, motor weakness, and foot deformities. There may be associations with other developmental abnormalities of the spine. MRI of the spinal canal demonstrates a high positioned and blunted or wedge-shaped conus, in addition to the aforementioned vertebral anomalies (Fig. 13.74).

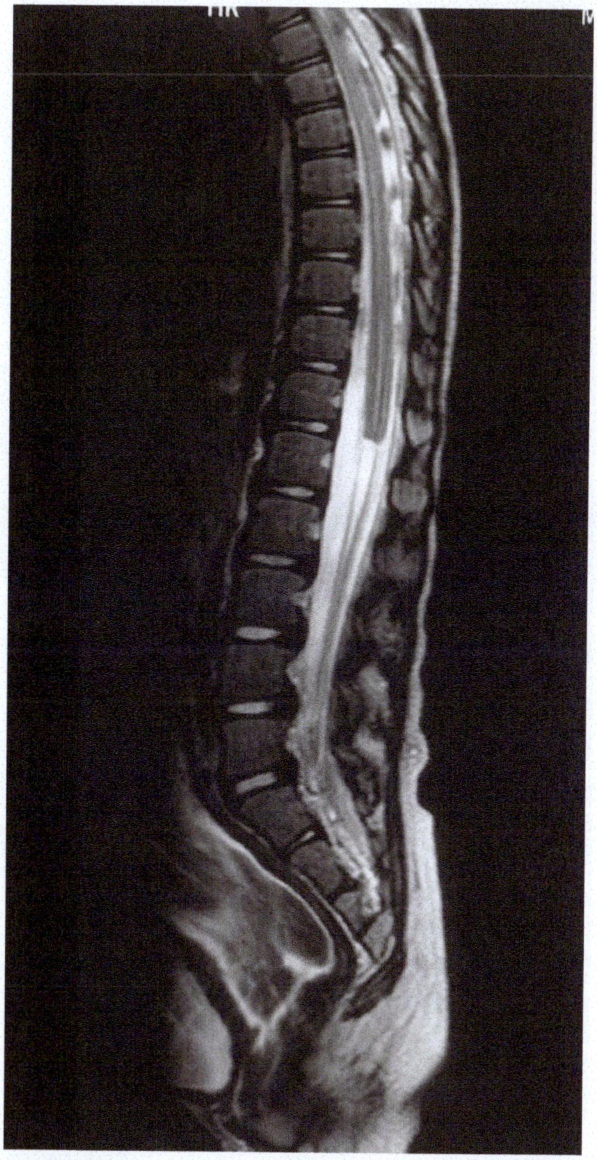

Fig. 13.74 Mild caudal regression. The spinal column is normal except for the sacrum. S3 and S4 are dysplastic. In addition, S5 and the coccyx are absent. The cord terminus is situated at the T12/L1 level and has the characteristic blunted shape of caudal regression

13.3.3.11 Anterior Sacral Meningoceles

Anterior sacral meningoceles are diverticula of the intraspinal thecal sac, which protrude anteriorly into the extraperitoneal presacral space. They occur sporadically or in association with NF, Marfan's syndrome, or the Currarino triad (Fig. 13.75). Patients with anterior sacral meningoceles may be asymptomatic, or suffer from disturbances secondary to the mass effect, ranging from back pain, constipation, and genitourinary problems to neurological symptoms. The spinal canal is widened, and a minor or major sacrum defect is almost always present. On MRI, these rounded masses may be unilocular or multilocular and demonstrate signal characteristics of CSF on all sequences, sometimes containing neural structures.

13.3.3.12 Currarino Triad

Currarino triad is an autosomal dominant inherited complex, consisting of an anorectal malformation,

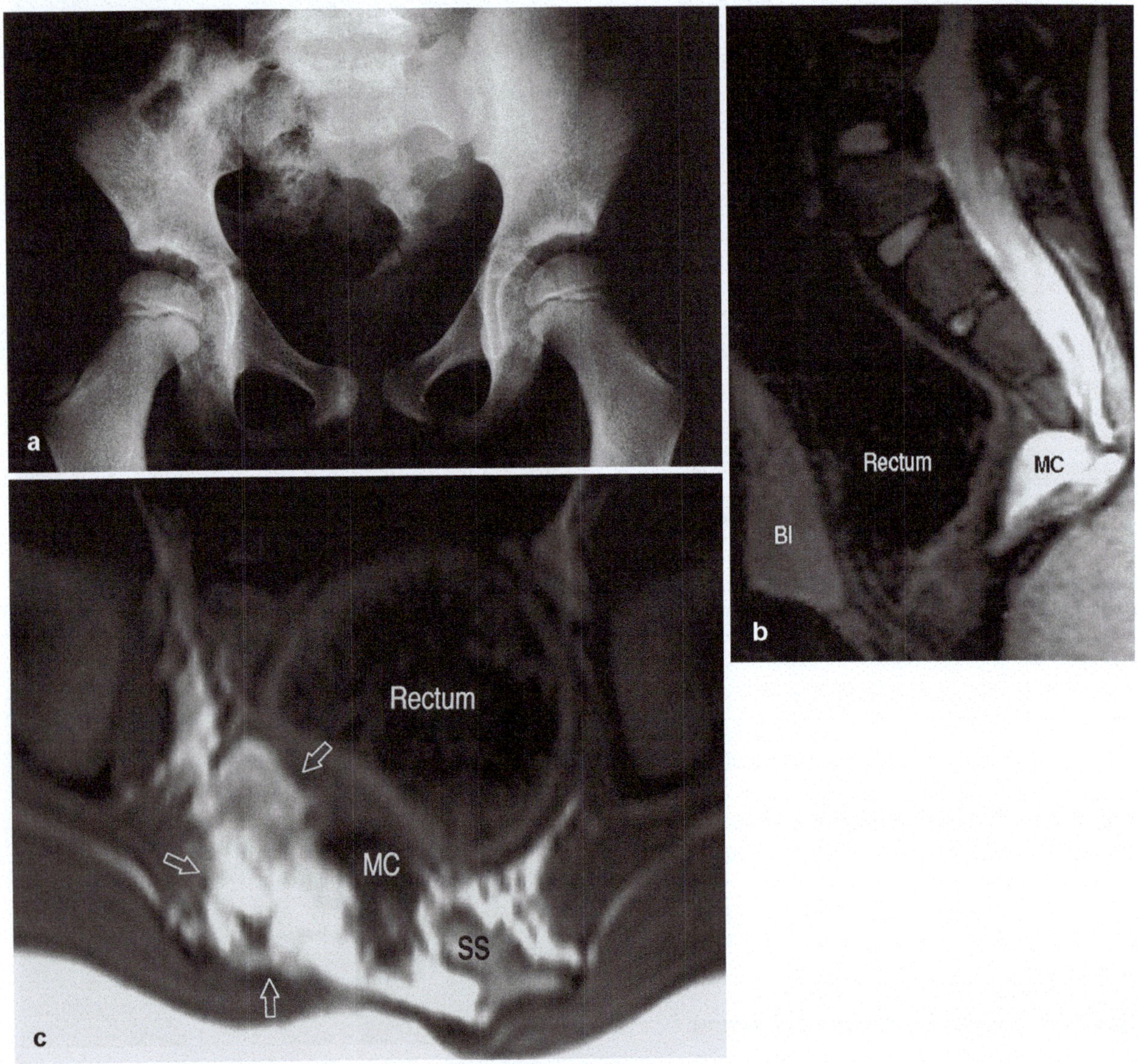

Fig. 13.75 Currarino triad. Conventional radiograph (**a**) shows sacral dysplasia with a curved deviation to the left, a so-called scimitar sacrum. Sagittal T2-WI (**b**) and transverse T1-WI (**c**) show a presacral meningocele, a left-sided scimitar sacrum, and a predominately right-sided fatty mass

sacral defects, and a presacral mass. Patients suffer from constipation from birth, and plain films reveal a scimitar sacrum. MRI is necessary to evaluate patients for concurrent anterior sacral meningocele, lipoma, dermoid, teratoma, and tethered cord (Fig. 13.75).

13.3.4 Spinal Infections

Inflammatory processes during childhood include spondylitis, discitis, spondylodiscitis, sacroiliac pyarthrosis, epidural abscess, meningitis, arachnoiditis, myelitis, and, finally, spinal cord abscess. All of these entities show the same appearance as in adults and should be examined with paramagnetic contrast. In this section, attention is paid to discitis and autoimmune demyelination due to MS.

13.3.4.1 Discitis and Spondylodiscitis

Discitis is an inflammatory process of the intervertebral disk space. The most common site is the lumbar region. Discitis occurs frequently in children from 6 months to 4 years of age, with a second peak at 10–14 years of age. Cultures of blood or biopsy material are positive in up to 50% of the patients; *Staphylococcus aureus* is almost always the organism involved. At first, radiographs of the spine are normal; bone scintigraphy shows increased uptake as early as 1–2 days after the onset of symptoms. On T1-WI, disk-space infection demonstrates poor delineation of the involved disk, with hypointense signal in the adjacent vertebrae reflecting marrow edema. On T2-WI, the disk and the adjacent vertebrae show abnormally increased SI. There may be contrast enhancement of the disk and the adjacent vertebral body, with or without disk extrusion, and epidural or paraspinal extension of the infection (Figs. 13.76 and 13.77).

13.3.4.2 Multiple Sclerosis

MS is rare in the pediatric age group, but as the mean age of presentation in children is 13 years, a radiologist dealing with children should be aware of its presentation within the spine. Additionally, spinal cord lesions due to MS in children may differ from the presentation in adults. MS in children tends to show more diffuse cord involvement (three or more vertebral levels) or even holocord involvement, with increased T2-W signal and decreased T1-W signal reflecting demyelination and cord edema (Fig. 13.78). Enhancement with paramagnetic contrast is variable and is associated with disease activity. The differential diagnosis includes ADEM, transverse myelitis, cord infarct, AIDS-related myelopathy, and neoplasm.

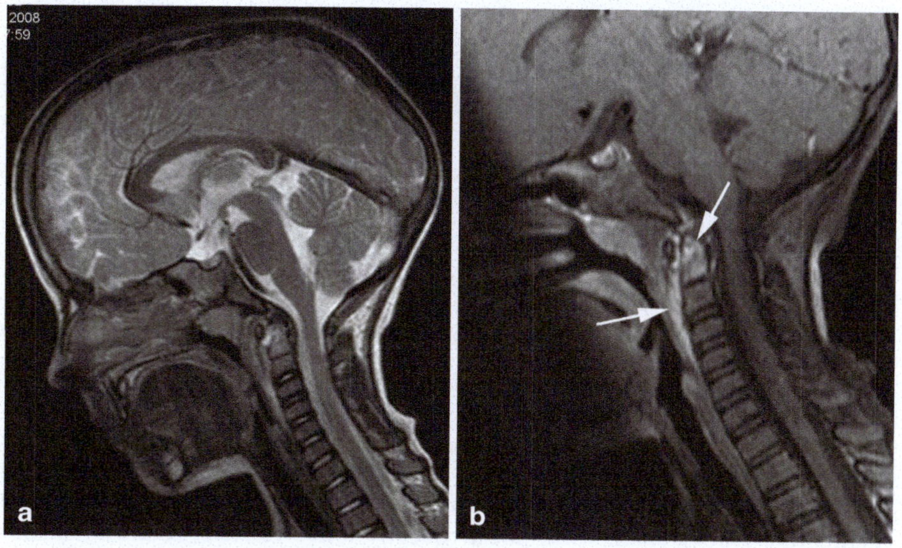

Fig. 13.76 Spondylitis of the dens. Sagittal T2-WI (**a**) shows high SI in the tip of the dens and in the adjacent prevertebral space. Contrast-enhanced fat-saturated sagittal T1-WI (**b**) demonstrates enhancement (*arrows*)

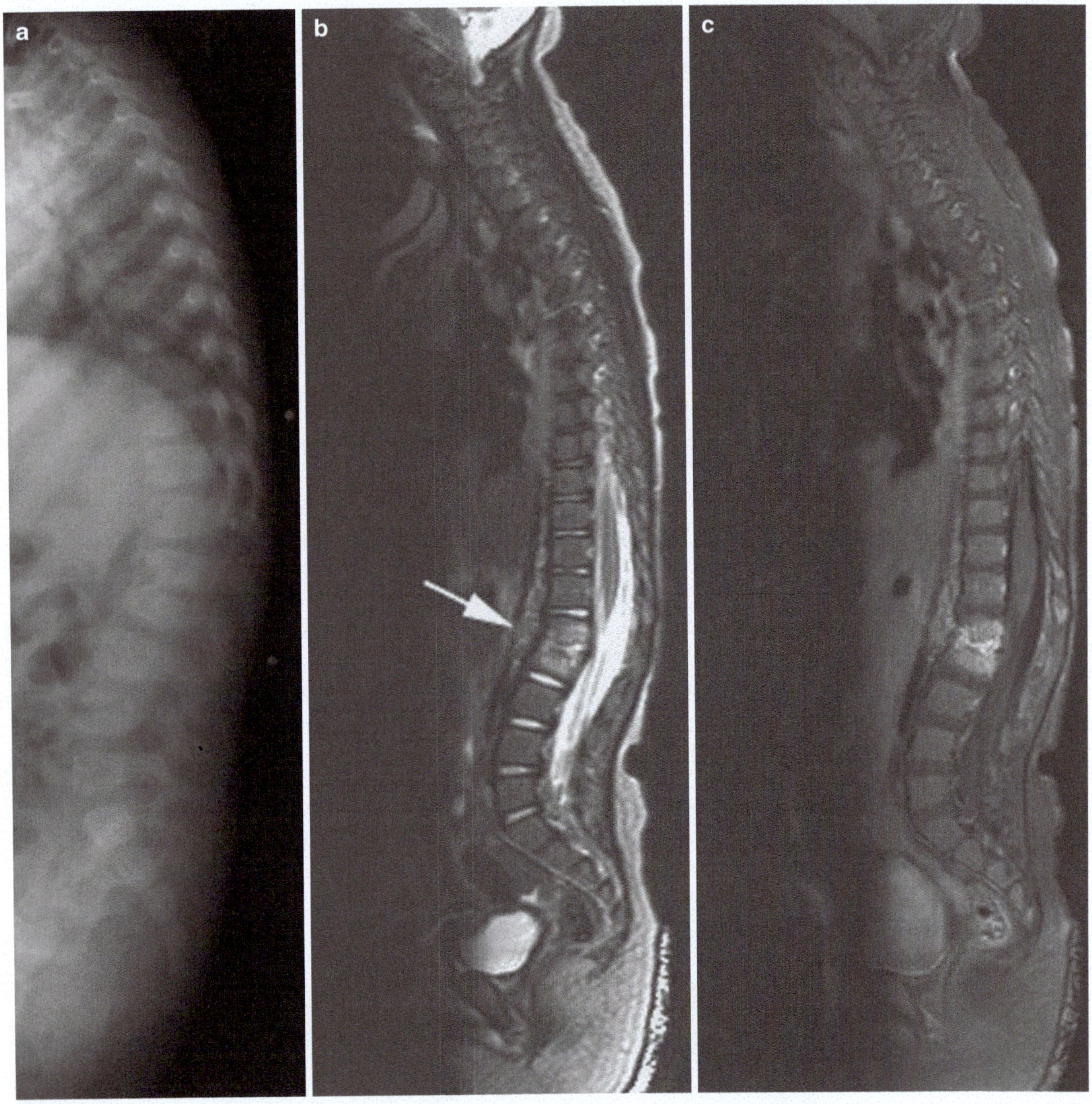

Fig. 13.77 Spondylodiscitis. Lateral plain film (**a**) shows an irregular contour of the endplates of L1 and L2, with narrowing of the disc space. Sagittal T2-WI (**b**) demonstrates hyperintense vertebral bodies and intervertebral disc, together with a ventral soft-tissue mass (*arrow*). Contrast-enhanced fat-saturated T1-WI (**c**) shows enhancement of the disc, the vertebral bodies, and the soft-tissue mass

13.3.5 Spinal Tumors in Childhood

13.3.5.1 Intradural-Intramedullary Tumors

Astrocytoma

Approximately 50–60% of intramedullary tumors in children are astrocytomas, which are frequently low grade (grade I or II) by histology. Occasionally, higher grade malignancies occur, such as malignant glioma or glioblastoma multiforme. Astrocytomas are most often located in the thoracic spine. On MRI, astrocytomas present with spinal cord enlargement, and are most commonly hypointense on T1-WI and hyperintense on T2-WI. However, they can also appear as mixed signal-intensity lesions, rarely hemorrhagic, that have variable contrast enhancement. They may contain cysts, either representing tumor-lined or gliotic-lined

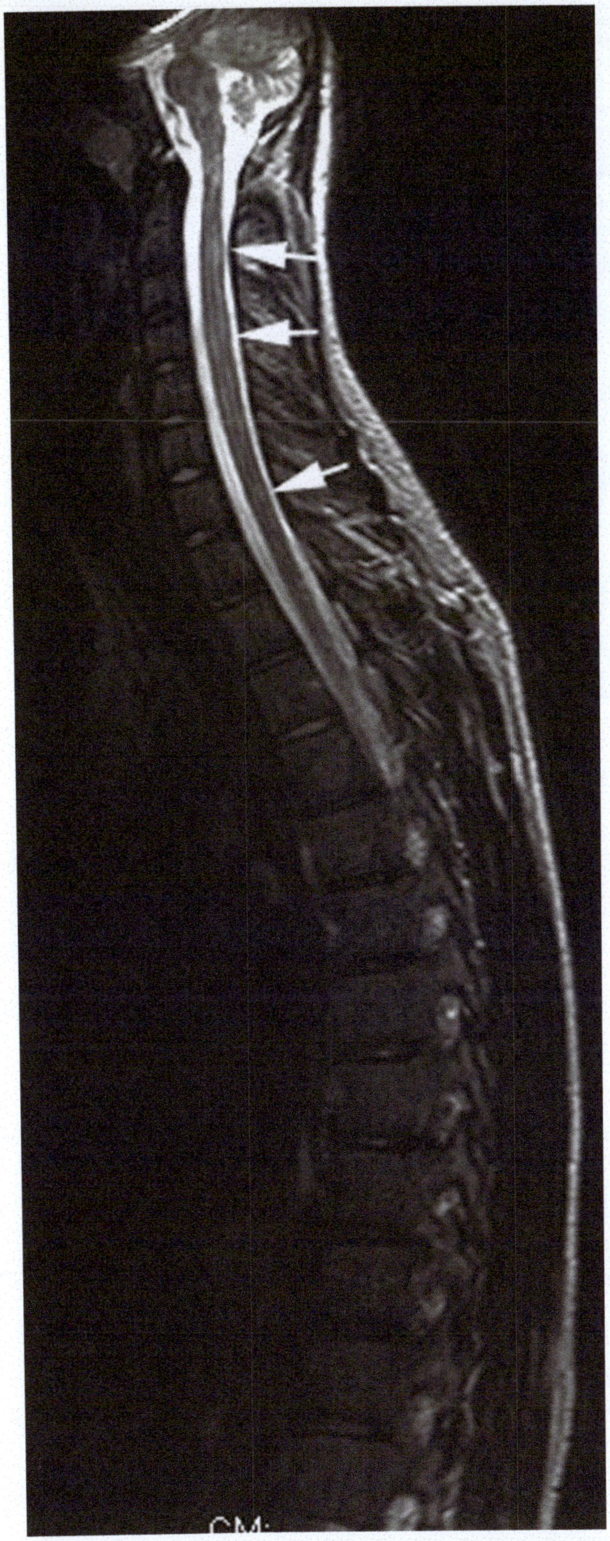

Fig. 13.78 Multiple sclerosis. Sagittal T2-WI shows numerous slightly hyperintense lesions (*arrows*) in the cervical segment of spinal cord

cystic cavities or syringomyelia above or below the tumor (Fig. 13.79).

Ependymoma

Ependymomas constitute 20–30% of intramedullary tumors in children. They typically arise in the lumbar region from ependymal cells within the spinal cord or filum terminale (Fig. 13.80). Ependymomas tend to be more sharply circumscribed hypointense or isointense masses, enhancing more heterogeneously on T1-W sequences than astrocytomas. Evidence of hemorrhage at their inferior and superior margins may be another helpful imaging finding in differentiating ependymoma from astrocytoma.

Hemangioblastoma

Hemangioblastomas may be associated with von Hippel-Lindau syndrome and occur anywhere along the spinal axis. They are difficult to distinguish from AVMs and present as well-demarcated, intense contrast-enhancing masses, with cysts, areas of hemorrhage, and flow voids, due to draining and feeding vessels.

13.3.5.2 Intradural Extramedullary Tumors

The four most common intradural extramedullary tumors in childhood comprise neurofibroma/schwannoma, drop metastasis from primary intracranial tumors, congenital lipomas, and epidermoids/dermoids.

Neurofibroma and Schwannoma

Neurofibromas and plexiform neurofibromas are typically associated with NF-1, whereas schwannomas may occur in patients without NF. Neurofibroma and schwannoma of the spine originate from the nerve roots, and typically present as well-demarcated, dumbbell-shaped, soft-tissue masses passing through a frequently enlarged neural foramen. Neurofibromas are commonly hypointense or isointense on both T1-WI and T2-WI, with variable enhancement after CM. They may be less frequently hyperintense on T2-WI. Plexiform neurofibromas are typically wavy, elongated masses, which are

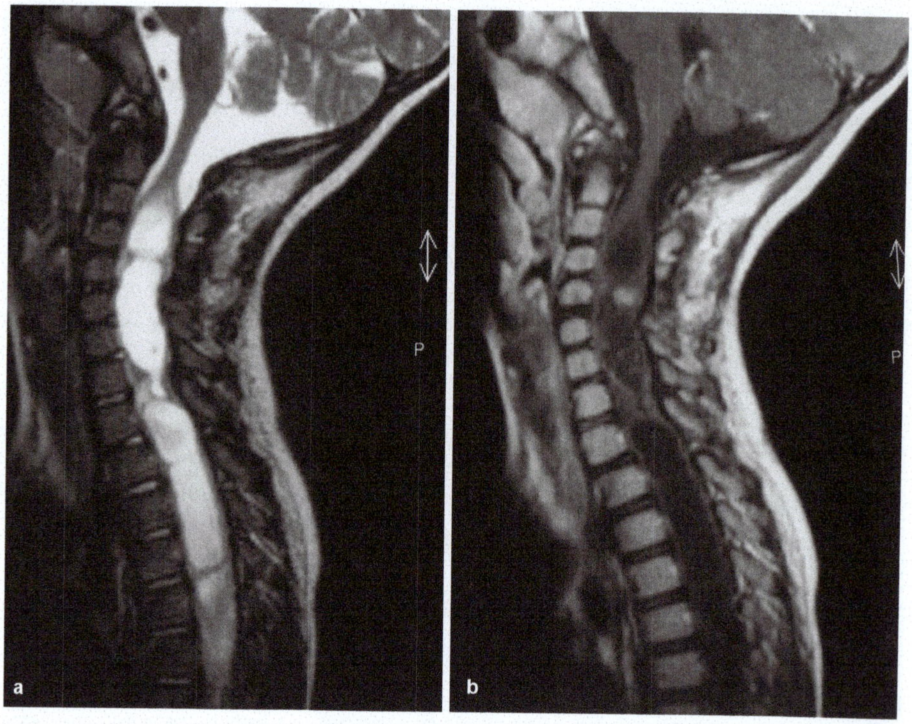

Fig. 13.79 Spinal astrocytoma. Sagittal T2-WI (**a**) and sagittal T1-WI (**b**) after administration of contrast show an enhancing nodule of tumor at the C4 level within the cervical cord. The cystic areas presumably represent necrotic regions within the tumor, and tumor-associated cysts (Courtesy of W. Michl)

hyperintense on T2-WI and heterogeneous on T1-WI, with variable contrast enhancement.

In contrast, schwannomas are well-demarcated masses, typically hyperintense on T2-WI, and usually enhance homogeneously with paramagnetic contrast (Fig. 13.81).

Drop Metastasis from CNS Neoplasms

CSF seeding from other CNS neoplasms is more common in children than in adults. The CNS neoplasms that most frequently metastasize in childhood are PNET and ependymoma. However, other tumors, such as germinomas, high-grade gliomas, lymphoma, choroid plexus tumors, and neuroblastomas, may present with metastatic subarachnoid disease (Fig. 13.82).

Epidermoid/Dermoid

The MR appearance of dermoids is variable, sometimes showing high intensity on T1-WI, but more commonly having low to intermediate SI on T1-WI and high SI on T2-WI. Dermoids are more common in the lumbar region, whereas epidermoids are distributed uniformly along the spinal canal. Epidermoids are most commonly isointense to CSF on both T1-WI and T2-WI. However, they are sometimes hyperintense on T1-WI, and consequently difficult to distinguish from dermoid or lipomas without the use of FS T1-W sequences (Fig. 13.83). Neither dermoids nor epidermoids enhance with paramagnetic contrast, unless they are infected. Infection is much more common if these lesions have developed in association with dermal sinuses.

13.3.5.3 Extradural Tumors

Extradural tumors in children are most commonly metastatic lesions from paravertebral soft tissue, with extension through the neural foramina into the spinal canal. Neuroblastoma is the most important extradural tumor in children (see Sect. 13.4.3). The most common newborn tumor arising from the extradural space is sacrococcygeal teratoma.

Sacrococcygeal Teratoma

Sacrococcygeal teratoma is defined as a congenital sacral tumor containing elements of all the three germ cell layers arising from the coccyx. The more correct

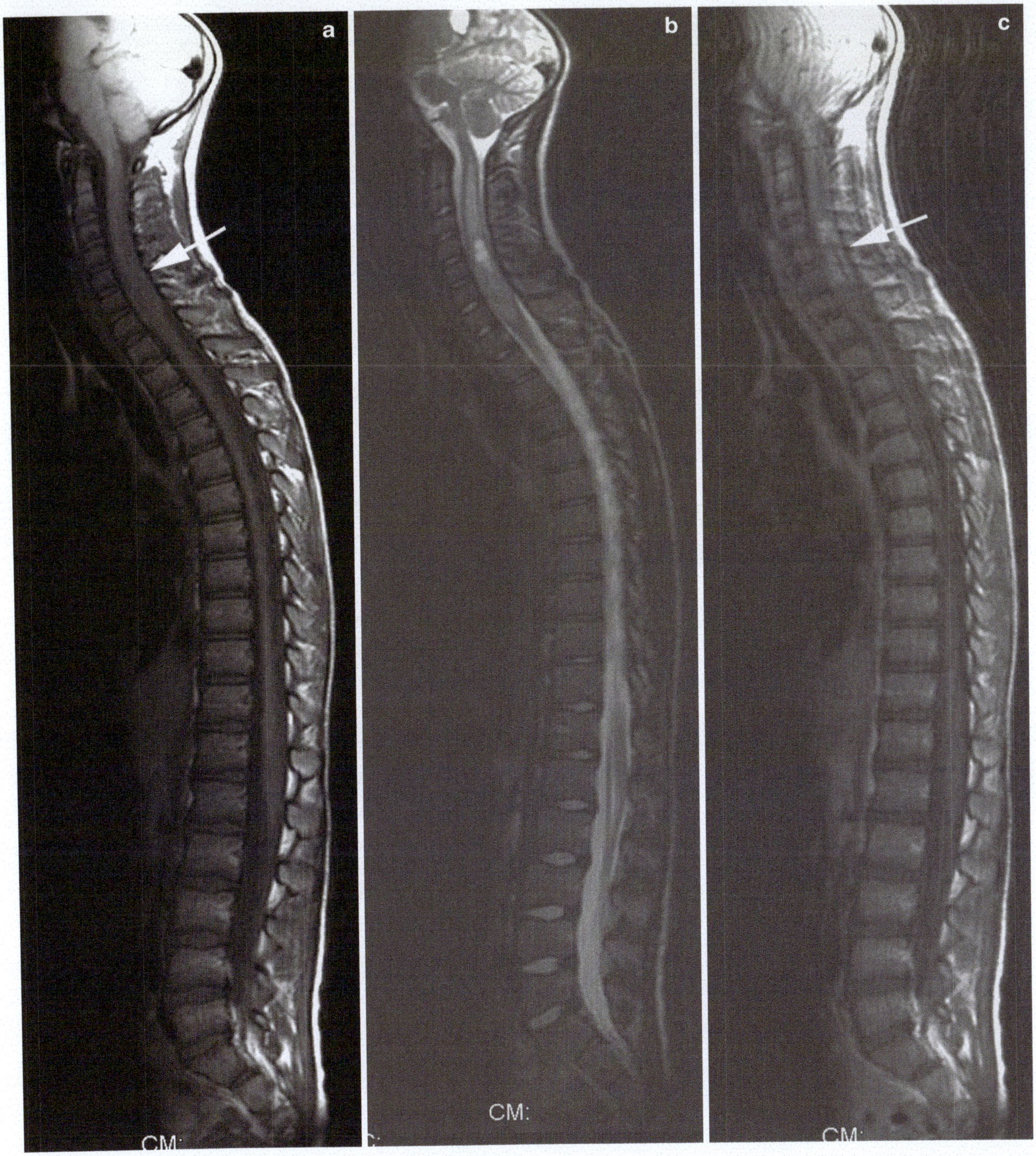

Fig. 13.80 Ependymoma (WHO grade 3). Sagittal T1-WI (**a**) shows enlargement of the cervical spinal cord (*arrow*). Sagittal T2-WI (**b**) and fat-saturated contrast-enhanced T1-WI (**c**) demonstrate enhancing tumor (*arrow*) with rostral and caudal vasogenic edema

synonym is sacral germ-cell tumor of the coccyx. Typically, a large sacral mass is noted prenatally or at the time of delivery (Fig. 13.84). Less commonly, the tumor is diagnosed in a newborn with buttock asymmetry or in an infant with a presacral tumor presenting with obstipation, urinary frequency, or incontinence. Generally, 80% of these tumors are mature, but 20% are immature and immature teratomas have a greater risk of malignancy. Malignant risk increases with age of diagnosis, higher surgical subtype, male gender, and

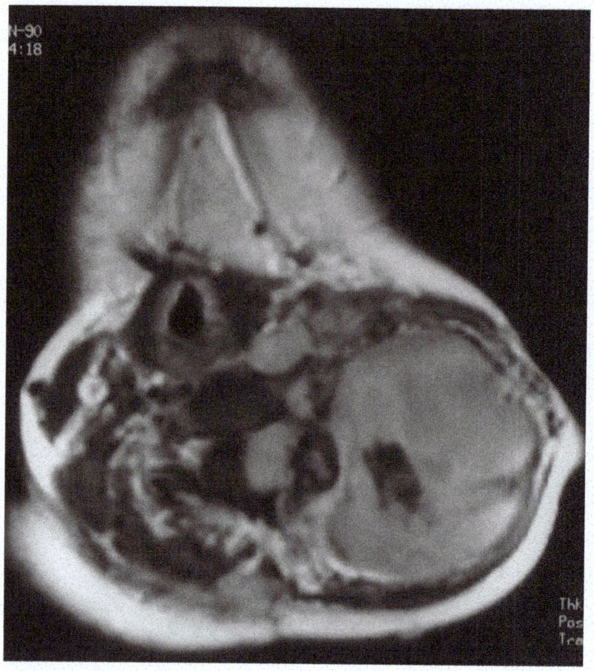

Fig. 13.81 Schwannoma. Transverse contrast-enhanced T1-WI demonstrates a huge, dumbbell-shaped mass with an area of tumor necrosis in the cervical spine and the left neck

presence of necrosis or hemorrhage. Four different subtypes are distinguished, according to the Altmann/AAP classification:

Type I	Primarily external (47%)	→	best prognosis
Type II	Dumbbell shape, equal internal/external portions (34%)		
Type III	Primarily internal, within the abdomen/pelvis (9%)		
Type IV	Entirely internal, with no visible external component (10%)	→	worst prognosis

Surgery alone is curative if the entire benign tumor and coccyx is removed (if the coccyx is not resected, tumor recurs). On MRI, a mature teratoma presents as a large sacral mass showing a heterogeneous mixed signal intensity, as it consists of fat (hyperintese on T1-WI and T2-WI), mixed solid (isointense on T1-WI and

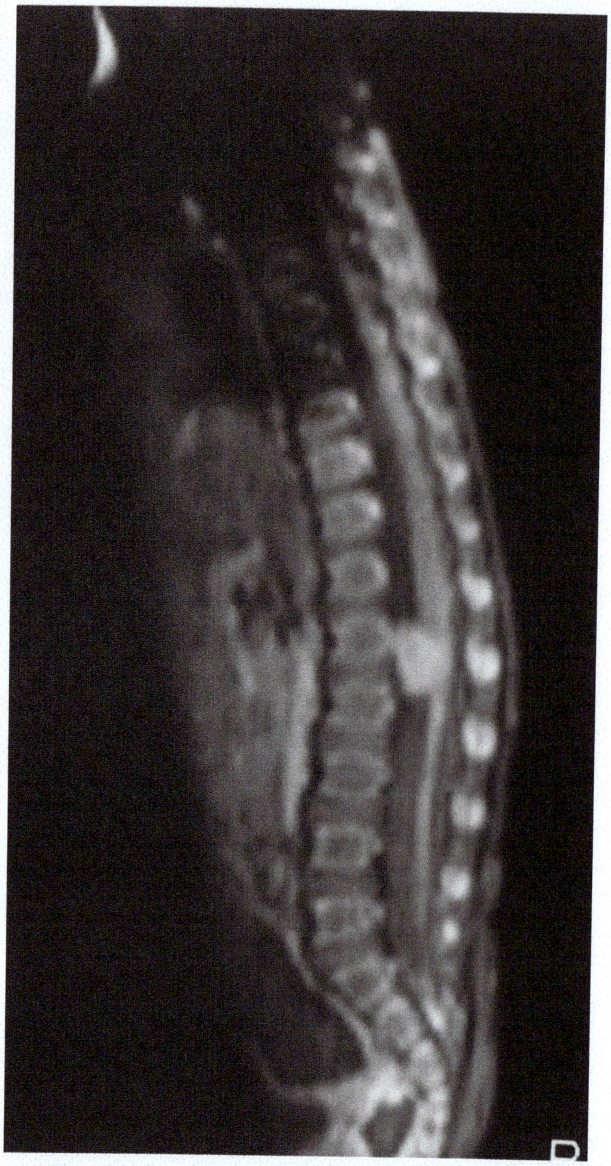

Fig. 13.82 Drop metastases. Sagittal FS contrast-enhanced T1-WI reveals drop metastases in the spinal canal from medulloblastoma (primitive neuroepithelial tumor) (Courtesy of W. Michl)

T2-WI) and cystic (hypointense on T1-WI and hyperintense on T2-WI) components, and calcifications (bone, teeth, and/or cartilage) (hypointense on T1-WI and T2-WI). After application of paramagnetic contrast, the solid portion and cyst walls will enhance. Hemorrhage and calcifications are best detected by T2* GRE sequences. It is crucial to examine these lesions in a sagittal and axial orientation with T2-W

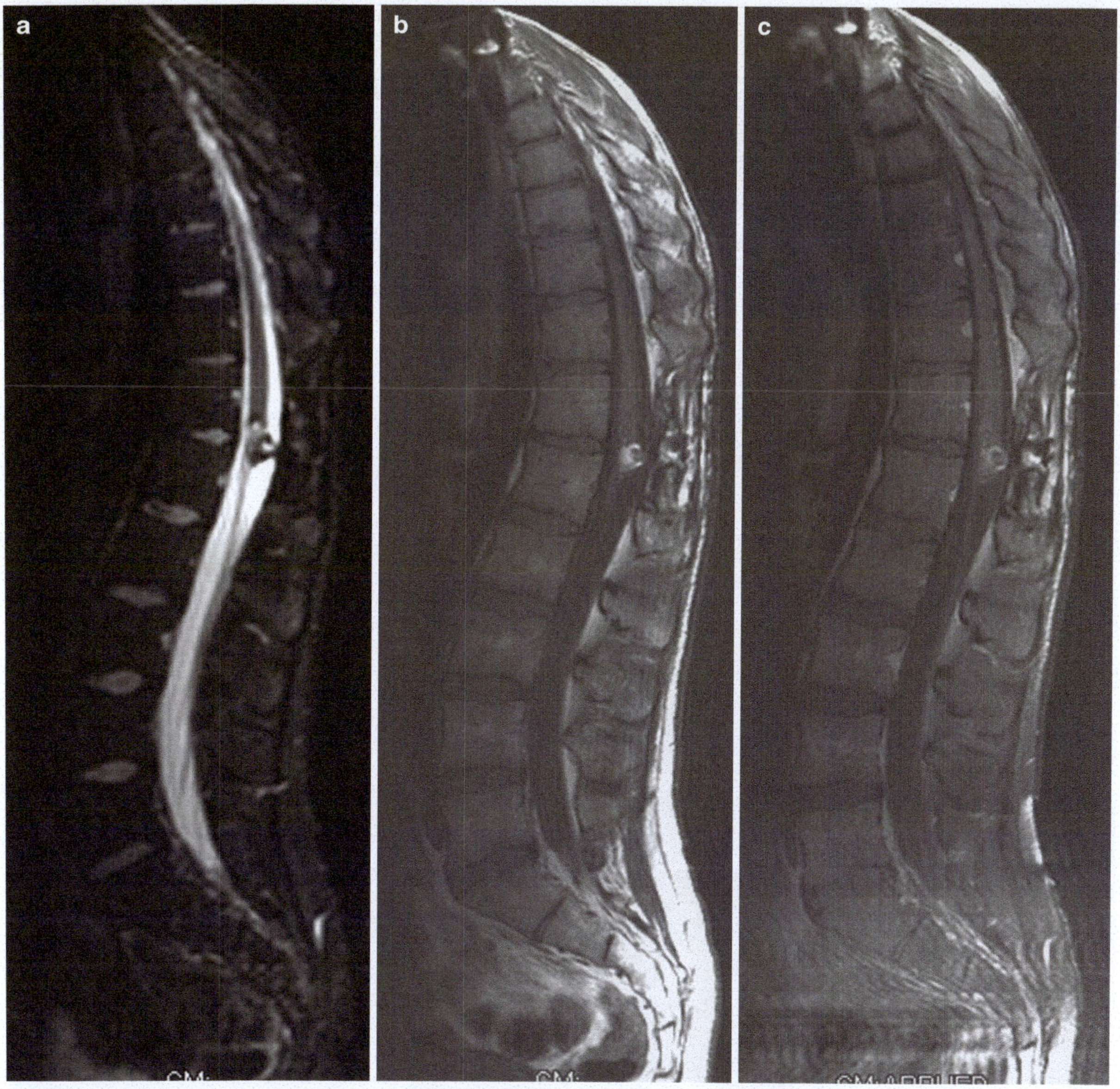

Fig. 13.83 Dermoid. Sagittal STIR (**a**) and T1-WI (**b**) show a rounded fat-containing lesion in the medullary cone in a 21-year-old boy with disturbance of micturition. Sagittal contrast-enhanced T1-WI (**c**) with insufficient fat saturation due to technical impairment demonstrates subtle enhancement

and T1-W sequences pre- and postadministration of paramagnetic contrast (Figs. 13.85 and 13.86).

Primary Neoplasms of the Spinal Column

Primary tumors of the spine are rare in children. Hemangioma, osteoid osteoma, osteoblastoma, aneurysmal bone cyst, osteochondroma, giant-cell tumor, osteosarcoma, Ewing's sarcoma, chondrosarcoma, and chordoma are included in this group. These lesions do not differ in radiographic and MR appearance from the same lesions in adults.

Secondary neoplasms of the spine in children comprise Langerhans cell histiocytosis, leukemia, lymphoma, rhabdomyosarcoma, neuroblastoma, Wilms' tumor, and PNET. The imaging findings of these tumors are discussed in Sect. 13.5.

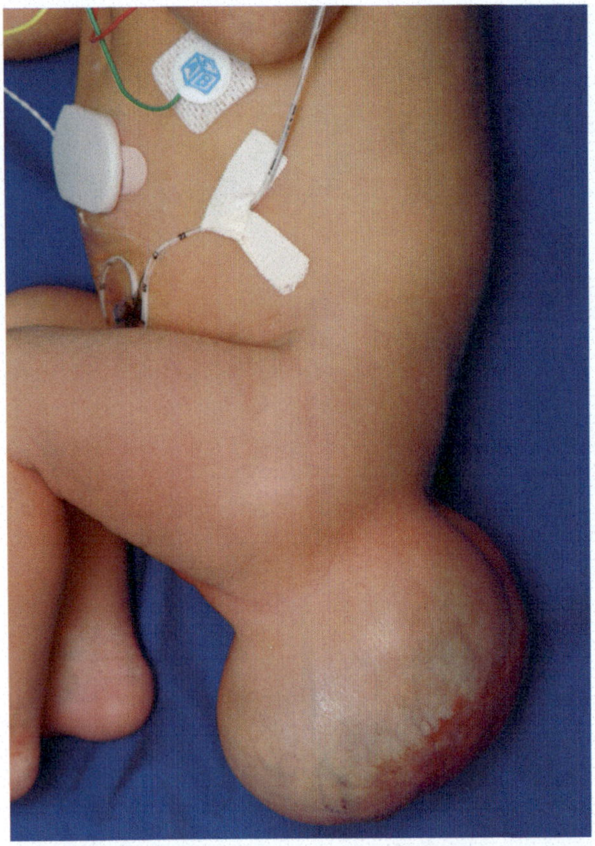

Fig. 13.84 Newborn with a sacrococcygeal teratoma

13.4 Pediatric Abdominal Imaging

13.4.1 Technique

13.4.1.1 Coils and Patient Positioning

For abdominal MR examinations of neonates and young infants, a phased-array surface coil (i.e., a multichannel round coil) or a cardiac coil is used. If not available, a head coil can also be utilized, as long as the coil is large enough for the child. Older children are positioned in the body phased-array coil, and the coil is fixed by a plastic tunnel to reduce artifacts caused by a moving coil due to breathing. A symmetric and comfortable posture should be arranged.

13.4.1.2 Sequence Protocol

With regard to the imaging strategy, it is important to consider that breath-hold techniques can only be applied in cooperative patients or during general anesthesia. Therefore, the sequence protocol differs from that for adults. For an overview, a mainly T2-T2*-W sequence (steady-state gradient echo) in transverse and

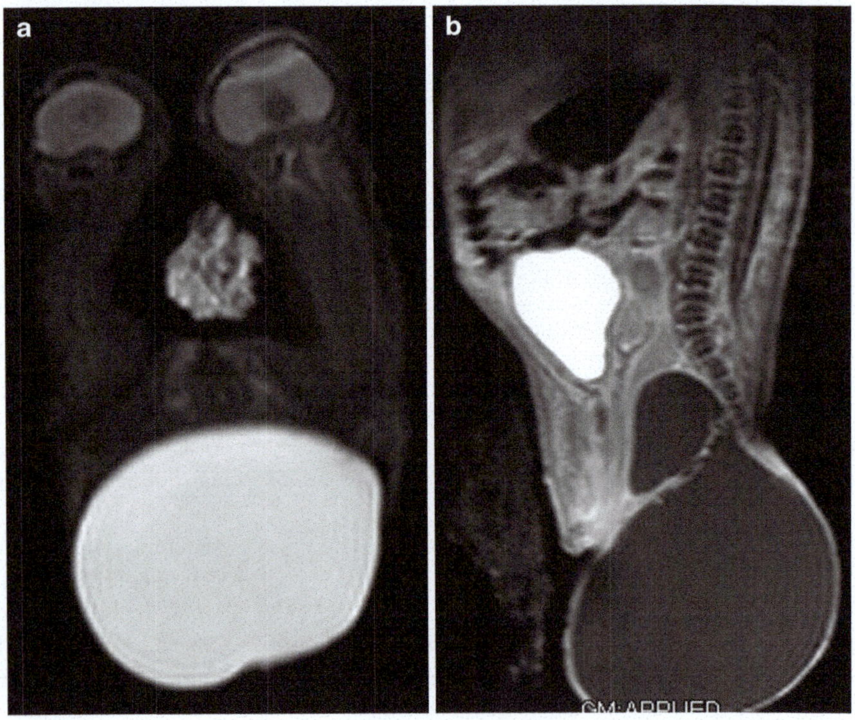

Fig. 13.85 Sacrococcygeal teratoma. Transverse STIR image (**a**) and sagittal contrast-enhanced fat-saturated T1-WI (**b**) show a large, completely cystic type 1 sacrococcygeal teratoma

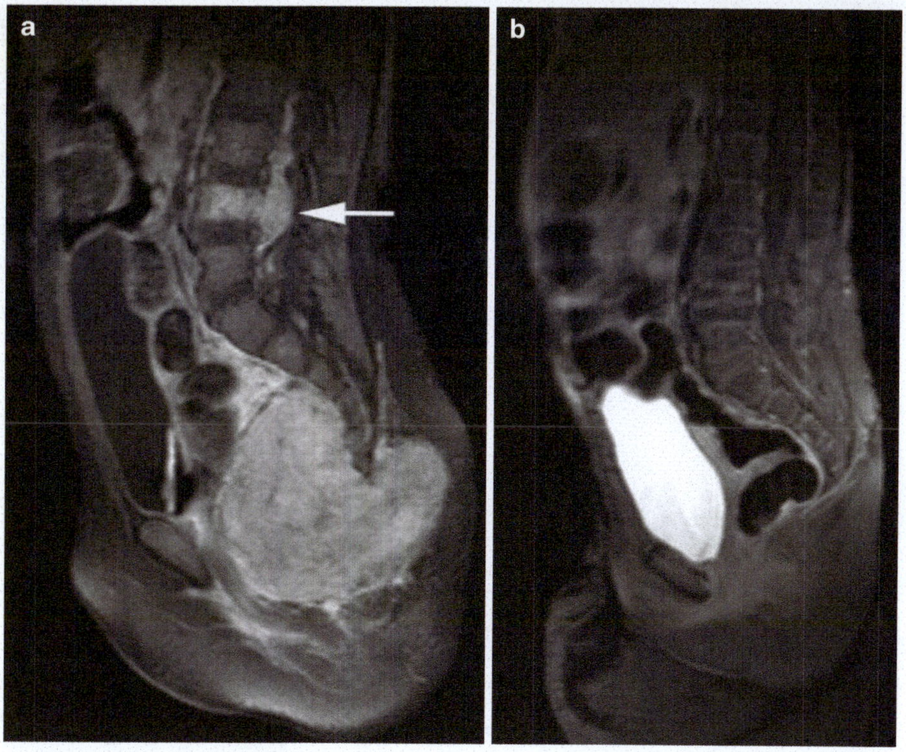

Fig. 13.86 Sacrococcygeal teratoma. Sagittal contrast-enhanced fat-saturated T1-WI (**a**) shows a malignant type IV sacrococcygeal teratoma, with metastasis in the spinal canal and L4 (*arrow*). AFP-level was markedly elevated (52,554 ng/mL) in this 14-month-old girl. Sagittal contrast-enhanced fat-saturated T1-WI (**b**) after chemotherapy and surgery 5 months later demonstrates decreased height of L4 but no residual tumor or metastases. This was a pathologically proven yolk-sac tumor.

coronal orientation is obtained. Secondly, a STIR or FSE-T2-W sequence in transverse and coronal view is acquired. T1-WIs can be either applied as an SE, an FSE, or a GR sequence in transverse plane. In addition, a 2D TOF venous MR angiography can be used, especially for assessment of involvement of renal vein, portal vein, liver veins, or inferior vena cava (IVC) by tumor. Contrast-enhanced images are acquired using a dynamic 3D spoiled-gradient echo T1-W sequence. This offers multiphasic imaging as well as contrast-enhanced MR angiography in MIP technique. Additionally, FS T1-WI is obtained in transverse and coronal orientation.

13.4.2 Liver Imaging

13.4.2.1 Normal Antomy

The liver is the largest of the abdominal organs, occupying most of the right upper quadrant and extending across the midline. The right liver lobe is bigger than the left, with the caudate and quadrate lobes being substantially smaller. The liver is relatively larger in neonates and infants than it is in older children and adults. The liver is divided into right and left hepatic lobes, each composed of two segments. The right lobe is divided into anterior and posterior segments, while the left lobe has medial and lateral segments. The caudate lobe is a separate smaller lobe that derives its arterial supply from both the right and left hepatic arteries and has venous drainage directly into the IVC. The separation into right and left lobes is defined by the middle hepatic vein superiorly and by the gallbladder fossa inferiorly. The division of the right lobe into anterior and posterior segments is defined by the right hepatic vein. The division of the left lobe into medial and lateral segments is defined superiorly by the left hepatic vein and inferiorly by the fissure for the ligamentum teres. For clinical purposes, the classification system by Couinaud (Fig. 13.87), which divides the liver into segments based on portal venous supply and hepatic venous drainage has widely been accepted, as it defines the liver into segments that are surgically resectable. This system introduces a plane to create superior and inferior subsegments of the anterior and posterior segments of the right lobe, defined by the right portal vein, and another plane to create superior and inferior subsegments of the lateral segment of the left lobe, defined by the left portal vein.

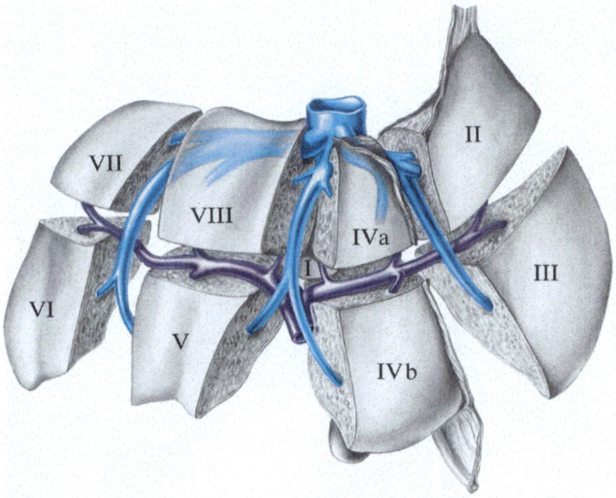

Fig. 13.87 Liver segments according to Couinaud. Segment I: caudate lobe; segments II and IV a: left liver lobe cranially to portal vein; segments III and IV b: left liver lobe caudally to portal vein; segments VII and VIII: right liver lobe cranially to portal vein; segments V and VI: right liver lobe caudally to portal vein

13.4.2.2 Normal Variations and Liver Anomalies

A number of normal variations in liver size and shape occur. Common variations include horizontal elongation of the lateral segment of the left lobe that may wrap around the spleen anteriorly, hypoplasia of the left lobe, and vertical elongation of segment V of the right lobe, termed Riedel's lobe. Variations of liver positioning are present in patients with Situs inversus (0.01%) (Fig. 13.88) and Situs ambiguous. Situs ambiguous (Fig. 13.89) is associated with other anomalies of the heart, lungs, spleen, and pancreas. In addition, abnormal position of liver occurs in Chilaiditi syndrome and in cases with herniation of the liver into the thorax through defects in the diaphragm or relaxation of the diaphragm. The spectrum of fibropolycystic liver diseases represents structural malformation of liver parenchyma and comprises simple liver cysts, congenital polycystic liver disease, biliary hamartomas (von Meyenburg complex), Caroli syndrome, and choledocheal cysts.

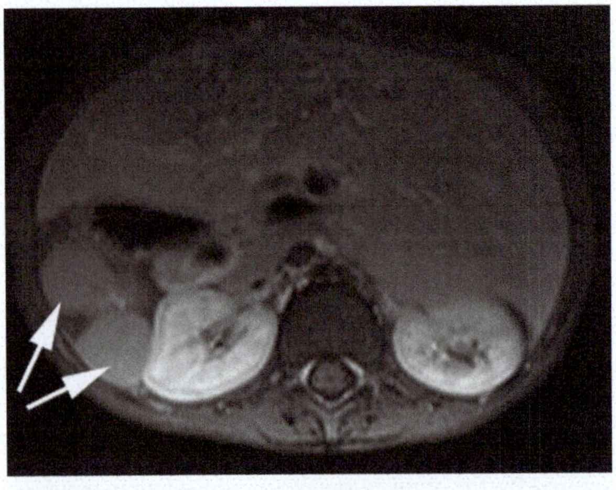

Fig. 13.88 Situs inversus. Transverse enhanced T1-WI shows situs inversus, with the liver positioned on the left side in concert with polysplenia (*arrows*) on the right side

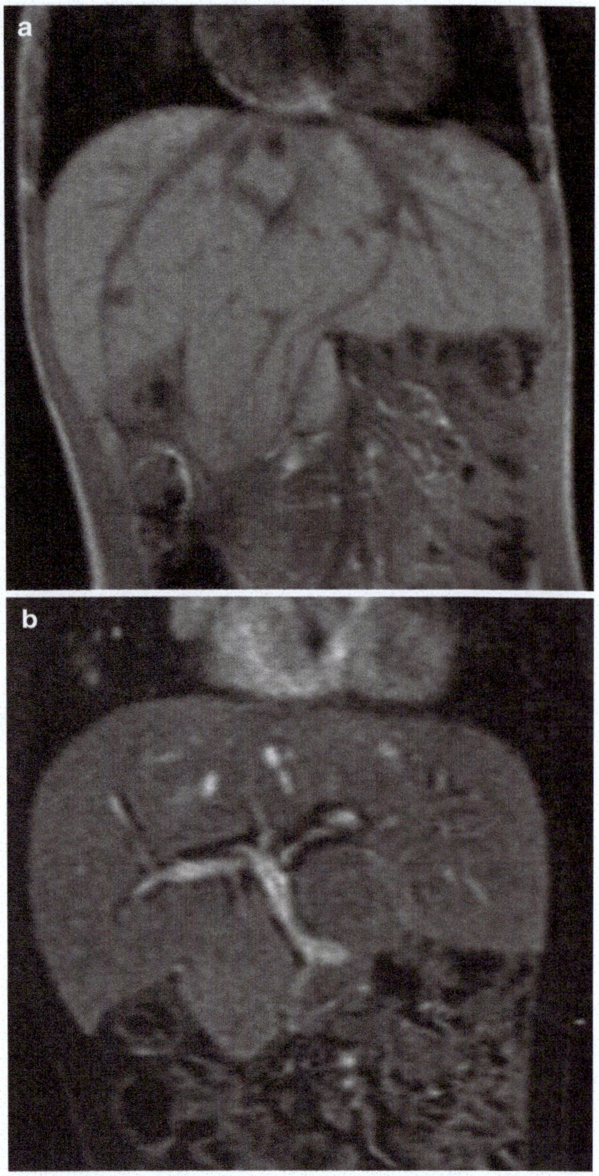

Fig. 13.89 Situs ambiguous. Coronal T1-WI precontrast (**a**) and postcontrast (**b**) administration show a trilobed liver in a patient with situs ambiguous

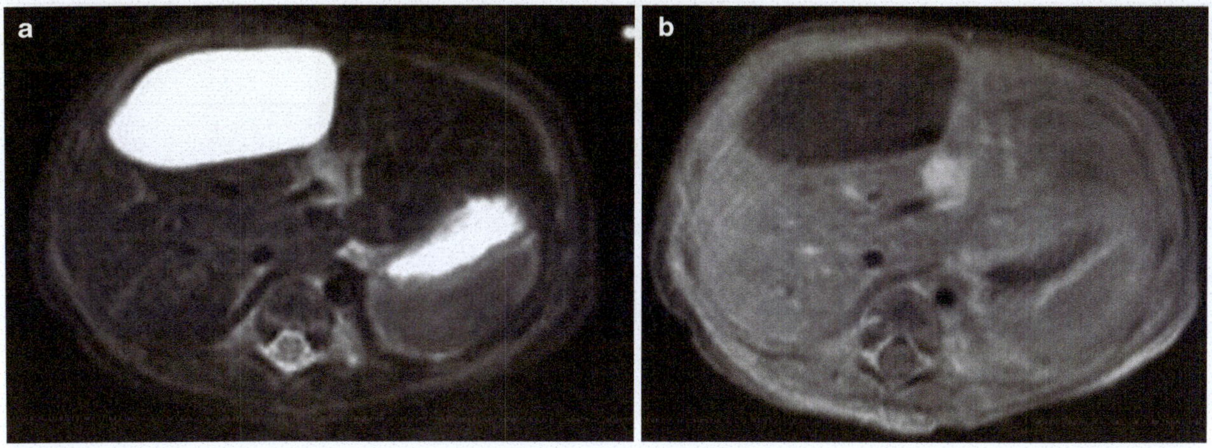

Fig. 13.90 Congenital liver cyst. Transverse STIR image (**a**) and fat-saturated contrast-enhanced T1-WI (**b**) show a cyst in the left lobe of the liver in a 3-day-old newborn

Liver Cysts

Liver cysts are benign focal liver lesions arising from the biliary epithileum that do not communicate with the biliary tree (Fig. 13.90). Incidence in the whole population is less than 5%. They may occur as solitary, multiple, or diffuse, and are usually discovered incidentally by US, CT, or MR imaging. The imaging features of liver cysts in children do not differ from those in adults. Most commonly, the cysts are small and asymptomatic, but they can be quite large (>10 cm) and become symptomatic by compression of surrounding tissue (obstructive jaundice, portal hypertension) or other complications, such as intracystic hemorrhage, rupture, and infection. In children presenting with liver cysts, careful evaluation of the kidneys is necessary to detect polycystic kidney disease. Liver cysts must be differentiated from parasitic, benign, and malignant lesions. Cystic liver lesions can result from a parasitic infection by *Echinococcus granulosus* or *multilocularis*. Cysts of *E. granulosus* or *cysticus* (Figs. 13.91 and 13.92) cause local displacement, whereas those of *E. multilocularis* or *alveolaris* grow in an infiltrative and destructive manner (Fig. 13.93). In addition, mesenchymal hamartoma and undifferentiated embryonal sarcoma of the liver may present as cystic liver lesions.

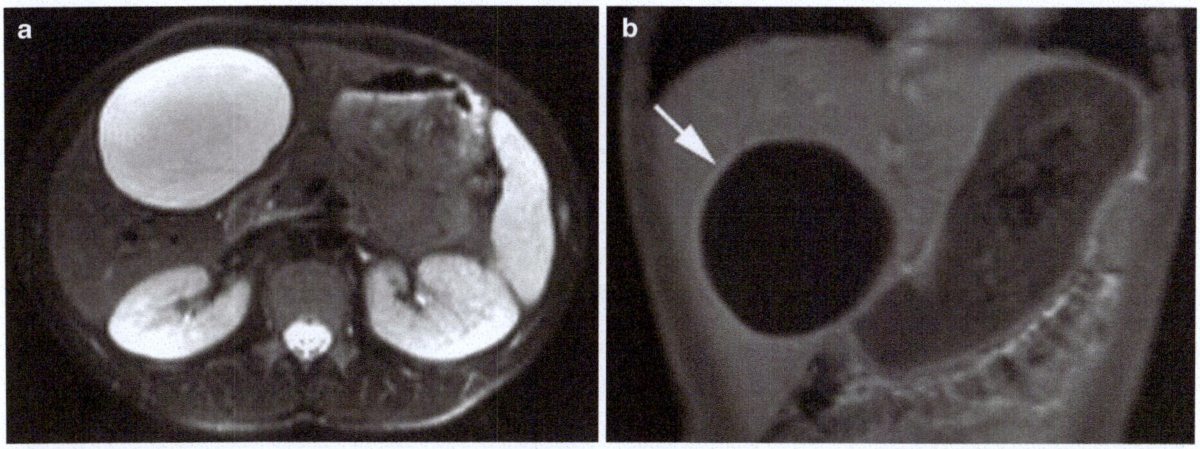

Fig. 13.91 *Echinococcus granulosus* cysts. Transverse STIR image (**a**) demontrates a well-circumscribed cystic liver lesion with wall thickening in a 13-year-old boy. Fat-saturated contrast-enhanced coronal T1-WI (**b**) image shows enhancement of cyst wall (*arrow*)

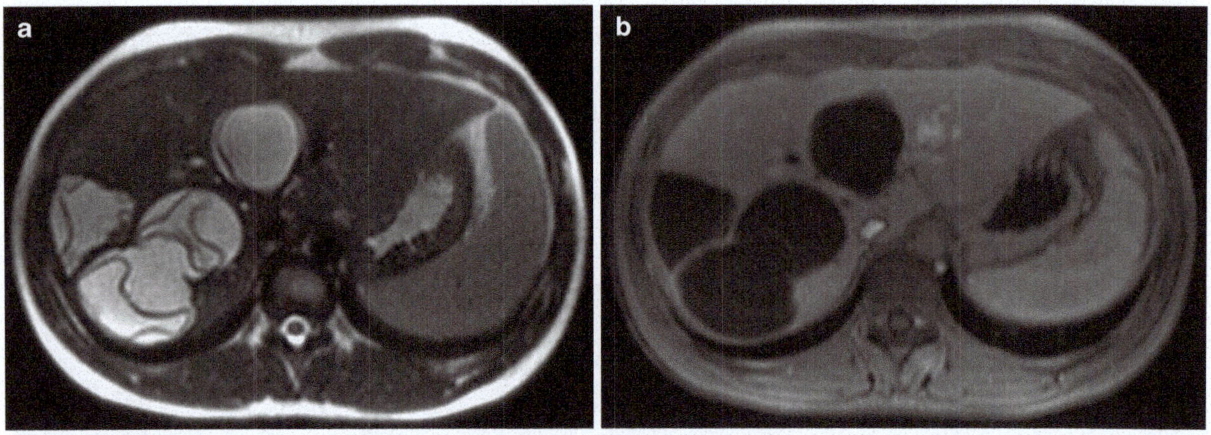

Fig. 13.92 *Echinococcus granulosus* cysts. Transverse T2-WI (**a**) and fat-saturated contrast-enhanced image T1-WI (**b**) show four well-circumscribed cystic liver lesions with detachment of scolices membranes in a 13-year-old boy after treatment with mebendazol

Choledochal Cysts

Choledochal cysts refer to the dilatation of the biliary duct system, which can be either saccular or fusiform. Most commonly (70–90%), the common bile duct is affected. A classification system suggested by Todani and Traverso has widely been accepted and describes five types, with several subtypes. The several types differ in etiology and pathogenesis as well as in appearance and presentation (Fig. 13.94 and Table 13.8). Choledochal cysts may present in newborns and infants with cholestatic jaundice, and may be clinically inseparable from neonatal hepatitis or biliary atresia. A characteristic triad of abdominal pain, obstructive jaundice, and fever has been reported, but only a minority of patients present with all three findings. Usually, US is the first imaging study requested, and sludge or stones may be identified in the dilated ducts. On MRI, SI of the saccular or fusiform cystic lesions is the same as that from bile in the gallbladder, on all pulse sequences. MR cholangiography (MRC) is excellent for the depiction of anatomical and pathological bile duct structures and enables exact classification (Fig. 13.95). Surgical excision is performed as therapy.

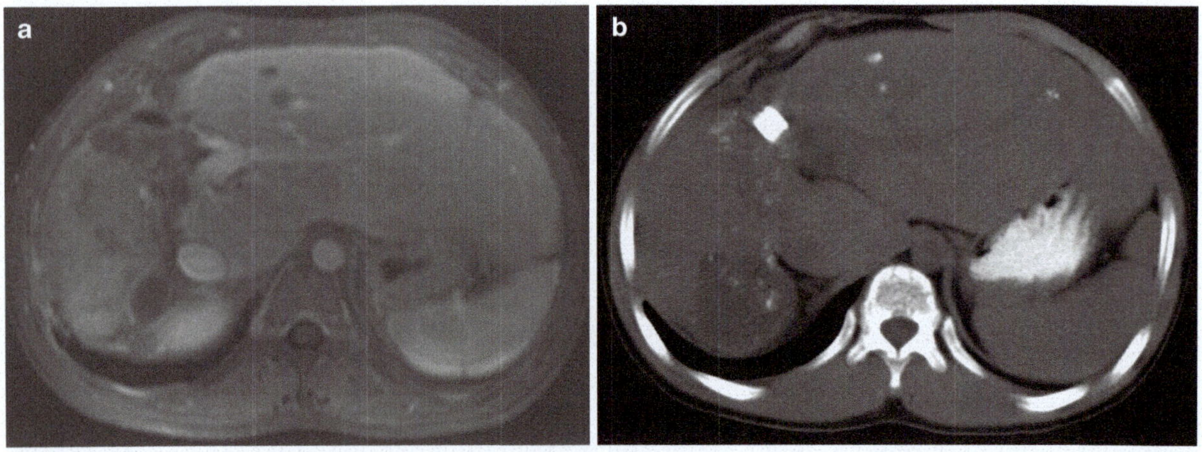

Fig. 13.93 *Echinococcus multilocularis* cysts. Transverse fat-saturated contrast-enhanced T1-WI (**a**) shows multiple cysts of different sizes in both liver lobes in a patient who had already had surgical resection of *Echinococcus multilocularis* cysts. CT (**b**) demonstrates multiple calcifications, which cannot be detected by MRI

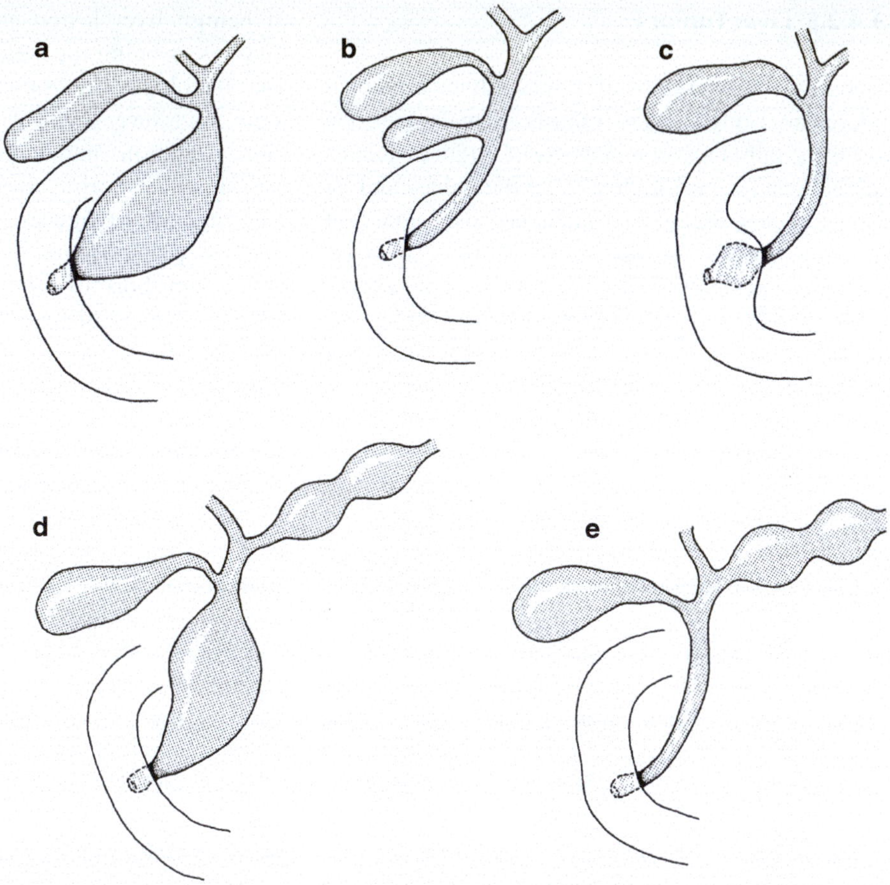

Fig. 13.94 Illustration of choledochal cysts according to Todani and Traverso. (**a**) Choledochal cyst, (**b**) Choledochal diverticula, (**c**) Choledocholcele, (**d**) Segmental intra- and extrahepatic bile duct cysts, (**e**) Intrahepatic bile duct cysts (Caroli syndrome)

Table 13.8 Classification of bile duct cysts according to Todani and Traverso

Type	Description	Frequency (%)
I	Choledochus cyst	70–90
Ia	Cystic dilatation of hepatic duct and common bile duct	
Ib	Segmental dilatation of common bile duct	
Ic	Diffuse dilatation of hepatic duct and common bile duct	
II	Choledochal diverticula	2
III	Choledochocele	3–5
IV	Multiple segmental intra- and extra-hepatic bile duct cysts	10–20
IVa	Intra- and extrahepatic bile duct cysts + cystic dilatation of extrahepatic bile ducts	
IVb	Extrahepatic bile duct cysts + normal intrahepatic bile ducts	
V	Caroli syndrome (intrahepatic cysts)	4–13

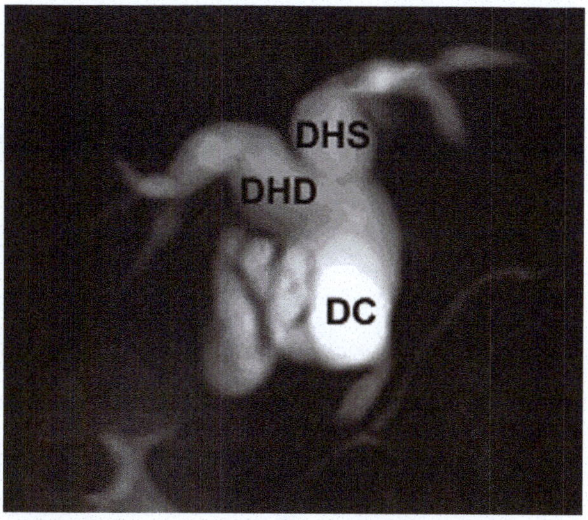

Fig. 13.95 Choledochal cyst type IVa. MRCP shows cystic dilatation of the right (DHD), left (DHS), and common bile duct (DC)

13.4.2.3 Liver Tumors

Approximately one-third of primary liver tumors in children are benign, and two-thirds are malignant. The liver is the third most common site of origin of abdominal malignancies in children, after the kidney and the adrenal glands. Benign and malignant liver tumors in children comprise hepatoblastomas (HBs, 43%), hepatocellular carcinomas (HCCs, 23%), benign vascular tumors (13%), mesenchymal harmatomas and sarcomas (6% each), adenomas and focal nodular hyperplasia (2% each), and other tumors (5%). Table 13.9 shows a survey of liver tumors in children along with the ages of presentation.

Infantile Hemangioendothelioma and (Cavernous) Hemangioma

Infantile or juvenile hemangioendothelioma (IH) is the most common benign liver tumor of mesenchymal origin in children. As with with other vascular anomalies, there is confusion of nomenclature (see text regarding vascular anomalies in the musculoskeletal section) and many authors use many different terms, such as hemangiomatosis, cavernous and capillary hemangiomas, and infantile (capillary) hemangioendothelioma for the same infantile vascular liver lesion. In addition, some authors consider this type of benign liver lesion and the differing histologic findings as being the same entity in different stages. Two histologic subtypes are described in the pathologic literature: Type 1 hemangioendothelioma is more common, and consists of a single layer, or occasionally several layers, of flat endothelial cells with rare mitotic figures. Type 2 has endothelial cells that are pleomorphic, larger and more hyperchromatic than those of type 1. Furthermore, the type 2 lesions are more disorganized and contain no stromal bile ductules when compared with type 1. It can be difficult to differentiate type 1I hemangioendothelioma from angiosarcomas. Fibrosis or thrombosis and calcifications are frequently seen in large lesions. From a clinical standpoint, IH typically manifests in 85–90% in the first 6 months of life, is more common in girls than in boys (1.4:1), and tends to involute spontaneously, without therapy, over months to years. Clinical presentations include hepatomegaly, high-output congestive heart failure, anemia, thrombocytopenia, respiratory distress, and jaundice. IH can be focal or multifocal, with the multifocal type being often associated with hemangiomas of the skin and other organs. The term "disseminated hemangiomatosis" is applied to patients with three or more organs involved. IHs are not a homogeneous group, either in terms of pathology or imaging. Multifocal lesions are fairly consistent in their imaging features, whereas focal lesions present with a spectrum of

Table 13.9 Neoplasias of the liver in children according to usual age of presentation

Age	Infancy (0–1 year)	Early childhood (1–3 years)	Later childhood (3–10 years)	Adolescence (10–16 years)
Benign tumors	Hemangioendothelioma Mesenchymal hamartoma Teratoma	Hemangioendothelioma Mesenchymal hamartoma Inflammatory myofibroblastic tumor	Angiomyolipoma	Adenoma FNH Biliary cystadenoma
Malignant tumors	Hepatoblastoma Rhabdoidtumor Yolk sac tumor Langerhans's cell histiocytosis Megakaryoblastic leukemia Disseminated neuroblastoma	Hepatoblastoma Rhabdomyosarcoma	HCC Embryonal sarcoma (undiff.) Angiosarcoma	Fibrolamellar HCC Hodgkin disease/ lymphoma Leiomyosarcoma

HCC hepatocellular carcinoma

imaging patterns. In both types, MR imaging shows the secondary features of high flow with tapering of the abdominal aorta, marked enlargement of the feeding arteries (hepatic artery, and sometimes superior mesenteric artery) and the hepatic veins and the right atrium. Multifocal IHs are hypointense on T1-WI and uniformly hyperintense on T2-WI, and vividly enhance after administration of paramagnetic contrast (Fig. 13.96). Focal IHs are more heterogeneous. Some have relatively little vascular enlargement, are hyperintense on T2-WI, and show a contrast enhancement along the periphery, with variable degrees of necrosis in the center (Fig. 13.97). On T1-WI, these lesions are hypointense, although some hyperintense areas may be present due to hemorrhage. Others have predominately large flow voids with surrounding signal abnormality. Arteriovenous and portovenous anastomoses, as well as large central varix can be identified in some of these lesions. Slow blood flow through the enlarged vascular spaces may also be noticed in other cases. Therapy is reserved for severely symptomatic lesions and may consist of treatment with high dose steroids, alpha interferon, hepatic artery ligation or embolization, or surgical resection.

Hepatoblastoma

Hepatoblastomas (HBs) comprise 43% of primary liver tumors and 15% of all pediatric abdominal tumors. HB is slightly more common in males, with a reported male to female ratio of 1.4–2.0:1.0, and usually children under the age of 3 years are affected. HBs arise from a precursor to the mature hepatocyte. Therefore, various histologic patterns are encountered, ranging from undifferentiated small cells to embryonal epithelial cells to well-differentiated fetal hepatocytes, and in the majority of cases the tumor is composed of different cell types. HB is associated with Glycogen storage diseases types I-IV, hereditary polyposis of the colon, Beckwith-Wiedemann syndrome and other syndromes with hemihypertrophy, Li-Fraumeni syndrome, trisomy 18, and prematurity. Clinically, HB presents as an asymptomatic abdominal mass, palpated either by a parent or pediatrician, with symptoms such as abdominal pain, weight loss, nausea, vomiting, and, rarely, dyspnea usually occurring in advanced disease. Jaundice resulting from compression of the major bile ducts is rare, and more typical for major bile duct invasion by rhabdomyosarcoma. In addition, HBs may produce hormones causing unusual clinical symptoms,

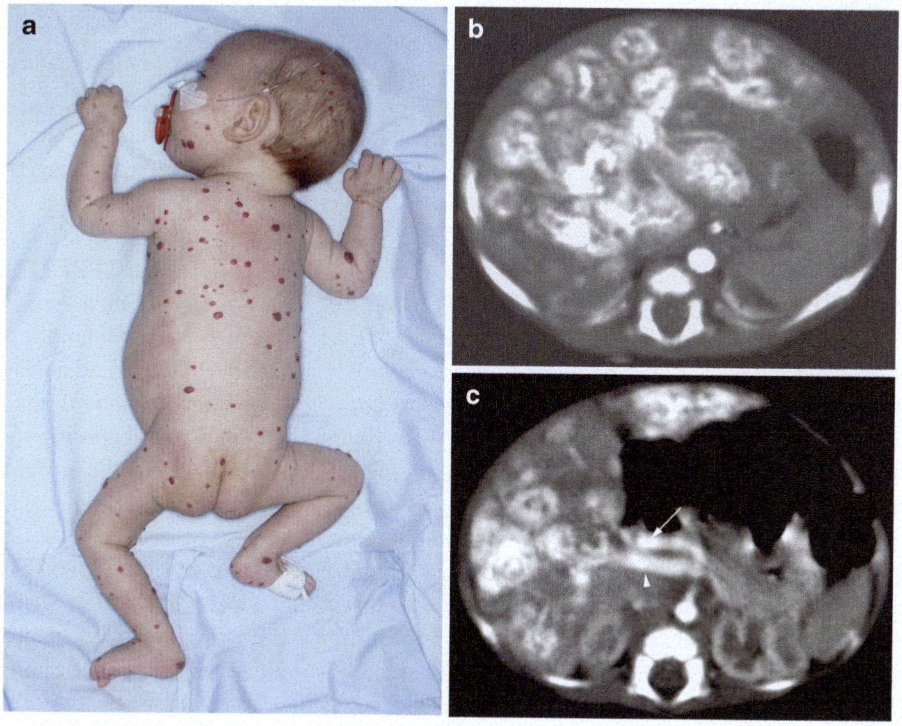

Fig. 13.96 Infantile hemangioendothelioma (multifocal type). Photography (**a**) of a newborn shows multiple cutaneous hemangiomas. CT (**b, c**) of this child shows multiple vividly enhancing liver lesions. Notice that the hepatic artery (*arrow*) has almost the same diameter as the portal vein (*arrowhead*)

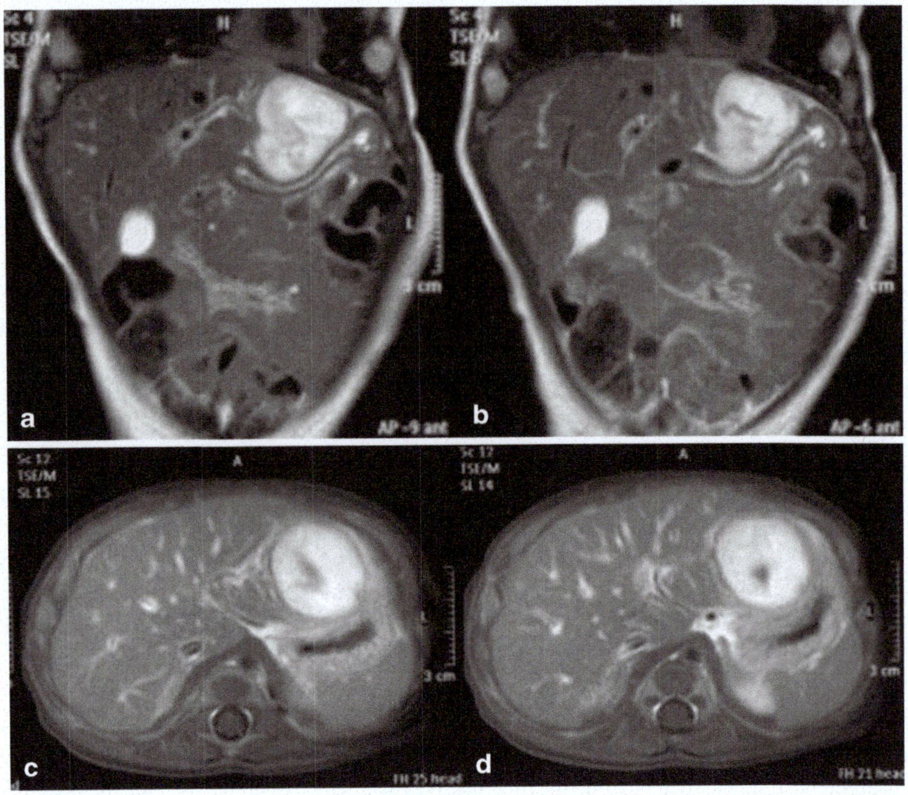

Fig. 13.97 Infantile hemangioendothelioma (focal type). Coronal T2-WI (**a, b**) show a hyperintense, slightly inhomogeneous lesion in the left liver lobe compressing the stomach. Transverse fat-saturated contrast-enhanced T1-WI (**c, d**) show contrast enhancement along the periphery, with a necrotic center

such as osteoporosis, virilization, precocious puberty, and hypercalcemia. In 90% of patients with HB, the serum levels of α-fetoprotein are elevated, and thus AFP (although being the major protein produced by the fetal liver) is a useful tumor marker, both for diagnosis and monitoring therapy. On imaging studies, HBs tend to present as solitary, well-defined masses, with a pseudocapsule and a tendency to invade the portal and hepatic veins. However, multifocal lesions or, rarely, diffuse infiltrative masses do also occur. On MRI, HB displays a hypointense SI on T1-WI, but may contain high SI due to hemorrhage. On T2-WI, SI is typically high, but may be variable due to necrosis, hemorrhage, or calcifications. After administration of CM, a heterogeneous enhancement on T1-WI is found (Fig. 13.98). The most important goal of imaging HB is to define the anatomic extent of disease and its relationship to hepatic lobar anatomy for guiding therapy. Therefore, it is of paramount importance to visualize portal and hepatic veins and hepatic arteries to detect variations of liver vessel anatomy and possible invasion by tumor. To achieve this, a highly recommendable practice is to use MR angiography and venography techniques. The most common sites for metastases of HBs are in the lung and periaortic lymph nodes. Brain metastases have been described on rare occasions. Traditionally, HBs and HCC are staged according to the Pediatric Oncology Group system (Table 13.10). In addition, the International Society of Pediatric Oncology developed a staging system based on the number of liver segments involved, as determined by preoperative imaging studies. This pretreatment classification scheme, called "PRETEXT," is shown in Fig. 13.99 and is useful in determining resectability preoperatively. In this system, the liver is divided into four sectors: an anterior and a posterior sector on the right, and a medial and a lateral sector on the left. Staging groups are assigned according to tumor extension within the liver, as well as the presence or absence of involvement of the hepatic vein, the portal vein, regional lymph nodes, or distant metastases. In contrast to the POG staging system, PRETEXT characterizes the tumor independently from therapeutical approach and has been proven to be of prognostic relevance. Surgery, either as the initial approach or after chemotherapy, is the mainstay for treatment of hepatoblastoma.

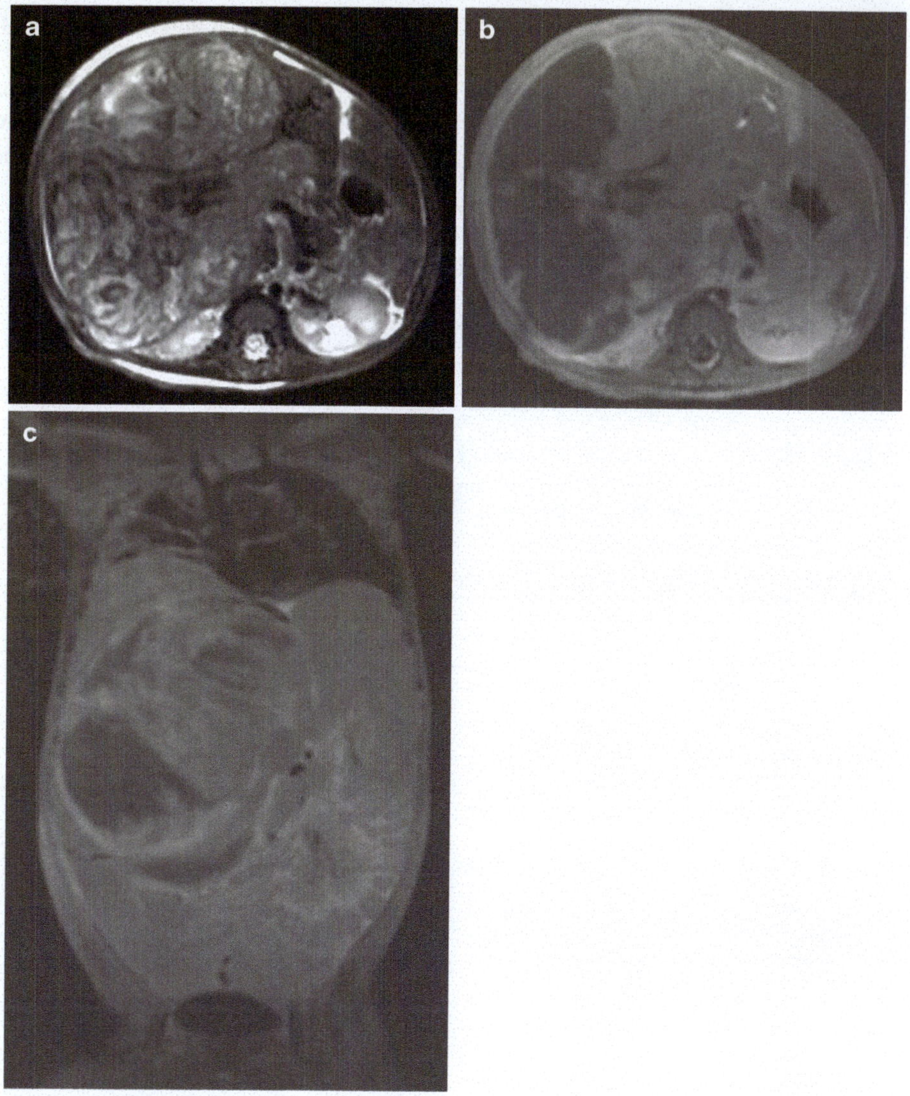

Fig. 13.98 Hepatoblastoma. Transverse T2-WI (**a**) and fat-saturated contrast-enhanced transverse (**b**) and coronal (**c**) T1-WI show a large liver tumor with necrosis involving both liver lobes in a 15-month-old boy

Cisplatin-based chemotherapy has markedly increased the number of patients who can be rendered disease-free through tumor resection after initial chemotherapy, and has increased the event-free survival rate from 25 to 30% in the 1980s to 60–80% currently, depending on risk factors. Liver transplantation is another therapeutic option, but is limited by the availability of donor livers.

Hepatocellular Carcinoma

Hepatocellular carcinomas (HCCs) comprise 23% of primary liver tumors and occur primarily after the age of 10 years. In children between 15 and 19 years, it accounts for 87% of all malignant liver tumors. Patients with the fibrolamellar variant of HCC are more likely to be older than 10 years. HCC is associated with multiple risk factors, and 70% HCCs arise from preneoplastic lesions, usually with the background of cirrhosis. Major etiologic factors associated with HCC include infection with hepatitis B and hepatitis C viruses, excessive alcohol intake, and aflatoxin B exposure. Furthermore, HCC is associated with hereditary tyrosinemia type 1, glycogen storage diseases types I-IV, deficiency of α-1-antitrypsin, familial adenomatous polyposis, Alagille syndrome, other familial cholestatic syndromes, neurofibromatosis, and

Table 13.10 Pediatric oncology group staging of hepatoblastoma (also used for HCC)

Stage I	*Favorable histology* Completely resected Pure fetal histology with low mitotic index (<2 per 10 high-power fields) *Other histology* Completely resected Histology other than purely fetal pattern with low mitotic index
Stage II	Grossly resected with evidence of microscopic residual Resected tumors with preoperative or intraoperative rupture
Stage III	Unresectable without undue risk to patient, including partially resected tumors with measurable tumor left behind Lymph node involvement
Stage IV	Measurable metastatic disease

ataxia telangiectasia. The fibrolamellar variant of HCC arises in otherwise normal livers. HCCs in children do not differ histologically from those in adults. However, occasionally malignant liver tumors in children are seen to have features of both HCC and HB. Clinical presentation of HCC does not differ from that of HB. AFP levels are markedly elevated in two-thirds of HCC cases, but are usually normal in the fibrolamellar variant of HCC. On imaging studies, HCCs present with four different growth patterns: the infiltrative type (33%), the expansive type (solitary or multiple nodes; 18%), the mixed infiltrative-expansive type (42%), and the diffuse type (5%). On MRI, HCC has a variable appearance, due to hemorrhage, necrosis, cystic areas, and calcifications, and may invade portal and hepatic veins, as does HB. After administration of paramagnetic contrast, a variable enhancement of the tumor is found (Fig. 13.100). Thus HCC cannot be differentiated from HB by imaging. However, the fibrolamellar

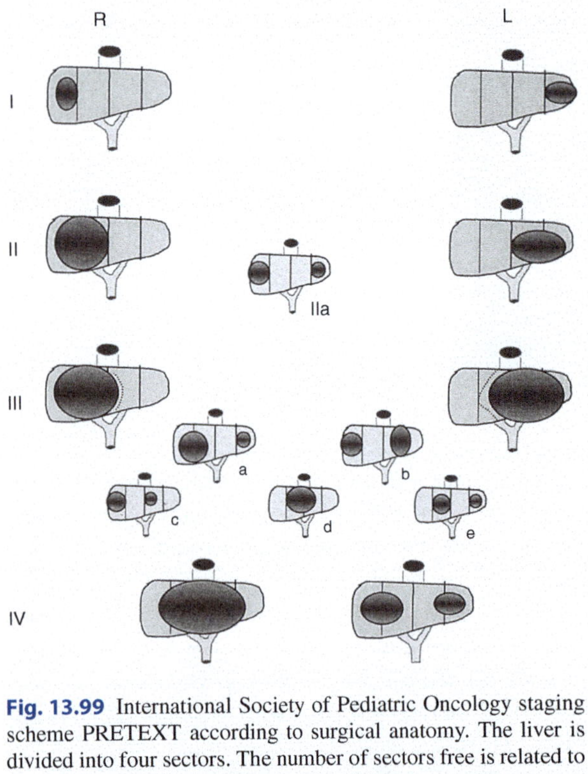

Fig. 13.99 International Society of Pediatric Oncology staging scheme PRETEXT according to surgical anatomy. The liver is divided into four sectors. The number of sectors free is related to stage as follows: PRETEXT I, three adjoining sectors free (tumor in only one sector); PRETEXT II, two adjoining sectors free of tumor (tumor involving two sectors); PRETEXT III, one sector or two nonadjoining sectors free of tumor (tumor involves two or three sectors); PRETEXT IV, no sector free of tumor (tumor in all four sectors)

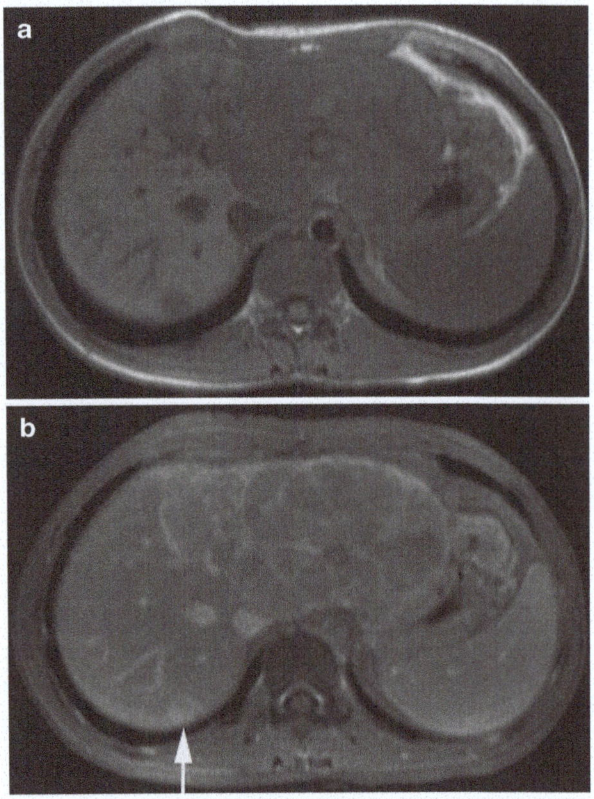

Fig. 13.100 HCC. Transverse T1-WI precontrast (**a**) and fat-saturated T1-WI postcontrast (**b**) shows an expansive type of HCC in the left liver lobe, with a nodule in the right liver lobe (*arrow*) in a 17-year-old boy

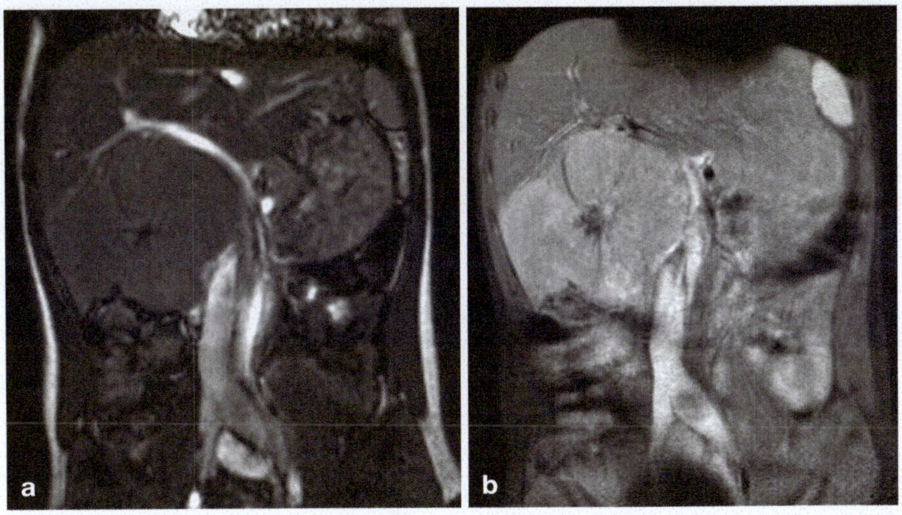

Fig. 13.101 Fibrolamellar HCC. Coronal T2-WI (**a**) and fat-saturated contrast-enhanced T1-WI (**b**) show a tumor in the right liver lobe in a 12-year-old boy, with a hypointense stellate scar in the center demonstrating no enhancement

variant of HCC may display a characteristic sign on MR imaging: a central stellate scar in the middle of the tumor, which is of low SI on both T1-WI and T2-WI and does not enhance after administration of paramagnetic contrast, whereas the tumor enhances heterogenously (a partial enhancement of the central scar may be seen in the late phase) (Fig. 13.101). As mentioned in the section above, two staging systems are used for HCC and HB (Table 13.10 and Fig. 13.99). In contrast to HB, HCC does not respond well to chemotherapy or radiotherapy, and thus surgical resection, if possible, is the only curative modality. Unfortunately, only between 30 and 50% of all HCCs are resectable at diagnosis and the event-free survival rate is currently approximately 20%. Limited experience is available in treatment of children with HB and HCC with TACE (transcatheter arterial chemoembolization) and TACE plus radiotherapy. Liver transplantation is another therapeutic option, but is limited by the availability of donor livers, as well as the fact that many patients present with metastatic disease, most often to the lungs and periaortic lymph nodes.

Mesenchymal Hamartoma

Approximately 6% of all liver tumors in childhood are mesenchymal hamartomas (MH), and children less than 2 years of age are typically affected. The male female ratio is 2:1. MH is a benign developmental cystic liver tumor, and results from a failure of the development of the ductal plate. Histologically, a disorganized mixture of loose mesenchymal cells with abnormal bile ducts, blood vessels, and well-differentiated hepatocytes is found. MH is more often located in the right hepatic lobe (65%) than in the left lobe (20%), but may also occur in both lobes or present as a pedunculated mass (20%). MHs are cystic, with a variable amount of stroma, and therefore imaging appearance depends on the amount of stromal tissue in the hamartoma. Consequently, MH may be composed of multi-septated cysts or may be completely solid. On MRI, the cysts appear hypointense on T1-WI and hyperintense on T2-WI. The septa and the stromal components can enhance after administration of paramagnetic contrast (Fig. 13.102). In rare cases, malignant transformation of MH into undifferentiated embryonal sarcoma occurs, and therefore biopsy of the tumor is always performed and complete resection is preferred. If the tumor cannot be completely resected, long-time follow-up is necessary.

(Undifferentiated) Embryonal Sarcoma

Undifferentiated embryonal sarcoma (UES) is a rare, malignant liver tumor of mesenchymal origin, and accounts for 6% of liver tumors in childhood. In contrast to MH, UES affects older children and adolescents and both genders with the same frequency. The histogenetic background of this tumor has not been completely eludicated yet, but a close relation to MH

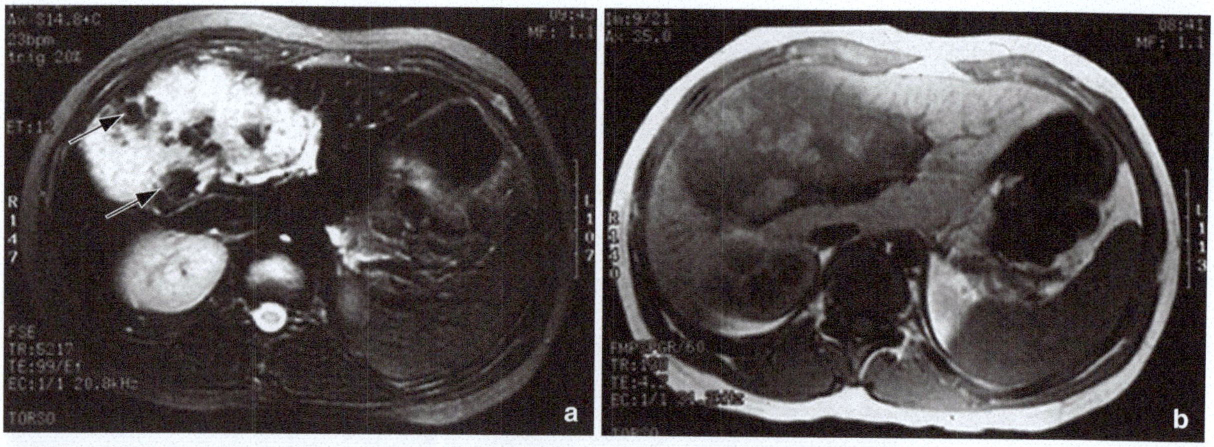

Fig. 13.102 Mesenchymal hamartoma. Transverse T2-WI (**a**) and T1-WI (**b**) show a heterogeneous liver lesion with islands of stromal tissue (*arrow*) in an otherwise predominantly necrotic/cystic tumor (Courtesy of D. von Schweinitz)

is discussed, as both tumors share the feature of a translocation in the long arm of chromosome 19. UES is composed of primitive spindle cells in a myxoid stroma, which consists of acidic mucopolysaccharides. Most commonly, a solitary well-defined tumor with a pseudocapsule located in the right liver lobe with a size ranging from 7 to 20 cm is found. A hallmark of UES is a discrepancy in appearance on US on the one hand, and CT and MRI on the other hand. On US, an iso- to hyperechoic solid-appearing lesion is delineated, while CT and MRI suggest a more cyst-like lesion with water aquivalent HU values, and high signal on T2-WI images and low signal on T1-WI. This phenomenon is thought to be caused by high water content due to the hydrophilic mucopolysaccharides in the myxoid component of this tumor. After administration of paramagnetic contrast, the solid tumor septa and the pseudocapsule will enhance (Fig. 13.103). UES is a highly malignant lesion, metastasising to lung and bones. Surgery and chemotherapy are the mainstay of therapy, but overall prognosis is bad.

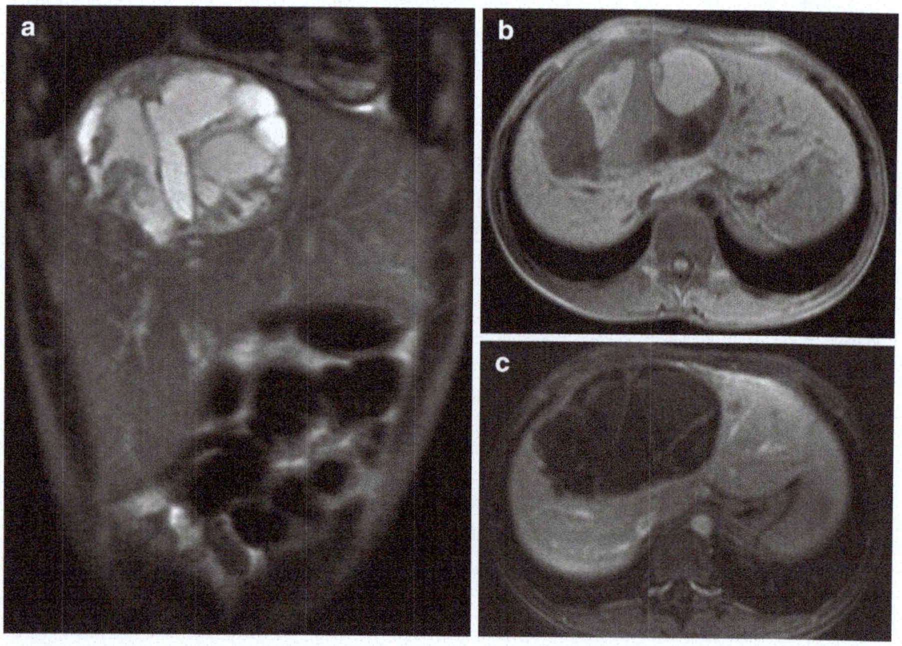

Fig. 13.103 Undifferentiated embryonal sarcoma. Coronal T2-WI (**a**) and transverse T1-WI (**b**) show a heterogeneous tumor with multiple septae involving both liver lobes. Fat-saturated contrast-enhanced T1-WI (**c**) shows enhancement of septae and pseudocapsule

Rhabdomyosarcoma

Rhabdomyosarcoma is a very rare tumor of mesenchymal origin, arising from the striated muscle cells of bile ducts. Most commonly, small children (peak incidence 3 years) are affected, and they typically present with a hepatic tumor, palpated by a parent or pediatrician, and jaundice. When the tumor arises in one of the large bile ducts, it is usually of the gross appearance of sarcoma botryoides, and dilatation of the affected bile ducts is present (Fig. 13.104). On MRI, RM shows a high SI on T2-WI and a low SI on T1-WI and enhances inhomogenously after administration of paramagnetic contrast. If bile duct dilatation is present, a grape-like tumor cluster on thin sliced T2-WI in the coronal plane may be depicted. If RM arises in an intrahepatic duct, it cannot be differentiated from other intrahepatic malignancies on imaging studies.

Hepatic Metastases

Many different tumors may metastasize to the liver, with neuroblastoma being the most common (Fig. 13.105). As in adults, the MR imaging appearance of hepatic metastases is variable.

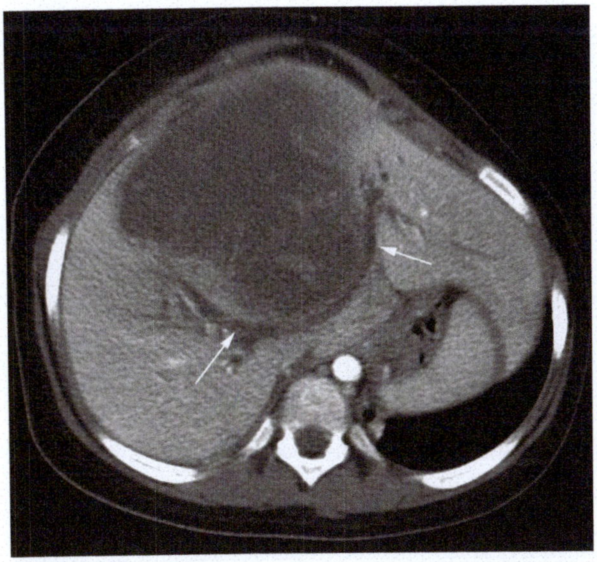

Fig. 13.104 Rhabdomyosarcoma. Contrast-enhanced CT shows a large hypodense liver tumor with dilatation of the bile ducts (*arrows*)

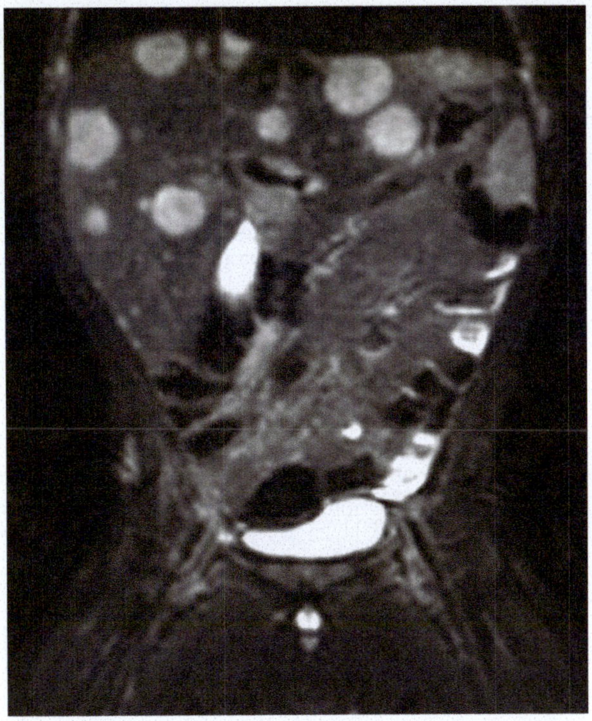

Fig. 13.105 Metastases of a neuroblastoma. Coronal STIR image demonstrates multiple liver metastases in a patient with a neuroblastoma of the right adrenal gland (same patient as in Fig. 13.107)

13.4.3 Adrenal Glands Imaging

13.4.3.1 Neuroblastoma

Neuroblastoma is the most common abdominal tumor in children, with an incidence of 8–10% of all pediatric malignant neoplasias (Fig. 13.42), and it is definitely the most mysterious tumor of childhood. On one hand, these tumors may regress spontaneously, particularly in infants, or may mature to into a benign ganglioneuroma. On the other hand, most children older than 1 year presenting with extensive or metastatic disease at the time of diagnosis have a poor overall prognosis. This incredible heterogeneity has been eludicated by molecular genetic and biologic analyses, and many genetic features of neuroblastomas have been identified that correlate with the clinical outcome. For instance, near triploidy is associated with favorable outcome, whereas MYCN oncogene amplification, unbalanced gain of 17q, or allelic loss at 1p or 11q are linked with more aggressive tumors and poor prognosis. It is far beyond the scope of this radiology textbook to go into deeper details, but it is important to understand that oncologists use various clinical and genetic features of neuroblastomas to guide therapy. Therefore, familiarity with the international neuroblastoma staging system (Table 13.11) is necessary, and description of imaging findings should take this into account.

Neuroblastoma is one of the small, round blue-cell neoplasms in childhood (such as Ewing sarcoma, non-Hodgkin lyphoma, PNET, and undifferentiated soft-tissue sarcomas) and presumable arises from the primitive neural crest cells. The sites in which neuroblastoma occurs correlate with normal tissues of the sympathic nervous system, including spinal sympathetic ganglia and adrenalchromaffin cells. Therefore, neuroblastoma may arise from the adrenal gland (35%) or anywhere along the sympathetic chain in the neck (1–5%), in the posterior mediastinum (20%), in the extraadrenal retroperitoneum (30–35%), and in the pelvis (2–3%). It is a disease of infancy and early childhood, with a mean age of 22 months at presentation.

Table 13.11 International neuroblastoma staging system (Brodeur et al. 1993, 1998)

Stage 1	Localized tumor with complete gross excision, with or without microscopic residual disease; representative ipsilateral lymph nodes negative for tumor microscopically (nodes attached to and removed with the primary tumor may be positive)
Stage 2A	Localized tumor with incomplete gross excision; representative ipsilateral nonadherent lymph nodes negative for tumor microscopically
Stage 2B	Localized tumor with or without complete gross excision, with ipsilateral nonadherent lymph nodes positive for tumor. Enlarged contralateral lymph nodes must be negative microscopically
Stage 3	Unresectable unilateral tumor infiltrating across the midline,[a] with or without regional lymph node involvement; or localized unilateral tumor with contralateral regional lymph node involvement; or midline tumor with bilateral extension by infiltration (unresectable) by lymph node involvement
Stage 4	Any primary tumor with dissemination to distant lymph nodes, bone, bone marrow, liver, skin, and/or other organs (except as defined for stage 4S)
Stage 4S	Localized primary tumor (as defined for stage 1, 2A, or 2B) with dissemination limited to skin, liver, and/or bone marrow,[b] limited to infants <1 year of age

Multifocal primary tumors (e.g., bilateral adrenal primary tumors) should be staged according to the greatest extend of disease, as defined previously, followed by a subscript "M" (e.g., 3_M)

[a]The midline is defined as the vertebral column. Tumors originating on one side and "crossing the midline" must infiltrate to or beyond the opposite side of the vertebral column

[b]Marrow involvement in stage 4S should be minimal, that is, less than 10% of total nucleated cells identified as malignant on bone marrow biopsy or on marrow aspirate. More extensive marrow involvement would be considered to be stage 4. The MIBG scan (if done) should be negative for the marrow

Clinical presentation depends on location of primary, regional, and metastatic disease. Primary thoracic tumors are often diagnosed coincidentally, when chest radiographs are obtained for evaluation of infections (Fig. 13.106). Cervical and high thoracic tumors may present with Horner syndrome (ptosis, myosis, and anhydrosis) and large thoracic neuroblastomas may lead to mechanical obstructions, with resultant superior vena cava syndrome or cardiac output failure. Symptomatology of paraspinal neuroblastomas invading into the spinal canal via neuroforamina may be radicular pain, (sub)acute paraplegia, bladder or bowel dysfunction, and, not surprisingly, cord compression can be a medical emergency. In abdominal disease, patients often present late, with large painless tumors, and complaints of fullness and discomfort, and bladder and bowel symptoms due to compression. Massive involvement of the liver in metastatic disease is particularly frequent in infants (e.g., stage 4S) and may lead to respiratory distress. In addition, primary or metastatic abdominal masses can cause compromise of venous and lymphatic drainage from the lower extremities, leading to scrotal and lower extremity edema. Furthermore, skin metastasis with nontender, bluish subcutaneous nodules (in infants with stage 4S) and skull base metastasis (racoon eyes) may be present (Fig. 13.107). Widespread bone and bone marrow disease causes bone pain and can lead to limping, or irritability in a younger child. Furthermore, neuroblastoma may present with two distinct paraneoplastic syndromes: opsoclonus-myoclonus syndrome (rapid eye movements, ataxia, and myoclonia) is observed in 2–4% of newly diagnosed neuroblastomas, and intractable watery diarrhea is caused by tumor secretion of vasoactive intestinal peptides. Due to their noradrenergic derivation, neuroblastomas have multiple components

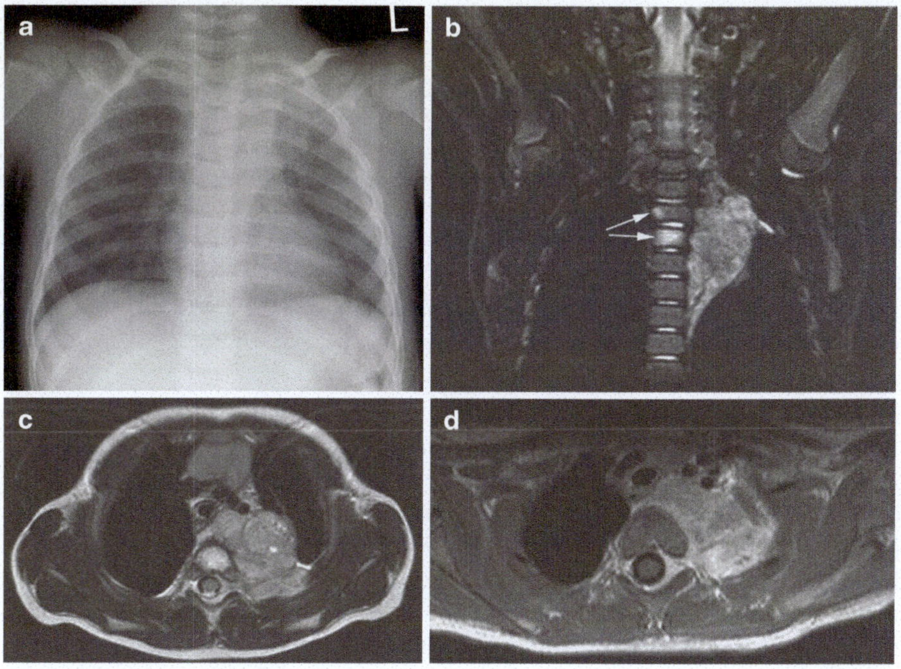

Fig. 13.106 Neuroblastoma. Chest X-ray (**a**) shows a mediastinal mass on the left side. Coronal STIR image (**b**), transverse T2-WI (**c**), and contrast-enhanced fat-saturated T1-WI (**d**) illustrate a left-sided paravertebral neuroblastoma of the sympathetic chain, with intraspinal infiltration and growth through intervertebral foramina. Note metastases in the thoracic spine (*arrows*)

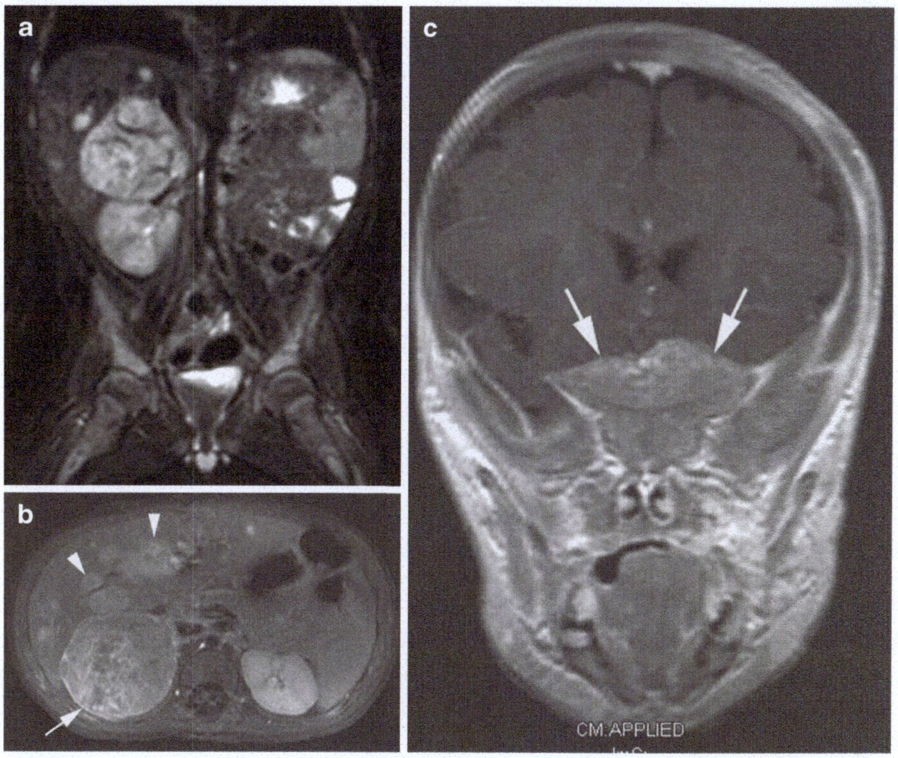

Fig. 13.107 Stage 4S Neuroblastoma. Coronal STIR image (**a**) and transverse contrast-enhanced T1-WI (**b**) show a neuroblastoma of the right adrenal gland (*arrow*), with multiple enhancing liver metastases (*arrowheads*). Coronal contrast-enhanced T1-WI (**c**) demonstrates skull base metastasis (*arrows*) in this 7-month-old boy presenting with racoon eyes

of catecholamine synthesis and metabolite pathways activated. Therefore, levels of chatecholamines, especially in homovanillic acid (HVA) and vanillylmandelic acid (VMA) in urine, are elevated in 95% of patients with neuroblastoma, and this is used for differential diagnosic work-up, monitoring response to therapy, and follow-up. Furthermore, 70% of neuroblastomas show an avid uptake of I^{123}-MIBG, which is related to catecholamine production. Hence MIBG scintigraphy is a very important tool that helps to differentiate neuroblastoma from Wilms' tumor, provides information about disease burden, and gives valuable information in follow-up studies.

As mentioned earlier, neuroblastoma may be an incidental finding on plain films, but after a clinical examiniation US is usually the first imaging modality performed. Further evaluation by CT or MRI has to be decided on clinical grounds and the basis of location of the tumor. MRI is the only imaging modality that allows sufficient assessment of any intraspinal involvement and lacks radiation exposure. In addition, MR imaging shows the extent of the mass, displacement, and encasement of vessels, direct spread into adjacent tissue, and metastatic disease to lymph nodes, liver, bone marrow, and other organs, and exactly defines the tumor origin. However, CT more sensitively depicts calcifications, which are much more frequent (60% gross, 90% microscopic) in neuroblastoma than in Wilms' tumor; especially in abdominal neuroblastoma, the small vessels in these young patients may be better visualized by CECT than on MRI, which is important prior to surgery. On MRI, neuroblastoma presents as a well-defined mass, with high SI on T2-WI, and low SI on T1-WI, which enhances after administration of paramagnetic contrast (Fig. 13.108). However, due to calcifications, hemorrhage, and necrosis, SI may be heterogeneous on both T1-WI and T2-WI. In abdominal disease, it typically extends behind the aorta and surrounds and engulfs vascular structures such as the aorta, IVC, celiac artery, superior mesenteric artery, and the renal vessels (Fig. 13.109).

Treatment of neuroblastoma comprises a watch-and-wait strategy, surgery, chemotherapy, and radiotherapy. The role of each is determined by the anticipated clinical behavior of the tumor in individual cases, considering the stage, age, and tumor pathobiology. Table 13.12 gives an overview of differential diagnosis of neuroblastoma.

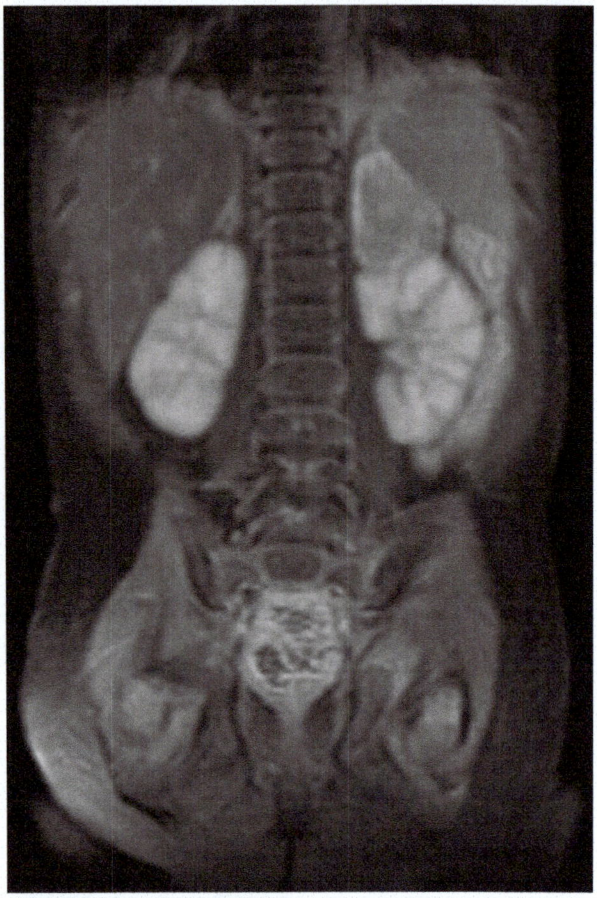

Fig. 13.108 Stage 1 neuroblastoma. Fat-saturated contrast-enhanced coronal T1-WI shows a well-defined mass of the left adrenal gland

13.4.3.2 Ganglioneuroblastoma and Ganglioneuroma

The fully differentiated benign counterpart of neuroblastoma is a ganglioneuroma, which is composed of mature ganglion cells, neutrophils, and Schwann cells. Ganglioneuroblastoma is a heterogeneous group of tumors with histopathologic features that range from a predominance of neuroblastic elements with rare maturing cells to neoplasms comprised almost exclusively of ganglioneuroma and containing occasional rests of neuroblasts. Therefore, some ganglioneuroblastomas may behave aggressively. In principle, the three classic histopathologic patterns of neuroblastoma, ganglioneuroblastoma, and ganglioneuroma reflect a spectrum of maturation and differentiation. Consequently, ganglioneuroblastomas and ganglioneuromas occur in the same

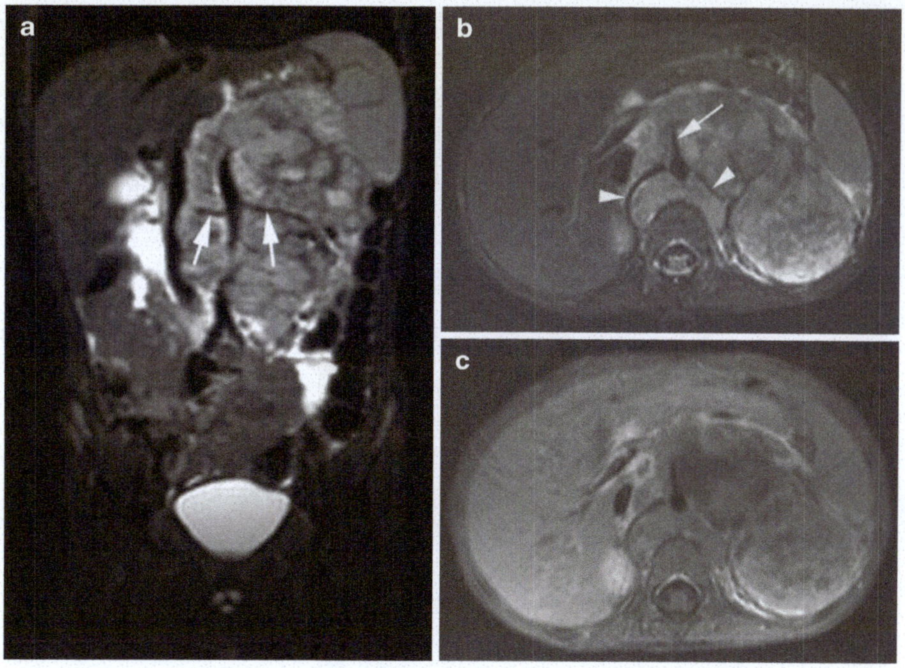

Fig. 13.109 Neuroblastoma. Coronal and transverse STIR images (**a, b**) show a large neuroblastoma extending behind the aorta and the diaphragmatic crus (*arrowheads*) on both sides. The tumor is engulfing the celiac trunk and both renal arteries (*arrows*). On transverse fat-saturated contrast T1-WI (**c**), the tumor demonstrates a very inhomogeneous enhancement

locations as neuroblastomas and symptoms depend on location, size, growth, and displacement of adjacent structures. Imaging features can be identical to that of low-stage neuroblastoma (Fig. 13.110). Differentiation can only be achieved by histology.

13.4.3.3 Pheochromocytoma

Pheochromocytoma is a very rare entity during childhood, and is predominantely diagnosed between 6 and 15 years of age, with a slight predominance in boys.

Table 13.12 Differential diagnosis of neuroblastoma

Wilms' tumor	Origin in the kidney, no increased catecholamines, no uptake of I^{123}-MIBG
Ganglioneuroma	No distinction possible between low stage neuroblastoma and ganglioneuroma
Adrenal hemorrhage	High SI on T1-W and T2-WI Hemorrhage and tumor shrink after 2–3 weeks, elevated catecholamines only in neuroblastoma
Pheochromocytoma	

Approximately 80–85% of pheochromocytomas are located in the adrenal medulla, and 15–20% arise from extra-adrenal (aortic) paraganglia or paravertebral sympathetic nervous ganglia. They may occur multifocally (in up to 30% of cases) and bilaterally (in 10% of cases), especially in hereditary tumor syndromes. Pheochromcytoma is associated with MEN IIa and IIb, von Hippel-Lindau disease, and, rarely, with von Recklinghausen's disease. Pheochromocytomas can turn malignant, and malignancy in these tumors is established by the presence of distant metastasis. Clinically, patients present with symptoms and signs of catecholamine excess: hypertension, palpitation, headache, sweating, flushing, anxiety, tremor, nausea and vomiting, abdominal or chest pain, and visual disturbances. Usually, the diagnosis is made by elevated catecholamine concentrations (including free metanephrine and normetanephrine) in urine and serum. After the diagnosis has been established, US, CT, or MRI and I^{123}-MIBG scintigraphy are performed. MRI usually demonstrates a well-defined mass of moderate size (2–5 cm in diameter), displaying very high SI (so high that it may mimic a cyst) on T2-WI. On T1-WI, the lesion shows a hypointense SI, with marked enhancement after administration of paramagnetic contrast (Fig. 13.111). After confirmation of diagnosis by imaging tests, therapy with adrenergic antagonists prior to surgery is initiated.

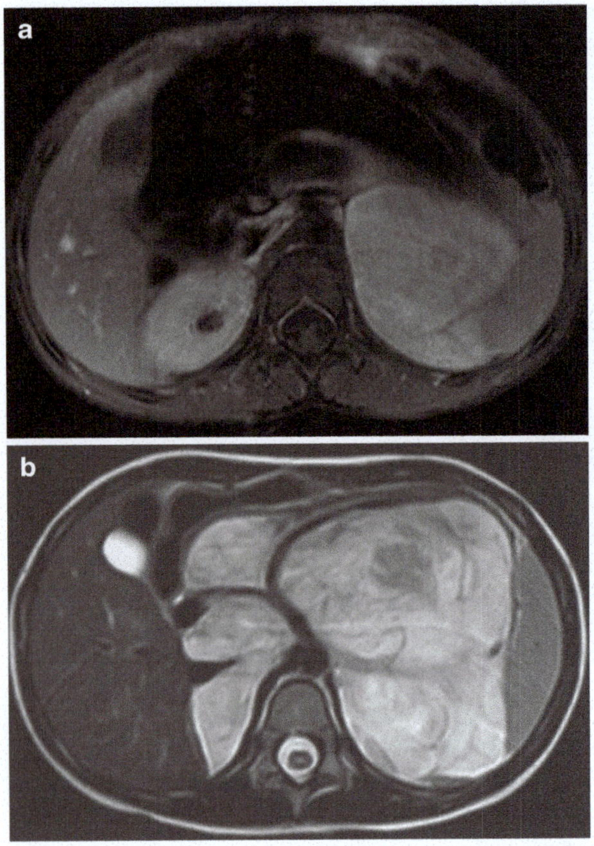

Fig. 13.110 Two examples of ganglioneuromas. Fat-saturated contrast-enhanced transverse T1-WI (**a**) show a large, left-sided, suprarenal tumor that displaces the left kidney. Transverse T2-WI (**b**) of another patient demonstrates a tumor engulfing the celiac trunk, the portal vein, and IVC. With respect to MR criteria, these masses are not distinguishable from a low stage neuroblastoma

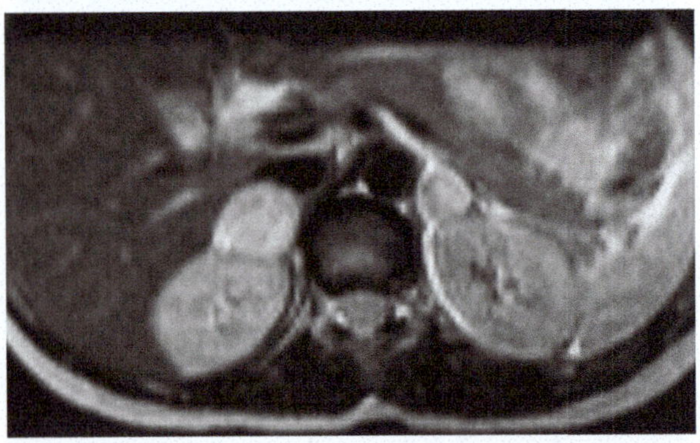

Fig. 13.111 Bilateral pheochromocytoma. Transverse T2-WI shows bilateral pheochromocytoma with high signal intensity

Prognosis after successful surgery is excellent, because fewer than 10% of intraadrenal pheochromocytomas are malignant. Treatment options for patients with unresectable malignant tumors or metastases include I^{131}-MIBG and, eventually, chemotherapy and/or tumor chemoembolization. Unfortunately, the 5-year overall survival rate is only approximately 36%.

13.4.4 Kidney Imaging

Urinary tract infection is the most common problem of the genitourinary system in children. Common congenital anomalies are vesicoureteral reflux, ureteropelvic junction obstruction, primary megaureter, ureteropelvic duplications, ureterocele, posterior urethral valves, and renal ectopia and fusion. In addition, renal cystic diseases such as autosomal recessive polycystic kidney disease, autosomal dominant kidney disease, solitary simple cysts, multicystic dysplastic kidney, syndrome-related cysts, and calyceal diverticulum are commonly encountered in children. Ultrasound, voiding cystourethrography (VCUG), IVP, fluoroscopy, and scintigraphy usually suffice to diagnose these entities, and evaluation with MRI is reserved for indistinct cases. However, MRI plays a very important role in diagnosing renal tumors, such as Wilms' tumor, multilocular cystic nephroma, congenital mesoblastic nephroma, angiomyolipoma, and renal cell carcinoma, and in differentiating them from suprarenal processes.

13.4.4.1 Normal Anatomy

Normally, the kidneys form at the sacral level and ascend to L1 into the retroperitoneal space by term. Initially, the renal pelvis is directed anteriorly, but rotates 90° medially as it ascends. In newborns and infants, the kidneys appear different on MRI (and US) than in older children and adults. They display a prominent undulating contour (Fig. 13.112), which represents fetal lobulation and should not be confused with scarring. On T1-WI, the renal cortex displays a higher SI than the medulla, and the pyramids are more prominent in neonates and young children than in older children and adults. Due to the rapid blood flow, flow

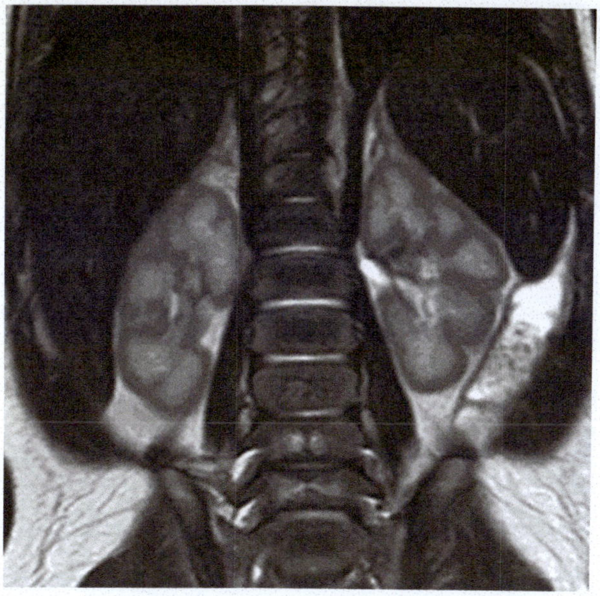

Fig. 13.112 Fetal lobulation. Coronal T2-WI of a 5-week-old boy shows undulating contours of both kidneys. In addition, SI of the liver, spleen, and spinal column is low due to hemosiderosis secondary to hemolysis

voids in the renal artery and vein are present. There is no high SI in the hilar region in young children, because of the lack of adipose tissue. Therefore, SI of renal hilum increases with age, and by puberty the kidneys have the same appearance as in adults. On T2-WI, cortex and medulla both exhibit high SI and less corticomedullary differentiation can be recognized. After administration of paramagnetic contrast, the renal cortex vividly enhances, while the SI of the medulla shows a gradual increase with time on T1-WI and dynamic contrast-enhanced 3D gradient-echo MR angiography.

13.4.4.2 Kidney Anomalies

MRI gives an excellent overall view of the abdominal and pelvic organs, and therefore facilitates the diagnosis of renal agenesis, ectopic kidney (intrathoracic or pelvic kidney), and fusion anomalies (crossed-fused ectopia or horseshoe kidney) (Fig. 13.113). A combination of axial and coronal T1-WI should be employed to visualize kidney ectopia or anomalies such as horseshoe kidney. Not surprisingly, in renal anomalies there is a high incidence of aberrant and multiple renal arteries and veins, and it might be necessary to perform

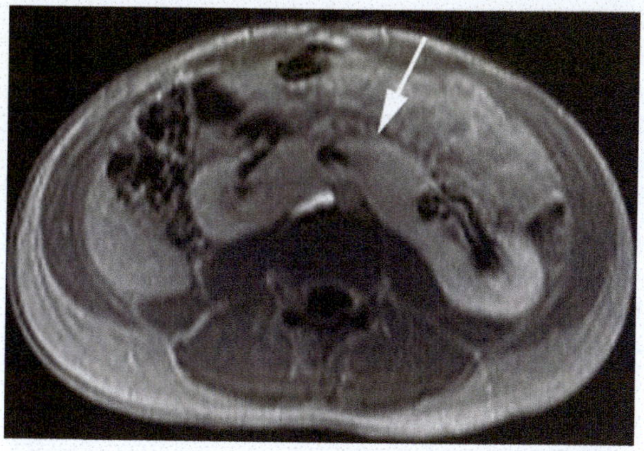

Fig. 13.113 Horseshoe kidney. Transverse contrast-enhanced fat-saturated T1-WI shows a broad parenchymal bridge (*arrow*)

MR angiography and venography prior to surgery. Generally, malpositioned kidneys are susceptiple to trauma, iatrogenic injury, obstruction, infection, and stones. Horseshoe kidneys are the most common fusion anomaly (1 in 400 births) and are associated with genital anomalies, VACTERL, Turner, and other syndromes. The midline junctional zone of a horseshoe kidney may be composed of normal parenchyma or fibrotic nonfunctional tissue. Cross-fused kidneys are less common and are also associated with syndromes. In cross-fused kidneys, the lower pole ureter inserts into the trigone on the contralateral side. Furthermore, MRI is helpful in concert with VCUG, IVP, and other fluoroscopic imaging studies in evaluation of complex anomalies associated with kidney anomalies such as the epispadias–exsthrophy complex.

13.4.4.3 Renal Cystic Disease

Renal cystic disease in children comprises solitary simple cysts, solitary complicated cysts (rarely), syndrome-related cysts, infantile (recessive) polycystic disease (RPKD), adult (autosomal dominant) polycystic disease (ADPKD), multicystic dysplastic kidney (MDK), multilocular cystic nephroma (MLCN), cystic neoplasms, and calyceal diverticulum. US usually suffices in diagnosing some of these entities, but MRI is helpful in indistinct cases. Solitary cysts and parapelvine cysts are relatively uncommon in childhood and, first and foremost, a solitary cyst must be differentiated from a calyceal diverticulum, which is easily done by IVP. If multiple cysts of different sizes are encountered in a child, they may be syndrome-related; for example, they may be associated with tuberous sclerosis. Generally, cysts are incidental findings, and must be differentiated from multilocular cystic nephroma and the cystic type of Wilms' tumor. MR imaging may help to clarify inconclusive cases, such as complicated cysts with hemorrhage. Small amounts of calcification in the wall of the cyst may not be identified by MR imaging, but larger amounts of calcifications may be seen as a rim of signal void. A reliable differentiation of hemorrhagic cysts, infected cysts, or neoplasms is not always possible. On MRI, cysts present as homogeneous, well-defined masses with clearly defined thin walls, with low SI on T1-WI and high SI on T2-WI (Fig. 13.114). After administration, the walls enhance to a variable extend. If there is high protein fluid or subacute hemorrhage in the cyst, both T1-WI and T2-WI show inhomogeneous high SI. Therefore, hemorrhagic cysts show a variable MR appearance, even within the same kidney.

Infantile (Recessive) Polycystic Disease

RPKD is inherited as an autosomal recessive disorder that shows a spectrum of abnormalities, including both microcystic and macrocystic renal disease, and variable degrees of hepatic fibrosis. It is a single gene disorder characterized by bilateral, symmetric cystic renal disease involving distal convoluted tubules and collecting ducts. The gene is called polycystic kidney and hepatic disease 1 (PKDH 1) and maps to chromosome 6p. The perinatal form has the worst prognosis, with a high mortality in the first month of life, and is characterized by severe renal disease, pulmonary hypoplasia, and minimal hepatic fibrosis. In the juvenile form, there is a milder course of renal disease but a more severe hepatic fibrosis, and therefore portal hypertension and gastrointestinal bleeding are the problem. Severity and outcome vary within affected families. Survival rate has increased for the milder form from 82% at 3 years of age and 79% at 15 years. Currently, long-time survivors have had combined renal and hepatic transplants. Numerous small cysts (1–2 mm in diameter) in both the cortex and the medulla and bilaterally enlarged kidneys are characteristic of infantile polycystic disease, although some bigger cysts may be present as well. MRI and MR urography demonstrates enlarged, lobular kidneys with radially arranged dilated tubules and absence of corticomedullary differentiation. On T2-WI, the kidneys show a uniform high SI and sometimes small discrete cysts are discernable; on T1-WI, a uniform or grainy hypointense signal is present (Fig. 13.115).

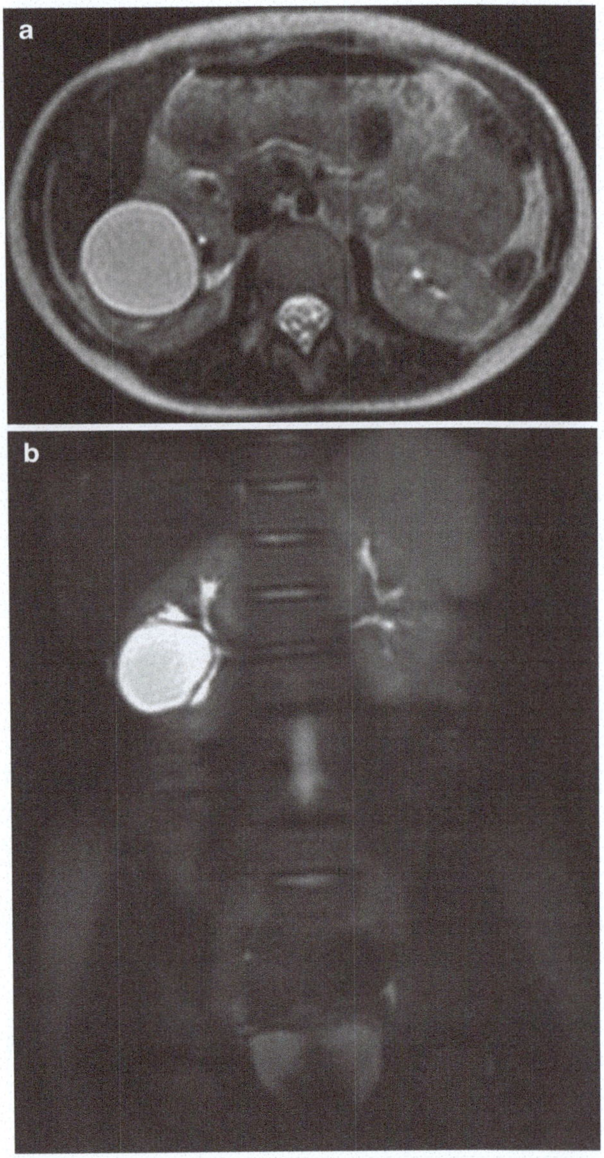

Fig. 13.114 Renal cyst. Transverse HASTE image (**a**) and coronal T2-WI (**b**) show an uncomplicated cyst in the lower pole of the right kidney

Adult (Autosomal Dominant) Polycystic Disease

ADPKD is a hereditary disorder characterized by multiple renal cysts and a variety of other systemic manifestations. Other systemic manifestations are cystic organ involvement of the liver (50%), pancreas (9%),

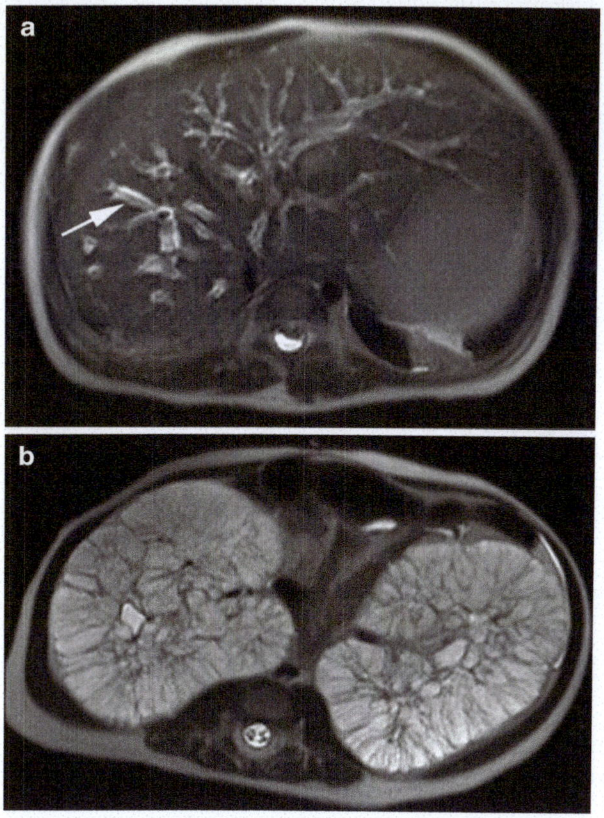

Fig. 13.115 RPDK. Transverse T2-WI (**a, b**) show periportal cuffing (*arrow*), consistent with liver fibrosis, and bilateral enlarged kidneys with multiple septated cysts (Courtesy of K. Hauenstein)

or brain/ovaries/testes (1%), and "noncystic" manifestations, such as cardiac valvular disorders, hernias, colonic diverticula, and cerebral "berry" aneurysms. Interestingly, it is one of the most common monogenetic disorders, with an incidence of 1:400–1,000, and thus more common than, for example, cystic fibosis, hemophilia, and sickle cell disease. In 90% of cases, the disease is autosomal dominant, and 10% are spontaneous mutations. Therefore, there is a 50% chance that a child could inherit a mutant gene from an ADPKD parent. Based on gene location, three different types of ADPKD are currently differentiated: PKD 1 (90% of cases, chromosome 16), PKD 2 (10%, chromosome 4), and PKD 3 (gene poorly defined). In ADPKD, the cysts tend to be larger than 1 cm in diameter, and cyst visibility increases with age: 54% of cysts occur in the first decade of life, 72% appear within the second decade, and 86% are visible in the third decade of life. Therefore, the kidneys may be completely normal in newborns and infants and, with increasing age, a growing number of cysts and and increasing size of kidneys will be found. On MRI, multiple, well-defined round or oval cysts of varying size, with hypotense SI within the thin cysts walls on T1-WI and high SI of cyst content on T2-WI are shown in case of uncomplicated cysts. In case of complicated cysts, the SI varies both on T1-WI and T2-WI, dependent on age of hemorrhage. Complicated infected cysts display marked thickening of cyst wall and adjacent renal fascia, with enhancement after administration of paramagnetic contrast.

13.4.4.4 Renal Abscess

Renal abscesses, xanthogranulomatous pyelonephritis (XPN), and carbuncles occur less frequently in children than in adults. However, they represent an important and difficult differential diagnosis to renal malignomas. XPN is an uncommon form of chronic pyelonephritis, most commonly caused by *Proteus mirabilis, E. coli*, and *S. aureus,* and is characterized by necrosis and destruction of the renal parenchyma. The affected part of the kidney is replaced by cystic necrotic areas of suppurative fibrogranulomatous tissue and soft yellow nodules composed of lipid-filled macrophages (foam cells, xanthoma cells). On MR imaging, an abscess, carbuncle, or XPN with a surrounding inflammatory reaction may mimic a necrotic malignoma with adjacent soft-tissue infiltration (Fig. 13.116). Therefore,

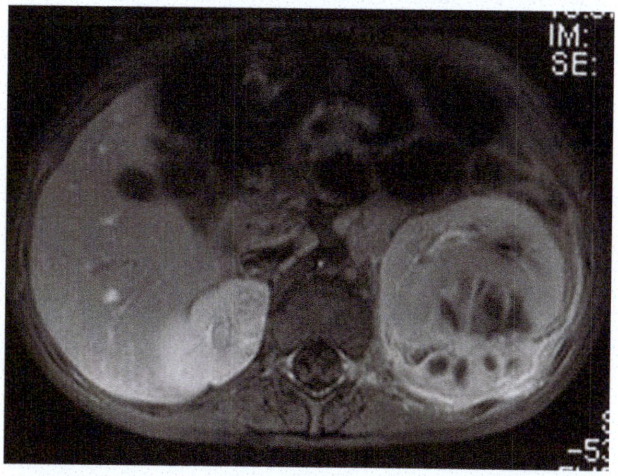

Fig. 13.116 Xanthogranulomatous pyelonephritis. Transverse fat-saturated contrast-enhanced T1-WI image shows an inhomogeneously enhancing mass in the left kidney. The irregular border of this process demonstrates strong contrast enhancement. Surrounding inflammatory reaction may mimic a necrotic Wilms' tumor

exact analysis of the patient's history, as well as clinical and laboratory findings (fever, other signs for inflammation), are mandatory. An irregular mass lesion with low to medium signal in the center is typical for a renal abscess on T1-WI. On corresponding T2-WI, the center shows high SI. The irregular border of the abscess enhances markedly with paramagnetic contrast. Perinephric abscesses may be caused by pyelonephritis or carbuncle rupture.

13.4.4.5 Tumors of the Kidneys

Multilocular Cystic Nephroma

Multilocular cystic nephroma (MLCN) is a rare benign cystic renal neoplasm that is best classified as one of two types of multilocular cystic renal tumors: cystic nephroma (MLCN) and cystic partially differentiated nephroblastoma (CPDN). The latter shows cysts with blastemal tissue as septa, whereas cystic nephroma does not have any blastemal tissue in its cysts. Both entities can only be distinguished by histology and not by imaging. There are two peak incidences: one in children at an age of 3 months to 2 years (with the males more commonly affected), and the other in adults at an age of 50–60 years (with the females more commonly affected). In children, histology mostly shows CPDN, while MLCN prevails in the adult population. Patients may present with a palpable mass in the abdomen, and sometimes with hematuria and/or back pain. On MR imaging, a well-demarcated, septated, multiloculated cystic mass with a thick fibrous capsule is observed, that may herniate into renal pelvis, distorts the collecting system, and may cause obstruction. The septa of the cysts may enhance with paramagnetic contrast (Fig. 13.117). MLCN must be distinguished from nephroblastomas, as the therapeutic management is completely different. Resection of the mass and preservation of the residual kidney is the therapy of choice. Preoperative chemotherapy, as in Wilms' tumor, must be avoided.

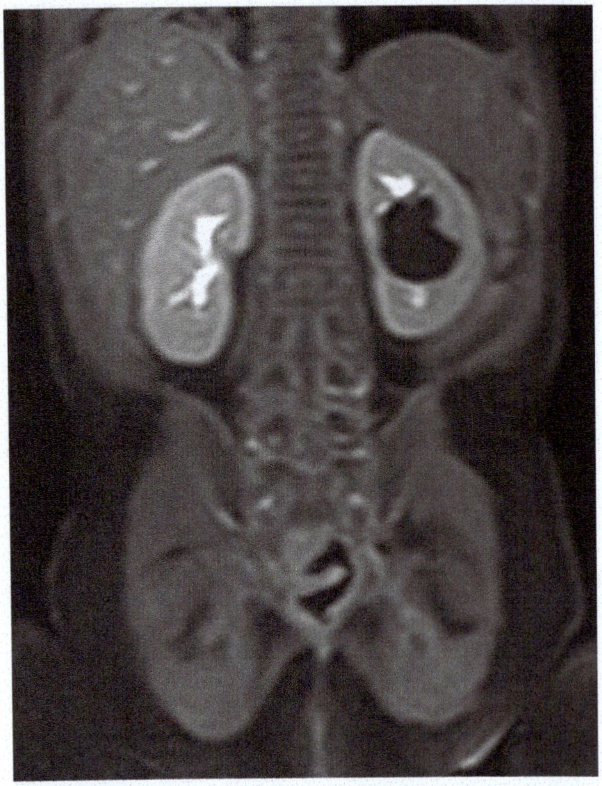

Fig. 13.117 Multilocular cystic nephroma. Coronal fat-saturated contrast-enhanced T1-WI shows a nonenhancing cystic lesion in the center of the left kidney

Congenital Mesoblastic Nephroma

Congenital mesoblastic nephroma (CMN) is a "benign" hamartomatous renal tumor composed of spindle cells, smooth muscle cells, and fibroblasts. Based on histology, three subtypes are distinguished: the "classical" (24% of cases), the "cellular" (most frequent, 66% of cases), and the "mixed" (10% of cases) type. The cellular subtype resembles congenital fibrosarcoma and the classical subtype resembles infantile fibromatosis. The most significant clinical and pathological feature of congenital mesoblastic nephromas is their tendency to grow into hilar and perirenal soft tissue, often in a subtle fashion. As a result, recurrence and metastasis is seen in up to 20% of patients. CMN typically presents as a solid, unilateral renal mass in a fetus or newborn. Size varies from 1 cm to more than 15 cm in diameter. Occasionally, hemorrhage, necrosis, and cystic areas are seen, whereas hydronephrosis is not usually present. On MRI, the solid tumor is hyperintense on T2-WI and hypointense on T1-WI, and enhances in a variable manner after administration of paramagnetic contrast (Fig. 13.118). CMN is successfully treated with nephrectomy alone, but a wide surgical margin is necessary, due to the infiltrative nature of the lesion. The prognosis is excellent if the tumor is diagnosed and resected before 6 months of age.

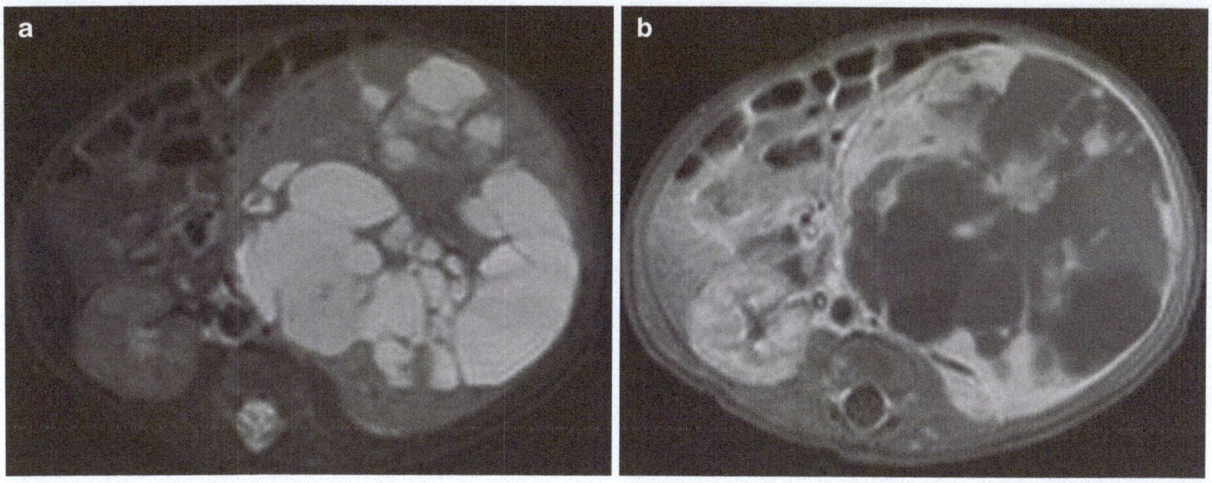

Fig. 13.118 Congenital mesoblastic nephroma. Transverse T2-WI (**a**) and contrast-enhanced fat-saturated T1-WI (**b**) shows a large tumor of the left kidney, composed of multiple cysts and vividly enhancing solid components in an 11-day-old boy

Nephroblastomatosis

Metanephric blastema normally disappears by 36 weeks gestational age, but it may persist in newborns and infants. The majority of nephrogenic rests become dormant or involute spontaneously, and only rarely do they persist after 7 years of age. Persistance of metanephric blastema is termed nephroblastomatosis, which is a premalignant lesion. In 30–40% of patients with nephroblastomatosis Wilms' tumor develops, and nephroblastomatosis is found in almost 100% of patients with bilateral Wilms' tumor (Fig. 13.121). Nephroblastomatosis often affects both kidneys, and two pathologic subtypes are distinguished: perilobar rests (90%), which are located in the renal cortex or at the corticomedullary junction, and intralobar rests (10%), which are situated deeper in the renal parenchyma. Perilobar nephroblastomatosis is found in Beckwith-Wiedemann syndrome, hemihypertrophy, Perlmann syndrome, and trisomy 18, while intralobar nephroblastomatosis is present in Drash syndrome, sporadic aniridia, and WAGR syndrome. Therefore, children with syndromes at risk to develop a Wilms' tumor have to be screened regularly by US. On MRI, nephroblastomatosis presents as unifocal or multifocal round or ovoid tumors or subcapsular rind-like renal masses that are homogeneous and iso- to hypointense compared with normal renal tissue (Fig. 13.119). On T2-WI, nephroblastomatosis is iso-to slightly hyperintense to renal parenchyma, and does not enhance significantly after administration of paramagnetic contrast. For the detection of nephroblastomatosis, T1-W sequences after application of CM are most important, and a time-resolved dynamic 3D gradient-echo sequence in coronal orientation with thin slices is recommendable. It is not possible to differentiate between nephroblastomatosis and Wilms' tumor by imaging alone, but, as a rule, nephroblastomatosis is homogeneous on all cross-sectional imaging modalities, while Wilms' tumor tends to be heterogenous.

Wilms' Tumor: Nephroblastoma

Wilms' tumor is a malignant tumor of primitive metanephric blastema and it is the most common primary renal neoplasm. In addition, it is the most common abdominal tumor in childhood and the third most frequently occurring malignancy in children after leukemia and CNS tumors. Wilms' tumor shows its peak incidence at an age of 1–3 years, with 90% of patients being younger than 7 years of age. Approximately 5–7% of Wilms' tumors are bilateral, and an additional 12% arise multifocally within a single kidney. Extrarenal Wilms' tumor occurs in the retroperitoneum adjacent to but unconnected with the kidneys, or in the pelvis, inguinal region, and chest. An increased incidence is seen in children with syndromes such as aniridia, hemihypertrophy, genitourinary anomalies (Drash syndrome), Beckwith-Wiedemann syndrome, trisomy 18, Sotos syndrome, WAGR syndrome (Wilms tumor, aniridia, genitourinary anomalies, and mental retardation). Therefore, children with syndromes that

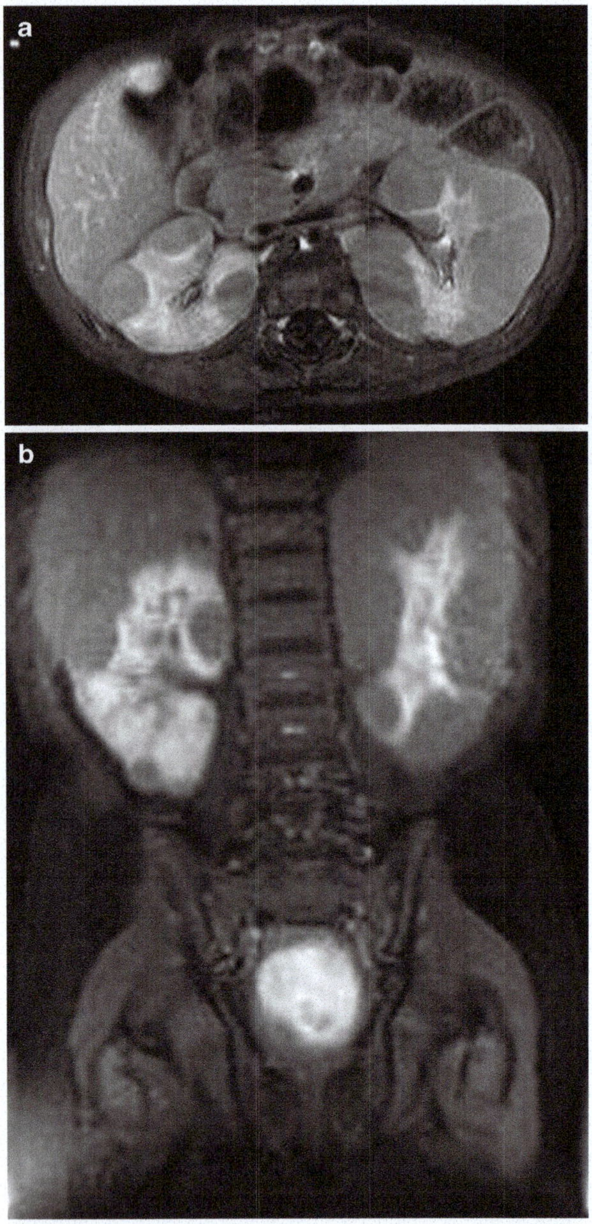

Fig. 13.119 Nephroblastomatosis. Transverse (**a**) and coronal (**b**) contrast-enhanced fat-saturated T1-WI show multiple homogeneous nonenhancing lesions in both kidneys

predispose to a risk of developing a Wilms' tumor have to be screened regularly by US. The first gene identified in the development of Wilms' tumor was a deletion on chromosome 11, and it was named WT 1. In the meantime, many alterations in multiple genes have been described. The classic Wilms' tumor is made up of varying portions of three cell types: blastemal, epithelial, and stromal. However, not all specimens show this triphasic histology; monophasic and biphasic patterns are frequently encountered. The National Wilms Tumor Study Group (NWTSG) distinguishes a "classic or favorable" (~90% of cases) and an "unfavorable" histology (~4–10% of cases). In the latter, anaplasia is present. In contrast, the histologic classification system of the International Society of Pediatric Oncology (SIOP) distinguishes between nephroblastomas of low, intermediate, and high malignancy. The difference between both classifications is based on a different therapeutic approach, because the SIOP criteria for nephroblastoma staging (Table 13.13) refer to histological examination of Wilms' tumors after neoadjuvant chemotherapy and surgical rersection, while the NWTSG criteria for nephroblastoma staging (Table 13.14) are

Table 13.13 SIOP criteria for nephroblastoma staging

Stage	Criteria
I	The tumor is limited to the kidney or surrounded with a fibrous pseudocapsule if outside the normal contours of the kidney; the renal capsule or pseudocapsule may be infiltrated with the tumor but it does not reach the outer surface, and it is completely resected The tumor may be protruding (bulging) into the pelvic system and dipping into the ureter, but it is not infiltrating their walls The vessels of the renal sinusare not involved Intrarenal vessels may be involved
II	The tumor extends beyond the kidney or penetrates through the renal capsule and/or fibrous pseudocapsule into the perirenal fat, but it is completely resected The tumor infiltrates the renal sinus and/or invades blood and lymphatic vessels outside the renal parenchyma, but it is completely resected The tumor infiltrates adjacent organs or vena cava, but it is completely resected The tumor has been surgically biopsied (wedge biopsy) prior to preoperative chemotherapy or surgery
III	Incomplete excision of tumor, which extends beyond resection margins (gross or microscopic tumor remains postoperatively) Any abdominal nodes are involved Tumor rupture before or during surgery (irrespective of other criteria of staging) The tumor has penetrated the peritoneal surface Tumor implants are found on the peritoneal surface Tumor thrombi present at resection, margins of vessels or ureter transected or removed piecemeal by surgeon
IV	Hematogenous metastases (lung, liver, bone, brain, etc.) or lymph node metastases outside the abdominopelvic region
V	Bilateral renal tumors at diagnosis. Each side has to be substaged according to above classifications

Table 13.14 NWTSG criteria for nephroblastoma staging

Stage	Criteria
I	The tumor is limited to the kidney or surrounded with a fibrous pseudocapsule if outside the normal contours of the kidney; the renal capsule or pseudocapsule may be infiltrated with the tumor but it does not reach the outer surface, and it is completely resected The tumor may be protruding (bulging) into the pelvic system and dipping into the ureter, but it is not infiltrating their walls The vessels of the renal sinus are not involved Intrarenal vessels may be involved
II	The tumor extends beyond the kidney or penetrates through the renal capsule and/or fibrous pseudocapsule into the perirenal fat, but it is completely resected The tumor infiltrates the renal sinus and/or invades blood and lymphatic vessels outside the renal parenchyma, but it is completely resected The tumor infiltrates adjacent organs or vena cava, but it is completely resected The tumor has been surgically biopsied (wedge biopsy) or there was spillage of tumor before or during surgery that is confined to the flank and does not involve the peritoneal surface
III	Residual nonhematogenous tumor is present and confined to the abdomen Any one of: Any abdominal lymph nodes are involved The tumor has penetrated through the peritoneal surface Tumor implants are found on the peritoneal surface Gross or microscopic tumors remains postoperatively The tumor is not resectable because of local infiltration into vital structures Tumor spill before or during surgery
IV	Hematogenous metastases (lung, liver, bone, brain, etc.) or lymph node metastases outside the abdominopelvic region
V	Bilateral renal tumors at diagnosis. Each side has to be substaged according to above criteria prior to biopsy or treatment

based on findings after surgical resection alone. Clinically, children very often present with a large, unilateral, abdominal mass. Less common signs are abdominal pain or hematuria. Specific laboratory findings do not exist. According to the SIOP therapy protocol, Wilms' tumor is treated with preoperative chemotherapy. Due to the danger of tumor rupture and intraperitoneal tumor spread, biopsy is not performed in Wilms' tumor. However, a fine needle biopsy is allowed in unusual and selected cases. Therefore, the diagnosis and indication for preoperative chemotherapy are primarily based on imaging. Benign masses and other malignant tumors (neuroblastomas) must be differentiated. The role of MRI in Wilms' tumor is: (1) precise definition of the tumor extent and its relationship to adjacent structures, (2) exact visualization of the tumor capsule, (3) assessment of the degree of vessel involvement and visualization of a tumor thrombus in the renal vein and IVC, (4) detection of lymph node metastases, liver and bone metastases, and (5) exclusion of contralateral lesions. On MRI, Wilms' has a variable appearance. Usually, a well-defined mass is present, with a pseudocapsule composed of collagen and compressed atrophic renal tissue that is hypointense on T1-WI, hyperintense on T2-WI, and enhances after administration of paramagnetic contrast. However, due to areas of necrosis, hemorrhage, and sometimes calcifications, the tumor may appear heterogenously on both T1-WI and T2-WI (Fig. 13.120). The best sequence to differentiate between tumor and residual kidney is a T1-W sequence after administration of CM. To further detect even small coexistent lesions in the same kidney and in the contralateral kidney (Fig. 13.121), a time-resolved dynamic 3D gradient-echo sequence in coronal orientation is recommendable. Furthermore, coronal images reveal decisive information about tumor origin (kidney: Wilms' tumor vs. adrenal gland: neuroblastoma) and craniocaudal extension. Lack of flow in venous MRA allows evaluation of possible tumor thrombus in the renal vein or IVC. In addition, tumor thrombus can be depicted on T1-WI after administration of paramagnetic contrast (Fig. 13.122). Wilms' tumor displaces rather than encases the abdominal aorta and IVC and seldom extends behind the aorta as a neuroblastoma does. Direction and position of displacement and course,

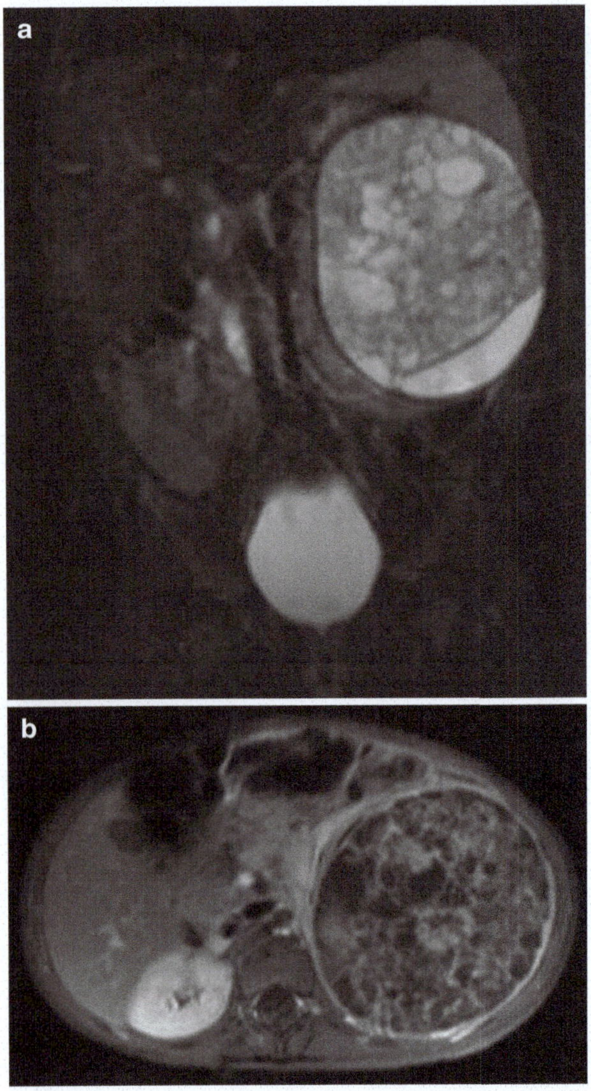

Fig. 13.120 Wilms' tumor. Coronal STIR image (**a**) and fat-saturated contrast-enhanced transverse T1-WI (**b**) show a tumor in the left kidney with inhomogeneous internal structure. Cystic and necrotic areas within the mass can be delineated

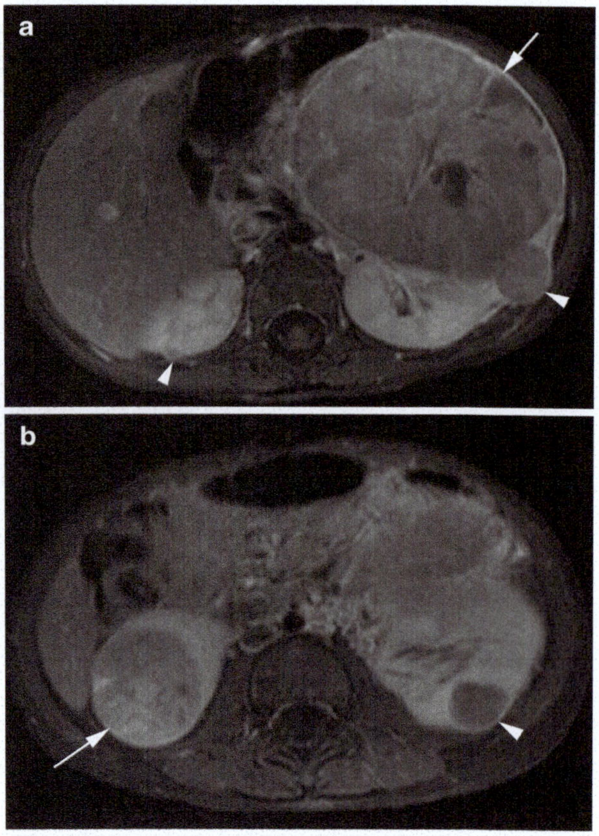

Fig. 13.121 Bilateral Wilms' tumor and nephroblastomatosis. Transverse contrast-enhanced fat-saturated T1-WI (**a, b**) demonstrate bilateral Wilms' tumor (*arrows*), with typical inhomogeneous internal structure. The nodules of nephroblastomatosis (*arrowheads*) show a homogeneous low signal

patency, and number of renal arteries and veins are of interest for the surgeons.

Clear Cell Sarcoma of the Kidney

Clear cell sarcoma is the second most common pediatric renal neoplasm and accounts for 4–5% of primary renal tumors in children. The peak incidence is at 1–4 years of age, and all documented cases have been unilateral. The tumor is characterized by its aggressive behavior, and is associated with a significantly higher rate of relapse and mortality than with Wilms' tumor. In 40–60% of patients, clear cell sarcoma metastazises to the bones, while only 2% of patients with nephroblastoma present with bone metastasis. However, metastatic disease may also occur in lymph nodes, brain, liver, and lungs - in some cases, long after nephrectomy. Imaging studies do not allow differentiation of clear cell sarcoma from Wilms' tumor (Fig. 13.123). Treatment consists of intensified chemotherapy and nephrectomy, with current long-term survival rates of 70–80%.

Rhabdoid Tumor of the Kidney

Rhabdoid tumor comprises 2% of pediatric renal tumors and is a highly aggressive malignancy of early

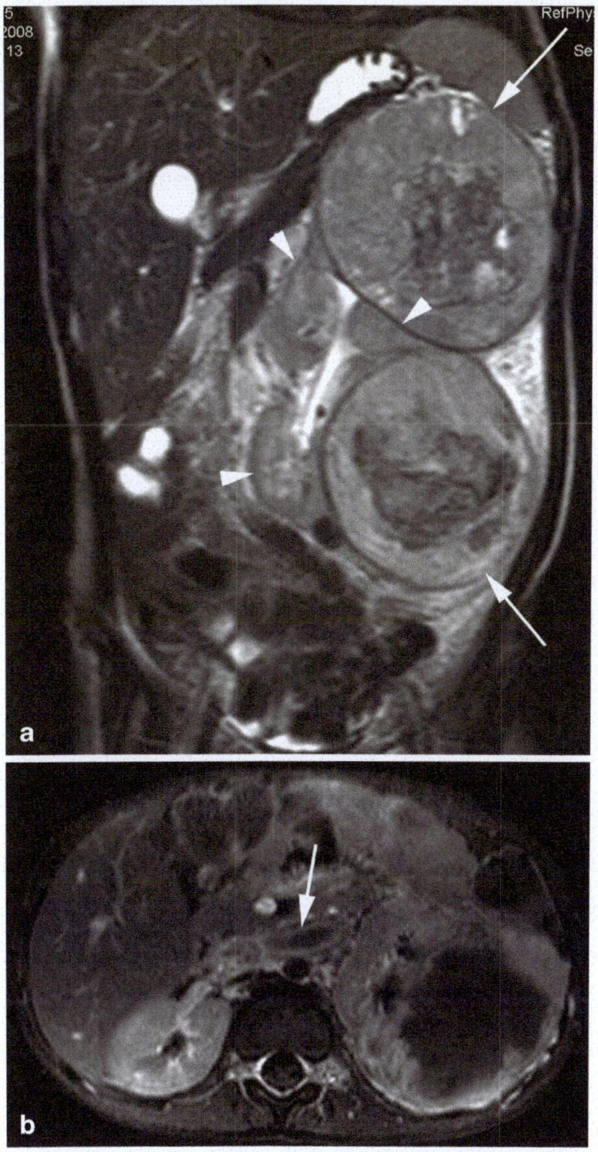

Fig. 13.122 Wilms' tumor and tumor thrombus. Coronal T2-WI (**a**) shows two large tumor nodules in the left kidney (*arrows*) compressing the normal renal parenchyma (*arrowheads*). Transverse contrast-enhanced fat-saturated T1-WI (**b**) demonstrates tumor thrombus in the left renal vein (*arrow*) extending into IVC (not shown)

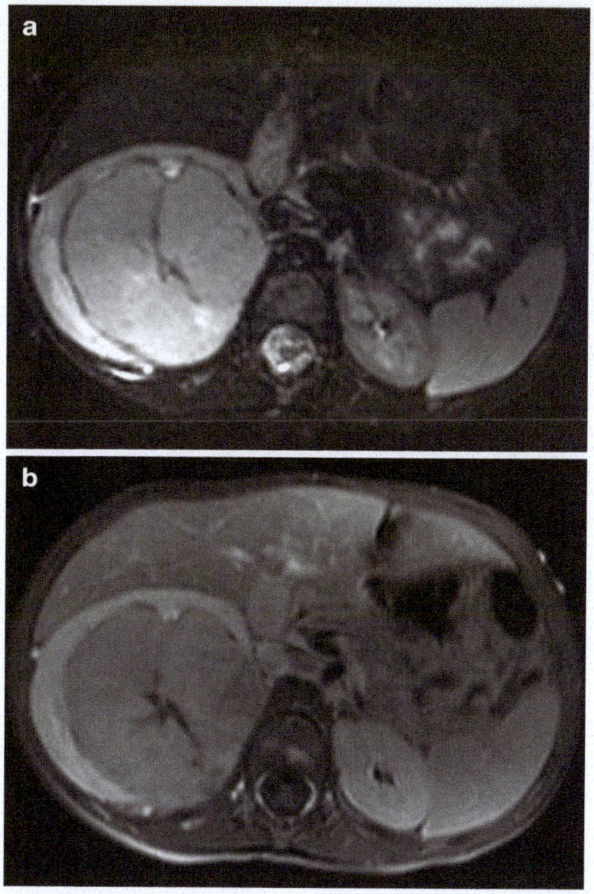

Fig. 13.123 Clear cell sarcoma. Transverse STIR image (**a**) and contrast-enhanced fat-saturated T1-WI (**b**) show a solid lesion in the right kidney

childhood, with the majority of cases being diagnosed between 6 and 12 months of age. Its name is derived from its histologic appearance, which resembles that of a tumor of skeletal muscle origin, although it has been proven that it is not related to myogenic cells. The cell of origin for this distinctive tumor is still unknown. Rhabdoid tumor does not arise exclusively in the kidney, but can occur in multiple other sites. Clinically, it may present with hematuria, but more frequently manifests with symptoms referable to widely metastatic diseases to lungs, liver, abdomen, brain, lymph nodes, or bone. A distinct feature is a synchronous or metachronous primary intracranial mass or brain metastasis. The brain lesion is often near the midline and often in the posterior fossa. Many of these brain lesions have been classified as medulloblastomas or PNET, although other histologies have also been described. Whether synchronous or metachronous renal and CNS lesions represent metastases or two primary sites in a patient with a predisposition to tumor development has not yet been clarified. Rhabdoid tumor is resistant to treatment and has a dismal prognosis, with an 18-month survival rate of only 20%. Imaging studies do not allow safe differentiation of rhabdoid tumor from Wilms' tumor (Fig. 13.124).

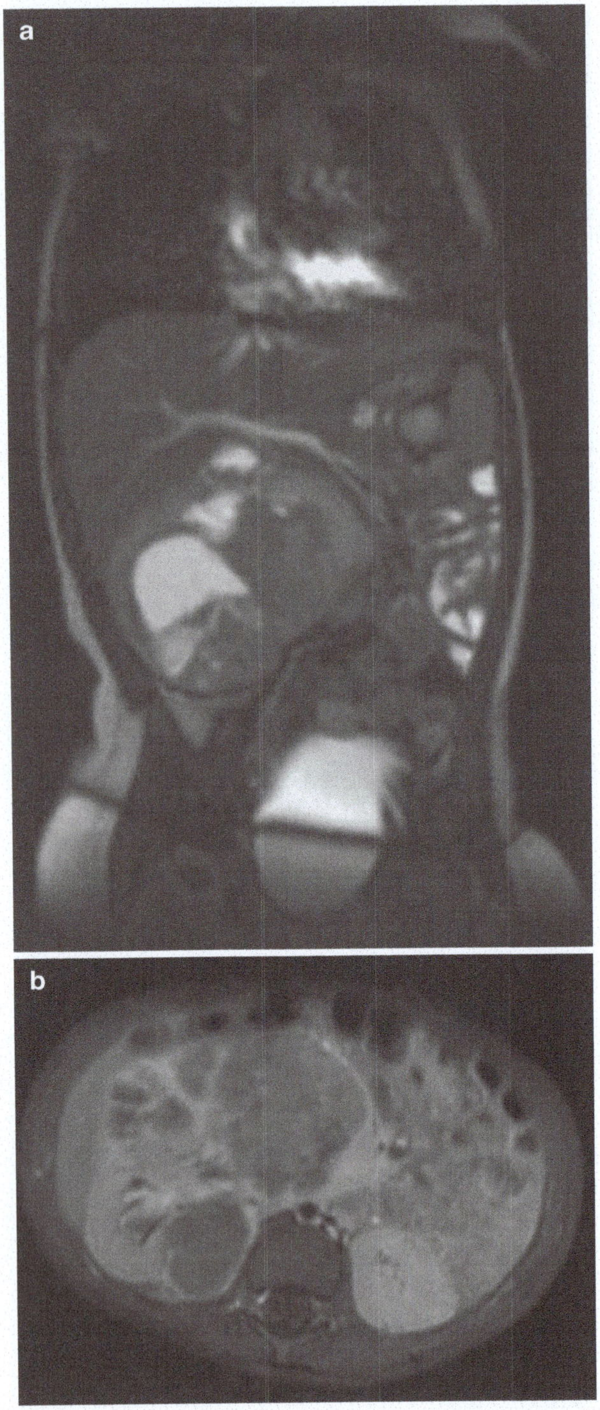

Fig. 13.124 Rhabdoid tumor. Coronal T2-WI (**a**) and transverse contrast-enhanced fat-saturated T1-WI (**b**) show a large, very heterogeneous lesion with cystic and solid parts in the right kidney

Renal Cell Carcinoma

Two different types of renal cell carcinoma may occur in children: renal papillary carcinoma and the rare renal medullary carcinoma, which is restricted to patients with sickle cell hemoglobinopathy (most commonly, sickle cell trait). Renal medullary carcinoma is a highly malignant tumor that almost exclusively occurs in adolescents and young adult blacks, but may present in children as young as 3 years. Renal medullary carcinoma is thought to arise at the renal pelvic-mucosal interface, and therefore imaging may show an infiltrative lesion invading the renal sinus, with peripheral caliectasis. In addition, peripheral satellite nodules may be present. The prognosis is extremely poor. In contrast, papillary carcinoma of the kidney has an excellent prognosis, if resected early (Fig. 13.125). Both types of renal cell carcinomas cannot be differentiated from other malignant renal masses by imaging.

Angiomyolipoma

Angiomyolipoma (AML) is an uncommon benign renal tumor consisting of a disordered arrangement of abnormal blood vessels, smooth muscle, and fat. These tumors most often occur sporadically, and can also be located in the liver and in other sites. However, they are found in 40–80% of patients with tuberous sclerosis, and are additionally associated with von Hippel-Lindau syndrome and neurofibromatosis. The mean age of presentation is 41 years, with a 4:1 female predominance. In children, AMLs are rare in the absence of tuberous sclerosis. Eighty percent of children with tuberous sclerosis develop angiomyolipomas by the age of 10 years. Symptoms are related to intralesional hemorrhage from aneurysms that develop due to the abundant and abnormal elastin-poor vascularity of the tumor. Lesions smaller than 4 cm in diameter are typically asymptomatic, whereas lesions of diameter larger than 4 cm are more prone to spontaneous bleeding, and patients may therefore present with flank or abdominal pain, hematuria, and even severe life-threatening hemorrhage. When enough fatty tissue is present within the mass, the CT and MRI appearances are virtually pathognomonic. However, intratumoral hemorrhage and predominant

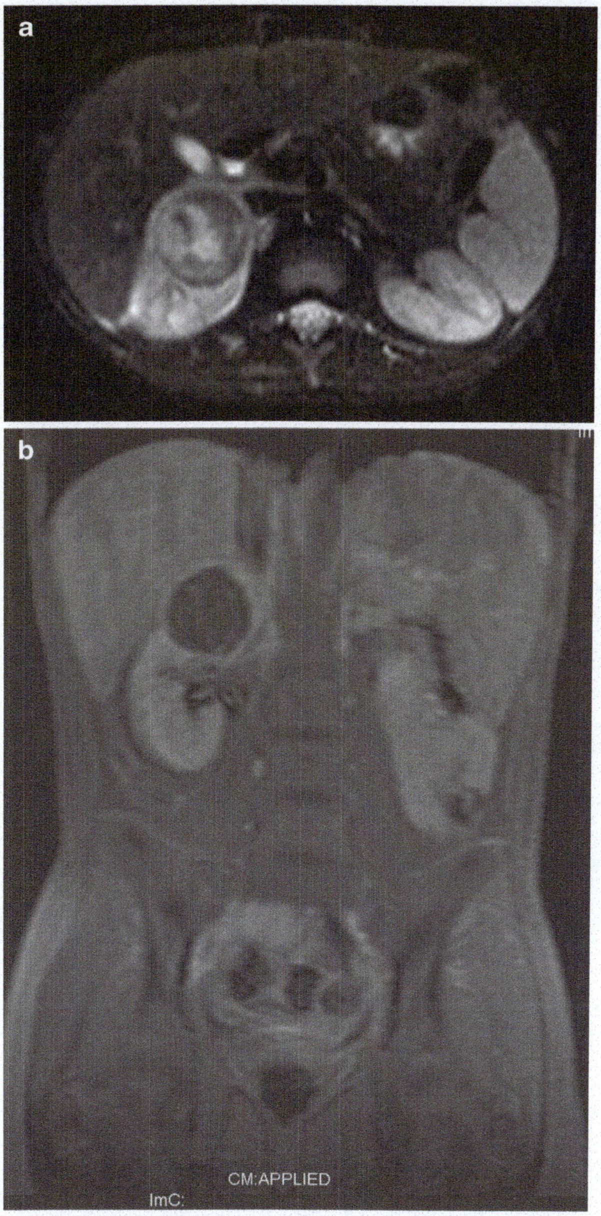

Fig. 13.125 Renal cell carcinoma. Transverse STIR image (**a**) shows a round heterogeneous tumor in the upper pole of the right kidney. Coronal contrast-enhanced fat-saturated T1-WI (**b**) demonstrates rim enhancement of the lesion. At pathology, this was a predominantly necrotic papillary renal cell carcinoma

muscle or vascular components may make differential diagnosis difficult. On MRI, a well-circumscribed intrarenal fatty mass is found, which displays varied SI due to variable amounts of vessels, muscle, and fat on T1-WI. Areas containing fat show high SI on T1-WI and low SI on fat-suppressed sequences. If the fat content is high, there is less enhancement of the lesion after administration of paramagnetic contrast; if there is high content of vascular elements, marked enhancement is present. On T2-WI, angiomyolipoma shows high SI, but may appear heterogenous due to hemorrhage (Fig. 13.126).

13.4.5 Miscellaneous Abdominal Diseases

13.4.5.1 Mesenteric Lymphatic Malformations

Mesenteric lymphatic malformations (MLM), also called mesenteric cysts, omental cysts, or mesenteric lymphangiomas, are relatively rare (1/20,000 pediatric hospital admissions). Approximately 40% of mesenteric cysts are seen in children less than 1 year of age and 80% in patients younger than 5 years of age. MLM are congenital, benign lesions and defined as dysplastic collection of lymph-containing cystic structures lined by epithelium that failed to communicate with the central lymphatic system arising from the mesentery. They range from small (few millimeters) to large (40 cm), and may be unilocular, multilocular, or multiple. Of the intraabdominal lymphatic malformations, 60% are located in the mesentery of the small bowel, 24% in the mesocolon, and 14.5% in the retroperitoneum. Patients may present with abdominal distension, pain, nausea, vomiting, a palpable tumor, or with complications such as obstruction, hemorrhage, and infection, or hydronephrosis caused by large cysts. MLMs, as all other types of cysts, are characterized by a very high SI on T2-WI (Fig. 13.127). Depending on the fluid content, SI varies from low (simple fluid) to high (blood) on plain T1-WI. Cystic lesions usually do not enhance after the application of CM, unless they are infected. Microcystic lymphatic malformations, however, may demonstrate a moderate to high contrast enhancement and appear as solid lesions. Therefore, differentiation from other tumors (i.e., neuroblastomas) may be difficult. Treatment may consists of laprascopic enucleation, bowel resection, or marsupialization. Recurrence rates range from 0 to 13%.

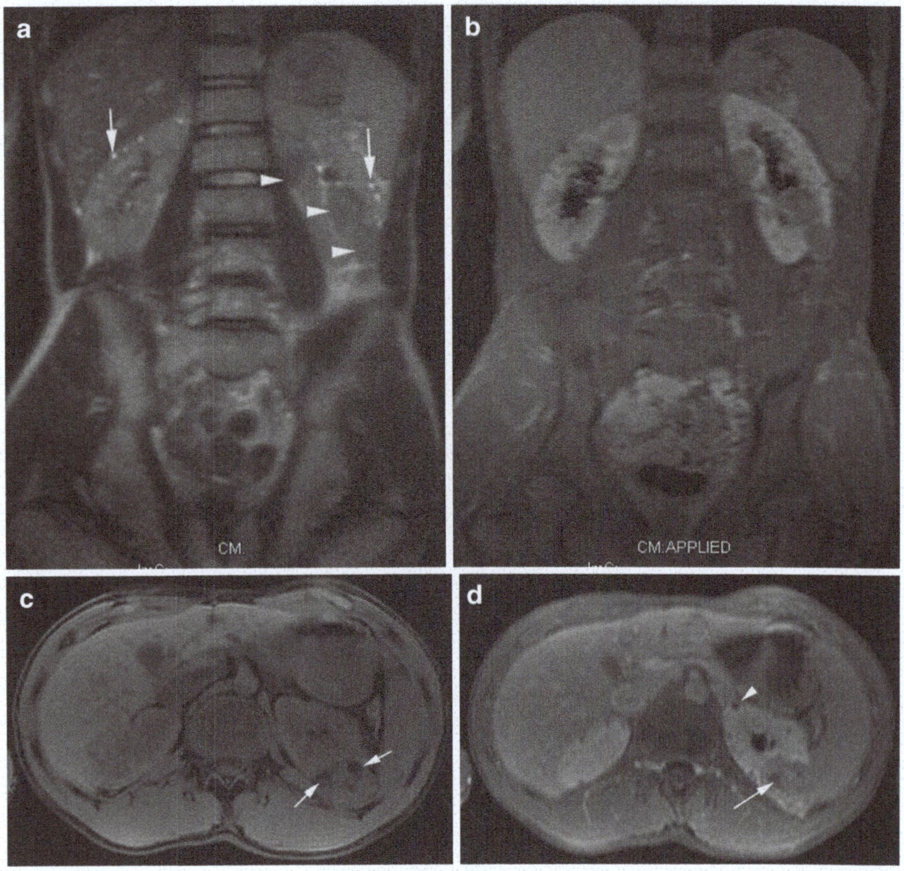

Fig. 13.126 Angiomyelolipoma. Coronal HASTE (**a**) and contrast-enhanced fat-saturated T1-WI (**b**) show multiple tiny cysts (*arrows*) and three angiomyolipomas in the left kidney (*arrowheads*). Transverse fat-saturated opposed-phase (**c**) and contrast-enhanced fat-saturated T1-WI (**d**) demonstrate the fat (*arrows*) in the enhancing angiomyolipoma and the tiny nonenhancing cysts (*arrowheads*) in an 18-year-old boy with tuberous sclerosis

13.4.5.2 Duplication Cysts

Duplication cysts result from failures of normal recanalization and can occur anywhere along the GI tract. Most commonly, they arise intraabdominally (75%), 20% occur in the chest, and 5% in a thoracoabdominal location. Unusual locations of enteric cysts include the floor of the mouth (1%), retrorectal (4%), retroperitoneal (<1%), and intrapancreatic (<1%). On US, duplication cysts have the characteristic bowel wall signature: echogenic mucosa, hypoechogenic muscular layer, and echogenic serosa. As duplication cysts are lined by epithelium representing some part of the alimentary tract, they may secrete alimentary tract substances such as gastric acid, pancreatic enzymes, and mucus. In fact, 50–60% of duplication cysts contain gastric mucosa or pancreatic tissue. Therefore, they are predisposed to inflammation, ulceration, hemorrhage, and rupture. Two types of duplications are possible: cystic duplication that usually does not communicate with the intestinal lumen, and tubular duplications that may communicate with the intestine at one or several points along the common wall. On MRI, the cyst wall appears with low SI on T2-WI, unless the wall is infected, in which case high SI on T2 will be seen. The cyst fluid itself shows a very high SI on T2-WI. Depending on the fluid content, the SI on T1-WI varies from very low signal in simple fluid, slightly higher signal due to infection, and high SI due to hemorrhage (Fig. 13.128). In 10–20%, synchronous lesions are found, and therefore survey of remaining chest or abdomen is recommended. They are treated by surgical excision.

13.4.5.3 Lymphoma

Lymphomas are the third most common group of malignancies in childhood after leukemias and brain tumors (Fig. 13.42) and account for 12.5–15% of malignant diseases. As imaging findings of lymphomas in children do not differ from those in adults, only

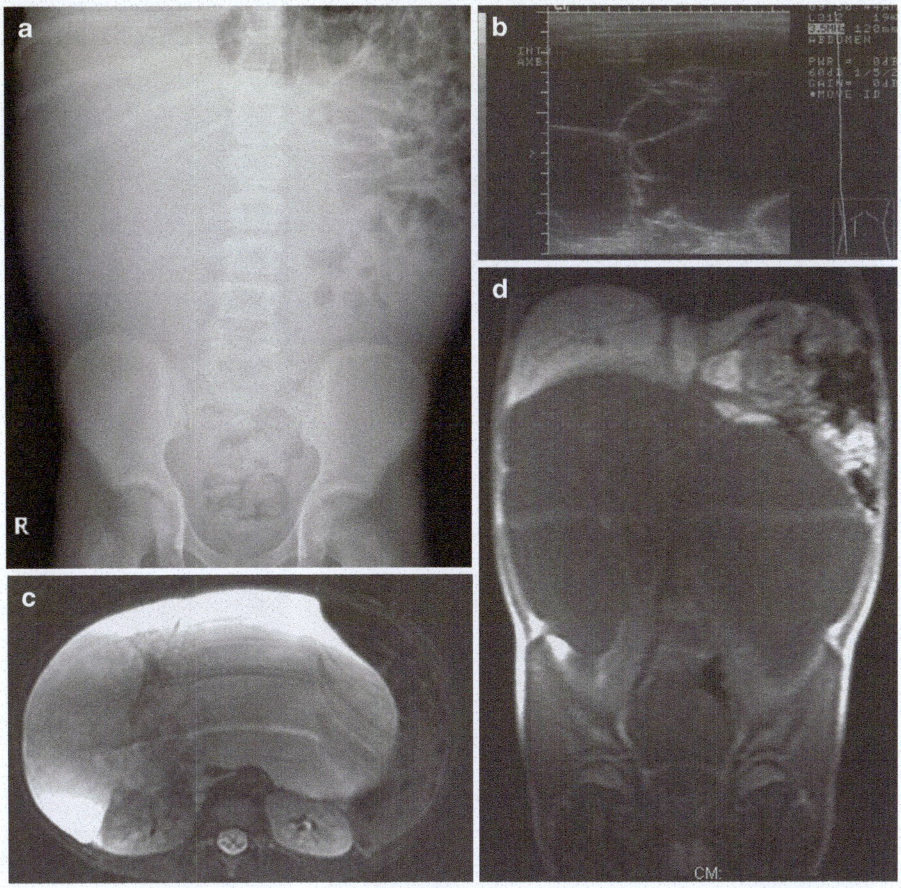

Fig. 13.127 Mesenteric lymphatic malformation. Radiography of the abdomen in AP projection (**a**) shows bowel loops being displaced to the left hemiabdomen by a mass lesion. Ultrasound (**b**) demonstrates multiple septa in this large cystic lesion. Transverse STIR image (**c**) and coronal T1-WI (**d**) depict a large, multiseptate, prevertebral cyst with high SI on T2 and low SI on T1

a few important key facts are briefly highlighted in the following paragraphs.

The most frequently encountered lymphomas in children are non-Hodgkin Lymphoma (NHL) (58%) and Hodgkin Lymphoma (41%). All types of lymphomas affect boys more often than girls (NHL, 2:1; and Hodgkin lymphoma, 1.8:1).

The classification of NHL has evolved dramatically in recent years, and includes a large number of distinct disease entities. However, the vast majority of lymphoid neoplasms listed in the WHO classification are extremely rare in children. Only four of the disease categories commonly occur in children: precursor T- and B-lymphoblastic leukaemia/lymphoma (Fig. 13.129), Burkitt cell leukaemia/lymphoma (Fig. 13.130), diffuse large B-cell lymphoma, and anaplastic large cell lymphoma. NHL is staged according to a classification system proposed by Murphy (Table 13.15), as the Ann Arbor staging classification does not adequately reflect prognosis of NHL in childhood and presence of often extensive extranodal disease in children further limits its usefulness. Clinical presentation of NHL varies according to location of the disease and according to the different entities. A mediastinal mass is typical (not specific) for a lymphoblastic T-cell lymphoma, whereas the classic scenario of a diffuse large B-cell lymphoma is an aggressively infiltrating mediastinal mass with pleural and pericardial effusions in concert with focal infiltrations of the kidneys (Fig. 13.131). The characteristic location of Burkitt lymphoma is the abdomen, and children present either with a small tumor in the bowel wall leading to invagination or ileus or present with huge abdominal tumors and ascites.

The pathologic classification of Hodgkin lymphoma is now separated into two main groups: classic Hodgkin lymphoma and lymphocyte predominance Hodgkin lymphoma. In childen, the first accounts for 95% of cases and the latter only for a minority of cases. Classic Hodgkin lymphoma (Fig. 13.132) usually presents with enlarged supradiaphragmatic lymph nodes,

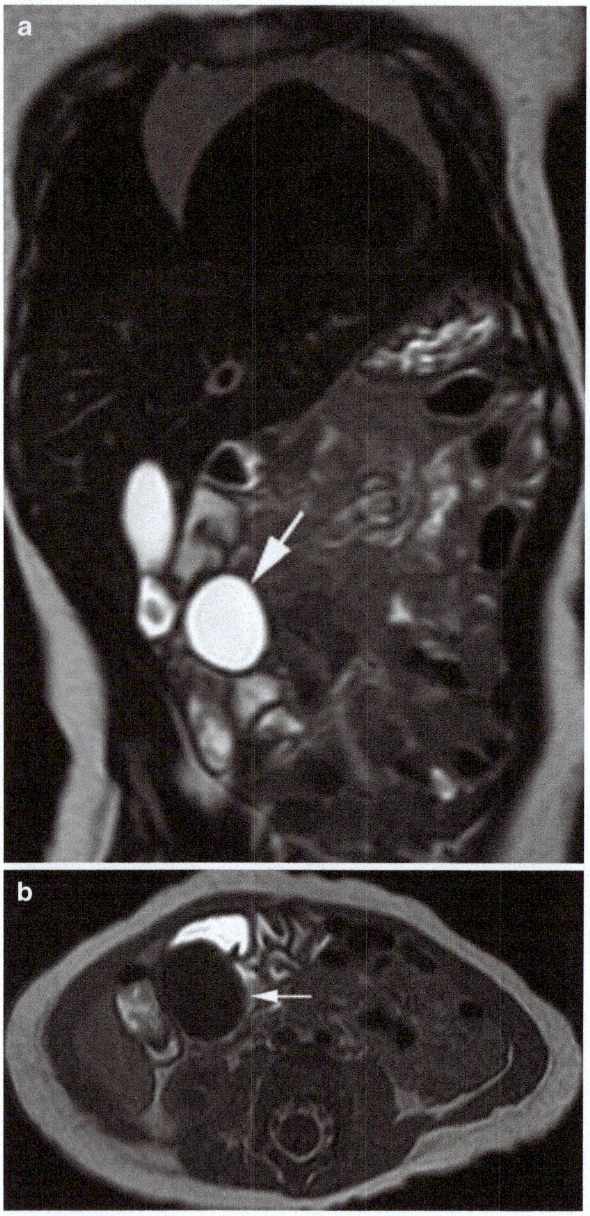

Fig. 13.128 Gastrointestinal duplication cyst. Coronal T2-WI (**a**) and transverse T1-WI (**b**) show a cystic lesion (*arrows*) in the right hemiabdomen, in close proximity to the ascending colon, in a 4-month-old girl

typically with regional rather than disseminated lymph node involvement, and is staged according to the Ann Arbor staging classification (Table 13.16).

For diagnosis and staging of abdominal lymphomas in childhood, a combination of US, MRI, and FDG-PET should be used to reduce radiation dose exposure. However, especially in Burkitt lymphoma,

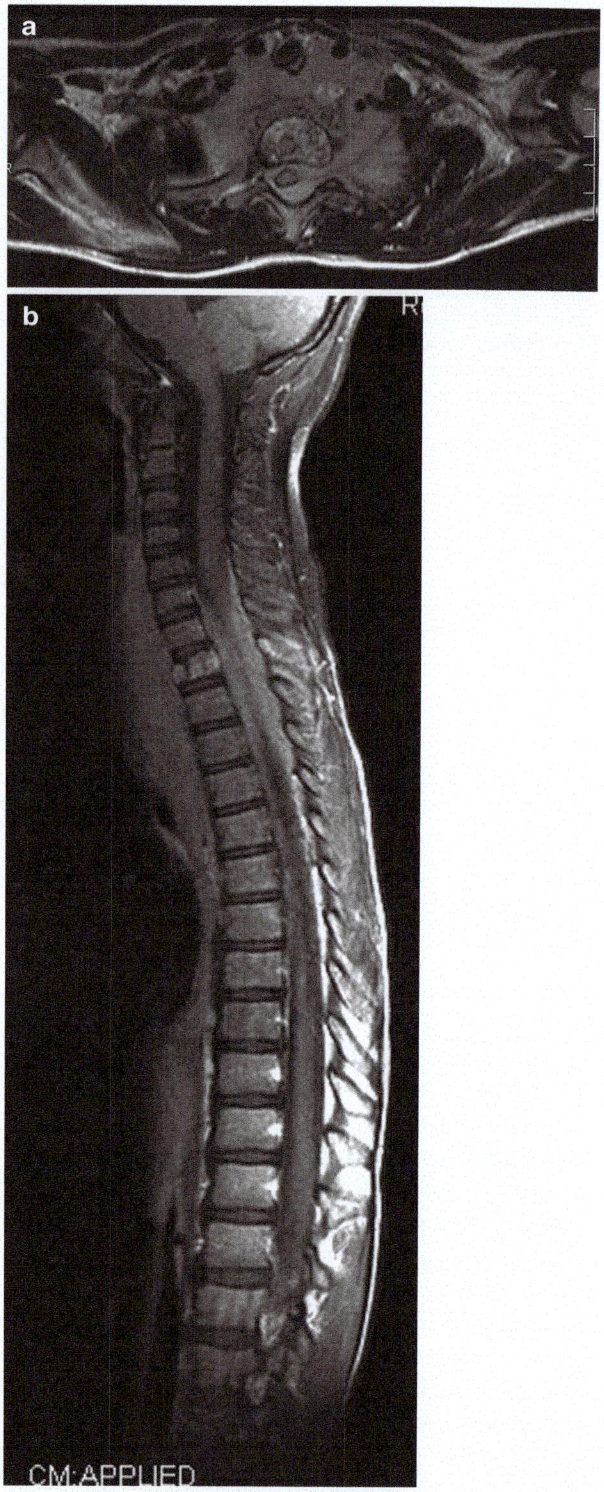

Fig. 13.129 B-lymphoblastic lymphoma. Transverse T2-WI (**a**) and sagittal fat-saturated contrast-enhanced T1-WI (**b**) show a large infiltrative growing mediastinal mass invading the spinal canal

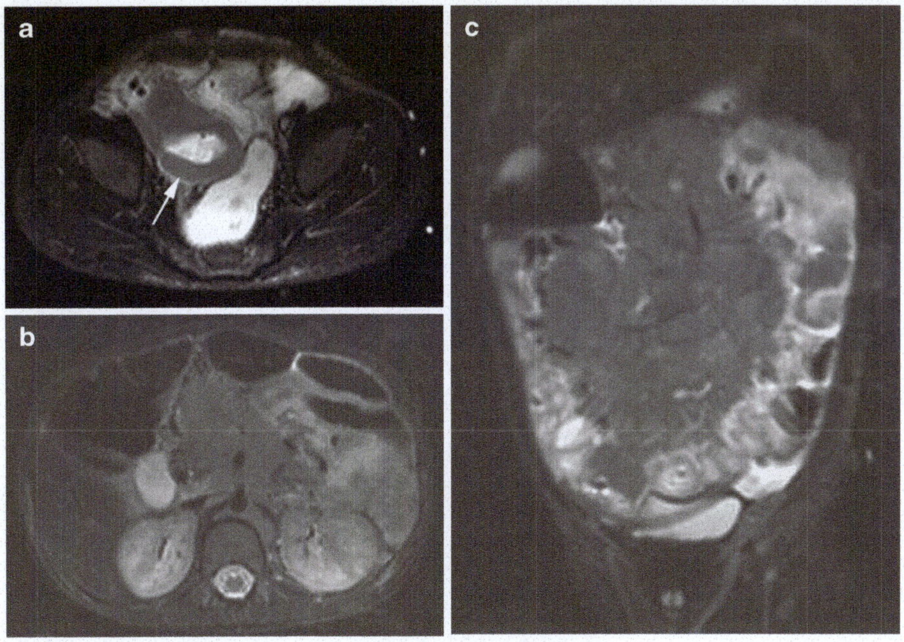

Fig. 13.130 Burkitt cell lymphoma. Transverse STIR image (**a**) shows bowel wall thickening of the distal ileum (*arrow*). Transverse (**b**) and coronal (**c**) STIR image demonstrate extensive mesenteric and retroperitoneal lymph node enlargement

Table 13.15 Murphy staging system for non-Hodgkin lymhoma (Adapted from Gadner 2006)

Stage I	A single tumor (extranodal) or single anatomic area (nodal) without local extension, with the exclusion of mediastinal, abdominal, and epidural localization
Stage II	A single tumor (extranodal) with regional lymph node involvement Two or more nodal areas on the same side of the diaphragm Two single (extranodal) tumors with or without regional node involvement on the same side of the diaphragm A localized resectable abdominal tumor Not: Mediastinal or epidural localization or extensive non-resectable abdominal tumors
Stage III	Two single tumors (extranodal) on opposite sides of the diaphragm Two or more nodal areas above and below the diaphragm All the primary intrathoracic tumors (medistinal, pleural, and thymic) All extensive primary intraabdominal tumors All epidural tumors
Stage IV	Any of the above with bone marrow (<25%)* and/or CNS involvement

*More than 25% bone marrow involvement is considered as acute B-cell leukemia

CT after administration of oral and rectal contrast may be superior to MRI for exact delineation of bowel wall involvement. For diagnosis and staging of supradiphagmatic lymphoma, CT of the chest after administration of contrast is recommended. In contrast, for staging of lymphoma of the neck, MRI should be employed to reduce exposure of the thyroid to radiation.

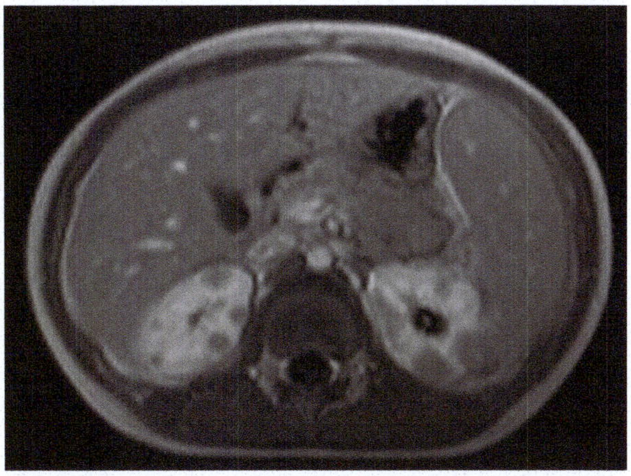

Fig. 13.131 Diffuse large B-cell lymphoma. Transverse contrast-enhanced T1-WI shows multiple rounded lesions in both kidneys

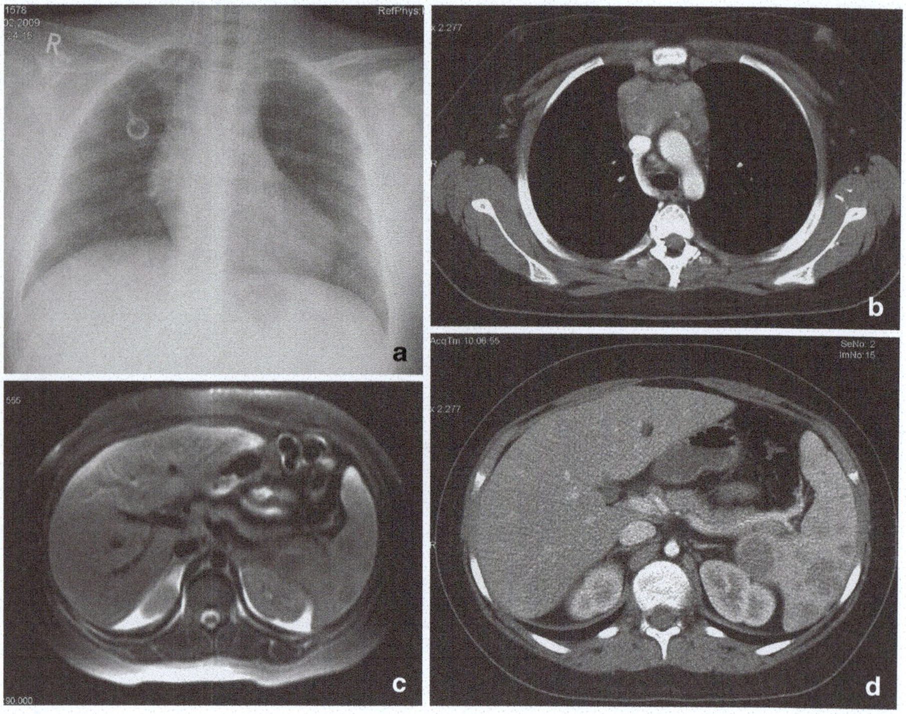

Fig. 13.132 Hodgkin lymphoma stage III_S. Chest X-ray (**a**) shows a broad mediastinum. On CT (**b**), mediastinal lymph node enlargement is present. Transverse STIR image (**c**) and CT (**d**) demonstrate multiple lesions in the spleen

13.4.5.4 Rhabdomyosarcoma

Rhabdomyosarcoma (RMS) is a mesenchymal sarcoma arising from primitive muscle cells (rhabdomyoblasts) that fail to differentiate into skeletal muscle. RMS belongs to the group of soft tissue sarcomas, which are the fourth most common tumors in children, and approximately 70% of children are younger than 10 years of age at the time of presentation. RMS can occur anywhere in the body, but the most common location is the head and neck region (28–40%), followed by the genitourinary tract (20%), the extremities (15–20%), the trunk (11%), and the retroperitoneum (6%). Two different histologic types are differentiated: alveolar (variant: solid-alveolar) and embryonal (variant: botroid, spindle cell). Embryonal RMS accounts for 60–70% of childhood RMS and is the most common type in children under 15 years of age, whereas alveolar RMS occurs in adolescents and accounts for 20% of RMS (also see the musculoskeletal system section). Rhabdomyosarcoma is the most common tumor of the lower urinary tract in children, and patients present with urinary obstruction and, less commonly, with hematuria. Unfortunately, abdominal rhabdomyosarcomas are typically very large in size at the time of presentation. RMS may originate from bladder, prostate, paratesticular tissues, vagina, cervix, uterus, and pelvic side walls. They spread by local extension, via lymphatics, and hematogeneous metastases to lungs, liver, and bone. On MRI, RMS may appear as a solid mass demonstrating hypointense or similar SI to muscle on T1-WI and hyperintense SI on

Table 13.16 Ann Arbor staging classification for Hodgkin lymphoma (Adapted from Pizzo and Poplack 2006)

Stage I	Involvement of a single lymph node region (I) or of a single extralymphatic organ or site (I_E)
Stage II	Involvement of two or more lymph node regions on the same side of the diaphragm (II) or localized involvement of an extralymphatic organ or site and one or more lymph node regions on the same side of the diaphragm (II_E)
Stage III	Involvement of lymph node regions on both sides of the diaphragm (III), which may be accompanied by involvement of the spleen (III_S), or by localized involvement of an extralymphatic organ or site (III_E), or both (III_{SE})
Stage IV	Diffuse or disseminated involvement of one or more extralymphatic organs or tissues, with or without associated lymph node involvement

The absence or presence of fever higher than 38°C for 3 consecutive days, drenching night sweats, or unexplained loss of 10% or more of body weight in the 6 months preceding admission are to be denoted in all cases by the suffix letters A or B, respectively

T2-WI, but may appear heterogeneously and enhance inhomogeneously with paramagnetic contrast, due to hemorrhage and necrosis (Fig. 13.133). However, the botryoid variety of embryonal RMS may present as a lesion with multiple cysts (bunch of grapes). After biopsy, neoadjuvant chemotherapy is employed prior to surgical resection.

13.4.5.5 Ovarian Tumors

Ovarian tumors are rare, accounting for only approximately 1% of childhood malignancies, and they may occur at any age. However, the incidence increases at 8–9 years and peaks at 19 years. In contrast to adult ovarian tumors, two-thirds of pediatric ovarian tumors are of germ cell origin, with tumors of epithelial and stromal origin occurring less frequently. Table 13.17 gives an overview of the histological classification of pediatric ovarian tumors. Among the ovarian germ cell tumors, teratomas are the most common ones. Teratomas are composed of well-differentiated tissues arising from the three germ layers (endoderm, ectoderm, and mesoderm), and usually contain tissues foreign to the anatomic site of origin. Teratomas can be classified according to their histologic composition as

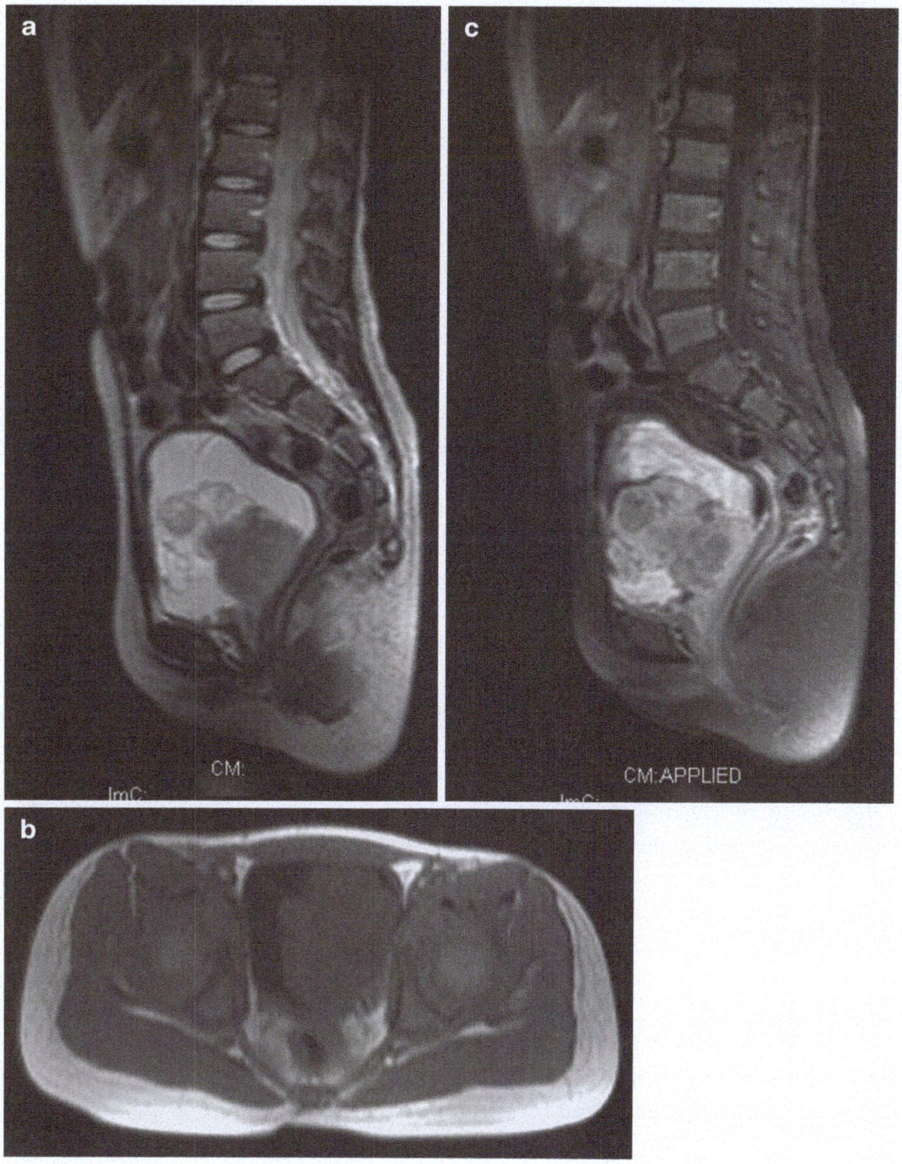

Fig. 13.133 Rhabdomyosarcoma. Sagittal T2-WI (**a**) shows a large lobulated tumor in the bladder extending into the urethra. Transverse T1-WI (**b**) and sagittal contrast-enhanced fat-saturated T1-WI (**c**) demonstrate an inhomogenously enhancing lesion

Table 13.17 Histologic classification of pediatric ovarian tumors (Adapted from Pizzo and Poplack 2006)

Germ cell	Non-germ cell
Teratoma • Mature • Immature: 0 = Mature tissue only 1 = Immature tissue, less than 1 low-power field per slide 2 = Immature tissue, 1–3 low-power fields per slide 3 = Abundant immature tissue • Teratoma with associated malignant germ cell tumor component • Teratoma with associated malignant somatic component (squamous carcinoma, glioblastoma, peripherial neuroectodermal tumor, etc.)	Epithelial (serous, mucinous) Sex cord-stromal (granulosa, Sertoli-Leydig, mixed)
Dysgerminoma	
Endodermal sinus tumor (yolk sac tumor)	
Embryonal carcinoma	
Mixed malignant germ cell tumor	
Choriocarcinoma	
Gonadoblastoma	
Polyembryoma	

mature (containing well-differentiated tissues, most often neuroectodermal), or immature (containing varying degrees of immature fetal tissues, most often neuroectodermal), or malignant (containing at least one of the malignant germ cell elements). Only the mature teratoma can be considered to be a benign lesion. The types of malignant ovarian germ cell tumors, in order of decreasing frequency, are: dysgerminoma, endodermal sinus tumor (yolk sac carcinoma), immature teratoma, and embryonal carcinoma. Patients with ovarian tumors may present with abdominal pain, a palpable abdominal mass, abnormal uterine bleeding, ovarian torsion, urinary symptoms, gastrointestinal complaints, and back pain. The role of clinical markers in the diagnosis of germ cell tumors is well established. The oncofetoproteins AFP and β-HCG, and in special cases the cellular enzymes LDH (lactate dehydrogenase) and PLAP (a fetal isoenzyme of alkaline phophatase), and other cytogenetic and molecular markers are used for diagnosis of germ cell tumors, monitoring treatment success, and indicating presence of residual or progressive disease. Table 13.18 summarizes typical clinical characteristics of pediatric ovarian tumors. On MRI, a mature teratoma presents as a mass showing a heterogeneous mixed signal intensity, as it consist of fat (hyperintense on T1-WI and T2-WI), mixed solid (isointense on T1-WI and T2-WI), and cystic (hypointense on T1-WI and hyperintense on T2-WI) components, and calcifications (bone, teeth, and/or cartilage; hypointense on T1-WI and T2-WI). After application of paramagnetic contrast, the solid portion and cyst walls will enhance. Hemorrhage and calcifications are best detected by T2* GRE sequences. All other germ cell tumors may appear similar to teratomas or present as solid masses (Fig. 13.134). As they cannot be differentiated by imaging alone, surgical resection is performed in tumors that can be resected without sacrificing vital structures. In unresectable tumors, debulking or biopsy is performed prior to chemotherapy and then followed by surgery.

13.4.5.6 Anorectal Anomalies

Anorectal anomalies include ectopic anus, imperforate anus, rectal atresia, and anal/rectal stenosis, with ectopic anus being the most common form (Table 13.19). In the latter condition, the hindgut fails to descend, and opens ectopically through a fistula into the perineum, vestibule, vagina, urethra, or bladder. Furthermore, associated abnormalities of the genitourinary system and spine are frequently present. Arrest of the hindgut can be high, intermediate, or low. In the case of high arrest, the colon ends at or above the puborectalis sling, which is hypoplastic, or even absent. In the case of low arrest, the ectopic hindgut passes through a usually well-developed puborectalis sling and demonstrates a superficial covering at the skin margin. Plain films and injection of contrast agent into the bladder and the female genital tract or male urethra are necessary for visualization of the rectum and fistulas. On MR imaging, fistulas are difficult to depict. However, MR imaging plays an important role in the evaluation of the associated anomalies and preoperative and postoperative assessment. T1-WI is required in all three imaging planes, for excellent anatomic resolution. The levator ani muscle and the residual external sphincter muscle

Table 13.18 Clinical characteristics of pediatric ovarian tumors (Adapted from Pizzo and Poplack 2006)

Tumor type	Relative frequency (%)	Median age (years)	Characteristics
Dysgerminoma	24	16	Rapid growth; 14–25% with other germ cell elements; very radiosensitive
Endodermal sinus tumor (yolk sac)	16	18	AFP; 75% stage I; all patients require chemotherapy because of high risk for relapse, even in low stage disease
Teratoma			
Mature	31	10–15	Neuroglial implants may occur with cystic or solid teratomas, but do not affect prognosis; surgery is mainstay of therapy
Immature	10	11–14	Grading system based on amount of neuroepithelium present; prognosis inversely related to stage and grade; 30% with AFP
Embryonal carcinoma	6	14	47% prepubertal; HCG and precocious puberty common; chemotherapy indicated
Mixed malignant germ cell tumor	10	16	40% premenarchal; 30% sexually precocious; AFP/HCG may be increased
Gonadoblastoma	1	8–10	Associated with dysgenetic gonads and sexual maldevelopment; removal of both gonads is treatment of choice
Other (polyembryoma, choriocarcinoma)	<1	–	Rare in children

AFP alpha-fetoprotein; *HCG* human chorionic gonadotropin

mass can be demonstrated well by MR imaging. Specifically, the identification and location of the external sphincter muscle mass are crucial for guiding the pull-through surgical procedure. High or intermediate ectopic anus is treated by decompression colostomy initially, with definite pull-through corrective surgery at an age of 1–2 years. Postoperatively, MR imaging may be necessary to prove malplacement of the rectum or inclusion of mesenteric fat within the sphincter ring.

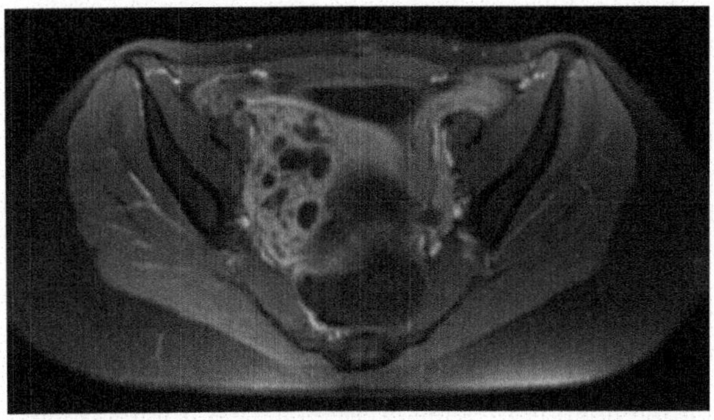

Fig. 13.134 Immature teratoma. Transverse fat-saturated contrast-enhanced T1-WI shows an enlarged right ovary with multiple cysts

Table 13.19 Anorectal anomalies (Modified from Swischuk 1997)

Ectopic anus	The hindgut opens ectopically at an abnormal high location (i.e., perineum, vestibule, urethra, bladder or vagina). There is a failure of normal descent of the hindgut
Imperforate anus	The terminal bowel ends blindly and there is no opening or fistula. Two types are distinguished: (a) membranous imperforate anus; and (b) anorectal or anal atresia
Rectal atresia	The anus is present and open, but a variable segment of rectum is atretic. No fistula is present
Anal and rectal stenosis	Incomplete atresia of either structure
Cloacal anomalies	Only in females; urethra, vagina, and uterus end in one opening tract. Often associated with hydrometrocolpos and duplication of vagina and/or uterus

13.5 Pediatric Musculoskeletal System and Bone Marrow Imaging

13.5.1 Technique

13.5.1.1 Coils and Patient Positioning

Depending on the scanner, there are different coil systems designed for adults that have to be used for children. Depending on the system and the available coils, it may be advisable to use the head coil not only for the head, but also for the spine, pelvis, and extremities, as long as the coil is large enough for the infant. If available, standard dedicated phased-array coils are recommended for evaluation of all joints. Depending on the size of the patient, the available surface coils must be adapted, especially if side-to-side comparison is useful. Therefore, the pelvis and/or hips are examined with the body-array coil. In general, the coil that provides highest spatial resolution in concert with the smallest field-of-view is most appropriate for imaging small joints. Optimal positioning in the center of the coil and immobilization of the patients with vacuum beds, sponges, sand bags, and blankets are mandatory.

13.5.1.2 Sequence Protocol

Basically, the sequence protocols used in children for evaluation of the bone marrow and musculoskeletal system do not differ from those used in adults. Slice thickness, field-of-view, and rectangular field-of-view are adapted to the patient's size. The basic imaging protocol includes FS intermediate-weighted sequences (FS PD-W) or T2-W sequences, STIR sequences, T1-W sequences, and FS T1-W sequences after the administration of paramagnetic contrast, if necessary. For evaluation of cartilage, an additional fluid-sensitive FS T2-W sequence is recommended. For imaging protocols of the different regions, the reader is referred to Chaps. 3 and 5 and hints in the following text.

13.5.2 Normal Appearance of Bone Marrow in Children

Knowledge of the normal appearance and expected marrow distribution in each age group is important for the diagnosis of diseases affecting the bone marrow in children. Normal yellow or fatty marrow consists of 15% water, 5% protein, and 80% fat. It is less vascularized than red or hematopoietic marrow, which is composed of 40% water, 20% protein, and 40% fat. At birth, the entire skeleton contains hematopoietic marrow, and there is a progressive transformation from red to fatty marrow, in a predictable pattern, from infancy to early adulthood (Fig. 13.135). In the extremities, the conversion progresses distally (fingers, toes) to proximally (shoulder, hips) within each bone, starting in the epiphysis. In the tubular bones, marrow transformation starts in the diaphysis and moves toward the metaphyses, which contain red marrow up to adulthood. This process is slower in the axial skeleton and the pelvis, where red marrow is present throughout life. On T1-WI, fatty marrow is of high SI, whereas red marrow is of low SI. On conventional T2-W SE sequences, fatty and red marrow are of intermediate SI. On STIR images, fatty marrow is of very low SI and red marrow is of intermediate to high SI. In general, coronal planes are most useful in the evaluation of bone marrow. As a consequence of anemia or other processes that cause an elevation of the level of the circulating hormone erythropoietin, yellow marrow reconverts to red marrow. Marrow reconversion proceeds in the reverse order of conversion.

13.5.3 Bone-Marrow Disorders

13.5.3.1 Sickle Cell Anemia

Marrow abnormalities related to sickle cell disease include red-marrow expansion due to chronic hemolytic anemia, infarction or avascular necrosis secondary to erythrocyte abnormality, and secondary hemosiderosis due to multiple transfusions. Red-marrow expansion results in decreased marrow SI on T1-WI and mixed SI on T2-WI, whereas hemosiderosis leads to a marked decrease in SI on all pulse sequences. Chronic bone infarcts typically present as sharply demarcated areas with irregular serpiginous low SI lines on all imaging sequences, and the central zone may be low SI on all imaging sequences or may follow fat SI (Fig. 13.136). Differentiation of acute bone infarction from osteomyelitis in sickle cell patients is very challenging, as both may occur in the diaphysis, show abnormal marrow, cortical involvement, juxtacortical soft tissue edema, and peripheral rim enhancement. Unfortunately, sickle

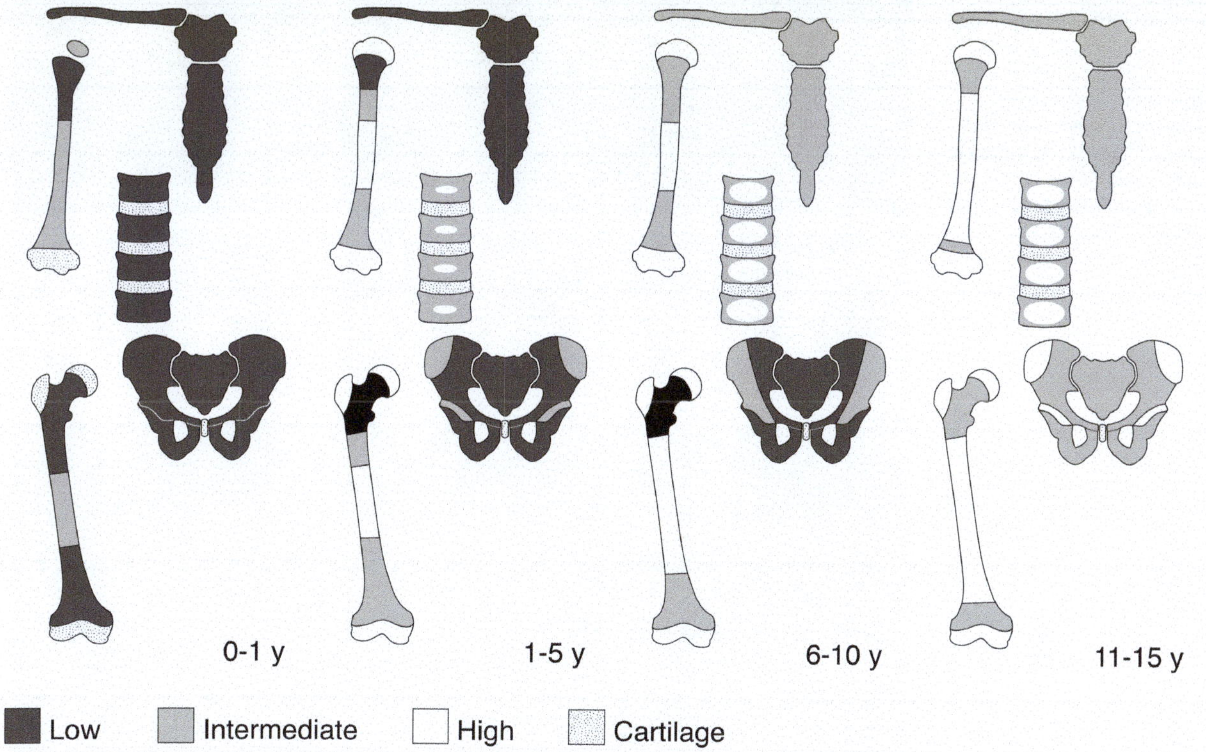

Fig. 13.135 Marrow transformation as depicted on T1-WI. In infants, most of the bones are of low signal intensity due to the presence of hematopoietic marrow. The vertebral bodies are hypointense compared with disks. In early childhood (1–5 years), the epiphysis and the diaphysis of the long bones are of high signal intensity, and the vertebral bodies are isointense with the disks. During late childhood (6–10 years) and early adolescence (11–15 years), the spine, iliac wings, and distal metaphyses become more and more hyperintense due to replacement of hematopoietic marrow by fatty marrow (Adapted from Kirks 1998)

cell patients have a higher incidence of osteomyelitis, especially from infection with Salmonella and other gram-negative bacilli, and therefore correlation with clinical and laboratory findings is essential.

13.5.3.2 Aplastic Anemia

Aplastic anemia is simple to recognize by MRI, as the extensive replacement of normal red marrow with fat results in bright SI on T1-WI, often including the axial skeleton as well. Especially in the vertebral column, patchy areas of decreased SI develop with treatment, reflecting regeneration of red marrow.

13.5.3.3 Gaucher Disease

Storage of glucocerebrosides in the bone marrow, due to a relative deficiency of β-glucocerebrosidase, produces patchy, heterogeneous, decreased SI on T1-WI and T2-WI and increased signal on STIR images, frequently with sparing of the epiphyses. Typical involvement of the distal femurs causes the characteristic Erlenmeyer flask deformity. Patients may additionally suffer from bone infarctions and conditions that clinically and radiographically are indistinguishable from osteomyelitis.

13.5.3.4 Iron-Storage Disorders

Iron storage of ferritin and hemosiderin, due to repeated blood transfusions, anemias, hemoglobinopathies, and hemochromatosis, causes decreased SI in both T1-W and T2-W sequences (Fig. 13.112).

13.5.3.5 Bone Infarction and Avascular Necrosis

Osteonecrosis is the term used to describe bone death due to ischemia. When osteonecrosis affects an epiphysis or subarticular bone, it may be referred to as avascular necrosis or ischemic necrosis or aseptic necrosis,

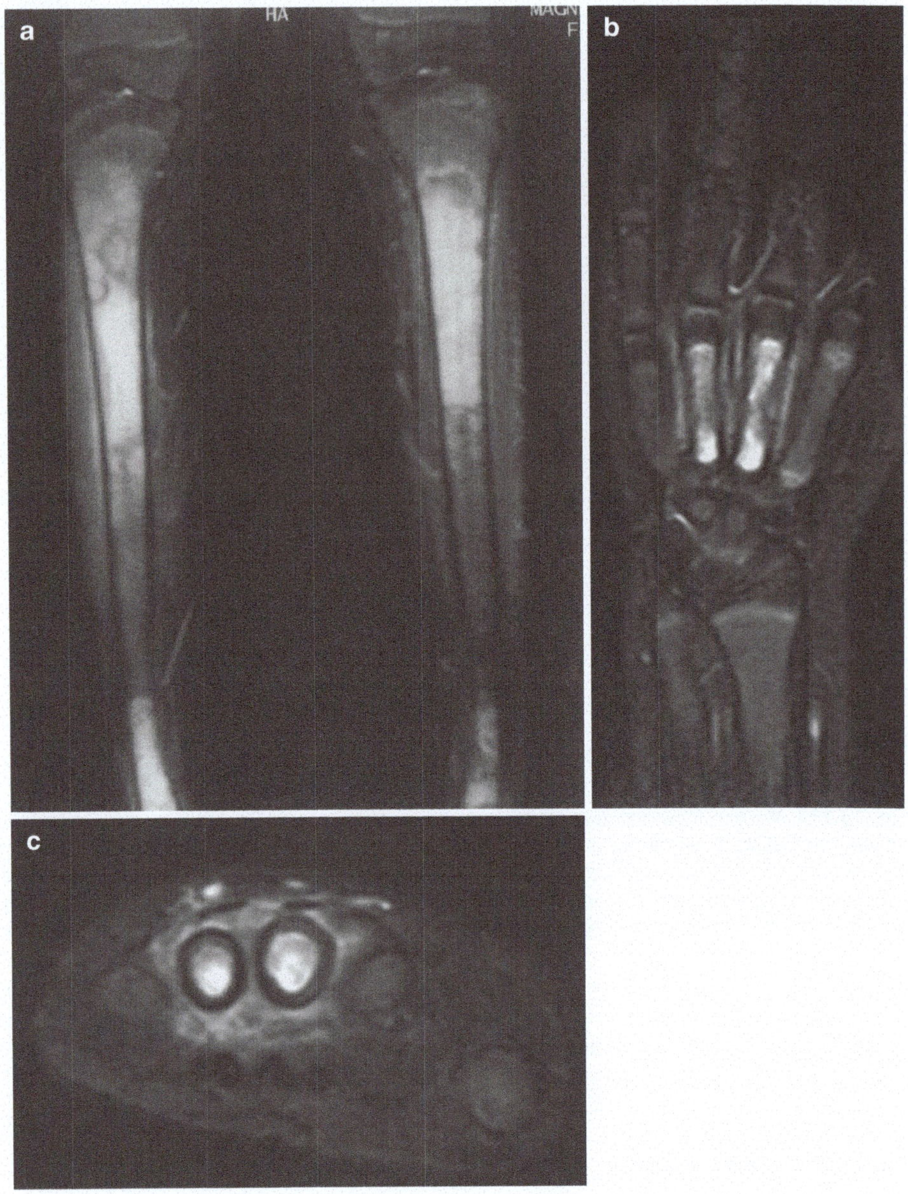

Fig. 13.136 Sickle cell anemia. Coronal STIR image (**a**) of both lower legs reveals bone infarctions with serpiginous low signal intensity rim and associated edema. Coronal STIR image (**b**) and transverse T2-WI (**c**) of the left hand in another patient with acute pain shows extensive bone marrow and soft-tissue edema

whereas osteonecrosis of the metaphysis or diaphysis is referred to as bone infarction. Bone infarction and avascular necrosis are associated with conditions such as sickle cell anemia and other hemoglobinopathies, metabolic conditions (including Gaucher's disease, chronic renal failure), vasculitidies (such as lupus erythematous, juvenile rheumatoid arthritis), and idiopathic diseases (including Legg-Calve-Perthes disease, Koehler's disease, Kienböck's disease, and Panner's disease) (Fig. 13.137). In addition, osteonecrosis may be a sequel of meningococcal infection, slipped capital epiphysis, steroid therapy, radiation, leukemia, and bone marrow transplantation. MRI appearance of bone infarction and avascular necrosis is very similar. In the acute setting, significant marrow and soft-tissue edema are nonspecific findings. In case of epiphyseal osteonecrosis, a reactive joint effusion may be associated. It is important to keep in mind that MRI findings of acute osteonecrosis may be indistinguishable from osteomyelitis, neoplasms such as lymphoma, and stress reaction. In addition, osteonecrosis complicated by insufficiency fracture may also be associated with significant marrow

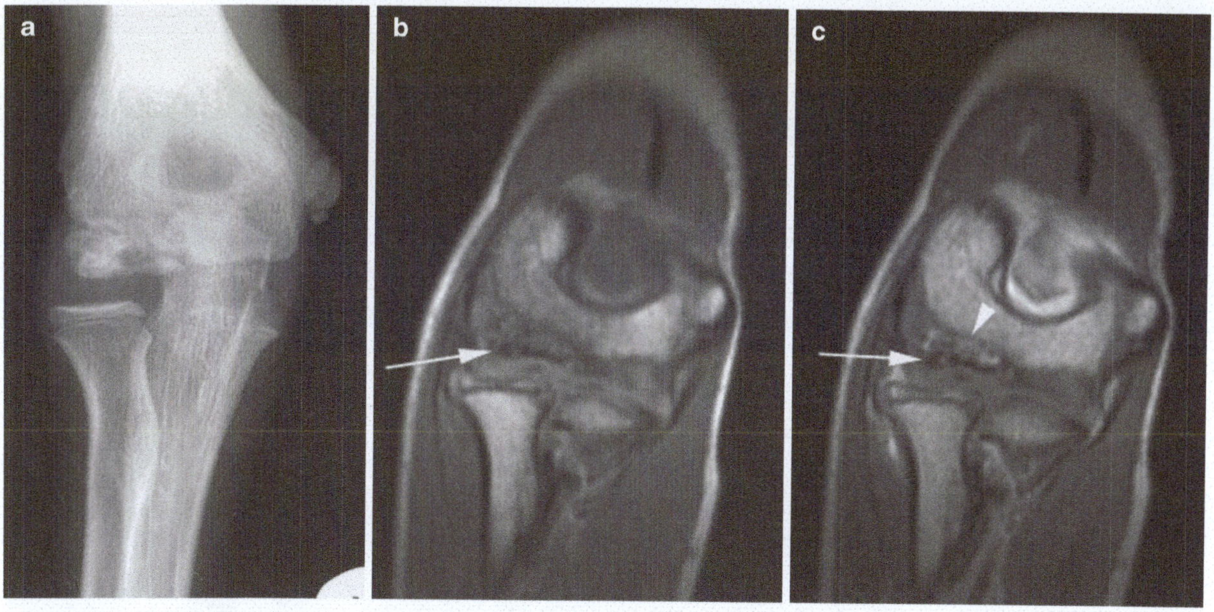

Fig. 13.137 Panner's disease (avascular necrosis of the capitellum). Radiography of the left elbow in AP projection (**a**) shows foci of increased density in the capitellum. Coronal precontrast (**b**) and postcontrast administration T1-WI (**c**) demonstrate hypointense foci in the capitellum on T1-WI, representing sclerosis or ischemic necrosis (*arrow*). Note that the part of the capitellum adjacent to ischemic necrosis (*arrowhead*) and synovium enhances

and soft-tissue edema. In the subacute and chronic setting, osteonecrosis is easier to differentiate from osteomyelitis, as MRI appearance is typically characterized by a serpiginous low SI rim on both T1-WI and T2-WI (Fig. 13.138); this corresponds to the rim of sclerosis sometimes detected on plain films. In more detail, some authors describe the so-called "double line sign" with the outer hypointense rim representing bony sclerosis and the inner T2 hyperintense zone reflecting granulation tissue. In the acute, subacute, and chronic stages, normal fat signal on all sequences of the central island of the infarct may be preserved. However, the center may be of low SI on all imaging sequences, due to sclerosis. Gadolinium is helpful to differentiate granulation tissue and necrotic bone. The most commonly affected site of avascular necrosis in the pediatric age group is the femoral head.

13.5.3.6 Legg-Calvé-Perthes Disease

Legg-Calvé-Perthes (LCP) disease is an idiopathic avascular necrosis of the immature proximal femoral epiphysis, and affects children between the ages of 3 and 12 years. There is a boy-to-girl ratio of 4:1, and a striking retardation of skeletal maturation in both sexes. In 20% of cases, LCP may metachronously occur bilaterally. Children may present with groin, thigh, or knee pain, and limitation of abduction and internal rotation. For the prognosis and treatment of LCP, it is necessary to perform a staging and a grading (extension of femoral head involvement). Probably the most commonly accepted classification based on radiographic findings is the one by Caterall, who divides patients into four prognostic groups based on seven radiographic findings. The prognosis depends on the stage at the time of presentation, the child's age, and the extent of femoral head, physeal, and metaphyseal involvement. Fortunately, 50% of children will do well without treatment. On plain-film radiography, four stages of LCP can be distinguished: initial, fragmentation, reparation, and healed stages. MRI has been used to identify both morphologic and signal characteristics of the proximal femur in early stages, with negative plain-film findings. MRI delineates the extent of physeal and marrow involvement, and thus helps with the prognosis and treatment planning. In advanced disease, MRI can help with preoperative assessment of femoral head coverage and articular integrity.

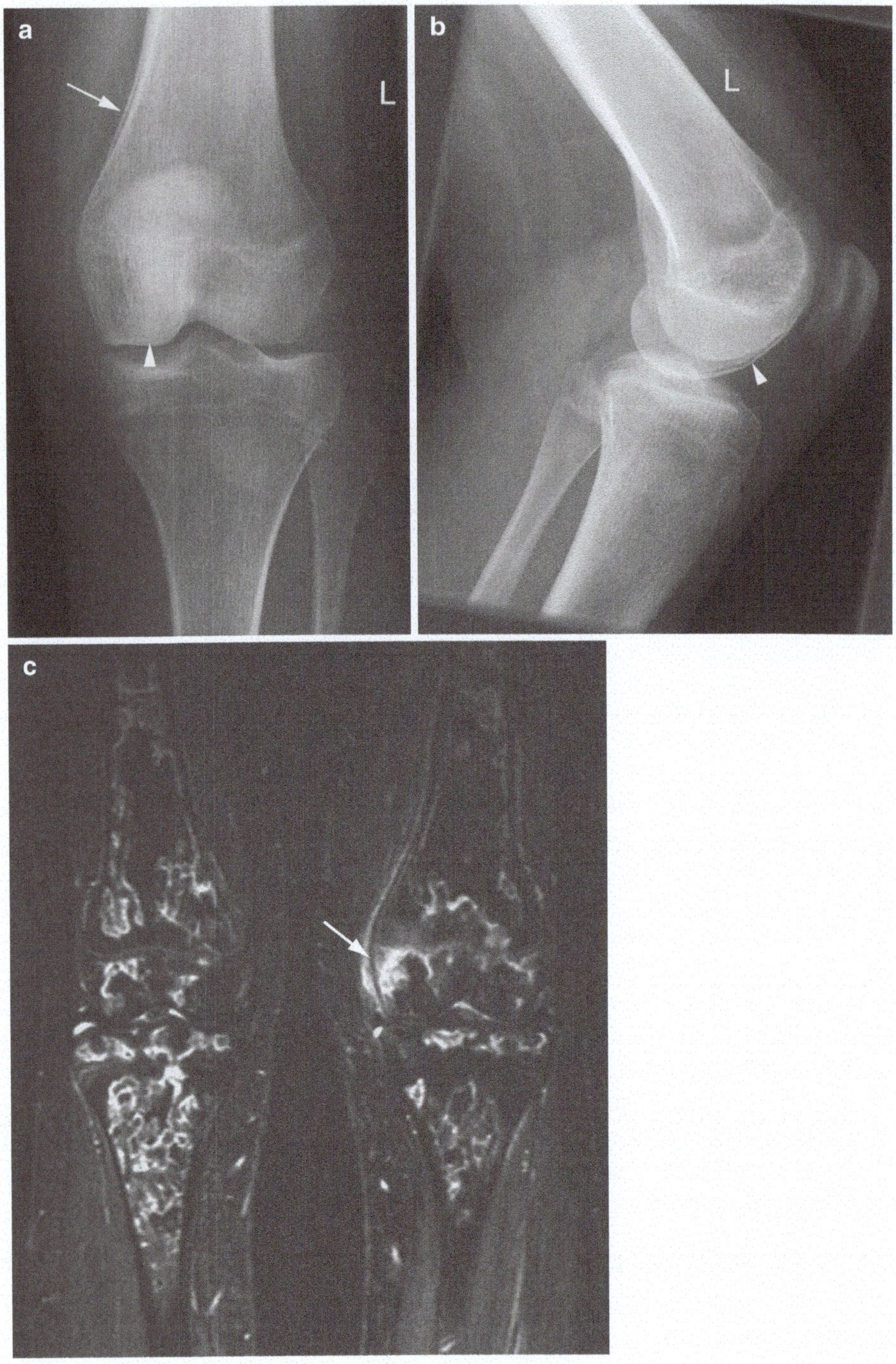

Fig. 13.138 Bone infarctions and avascular necrosis in a 14-year-old girl with lupus erythematous under steroid therapy. Radiography of the left knee in AP (**a**) and lateral projection (**b**) show a unilamellated periosteal reaction medially (*arrow*) and a linear lucency in the medial femoral condyle (*arrowhead*). Coronal STIR (**c**), T1-WI (**d**), and contrast-enhanced fat-saturated T1-WI (**e**) of both knee joints demonstrate bone infarctions and avascular necrosis with serpiginous low signal intensity rim on both T1-WI and T2-WI, and edema in the medial femoral condyle (*arrow*). Transverse T2-WI (**f**) shows reactive joint effusions on both sides

For evaluation of the LCP, coronal T2-WI and T1-WI, precontrast and postcontrast, and additional T1-WI in sagittal orientation are necessary. Slice thickness should be 3–4 mm. MR findings vary with the stage and extent of the disease. In the initial stage, low SI within the epiphyseal marrow on T1-WI and high SI on T2-WI, affecting either the subchondral region or the whole femoral epiphysis, are observed, reflecting bone marrow edema. In the early beginnings of LCP, joint effusions are always present. In this stage, plain-film findings are negative or show subchondral lucency in the femoral head.

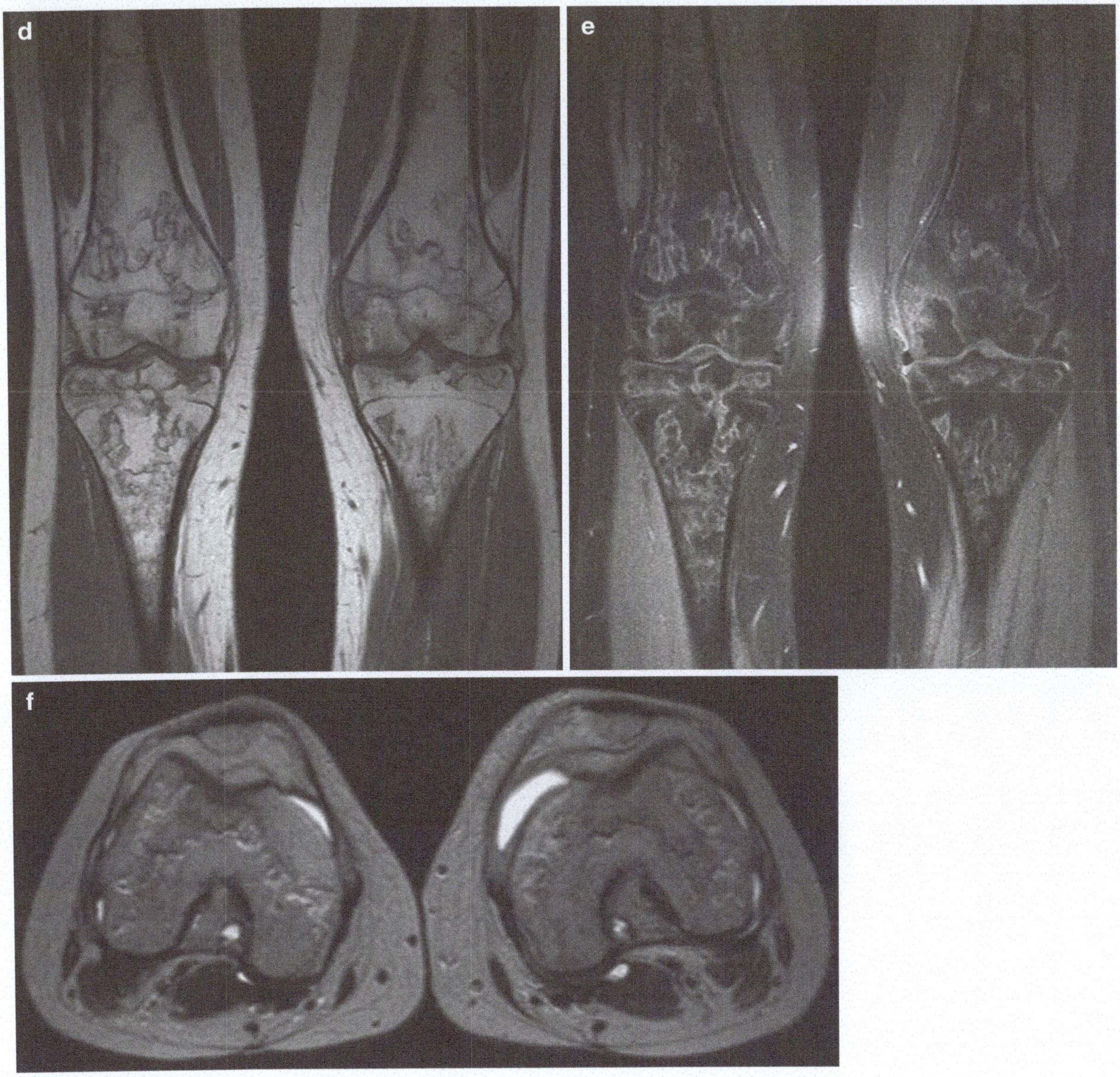

Fig. 13.138 (continued)

In the late initial and fragmentation stages, areas affected by avascular necrosis demonstrate complete loss of signal on T1-WI and T2-WI and show no enhancement after the administration of CM. Metaphyseal involvement with loss of signal on T1-WI may be observed as well. Plain-film radiography in these stages shows either increasing sclerosis, flattening of the femoral head, and/or fragmentation (Fig. 13.139).

During reparation, there is femoral and acetabular cartilaginous hypertrophy, and the normal SI of bone marrow reappears first, medially and laterally; the proximal femur remodels, and deformities of the femoral head become evident.

In the healed stage, the proximal femur is remodeled by trabecular bone, and residual shape alterations may or may not be seen. There may be complete restoration to a normal appearance, or the final stage may be a physeal arrest, a flattened misshapen femoral head, a short femoral neck, or coxa magna. Important items in the differential diagnosis of LCP include

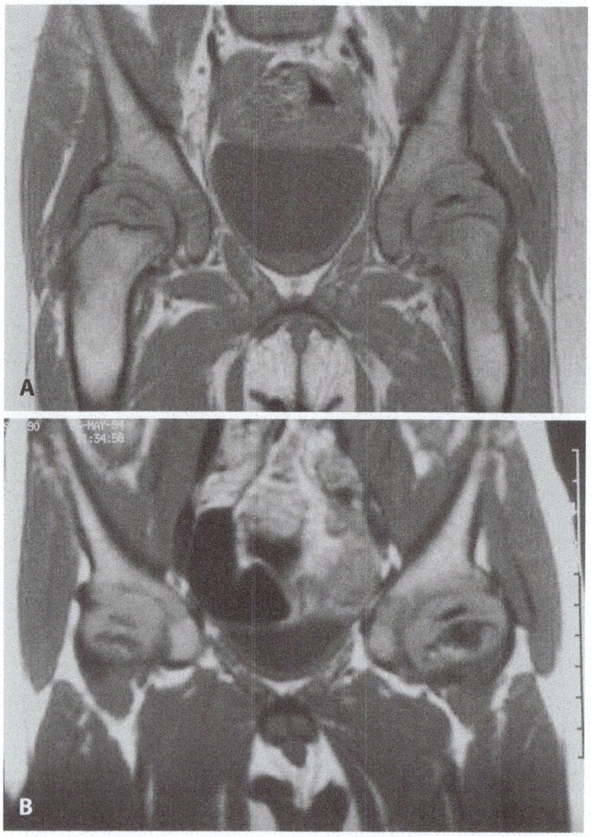

Fig. 13.139 Legg-Calvé-Perthes disease. Coronal T1-WI (**a**) shows complete loss of signal in the left femoral epiphyses and less severe physeal and metaphyseal involvement. Coronal T1-WI (**b**) shows extensive avascular necroses involving epiphyses, physis, and metaphyses on the left side

normal variants (femoral head dysplasia of Meyer in patients less than 4 years of age) and other reasons for avascular necrosis, such as treatment with steroids, trauma, osteomyelitis, hemoglobinopathies, and Gaucher disease. Femoral head deformity is also seen in multiple epiphyseal dysplasias (Fairbank disease), mucopolysaccharidoses, and after developmental dysplasia of the hip. Coxitis fugax can be distinguished from LCP by US showing synovitis, joint effusion, and clinical course, as clinical symptoms of coxitis fugax resolve in less than 4 weeks.

13.5.3.7 Osteochondritis Dissecans

Osteochondritis dissecans (OCD) of the knee most commonly involves, in order of decreasing frequency, the medial femoral condyle, the lateral femoral condyle, the femoral trochlea, and the patella. However, it also occurs in children in the capitellum and the talus (Fig. 13.140). Bilateral involvement of the knees is encountered in 20% of the cases. The exact etiology of OCD is presently unknown, but repetitive microtrauma is probably the primary mechanism leading to development of OCD. However, acute trauma, ischemia, ossification abnormalities, and genetic factors have also been proposed. A staging system for OCD has been developed, based on the arthroscopic findings. An osseous lesion of 1–3 cm in size and an intact articular cartilage characterize stage 1. In stage 2, an articular cartilage defect is present without a loose body. Stage 3 is defined by a partially detached osteochondral fragment with or without interposition of fibrous tissue. In stage 4, a loose body and a defect filled with fibrous tissue are found. OCD of the knee is divided into juvenile and adult forms on the basis of skeletal maturity (open or closed growth plates). Adult OCD may arise de novo, but it is more commonly the result of an incompletely healed previous asymptomatic lesion from juvenile OCD. The separation of OCD of the knee into juvenile and adult forms is clinically relevant, as the two pathologic conditions have distinctly different courses. Juvenile OCD has a much better prognosis than does adult OCD. The focus of OCD shows low SI on both T1-WI and T2-WI. STIR sequences or fluid-sensitive T2*-WIs help to decide whether cartilage is intact or not. Areas of high SI on these sequences reflect subchondral fluid or cystic lesions secondary to fissuring of the overlying cartilage. Administration of CM provides information about the degree of vascularization of the focus. Healed lesions do not demonstrate a bright SI interface between the fragment and the bone, and show return of normal fat-marrow signal. A high T2 signal rim or cysts surrounding an adult osteochondritis dissecans lesion are unequivocal signs of instability. However, a high intensity rim surrounding a juvenile OCD lesion indicates instability only if it has the same SI as adjacent joint fluid, is surrounded by a second outer rim of low T2 signal intensity, or is accompanied by multiple breaks in the subchondral bone plate on T2-WI. Cysts surrounding a juvenile OCD lesion indicate instability only if they are multiple or large in size.

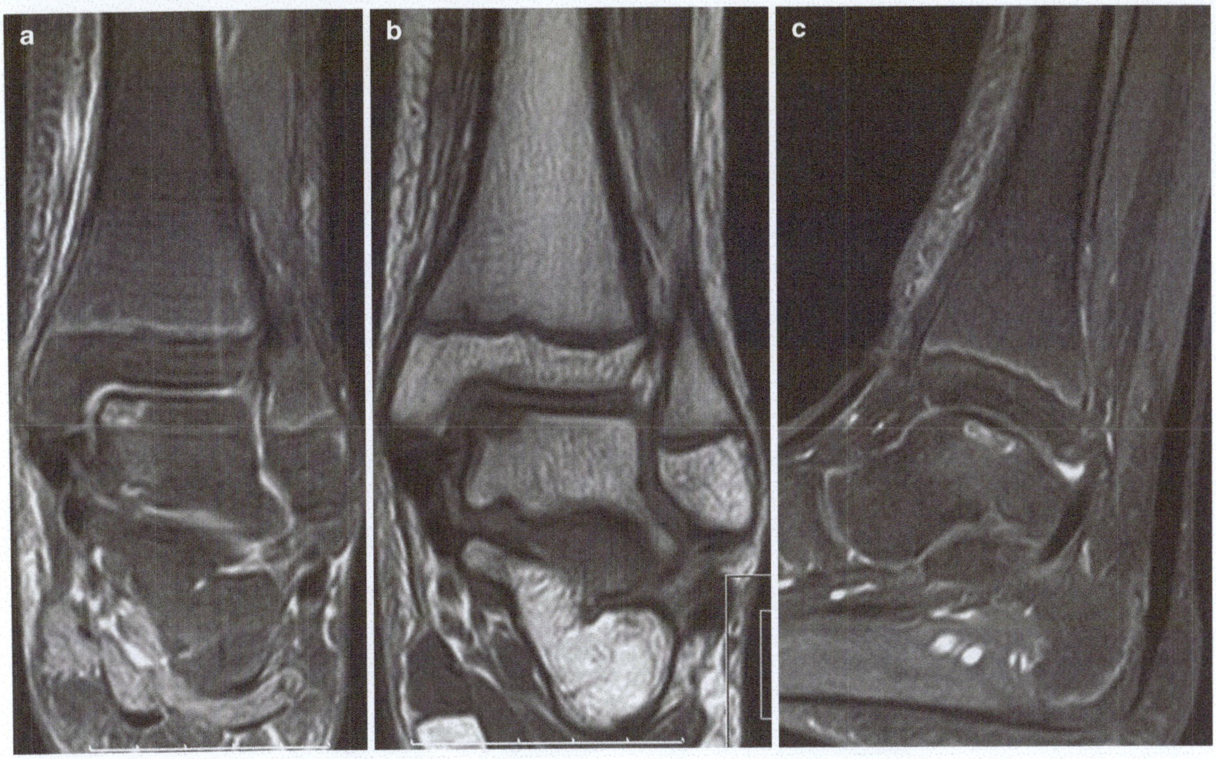

Fig. 13.140 Osteochondritis dissecans. Coronal fat-saturated PD-WI (**a**) and T1-WI (**b**) show an osteochondral lesion of the medial talar dome. The overlying cortex and cartilage are intact. Sagittal fat-saturated contrast-enhanced T1-WI (**c**) demonstrates inhomogeneous enhancement of the lesion

13.5.4 Synovial Disorders

13.5.4.1 Juvenile Rheumatoid Arthritis

The diagnosis of juvenile rheumatoid arthritis (JRA) may be made when a patient presents under the age of 16 years with arthritic symptoms for at least 6 weeks. The alternative nomenclature for JRA accepted by the ILAR (International League of Associations of Rheumatologists) is juvenile idiopathic arthritis (JIA). JRA/JIA is divided into four subtypes. The negative rheumatoid factor subtypes include: oligoarticular (four joints or less are involved), polyarticular (more than four joints involved), and systemic disease (Still's disease – polyarticular disease with characteristic fever, hepatosplenomegaly, lymphadenopathy, pericarditis, pleuritis, peritonitis, interstitial lung disease, evanescent rash, and macrophage activation syndrome). The positive rheumatoid factor subtype usually occurs in older children, more often in females, and is polyarticular. Clinical symptoms are analogous to its adult counterpart. Generally, MRI appearance of JRA does not differ from rheumatoid arthritis in adults, and the pattern of distribution of inflammatory changes within the hand and wrist are basically the same. A rather characteristic finding in JRA is periostitis, which is not seen in adult patients with rheumatoid arthritis unless there has been trauma or infection. In the early stage of JRA, plain-film findings in children are negative or show osteopenia and periarticular soft-tissue swelling. Localized hyperemia leads to osteopenia on the one hand and, on the other hand, to an advanced bone age of the involved joint or joints. Therefore, JRA may be the only indication for acquisition of a contralateral plain film. Erosions and joint space narrowing are late manifestations of the disease in children, as they have relatively thick articular and epiphyseal cartilage protecting the subchondral bone from synovial inflammation (Fig. 13.141a, b). Hyperemia and disuse are the reasons for epiphyseal overgrowth associated with gracile diaphyses, but these

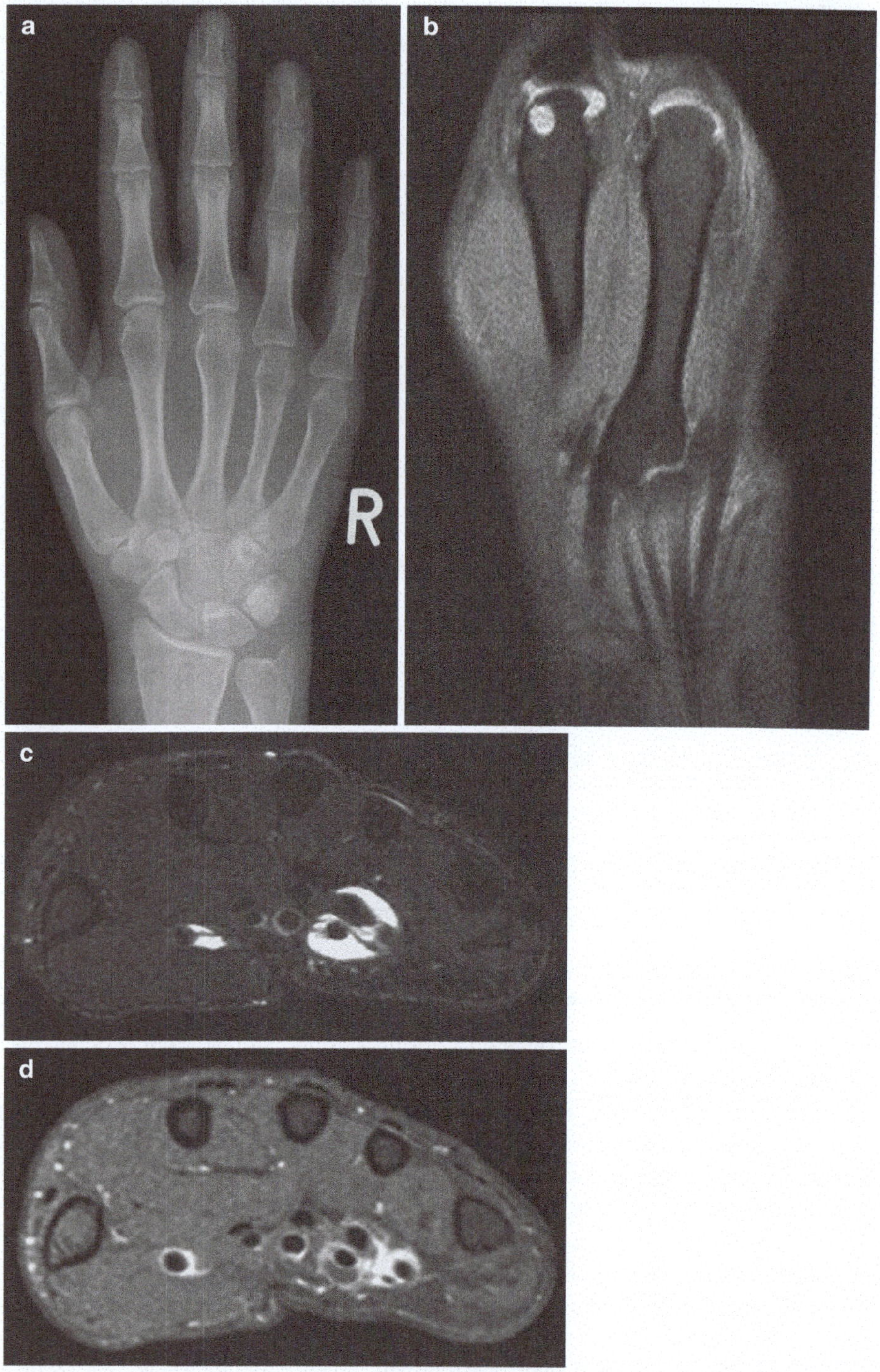

Fig. 13.141 Juvenile rheumatoid arthritis. Radiograph of the right hand (**a**) and coronal T2-WI (**b**) show erosion in the second metacarpal bone and fluid in the MCP II and III joints. Transverse STIR image (**c**) and fat-saturated contrast-enhanced T1-WI (**d**) demonstrate fluid in the flexor tendon sheaths and diffuse tendon sheath enhancement in a 15-year-old girl with RF positive polyarticular JRA. Note acceleration of bone age

are also findings in late disease. Chronic synovitis leads to synovial hypertrophy, pannus formation, and rice bodies, followed by cartilage and bone destruction, eventually ending in ankylosis or joint instability. Intraarticular rice bodies are composed of necrotic cellular debris encapsulated by fibrin and/or collagen, and are usually hypointense on T1-WI and T2-WI. Pannus is composed of reactive granulation tissue in the joint. Fibrous pannus is hypointense on T1-WI and hypointense to intermediate on T2-WI, and shows minimal enhancement, whereas hypervascular pannus is hypointense on T1-WI and intermediate to hyperintense on T2-WI, and enhances significantly after administration of paramagnetic contrast. As it is difficult to distinguish synovial hypertrophy from joint fluid on both T1-WI and T2-WI, the administration of CM is crucial to delineate enhancing synovium (Fig. 13.142). On FS PD-WI, synovial hypertrophy tends to be less hyperintense compared to joint fluid. If paramagnetic contrast is not applied in a child with unexplained joint pain and swelling, the proper diagnosis may be missed or made with delay. In addition, MRI is ordered by the clinician in patients with known JRA, to determine the level of disease activity prior to changes in medical therapy. The MRI features useful in evaluating response to therapy and predicting future articular destruction and erosions are subchondral bone edema seen on fluid-sensitive sequences, subchondral bone enhancement, and extent of synovial hypertrophy and enhancement. In a given joint, subchondral bone edema correlates with future sites of erosion and degrees of synovial hypertrophy show a relationship with future number of erosions. Active and inactive erosions, subchondral cysts, and pre-erosive osteitis should always be evaluated on MRI, in correlation with plain films. Both, pre-erosive osteitis and active erosions show increased SI on T2-WI and contrast enhancement after administration of paramagnetic contrast on T1-WI, but can be differentiated by the presence of normal bony cortex and cartilage overlying the area of subchondral edema. Longstanding JRA may also lead to lipoma arborescens, which represents synovial metaplasia that may be primary or secondary to trauma or inflammatory arthritis and follows fat on all imaging sequences. Tenosynovitis and myositis may be primary manifestations of JRA or may be secondary to an adjacent arthritis (Fig. 13.141c, d). MRI features of tenosynovitis include tendon thickening, enhancement and edema, and fluid within the surrounding tendon sheath. As tendon rupture may be a sequel of tenosynovitis, careful evaluation of tendon integrity on sagittal or coronal sequences is necessary. Most importantly, when a single joint is involved, the possibility of aseptic arthritis must always be excluded.

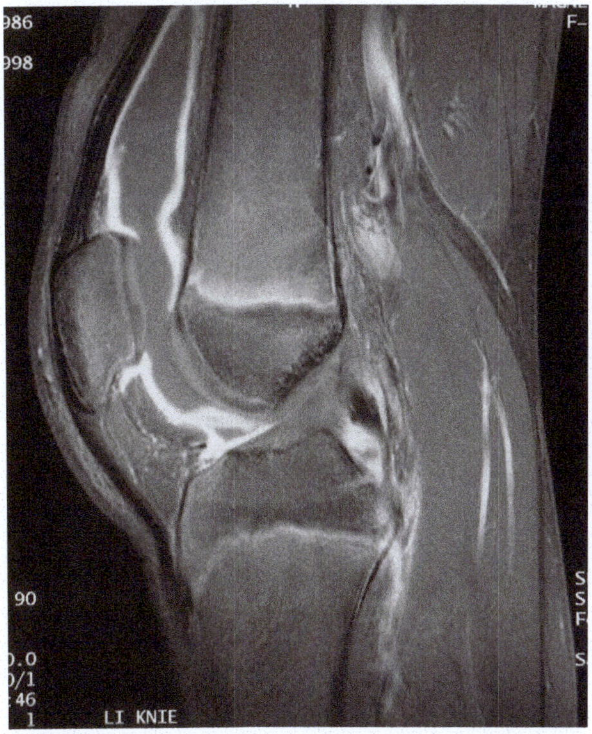

Fig. 13.142 Juvenile chronic polyarthritis. Sagittal contrast-enhanced fat-saturated T1-WI shows marked synovial enhancement and joint effusion

13.5.4.2 Lyme Arthritis

Lyme arthritis is a late sequel of a systemic infection by *Borrelia burgdorferi*, which is a tick-borne disease, and can occur weeks to years after initial infection. The knee is affected in 80% of the cases, and usually only a single joint is involved (Fig. 13.143). However, the shoulders, elbows, ankles, hips, wrists, temporomandibular joint, and even the small bones of the extremities can be affected. Lyme arthritis may present acutely with knee pain that is indistinguishable clinically from septic arthritis or a new onset of juvenile rheumatoid arthritis. It is not possible to differentiate Lyme arthritis from oligoarticular JRA or septic arthritis by MRI, but MRI is helpful to rule out osteomyelitis with secondary septic arthritis, abscess, neoplasm, or pigmented villonodular synovitis (PVNS).

13.5.4.3 Hemophilia

In hemophilia, deficiency of factor VIII (hemophilia A) or factor IX (hemophilia B) causes repeated hemarthrosis, leading to synovial inflammation, pannus and fibrous-tissue formation, focal or diffuse cartilage

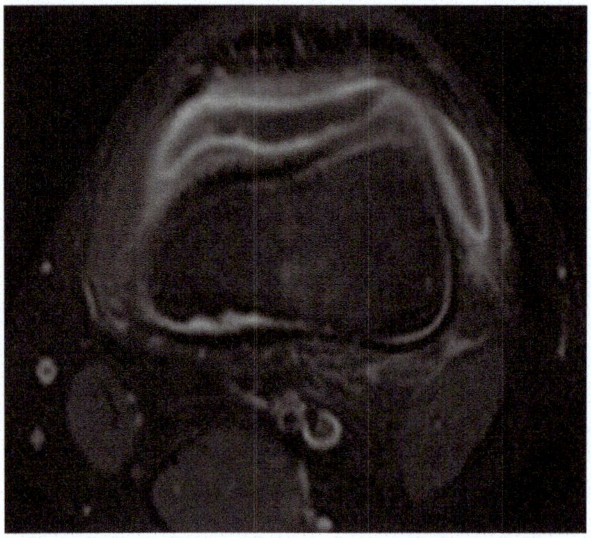

Fig. 13.143 Lyme arthritis. Transverse contrast-enhanced fat-saturated T1-WI shows synovial enhancement and joint effusion (Courtesy of O. Rompel)

destruction, and subchondral cysts with variable signal contents. Due to hemosiderin deposition, the hypertrophic synovium demonstrates low SI on T1-WI and T2-WI. This susceptibility artifact is best appreciated on GRE sequences. Fibrous tissue also presents with low SI on T1-W and T2-W sequences. Additional typical findings are thickened, irregular fat pads, and joint effusions with variable SI, depending on the presence of various blood breakdown products. The most commonly involved joint is the knee, followed by the ankle (Fig. 13.144), elbow, and shoulder. MRI in hemophilic arthropathy is performed to detect degenerative changes before they are visible on plain films, in order to determine whether the patient will benefit from synovectomy.

13.5.5 Acute Osteomyelitis and Septic Arthritis

The majority of pediatric cases of osteomyelitis are due to hematogenous spread from acute sepsis with bacterial, viral, or other infectious agents. *Staphylococcus aureus* is responsible for up to 70% of hematogenous osteomyelitis, and 30% of the patients have a history of upper respiratory infection, otitis media, or other infections. Osteomyelitis may also result from a direct penetrating wound, or spread to bone by extension from other adjacent structures. The majority of cases of hematogenous osteomyelitis

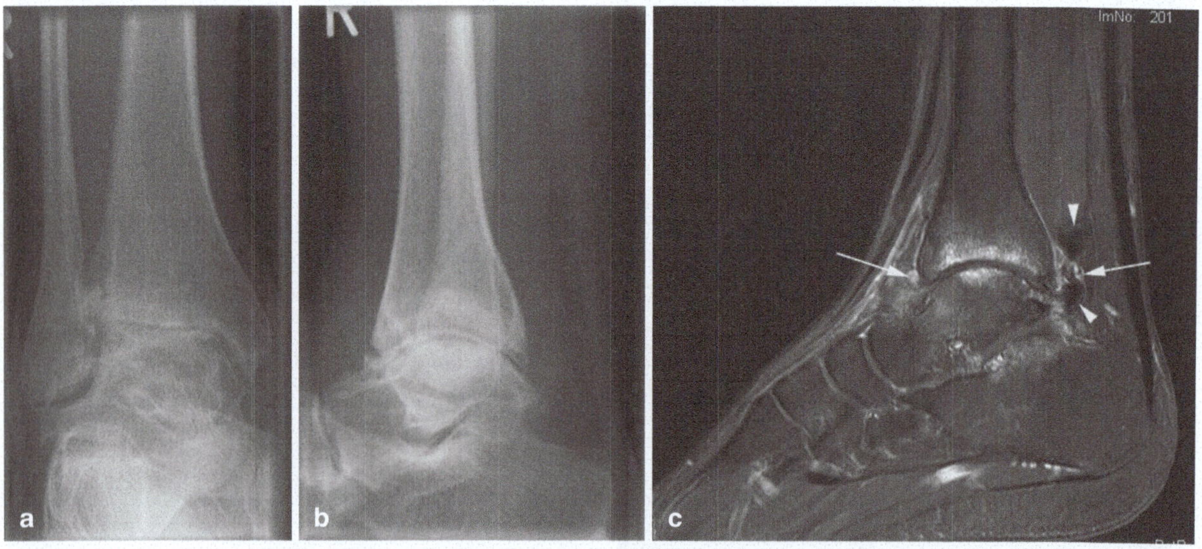

Fig. 13.144 Hemophilic arthropathy. Radiography of the right ankle in AP (**a**) and lateral projection (**b**) show severe secondary osteoarthritis due to recurrent bleeding into the joint in a 21-year-old boy with hemophilia A. Sagittal contrast-enhanced fat-saturated T1-WI (**c**) demonstrates cartilaginous destruction, joint space narrowing, marrow edema in the talus, and subchondral tibial plafond. The synovium is thickened and shows diffuse enhancement (*arrow*). In addition, hemosiderin depositions in the posterior recessus (*arrowheads*) are present

involve the tubular bones and the metaphysis. In children younger than 18 months, transphyseal vessels still exist, and infection can therefore spread to the physis, epiphysis, and the adjacent joint. In older children, avascular physeal cartilage acts as a relative barrier (Fig. 13.145). Spread to the medullary cavity and diaphysis easily occurs. In children, most cases of septic arthritis are due to spread from an adjacent focus of osteomyelitis, leading to synovitis and joint effusions, possibly being complicated by epiphyseal infarction and joint destruction. Osteomyelitis is difficult to diagnose in the first years of life, as it is usually silent, and is often detected only 2–4 weeks after onset of infection. Plain-film radiographs obtained during the first week of disease may show nothing but soft-tissue swelling. Later on, destructive bone changes appear as focal or confluent radiolucencies in bone (Fig. 13.146a,b). After approximately 10 days, early periosteal new bone formation is observed. MRI is the method of choice to diagnose osteomyelitis and primary or secondary arthritis, as differentiation between isolated periostitis, medullary infection, periosteal abscess, and involvement of joints can be excellently depicted. On MRI, osteomyelitis appears as a defined focal lesion in the metaphysis (Fig. 13.147) (and/or epiphysis in children under 18 months of age, Fig. 13.146c, d), with low SI on T1-WI and high SI on T2-WI, accompanied by edema extending into the marrow and adjacent soft tissues. After administration of CM, infected tissues vividly enhance and nonenhancing areas of necrosis can be detected. Joint effusion in the setting of intraarticular osteomyelitis may be due to a sympathetic effusion or secondary to septic arthritis. A feature suggesting sympathetic effusion is a modest thin synovial enhancement, whereas secondary septic arthritis is characterized by thick and irregular synovial enhancement, the presence of a cloaca, a direct intraarticular communication with osteomyelitis via a cortical breach. Primary septic arthritis usually presents with symmetric marrow edema on both sides of the joint, whereas asymmetric marrow edema on both sides of the joint is more typically for secondary septic arthritis caused by intraarticular osteomyelitis. The alternative diagnoses of joint effusion with juxtaarticular marrow edema are primary septic arthritis, Lyme arthritis, JRA, spondylarthropathy such as psoriatic arthritis, or trauma. Finally, osteomyelitis may be indistinguishable from Ewing's sarcoma on radiographic and MR findings.

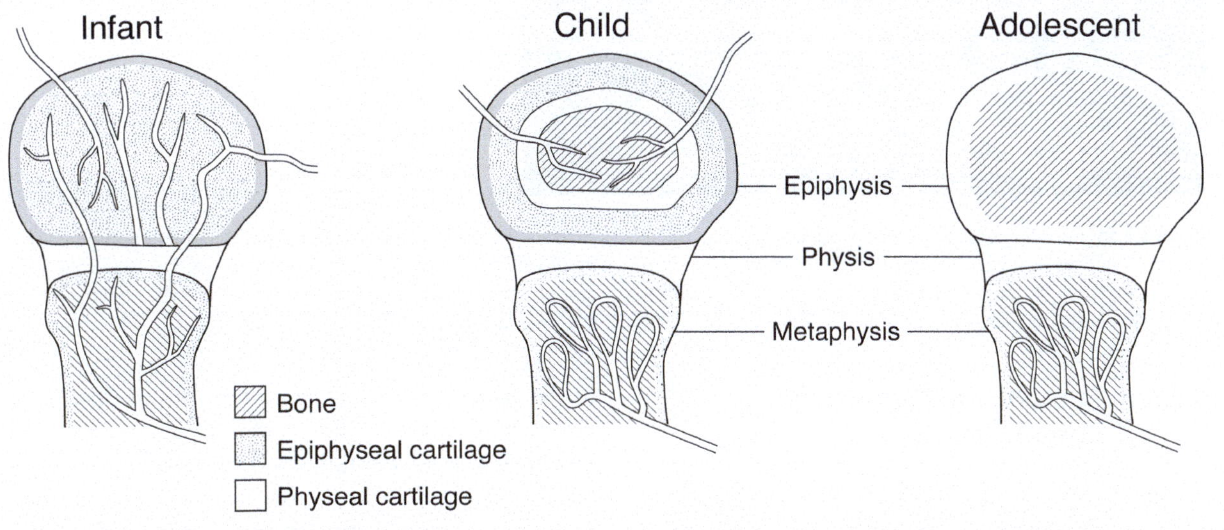

Fig. 13.145 Age-related changes in the anatomy of a growing long bone. *Infant*: the epiphysis is completely or almost completely cartilaginous. Epiphyseal and metaphyseal vessels communicate across the physis. *Child*: the ossification center in the epiphysis is well formed. The physis acts as a relative barrier between epiphyseal and metaphyseal vessels. *Adolescent*: the epiphysis is ossified, but the physis remains cartilaginous. The epiphysis has fewer vessels than the metaphysis (Adapted from Kirks 1998)

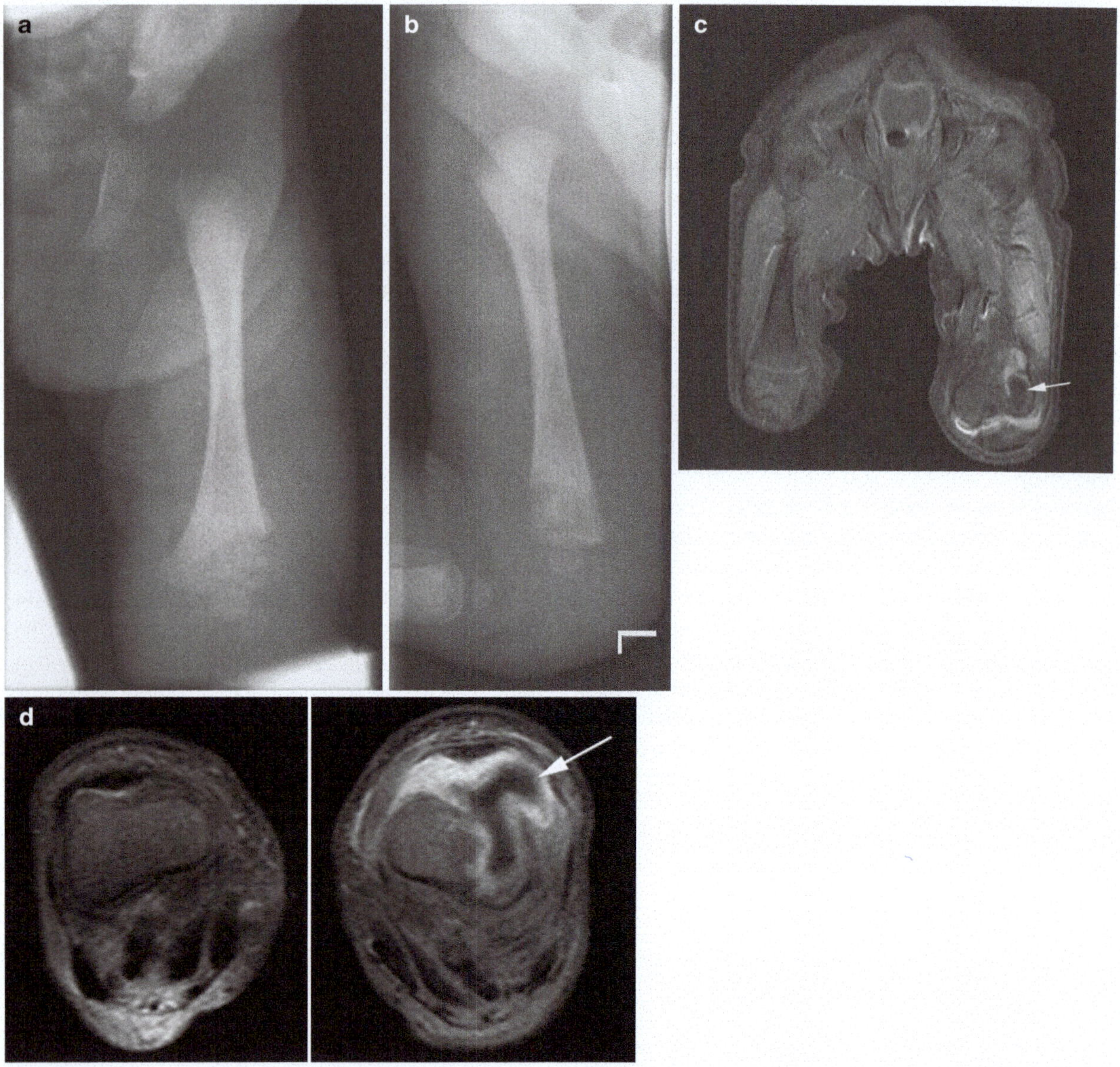

Fig. 13.146 Osteomyelitis in a neonate. Radiography of the left femur in AP (**a**) and lateral projection (**b**) demonstrate a large osteolytic defect in the distal metaphysis. Coronal (**c**) and transverse (**d**) contrast-enhanced fat-saturated T1-WI show an abscess (*arrows*) in the physis of the left distal femur extending into the epiphysis as well as into the metaphysis, in a 4 week-old girl. Her mother suffered from vaginal infection with *Staph. aureus*, which was insufficiently treated

13.5.6 Tumors and Tumor-Like Conditions

The diagnosis of musculoskeletal tumors is still primarily based on plain-film radiographs, and confirmed by biopsy. As a rule, MR examinations of tumors and tumor-like conditions should not be performed without plain-film radiography. Due to advances in neoadjuvant therapy and surgical techniques, approximately 80% of the patients with malignant bone lesions are now potential candidates for limb-salvage procedures. Determination of the tumor extent, detection of skip lesions, and evaluation of vital structure involvement, such as neurovascular bundles, adjacent muscle groups, joint and transphyseal extension, is best accomplished by MRI. In addition, assessment of successful therapy, completeness or complications of surgery, and detection of recurrent disease can be monitored by MRI.

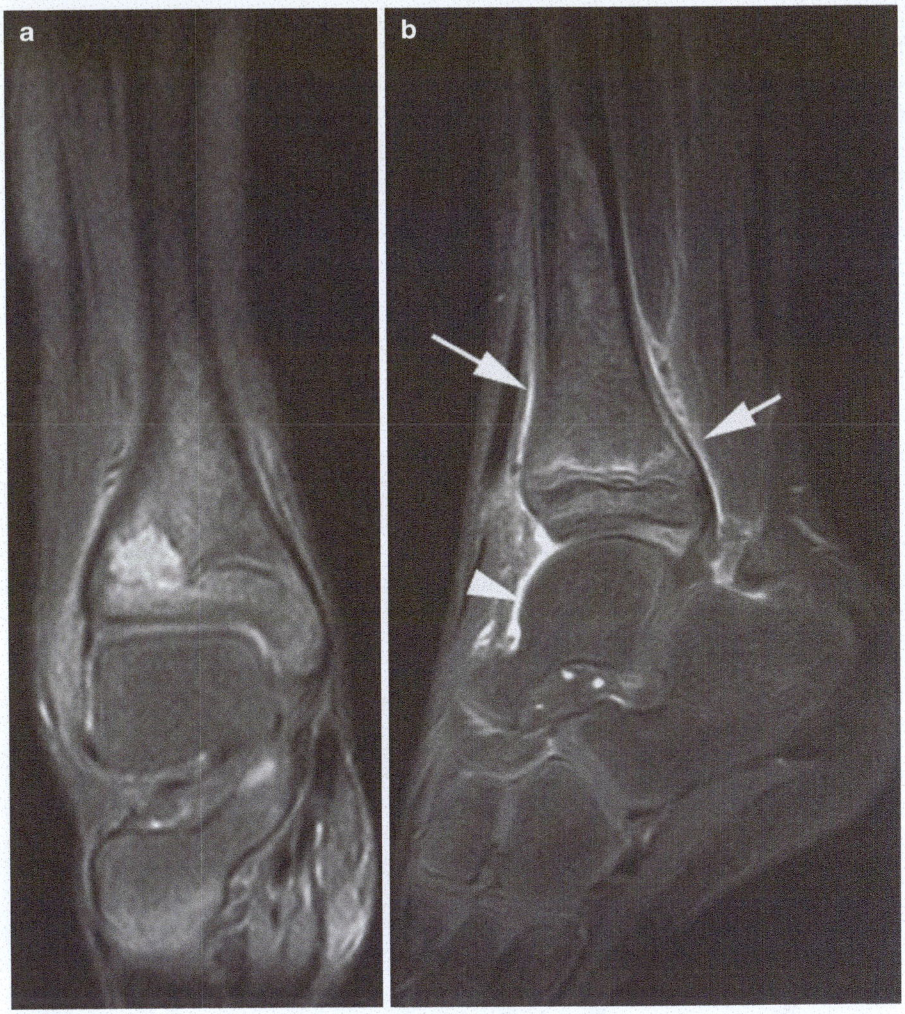

Fig. 13.147 Osteomyelitis in an older child. Coronal fat-saturated T2-WI (**a**) demonstrates increased signal intensity in the metaphyses of the distal tibia medially. Sagittal fat-saturated contrast-enhanced T1-WI (**b**) demonstrates enhancement of the adjacent soft tissues (*arrows*) and synovium (*arrowhead*)

Indicators suggesting a response to therapy include decrease of tumor size and peritumoral edema with better demarcation and recurrence of normal fatty marrow signal. However, in many cases, the presence or absence of vital tumor cells may only be proven by biopsy.

When evaluating an extremity tumor, obtaining a combination of transverse and coronal or sagittal images, including the entire length of an involved bone, is recommended. Whether coronal or sagittal planes should be obtained depends on the location of the lesion. A process located ventrally or dorsally should be examined in the sagittal plane, whereas a process located medially or laterally is better evaluated by coronal plane imaging. Contrast should be administered for better delineation of the tumor and for distinction between tumor and necrosis.

T1-W SE sequences in a coronal plane are best for judgment of intramedullary extent, whereas T2-W transverse images are suitable for the evaluation of invasion into adjacent musculature and neurovascular bundles. Dynamic MRI and FS T1-WI after the administration of CM are recommended, to make a distinction between tumor, peritumoral edema, and necrosis. In the following paragraphs, attention is given to the most common pediatric tumors. The role of DWI in these cases is currently under debate.

13.5.6.1 Benign Bone and Soft-Tissue Tumors

There are no generally accepted indications for the performance of MR imaging of benign bone tumors such as unicameral bone cyst, osteochondroma, enchondroma, and chondroblastoma, as they show typical findings on conventional plain-film radiographs. However, in indistinct cases, MRI may be helpful either in assuring the diagnosis or determining whether a given lesion should be biopsied.

Osteoid Osteoma

Patients with osteoid osteoma typically present with a history of pain, especially at night, which is relieved by aspirin. However, osteoid osteoma can also cause a variety of different symptoms, such as joint effusion, painful scoliosis, limb-length discrepancy, or local gigantism in a digit. The majority of osteoid osteomas arise from the diaphysis or metaphysis of the femur, followed by the tibia, these being the most common locations. There are four different types of osteoid osteomas: cortical, medullary, subperiosteal, and intraarticular. When greater than 1.5 cm in diameter, the lesions are generally considered osteoblastomas, which have an identical histology but a greater predilection for the axial skeleton. The cortical type is the most frequent (80–90%). The lesion is characterized by a central, often calcified, nidus surrounded by reactive bone sclerosis and cortical thickening. On MRI, the nonossified nidus has high SI on T2-WI and is almost always invisible on T1-WI prior to the administration of paramagnetic contrast (Fig. 13.148). The ossified nidus is hypointense on both T1-WI and T2-WI, but surrounded by a rim, which is hypointense on T1-WI and hyperintense on T2-WI. Associated bone marrow, periosteal reaction, and extraosseous soft-tissue edema enhancing with paramagnetic contrast are frequently observed. MRI is limited as a primary investigative tool for the evaluation of osteoid osteoma because it may suggest other neoplastic or inflammatory processes, as the nidus may be inconspicuous and

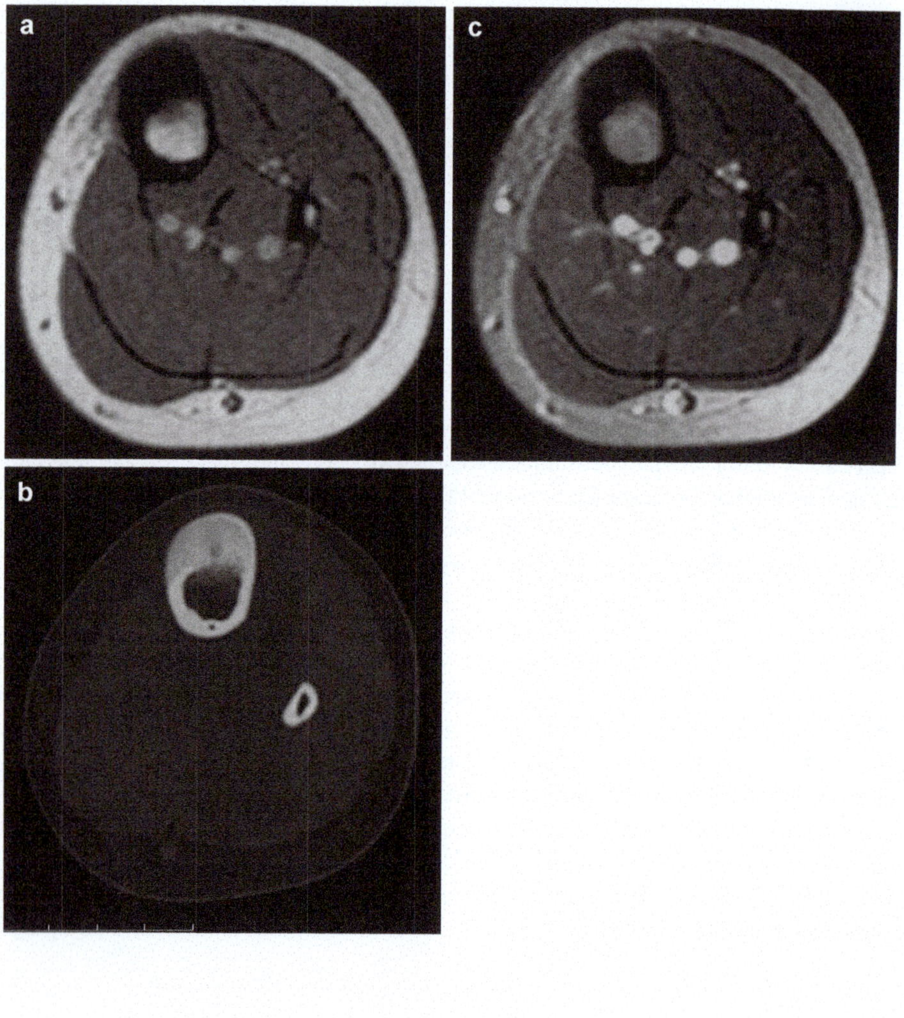

Fig. 13.148 Cortical osteoid osteoma. Transverse T1-W precontrast (**a**) and postcontrast (**b**) images demonstrate enhancing nidus in the left tibia, with marked reactive bone sclerosis. Corresponding transverse CT (**c**) depicts a nonossified nidus

soft tissue and marrow edema are nonspecific. Therefore, CT may be superior to MRI in evaluating patients with suspected osteoid osteoma. The MRI diagnosis of an intraarticular osteoid osteoma is even more challenging, as synovitis and joint effusions are encountered and periosteal reaction and bony sclerosis may be absent. Intraarticular osteoid osteoma may mimic chondroblastoma, epiphyseal osteomyelitis, and pyogenic and non-pyogenic arthritis.The main differential considerations for osteoid osteoma in the absence of a discrete mass are stress injury and osteomyelitis.

Aneurysmal Bone Cyst

Aneurysmal bone cysts (ABCs) are most commonly found in the posterior osseous elements of the spine and in the long bones, where they appear as expansile, lytic, and eccentric metaphyseal lesions. However, ABCs may also arise from the cortex, the surface (between the periosteum and cortex), or both. In children, the five most common locations, in order of frequency, are the femur, tibia, spine, humerus, and pelvis. On MRI, ABCs present as well-defined lesions, with lobulated margins, and areas of mixed SI on T1-W and T2-W sequences, reflecting chronicity of the associated hemorrhage. ABCs may have multiple cavities containing fluid-fluid levels, probably representing layering of uncoagulated blood within the lesion, separated by enhancing internal septations (Fig. 13.149). Fluid-fluid levels were initially believed to be highly suggestive of ABCs, but they have also been described in lesions such as simple bone cysts, fibrous dysplasias, giant cell tumors, chondroblastomas, telangiectatic osteosarcomas, vascular malformations, and malignant fibrous histiocytomas. One third of ABCs are secondary to preexisting lesions, such as giant-cell tumors, osteoblastomas, chondroblastomas, fibrous dysplasias, nonossifying fibromas, chondromyxoid fibromas, and osteosarcomas. The presence of solid tumor and/or enhancing components as well as cortical destruction in an ABC should always raise the consideration of an underlying primary lesion. Due to the aforementioned association with osteosarcoma and the fact that the telangiectatic variant of osteosarcoma, in particular, may be indistinguishable from ABCs, close clinical follow-up and biopsy are mandatory in these lesions. Once the diagnosis of a primary ABC is established, it is important, for planning of the treatment, to describe exactly the extent of the lesion and its relationship to the growth plate. Additionally, MRI is very useful to monitor therapy, as ABCs have a high local recurrence rate following curettage.

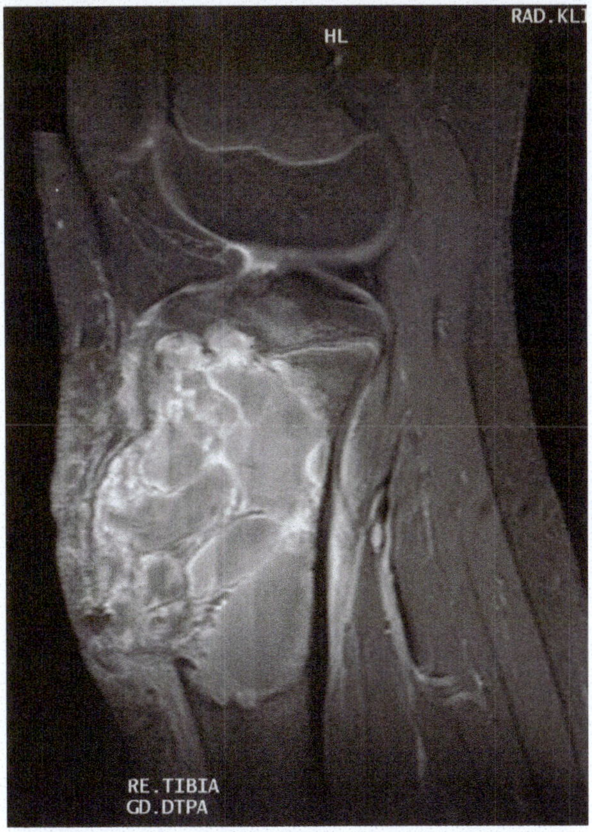

Fig. 13.149 Aneurysmal bone cyst. Sagittal contrast-enhanced fat-saturated T1-WI shows multiple fluid-fluid levels in this expansile growing lesion in the left tibia

Langerhans' Cell Histiocytosis

Langerhans' cell histiocytosis (LCH) is a disease of unknown etiology and is characterized by an abnormal proliferation of Langerhans' cells (LC), with either focal or systemic manifestation. LCH clinically presents in three different types: eosinophilic granuloma (EG), Letterer-Siwe disease (LS), and Hand-Schüller-Christian disease (HSC) (Table 13.20). Many cases of LCH cannot be categorized into one of the aforementioned groups, as there is considerable overlap and evolution from one syndrome to the other. The prognosis of EG is excellent, whereas the prognosis of the disseminated forms strongly depends on the number of

Table 13.20 Manifestations of Langerhans' cell histiocytosis

	LS	HSC	EO
Type	Acute disseminated	Disseminated	Localized
Age range (year)	<1	3–6	10–14
Frequency (%)	10	20	80
Involved organs	Skin, liver, spleen, lymph nodes, bone marrow	Classic triad: diabetes insipidus, exophthalmus, calvarial destruction	Bone or lung

LS Letterer-Siwe; *HSC* Hand-Schüller-Christian; *EO* eosinophilic granuloma

involved organs and the extent of organ infiltration. The therapy for LCH depends on the histologic classification and the extent of disease. It may consist of observation without intervention, intralesional steroid injection or curettage of the involved bone in EG, or even chemotherapy.

The most common sites of skeletal involvement in LCH are the skull (28%) (Fig. 13.150), the ribs (14%), the femur (13%), the pelvis (10%), the spine (7%), the mandible (7%), and the humerus (6%). LCH can have many different radiographic appearances. Lesions in flat bones tend to be well-defined lytic lesions, whereas lesions in long bones more often present as lytic lesions with reactive sclerosis and periosteal reaction, most commonly located in the diaphysis. LCH of the skull presents with uneven destruction of the inner and outer tables or other peculiar calvarial lesions in children, involving the sella turcica, mastoids, orbits, and mandible (floating teeth). Involvement of the spine typically manifests as vertebra plana (Fig. 13.151) and a soft-tissue paravertebral mass. On MRI, the area of abnormal SI is usually larger than suggested by plain-film radiography. The lesions are hyperintense on T2-WI and STIR images and hypointense on T1-WI, with homogeneous enhancement after CM. However, MRI cannot distinguish actual LCH involvement from edema in soft tissues and bone marrow. The MRI features of LCH are nonspecific during the active phase and may mimic other aggressive-appearing entities such as osteomyelitis, Ewing's sarcoma, and lymphoma. LCH involving tubular bones arises from the medullary cavity and may demonstrate cortical destruction with extraosseus soft tissue extension. A clue that favors the diagnosis of LCH on MRI is sharply marginated cortical destruction, correlating with a narrow zone of transition on plain film radiography and CT. Even in the absence of a pathologic fracture, very often adjacent marrow and juxtacortical soft-tissue edema can be observed (Fig. 13.152). In the healing phase, low SI on both T1-WI and T2-WI may be seen. More

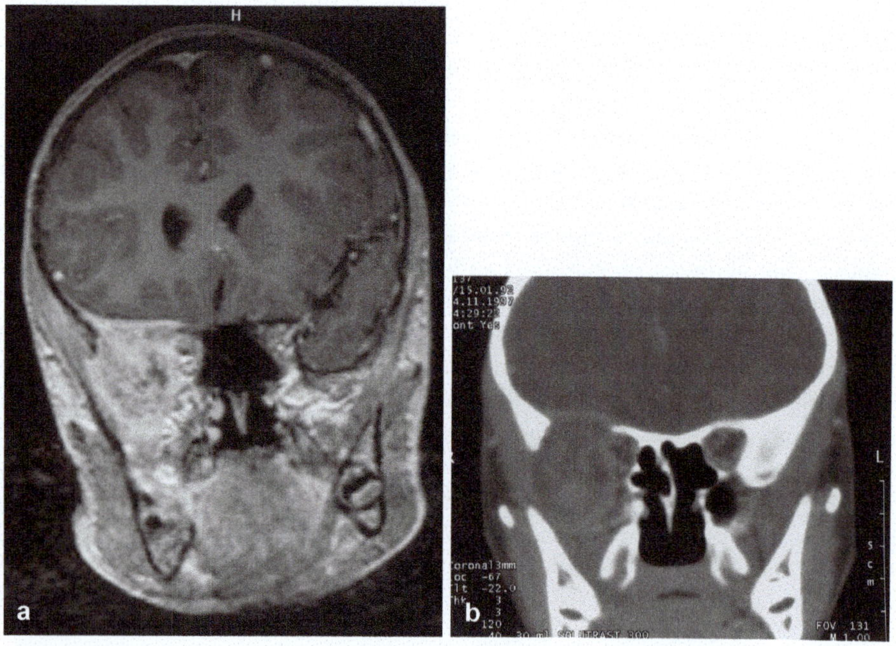

Fig. 13.150 Langerhans' cell histiocytosis of the skull base. Coronal contrast-enhanced T1-WI (**a**) shows a uniformly enhancing mass in the right orbit, with a sharply demarcated defect in the sphenoid bone. Coronal CT (**b**) clearly depicts the osseous defect

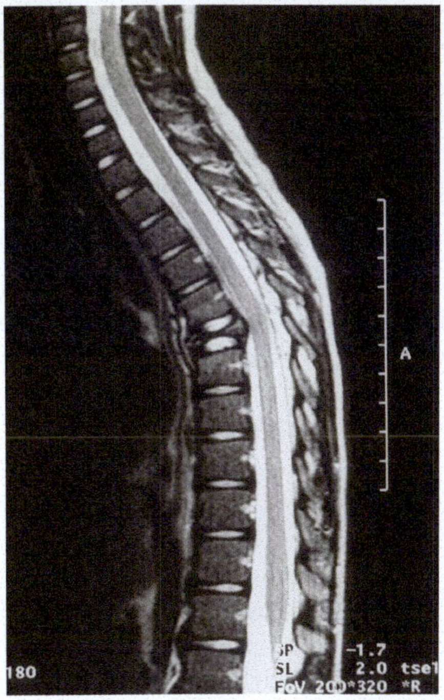

Fig. 13.151 Langerhans' cell histiocytosis of the spine. Sagittal T2-WI shows vertebra plana of Th6 with resulting gibbus

important, whole body STIR MRI probably will be the method of choice to assess the presence of multiple lesions in LCH, as some lesions may not be detected either on radionuclide bone scans or on skeletal survey, and there is no general agreement on whether a scintigraphy, a skeletal survey, or both should be performed. For evaluation of pulmonary involvement, chest radiograph and (high resolution) CT of the lung is recommended.

Vascular Anomalies

In 1982, Mulliken and Glowacki proposed a classification of vascular anomalies that separates vascular tumors from vascular malformations based upon cellular features and clinical course (Table 13.21). This system has been widely accepted, and has been adopted by the International Society for the Study of Vascular Anomalies (ISSVA). Based on this classification system, the vast majority of symptomatic vascular anomalies found in patients older than 12 months are vascular malformations, not hemangiomas as often stated in the literature. It

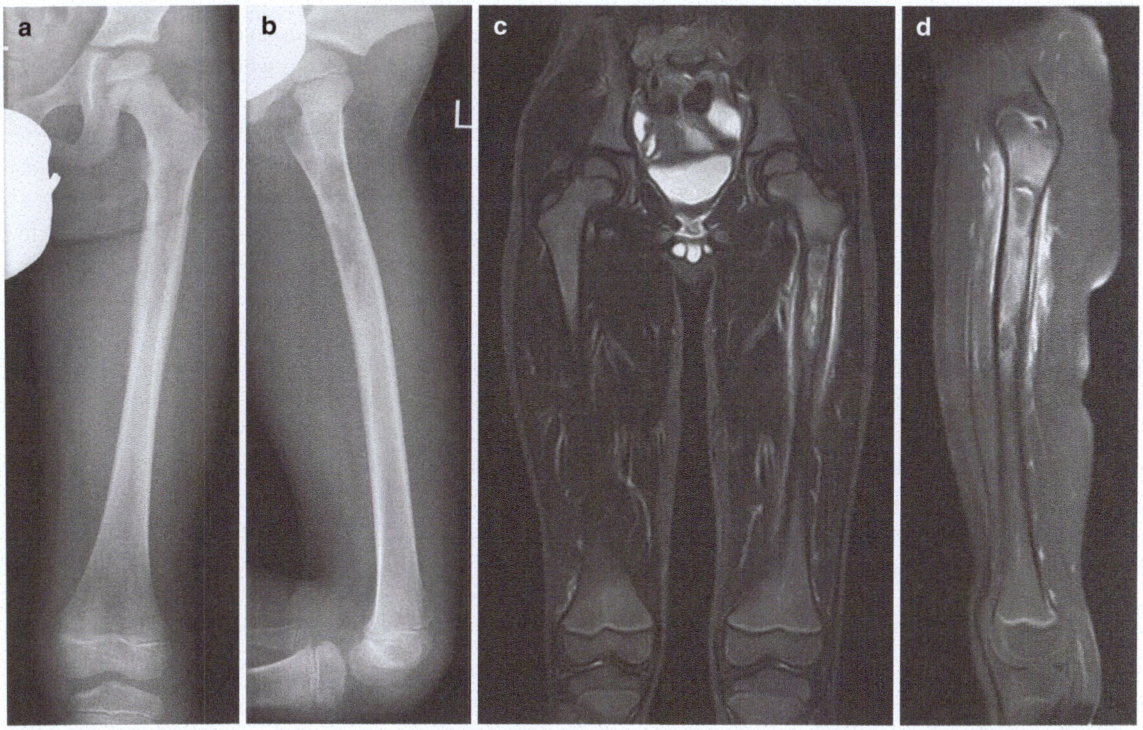

Fig. 13.152 Langerhans' cell histiocytosis of the left femur. Radiography of the left upper leg in AP (**a**) and lateral projection (**b**) show a nonsclerotic geographic osteolytic lesion, with a relatively narrow zone of transition in the metadiaphysis of the femur, and a lamellated periosteal reaction. Coronal fat-saturated T2-WI (**c**) and sagittal contrast-enhanced fat-saturated T1-WI (**d**) demonstrate a heterogeneous lesion with juxtacortical soft-tissue edema

Table 13.21 Classification of vascular anomalies

Vascular tumors	Hemangioma	Infantile (usually present at approximately 3 months) Congenital hemangioma (present at birth) – RICH (rapidly involuting congenital hemangioma) – NICH (noninvoluting congenital hemangioma)
	Other vascular tumors	Kaposiform hemangioendothelioma Tufted angioma Angiosarcoma
Vascular malformations	High flow	Arteriovenous fistula (AVF) Arteriovenous malformation (AVM)
	Low flow	Capillary malformation Venous malformation Lymphatic malformation Macrocystic Microcystic Combined

is of paramount importance to establish the correct diagnosis in order to decide the appropriate treatment and to inform the parent of the prognosis. The majority of hemangiomas and vascular malformations can be recognized on clinical grounds. However, some cases remain a challenge, either because of difficulties in classification or because of an atypical presentation. Generally, infantile hemangiomas are proliferative endothelial cell tumors, which typically present in early infancy, grow rapidly in the first 6 months of life, and then slowly involute. Vascular malformations are always present at birth, have a normal cellular turnover, grow commensurately with the child, and are further classified according to channel abnormalities (arteriovenous, capillary, venous, lymphatic, mixed) and flow characteristics (high-flow, low-flow). Furthermore, infantile hemangioma must be differentiated from congenital hemangioma (incidence 10%). Infantile hemangioma, by definition, is not evident at birth, whereas congenital hemangioma is present at birth and defined as rapidly involuting congenital hemangioma (RICH) if it involutes by approximately 1 year of age, and classified as non-involuting congenital hemangioma (NICH) if it persists after 1 year of age. To date, it has not been clarified whether there is a biologic relationship between common infantile hemangioma and the rare congenital vascular tumors, RICH and NICH. In addition, other vascular tumors such as kaposiform hemangioendothelioma, tufted angioma, and angiosarcoma occur in children and must be diffentiated from the abovementioned entities. Ultrasound and MRI are the imaging tests of choice for making a diagnosis and evaluating the extent of these diseases. However, arteriography and phlebography are still necessary, and very helpful in selected cases of vascular malformations. MRI protocols should include T1-WI and (fat-saturated) T1-WI after administration of paramagnetic contrast, fat-saturated T2-WI, and gradient echo imaging sequences, to determine the presence or absence of high (arterial) flow through a given lesion. For the MR appearance of hemangiomas and arteriovenous, venous, and lymphatic malformations ("lymphangiomas"), see Table 13.22.

Infantile Hemangioma

Infantile hemangiomas occur in 1–2% of neonates, and in up to 12% of infants by 2 months. Females predominate in a ratio of 3–5:1. There is a higher incidence (15%) in premature infants weighing less than 1,000 mg. The median age of the child when the hemangioma appears is 2 weeks; however, approximately – one third of infantile hemangiomas are discovered at birth, presenting either as an erythematous macular patch, a blanched area, a teleangiectasia, or a pseudo-ecchymotic patch. Infantile hemangioma can occur anywhere in the body and is frequently located at the head and neck (60%), trunk (25%), and extremities (15%). Visceral hemangiomas are more common in children with multiple cutaneous lesions (so-called hemangiomatosis) (Fig. 13.96a–c). Most hemangiomas are recognized clinically and do not require any investigation or any treatment, for they will subside spontaneously. However, imaging is needed in cases of subcutaneous hemangiomas with normal overlying skin, cases of clinically atypical soft-tissue masses, when the evaluation of extension of obvious hemangiomas is necessary, cases of hemangiomas leading to complications, and for guiding therapy. The typical common infantile hemangiomas are true neoplasms and show a three-stage process of growth, stagnation, and regression. They grow rapidly during the first 6 months of life (proliferating phase), remain stable in size till the end of the first year of life, and then involute slowly from 1 to 10–12 years (involuting phase). Infantile hemangiomas typically become evident during the proliferative phase, in the first months of life. On MRI, a discrete, lobulated, well-defined mass is seen, with marked hyperintense SI on T2-WI ("light-bulb" bright) and hypointense SI on T1-WI, showing a uniformly

Table 13.22 Magnetic resonance imaging findings in pediatric vascular anomalies (Adapted from Kirks 1998)

Lesion	T1-WI	T1-W + contrast	T2-W	Gradient
Hemangioma				
Proliferating	STM iso- or hypo-intense to muscle, flow voids	Uniform intense enhancement	Increased SI	HFV within and around STM, flow voids
Involuting	Variable fat content	As above	Variable fat	As above
Involuted	High SI (fat)	No enhancement	Decreasd SI	No HFV
Vascular malformation				
Arteriovenous MF	STT, mixed SI, flow voids	Diffuse enhancement	Variable increased SI, flow voids	HFV throughout abnormal tissue
Venous MF	Septated STM, isointense to muscle, high signal thrombi	Diffuse or inhomogeneous enhancement	High SI, signal voids (phleboliths)	No HFV, signal voids (phleboliths)
Lymphatic MF, macrocystic	Septated STM, low SI	Rim or no enhancement	High SI, fluid-fluid levels	No HFV
Lymphatic MF, microcystic	STT, hypo- or isointense to muscle	No or minimal enhancement	Diffuse increased SI, subcutaneous stranding	No HFV

STM soft tissue mass; *STT* soft tissue thickening; *SI* signal intensity; *HFV* high flow vessels; *MF* malformation; *WI* weighted image

intense enhancement after administration of paramagnetic contrast. In addition, prominent draining veins within and adjacent to the mass, seen as flow voids or showing high flow on GRE images, can be depicted (Fig. 13.153). During this phase, the presence of flow voids in a hemangioma may be mistaken for an AVM. However, a soft-tissue mass is not a feature of an AVM. When the characteristic MRI features of an infantile hemangioma are present in the appropriate clinical context, the diagnosis is usually secure. However, if the margins are unsharp or the lesion is multicompartimental, hemangioendothelioma, rhabdomyosarcoma, fibrosarcoma, and infantile myofibromatosis may also be considered. In the involutional phase, decreasing size

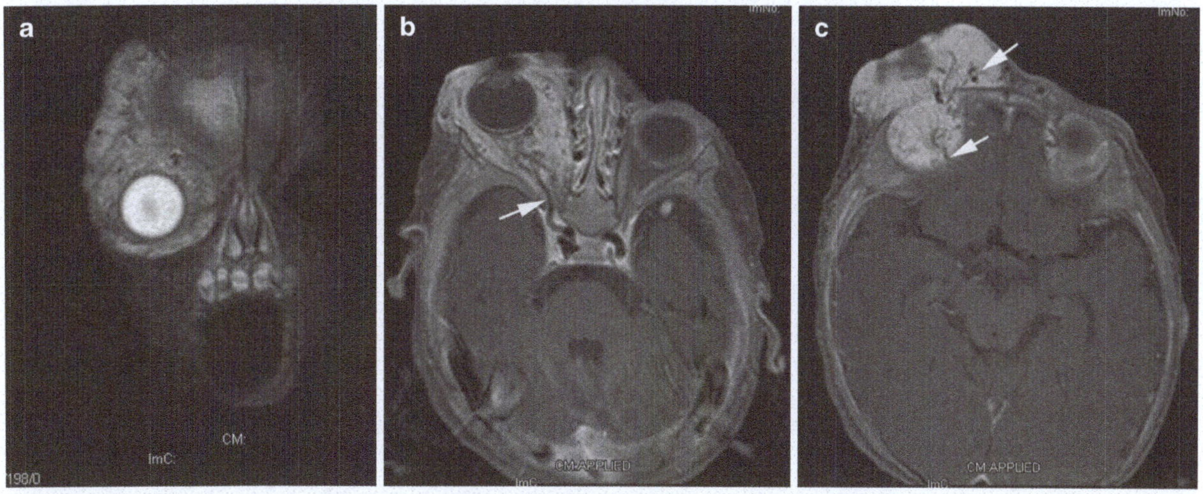

Fig. 13.153 Infantile hemangioma. Coronal STIR image (**a**) and transverse fat-saturated contrast-enhanced T1-WI (**b, c**) show a lobulated, sharply confined enhancing mass in the right orbit and face, with multiple flow voids arising from the ophthalmic artery (*arrows*)

and fatty replacement is observed. Therefore, the lesion becomes more heterogeneous, tumor enhancement pattern decreases, and calcification and blood breakdown products may be detected. In most patients, complete involution is seen by 9–10 years of age and fibrofatty tissue may be the only remnant of a hemangioma. Potential complications are compression of vital structures (airway, orbit), heart failure, fissure formation, ulceration, bleeding, and psychological issues, particularly in cases with massive facial disfigurement. As most hemangiomas require no treatment, therapy is reserved for hemangiomas with potential for complications. Treatment may consist of cryotherapy, laser therapy (dye and Nd-YAG) for skin involvement, or systemic steroids and/or surgical removal. An important associated abnormality is PHACE syndrome (posterior fossa brain anomalies, hemangioma, arterial and cardiac anomalies, eye defects) (Fig. 13.154a–d).

Congenital Hemangioma

Congenital hemangiomas are clinically and biologically different from infantile hemangiomas. They are present at birth, and rapidly decrease rather than increase in size at presentation, compared with infantile hemangiomas. They present as masses, often associated with dilated draining channels, arterial aneurysms, and/or arteriovenous fistulas. Unlike infantile hemangiomas, congenital hemangiomas may be infiltrative and occupy multiple compartments. Most of these are classified as rapidly involuting congenital hemangiomas (RICHs), and will completely involute by 1 year of age. Rarely, congenital hemangiomas do

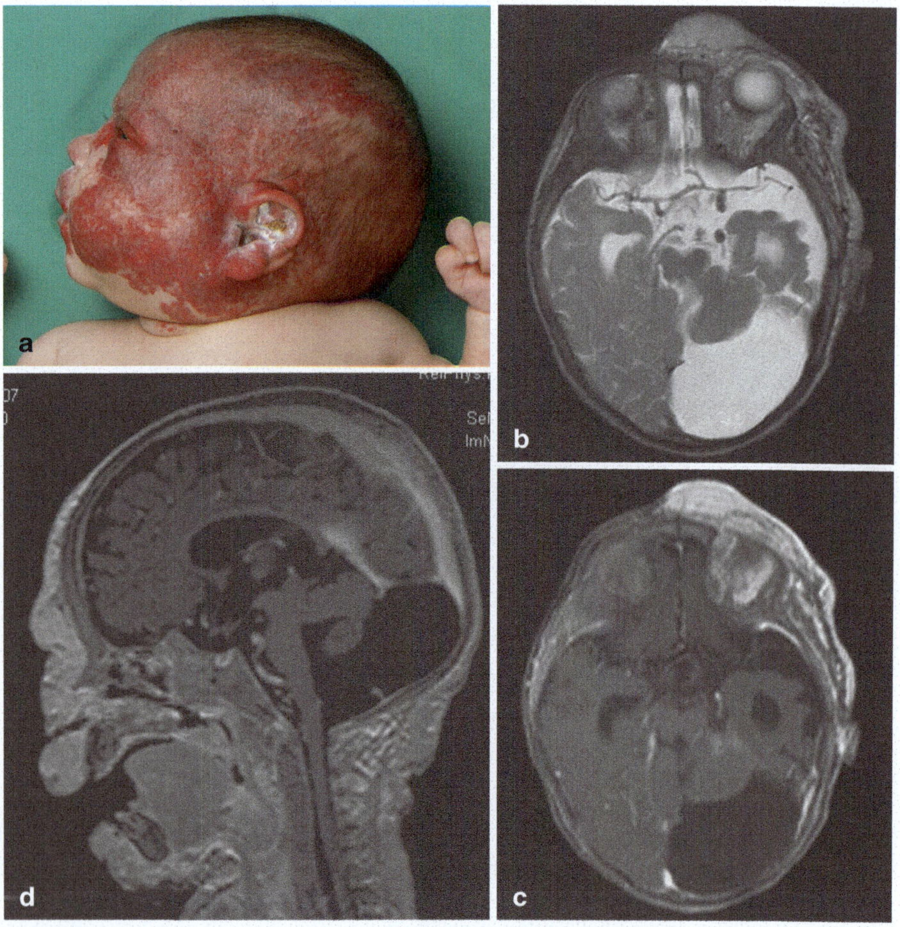

Fig. 13.154 Infantile hemangioma in a patient with PHACE syndrome. Photograph of a female newborn (**a**). Transverse T2-WI (**b**) and fat-saturated contrast-enhanced transverse (**c**) and sagittal T1-WI (**d**) demonstrate hypoplasia of the left cerebellum and a large hemangioma of the left face with extension into the left orbit

Table 13.23 Comparison of infantile hemangioma, RICH, and KHE (Adapted from Kan 2007)

	Margins	Clincal course	Other
Infantile hemangioma	Well-defined	Initially enlarges during the first year of life, then slowly regresses	Glucose transporter protein isoform 1 (GLUT1) positive
Congenital hemangioma (RICH, NICH)	Infiltrative	Present at birth, then rapidly involutes If it grows with the child or does not involute by approximately 1 year of age, then NICH (noninvoluting congenital hemangioma)	May develop heart failure due to AV shunting (typically seen with liver lesions); may develop mild thrombocytopenia
Kaposiform heman-giomaendothelioma (KHE)	Infiltrative	50% present at birth, rapidly enlarges, may spontaneoulsly shrink, but never disappears	No heart failure, it may develop significant thrombocytopenia

not involute, and grow proportionally with the child. These lesions are classified as non-involuting congenital hemangiomas (NICHs) (Table 13.23).

Kaposiform Hemangioendothelioma

Kaposiform hemangioendothelioma (KHE) is a unique entity that is clinically and biologically distinct from infantile and congenital hemangioma (Table 13.23). The diagnosis is only based on the histologic pattern showing infiltrating nodules, spindled cells lining slitlike or crescentic vessels containing hemosiderin, whereas proliferating infantile hemangioma is composed of distinct nodules of well-formed capillaries. The second difference is associated "lymphangiomatosis" and KHE growing into lymphatic spaces. KHE is usually larger than infantile hemangiomas at presentation, and does not completely involute. It may be associated with Kasabach-Meritt syndrome (cutaneous vascular lesions and thrombocytopenia). Approximatly 50% of KHE are present at birth and the remainder present during the first year of life. KHE typically occurs in the proximal arms and legs and the trunk, including the retroperitoneum, whereas craniofacial lesions are uncommon. It is unclear whether KHE arises in the viscera, but it can invade nearby organs; for example, retroperitoneal involvement of the pancreas, mesentery, porta hepatis, or mediastinal extension into the pericardium, pleura, and thymus. These tumors are infiltrative, growing lesions and have ill-defined margins, cross planes of tissue into muscle and bone, and show a diffuse and inhomogeneous or homogeneous enhancement pattern (Fig. 13.155). Although KHE may be present at birth, it disproportionately increases in size, rather than rapidly involuting like a congenital hemangioma. KHE neither completely regresses spontaneously nor does it metastize.

Arteriovenous Malformation

Arteriovenous malformations (AVM) are congenital malformations that are not true neoplasms, as stated above. They are present at birth and enlarge proportional to the child, do not involute, and remain throughout life. In AVMs, there are abnormal direct connections between arterial and venous structures, bypassing the capillary bed. They are much less common than venous malformations, lymphatic malformations, and hemangiomas, and can occur in any location. Clinical findings include a pulsatile mass with thrill, bruit, and, occasionally, local hyperthermia. On MRI, the characteristic imaging finding is a tangle of vessels without an associated soft-tissue mass, showing flow voids on T1-WI and T2-WI in multiple vessels (arterialization of veins). On T2-WI, a hyperintese surrounding edema may be depicted. After administration of paramagnetic contrast, intense enhancement of multiple vessels can be seen, and the enlarged draining veins are typically much larger than the feeding arteries (Fig. 13.156). Conventional angiography is vital for planning and performing embolization therapy and is frequently performed 24 h prior to surgery, in order to limit hemorrhage.

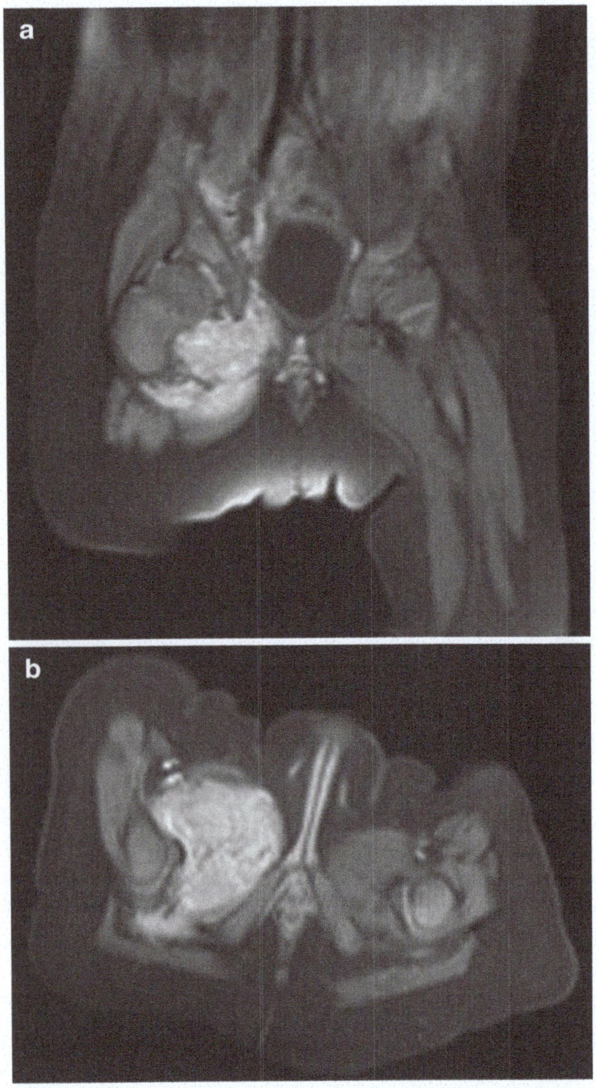

Fig. 13.155 Kaposiform Hemangioendothelioma. Coronal (**a**) and transverse (**b**) contrast-enhanced fat-saturated T1-WI show a homogenously enhancing mass in the right pelvis extending into the hip joint, with infiltration of the adjacent muscle groups

Incomplete resection results in collateral forming and recurrence of the lesion. AVMs can enlarge due to various stimuli, such as trauma, puberty, pregnancy, or after biopsy, proximal ligation, or a subtotal excision. Potential complications are skeletal overgrowth (limb length discrepancy), trophic changes, pain, congestive heart failure, steal phenomenon, ulceration and bleeding, embolism, rapid enlargement related to hemorrhage, and thrombosis. When the malformation involves the entire extremity, the condition is described as Parkes-Weber syndrome. AVMs involving the lungs, brain, or GI system are common in Rendu-Osler-Weber syndrome.

Venous Malformation

Venous malformations (VMs) are the most common symptomatic vascular malformations, and are characterized by dysplasias of small and large venous channels. The characteristic physical findings are a soft, compressible, nonpulsatile mass or swelling, usually of bluish color, occasionally with normal overlying skin. However, VMs can also present as a diffuse abnormality of extremity venous structures (multiple varicosities). VMs expand following compression, when the limb is dependent, or after Valsalva maneuver, and can be small and localized or extensive, involving the entire extremity or body part. They may be associated with muscular athrophy, and often do not respect tissue/fascial planes and may involve multiple tissue types, such as muscle, subcutaneous tissues, and bone. Main localizations are head and neck (40%), extremities (40%), and the trunk (20%). On plain films, VM shows a soft-tissue mass, with occasional phleboliths and adjacent skeletal anomalies. On MRI, VM are hyperintense on T2-WI and intermediate in SI on T1-WI, and present as either focal multilocular or septated masses, with serpentine channels being a characteristic pattern. Phleboliths may appear dark in signal, and acute thrombus in venous channels may be high or low in SI, depending upon age. Channels and "cystic" areas enhance diffusely (Fig. 13.157). In some VMs, there may be an associated nonvascular hamartomatous connective tissue component that contain fat and may not enhance. Dynamic contrast-enhanced 3D gradient-echo MR angiography is very useful to document slow-flowing blood and to rule out a fast-flow vascular anomaly. As VMs contain dilated slow-flow vascular spaces, enhancement of the channels is typically seen after administration of paramagnetic contrast. This allows differentiation of VMs from other nonenhancing cystic malformations, including lymphatic malformations, brachial cleft cysts, foregut duplication cysts, and similar malformations. However, if scanning is done too soon after administration of paramagnetic contrast, contrast-enhanced imaging may falsely suggest a lymphatic malformation. Extremity venous malformations

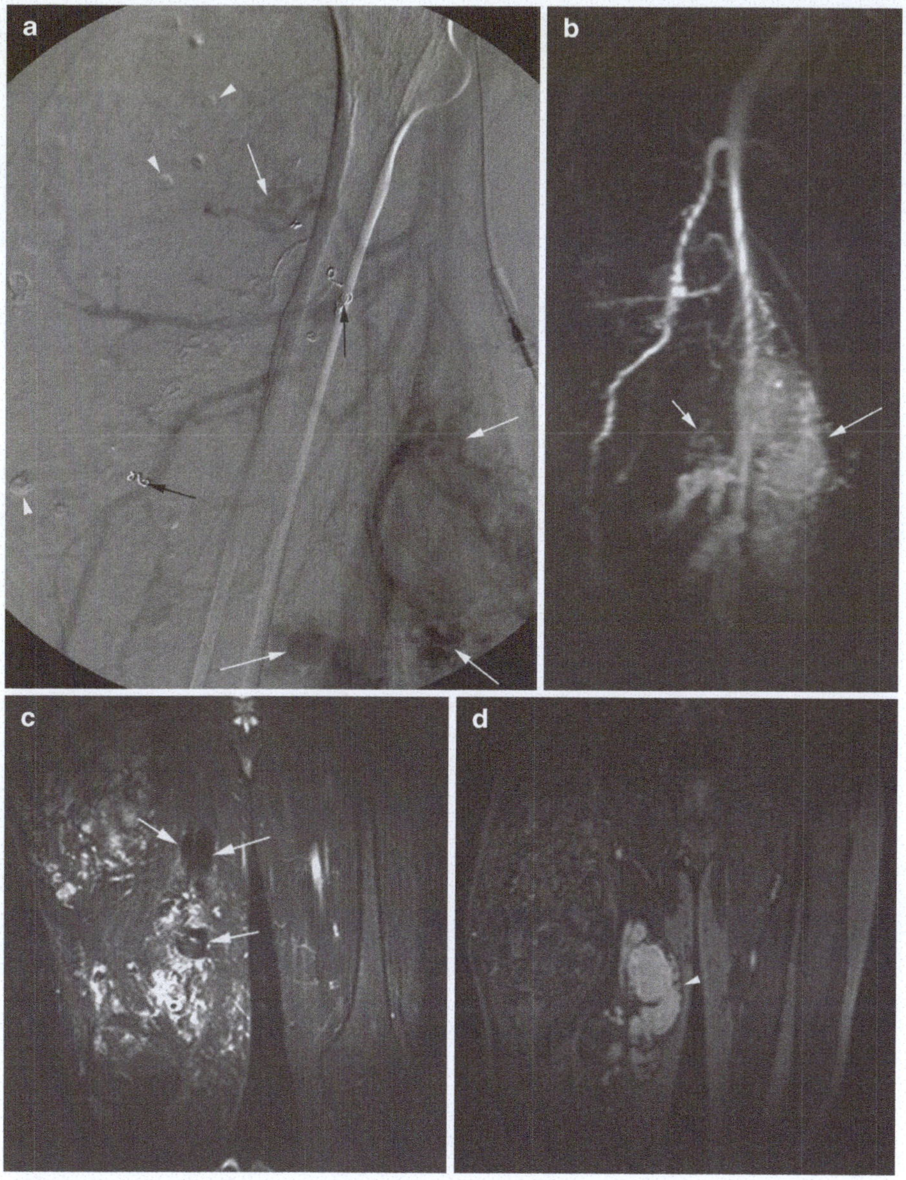

Fig. 13.156 Arteriovenous malformation. Digital subtraction angiography (**a**) and MIP (**b**) of the right upper leg show enlarged and tortuous arteries given off the superficial and profound femoral artery, and a large aneurysmatic dilatated vein (*arrows*). Note multiple phleboliths (*arrowheads*) and coils (*black arrows*) after embolization therapy of a part of the lesion. In addition, flow-voids indicating fast flow in the superficial femoral artery and superficial femoral vein (*arrows*) and in the large aneurysmatic dilatated vein (*arrowhead*) are present on coronal STIR image (**c**). Coronal time-resolved MRA (**d**) and transverse contrast-enhanced fat-saturated T1-WI (**e, f**) with insufficient fat suppression demonstrate thrombi (*arrow*) and complete filling of the dilated venous vessel (*arrowhead*). The involvement of the lateral musculature of the right upper leg shows features of a venous malformation, whereas involvement of the medial musculature is typical for arteriovenous malformation

may be associated with limb length discrepancy, especially if the malformation is diffuse. Most patients with diffuse VM have undergrowth of the affected limb. In VM and associated syndromes such as Klippel–Trenaunay syndrome (which is associated with overgrowth of the affected limb and intracutaneous capillary malformation), imaging is performed to ensure patency or existence of the deep venous system on the one hand and, on the other hand, to visualize abnormalities of the venous structures, for example, marginal veins (Fig. 13.158). This may be a challenging task in extensive disease, and phlebography or direct injection of contrast media in abnormal veins may be necessary. Intraarticular location of VM may lead to hemosiderin-arthropathy due to repeated bleeding, and therefore MRI evaluation of articular cartilage and extension of joint involvement is crucial (Fig. 13.159). Intraarticular VMs are best managed by excision, if possible. Head

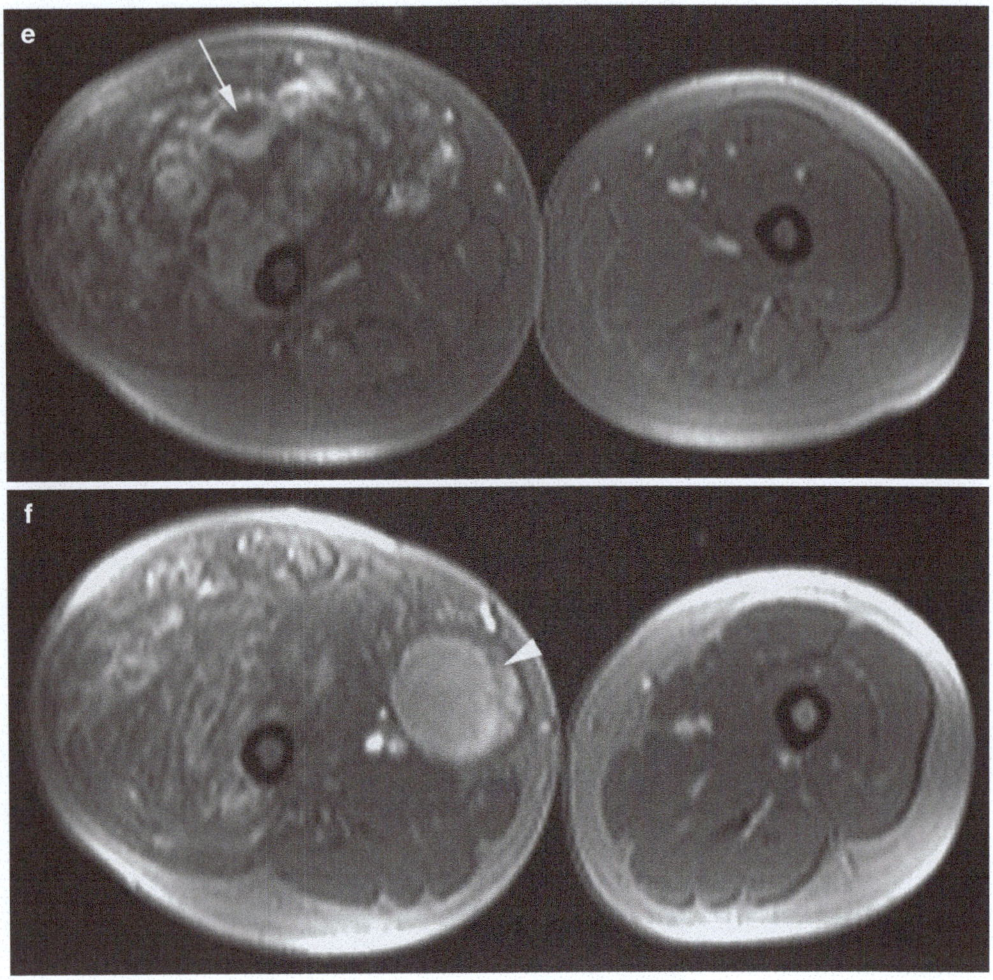

Fig. 13.156 (continued)

and neck venous malformations vary in size, can lead to airway obstruction, and large malformations of the face and scalp can be associated with sinus pericranii and other intracranial venous anomalies. VMs of the GI tract most commonly present with chronic bleeding and anemia, and may be part of the Blue rubber bleb nevus syndrome (venous malformation seen in skin, GI, and musculokeletal systems). Generally, potential complications of VM are sudden enlargement due to hemorrhage, thrombosis or growth during puberty, skin necrosis, nerve damage, muscle atrophy, pulmonary embolism, disseminated intravascular coagulation, and death. Venous malformations are a lifetime problem, with treatment aimed at reducing symptoms rather than eliminating disease.

Lymphatic Malformation

Lymphatic malformation (LM) is defined as dysplastic collection of lymph-containing cystic or capillary structures lined by epithelium. Like the other abovementioned vascular malformations, they are usually apparent in early childhood. These malformations range from small, localized lesions to large masses that may diffusely involve an extremity or other body part or multiple organ

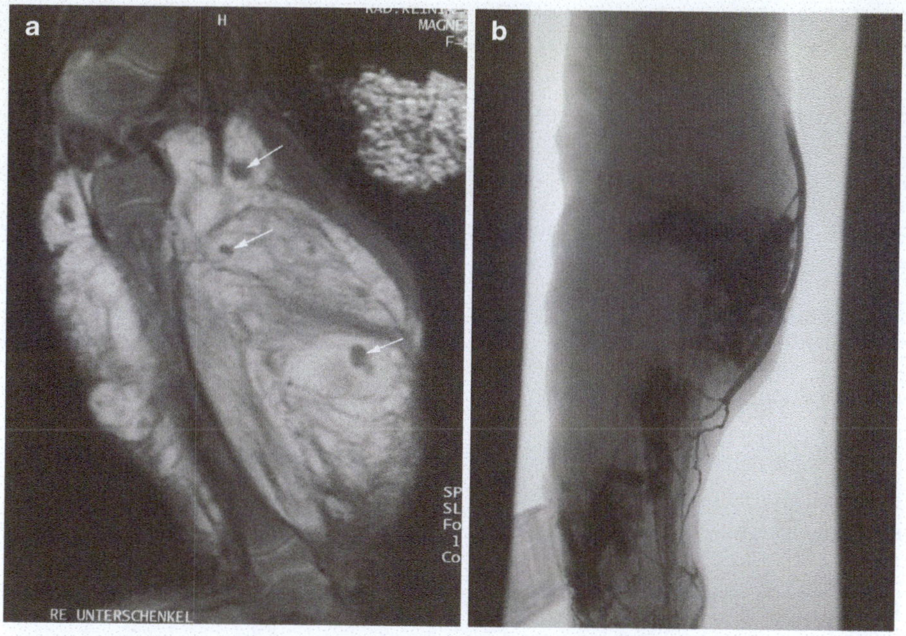

Fig. 13.157 Low-flow venous malformation of the right lower leg. STIR image (**a**) demonstrates large, hyperintense, septated, cystic, soft-tissue mass with signal voids due to phleboliths (*arrow*). Phlebography performed 2 years later (**b**) (early filling) shows complete infiltration of subcutaneous fat and muscles by anomalous veins in the lower leg

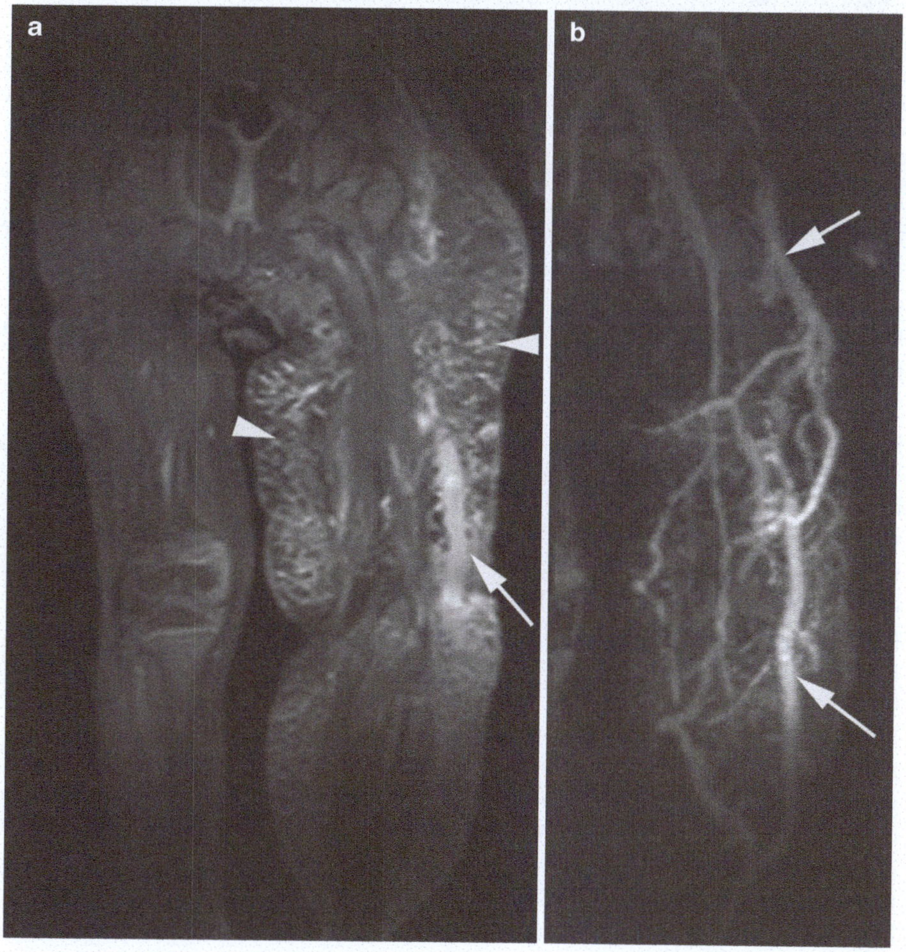

Fig. 13.158 Klippel–Trenaunay syndrome with marginal vein. Fat-saturated contrast-enhanced T1-WI (**a**) and 2D TOF MRV (**b**) show hypertrophy of the buttock and left leg with diffuse infiltration of the subcutaneous fat compatible with microcystic and /or capillary malformation (*arrowheads*). On MRV, a marginal vein (*arrows*) along the lateral aspect of the leg and thigh, and multiple other anomalous veins are identified. The deep venous system is existent and patent

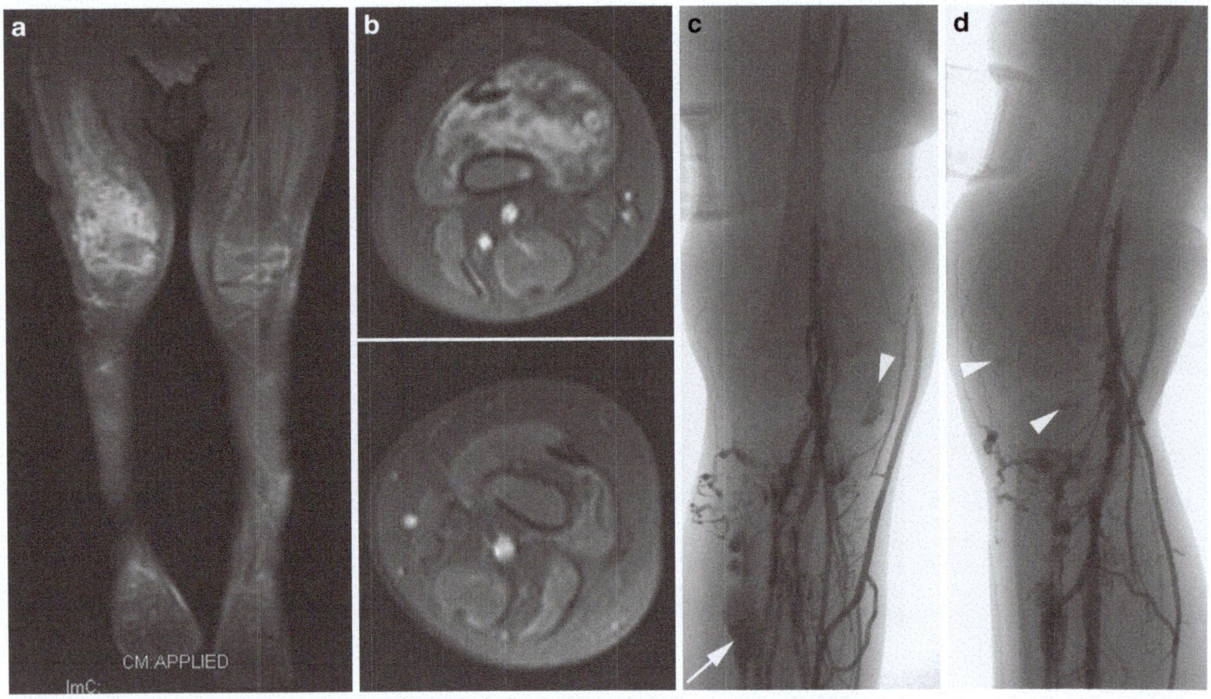

Fig. 13.159 Low-flow venous malformation. Coronal (**a**) and transverse (**b**) contrast-enhanced fat-saturated T1-WI show a large inhomogeneously enhancing mass in the right upper leg extending into the knee joint. Phlebography in AP (**c**) and lateral (**d**) projection demonstrates anomalous veins in the lower leg, aneurysmatic dilatation of the anterior tibial veins (*arrow*), and some anomalous branches extending into the joint space in a 2-year-old boy (*arrowheads*)

systems. Furthermore, LM often does not respect tissue/facial planes and may involve multiple tissue types, such as muscles, subcutaneous tissues, and bone. Lymphatic malformations are classified as microcystic, macrocystic, or combined. Approximately 60–70% of the LMs are located in the cervicofacial region, 20% in the axilla, and the remainder occur in a varity of other sites, such as the trunk, extremities, mesentery, retroperitoneum, and pelvis. On MRI, LMs have a rather characteristic appearance, which varies with the size of the cystic components. Macrocystic LMs have clearly defined cysts and septa. The cysts are hyperintense on T2-WI, hypointense on T1-WI, and the septations and walls of the cysts enhance after administration of paramagnetic contrast, giving a characteristic pattern ("rings and arcs") (Fig. 13.160). Fluid–fluid levels within the cysts are a common finding, due to protein or blood content. More important, no high–flow vascular signal voids or flow-related enhancement is detectable. Cysts in the microcystic LM are usually too small to be identified as discrete structures on MRI; therefore, they mostly appear as diffuse areas, of low SI on T1-WI and high SI on T2-WI, that may show mild diffuse enhancement or no enhancement at all, after administration of paramagnetic contrast. Hence, microcystic LM may easily be confused with other

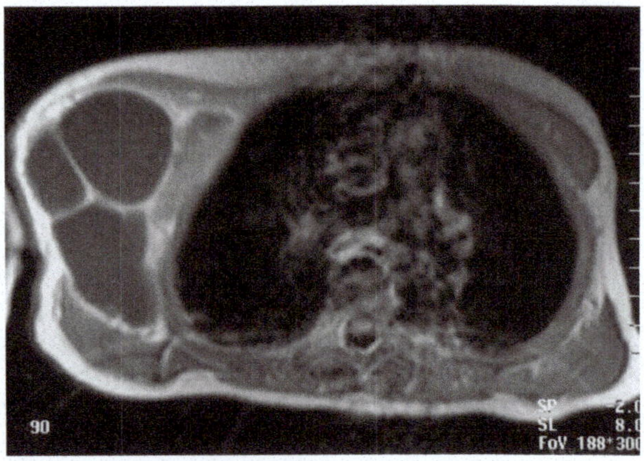

Fig. 13.160 Macrocystic lymphatic malformation. Transverse contrast-enhanced T1-WI shows large, septated, cystic, soft-tissue mass with rim enhancement in the right axilla

soft-tissue disease entities, and distinguishing capillary malformations from microcystic LM, which often coexist in the same area, may be impossible, both on MRI and by histology. Interestingly, LM of the floor of the mouth are usually microcystic and diffuse and display minimal or no contrast enhancement. Gorham–Stout syndrome is characterized by LM involving the bone. On plain films, Gorham–Stout syndrome shows a spectrum from permeative osteolysis to vanishing bone. On MRI, diffuse intraosseous enhancement may be seen, representing a combination of vascular channels, including microcystic LM and hypervascular fibrous tissue. Extraosseous extension into the adjacent tissues is often present. The most common potential complications of LM are compression of airways or other vital structures, rapid increasement due to hemorrhage, or inflammation with pain, extremity swelling, and muscle atrophy. Treatment of lymphatic malformation is either surgical resection or percutaneous sclerosis.

Combined Vascular Malformations

Combined Vascular Malformations are characterized by overgrowth of involved body parts, and can be categorized as slow-flow vascular malformations such as Klippel–Trenaunay syndrome (Figs. 13.158 and 13.161) (capillary-lymphaticovenous malformation of lower extremity, dermal capillary strain with lymphatic vesicles, varicosities of superficial veins, anomalies and occasional absence of deep venous system), Maffucci syndrome (venous malformation seen in association with multiple enchondromatosis), and fast-flow combined vascular malformations such as Parkes-Weber syndrome (port-wine stain, multiple arteriovenous fistulas, and overgrowth of the affected limb).

Dermatomyositis

Dermatomyositis is an idiopathic inflammatory myopathy with diffuse nonsuppurative inflammation of striated muscle and skin. Females are more commonly affected, and age range at presentation is 5–14 years. Patients with juvenile dermatomyositis tend to develop soft-tissue calcifications, skin ulcerations, and arthritis, and suffer from vasculitis like problems (e.g., skin and mucosal ulceration), compared with adult patients with dermatomyositis. In contrast to adults, polymyositis and inclusion myositis are rare in children. On MRI, increased SI on (FS) T2-WI in the affected muscle groups, superficial and deep fascia, skin and subcutaneous fat can be depicted. Typically, there is a bilateral, symmetric, and proximal appendicular distributon of muscle inflammation.The proximal lower extremity (especially the adductor, gluteus,

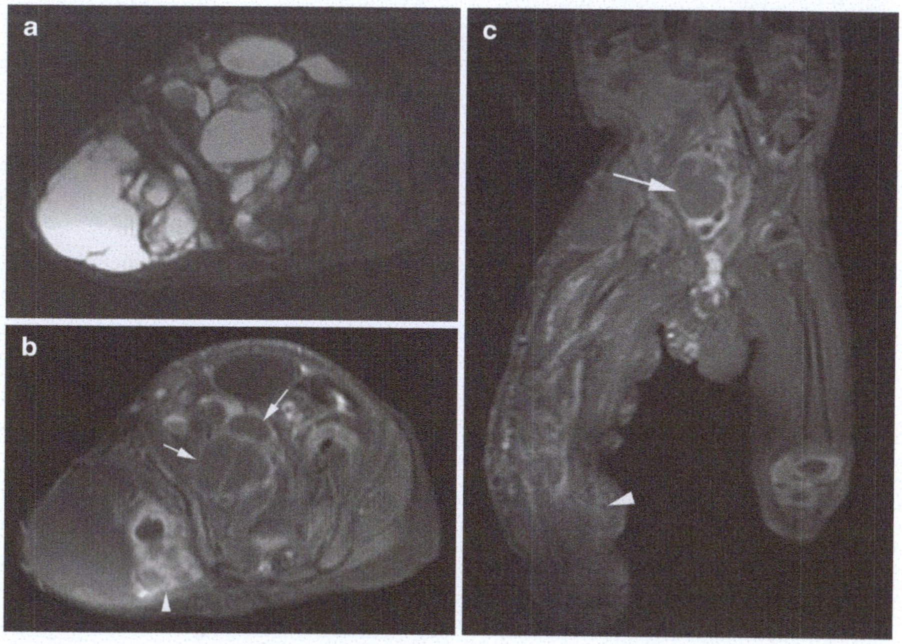

Fig. 13.161 Mixed capillary-lymphaticovenous malformation in a patient with Klippel–Trenaunay syndrome. Transverse STIR image (**a**) and transverse (**b**) and coronal (**c**) fat-saturated contrast-enhanced T1-WI show hypertrophy of the buttock and right leg, multiple cysts enhancing with "rings-and arcs pattern" (*arrows*), more solid components with inhomogeneous enhancement consistent with microcystic and/or capillary components and anomalous venous vessels (*arrowhead*)

and quadricep groups) is usually affected first, followed by the proximal upper extremity muscles. Therefore, for evaluation of dermatomyositis, coronal, and axial planes are recommended. As abnormalities will enhance after administration of paramagnetic contrast, contrast administration is usually not necessary in probable dermatomyositis. On follow-up studies, complications including calcifications, muscle necrosis, and muscle atrophy with fatty replacement are observed. In addition, MRI is performed to determine biopsy site when the clinical presentation and MR features are atypical.

13.5.6.2 Malignant Bone and Soft-Tissue Tumors

Osteosarcoma

Osteosarcoma is the most common primary malignant bone tumor of childhood, and is a malignant tumor with the ability to produce osteoids directly from neoplastic cells. The peak incidence is between the ages of 10 and 20 years. Osteosarcomas may be divided based on their location: medullary, surface, or extraskeletal. The majority of osteosarcomas are either conventional (high-grade intramedullary) osteosarcomas (75–85%) or teleangiectatic osteosarcomas (5–11%). Multicentric osteosarcomas, periosteal osteosarcomas, parosteal osteosarcomas, and secondary osteosarcomas account for 1, 1, 3 and 5% of cases, respectively. Furthermore, four subtypes of surface osteosarcomas are discriminated: periosteal (25%), intracortical (rare), parosteal (65%) and high grade surface (10%). Conventional osteosarcoma most commonly occurs in decreasing order of frequency in the femur (40%; 75% distal), the tibia (20%; 80% proximal), and the proximal humerus (15%). Conventional osteosarcoma arises from the medullary cavity, often eccentrically in the metaphysis, and presents as a poorly defined mass extending through the cortex. In 75% of the cases, extension into epiphysis is present. On conventional radiographs, usually a considerable permeative bony destruction, with a wide or narrow zone of transition in concert with various irregular periosteal reactions (layered periosteal new bone deposition, spicules, sunburst, Codman triangle), is present. Occasionally, osteosarcoma presents with uniform sclerosis of the affected bone, without periosteal reaction, a soft-tissue mass, or destruction of the cortex. Teleangiectatic osteosarcoma is an osteolytic variant of osteosarcoma, and more than 90% of the tumoral mass must contain hemorrhagic, cystic, or necrotic components prior to treatment, to be considered a teleangiectatic osteosarcoma. On MRI, conventional osteosarcoma presents with low SI on T1-WI and variable high SI in T2-WI, and demonstrates heterogeneous enhancement after administration of paramagnetic contrast (Fig. 13.162). Areas of tumor osteoid formations are of low SI in all sequences (Fig. 13.163). An alternative consideration for low SI within an osteosarcoma is blood products due to intratumoral hemorrhage. Fluid–fluid levels within cystic components may be seen with conventional and teleangiectatic osteosarcoma, and may develop after chemotherapy. However, fluid–fluid levels are much less commonly seen compared with ABC, and the presence of extensive cortical destruction, osteoid matrix calcification, and an enhancing soft-tissue mass, and/or thick nodular septal enhancement favors teleangiectatic osteosarcoma over a primary ABC. MRI is ordered at initial presentation to evaluate the extent of tumor, including the degree of marrow replacement, cortical destruction, skip lesions (seen in 3% of osteosarcomas at time of presentation), regional metastases, extraosseus soft-tissue extent, intraarticular spread, and involvement of neurovascular structures. Therefore, MRI should include a large FOV to image the entire extremity, with T1 W and fluid sensitive sequences to rule out skip lesions and define intraosseus tumor extent. Images with a smaller FOV centered on the lesion should then be aquired with an appropriate surface coil, to assess for transphyseal, intraarticular, and extracompartmental soft-tissue extension. Axial images are useful to assess integrity of adjacent neurovascular structures, as well as tumor seeding of the needle tract or surgical biopsy site. After chemotherapy, MRI is performed to evaluate tumor response and tumor margins, prior to resection. Determining response to chemotherapy is demanding, because the osteoid matrix may regress slowly despite extensive tumoral necrosis, and intra-tumoral hemorrhage, cystic change, and juxta-tumoral edema exaggerate the true size of viable tumor. T1 W sequences tend to be more accurate for determining true tumor margins, whereas STIR sequences often exaggerate tumor extent. Dynamic enhanced MRI is recommended, as it may be helpful in identifing residual

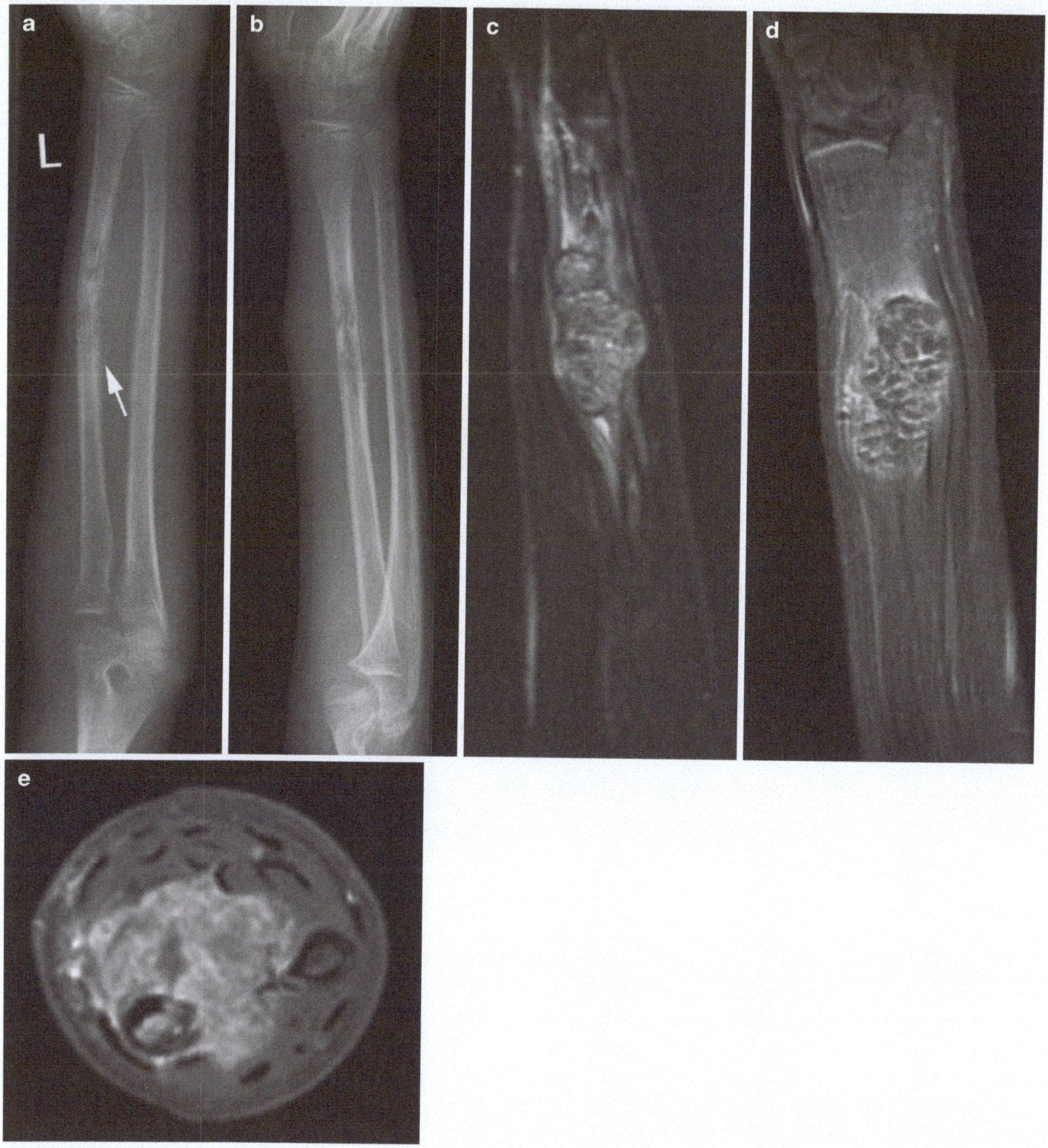

Fig. 13.162 Intramedullary osteosarcoma. Radiography of the left forearm in AP (**a**) and lateral projection (**b**) show a permeative bony destruction with a narrow zone of transition, layered periosteal new bone deposition, and Codman triangle (*arrow*). Sagittal STIR image (**c**) and coronal (**d**) and transverse contrast-enhanced fat-saturated T1-WI (**e**) demonstrate a large mass with infiltration of the deep flexors, the interosseous membrane, and extensor digitorum muscle

tumor. Van der Woude et al. observed that viable tumor enhanced within 6 s after arterial enhancement, while peritumoral edema and fibrosis enhanced at 6 s or longer after chemotherapy. For surgical considerations, a 1 cm tumor-free soft-tissue resection margin and a 2–3 cm bony margin is considered necessary.

Periosteal osteosarcoma most often occurs in patients 20–30 years of age, arises like conventional

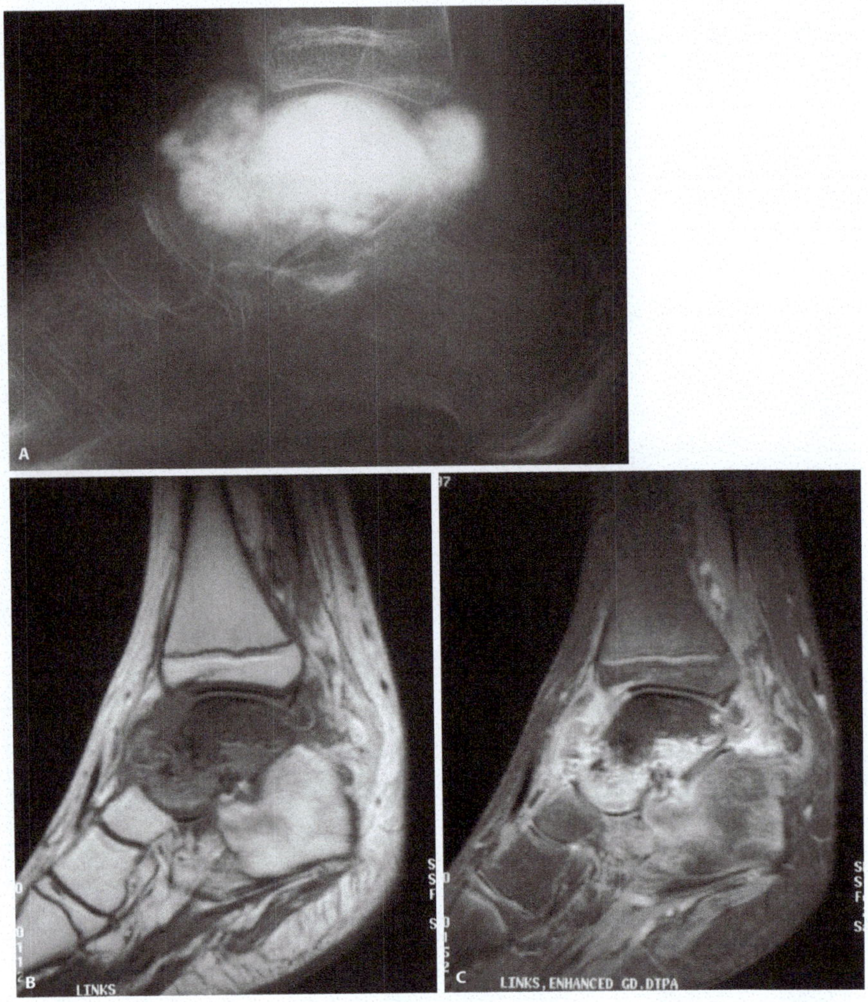

Fig. 13.163 Osteoblastic osteosarcoma. Lateral conventional radiograph (**a**) of the right foot shows considerable new bone formation in the talus. Sagittal T1-WI (**b**) and contrast-enhanced fat-saturated T1-WI (**c**) demonstrate markedly enhancing marrow involvement and soft-tissue component

osteosarcoma, in the majority of cases in the femur and the tibia, and is characteristically located in the diaphysis or metadiaphysis. On conventional radiographs, periosteal osteosarcoma most often shows cortical thickening with cortical scalloping, but hair-on-end periosteal reaction extending to an extraosseous soft tissue mass may also be present. On MRI, a well-defined surface-based extraosseous soft-tissue mass without medullary involvement, displaying heterogeneous isointense SI on T1-WI and heterogeneously high SI on T2-WI with heterogeneous contrast enhancement, can be depicted (Fig. 13.164). Parosteal osteosarcoma usually occurs in the age group between 30 and 50 years, is predominantely located in the posterior aspect of the distal femoral metaphysis, and is covered more extensively in the chapter on the musculoskeletal system. The most common locations for metastasis of osteosarcomas are the lung and the skeleton.

Ewing's Sarcoma

Ewing's sarcoma is the second most common primary bone tumor in children, occurring at between 5 and 25 years of age, and is exceedingly rare before 5 years of age. Ewing's sarcoma of bone belongs to the Ewing's family of tumors, which comprises primitive neuroectodermal tumor (PNET), extraosseous Ewing's sarcoma, and Askin's tumor, which are all aggressive small, blue, round cell tumors. In patients with Ewing's sarcoma, chromosomal translocations of chromosome 11 and 22 have been descibed. Ewing's sarcoma may

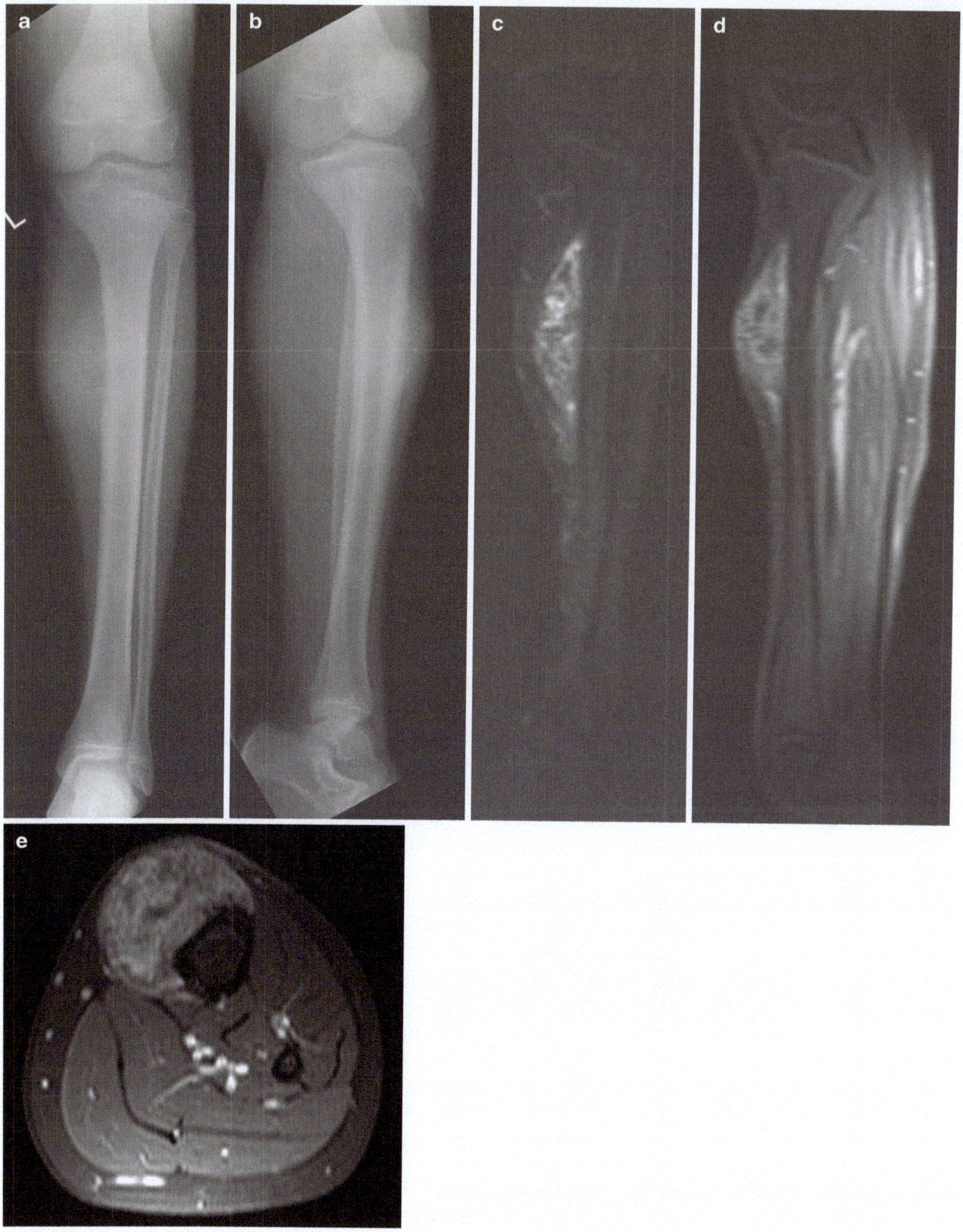

Fig. 13.164 Periosteal osteosarcoma. Radiography of the left tibia in AP (**a**) and lateral (**b**) projection show a crescent-shaped lesion along the medial and anterior surface of the tibial meta-diaphysis, with destruction of the cortex and ossifying tumor matrix. Coronal STIR image (**c**), contrast-enhanced fat-saturated sagittal (**d**) and transverse T1-WI (**e**) demonstrate a heterogeneously enhancing mass without involvement of the medullary cavity

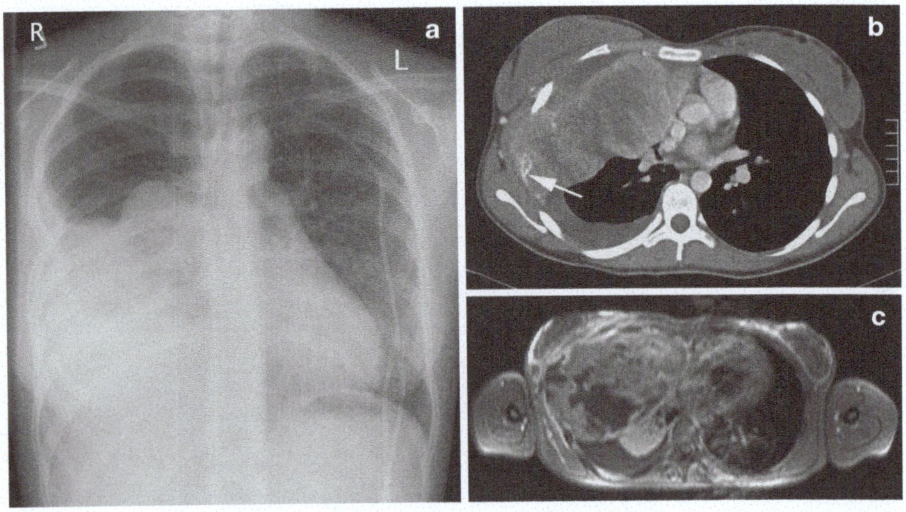

Fig. 13.165 Ewing's sarcoma. Chest X-ray (**a**) and contrast-enhanced CT (**b**) of the chest shows a large soft-tissue mass arising from a destroyed fifth rib (*arrow*), and pleural effusion. Transverse contrast-enhanced fat-saturated T1-WI (**c**) demonstrates the partially necrotic soft-tissue mass in an analogous manner

affect any bone in the body, but most commonly occurs, in decreasing order of frequency, in the femur, pelvis, tibia, humerus, and ribs (Fig. 13.165). The tumor is more frequently located in the metaphysis (59%) of the long bones, but diaphyseal involvement (35%) is more common than with other bone malignancies such as osteosarcoma. Ewing's sarcoma has a greater propensity for flat bones such as pelvis and scapula, especially in children older than 10 years. On conventional radiographs, Ewing's sarcoma shows extensive and lytic bone destruction, with a permeative or moth-eaten appearance or poorly marginated ill-defined intramedullary lucencies. Lesions in the diaphysis are usually central, whereas those in the metaphysis are eccentric. Codman's triangle, onion-skin and hair-on-end (perpendicular), and spiculated aggressive periosteal reaction are common. In 15% of cases, Ewing's sarcoma may appear as a very sclerotic lesion, especially in flat bones. If sclerosis is present, it is confined to bone in contrast to osteosarcoma. Although Ewing's sarcoma may be osteoblastic or mixed, it does not produce mineralized osteoid matrix. On MRI, Ewing's sarcoma demonstrates high SI on T2-WI compared to skeletal muscle, and low to intermediate SI on T1-WI compared to fatty marrow, with prominent, sometimes heterogeneous enhancement after contrast administration (Fig. 13.166). Occasionally, Ewing's sarcoma is iso- to hypointense on T2 WI compared to muscle because of dense cellularity. Especially in flat bones, the extraosseous soft-tissue component of Ewing's sarcoma tends to be larger, as its intramedullary component. As in osteosarcomas, skip metastasis (4%) may be present at the time of presentation; therefore, imaging recommendations are the same as in osteosarcoma (see above). Ewing's sarcoma is a great mimic, and may be indistinguishable from osteomyelitis by radiographic and MR findings, and must be differentiated from osteosarcoma, LCH, lymphoma/leukemia, and metastasis.

Leukemia

Leukemia is a malignancy of hematopoetic stem cells with diffuse infiltration or replacement of the bone marrow by malignant cells, and it is the leading cause of malignancy and death in childhood. Leukemias are basically classified as either lymphocytic or myelogenous. In the pediatric population, acute lymphoblastic leukemia (ALL) accounts for 75%, AML for 15–20%, and chronic myelogenous leukemia (CML) for 5% of cases. The peak incidence of ALL is 2–10 years, whereas AML occurs in children younger than 2 years and shows a smaller peak in later childhood. In the pediatric population, the long bones are most commonly affected. On plain films, a spectrum of different findings can be encountered. Plain films may be normal, or show diffuse osteopenia due to bone marrow packing. In approximately 50% of ALL cases, transverse, radiolucent metaphyseal bands with variable sclerotic margins involving the large joints, the so-called "leukemic lines," can be depicted (Fig. 13.167). In other cases, multiple well-defined osteolytic lesions, moth-eaten appearance, or a permeative pattern may be encountered. Periostitis may be seen after fracture or

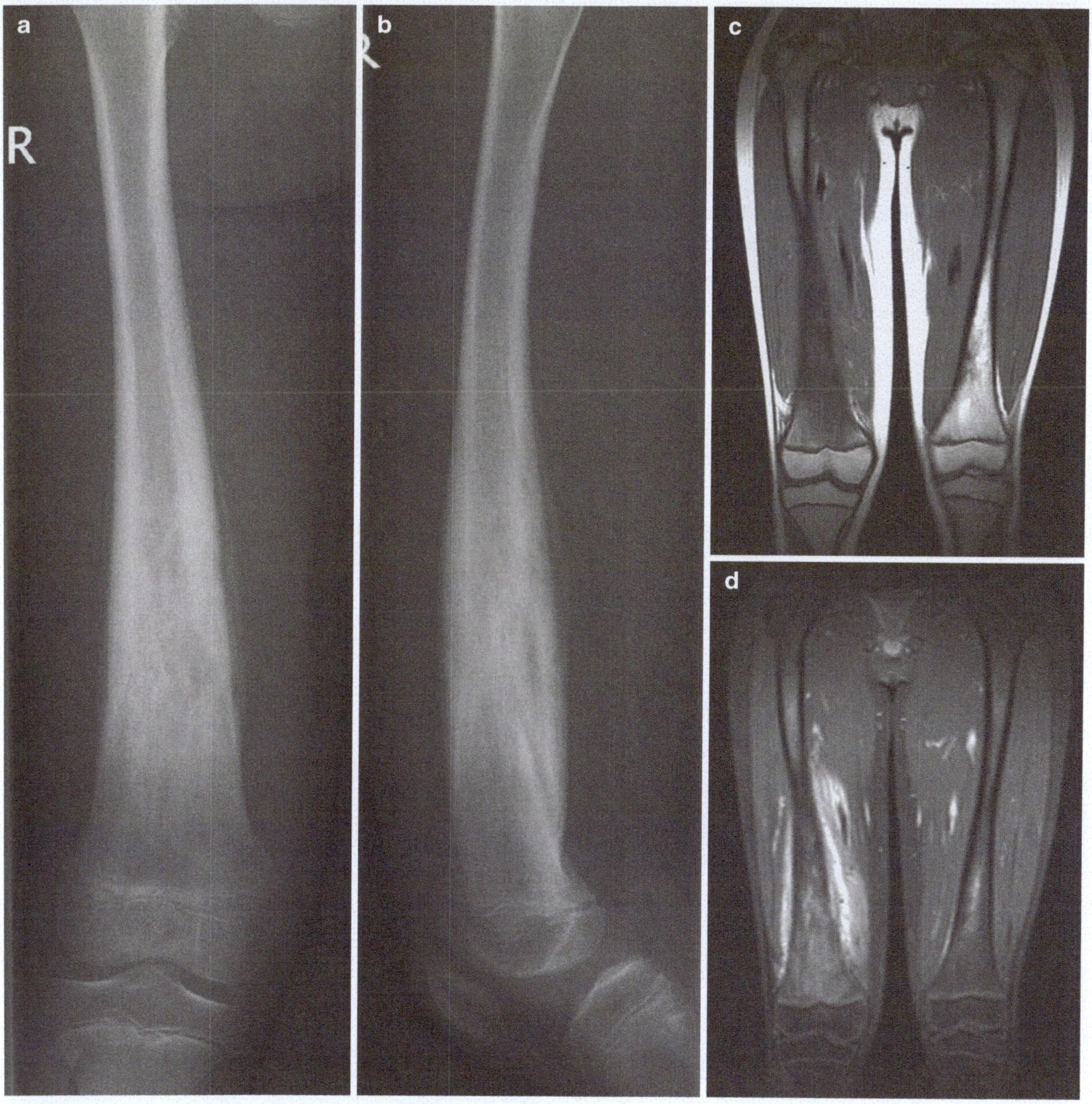

Fig. 13.166 Ewing sarcoma. Radiography of the right upper leg in AP (**a**) and lateral projection (**b**) shows fine permeated pattern involving the medullary space and cortex in concert with multilamellated periosteal reaction of the diametaphysis. Coronal T1-WI (**c**) and contrast-enhanced fat-saturated T1-WI (**d**) demonstrate extensive soft-tissue mass and diametaphyseal marrow infiltration

when leukemic infiltration is present. On MRI, leukemic infiltration is hypointense on T1 (hypointense leukemic infiltrate replaces the normal high signal intensity marrow fat) and markedly hyperintense on fluid-sensitive sequences compared to muscle. Normal red marrow may be slightly hyperintense on fluid-sensitive sequences, has a typical flame shaped appearance (Fig. 13.168), and follows the characteristic pattern of conversion (see Fig. 13.135 and Table 13.24). Leukemic arthritis is much more common in children than it is in adults and it may mimic all other forms of inflammatory arthridities. Therefore, in a child presenting with

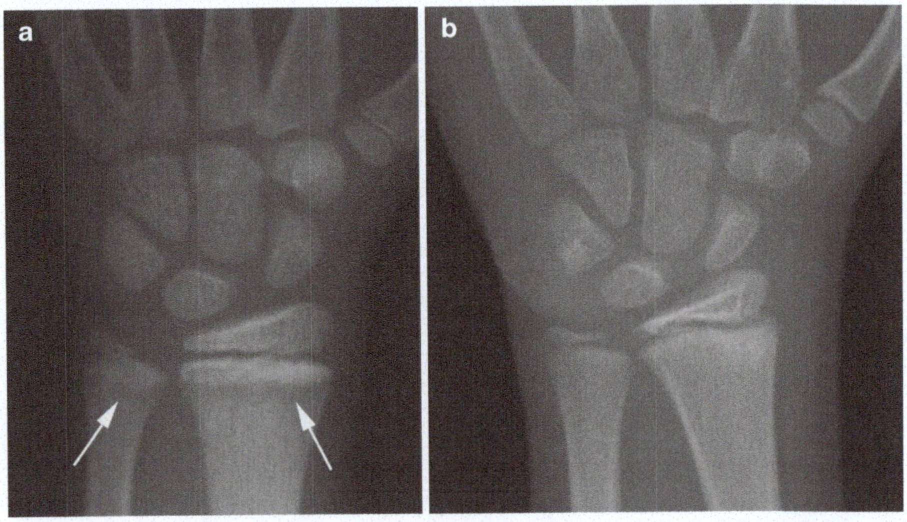

Fig. 13.167 ALL. Radiography (**a**) of the left wrist in AP projection shows metaphyseal radiolucent bands (*arrows*) with sclerotic margins paralleling the physis in the distal ulna and radius (Courtesy of O. Rompel). Compare to normal radiography (**b**) of another child of the same age

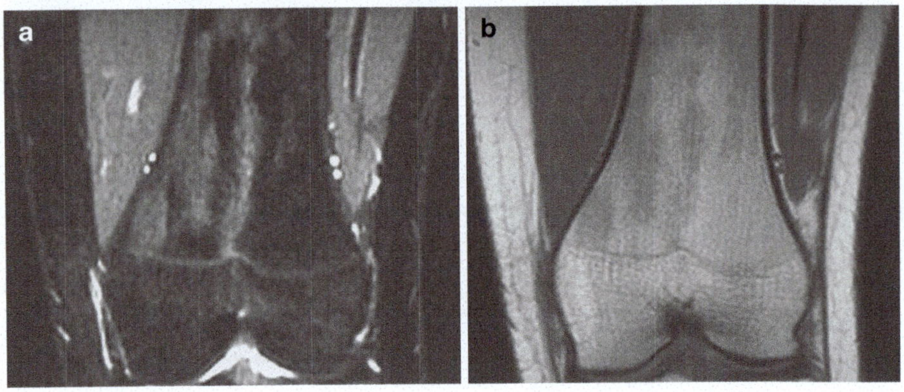

Fig. 13.168 Normal red marrow. Coronal STIR image (**a**) and T1-WI (**b**) show flame-shaped or paint brush appearance of normal red marrow in a 14-year-old girl

"osteomyelitis" or "septic arthritis," one should always look for other symptoms like paleness, anemia, and bruising, and rule out leukemia by complete blood count (CBC) with smear, and consider bone marrow biopsy. Chloroma (granulocytic sarcoma) is typically encountered in the setting of AML, and can occasionally be seen in myelodysplastic or myeloproliferative disorders. These are focal, solid tumors composed of immature myeloid cells that most commonly occur in subcutaneous soft tissues, bone, or head and neck, where they can simulate menignoma or epidural hematoma. Generally, on plain films, sclerosis is typically encountered in myelogenous leukemia, and chloroma may present as a sclerotic lesion. On MRI, granulocytic sarcomas have a nonspecific appearance and are isointense on T1-WI, hyperintense on T2-WI, and show variable enhancement after administration of paramagnetic contrast. Granulocytic sarcomas may demonstrate rim enhancement with a hypointense center, mimicking abscess (Fig. 13.169a–c).

Table 13.24 Various MRI appearance of yellow and red marrow and tumor (Adapted from Kan 2007)

Sequence	Yellow marrow	Red marrow	Tumor
T1	Moderately hyperintense to muscle	Mildly hyperintense to isointense to muscle	Hypo- to isointense to muscle
T2-FS or STIR	Hypointense to muscle	Iso- to slightly hyperintense to muscle	hyperintense to muscle
Diffusion (echoplanar)	– Restricted diffusion	– Restricted diffusion	+ Restricted diffusion
Chemical shift (out of phase)	Hypointense	Hypointense	Hyperintense

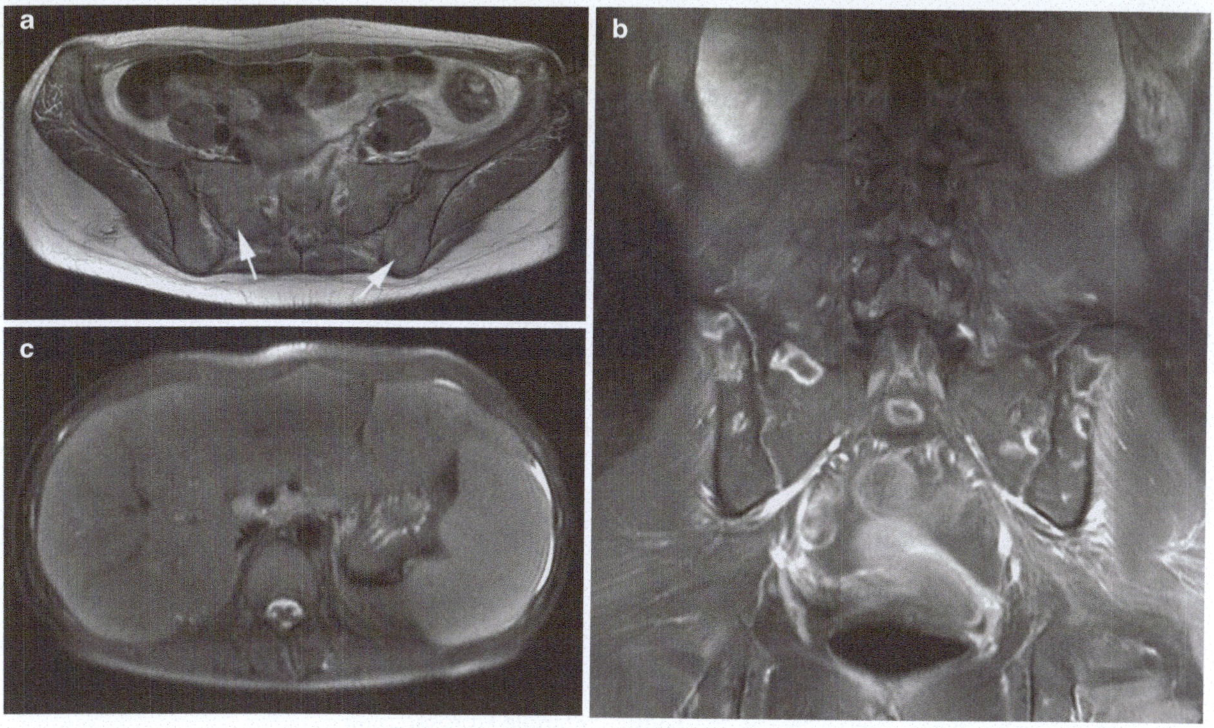

Fig. 13.169 AML with granulocytic sarcomas. Transverse T2-WI (**a**) shows multiple lesions in the sacrum and iliac wings, with a hyperintense center and a hypointense rim (*arrows*). Contrast-enhanced fat-saturated T1-WI (**b**) demonstrates rim enhancement of these lesions with a hypointense center mimicking abscesses. Transverse fat-saturated T2-WI (**c**) shows enlargement of the liver and spleen and ascites in a 16-year-old girl

The musculoskeletal findings in acute leukemia and complications of treatment comprise a wide range of findings, such as marrow infiltration, permeative lytic bone destruction, periosteal new bone formation, chloroma, insufficiency and pathologic fracture, osteonecrosis, spontaneous hemmorrhage, osteomyelitis, infectious arthritis, leukemic arthritis, and secondary neoplasms.

Lymphoma

Primary bone lymphoma (PBL) is diagnosed if the pathologic diagnosis of lymphoma without evidence of nodal or distant disease within 6 months of presentation is assured. Primary NHL of bone may occur at any age, although it is rare in children younger than 10 years. It frequently involves the lower extremities, and tumor most often occurs in the metadiaphyseal region, but can occur in the epiphysis as well. Plain-film findings of PBL show a wide spectrum and may be normal or display permeative osteolysis, moth-eaten osteolysis, or mixed osteolytic/blastic destruction. Aggressive periosteal reaction, cortical destruction, juxtacortical soft-tissue mass, sequestra, pathologic fractures, and transphyseal extension may also be seen. Therefore, a wide spectrum of signal alterations and findings can be encountered on MRI. PBL may be hypointense to hyperintense both on T1-WI and T2-WI, and shows a heterogeneous enhancement after administration of paramagnetic contrast. If PBL extends from or originates in the epiphysis, it may mimic ostemyelitis or chondroblastoma. As PBL may mimic many other benign and malignant lesions on both plain films and MRI, biopsy is necessary for diagnosis.

Metastatic Disease

Metastatic skeletal lesions in children most commonly arise from small round-cell tumors, such as leukemia, lymphoma, or neuroblastoma (Fig. 13.106), but may also be due to osteosarcoma, Ewing's sarcoma, PNET, rhabdomyosarcoma, retinoblastoma, cerebellar medulloblastoma, and Wilms' tumor (5%). In general, metastatic disease appears as focal lesions, involving both cortical bone and marrow, demonstrating low SI on T1-W sequences and bright SI on STIR and T2-W sequences. However, diffuse metastatic disease may be difficult to distinguish from normal marrow on MRI, especially in children. Generally, whole body STIR and/or PET or PET/CT are increasingly performed for evaluation in pediatric oncology.

Aggressive Fibromatosis

Aggressive fibromatosis (infantile fibromatosis) is a group of benign disorders, with locally invasive growth of fibrous tissue that may recur after initial resection but lacks metastatic disease. This tumor can involve subcutaneous tissues, muscles, nerves, vessels, and bone, and can occur almost everywhere in the body, and may be multicentric. On plain films, erosion or bowing of bones can be observerd. On MRI, fibromatosis demonstrates hypointense SI to muscle on T1-WI, and enhances after the administration of paramagnetic contrast. On T2-WI, hypointense to hyperintense SI compared to muscle is observed. Compared to collagen components, the more a cellular component is present, the more hyperintense is the SI on T2-WI (Fig. 13.170). Infantile myofibromatosis is the most common subtype occurring in infancy, and approximately 50% of these tumors are present at birth or are detected by 2 years of age. Three different types are discriminated: solitary, multricentric with visceral involvement, and multricentric without visceral involvement. The multricentric type with visceral involvement has a poor prognosis, whereas the other types undergo spontaneous involution within 1 or 2 years. On plain films, infantile myofibromatosis often has a characteristic metaphyseal osseus lesion with bowing of bone, and sometimes central calcifications can be present. On MRI, the so-called target appearance is observed, referring to the peripheral contrast enhancement without central enhancement on T1-WI after administration of paramagnetic contrast. As a lesion in this age group has to be differentiated from vascular lesions, congenital leukemia/lymphoma, or a sarcoma, biopsy is always necessary.

Infantile Fibrosarcoma

Infantile fibrosarcoma (IF) is the most frequent soft-tissue malignancy in neonates and young infants. It most commonly occurs in the extremities, and distant metastases are present in up to 25% of cases. This soft-tissue mass may be well defined or infiltrative, and has large feeding vessels. On MRI, it shows hypointense to

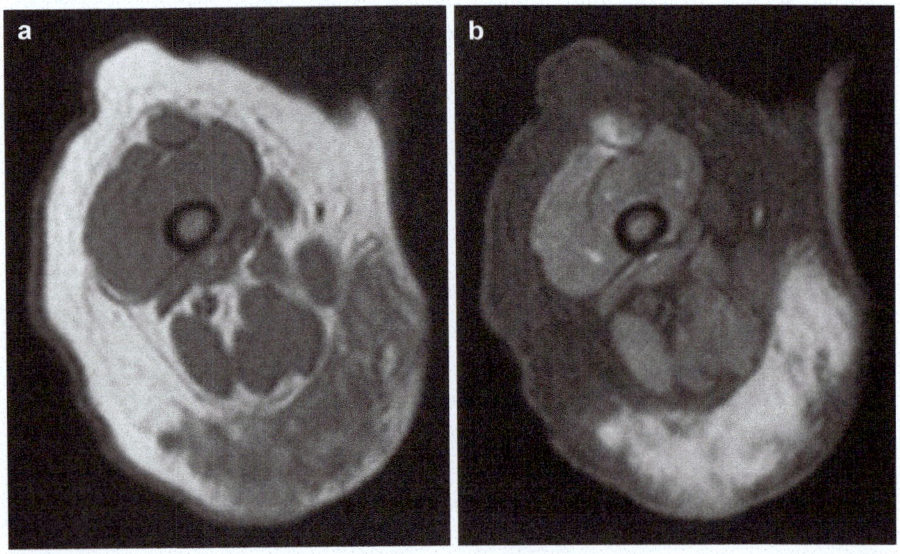

Fig. 13.170 Juvenile fibromatosis. Transverse T1-W (**a**) and FS T1-W (**b**) images show homogeneously enhancing tissue within the subcutaneous fat dorsally and in the rectus femoris muscle of the right upper leg

isointense SI on T1-WI and hyperintense SI on T2-WI, with demarcation of areas of necrosis after the administration of CM. Because of the high-flow vasculature, IF may be mistaken for congenital hemangioma, kaposiform hemangioendothelioma, or other vascular tumors and malformations. Further differential diagnoses for a large soft-tissue mass in newborns comprise infantile myofibromatosis, rhabdomyosarcoma, and, rarely, infantile leukemia. Therefore, biopsy is mandatory to establish the diagnosis. The adjacent bones are often splayed rather than destroyed. Infantile fibrosarcoma responds to chemotherapy with a greater than 90% 5-year disease-free survival rate when disease is localized. Fortunately, response allows a more limited resection.

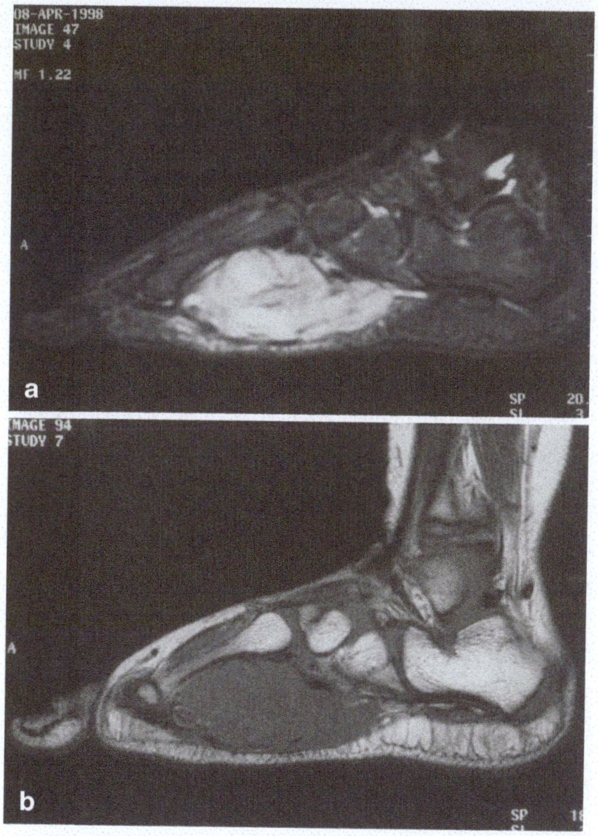

Fig. 13.171 Rhabdomyosarcoma. Sagittal STIR image (**a**) and T1-W (**b**) images show a mass in the sole of the left foot

Rhabdomyosarcoma

Rhabdomyosarcoma (RMS) is a mesenchymal sarcoma arising from primitive muscle cells (rhabdomyoblasts) that fail to differentiate into skeletal muscle. RMS belongs to the group of soft tissue sarcomas, which are the fourth most common tumors in children, and approximately 70% of affected children are younger than 10 years of age at time of presentation. RMS can occur anywhere in the body, but the most common location is the head and neck region (28–40%), followed by genitourinary tract (20%), extremities (15–20%), the trunk (11%), and the retroperitoneum (6%). Two different histologic types are differentiated: alveolar (variant: solid alveolar) and embryonal (variant: botroid, spindle cell). Embryonal RMS accounts for 60–70% of childhood RMSs and is the most common type in children under 15 years of age, whereas alveolar RMS occurs in adolescents and accounts for 20% of RMSs. According to the German guidelines of pediatric oncology and hematology, embryonal RMS with a size ≤5 cm in a child <10 years, arising from the head and neck region (but not parameningeal) or genitourinary locations (nonbladder/prostate) have a more favorable prognosis than alveolar RMSs >5 cm in children >10 years with tumors arising in the head and neck region, from the bladder, prostate or extremities, or parameningeal RMS. On MRI, RMSs tend to be solid masses demonstrating hypointense or similar SI to muscle on T1-WI and hyperintense SI on T2-WI, but may appear heterogeneously and enhance inhomogeneously with paramagnetic contrast, due to hemorrhage and necrosis (Fig. 13.171). After biopsy, neoadjuvant chemotherapy is employed prior to surgical resection.

13.5.7 Trauma

Fractures in children differ from those in adults because, on the one hand, children's bones are more porous and can tolerate a greater deformation than the bone of an adult, and, on the other, the epiphysis is not fused. Typical childhood fractures are bowing fractures, torus fractures, greenstick fractures, and complete fractures, which can be easily diagnosed by plain-film radiographs.

Stress fractures are rare, and occur mostly in the proximal tibia in older children. They demonstrate a zone of sclerosis along a fracture line and periosteal new bone deposition, findings which should not be misinterpreted as a malignant process. On MRI, periosteal edema, endostal edema, and marrow edema are present, and the fracture line is usually perpendicular to the shaft and appears hypointense on T1-WI and may be hypo- to hyperintense on T2-WI. When marrow edema is present without a discrete fracture line, the term stress reaction is more appropriate (Fig. 13.172 and Table 13.25).

More complex are those fractures involving the physis. The standard classification for physeal fractures is that of Salter and Harris. This classification categorizes injuries of the epiphyseal–metaphyseal complex according to the course of the fractures:

- SH I fracture: widened physis
- SH II fracture: widened physis with metaphyseal fragment
- SH III fracture: widened physis with epiphyseal fracture
- SH IV fracture: fracture extending through epiphysis and metaphysis
- SH V fracture: crush injury of the physis (rarely seen on plain-film radiographs)
- SH VI fracture: injury of the perichondral ring

In most cases, plain-film radiography is sufficient to diagnose these lesions. There are no generally established indications for the performance of MR examinations in the case of uncomplicated or physeal fractures, as immobilization and follow-up radiographs are sufficient for treatment. However, MRI can be helpful in selected cases, such as fractures of the femoral neck with risk of developing femoral-head necrosis, or complex injuries of the elbow and ankle, frequently necessitating surgery. On MRI, fracture lines can be identified as lines or zones of low SI in T1-WI, with high SI on T2-WI, reflecting concurrent bone bruise and edema. In contrast to CT, MRI is appropriate to depict the area of bridging exactly in the case of premature closure of the epiphysis caused by physeal bridging.

Joint dislocations occur almost exclusively in older children, as the epiphyseal–metaphyseal junction is a weak zone, and physeal fractures are therefore more frequently encountered than joint dislocation. In young children, the joint most commonly injured is the elbow, whereas the ankle and knee are frequently affected in older children. A severely injured knee joint should be evaluated by MRI (Fig. 13.173).

Acute or chronic avulsion fractures in older children occur along the crest of the iliac wing, the greater and lesser trochanters, along the inferior aspect of the ischium, the medial supracondylar ridge of the femur, and the medial epicondyle of the humerus. MRI is very helpful in evaluating the extent of avulsion fractures (Fig. 13.174). The bones can be strikingly irregular, and a pseudomalignant appearance can result in the course of healing.

13.5.7.1 Slipped Capital Femoral Epiphysis

The etiology for slipped femoral capital epiphysis (SCFE) has not been completely clarified yet, and is probably a combination of repetitive microtrauma predisposing to epiphyseal displacement and delayed metaphyseal endochondral ossification. Children that are obese, marfanoid, of African descent, or suffer from endocrinopathies such as growth hormone deficiency, hypothyroidism, or hypogonadism, metabolic disorders such as rickets and malnutrition, or renal failure are at the risk of developing SCFE. Furthermore, radiation therapy, chemotherapy, Down syndrome, and developmental dysplasia of the hip are other predisposing factors. Children present with pain, primarily in the hip, groin, or proximal thigh (85%), or in the distal thigh or knee (15%). The average age of presentation is 11–12 years in girls and 13–14 years in boys, with the males being affected more often (M:F = 2.5:1). SCFE can affect both hips, and in 22% of cases, it is bilateral at time of presentation. If both hips are involved, this usually occurs within 2 years. Clinically, SCFE is classified based on chronicity: acute (<3 weeks) vs. chronic (>3 weeks); stability: stable (able to bear any weight) vs. unstable (unable to bear weight); and severity based on slip angle (mild, moderate, severe). Occurrence of femoral-head necrosis is more dependent on unstability than on the severity of the slip. In SCFE, there are classical radiographic findings. On the anteroposterior radiograph, the epiphysis drops

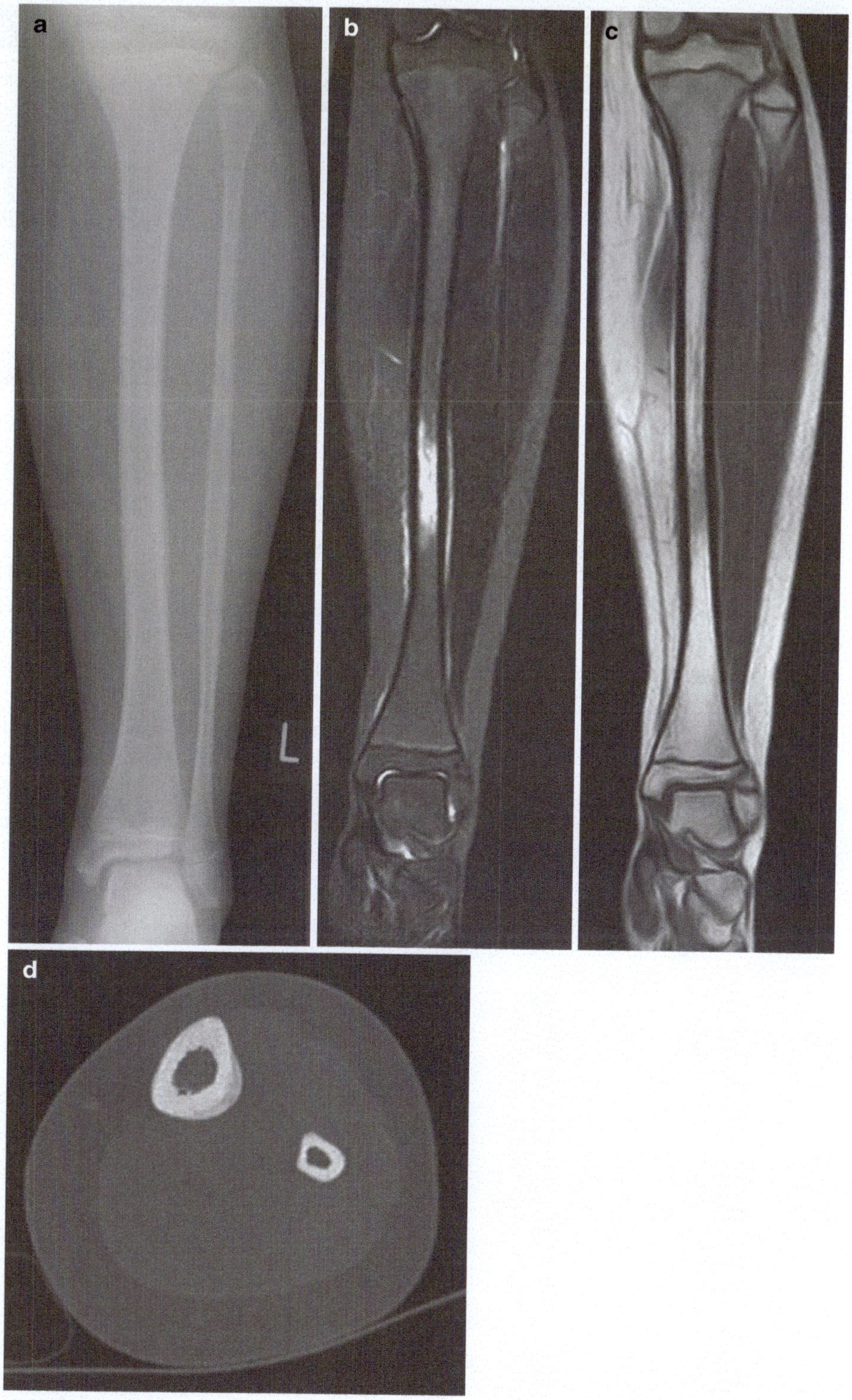

Fig. 13.172 Tibial stress reaction grade 3. Radiography of the left lower leg (**a**) and CT (**d**) show a thick unilamellated periosteal reaction at the lateral tibia. Coronal STIR (**b**) and T1-WI (**c**) demonstrate intramedullary and periosteal STIR hyperintensity together with a mild T1 hypointensity. A discrete fracture line is not seen

Table 13.25 MRI grading system for tibial stress reaction (Adapted from Kan 2007)

Grade	Periosteal edema T2	Marrow edema T2	Marrow edema T1	Other
1	+	None	None	
2	+	+	None	
3	+	+	+	
4	+	+	+	Fracture line present through marrow and cortex

+ hypointense T1 S1 or hyperintense T2 S1

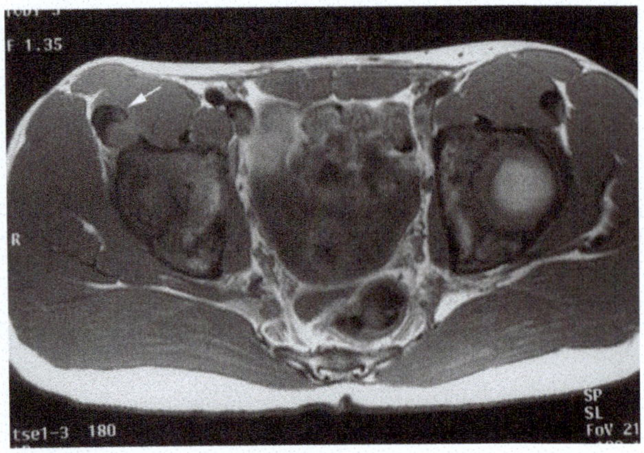

Fig. 13.174 Avulsion fracture. Transverse T1-WI shows avulsion of the rectus femoris tendon from the anterior inferior iliac spina (*arrow*) on the right side

toward or below Klein's line, which is a line drawn along the top of the femoral neck and continued toward the acetabulum (Fig. 13.175a, b). This line normally crosses a small portion of the capital femoral epiphysis. SCFE is more easily depicted on frog-lateral radiographs, as medial displacement of epiphysis relative to metaphysic, or on cross-table lateral radiographs, with 25° flexion as posterior displacement. On MRI, focal or diffuse widening of the physis, periphyseal edema, joint effusion, synovitis, and a variable extend of slippage can be observed in SCFE (Fig. 13.175c, d). Images should be aquired in all three planes to illustrate degree and direction of slippage. The role of MRI is to detect SCFE in the preslip or early slip stage in patients with normal plain-film findings or physeal widening, to illustrate the degree of slippage and femoral neck angulation prior to surgical treatment by pin fixation, and to evaluate complications of SCFE and its treatment, such as femoral-head necrosis, premature degenerative changes, labral tears related to CAM-type femoroacetabular impingement, chondrolysis, and coxa vara deformity.

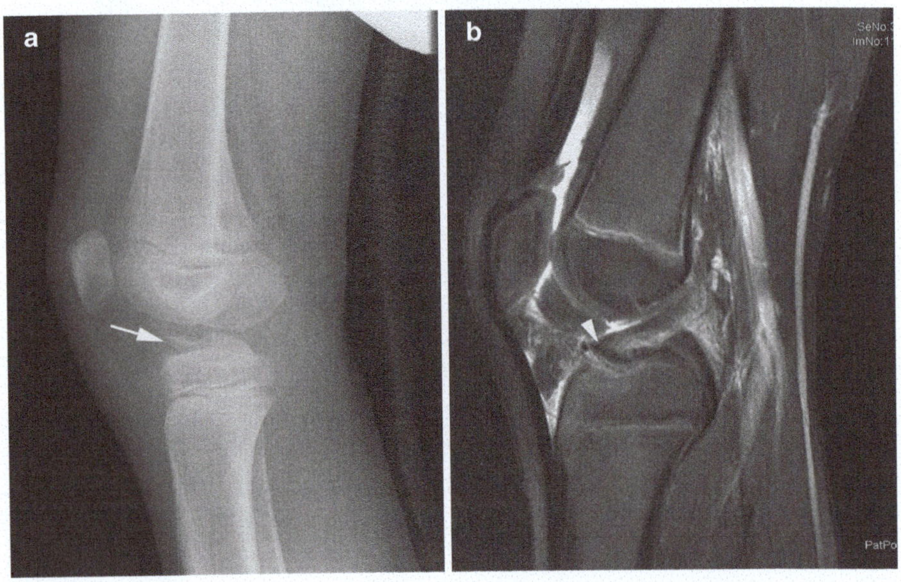

Fig. 13.173 Tibial eminence fracture. Radiography in lateral projection (**a**) clearly shows the tibial eminence fracture fragment (*arrow*). Sagittal contrast-enhanced fat-saturated T1-WI (**b**) demonstrates the anterior cruciate ligament fibers (*arrowhead*) inserting onto the fracture fragment, with the ligamentous morphology being preserved. A hemarthrosis is present

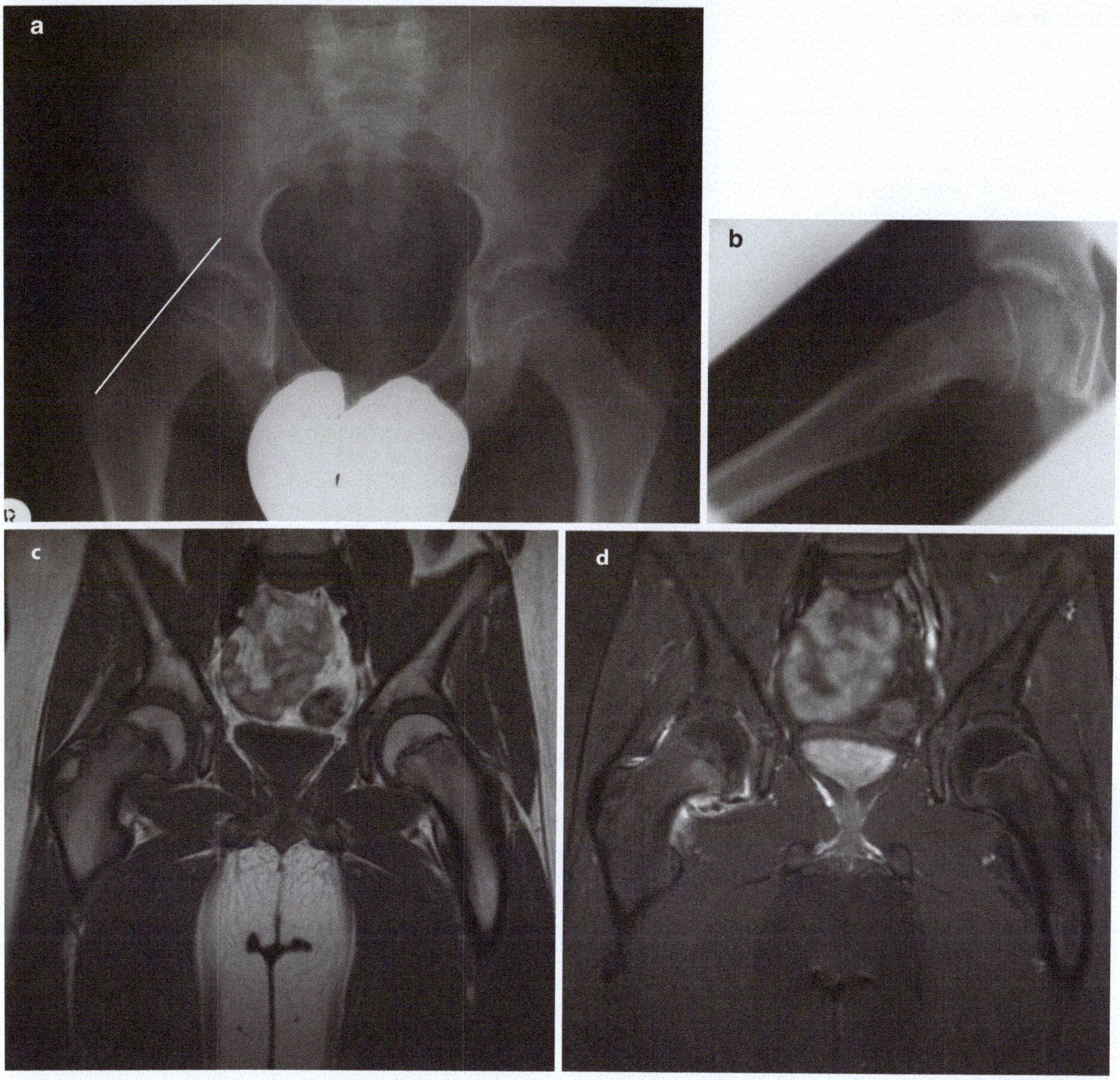

Fig. 13.175 Slipped capital femoral epiphysis. Radiography of the pelvis (**a**) shows mild physeal widening on the right side. Klein's line (white) does not bisect the capital femoral epiphysis. Frog-lateral radiography (**b**) clearly depicts posterior and medial displacement of the capital femoral epiphysis relative to metaphysis. Coronal T1-WI (**c**) shows physeal widening, diminished SI in the epiphyseal marrow and the metaphyseal marrow medially, in concert with displacement of epiphysis. Contrast enhanced fat-saturated coronal T1-WI (**d**) demonstrates enhancement of marrow and synovium

Further Reading

Argyropoulou MI et al (2007) MRI evaluation of tissue iron burden in patients with beta-thalassaemia major. Pediatr Radiol 37(12):1191–1200

Atlas SW (1996) Magnetic resonance imaging of the brain and spine, 2nd edn. Lippincott-Raven, Philadelphia, PA

Azouz EM (2008) Juvenile idiopathic arthritis: how can the radiologist help the clinician? Pediatr Radiol 38(suppl 3): S403–S408

Ball WS Jr (1997) Pediatric neuroradiology. Lippincott-Raven, Philadelphia, PA

Barkovich AJ (2005) Pediatric neuroimaging, 4th edn. Lippincott Williams & Wilkins, Philadelphia, PA

Barkovich AJ (2007) Diagnostic imaging pediatric neuroradiology, 1st edn. Amirsys, Salt Lake City, UT

Brisse HJ et al (2008) Imaging in unilateral Wilms tumour. Pediatr Radiol 38(1):18–29

Brodeur GM, Seeger RC, Barrett A et al (1988) International criteria for diagnosis, staging, and response to treatment in patients with neuroblastoma. J Clin Oncol 6:1874–1881

Brodeur GM, Pritchard J, Berthold F et al (1993) Revisions in the international criteria for neuroblastoma diagnosis, staging, and response to treatment. J Clin Oncol 11:1466–1477

Burrows PE, Laor T, Paltiel H, Robertson RL (1998) Diagnostic imaging in the evaluation of vascular birthmarks. Dermatol Clin 16:455–488

Cauley KA et al (2009) Diffusion tensor imaging and tractography of Rasmussen encephalitis. Pediatr Radiol 39(7):727–730

Chaudry G et al (2009) Imaging of congenital mesoblastic nephroma with pathological correlation. Pediatr Radiol 39(10): 1080–1086

DiVito A et al (2008) Juvenile idiopathic arthritis with rice bodies. Pediatr Radiol 38(11):1263

Donnelly LF (2005) Diagnostic imaging pediatrics, 1st edn. Amirsys, Salt Lake City, UT

Enjolras O, Mulliken JB (1998) Vascular tumors and vascular malformations (new issues). Adv Dermatol 13:375–423. Mosby-Year Book Inc

Gadner H, Gaedicke G, Niemeyer Ch, Ritter J (2006) Pädiatrische Hämatologie und Onkologie. Springer Medizin Verlag, Heidelberg

Helmberger H, Kammer B (2007) In Freyschmidt J Handbuch diagnostische Radiologie: Feuerbach ST Gastointestinales System. Springer, Berlin/Heidelberg/New York

Huang IH et al (2008) Fast-recovery fast spin-echo T2-weighted MR imaging: a free breathing alternative to fast spin-echo in the pediatric abdomen. Pediatr Radiol 38(6):675–679

Jaramillo D et al (2008) Pediatric musculoskeletal MRI: basic principles to optimize success. Pediatr Radiol 38(4):379–391

Kaatsch P (2009) Jahresbericht 2006/2007 des Deutschen Kinderkrebsregisters. www.kinderkrebsregister.de.

Kan JH (2007) Pediatric and adolescent musculoskeletal MRI. Springer Science + Business Media LLC, New York

Kan JH (2008) Major pitfalls in musculoskeletal imaging-MRI. Pediatr Radiol 38(suppl 2):S251–S255

Kan JH et al (2008) MRI diagnosis of bone marrow relapse in children with ALL. Pediatr Radiol 38(1):76–81

Karimova EJ et al (2007) MR imaging of osteonecrosis of the knee in children with acute lymphocytic leukemia. Pediatr Radiol 37(11):1140–1146

Kellenberger CJ (2009) Pitfalls in paediatric musculoskeletal imaging. Pediatr Radiol 39(suppl 3):372–381

Kerssemakers SP et al (2009) Sport injuries in the pediatric and adolescent patient: a growing problem. Pediatr Radiol 39(5):471–484

Kirks DR (1998) Practical pediatric imaging, 2nd edn. Lippincott-Raven, Philadelphia, PA

Kitagawa N et al (2007) Biliary rhabdomyosarcoma. Pediatr Radiol 37(10):1059

Knaap MS, van der Valk J (1995) Magnetic resonance of myelin; myelination and myelin disorders, 2nd edn. Springer, Berlin/Heidelberg/New York

Kuhn JP, Slovis TS, Haller JO (2004) Caffey's pediatric diagnostic imaging, 10th edn. Mosby, Philadelphia, PA

Kumar J et al (2008) Whole body MR imaging with the use of parallel imaging for detection of skeletal metastases in pediatric patients with small-cell neoplasms: comparison with skeletal scintigraphy and FDG PET/CT. Pediatr Radiol 38(9):953–962

Merrow AC et al (2008) Leukemia and treatment: imprint on the growing skeleton. Pediatr Radiol 38(5):594

Mulliken JB, Glowacki J (1982) Hemangiomas and vascular malformations in infants and children: a classification based on endothelial characteristics. Plast Reconstr Surg 69:412–422

Obeid M et al (2007) Diffusion-weighted imaging findings on MRI as the sole radiographic findings in a child with proven herpes simplex encephalitis. Pediatr Radiol 37(11):1159–1162

Osborn AG (1993) Diagnostic neuroradiology. Mosby, New York

Owens CM et al (2008) Bilateral disease and new trends in Wilms tumour. Pediatr Radiol 38(1):30–39

Phelan JA et al (2008) Pediatric neurodegenerative white matter processes: leukodystrophies and beyond. Pediatr Radiol 38(7):729–749

Pizzo PA, Poplack DG (eds) (2006) Principles and practice of pediatric oncology, 5th edn. Lippincott Williams & Wilkins, Philadelphia, PA

Roebuck D (2008) Focal liver lesion in children. Pediatr Radiol 38(suppl 3):S518–S522

Swischuk LE (1997) Imaging of the newborn, infant, and young child, 4th edn. Williams & Wilkins, Philadelphia, PA

Turkbey B et al (2009) Autosomal recessive polycystic kidney disease and congenital hepatic fibrosis (ARPKD/CHF). Pediatr Radiol 39(2):100–111

Van der Meijs BB et al (2009) Neonatal hepatic haemangioendothelioma: treatment options and dilemmas. Pediatr Radiol 39(3):277–281

Van Rijn RR et al (2008) Imaging findings in noncraniofacial childhood rhabdomyosarcoma. Pediatr Radiol 38(6):617–634

Whole-Body MRI

14

Gerwin Schmidt, Dietmar Dinter, Stefan Schoenberg, and Maximilian Reiser

Contents

14.1 Introduction

The introduction of whole-body magnetic resonance imaging (WB-MRI) has fundamentally changed diagnostic concepts for imaging of various systemic diseases in recent years. As an alternative to multi-modality imaging approaches, whole-body techniques are now increasingly applied in clinical routine, especially for an integrated imaging of malignant disease. However, the crucial problem for implementing WB-MRI in the past has been to integrate substantially different requirements in coil setup, contrast media application, slice positioning, and sequence design into one single comprehensive scan. Significant improvements in hardware, from pioneering approaches using a rolling platform system mounted on top of a conventional MRI scanner to the essential introduction of state-of the-art multi-channel whole-body scanners with automated free table movement, have cleared the way for clinically feasible and efficient total body imaging concepts. Furthermore, important innovations in sequence design and image acquisition physics, such as parallel acquisition techniques (PATs), have helped to significantly reduce overall examination times without compromising spatial resolution, and have increased patient comfort and acceptance. Now a dedicated assessment of various organs by sequences with adequate soft tissue contrast, image orientation, spatial

G. P. Schmidt (✉)
Department of Clinical Radiology,
LMU-University of Munich, Grosshadern Campus,
Marchioninistrasse 15, 81377 Munich, Germany
e-mail: gerwin.schmidt@med.uni-muenchen.de

P. Reimer et al. (eds.), *Clinical MR Imaging*,
DOI: 10.1007/978-3-540-74504-4_14,

resolution, and contrast media dynamics can be combined with whole-body anatomic coverage.

Various useful applications have emerged for an integrated diagnostic approach to cancer as a systemic disease, especially in the field of tumor imaging. WB-MRI has been introduced for primary tumor staging and surveillance of various neoplastic entities, as well as a potential new tool for secondary prevention and screening of asymptomatic patients. Furthermore, WB-MRI has been implemented as a diagnostic concept for imaging of different hematologic- and bone marrow disorders such as lymphoma or multiple myeloma. Finally, WB-MRI has found its way into clinical imaging as a useful new approach to describe various benign systemic diseases. These include inflammatory diseases including rheumatoid arthritis (RA) or long term-diabetes, as well as musculoskeletal disease such as multiple cartilaginous exostoses or systemic muscle dystrophy.

The following chapter outlines prerequisites, technical concepts, and developments for total body imaging, and highlights various established and future clinical application within the field of oncologic imaging and imaging of various benign systemic diseases.

14.2 Protocol Design, Technical Concepts and Advances in WB-MRI

14.2.1 Protocol Design

With its excellent tissue contrast and detailed morphological information, MRI is an ideal candidate for total body imaging. At the same time, MRI with a whole-body approach has to guarantee a high standard image resolution and quality in all anatomic regions, comparable to a dedicated MRI exam, within a reasonable total scan time.

An ideal WB-MRI concept for oncologic imaging purposes should include various sequence types and tissue contrasts, as well as different contrast media dynamics within a multi-planar imaging approach, and cover all possible routes of locoregional and hematogenic spread. A state-of-the-art tumor protocol may imply T1-weighted (W) turbo spin-echo sequence (TSE) and short tau inversion recovery sequence (STIR) imaging for the assessment of musculoskeletal pathologies and fast high resolution imaging of the lung. For the assessment of lung pathologies, fast spin echo imaging (e.g., half Fourier acquired single-shot turbo spin-echo sequence, HASTE) has been proved useful for a detailed reproduction of lung parenchyma and hilar structures with less blurring and signal decay. Additionally, contrast-enhanced studies of the brain, abdomen, and pelvis, including dynamic contrast media application (e.g., T1-weighted 3D- gradient echo sequences) in the upper abdomen for an accurate assessment of parenchymal lesions are indispensable (Fig. 14.1). An example of an "all-round" whole-body tumor protocol for a multi-planar imaging approach within a total scan time of 52 min (without localizers) is presented in Table 14.1. In Table 14.2, sequence parameters of the protocol are summarized for different field strengths. Alternatively, the protocol may be reduced for a noncontrasted total bone marrow screening approach, comprising T1-W TSE and STIR imaging of the body combined with dedicated imaging of the complete spine, at a total scan time of 45 min (see Fig. 14.6). The described protocol can, naturally, only be a representative example of an integrated WB-MRI concept, and obviously a sensible WB-MRI concept has to be individually adapted to the clinical problem and nature of the examined pathology. Specifically adapted whole-body MRI protocols for non-oncologic applications such as systemic imaging of rheumatic disease and diabetes are discussed in the following sections (see Sects. 14.5.1.1 and 14.5.2).

Finally, it has to be stressed that up to now it remains difficult to integrate complex dedicated coil setups for imaging of specific entities such as breast- or prostate cancer (which represent two of the four most frequent cancers) into a time-effective whole-body protocol. The aspect of tailoring different protocols to certain tumor types or to a specific risk profile of the patient to further increase both sensitivity and feasibility certainly remains an important matter concerning the development of WB-MRI concepts in the coming future.

14.2.2 Technical Approaches

All WB-MRI concepts are limited by two geometrical restrictions inherent to every MRI system: the maximum possible field of view (FoV) along the *z*-axis and the possible range of table movement within the magnet. These two system properties influence the choice of the most adequate or efficient acquisition technique.

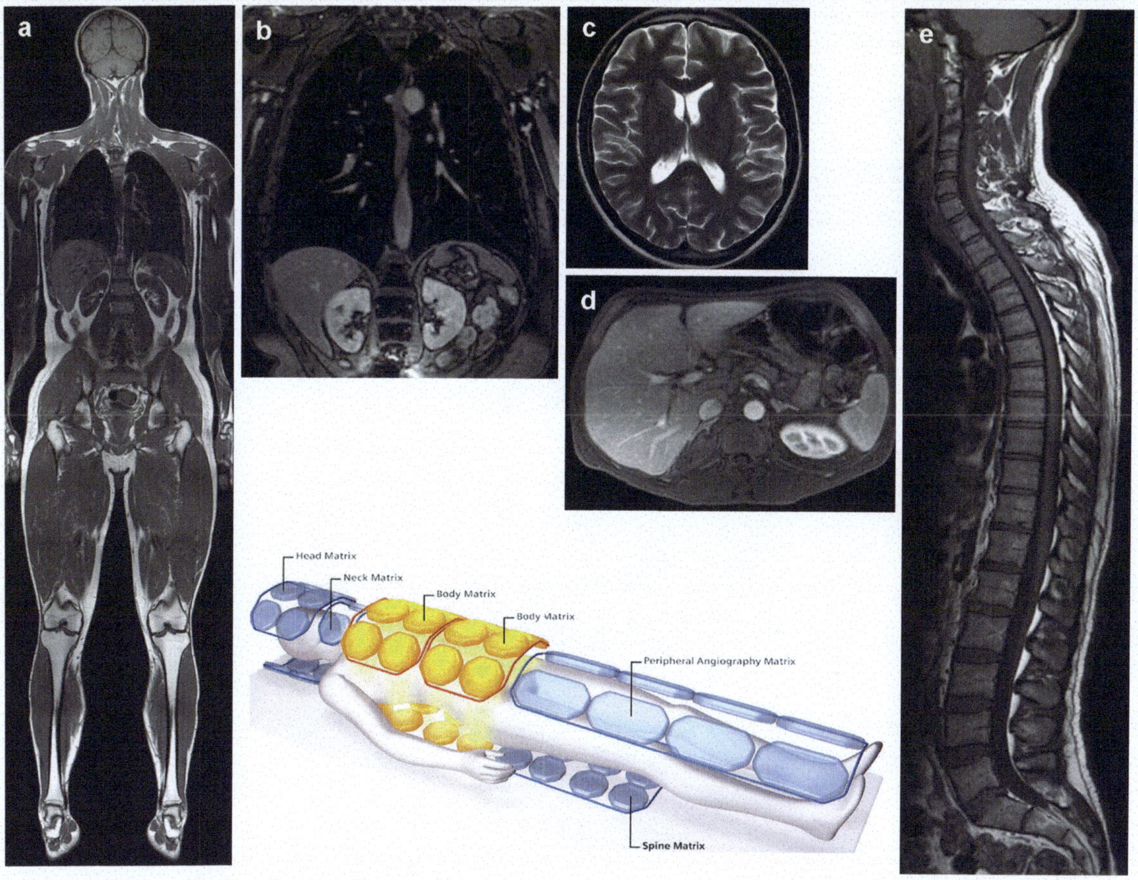

Fig. 14.1 Total body matrix coil system with a combination of head, neck, body, spine, and peripheral angio-coils, equipped with multiple receiver coil elements. Either WB-MRI from head to toe or dedicated imaging of special areas of interest is possible, using parallel imaging (PI) in all three spatial orientations. (**a**) Coronal T1-W TSE WB-MRI at five body levels. (**b**) Coronal contrast-enhanced 3D-GRE sequence of the chest and upper abdomen. (**c**) Axial T2-W TSE of the brain. (**d**) Axial T1-W fat sat GRE of the abdomen. (**e**) Sagittal T1-W TSE of the whole spine at two body levels

14.2.2.1 Multi-Step Approach

Initially, WB-MRI was performed with a sequential scanning approach on conventional MRI scanner systems using standard head, neck, body, and spine array coils. First, the patient was examined head first with coronal scans of the skull/neck and the thorax using a combination of head coil, neck array coil, and one to two body array coils. Sagittal images of the spine were acquired using the spine array coil. In order to acquire image data from the pelvis and distal extremities, however, on most scanners, the subject had to be repositioned from the head-first to the feet-first position because of the limited range of table movement (including a time-consuming rearrangement of the coil setup). Therefore, a total examination time beyond an hour had to be taken in account, restricting clinical feasibility and patient acceptance. This pioneering approach has initially been only used for imaging of skeletal metastases using T1-W TSE and STIR sequences.

14.2.2.2 Rolling Table Concept

The introduction of the AngioSURF or BodySURF™ technique was an important first step to overcome FoV restrictions and perform WB-MRI within a one-step examination. The setup consists of a rolling table (length 270 cm, width 33–50 cm) mounted on top of a conventional scanner table, allowing free movement in the *z*-direction. The signal is acquired using the

Table 14.1 WB-MRI protocol for oncologic imaging on a 32-receiver channel whole-body scanner at 1.5 or 3 T, with the use of total body matrix technology and PI. Total imaging time is 52 min at 1.5 T and 43 min at 3 T, with unchanged image resolution. Total field of view along the *z*-axis is a maximum of 205 cm

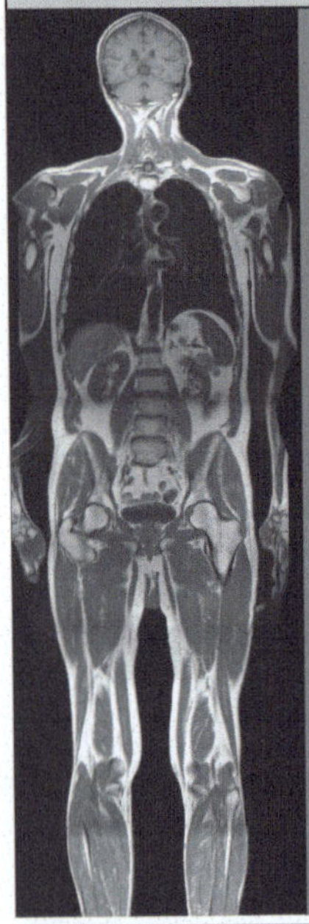

Whole-body MRI at 1.5 or 3 T				
Min	**Head/neck**	**Thorax**	**Abdomen/pelvis**	**Lower extremity**
	STIR cor	STIR cor	STIR cor	STIR cor
		HASTE ax	HASTE ax	
			T2 TSE fs ax	
20	T1 SE cor	T1 TSE cor	T1 TSE cor	T1 TSE cor
	Contrast media application			
		T1 TSE sag	T1 TSE sag	
40		STIR sag	STIR sag	
		T1 fs 3D-GRE ax	T1 fs 3D-GRE ax	
			T1 TSE fs ax	
50	T1 TSE ax			
	T2 TSE ax			
Total scan time at 1.5 T = 52 min, at 3 T = 43 min, PAT 2-3				

Table 14.2 Sequence protocol for high resolution total body imaging at 1.5 and 3 T using a high resolution approach with various contrast dynamics

Sequence	Image plane	Matrix/resolution (mm^3)	1.5 T Acquisition time (min)	3 T Acquisition time (min)
STIR-WB	Coronal	384/1.8 × 1.3 × 5.0	9:43	6:40
HASTE-abdo	Coronal	384/1.4 × 1.3 × 5.0	0:38	0:33
HASTE-lung	Axial	320/1.3 × 1.2 × 6.0	0:44	0:42
T2wfs TSE-liver (free-breathing)	Axial	320/1.6 × 1.2 × 5.0	3:41	3:41
T1w TSE-WB	Coronal	384/1.7 × 1.3 × 5.0	10:30	7:53
T1w TSE-spine	Sagittal	384/1.0 × 1.0 × 3.0	7:46	6:15
STIR-spine	Sagittal	384/1.0 × 1.0 × 3.0	7:22	7:00
Dynamic T1wfs 3D-GRE liver	Axial	384/1.9 × 1.5 × 3.0	2:20	2:20
Static VIBE thorax	Axial	380/1.6 × 1.6 × 1.5	0:25	0:25
T1wfs GRE pelvis	Axial	320/1.5 × 1.2 × 6.0	1:17	1:10
T1w TSE-brain	Axial	320/0.7 × 0.7 × 5.0	3:11	–
T1w GRE-brain	Axial		–	3:17
T2w TSE-brain	Axial	512/0.5 × 0.5 × 5.0	3:11	2:52
Total			51:49	42:48

integrated spine array and a flexible phased array body coil, which remains fixed in the center of the gantry. During the examination, the patient is manually moved in between both coils through the isocenter of the magnet at different body levels. Despite an important increase in patient comfort and significant reduction of total scan time, several restrictions of this concept had to be taken into account. First, practicability of this concept is mainly restricted to slimmer patients; second, significant compromises in spatial resolution will have to be taken into account when using the phased array body coil (designed for abdominal imaging) in the head/neck region or on peripheral body parts.

Yet, this pioneering approach has been successfully introduced for whole-body MRI screening for metastatic disease, especially bone metastases, using coronal scans at five different body levels. T1-W-gradient echo pre- and postcontrast, as well as fast spine echo T2-weighted sequences (e.g. HASTE) and STIR sequences were acquired within a total scan time of 40 min. It has also been demonstrated for whole-body MR-angiography (MRA) using an initial approach for image acquisition during continuous table movement (CTM). With a real-time, axial 2D TrueFISP sequence at a table speed of 5 cm/s, total acquisition time was approximately 30 s.

14.2.2.3 Total Body Matrix Technology

An important technological advance for an enduring introduction of WB-MRI into clinical routine was the development of multi-receiver channel scanners using total body matrix coil setups (TIM, total imaging matrix, Siemens Medical Solutions/Erlangen, Germany). Scanners equipped with up to 32 independent receiver channels combined with a multiple phased-array coil system of 76–102 elements covering the whole body have realized imaging of the total body from head to feet without compromises in spatial resolution. Figure 14.1 gives a schematic overview of the coil setup. Once the patient is placed in a supine position, either imaging of specific organ regions of interest or imaging of the whole body with a maximum FoV of 205 cm along the *z*-axis is possible using free table movement. Additionally, various combinations of the individual coil elements enable use of parallel imaging acquisition techniques (PI) in three spatial orientations, which results in substantially shorter room time. Now, tailored and flexible sequence protocols with high resolution imaging similar to dedicated MRI are possible, including various sequence types and tissue contrast, as well as different contrast media dynamics into a multi-planar imaging approach. Further evident advantages of PI for WB-MRI are shorter individual scan times, which can be used either for image enhancement by use of multiple averaging or for shorter breath holds, an important aspect for oncologic WB-MRI, often performed on multi-morbid patients in impaired physical condition. Also, PI has important advantages in single shot applications, e.g., echo planar imaging (EPI) diffusion weighted imaging for the brain or HASTE imaging of the lung. On one hand, it reduces blurring and image distortion; on the other hand, it leads to shorter echo times and length of echo train, which is especially useful in tissue with high T2* decay, such as lung parenchyma, thereby avoiding loss of SNR. An advantage of PI for dynamic contrast-enhanced sequences such as 3D gradient echo volume interpolated breathold exams (VIBE) is the larger anatomical coverage in one image stack during contrast media transit. When free-breathing T2-W imaging of the liver is performed, PI reduces scan time by half, from 8 min down to 4 min acquisition time, with higher spatial resolution.

14.2.2.4 WB-MRI Application at Higher Field Strength

Recently, approved clinical WB-MRI scanners with a field strength of 3 T have become commercially available, equipped with the previously described technique of multiple phased array coils and receiver channels. This has opened the way for a migration of multi-organ and whole-body applications to higher field strength. The gain of SNR can be used to reduce overall scan time, especially for the acquisition of T2-W fat suppressed sequences at a constant image resolution. The proposed sequence protocol for high contrast WB-MRI (see Sect. 14.2.1, Table 14.1) at 3 T results in a shortened total scan time of 43 min (compared to 52 min at 1.5 T), using identical image resolution parameters, which potentially can increase patient comfort and acceptance. Yet, further time savings within large FoV applications at 3 T are limited due to high field-specific conditions. Because of the increase in T1 relaxation times, T1-W SE/TSE sequences with longer repetition time (TR) have to be applied, if contrast parameters are meant to be kept constant. This consecutively limits reduction of acquisition time. Especially, TSE imaging, which is an important part of a whole-body examination protocol, is markedly influenced by specific absorption rate (SAR) limitations. Recently, the advent of hyperechoes and variable flip angle techniques have been proved useful for acceptable SAR values for larger anatomic coverage with TSE sequences. Finally, image resolution can further be increased at 3 T to potentially gain higher diagnostic sensitivity. The increased SNR with the use of PI allows recording of large, highly resolved isotropic 3D data sets (e.g., 3D turbo spin echo sequences with variable flip angle distribution/SPACE) within short acquisition times, which can further improve diagnosis of soft tissue or bone marrow pathologies in complex anatomic structures such as the pelvis, the shoulder girdle, or the rib cage. Nevertheless, image quality at 3 T is still somewhat limited by a variety of artifacts. This includes B_0-related susceptibility and off-resonance/banding artefacts, B_1-related standing wave effects, and increased chemical shift.

14.2.3 Postprocessing and Further Technical Concepts

14.2.3.1 Postprocessing

After data acquisition, different methods can be applied for postprocessing of the images. Basic techniques comprise the subtraction of post and precontrast images or maximum intensity projection, as used in MRA, or quantification of the apparent diffusion coefficient (ADC) from diffusion-weighted EPI sequence raw data. Furthermore, semiquantitative and quantitative parameters of organ perfusion can be calculated, and tumor-related angiogenesis or vessel immaturity can be assessed by wash-in/out parameters using pharmacokinetic modeling, e.g., for differentiation of breast cancer from benign breast tumors.

A pivotal postprocessing method of whole-body imaging is to combine the data sets that have the same sequence parameters and contrast weighting but were acquired at different table positions of the body in one single series of images. This so-called composing technique also carries out a distortion correction of the images, which are usually deformed at the edges of large FoV because of magnetic field inhomogeneities. Minor errors of the composing software can also be manually corrected. The composed images have the same matrix size as the original data, which allows zooming in without a loss of quality.

14.2.3.2 Further Technical Concepts

Further technical concepts in WB-MRI, which so far have only partly been implemented into clinical workflow, include computer-aided labeling of tumorous nodules in different organs (e.g., lung, breast), combined with the possibility to create a structured report to describe and store lesions and highlight important findings. Furthermore, these reports can be recalled during the next evaluation, which is helpful in oncological patients, to consistently report findings according to the RECIST criteria. Future challenges are the handling of large amounts of image data, and "filtering" the essential information for the radiologists by development of integrated computed aided diagnosis (CAD) concepts within clinical workflow. This already has been applied in the lung with semi-automatic detection and segmentation of nodules and tumors by computed tomography (CT), but it has remained difficult to implement automatic segmentation into a WB-MRI concept.

14.2.4 Outlook: Continuous Table Movement

The latest step after the established multi-step techniques has been the so-called "move during scan" or "CTM" technique. Disadvantages of multi-step techniques are the considerable amount of time required to reposition the table in-between the different anatomic stations, and the overlap of the single coronal FoV's with redundant image contents, which lead to signal reduction artefacts and geometric distortions at the image borders due to the nonlinearity of the gradient fields in composed images. To solve these problems, different approaches were undertaken: a fast axial 2D sequence can be performed while the table moves continuously at low speed, so that the movement of the table in z-axis undercuts the slice thickness. The limitations are the restricted matrix size as well as relative thick image slices so that these images cannot sufficiently be reformatted in three dimensions. Using newer approaches, the phase encoding direction or the frequency encoding direction is orientated along the movement axis during table movement, so that a 2D and 3D acquisition of the data is possible. The main problem with this technique is the fact that the excited spin has a different location than in the read-out spin while the table moves between transmitting and receiving.

There are some further challenges to overcome: inhomogeneity of the B_0 field and nonlinearity of the gradients lead to distortion artefacts as a function of time at the borders of the images. Furthermore, a number of adjustment parameters, which are normally once set at a fixed table position, must be adapted automatically during table movement. These parameters include calibration of the transmitter and the receiver coil, adaptation of the transmitter/receiver frequency, HF transmitting power and amplification, as well as shimming of the system, which all directly influence image quality. Using variable flip angle 3D sequences, these problems are now addressed. The potential for whole-body MRI is manifold: with significantly faster examinations with the use of 3D sequences, the possibility to reformat isotropic images and to gain "seamless" images boosts the clinical utility of WB-MRI to that of CT.

14.3 WB-MRI Applications for the Oncologic Patient

14.3.1 *WB-MRI for Cancer Staging*

Precise tumor staging and accurate tumor monitoring is a fundamental precondition when assessing prognosis and therapeutic options in a patient with a neoplastic disease. The TNM staging system proposed by the American Joint Committee on Cancer (AJCC) has become the international standard for this purpose. MRI, with its lack of ionizing radiation, high soft tissue contrast, and spatial resolution, is a useful application for tumor detection and staging of malignant disease. Multi-modality approaches are still widely used in clinical routine for the diagnostic assessment of cancer. However, the advent of WB-MRI into clinical practice has substantially expanded diagnostic options for cancer patients, and this method is increasingly considered as a first-line systemic imaging tool for neoplastic diseases.

14.3.1.1 WB-MRI for Local Tumor Staging

Various studies have been conducted, mainly comparing WB-MRI with either MS-CT or PET–CT for initial tumor staging. An initial comparative pilot study performed on 98 patients with various primary cancers using the "rolling table concept" has shown an advantage in diagnostic accuracy of PET–CT (80%) over WB-MRI (52%) for the assessment of T-stage. This may reflect the ability of PET–CT to differentiate viable tumor from adjacent structures due to the additional metabolic information (Fig. 14.2). However, other results performed on previously described state-of-the art multi-channel scanners indicate a balanced and robust performance of WB-MRI and PET–CT for primary T-staging and advantages of WB-MRI compared to MS-CT. However, WB-MRI cannot replace dedicated MRI examinations for T-staging in specific organs such as the breast or prostate, in which MRI with adequate organ compression in prone position or the use of an endorectal coil and MR spectroscopy remain the gold standard.

14.3.1.2 WB-MRI for the Assessment of Nodal Status

The benefit of metabolic information provided by hybrid techniques such as PET–CT over size criteria alone may become even more obvious in the assessment of N-stage. False-positive findings due to enlarged nodes in inflammatory processes or normal-sized nodes harboring micrometastases can impair sensitivity and specificity of MRI or CT. There have been promising reports on WB-MRI for the assessment of lymphoma patients as an alternative to MS-CT. WB-MRI showed an adequate performance by detecting 92% of lymph node stations diagnosed positive in CT for node sizes larger than 12 mm. However, detection dropped significantly, down to 67%, for nodes measuring between 6 and 12 mm. Borderline-sized lymph nodes located in areas prone to motion and pulsation artefacts, such

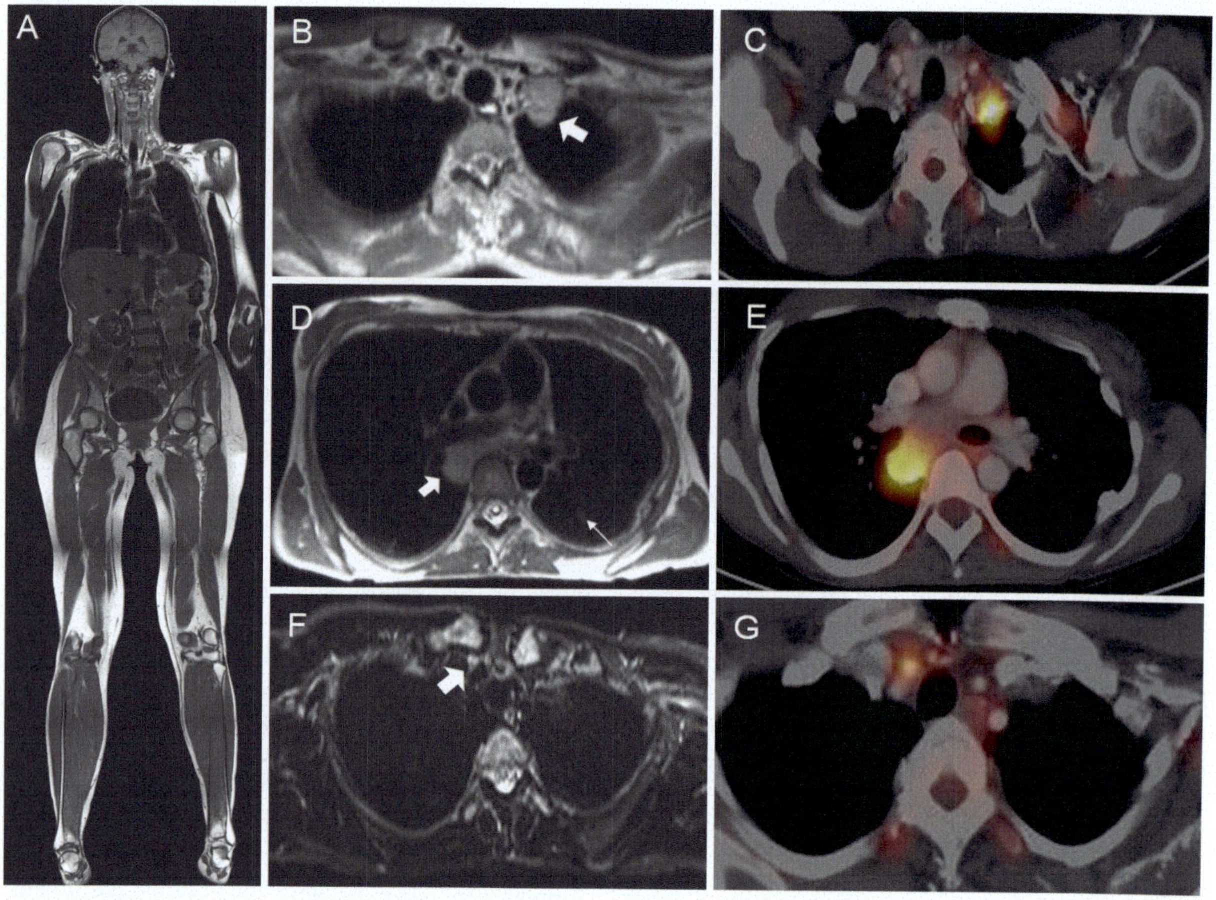

Fig. 14.2 Forty-two-year-old female, s/o bronchial carcinoma. (**a**) Whole-body T1-W TSE imaging at 1.5 T. (**b**) Axial fast T2-W turbo spin echo imaging of the lung reveals a tumor in the left apex (*arrow*). (**c**) PET–CT reveals a pathologic FDG uptake, indicating malignancy. (**d**) HASTE MRI of the lung reveals a large right hilar soft-tissue mass with accurate delineation (*short arrow*), and a suspicious lung nodule in left upper lobe (*long arrow*). (**e**) PET–CT confirms a hilar lymph node metastasis with highly increased uptake values. (**f**) Axial STIR imaging shows an undefined round structure with hyperintense signal in the right upper mediastinum, which could potentially be interpreted as a vessel cut (*arrow*). (**g**) PET–CT reveals another lymph node metastasis less than 1 mm in size at the same location

as the mediastinal, hilar, and diaphragmal regions, may potentially be missed by MRI (Fig. 14.2). Studies comparing WB-MRI with PET–CT for N-staging have reported diagnostic accuracies ranging between 91 and 97% for PET–CT and 79 and 82% for WB-MRI. Recent attempts to overcome these limitations were the introduction of whole-body diffusion MRI for enhanced display and detection of pathologic lymph nodes on the basis of fat suppressed STIR echo-planar imaging. The underlying rationale of this approach is the diffusion restriction in lymph nodes compared to surrounding tissue. It is hypothesized that this diffusion restriction is higher in malignant nodes compared to benign ones. A further development of this concept is the so-called "virtual PET–MRI," which is based on the fusion of a morphologic image (e.g., STIR) and diffusion MRI with the use of different *b*-values. As a result, a PET-like image is produced, indicating higher diffusion restriction in lymph node tissue with tumorous infiltration. However, despite encouraging reports, this new method is still the subject of research, and large patient cohort studies have to prove its efficacy in a clinical setting. In particular, the calculated ADC values for whole-body diffusion applications so far have not been shown to ensure reliable differentiation between benign and malignant nodes in larger clinical trials. Yet, within focused anatomic areas of interest like the neck or abdomen, significant differences in ADC values for a more accurate differentiation of benign and metastatic lymph nodes have been described in recent studies.

14.3.1.3 WB-MRI for the Detection of Distant Organ Metastases

Due to its excellent contrast in soft tissue and parenchymal structures, the main indication for WB-MRI certainly lies within the detection of distant metastatic disease. Reported diagnostic accuracies for M-staging compared to PET–CT as a competing whole-body staging modality range between 82 and 94% for PET–CT and 92 and 93% for WB-MRI. Advantages for WB-MRI have been reported in lesion-by-lesion analyses for the detection of liver, brain, and bone metastases. The implementation of, especially, a dynamic 3D-gradient echo sequence allows a reliable diagnosis of even small liver metastases below 5 mm. These can be invisible in MS-CT or PET–CT due to the low soft-tissue contrast and the frequently normal FDG uptake in small-sized lesions.

The examination of the thorax seems to be a challenge for MRI, especially within a whole-body approach. However, the implementation of fast T2-weighted turbo spinecho sequences in combination with PI has minimized the limitations of MRI in the assessment of lung pathologies, now enabling the detection of small lung nodules down to a size of 5 mm, coming close to resolution achieved with a conventional spiral CT scanner. Using T2-HASTE (half-fourier acquisition sinlge shot technique) with navigation technique or trigger technique, examination time for the thorax is reduced to 2 min; axial T2 fat saturated images with an excellent lesion-to-lung signal are acquired within less than 3 min. In a recent study, Frericks et al. have described a high accuracy of axial STIR imaging of the lung within a whole-body approach for lesions down to 3 mm, compared to MS-CT.

WB-MRI, with its anatomical coverage from head to toe, compared to a standard MS-CT or PET–CT protocol (which usually ranges from the skull base to the pelvis) potentially reveals additional findings of therapeutic and prognostic importance. Detection of previously unknown metastases to the brain and extremities in up to 17% of cases has been reported, with a consecutive change of patient management in up to 10% of patients.

Finally, the introduction of new whole-body diffusion techniques (as described in the previous section) has significantly enhanced detection and characterization of metastatic lesions for lymph node and organ metastases. Recent studies confirm the useful implementation for distant metastatic disease, especially to the liver, bone marrow, and soft tissue, in various tumor entities (Fig. 14.3).

14.3.1.4 Staging in Pediatric Oncology

Pediatric oncologic patients often require whole-body imaging as a baseline examination before the initiation of therapy and in the following weeks to objectively verify therapy response. Because of their relatively shorter body extension along the *z*-axis, they represent an attractive patient group for whole-body examinations as a single diagnostic approach. The overall examination protocol is reduced in total time, so that an examination of a pediatric patient only takes about 35–45 min. It is obvious to reduce examinations with high doses of ionizing radiation inherent to whole-body CT or PET–CT, especially within repeated follow-up examinations of young patients after therapy. Further advantages of a single comprehensive examination wherein all body parts are investigated are obvious. The pediatric patient only requires a single sedation, resulting in increased safety; furthermore, only a singular contrast media injection is required.

The sequence protocol should be based on the general protocol for metastatic disease, with special focus on speed and reduced sensitivity to motion, as involuntary motion occurs more frequently than in the adult population.

There are a number of oncological diseases for which a whole-body examination seems to be useful in children: in all cases of lymphatic diseases including Hodgkin's and Non-Hodgkin's disease, in children with solid tumors (juvenile rhabdomyosarcoma, Ewing's sarcoma, malignant osseous tumors, nephroblastoma, neuroblastoma, hepatoblastoma), and in mixed tissue tumors such as teratomas or dermoid tumors. At the moment, all these children undergo guideline-orientated standard imaging protocols, often as a combination of ultrasound of the abdomen, CT scan of the thorax, and MRI of the brain. Yet, recent studies have described

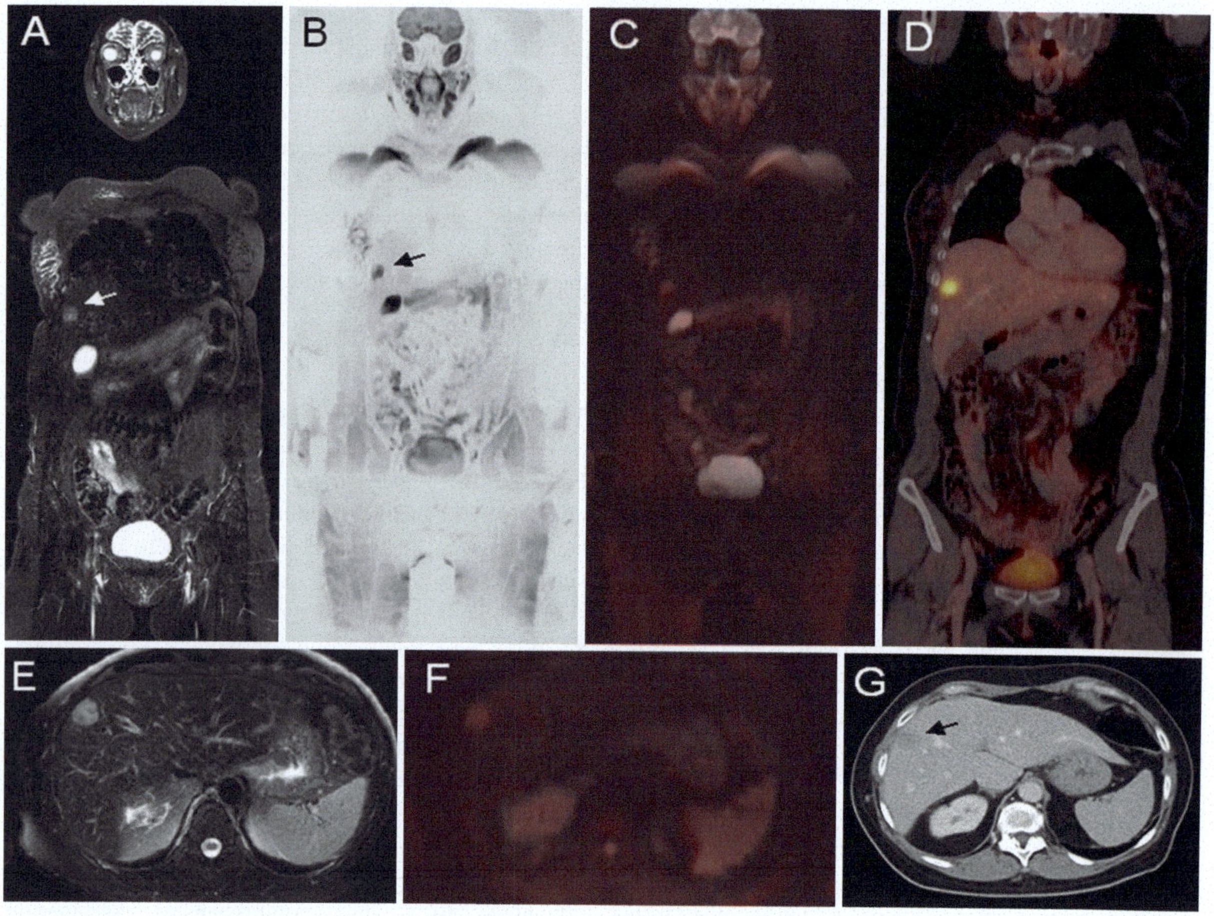

Fig. 14.3 Sixty-five-year-old female, post breast cancer, with pathologic tumor marker increase (CEA). (**a**) Coronal whole-body STIR imaging. A suspicious hyperintense liver lesion (*arrow*) is depicted. (**b**) Corresponding WB-diffusion imaging shows increased diffusion signal within the lesion. (**c**) Fused WB-STIR and WB-diffusion (so-called "virtual PET-MRI") shows the lesion with high contrast similar to a MR PET image. (**d**) PET–CT in the same patient shows pathologic tracer uptake, confirming metastasis. (**e, f**) Axial STIR and fused STIR/ diffusion image of the lesion. (**g**) MS-CT depicts the lesion with only mild hypointense contrast

MRI as the most suitable and objective method for tumor imaging of the brain, spine, abdomen, and pelvis. The concurrent whole-body method remains PET–CT and, in some instances, bone scan. PET–CT visualizes the metabolism within a tumor - this remains an advantage that cannot be addressed by WB-MRI. As a limitation, besides radiation exposure, PET and PET–CT suffer from limited spatial resolution, misregistration of tumors in some instances because of patient movement, and lack of FDG uptake in certain tumor entities and osteoblastic metastases. Also, radiation exposure is about 4–30 mSv and repetitive examinations may increase the risk of a secondary neoplasia.

Imaging of the extremities has not yet been integrated into the guidelines. Until now, only a dedicated examination, combined with MS-CT, is considered for work-up of soft tissue and osseous tumors of the extremities. Using WB-MRI, the extremities can be evaluated with T2 STIR and T1 SE sequences within 6–10 min. A recent study comparing different methods for tumor staging in pediatric patients resulted in better visualization of skeletal metastases and detected more extraskeletal metastases (e.g., in neuroblastomas) than with conventional guideline-orientated methods. On the other hand, a study of Daldrup-Link et al. highlighted the higher sensitivity of WB-MRI, in children, for bone marrow metastases, compared to bone scintigraphy (82 vs. 71% in a group of 39 children with 51 bone metastases), but a lower sensitivity compared to PET–CT (90 vs. 82%).

Finally, analogous to adult patient populations, whole-body diffusion techniques are getting a more important role in WB-MRI tumor imaging as a competitor for PET–CT for better discrimination between benign and malignant lymph nodes and organ lesions.

14.3.2 WB-MRI for Surveillance of Recurrent Disease

WB-MRI has great potential as application within tertiary prevention in previously cured cancer patients or for monitoring of a neoplastic disease. Here, WB-MRI can be especially useful in tumors with a high probability of organ metastases into the brain, liver, bone, or soft tissue, like breast cancer or malignant melanoma (Fig. 14.4). WB-MRI has been successfully introduced on 1.5 T as well as 3 T scanners for detection of tumor recurrence in breast cancer patients with a high risk profile for tumor recurrence (e.g., elevated tumor marker levels, clinical symptoms). In this population, a 61% prevalence of recurrent disease was found, and a lesion-by-lesion analysis demonstrated a diagnostic accuracy of 91% for WB-MRI. Yet, in one patient a false-positive local recurrence was reported. Note that for a clinically feasible whole-body exam in this setting, the primarily supine position of the patient without breast compression cannot replace a dedicated breast MRI exam in terms of local resolution and tissue coverage.

WB-MRI using high resolution coronal 3D-gradient echo (GRE) sequences pre- and post-contrast has proved useful for restaging of malignant melanoma, yielding a diagnostic accuracy of 80%, with high sensitivity for liver, bone, and brain metastases. Surprisingly, diagnostic accuracy was lowest for soft-tissue and subcutaneous metastases, explained by the fact that a primarily coronal approach is prone to miss smaller lesion located peripherally or superficially in the body. As a result, it is recommended to additionally scan the lower extremities in axial planes when examining tumor entities that frequently metastasize into soft tissue. WB-MRI led to treatment change in 23% of patients, most often through detection of cerebral metastases.

14.3.3 WB-MRI in Guideline-Orientated Staging and Surveillance Concepts

A medical or clinical guideline is a document to suggest criteria in specific areas of healthcare, as defined by an authoritative statement of current evidence, which is also known as "evidence-based medicine." A summary of the internationally accepted guidelines can be found online (e.g., at ebmg.wiley.com). In most cases, guidelines include summarized consensus statements, but they also address practical issues. In a more detailed definition, clinical guidelines briefly identify, summarize, and evaluate the best evidence and most current data on prevention, diagnosis, prognosis, and therapy, including dosage of medications, as well as risk/benefit and cost-effectiveness of a given therapy.

Regarding breast cancer screening for example, the recently-published "European guidelines for quality assurance in breast cancer screening and diagnosis" (fourth edition) addresses the important role of mammography, ultrasound, and MRI of the breast. For staging reasons, patients with tumors suitable for primary surgery are suggested to undergo an X-ray of the chest. Only in patients with pretherapeutic confirmed lymph node infiltration of the axilla and/or neoadjuvant therapy, a CT or ultrasound of the liver and skeletal survey (bone scan) is considered. As described in recent studies, potential additional findings in pre-therapeutic evaluated patients are found by means of whole-body imaging. In this setting, PET–CT and WB-MRI show comparable diagnostic accuracy for lung and lymph node pathologies. However, WB-MRI shows a higher sensitivity for bone, brain, and liver. As a consequence, especially WB-MRI can be considered as a pre-therapeutic method to detect silent metastasis.

14.3.4 WB-MRI for Secondary Prevention and Screening of Asymptomatic Patients

14.3.4.1 Definition of Prevention Types

Screening is defined as the presumptive identification of unrecognized disease or defects by the application of tests, examinations, or other procedures.

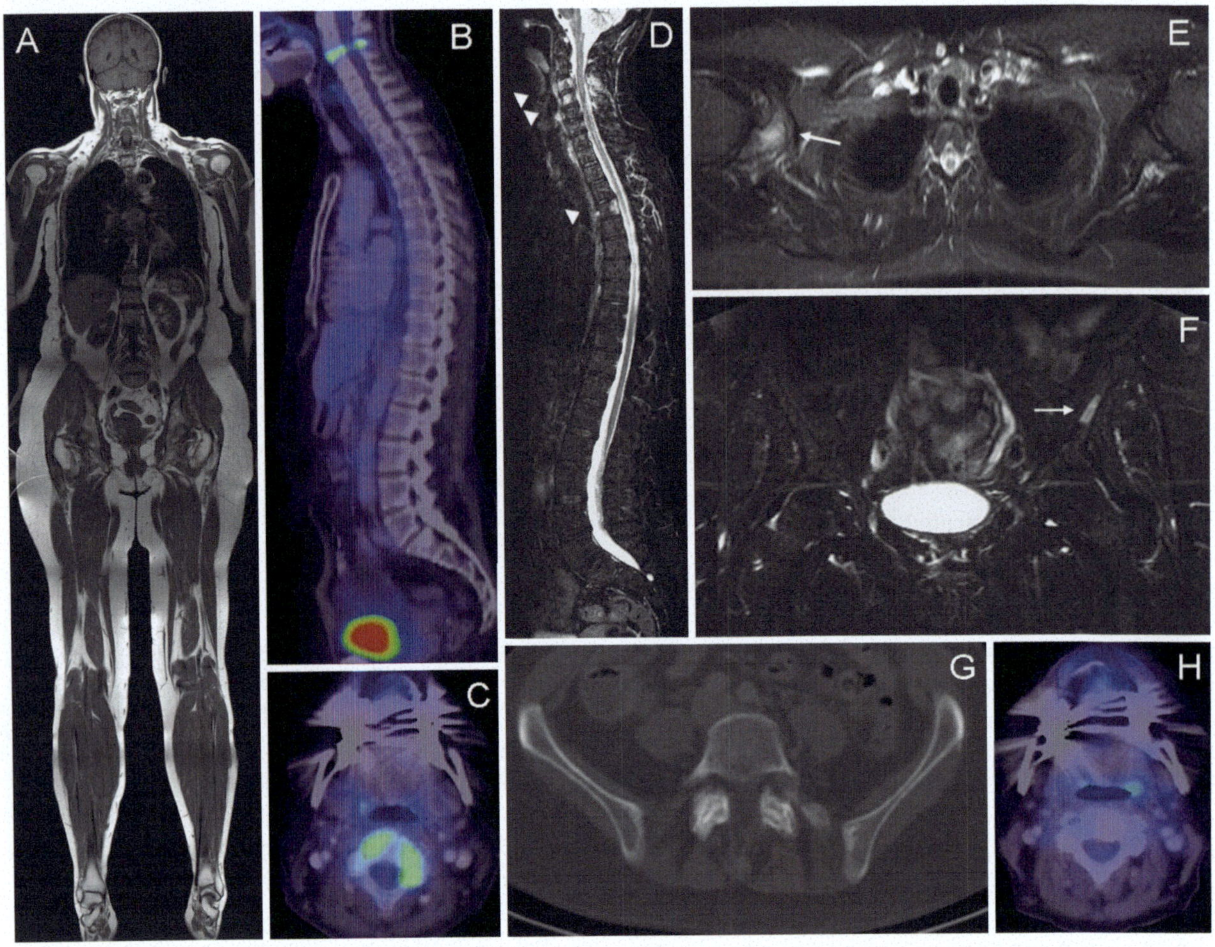

Fig. 14.4 (**a**) T-weighted (W) TSE WB-MRI at 1.5 T. (**b**, **c**) Sagittal PET–CT correlation of the spine depicts a singular, extensive bone metastasis (SUV 5,0) in C3. (**d**) WB-MRI shows multiple bone metastases in C3, C4, and TH5 (*arrowheads*). (**e**, **f**) More malignant lesions are found in the right coracoid and left iliac bone (*arrows*). (**g**) CT correlation of the pelvis is morphologically inconspicuous. (**h**) PET–CT follow-up of the spine after 2 months radiation therapy shows a significant decrease in FDG uptake by 50% (SUV = 2,5), indicating therapy response

Prevention can be subdivided into primary, secondary, and tertiary prevention. Primary prevention is directed toward preventing the initial occurrence of a disorder. Examples of primary prevention include avoidance of risk factors, e.g., with programs for healthy alimentation or increased body activity, as well as internal health control and prevention.

By definition, a screening examination is conducted within the scope of either secondary or tertiary prevention. Secondary tumor prevention aims at filtering cancerous disease from a primarily healthy population. The primary goal of screening in tertiary prevention is to obviate aggravation of a preexisting chronic disease in a patient by early interventional measures or therapy changes. The main focus in the oncologic patient is to detect tumor recurrence or metastatic disease within restaging procedures and to exclude secondary complications due to disease progression.

14.3.4.2 Prevalence of Disease and Effectivity of Treatment; Problems in Screening

The main problem in screening large populations is prevalence of disease. Screening often takes place in a potentially healthy environment, meaning that it mainly benefits a small percentage of ill patients, while negative side effects affect the whole examined population. Therefore, a minimal incidence of side effects and strict selection criteria are indispensable to focus secondary screening on a preselected population with an increased risk profile.

An important inherent problem of screening is false-positive test results, which increase the anxiety of the screened person and may require further diagnostic investigations, which again may produce side effects and additional expenses. Another aspect is overdiagnosis and overtreatment in screened persons, which may induce false-positive diagnosis of cancer and possibly lead to unnecessary treatment, with further treatment-related side effects.

As a result, screening is ethically justifiable only if evidence is available that these risks are counterbalanced by a screening-related benefit that potentially carries more weight than the potential risks. Thus, a screening procedure is only justifiable with a continuous risk-benefit analysis.

14.3.4.3 Different Diseases for Screening

In a population with a normal risk profile, there is good evidence for screening for breast, colorectal, and cervical cancer to reduce cancer-related mortality. Other types of cancer, such as prostate or ovarian cancer, are not supported by results from randomized trials. On the other hand, there is a controversial discussion about the benefit in a patient population with elevated cancer risk.

Colorectal cancer (CRC) is the third most common cancer type, and is the fourth most common cause of cancer deaths worldwide. Although this cancer type is ideal for screening (high incidence, long term interval to malignant degeneration, easily treatable precancer types, and improved prognosis after removal), a fecal occult blood test (FOBT), colonoscopy, and rectosigmoidoscopy are still the only established screening procedures. Although results are encouraging, virtual colonoscopy has not yet been established as a standard procedure. The implementation of a virtual colonoscopy combined with a WB-MRI approach has been investigated by some authors in the setting of a screening protocol within atherosclerosis screening. As technical prerequisites, it is mandatory to examine the patients in a high-field MR system with at least 1.5 T multi-channel technology and the option for PATs to obtain a matrix of at least 256 × 256 within an adequate examination time (<60 min), as formerly described. Also, a bowel cleansing, rectal filling of the bowel with 1–2 L of water, and the administration of *N*-butylscopalamine – if possible – to minimize bowel motion are necessary. The protocol starts with the examination of the head including time-of-flight angiography (scan time ~10 min), includes an angiography of the arteries at different table stations (~2 min), is followed by the investigation of the thorax and the heart (with functional imaging and delayed enhancement/~15 min), and ends with the evaluation of the bowel by repetitive T1W 3D GRE sequences wit fat suppression to assess contrast media uptake. In a recent study with this examination protocol by Goehde et al., the authors reported one false-positive result in 298 patients, from whom 169 patients had been controlled by further investigations or by follow-up. Besides revealing manifestations of atherosclerotic disease in 21% of patients (including cerebral and myocardial infarctions), colonic polyps ($n = 12$) and one renal cell carcinoma were detected. The mean room time was 63 min.

Though prostate cancer has a much higher prevalence, indolent disease is expected in up to 50–88% of detected cancers. Accordingly, it has been questioned whether screening truly has an impact on mortality. The main problem will be to separate the high-risk patient from the low-risk patient. One option is to take the PSA doubling time as a pragmatic tool to stratify patients according to the risk of tumor progression, and to apply either watchful waiting or radical therapy. The value of MRI in future could be to propagate a WB-protocol, e.g., in patients with high risk of lymph node metastasis or of bone metastasis (the risk is <1% in PSA levels <10), with additional focus on the pelvis, e.g., with the use of contrast-enhanced isotropic 3D-GRE imaging of the pelvis for the assessment of local lymph node status.

Lung cancer can be screened by repetitive CT of the chest, leading to the potential risk of inducing lung cancer itself. While sensitivity for tumor detection has greatly increased, the true impact of these procedures on mortality in specified risk groups remains unclear. The problem is the high rate of false-positive findings (5–50%), leading to unnecessary lung biopsies. WB-MRI is an option for the detection of lung cancer without ionizing radiation, with good and comparable results down to a lesion size of 3 mm, as described in the subgroup analysis of WB-MRI study populations, but has not been recommended yet.

14.3.4.4 WB-Imaging Strategies in Screening

Various studies have been performed for the evaluation of screening protocols using WB-MRI. Regarding these studies, the main focus was put on cardiovascular and oncological questions, or on both. The studies on cardiovascular diseases pointed out that there is an increased risk of having yet undiagnosed atherosclerotic changes, stenoses, and even stroke and/or myocardial infarction, which can be visualized using a WB-MRI screening protocol. Also, WB-MRI tumor screening may lead to a potentially life-changing diagnosis like a previously unknown malignancy.

The proposed sequence protocols should include a matrix size of at least 320, while 384 is preferable, and the maximum examination time should not exceed the limit of 50–60 min. Even using 1.5 T scanners, this time-line can be kept by using 3D GRE sequences and breath-hold sequences for the thorax and upper parts of the abdomen only, and by using a fast cardiovascular screening protocol, as shown in Tables 14.2–14.4.

14.3.4.5 Diagnostic Value, Positive Predictive Value, Cost of the Examination and of Further Examinations, Psychological Effects

Despite encouraging reports concerning diagnostic accuracy and important findings, it must be emphasized that an unsighted adoption of multi-organ whole-body examinations cannot be recommended.

As the exact positive and negative predictive values for potentially detectable diseases are not known, it is difficult to compare the results of these screening examinations with those of clinical examinations. A cost-benefit analysis must be performed, although only limited knowledge about it exists. It is necessary to define an intelligent preselection to increase the prevalence of findings and therewith the cost effectivity of this method. Within nononcologic screening programs, an interesting group could be patients with a coronary heart disease, having, in up to 50% of cases, stenosis of the renal arteries or the carotid arteries. Another group may consist of patients with diabetes mellitus, in which the rate of silent myocardial infarcts is elevated and the rate of glomerulopathy and renal diseases as well as peripheral vessel disease is high.

Another question to address is the cost of further examinations in patients with positive findings, potential invasive diagnostic procedures for clarification, the rate of morbidity and mortality, as well as the psychological consequences of positive and negative findings. Before a health insurance will pay for the WB-examination as a screening examination, the diagnostic value must be clarified by further studies.

The last important aspect is the support of the screenes. The referring institution (physician or screene itself) must be extensively informed before the examination about the possible advantages and disadvantages of the method. It is important that the physician knows the limitations of the procedure and knows comparable or more evaluated investigation methods.

14.4 Whole-Body Bone Marrow Imaging

MRI is the only imaging technique that allows direct visualization of the bone marrow and its components. The unique soft-tissue contrast of MRI enables for a precise assessment of tumor infiltration within the bone marrow and adjacent paraosseous structures such as the spinal canal. For an MRI bone marrow screening, the combination of non-contrasted T1-W Spinecho and Turbo STIR sequences proved to be most sensitive, and it allows reliable discrimination of benign from malignant marrow disorders. Using PAT acceleration, whole-body STIR imaging is possible within 12:28 min, and T1-W imaging within 16:10 min at a 1.8 × 1.3 and 1.3 × 1.1 mm in-plane-resolution, respectively. A proposed protocol is described in Table 14.5.

Table 14.3 Sequence parameters for optional dedicated pelvic imaging in the assessment of a patient with prostate cancer

Region	Sequence	Image plane	Matrix/resolution (mm^3)	Acquisition time	No. of slices
Pelvis	T1w fs 3D-GRE	Coronal	320/0.9 × 0.9 × 0.9	3.22	144

Table 14.4 Proposed screening examination protocol for WB-MRI with a special focus on cardiovascular disease

WB-MRI cardiovascular screening protocol at 1.5 T					
Min	**Brain**	**Cardiac**	**Thorax**	**Abdomen**	**MRA**
20	TOF EPI-DWI ax T2 TSE ax	Function perfusion	HASTE cor + ax	HASTE ax T2 TSE fs ax	
40	Contrast media application				
70	T1 TSE ax	DCE	T1w fs 3D GRE ax	T1 fs ax	Carotids / calf Abdomen / thigh
Total scan time = 60 min, PAT 2-3					

Table 14.5 Proposed examination protocol for the assessment of patients with bone marrow diseases (e.g., multiple myeloma, bone marrow expansion, lymphoma) with optional expansion to detect organ metastases (e.g., in breast cancer). Complete examination time for metastasis screening: 58.17 min, bone marrow evaluation without contrast media: 39.30 min, bone marrow evaluation with contrast media (spine): 43.26 min.

Region	Sequence	Image plane	Matrix/resolution (mm^3)	Acquisition time	Contrast media
Brain	T1 T2 FLAIR	Axial Axial Axial	384/1.1 × 1.1 × 5 384/1.1 × 1.1 × 5 320/1.2 × 1.1 × 5	2.11 2.43 3.21	– – –
WB	STIR	Coronal	512/2 × 1 × 5	3.2/region	–
WB	T1	Coronal	384/1.6 × 1.3 × 5	2.58/region	–
Spine	STIR	Sagittal	448/1.1 × 1 × 3	2.04 × 2	–
Spine	T1	Sagittal	512/1 × 0.9 × 3	1.58 × 2	–
Liver	Dyn.T1 fs 3D GRE	Axial	384/1.9 × 1.5 × 3	2.2	+
Spine	T1	Sagittal	448/1.1 × 1 × 3	1.58 × 2	+
Brain	T1	Axial	384/1.1 × 1.1 × 5	2.11	+
Brain	T1	Coronal	384/1.1 × 1.1 × 5	2.11	+

14.4.1 WB-MRI for Imaging of Hematologic Disease

Frequently encountered primary hematologic bone marrow disorders include lymphoma, especially in young adults, and multiple myeloma. The diagnosis of malignant lymphoma of the bone is delayed in many cases because of unspecific clinical signs and inapparent findings on radiographs. Additionally, extraskeletal involvement can significantly decrease patient survival. WB-MRI has been used in assessing bone marrow infiltration and extramedullary involvement by lymphoma. Although the modality of choice used in primary staging of this malignancy is ^{18}F-FDG-PET, whole-body MRI may represent an alternative, especially to bone or ^{67}Ga scintigraphy. In a study performed on 34 patients with non-Hodgkin's lymphoma using WB-MRI, significantly more malignant lesions were detected with MRI ($n = 89$) than with bone ($n = 14$) or ^{67}Ga scintigraphy ($n = 5$). Another group has analyzed the performance of WB-MRI vs. MS-CT, bone-, and ^{67}Ga scintigraphy using only WB STIR imaging for staging of lymphoma in children, and reported a higher sensitivity for MRI for detection of different sites of marrow and non-marrow involvement. Following treatment, however, residual and therapy-induced bone marrow signal abnormalities could not be differentiated from lymphomatous involvement. Therefore, WB-MRI seems primarily suitable for initial staging of the disease.

The initial diagnostic work-up for multiple myeloma in many institutions still consists of conventional radiographs of the axial skeleton and proximal extremities. This approach is still accepted as an important component of the clinical staging system of the disease according to Salmon and Durie, which defines selection of adequate therapy regime. Sensitivity of radiography in the detection of myeloma manifestations, however, is rather low, and MRI enables visualization of focal or diffuse myeloma infiltration of the marrow with high sensitivity and specificity. However, MRI protocols often do not include the skull, sternum, ribs, and proximal extremities, which represent frequent sites of infiltration. Thus, WB-MRI represents an efficient tool to increase sensitivity by detecting infiltration at these sites. Several reports have described the superior performance of WB-MRI compared to conventional radiographs as well as MS-CT for diagnostic accuracy and correct staging of the disease (Fig. 14.5a, b). Diffuse infiltration patterns may easily be missed or confused with benign osteoporosis. Also, MRI diagnosis was found to have a significant influence on patients' prognosis and therefore an extended staging system of Salmon and Durie, including MRI assessment, was introduced into clinical assessment of the disease.

14.4.2 WB-MRI for the Detection of Bone Metastases

The predominantly hematogenous spread of bone metastases explains its frequent distribution in active hematopoetic bone marrow, especially in the axial skeleton. However, it has been reported that up to 40% of bone metastases may occur in the appendicular skeleton, underlining the importance of whole-body anatomic coverage. At present, ^{99m}Tc-phosphonate-based skeletal scintigraphy is the standard method for initial staging. However, at the early stage of disease, lesions may remain invisible in the absence of an osteoblastic response. The diagnostic performance of WB-MRI compared to bone scintigraphy for the detection of skeletal metastases has been examined in various studies, and a higher specificity and sensitivity in the early detection of skeletal metastases has been reported. In a recently-published lesion-by-lesion analysis between WB-MRI and PET–CT as alternative screening methods for the detection of skeletal metastases, WB-MRI showed a significantly higher overall diagnostic accuracy (91 vs. 78%). Also, numerous additional skeletal metastases were found in the distal extremities.

However, diagnostic problems in MRI leading to a consecutive decrease of sensitivity may arise in younger patients where the differentiation of highly cellular hematopoietic marrow and neoplasia can be difficult, and knowledge of age-dependent conversion patterns is required. Also, additional metabolic information of, e.g., PET–CT can be helpful to reliably discriminate between malignant and benign focal lesions (e.g., atypical hemangioma).

WB-MRI, especially when performed in coronal orientation, is prone to miss lesions in small curved flat bones like the rib cage, a problem that is certainly reinforced by motion artefacts of respiration. This problem might be overcome using fast turbo spin echo sequences for thoracic imaging to reduce artefacts, in combination with axial slicing for more accurate assessment of the rib cage and sternal bone.

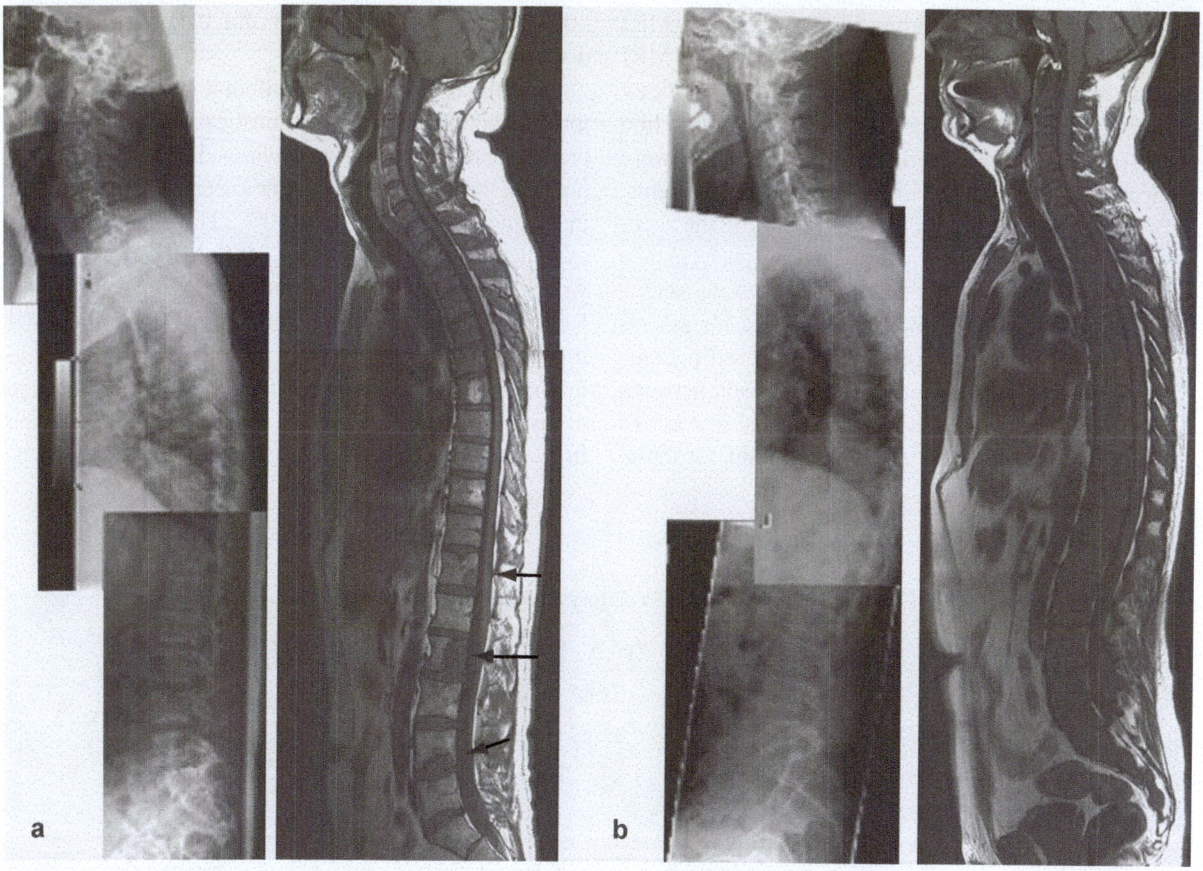

Fig. 14.5 (**a**) Fifty-six-year-old patient with X-ray and MRI of the spine: In the X-ray survey, degenerative changes in the spine were detected, as well as general osteoporosis (stage II according to Salmon and Durie). MRI of the spine shows multiple lytic lesions, especially in the lumbar spine, suggesting a stage III disease (*arrows*). (**b**) Sixty-two-year-old patient with X-ray and MRI of the spine. X-ray survey demonstrates no relevant changes in the bone structures of the spine. However, MRI of the spine leads to the diagnosis of a medullary expansion in the spongious parts of the vertebral column (loss of signal in the whole spine). Thus, a stage III disease was diagnosed, while X-ray only shows stage I disease

14.4.3 Guidelines

14.4.3.1 Guidelines in Malignant Bone Marrow Diseases

There are no existing guidelines for diagnostic strategies in benign or malignant bone marrow infiltration. The only accepted staging system is the Durie and Salmon PLUS system, which combines findings from peripheral venous blood sampling and the number of osteolytic lesions in conventional X-ray with MRI of the spine and pelvis. No dedicated guidelines exist for WB-MRI imaging protocols. For diagnosis of bone metastasis, a guideline from the "National Guideline Clearinghouse" can be found at http://www.guideline.gov, in which recommendations from the American College of Radiology are described.

The guidelines regarding the most important and frequent oncological diseases address similar and comparable imaging strategies, only modified by the time point of imaging. The main cancer types include prostate cancer in male patients and breast cancer in female patients, CRC, lung cancer, cancer of the bladder, cancer of the ovaries and uterus, and gastric, renal, and pancreatic cancers. In these diseases, a bone scan and dedicated X-ray scans are generally recommended in high-risk patients and in case of symptomatic disease. It is only in a few oncological diseases that a comparison of guideline-orientated imaging vs. WB-MRI has been performed. Schmidt et al. examined patients suffering from different oncological diseases with suspected bone metastases in a PET–CT vs. WB-MRI setting and found a higher sensitivity with WB-MRI than with PET–CT (94 vs. 78%), while the specificity was comparable in both modalities (76 vs. 80%). In a study by Ohno et al., WB-MRI and PET–CT were compared for M-staging in lung cancer in 90 patients. WB-MRI was superior to PET–CT regarding the accuracy (94 vs. 88%), also when evaluating performance on a per-patient basis (80 vs. 73%). In prostate cancer, bone scintigraphy is the method of choice for assessment of bone metastasis in newly diagnosed patients with a PSA level >10. In a recent comparison between 11C-Choline PET and WB-MRI, in a total number of 42 patients, 44 bone metastases were found. Of these, 40 were revealed by 11C-Cholin PET, and 39 were detected by WB-MRI.

In general, costs of the different imaging methods must be counterbalanced. In most cases, a bone scan is recommended in malignant diseases. In case of high-risk patients, the probability of bone metastasis is increased in a range between 5 and 30%. Therefore, a further examination (dedicated X-ray, CT, MRI or PET–CT) will be proposed in cases of nuclear tracer accumulation. Regarding the time expense and cost of this multi-modal imaging strategy, WB-MRI represents an alternative to this algorithm. Yet, further evaluation on a broader range of diseases will be mandatory. An example for a change in the diagnostic procedure is demonstrated in Fig. 14.6.

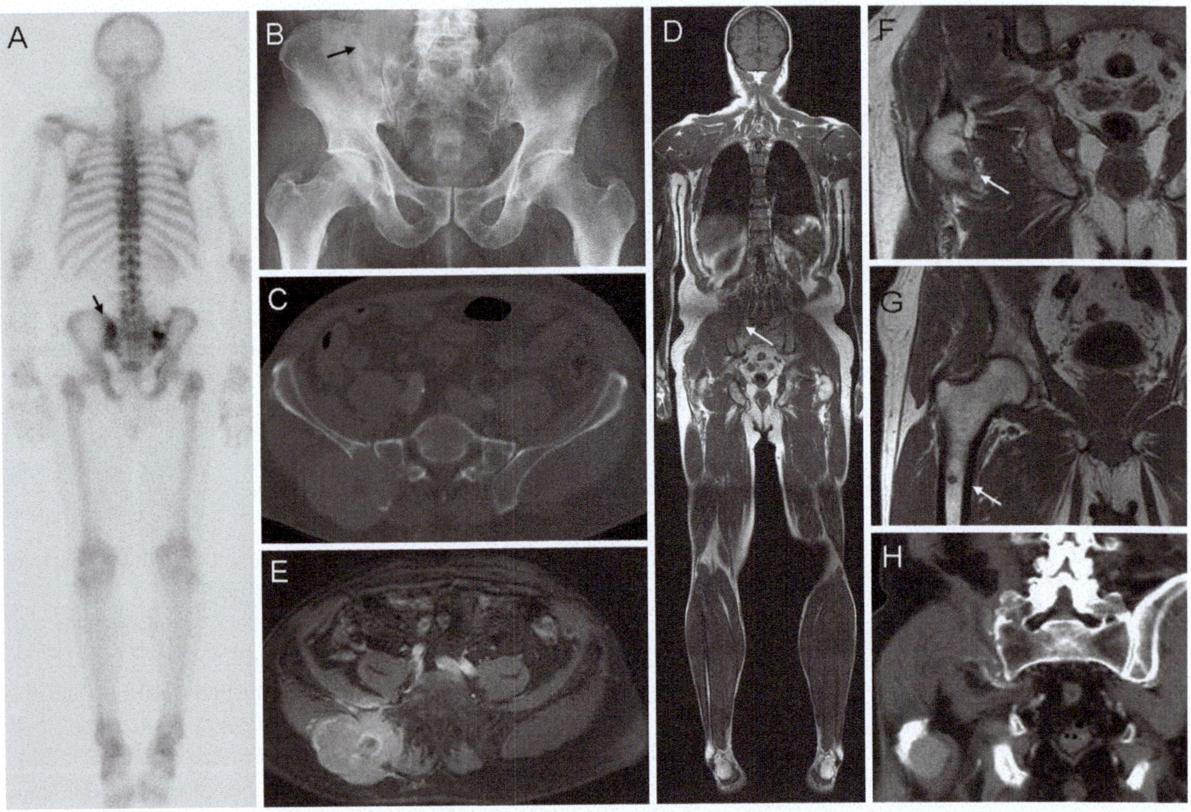

Fig. 14.6 Seventy-year-old patient, post left renal cell carcinoma/nephrectomy and newly occurred sacral pain: multi-modal restaging and WB-MRI. (**a**) Scintigraphy indicates a suspicious tracer uptake in the right iliosacral region (*arrow*). (**b**) X-ray shows osteolytic destruction of right medial iliac crest (*arrow*). (**c**) MS-CT confirms a large osteolytic metastasis of the iliac bone and iliosacral joint, with a soft-tissue component invading the right gluteal muscle. (**d**) In T1-W TSE WB-MRI, the hypointense mass is already discernible in the overview (*arrow*). (**e**) Axial contrast-enhanced MRI of the pelvis accurately delineates bony infiltration by the metastasis and its extent into surrounding gluteal soft tissue structures. (**f**, **g**) Enlargement shows more bone metastases in the right major trochanter and proximal femur shaft. (**h**) MS-CT follow-up after 3 months shows clear progression of the right trochanteric bone metastasis

14.4.3.2 Guidelines in Benign Bone Marrow Diseases

For benign diseases no guidelines exist, but it should be considered that MRI has a great diagnostic potential by differentiating fatty bone marrow structures from infiltrative lesions. However, the degree of osteoporosis or the differentiation of different types of bone marrow infiltration, whether it is metastatic or only due to expansion of blood-producing bone marrow, cannot be performed with certainty. Here, analysis of the geographical pattern is helpful: systemic diseases such as osteomyelofibrosis or polycythemia vera result in a more diffuse infiltration pattern with expansion of bone marrow. Osteomyelofibrosis is also quite distinctive due to signal drop in T1- and T2-W sequences (Fig. 14.7). On the other hand, patients with lymphoma or metastatic tumors reveal a more circumscriptive pattern.

14.5 WB-MRI Applications for Benign Disease

Image acquisition acceleration techniques like PAT and the introduction of high field whole-body scanners have opened the way for more complex and tailored WB-MRI protocols. Beyond the assessment of malignant neoplasms, WB-MRI has been introduced for imaging of various benign diseases potentially affecting the whole body, such as systemic imaging of inflammatory diseases and congenital skeletal diseases predisposing for malignancies, like multiple cartilaginous exostoses or histiocytosis X. Furthermore, WB-MRI applications have successfully been introduced for an evidence-based screening of patients suffering from long-term diabetes.

14.5.1 WB-MRI for the Assessment of Systemic Inflammatory Diseases

14.5.1.1 Rheumatic Disease

Rheumatoid arthritis (RA) is a common disease, affecting approximately 1% of the population. With the introduction of new disease-modifying therapeutic approaches, it has become increasingly important to detect RA as early as possible. Due to its high soft-tissue and bone marrow contrast, MRI shows the highest sensitivity for detecting and monitoring bone erosions, when compared to conventional radiographs or CT. MRI is also helpful in depicting pre-erosive changes in RA, such as synovitis, bone marrow edema, or osteitis, as well as tendinous and ligamentous abnormalities. As a disease potentially affecting the whole body anatomy, including small joints of the extremities and larger joints of the axial skeleton, RA is a suitable candidate for WB-MRI applications. A standard protocol for imaging of RA should include T2-W imaging (such as fat saturated T2 TSE or STIR) for depiction of synovial inflammation and joint effusion. Furthermore, T1-W 3D GRE imaging with adequate fat suppression pre- and post-contrast is essential for the assessment of bone marrow edema and pannus tissue. Table 14.6 shows a possible whole-body approach for RA on a multi-channel matrix coil system scanner at 1.5 T. An important challenge is to find an adequate compromise between large FoV imaging (e.g., in coronal orientation on five body levels) and adequate SNR/resolution for the extremities, especially the hands. Also, additional dedicated imaging of the complete spine in another plane is mandatory; optionally, a time-resolved contrast-enhanced sequence may be added in areas of strongest pain. Yet, in some cases, further examination of peripheral joints with a dedicated coil system may be necessary. Recently, the described protocol has successfully been evaluated for systemic imaging of psoriatic arthritis, within a total imaging time of 60 min, and image quality was rated as excellent in 22/25 examined patients. Also, significantly more regions affected by synovialitis and enthesitis were depicted by WB-MRI compared to a clinical exam (Fig. 14.8).

14.5.1.2 Osteomyelitis and Chronic Recurrent Osteomyelitis

The term osteomyelitis implies an infection of the bone and the bone marrow. Three routes of infection are possible and may occur: hematogenous spread, direct implantation, and infection by contiguity.

The best method to demonstrate infection of the bones and the surrounding soft tissues is MRI, especially with the use of fat-suppressed sequences before

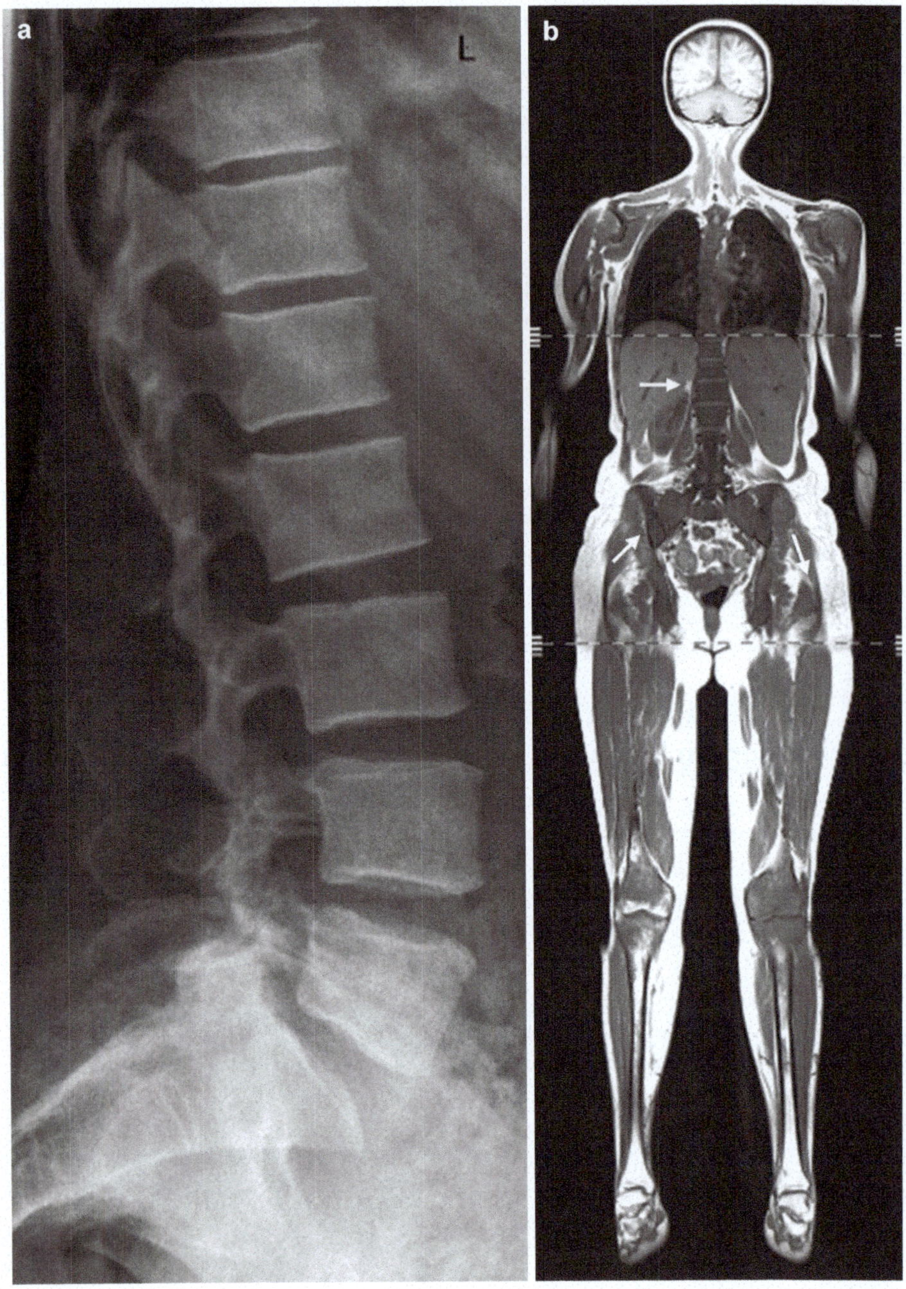

Fig. 14.7 Fifty-three-year-old female patient with a history of long-lasting osteomyelofibrosis. Conventional X-ray of the lumbar spine (**a**) demonstrates a normal finding. WB-MR T1-W sequences (**b**) demonstrate a pathological hypointense signal of the bone marrow structure in the spine, pelvis, and the proximal parts of the long extremity bones (*arrows*)

(T2 STIR, T2 fs) and after application of contrast media (T1 fs). CT can depict important details such as sequestered bone fragments and intraosseous fistula tracts, which are signs of chronic ostemyelitis. Three-phase bone scintigraphy is the radionuclide procedure of choice for the early diagnosis of osteomyelitis, as it is highly sensitive for the detection of bone and joint infections. However it is nonspecific in patients with traumatized bone, in the presence of prosthetic replacement, and in the neuropathic joint. If ^{18}F-FDG PET/CT is employed in the diagnosis of acute osteomyelitis; sensitivities of 98% and specificities between 75 and 99% are reported. In chronic osteomyelitis, PET is useful because FDG is avidly taken up by activated macrophages, which predominate in the chronic phase of an infection. In these patients, sensitivities

Table 14.6 WB-MRI protocol for imaging of rheumatic disease on a 32-receiver channel whole-body scanner at 1.5 T with the use of total body matrix technology and PI. Total imaging time is 60 min

WB-MRI protocol for rheumatic disease at 1.5 T					
	Shoulder (GH-, SC-, AC-joints, spine)	**Abdomen** (hands, spine)	**Pelvis** (hips, symphysis, SI-joints, spine)	**Knees**	**Ankles/feet**
	STIR cor	STIR cor	STIR cor	STIR cor	STIR cor
20	STIR sag	STIR sag	STIR sag		
	T1 fs 3D GRE sag	T1 fs 3D GRE sag	T1 fs 3D GRE sag		
	T1 fs 3D GRE cor	T1 fs 3D GRE cor	T1 fs 3D GRE cor	T1 fs 3D GRE cor	T1 fs 3D GRE cor
40	Contrast media application				
	Time resolved sequence (most painful region)				
	T1 fs 3D GRE sag	T1 fs 3D GRE sag	T1 fs 3D GRE sag		
60	T1 fs 3D GRE cor	T1 fs 3D GRE cor	T1 fs 3D GRE cor	T1 fs 3D GRE cor	T1 fs 3D GRE cor
Total scan time = 60 min, PAT 2-3					

and specificities of 100 and 92% are described, and in case of a negative PET finding can almost be excluded with high probability. Chronic recurrent multifocal osteomyelitis is a rare variant of osteomyelitis, accounting for 2–5% of cases of osteomyelitis. Often, bacteriologic investigation of the biopsy specimen is negative, suggesting that the inflammatory process might have become independent of the initial bacterial infection. Typical locations of CRMO are the metaphyses of the long bones, typically the distal femoral metaphyses, followed by the clavicles and the vertebrae. Involvement of the ribs, sternum, and pelvis is rare. Differential diagnoses of CRMO include Ewing sarcoma, histiocytosis X, metastatic neuroblastoma, leukaemia, and bone tuberculosis.

MRI and, in this setting especially, WB-MRI is the method of choice if negative scintigraphic or radiographic findings in a patient with clinical symptoms need further diagnostic work-up. The extent of bone marrow inflammation can be best assessed on T1-W images, due to the decreased bone marrow signal. With its lack of ionizing radiation, MRI is the method of choice for examinations of children, and follow-up investigations.

Overall, WB-MRI can be recommended for all children with suspected unifocal osteomyelitis to exclude further localizations, as well as for CRMO to assess the different possible localizations of the disease.

14.5.2 Systemic Imaging of Diabetes

Recently, tailored protocols for surveillance of patients suffering from longstanding diabetes have been introduced into clinical routine. The protocol implies dedicated imaging of the brain, including time-of-flight MR angiograms of the cerebral arteries, a contrast-enhanced 3D MRA of the whole body, dynamic assessment of cardiac function and viability, as well as high-resolution pre/postcontrast imaging of the feet. Table 14.7 gives a schematic overview of the sequence setup. Preliminary experience on asymptomatic patients suffering from type-1 or type-2 diabetes for more than 10 years showed

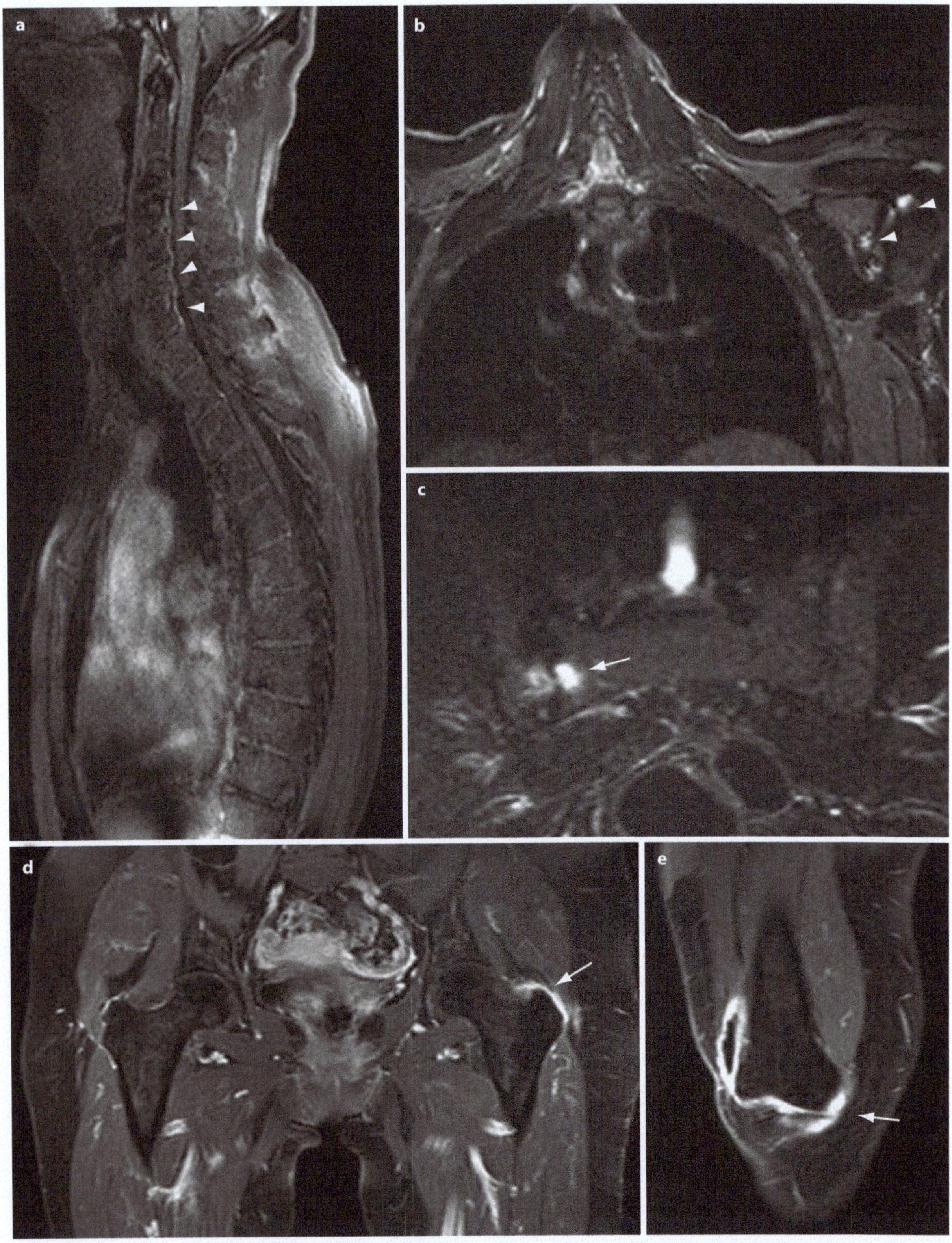

Fig. 14.8 WB-MR images from two patients with psoriatic arthritis. There is enthesitis (*arrowheads*) of the interspinal ligaments of cervical spine (**a**), destructive changes of the left glenoid with mild joint effusion (*arrowheads*) in the left shoulder (**b**), sacroileitis (*arrow*) of the right sacroiliac joint (**c**), trochanteric bursitis with enthesitis (*arrow*) of the left hip joint (**d**), and synovialitis (*arrow*) of the right knee joint (**e**, CE-3D-GRE-image)

Table 14.7 WB-MRI protocol for systemic diabetes imaging on a 32-receiver channel whole-body scanner at 1.5 T with the use of total body matrix technology and PI. Total imaging time is 65 min

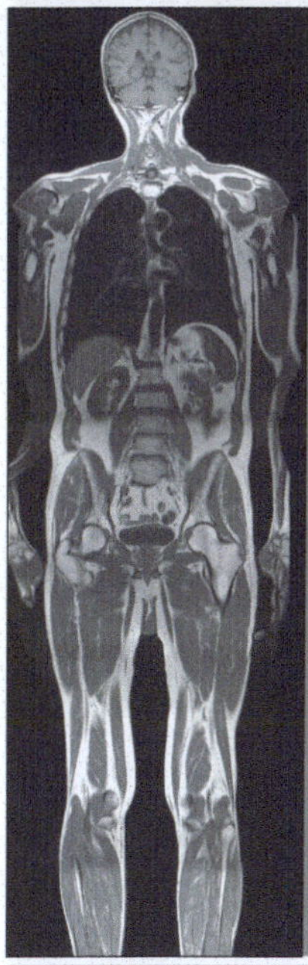

WB-MRI diabetes protocol at 1.5 T				
Min	**Brain**	**Cardiac**	**Feet**	**MRA**
			T1 TSE cor STIR cor	
	Epi-DWI ax T2 TSE ax			
20	FLAIR ax T2* TSE ax			
	TOF	Function		
	Contrast media application			
40	T1 TSE ax			carotids lower leg abdominal upper leg
50		DCE	T1 TSE fscor	
		TR MRA		
Total scan time = 65 min, PAT 2-3				

significantly more vascular pathologies, like stenosis of the carotid arteries (54 vs. 6%), renal arteries (25 vs. 0.25%), or peripheral arteries (51 vs. 14%), compared to a healthy population. Additionally, the incidence for silent myocardial infarctions in the diabetes group was 18%, compared to 1% in healthy patients. Also, skeletal pathologies, like neuropathic foot disease, were reliably detected. Diagnosis was followed by intervention in nine patients (Fig. 14.9). These results present a promising new method for comprehensive imaging of this systemic disease, which potentially may lead to a more effective therapy by earlier diagnosis of secondary complications.

14.5.3 Systemic Imaging of Benign Tumors (MCE, Enchondromatosis, Langerhans Cell Histiocytosis, Polyostotic Fibrous Dysplasia)

In patients with benign bone tumors (multiple cartilaginary exostoses, Langerhans cell histiocytosis (LCH), or polyostotic fibrous dysplasia), WB-MRI can be recommended for the primary diagnostic of location, as well as for follow-up examinations of identified pathologies. Furthermore, it is possible to define the best region for a histological verification of the disease. A proposed protocol with special attention to the cartilage is described in Table 14.8, followed by an example of a patient with multifocal osteochondromas (Fig. 14.10).

The usually benign lesion "Eosinophilic granuloma" is the most common and the mildest variant of the broad range of tumors subsumed under the term histiocytosis X, which is defined by the presence of Langerhans cells and thus called LCH. Eosinophilic granuloma typically occurs in the first and second decade of life. The skull, ribs, spine, pelvis, and femur are the most frequent locations, but potentially every bone can be involved. In most cases, the lesion is monostotic, but polyostotic forms are seen in up to 20% of cases. In the early stage, the osteolyses can appear aggressive, sometimes with poorly-defined margins, without a sclerotic rim, and are typically surrounded by an extensive, ill-defined edema. Later stages show a more benign appearance, as the lesion becomes sharply demarcated, with a well-defined sclerotic border and

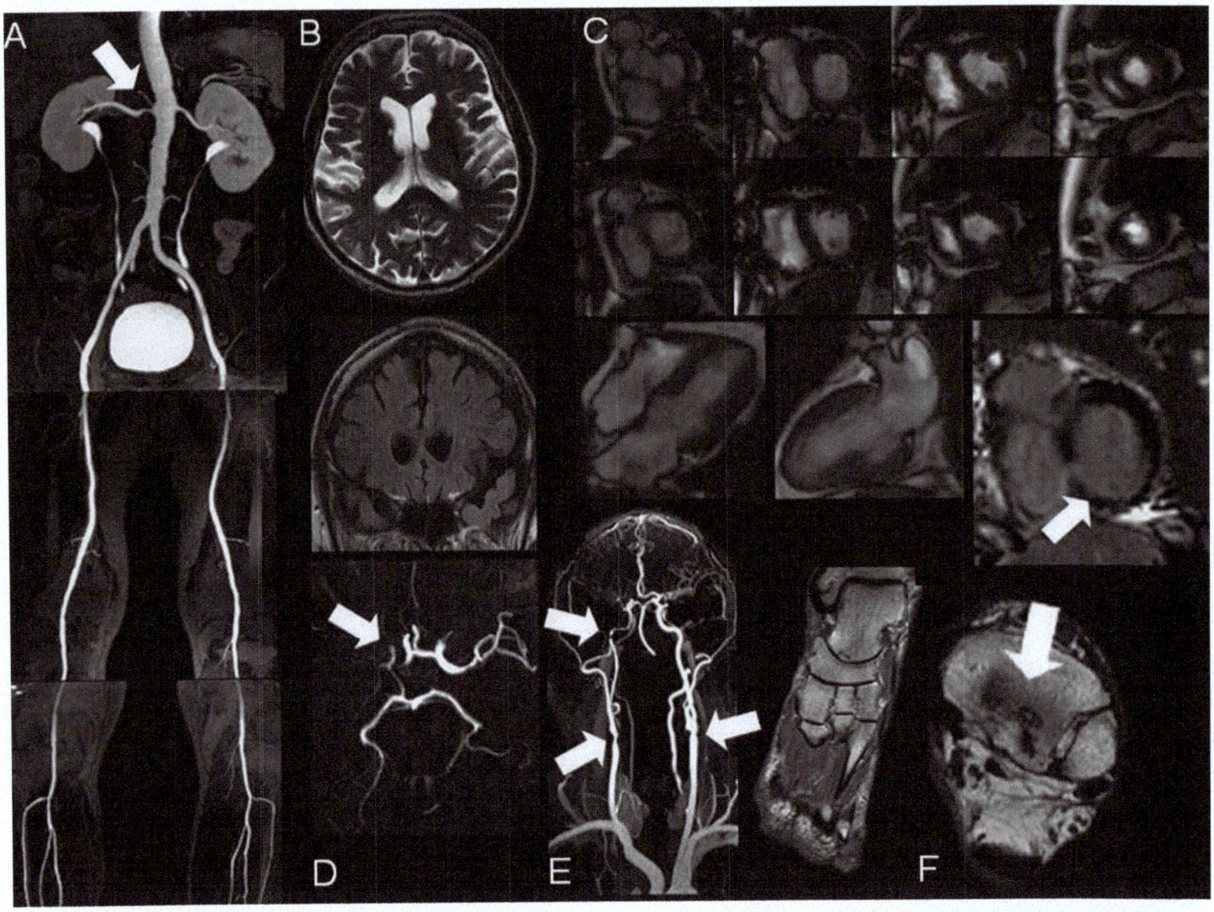

Fig. 14.9 (**a**) WB-MR exam of a 70-year-old male patient with type-2 diabetes for 33 years, including whole-body MRA. (**b**) The images of the brain are unremarkable. (**c**) DCE shows an inferior wall infarct without any signs of myocardial wall thinning or wall motion abnormalities. (**d, e**) MRA reveals an occlusion of the right middle cerebral artery, high grade stenoses of both common carotid arteries, and a stenosis of the right internal carotid artery within its intracranial portion, as well as a low-grade stenosis of the right renal artery and irregularities of the abdominal aorta (*arrows*). (**f**) Pedal MR images demonstrate a small bone marrow infarct of the anterior portion of the talus

Table 14.8 WB-MRI protocol in children with osteochondroma (1.5 T) with four examination regions

Region	Sequence	Image plane	Matrix/resolution (mm^3)	Acquisition time (min)	Contrast media
WB	STIR	Coronal	512/2 × 1 × 5	3.20/region	–
WB	T1	Coronal	384/1.6 × 1.3 × 5	2.58/region	–
Findings*	PD SE fs	Axial	256/1.3 × 1.3 × 5	3.14	–
Findings*	T1 fs 3D GRE	Axial	384/1 × 1 × 1	2.08	+

* proposed additional sequences, if findings are present

either a thick or no periosteal reaction. Healing lesions also can become sclerotic. Button sequester and soft tissue reactions can occur. Differential diagnoses include Ewing sarcoma (in cases of a moth-like growth pattern, periosteal reaction, extensive edema, and soft tissue involvement – the flare phenomenon – in the early stage of eosinophilic granuloma), lymphoma, and infection (also showing numerous inflammatory cells). Finally, often histology is needed to reliably differentiate between these entities.

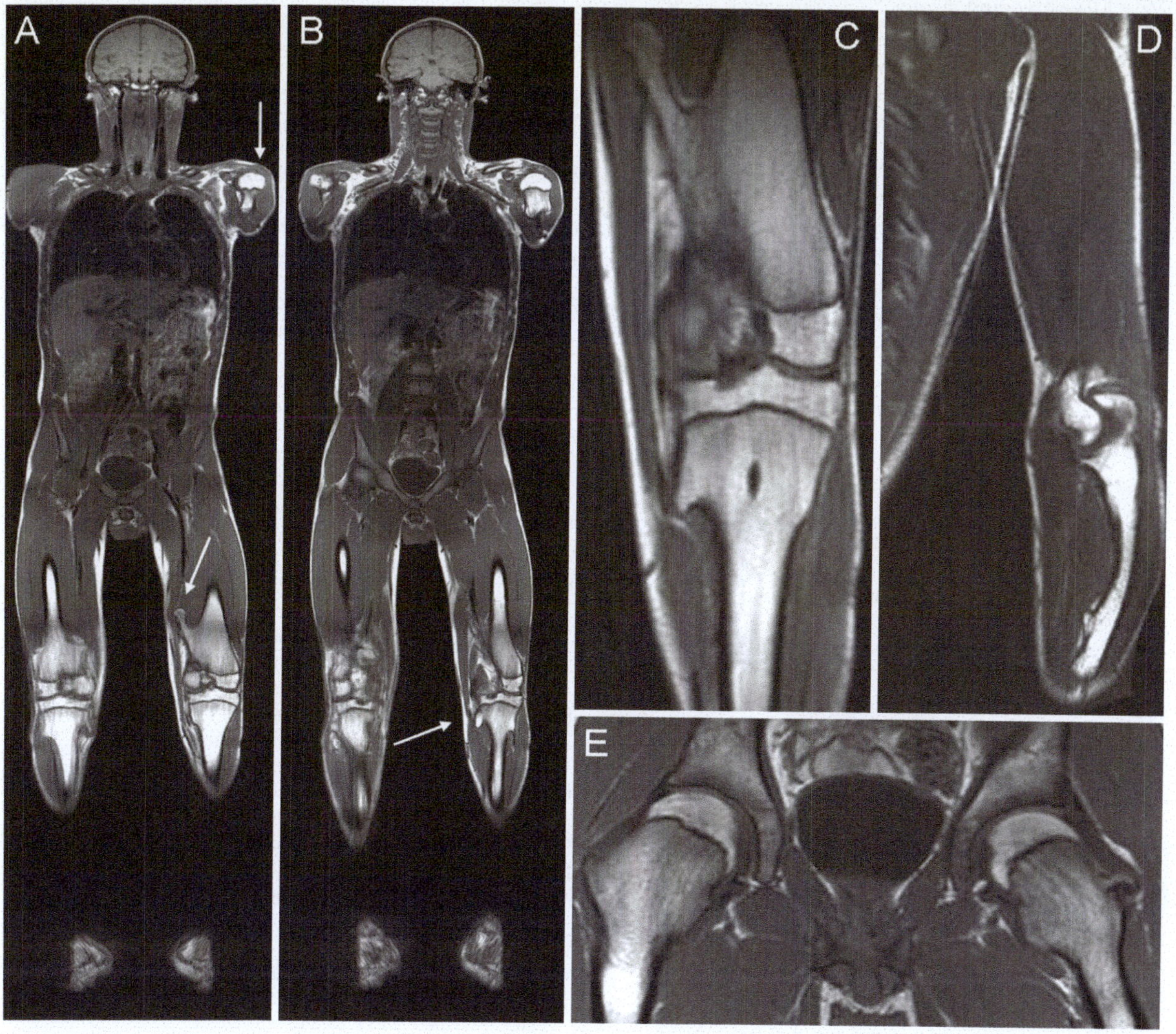

Fig. 14.10 Thirty-five-year-old male with multiple cartilaginous exostoses. (**a**, **b**) WB-MRI shows typical manifestations in the metaphyseal parts of the long bones of the upper and lower extremity. (**c**) Enlargement of the left knee joint shows an exostosis at the medial side of the femur and at the proximal tibia. (**d**) Exostosis at the radius. (**e**) Exostoses and deformation of both femoral necks. In summary, no exostosis wider than 2.5 cm was found in this patient, thus making a malignant transformation unlikely

Little data from literature exists comparing CT/PET–CT/scintigraphy and WB-MRI for these entities. A recent study analyzing eight children with multifocal LHC with radiography, bone scintigraphy, and WB-MRI reported more lesions detected by WB-MRI than radiography (in an additional three patients) and bone scan (in an additional two patients). Initial results demonstrate the potential of this method in young patients to also identify early signs of malignancy as well as organ-related complications of the diseases.

14.5.4 Arising Clinical Applications

WB-MRI, with new techniques to examine the whole body anatomy in significantly shorter scan time ("move-during-scan," "continuous table move acquisition"), faster sequence protocols and enhanced contrasts similar to those of PET ("WB-DWI with morphologic image fusion," "virtual PET-MRI," see Fig. 14.3) will become a strong competitor to PET–CT as an established whole-body modality for tumor staging. The advantage of having an examination without radiation exposure is counterbalanced by the disadvantage of having only restricted information about functional and metabolic parameters of the tumor. The next innovative diagnostic WB-imaging method may become PET MRI, which allows assessment of morphologic structures in high quality, in combination with metabolic parameters, while decreasing radiation exposure compared to PET–CT at the same time (about 4–7 mSv/PET vs. 20–25 mSv for PET–CT).

Further Reading

Akduman EI, Momtahen AJ, Balci NC, Mahajann N, Havliouglu N, Wolverson MK (2008) Comparison between malignant and benign abdominal lymph nodes on diffusion-weighted Imaging. Acad Radiol 15:641–646

Al-Shahi Salman R, Whiteley WN, Warlow C (2007) Screening using whole-body magnetic resonance imaging scanning: who wants an incidentaloma? J Med Screen 14(1):2–4

Antoch G, Vogt FM, Freudenberg LS, Nazaradeh F, Goehde SC, Barkhausen J et al (2003) Whole-body dual-modality PET/CT and whole-body MRI for tumor staging in oncology. JAMA 290:3199–3206

Appel H, Hermann KG, Althoff CE, Rudwaleit M, Sieper J (2007) Whole-body magnetic resonance imaging evaluation of widespread inflammatory lesions in a patient with ankylosing spondylitis before and after 1 year of treatment with infliximab. J Rheumatol 34:2497–2498

Barth MM, Smith MP, Pedrosa I, Lenkinski RE, Rofsky NM (2007) Body MR imaging at 3.0 T: understanding the opportunities and challenges. Radiographics 27:1445–1462

Baur A, Stäbler A, Bartl R, Lamerz R, Scheidler J, Reiser M (1997) MRI gadolinium enhancement of bone marrow: age related changes in normals and in diffuse neoplastic infiltration. Skeletal Radiol 26:414–418

Baur A, Stäbler A, Nagel D, Lamerz R, Bartl R, Hiller E, Wendtner C, Bachner F, Reiser M (2002) Magnetic resonance imaging as a supplement for the clinical staging system of Durie and Salmon? Cancer 95:1334–1345

Baur-Melnyk A, Buhmann S, Becker C, Schoenberg SO, Lang N, Bartl R, Reiser MF (2008) Whole-body MRI versus whole-body MDCT for staging of multiple myeloma. Am J Roentgenol 190:1097–1104

Becker N (2008) Epidemiology and statistics. In: Reiser MF, van Kaick G, Fink C, Schoenberg SO (eds) Screening and preventive diagnosis with radiological imaging. Medical radiology – diagnostic imaging and radiation oncology. Springer, Berlin, pp 3–13

Blomqvist L, Torkzad MR (2003) Whole-body imaging with MRI or PET/CT: the future for single-modality imaging in oncology? JAMA 24:3248–3249

Bolte H, Jahnke T, Schäfer FK, Wenke R, Hoffmann B, Freitag-Wolf S, Dicken V, Kuhnigk JM, Lohmann J, Voss S, Knöss N, Heller M, Biederer J (2007) Interobserver-variability of lung nodule volumetry considering different segmentation algorithms and observer training levels. Eur J Radiol 64:285–295

Börnert P, Keupp J, Eggers H, Aldefeld B (2007) Whole-body 3D water/fat resolved continuously moving table imaging. J Magn Reson Imaging 25:660–665

Brennan DD, Gleeson T, Coate LE, Cronin C, Carney D, Eustace SJ (2005) A comparison of whole-body MRI and CT for the staging of lymphoma. AJR 185:711–716

Buck FM, Treumann TC, Winiker H, Strobel K (2007) Chronic recurrent multifocal osteomyelitis (CRMO) with symmetric involvement of both femora: x-ray, bone scintigram, and MR imaging findings in one case. J Magn Reson Imaging 26:422–426

Busse RF (2004) Reduced RF power without blurring: correcting for modulation of refocusing flip angle in FSE sequences. Magn Reson Med 51:1031–1037

Daldrup-Link HE, Franzius C, Link TM, Laukamp D, Sciuk J, Jürgens H, Schober O, Rummeny EJ (2001) Whole-body MR imaging for detection of bone metastases in children and young adults: comparison with skeletal scintigraphy and FDG PET. Am J Roentgenol 177:229–236

Delorme S, van Kaick G (2008) General oncological aspects of screening. In: Reiser MF, van Kaick G, Fink C, Schoenberg SO (eds) Screening and preventive diagnosis with radiological imaging. Medical radiology – diagnostic imaging and radiation oncology. Springer, Berlin, pp 39–45

Dietrich O, Reiser MF, Schoenberg SO (2008) Artifacts in 3-T MRI: physical background and reduction strategies. Eur J Radiol 65:29–35

D'Sa S, Abildgaard N, Tighe J, Shaw P, Hall-Craggs M (2007) Guidelines for the use of imaging in the management of myeloma. Br J Haematol 137:49–63

Durie BG (2006) The role of anatomic and functional staging in myeloma: description of Durie/Salmon plus staging system. Eur J Cancer 42:1539–1543

Durie BGM, Salmon SE (1975) A clinical staging system for multiple myeloma: correlation of measured myeloma cell mass with presenting clinical features, response to treatment and survival. Cancer 36:842–854

Eibel R, Herzog P, Dietrich O et al (2006) Detection of pulmonary abnormalities in immunocompromised patients: fast single-shot MRI with parallel imaging in comparison to thin-section helical CT. Radiology 241:880–891

El-Shanti HI, Ferguson PJ (2007) Chronic recurrent multifocal osteomyelitis: a concise review and genetic update. Clin Orthop Relat Res 462:11–19

Engelhard K, Hollenbach HP, Wohlfart K, von Imhoff E, Fellner FA (2004) Comparison of whole-body MRI with automatic moving table technique and bone scintigraphy for screening for bone metastases in patients with breast cancer. Eur Radiol 14:99–105

Frericks BB, Meyer BC, Martus P, Wendt M, Wolf KJ, Wacker F (2008) MRI of the thorax during whole-body MRI: evaluation of different MR sequences and comparison to thoracic multidetector computed tomography (MDCT). J Magn Reson Imaging 27:538–545

Ghanem N, Kelly T, Altehoefer C, Winterer J, Schäfer O, Bley TA, Moser E, Langer M (2004) Whole-body MRI in comparison to skeletal scintigraphy for detection of skeletal metastases in patients with solid tumors Radiologe 44:864–873

Ghanem N, Uhl M, Brink I, Schäfer O, Kelly T, Moser E, Langer M (2005) Diagnostic value of MRI in comparison to scintigraphy, PET, MS-CT and PET/CT for the detection of metastases of bone. Eur J Radiol 55:41–55

Ghanem N, Altehoefer C, Kelly T, Lohrmann C, Winterer J, Schäfer O, Bley TA, Moser E, Langer M (2006a) Whole-body MRI in comparison to skeletal scintigraphy in detection of skeletal metastases in patients with solid tumors. In Vivo 20:173–182

Ghanem N, Lohrmann C, Engelhardt M, Pache G, Uhl M, Saueressig U, Kotter E, Langer M (2006b) Whole-body MRI in the detection of bone marrow infiltration in patients with plasma cell neoplasms in comparison to the radiological skeletal survey. Eur Radiol 16:1005–1014

Goebel M, Rosa F, Tatsch K, Grillhoesl A, Hofmann GO, Kirschner MH (2007) Diagnosis of chronic osteitis of the bones in the extremities. Relative value of F-18 FDG-PET. Unfallchirurg 110:859–866

Goehde SC, Hunold P, Vogt FM, Ajaj W, Goyen M, Herborn CU et al (2005) Full-body cardiovascular and tumor MRI for early detection of disease: feasibility and initial experience in 298 subjects. AJR 184:598–611

Goo HW, Choi SH, Ghim T, Moon HN, Seo JJ (2005) Whole-body MRI of paediatric malignant tumours: comparison with conventional oncological imaging methods. Pediatr Radiol 35:766–773

Goo HW, Yang DH, Ra YS, Song JS, Im HJ, Seo JJ, Ghim T, Moon HN (2006) Whole-body MRI of Langerhans cell histiocytosis: comparison with radiography and bone scintigraphy. Pediatr Radiol 36:1019–1031

Goyen M, Schlemmer HP (2007) Whole body MRI-diagnostic strategy of the future? Radiologe 47:904–914

Hargaden G, O'Connell M, Kavanagh E, Powell T, Ward R, Eustace S (2003) Current concepts in whole-body imaging using turbo short tau inversion recovery MR imaging. Am J Roentgenol 180:247–252

Heinemann V (2008) Oncological diseases. In: Reiser MF, van Kaick G, Fink C, Schoenberg SO (eds) Screening and preventive diagnosis with radiological imaging. Medical radiology - diagnostic imaging and radiation oncology. Springer, Berlin, pp 13–23

Iizuka-Mikami M, Nagai K, Yoshida K, Sugihara T, Suetsugu Y, Mikami M et al (2004) Detection of bone marrow and extramedullary involvement in patients with non-Hodgkin's lymphoma by whole-body MRI: comparison with bone and 67Ga scintigraphies. Eur Radiol 14:1074–1081

Johnston C, Brennan S, Ford S, Eustace S (2006) Whole body MR imaging: applications in oncology. Eur J Surg Oncol 32:239–246

Kalish GM, Bhargavan M, Sunshine JH, Forman HP (2004) Self-referred whole-body imaging: where are we now? Radiology 233:353–358

Kellenberger CJ, Epelman M, Miller SF, Babyn PS (2004a) Fast STIR whole-body MR imaging in children. Radiographics 24:1317–1330

Kellenberger CJ, Miller SF, Khan M, Gilday DL, Weitzman S, Babyn PS (2004b) Initial experience with FSE STIR whole-body MR imaging for staging lymphoma in children. Eur Radiol 14:1829–1841

Klotz LH (2005) Active surveillance for good risk prostate cancer: rationale, method, and results. Can J Urol 12:21–24

Koh DM, Takahara T, Imai Y, Collins DJ (2007) Practical aspects of assessing tumors using clinical diffusion-weighted imaging in the body. Magn Reson Med Sci 6:211–224

Kramer H (2008) Screening and preventive diagnosis with radiological imaging. Diagnostic algorithms for whole-body-exams. In: Reiser MF, van Kaick G, Fink C, Schoenberg SO (eds) Screening and preventive diagnosis with radiological imaging. Medical radiology – diagnostic imaging and radiation oncology. Springer, Berlin, pp 53–63

Kramer U, Schlemmer HP (2007) Remote control for magnetic resonance imaging as a part of daily routine examinations. Rofo 179:739–742

Krishnamurthy GT, Tubis M, Hiss J, Blahd WH (1977) Distribution pattern of metastatic bone disease. A need for total body skeletal image. JAMA 237:2504–2506

Ladd SC, Ladd ME (2007) Perspectives for preventive screening with total body MRI. Eur Radiol 17:2889–2897

Ladd SC, Zenge M, Antoch G, Forsting M (2006) Whole-body MR diagnostic concepts. Rofo 178:763–770

Laffan EE, O'Connor R, Ryan SP, Donoghue VB (2004) Whole-body magnetic resonance imaging: a useful additional sequence in pediatric imaging. Pediatr Radiol 34: 472–480

Lauenstein TC, Semelka RC (2006) Emerging techniques: whole-body screening and staging with MRI. J Magn Reson Imaging 24:489–498

Lauenstein TC, Goehde SC, Herborn CU, Goyen M, Oberhoff C, Debatin JF, Ruehm SG, Barkhausen J (2004) Whole-body MR imaging: evaluation of patients for metastases. Radiology 233:139–148

Lenk S, Fischer S, Kötter I, Claussen CD, Schlemmer HP (2004) Possibilities of whole-body MRI for investigating musculoskeletal diseases. Radiologe 44:844–853

Li S, Sun F, Jin ZY, Xue HD, Li ML (2007) Whole-body diffusion-weighted imaging: technical improvement and preliminary results. J Magn Reson Imaging 26:1139–1144

Lichy MP, Aschoff P, Plathow C, Stemmer A, Horger W, Mueller-Horvath C et al (2007) Tumor detection by diffusion-weighted MRI and ADC-mapping – initial clinical experiences in comparison to PET–CT. Invest Radiol 42:605–613

Manser RL, Irving LB, Byrnes G, Abramson MJ, Stone CA, Campbell DA (2003) Screening for lung cancer: a systematic review and meta-analysis of controlled trials. Thorax 58:784–789

Mazumdar A, Siegel MJ, Narra V, Luchtman-Jones L (2002) Whole-body fast inversion recovery MR imaging of small cell neoplasms in pediatric patients: a pilot study. Am J Roentgenol 179:1261–1266

Mellado Santos JM (2006) Diagnostic imaging of pediatric hematogenous osteomyelitis: lessons learned from a multi-modality approach. Eur Radiol 16:2109–2119

Mentzel HJ, Kentouche K, Sauner D, Fleischmann C, Vogt S, Gottschild D, Zintl F, Kaiser WA (2004) Comparison of whole-body STIR-MRI and 99mTc-methylene-diphosphonate scintigraphy in children with suspected multifocal bone lesions. Eur Radiol 14:2297–2302

Mulshine JL (2005) New developments in lung cancer screening. J Clin Oncol 10:3198–3202

Nakanishi K, Kobayashi M, Takahashi S, Nakata S, Kyakuno M, Nakaguchi K, Nakamura H (2005) Whole body MRI for detecting metastatic bone tumor: comparison with bone scintigrams. Magn Reson Med Sci 4:11–17

Nakanishi K, Kobayashi M, Nakaguchi K, Kyakuno M, Hashimoto N, Onishi H, Maeda N, Nakata S, Kuwabara M, Murakami T, Nakamura H (2007) Whole-body MRI for detecting metastatic bone tumor: diagnostic value of diffusion-weighted images. Magn Reson Med Sci 6:147–155

Nöbauer I, Uffmann M (2005) Differential diagnosis of focal and diffuse neoplastic diseases of bone marrow in MRI. Eur J Radiol 55:2–32

Ohno Y, Koyama H, Onishi Y, Takenaka D, Nogami M, Yoshikawa T (2008) Non-small cell lung cancer: whole-body MR examination for M-stage assessment – utility for whole-body diffusion-weighted imaging compared with integrated FDG PET/CT. Radiology 248:643–654

Pastorino U, Bellomi M, Landoni C, De Fiori E, Araldi P, Picchio M et al (2003) Early lung-cancer detection with spiral CT and positron emission tomography in heavy smokers: 2-year results. Lancet 23:593–597

Pfannenberg C, Aschoff P, Schanz S, Eschmann SM, Plathow C, Eigentler TK, Garbe C, Brechtel K, Vonthein R, Bares R, Claussen CD, Schlemmer HP (2007) Prospective comparison of 18F-fluorodeoxyglucose positron emission tomography/computed tomography and whole-body magnetic resonance imaging in staging of advanced malignant melanoma. Eur J Cancer 43:557–564

Plathow C, Meinzer HP, Kauczor HU (2006) Visualization of pulmonary nodules with magnetic resonance imaging (MRI) Radiologe 46:260–266

Rahmouni A, Luciani A, Itti E (2005) MRI and PET in monitoring response in lymphoma. Cancer Imaging 5:S106–S112

Sabati M, Lauzon ML, Mahallati H, Frayne R (2006) Interactive continuously moving table (iCMT) large field-of-view real-time MRI. Magn Reson Med 55:1202–1209

Schaefer JF, Schlemmer HP (2006) Total-body MR-imaging in oncology. Eur Radiol 16:2000–2015

Schäfer JF, Fischmann A, Lichy M, Vollmar J, Fenchel M, Claussen CD, Schlemmer HP (2004) Oncologic screening with whole-body MRI: possibilities and limitations. Radiologe 44:854–863

Schlemmer HP, Schäfer J, Pfannenberg C, Radny P, Korchidi S, Müller-Horvat C (2005) Fast whole-body assessment of metastatic disease using a novel magnetic resonance imaging system: initial experiences. Invest Radiol 40: 64–71

Schmidt GP, Baur-Melnyk A, Herzog P, Schmid R, Tiling R, Reiser MF et al (2005a) High-resolution whole-body MRI tumor staging with the use of parallel imaging versus dual modality PET–CT: experience on a 32-channel system. Invest Radiol 40:743–753

Schmidt GP, Schoenberg SO, Reiser MF, Baur-Melnyk A (2005b) Whole-body MR imaging of bone marrow. Eur J Radiol 55(1):33–40

Schmidt GP, Schoenberg SO, Schmid R, Stahl R, Tiling R, Becker CR, Reiser MF, Baur-Melnyk A (2007a) Screening for bone metastases: whole-body MRI using a 32-channel system versus dual-modality PET–CT. Eur Radiol 17: 939–949

Schmidt GP, Wintersperger B, Graser A, Baur-Melnyk A, Reiser MF, Schoenberg SO (2007b) High-resolution whole-body magnetic resonance imaging applications at 1.5 and 3 Tesla: a comparative study. Invest Radiol 42:449–459

Schmidt GP, Kramer H, Reiser MF, Glaser C (2007c) Whole-body magnetic resonance imaging and positron emission tomography-computed tomography in oncology. Top Magn Reson Imaging 18(3):193–202

Schmidt GP, Baur-Melnyk A, Haug A, Heinemann V, Bauerfeind I, Reiser MF, Schoenberg SO (2008) Comprehensive imaging of tumor recurrence in breast cancer patients using whole-body MRI at 1.5 and 3 T compared to FDG-PET–CT. Eur J Radiol 65:47–58

Schoenberg SO (2008) Personnel and structural prerequisites for screening-programs. In: Reiser MF, van Kaick G, Fink C, Schoenberg SO (eds) Screening and preventive diagnosis with radiological imaging. Medical radiology - diagnostic imaging and radiation oncology. Springer, Berlin, pp 63–77

Steinborn M, Heuck AF, Tiling R, Bruegel M, Gauger L, Reiser MF (1999) Whole body bone marrow MRI in patients with metastatic disease to the skeletal system. J Comput Assist Tomogr 23:123–129

Sumi M, Sakihama N, Sumi T, Morikawa M, Uetani M, Kabasawa H (2003) Discrimination of metastatic cervical lymph nodes with diffusion-weighted MR imaging in patients with head and neck cancer. Am J Neuroradiol 24:1627–1634

Walker R, Kessar P, Blanchard R, Dimasi M, Harper K, DeCarvalho V, Yucel EK, Patriquin L, Eustace S (2000) Turbo STIR magnetic resonance imaging as a whole-body screening tool for metastases in patients with breast carcinoma: preliminary clinical experience. J Magn Reson Imaging 11:343–350

Weckbach S, Kramer H, Parhofer KG, Reiser MF, Schoenberg SO (2006) Comprehensive diabetes imaging with whole body MRI at 1.5 and 3T in patients with longstanding diabetes. In: Fourteenth Scientific Meeting of the International Society for Magnetic Resonance in Medicine (ISMRM). Book of Abstracts, p 389

Weckbach S, Michaely HJ, Friedrich D, Schewe S, Reiser MF, Glaser C (2007) Whole body MR Imaging in psoriatic arthritis: development of an imaging protocol and evaluation in 25 patients. Eur Radiol 17(suppl 1):139

Zech CJ, Herrmann KA, Huber A, Dietrich O, Stemmer A, Herzog P, Reiser MF, Schoenberg SO (2004) High-resolution MR-imaging of the liver with T2-weighted sequences using integrated parallel imaging: comparison of prospective motion correction and respiratory triggering. J Magn Reson Imaging 20:443–450

Index

E

I

P

The manufacturer's authorised representative in the EU is Springer Nature Customer Service Centre GmbH, Europaplatz 3, 69115 Heidelberg, Germany. If you have any concerns regarding our products, please contact ProductSafety@springernature.com

Printed and bound by CPI Group (UK) Ltd, Croydon, CR0 4YY
25/09/2026
02222883-0002